Biomedical Library
Queen's University Belfast
Tel: 028 9097 2710
E-mail: biomed.info@qub.ac.uk

For due dates and renewals see
'My Account' at
http://qu-prism.qub.ac.uk/TalisPrism/

This book must be returned not later than
its due date, but is subject to recall if in
demand

Fines are imposed on overdue books

ESSENTIALS OF NEUROSURGERY

ESSENTIALS OF NEUROSURGERY
A Guide To
Clinical Practice

Editors

Marshall B. Allen, Jr., M.D.

Chief of Neurosurgery
Medical College of Georgia
Hospital and Clinics
Professor of Surgery (Section of Neurosurgery)
Medical College of Georgia
Augusta, Georgia

Ross H. Miller, M.D.

Clinical Professor of Surgery (Section of Neurosurgery)
Medical College of Georgia
Augusta, Georgia
Clinical Professor of Surgery (Section of Neurosurgery)
Medical University of South Carolina
Charleston, South Carolina

McGRAW-HILL, INC.
Health Professions Division

New York   St. Louis   San Francisco   Auckland   Bogotá   Caracas
Lisbon   London   Madrid   Mexico City   Milan   Montreal
New Delhi   San Juan   Singapore   Sydney   Tokyo   Toronto

ESSENTIALS OF NEUROSURGERY

1 2 3 4 5 6 7 8 9 0   KGPKGP   9 8 7 6 5 4

ISBN 0-07-001116-8

This book was set in Times Roman by J. M. Post Graphics,
    a division of Cardinal Communications Group, Inc.
The editors were Jane E. Pennington and Lester A. Sheinis.
The production supervisor was Richard C. Ruzycka.
The cover designer was Marsha Cohen/Parallelogram.
The indexer was Elizabeth Babcock-Atkinson.
Arcata Graphics/Kingsport was printer and binder.

This book is printed on acid-free paper.

Library of Congress Cataloging-in-Publication Data

Essentials of neurosurgery: a guide to clinical practice / editors.
    Marshall B. Allen. Ross H. Miller.
        p.   cm.
    Includes bibliographical references and index.
    ISBN 0-07-001116-8
    1. Nervous system—Surgery.   I. Allen, Marshall B, date.
II. Miller, Ross H.
    [DNLM: 1. Nervous System Diseases—surgery. 2. Neurosurgery—
methods.   WL 368 E78]
RD593.E87   1995
617.4'8—dc20
DNLM/DLC   92-10297
for Library of Congress

Contents

Contributors

NOTE: **The numbers in brackets refer to the chapters written or co-written by the contributor.**

Marshall B. Allen, Jr., M.D., F.A.C.S.
  [3,12,14,15,16,18,19,20,28]
Chief of Neurosurgery
Medical College of Georgia Hospital and Clinics
Professor of Surgery (Section of Neurosurgery)
Medical College of Georgia
Consultant in Neurosurgery
University Hospital
Consultant in Neurosurgery
Augusta Veterans Administration Hospital
Augusta, Georgia
Consultant in Neurosurgery
Dwight D. Eisenhower Army Medical Center
Fort Gordon, Georgia
Consultant in Neurosurgery
Central State Hospital
Milledgeville, Georgia

José A. Bauzá, M.D. [17]
Assistant Professor of Neuroradiology
Medical College of Georgia Hospital and Clinics
Consultant in Neuroradiology
Augusta Veterans Administration Hospital
Augusta, Georgia

Geoffrey P. Cole, M.D. [21]
Attending Physician
Athens Regional Medical Center
Attending Physician
Saint Mary's Hospital
Athens, Georgia

Ramón E. Figueroa, M.D. [6]
Chief of Neuroradiology
Associate Professor of Radiology
Medical College of Georgia Hospital and Clinics
Consultant in Neuroradiology
Augusta Veterans Administration Hospital
Consultant in Neuroradiology
University Hospital
Augusta, Georgia

Herman F. Flanigin, M.D.
  [5,10,11,13,22,23,24,25]
Senior Consultant
Neurology and Neurosurgery
Medical College of Georgia
Director Emeritus
Physiological Neurosurgery and
  Epilepsy Surgery Program
Medical College of Georgia Hospital
  and Clinics
Augusta, Georgia

Ann Marie Flannery, M.D.
  [7,8,9,18]
Assistant Professor of Surgery
  (Sections of Neurosurgery and Pediatrics)
Medical College of Georgia
Attending in Neurosurgery and Pediatrics
Medical College of Georgia Hospital
  and Clinics
Attending in Neurosurgery
Augusta Veterans Administration Hospital
Augusta, Georgia

J. Allan Goodrich, M.D. [19,20]
Assistant Professor of Surgery
  (Section of Orthopedics)
Attending in Orthopedics
Medical College of Georgia Hospital
  and Clinics
Attending in Orthopedics
Augusta Veterans Administration Hospital
Augusta, Georgia
Consultant in Orthopedics
Dwight D. Eisenhower Army Medical Center
Fort Gordon, Georgia

Martin Greenberg, M.D. [1,2,13]
Associate Professor of Surgery
  (Section of Neurosurgery)
Medical College of Georgia
Attending in Neurosurgery
Medical College of Georgia Hospital and Clinics
Chief of Neurosurgery
Augusta Veterans Administration Hospital
Augusta, Georgia
Consultant in Neurosurgery
Dublin Veterans Administration Hospital
Dublin, Georgia
Consultant in Neurosurgery
Columbia Veterans Administration Hospital
Columbia, South Carolina

Gregory P. Lee, Ph.D. [4]
Associate Professor of Surgery (Section of Neurosurgery)
Medical College of Georgia Hospital and Clinics
Staff Neuropsychology
Medical College of Georgia Hospital and Clinics
Augusta, Georgia

David W. Loring, Ph.D. [4]
Professor of Neurology
Medical College of Georgia Hospital and Clinics
Augusta, Georgia

Edward K. Mark, Jr., M.D. [6]
Assistant Professor of Surgery (Section of Neurosurgery)
Medical College of Georgia
Attending in Neurosurgery
Medical College of Georgia Hospital and Clinics
Attending in Neurosurgery
Augusta Veterans Administration Hospital
Augusta, Georgia

Dennis E. McDonnell, M.D., F.A.C.S.
  [10,11,13,14,15,16]
Associate Professor of Surgery (Section of Neurosurgery)
Medical College of Georgia
Attending in Neurosurgery
Medical College of Georgia Hospital and Clinics
Attending in Neurosurgery
Augusta Veterans Administration Hospital
Augusta, Georgia

Ross H. Miller, M.D. [26,27]
Clinical Professor of Surgery (Section of Neurosurgery)
Medical College of Georgia
Augusta, Georgia
Clinical Professor of Surgery (Section of Neurosurgery)
Medical University of South Carolina
Charleston, South Carolina

Anthony M. Murro, M.D. [5]
Associate Professor of Neurology
Medical College of Georgia Hospital and Clinics
Director of EEG Laboratory
Augusta Veterans Administration Hospital
Augusta, Georgia

Alexis Norelle, M.D. [6]
Attending in Neurosurgery
Gundersen Clinic/Lutheran Hospital
Attending in Neurosurgery
Saint Francis Medical Center
La Crosse, Wisconsin

Joseph R. Smith, M.D., F.A.C.S. [21,22,23,24,25]
Director of Physiological Neurosurgery
Medical College of Georgia
Director of Epilepsy Surgery Program
Medical College of Georgia
Professor of Surgery (Section of Neurosurgery)
Medical College of Georgia
Attending in Neurosurgery
Medical College of Georgia Hospital and Clinics
Consultant in Neurosurgery
Augusta Veterans Administration Hospital
Augusta, Georgia

Farivar Yaghmai, M.D. [9,10,11,12]
Associate Professor of Pathology
Medical College of Georgia
Consultant in Pathology
University Hospital
Consultant in Pathology
Augusta Veterans Administration Hospital
Augusta, Georgia
Consultant in Pathology
Dwight D. Eisenhower Army Medical Center
Fort Gordon, Georgia
Consultant in Pathology
Aiken Hospital
Aiken, South Carolina

Foreword

It is difficult for editors and authors to arrive at the appropriate content for an introductory text on any subject. The level of the text, illustrations, and references must be chosen carefully to avoid either talking down to the reader or talking over the reader's head. Likewise, the volume of material should be sufficient but not overpowering. The editor must balance the contributions of the various authors in these regards and must ensure that the intended topics are covered, without overlap or repetition. The material should be organized in a way to permit the student to read the book from cover to cover, but this same organization, as well as the index, should permit easy access to individual topics. Finally, the finished book should be affordable and easy to carry and use.

Dr. Allen and his associates have satisfied these criteria. Their work is meant to be informative, not encyclopedic, and they have succeeded in achieving the right level and volume of information about neurosurgery for the intended audience. This book is a useful addition to the neurosurgical literature; I believe it will be read widely.

Robert H. Wilkins, M.D.
Durham, North Carolina

Preface

Essentials of Neurosurgery has been compiled by the combined efforts of the faculty of clinical neurosurgery at the Medical College of Georgia. We have consulted with housestaff in neurosurgery and with colleagues from the allied disciplines of orthopedics, neuroradiology, and neuropathology.

The purpose of the book is to provide accessible and practical information for busy housestaff, residents, and practitioners in neurosurgery. We hope that this book will provide a quick reference to identify and to manage specific neurosurgical disorders. It is not our intention to compete with more comprehensive texts in neurosurgery but rather to provide a concise and practical reference.

The scope of this text is intended to be broad, covering routine neurosurgical diagnoses and corresponding procedures. Although this book has been compiled by the faculty of the Medical College of Georgia, we believe that the text reflects routine practice elsewhere and not just the methods used at this institution. Where our experience has been limited, we have attempted to include comments on alternative methods that may be practiced in other departments. In particular, our faculty has special interests in vascular lesions of the brain, pediatric neurosurgery, structural disorders of the spine, and functional neurosurgery (stereotactic surgery, surgical treatment of intractable pain, and surgical treatment of seizures). This is reflected in the contents of the book.

The text begins by reviewing basic information on neurological and related anatomy and the principles of basic clinical examination. This is followed by chapters covering the common and currently used clinical investigations to diagnose and manage neurosurgical disorders. Then the text provides more detailed reviews of the management of specific lesions affecting the nervous system. The reader will find study questions throughout the book, and we hope that these will be a useful resource to determine overall comprehension and understanding of clinical problems arising in routine neurosurgical practice.

As with all areas in medicine, techniques to diagnose and manage disorders in neurosurgery are advancing all the time. It is inevitable that many of the procedures described in our book will eventually be superseded by further technological improvements. At the time of publication, however, it is our intention to present what we believe are to be the most current and routine procedures in neurosurgical practice. We hope this will become a standard reference for those entering the field of neurosurgery.

The staff is extremely grateful to Dr. J. Allan Goodrich of Orthopedics Service, Dr. Farivar Yaghmai of Neuropathology, and Dr. Ramón Figueroa and Dr. José Bauzá of Neuroradiology for their support.

We express our most heartfelt thanks to Mrs. Beulah A. Collins for the tireless efforts she has put into the preparation of this manuscript.

Finally, the authors and editors would like to express our sincerest appreciation to Dr. Jane E. Pennington and the staff of McGraw-Hill, Inc., for the tolerance and support they have provided in the preparation of this work. Without their support, this work would not have been possible.

1 Neuroanatomical Basis for Surgery on the Cranium

Martin Greenberg

Scalp

☐ SURGICAL ANATOMY OF THE SCALP

The *scalp* is composed of five layers: the *skin; subcutaneous tissue; epicranial aponeurosis,* or *galea; loose areolar tissue;* and *pericranium* (Fig. 1-1).[1] The skin is thick and contains hair and sebaceous glands. The subcutaneous tissue is fibrofatty, has a network of fibrous septae, and is richly vascular as branches of the external and internal carotid arteries anastomose in this layer. The epicranial aponeurosis, or galea, is a strong, tendinous sheet with three attachments: anteriorly to the frontalis muscle, posteriorly to the occipitalis muscle, and laterally to the small temporoparietalis muscles. The galeal closure is the key for ensuring scalp flap integrity in the postoperative neurosurgical patient.

Loose areolar tissue connects the galea to the *pericranium,* or *periosteum* of the skull. The *areolar layer* contains the valveless *emissary veins,* which connect the scalp veins with the diploic veins of the skull and, ultimately, the *intracranial venous sinuses* (e.g., the superior sagittal sinus).[2]

The *pericranial layer* is the periosteum covering the skull. At the skull suture lines, the periosteum becomes continuous with the *endosteum* on the inner skull surface (Fig. 1-1). Further, the outer layer of the dura mater, or *endosteal layer,* is continuous with the periosteum of the inner surface of the skull. Thus, a traumatic fracture of the skull extending through the suture line may implicate an underlying intracranial pathological process or lesion (e.g., epidural or subdural hematoma or pneumocephalus).[3–7]

The inner layer of the dura mater, or *meningeal layer,* separates from the outer or endosteal layer at the midline to form the *superior sagittal sinus,* before continuing inferiorly to join and form the *falx cerebri* (Fig. 1-1).[1] A compound fracture of the skull along the midline or vertex may invoke massive bleeding from the scalp resulting from a tear in the superior sagittal sinus, or there may be nothing more than an underlying tear in the sagittal sinus, with tamponade.[3–7]

☐ VASCULARITY OF THE SCALP

ARTERIAL SUPPLY[2]

The *arterial supply* of the scalp lies in the second, or subcutaneous tissue, layer. The scalp is richly vascular because of anastomotic supply from both the *external carotid arteries* (ECA) and *internal carotid arteries* (ICA)—but predominantly from the ECA (Fig. 1-2). The *occipital artery,* fourth branch of the ECA, arises from the latter's posterior surface opposite the origin of the *facial artery,* passes through the posterior triangle of the neck and supplies the back of the scalp as high as the vertex of the skull. The *posterior auricular artery,* fifth branch of the ECA, also arises posteriorly and supplies the territory above and between the auricle and back of the scalp. The *superficial temporal artery* (STA), the smaller terminus of the ECA, courses in front of the auricle and divides into anterior and posterior branches supplying the frontal and temporal scalp regions, respectively. The *internal maxillary artery,* the larger terminus of the ECA, may also contribute to scalp vascularity via its numerous branches, including the mandibular, the middle meningeal, the pterygoid, and pterygopalatine segments. In this way, the ECA branches provide most of the blood supply to the scalp.

The ICA contributes to scalp vascularity solely through the *ophthalmic artery,* the first branch of the ICA after it exits the cavernous sinus. The ophthalmic artery enters the orbit through the optic canal below and lateral to the optic nerve. Its branches, the *supratrochlear* and *supraorbital arteries,* supply the scalp of the forehead and anastomose with branches of the STA, thus enhancing the vascularity of the scalp. Anteriorly, it anastomoses with the angular branch of the *internal maxillary artery.*

VENOUS DRAINAGE[2]

Venous drainage of the scalp can occur through two pathways. The *superficial veins* in the subcutaneous tissue drain

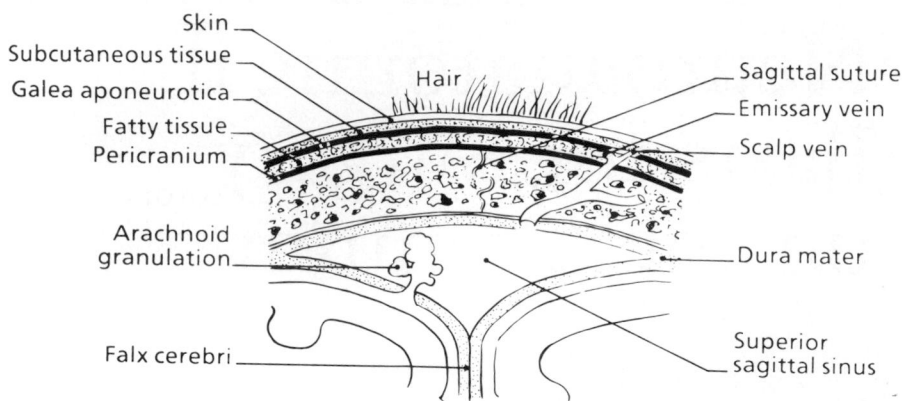

Figure 1–1 A coronal section of the scalp, skull, and superior sagittal venous sinuses (SSS).

directly into (1) the *internal* or *external jugular veins* or (2) the *emissary veins* in the loose areolar tissue layer and, finally, through the *diploic veins* of the skull into the *intracranial venous sinuses:* the *superior sagittal sinus* (SSS), *inferior sagittal sinus* (ISS), and *sigmoid sinus* (SS). For example, the mastoid emissary vein, frequently encountered during the course of surgery in the posterior fossa—especially in the cerebellopontine angle—drains into the SS.

☐ SCALP INCISIONS

Because of the rich vascularity of the scalp, several types of scalp incisions yield generously wide exposures for craniotomy with excellent cosmetic results.[3–10]

The *bicoronal flap* is ideal for treatment of large basal anterior frontal meningiomas and malignant tumors invading the anterior skull base, such as esthesioneuroblastomas, squamous cell carcinomas, or suprasellar lesions, as well as cerebrospinal fluid (CSF) leaks through the cribriform plate or frontal bone, and giant aneurysms of the anterior communicating artery. The *Soutar flap* is a modification of the bicoronal flap, wherein the skin incision closely follows the hairline and resembles a Turkish hat in outline (Fig. 1-3*A*).

Classically, the *coronal incision* allows access to both the frontal and temporal regions (Fig. 1-3*A*). The scalp incision

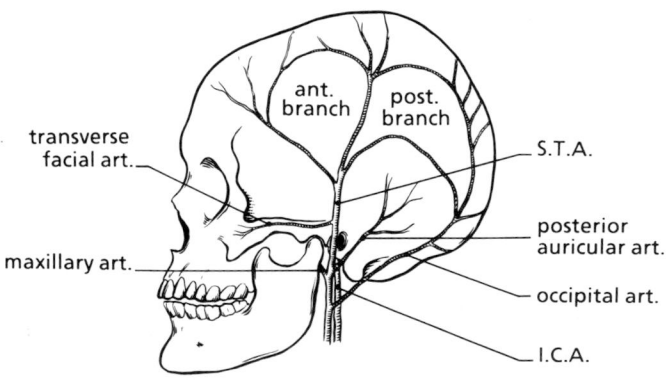

Figure 1–2 A diagram of the external carotid artery and key branches of neurosurgical interest.

is made behind the hairline, 1 cm anterior to the tragus of the ear, and extends from one zygomatic arch to the contralateral side. The skin, subcutaneous tissue, and galea are incised and mobilized as a single unit, and the pericranium can then be dissected with a scalpel or with cautery.

Great care is taken not to injure the *facial nerve,* which courses below the zygoma and has a key temporal branch supplying the *frontalis* and *orbicularis oculi muscles* (Fig. 1-3*B*). The STA should be preserved during the skin incision to ensure scalp viability. Full mobilization in length of the STA is necessary for external carotid to internal carotid (EC-IC) anastomoses involved in trapping and bypassing giant cavernous and other intracranial aneurysms, such as giant aneurysms of the anterior or middle cerebral arteries.

Hemostasis of the scalp is secured either with Raney or Michel clips applied to the scalp skin and galeal edges or with Dandy clamps applied to the galea. Infiltration with lidocaine with epinephrine 1:100 prior to incision decreases bleeding from the wound. Digital pressure applied by a surgeon's widely spaced fingertips controls bleeding from the scalp during the incision.

Scalp hair should be clipped and shaved in a wider circumferential area than the skin incision site in order to obviate troublesome hair from the prepping and draping procedures and to reduce the chance of infection. This preparation should precede the neurosurgical procedure by less than 2 to 3 hours. Weck blades held in a barber's handle serve as a useful tool for shaving.

The frontotemporal scalp flap allows access to the ipsilateral frontal and temporal lobes (Fig. 1-3*A*). Similarly, the skin incision is above the zygoma and anterior to the external ear, stays behind the hairline, and curves medially to end in the midline of the forehead. The scalp, underlying temporalis muscle, and pericranium can be incised and mobilized as a single unit, with the muscle being dissected with scalpel or cautery from the superior temporal line, leaving a small cuff for closure. The temporalis muscle may be incised and reflected anteriorly or inferiorly depending upon the surgeon's preference.

The *pterional approach* combines the frontotemporal flap with a sphenoid bone dissection and gains access to the sellar and parasellar regions through the Sylvian fissure. This sphenoidal approach is ideal for carotid-cavernous aneurysms and tumors of the anterior skull base, including meningiomas, craniopharyngiomas, optic gliomas, and so forth.[8]

The *question-mark scalp flap,* or its inverse, can be used for gaining access to ipsilateral lesions adjacent to or involving the anterior temporal lobe—including tumors, epidural or subdural hematomas—and for temporal lobectomy for epilepsy surgery (Fig. 1-3*B*). The scalp incision starts above the zygoma, curves posteriorly to 3.5 cm behind the external acoustic meatus, and curves anteriorly along the superior temporal line. Care is taken to preserve the temporal branch of the facial nerve and the STA.

The *horseshoe-shaped scalp flap,* often paramedian, is made in an inverted U shape which can be used for frontal, temporal, parietal, occipital, and even suboccipital exposures. The base of the flap should be as broad as its height to ensure vascularity. A horseshoe-shaped flap, centered over the coronal suture, can be used for the transcallosal approach to third ventricle tumors (Fig. 1-3*C*).[4] An inverted U-shaped incision based on the inion (external occipital protuberance) from mastoid tip-to-tip will allow ready access for posterior fossa surgery.[3]

The *linear transverse* and *curvilinear S-shaped incisions* are shortened modifications of scalp openings (Fig. 1-3*D*). These are ideal for closed and open head trauma and will easily incorporate contused scalp into the incision prior to debridement of devitalized skin. As an example, the linear transverse incision may be used in the temporal region for a subtemporal approach to low-lying basilar tip and posterior circulation aneurysms;[5] or, for the posterior fossa, a linear or curvilinear incision may be used for access to acoustic neuromas, vertebrobasilar aneurysms, or cerebellar hematomas (Fig. 1-3*D*). Thus, the linear and curvilinear scalp incisions provide for versatile exposure of the skull with excellent wound healing because of minimal interruption of blood supply.

☐ SAGITTAL SINUS AND VENOUS SINUSES[1,2]

The *venous sinuses* of the cranial cavity are formed from a split in the inner (*meningeal*) and outer (*endosteal*) layers of the *dura mater* (Fig. 1-1). The sinuses are lined by *endothelium,* devoid of smooth muscle, and are valveless.

The *superior longitudinal sinus,* or *sagittal sinus, is the major venous sinus implicated in neurosurgical pathology.* It begins in front at the foramen cecum and runs posteriorly along the skull vault to the *internal occipital protuberance,* where at the *torcular Herophili,* or *sinus confluens,* it forms the statistically more dominant *right transverse* and less dominant *left transverse sinuses,* respectively. Anatomically, the location of the transverse sinus is usually in a horizontal plane with the helix of the external ear (Fig. 1-3*E*). The transverse sinus ends by turning downward as the *sigmoid sinus,* which grooves the mastoid part of temporal bone (Fig. 1-3*E*). The sigmoid sinus turns forward and downward to become con-

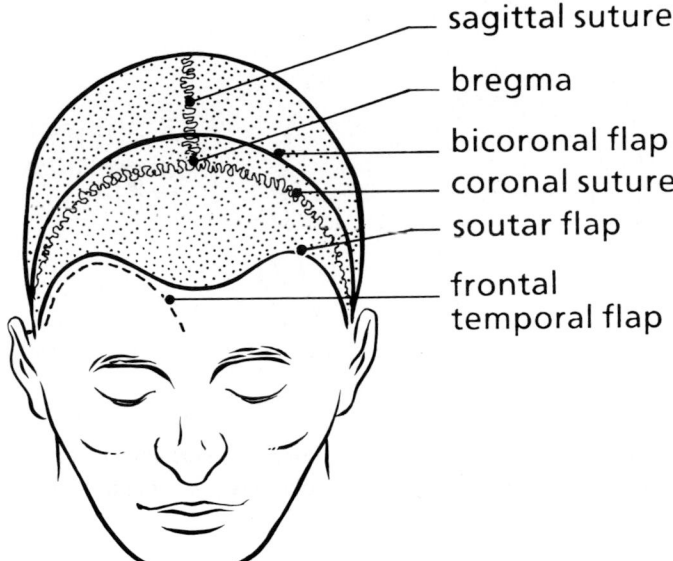

Figure 1–3A A diagram of relevant neurosurgical scalp flaps.

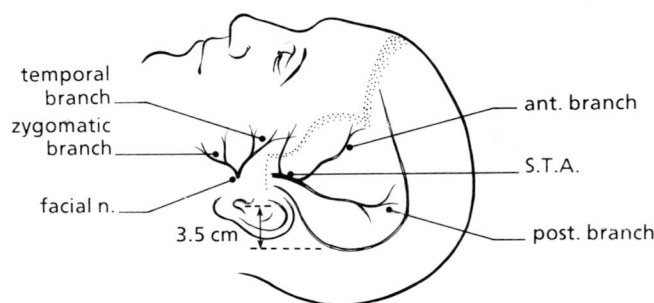

Figure 1–3B The scalp flap for temporal lobectomy, with attention to the facial nerve and superficial temporal artery.

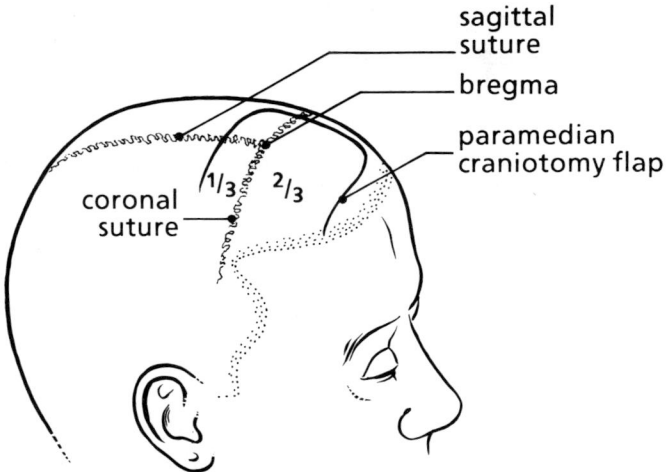

Figure 1–3C Diagram of the paramedian or central craniotomy flap.

tinuous with the *internal jugular vein.* The *occipital sinus,* often a vestigial remnant, begins near the foramen magnum and drains into the torcular Herophili.

Because of its anatomical length, the sagittal sinus is often injured traumatically or compromised by tumor growth, or it

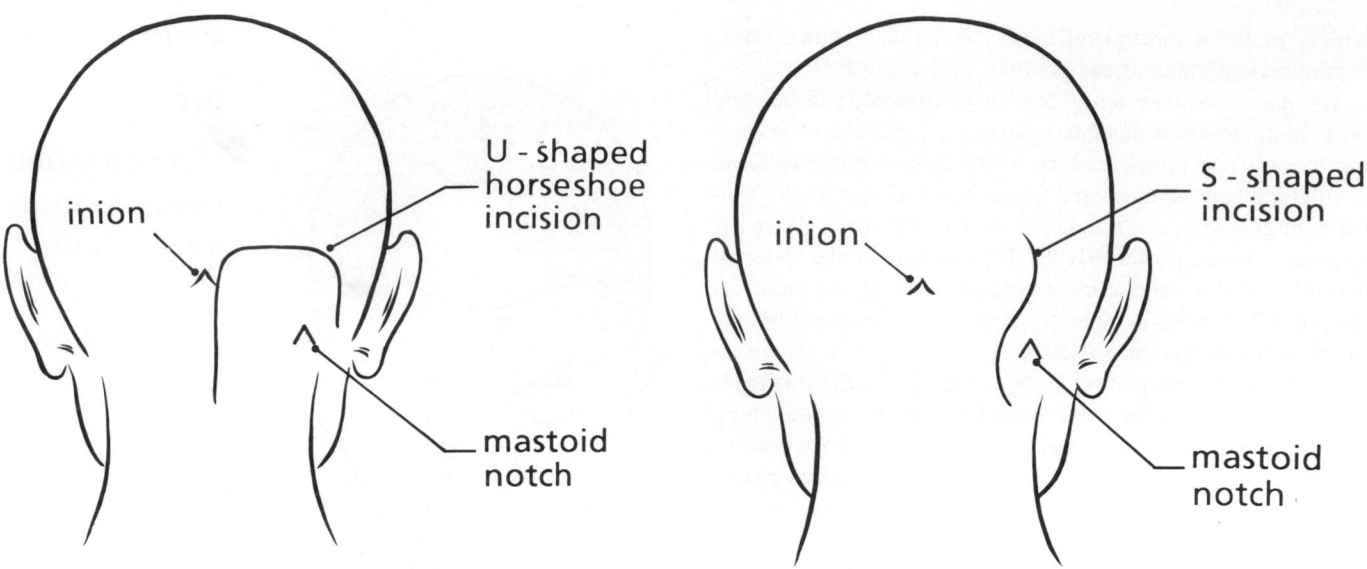

Figure 1–3D1 and 1–3D2   A diagram of the U-shaped horseshoe and S-shaped incisions.

may be functionally altered by draining veins of an arterio-venous malformation (AVM) under increased pressure.

The *length of the sagittal sinus* can be divided conveniently into thirds, based on local skull anatomy.[5-7] The first, or anterior, third of the sinus extends from the crista galli to the coronal suture; the middle third extends between the coronal and lambdoid sutures; and the posterior third runs from the lambdoid suture to the torcular Herophili. Occlusion of the anterior one-third causes minimal focal neurological damage, whereas occlusion to the middle third may result in damage to the sensorimotor cortex and produce severe neurological deficits due to thrombosis of feeding veins. Injury to the posterior third may cause visual field deficits by involving the visual cortex, or in some instances death from cerebral edema if the torcular Herophili is disrupted or thrombosed.

The sagittal sinus is a high-flow venous system under low pressure. Traumatic fractures indenting the sinus may tamponade any local bleeding.

A key to understanding the sagittal sinus is obtained from a review of its microscopic neuroanatomy (Fig. 1-1). The sagittal sinus is trefoil, or triangular, in shape, and has three edges. Thus a closed, depressed skull fracture may only com-

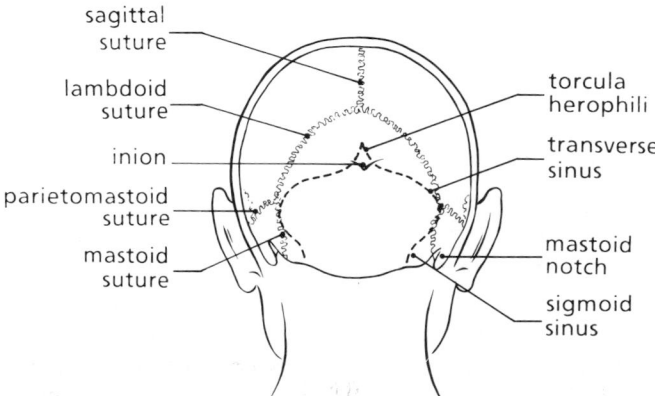

Figure 1–3E   A diagram of the transverse sinus and relevant anatomic landmarks.

press or tear one of the three edges and cause local hemorrhage. An open depressed skull fracture may tear one or all three edges and result in a massive hemorrhage from the wound.

The *surgical handling of injuries to the sagittal sinus is often first managed by local tamponade.*[5-7] Digital compression and raising the head of the operating room table above the heart will reduce hemorrhage. Local hemostatic agents including Gelfoam or Surgicel that has been immersed in a solution containing thrombin or dry Avitene may be applied locally, followed by cottonoids or cotton patties to lessen bleeding. If these maneuvers are inadequate, patches of dura, pericranium, or fascia lata may be applied or oversewn directly or overlapping the sinus. Large tears in the lateral sinus wall usually can be repaired directly with suture material. Reconstruction of the sinus can be performed with dural tunnels, venous replacement grafts, siliconized T-tube stents placed within the sinus lumen, or simply Foley catheters introduced to reconstruct the lumen and allow oversewing the sinus with dural patches.

With massive, uncontrolled bleeding, the sagittal sinus may be sacrificed by ligation with suture or Weck clips. The *key to ligation* is suturing all three corners of the sinus with tandem sutures, and then incising the sinus and falx between the sutures. This maneuver may be performed with impunity along the anterior one-third of the sinus, but ligation in the posterior two-thirds, especially behind the rolandic fissure and motor cortex, may lead to permanent neurological deficits and/or massive brain swelling.

Similarly, traumatic injury to the transverse or sigmoid sinus can be tested intraoperatively. Temporary occlusions of the nondominant (usually left) transverse or sigmoid sinus may be made with Weck or aneurysm clips as a test, with special attention focused on any resultant brain swelling to assess the adequacy of collateral flow.

Tumors of the parasaggital meninges, falx, or tentorium may invade any of the major sinuses.[3-10] Similarly, dural

AVMs may cause hypertension in the venous sinuses, thus impairing cerebral venous flow. Cerebral angiography or magnetic resonance imaging (MRI) flow studies with gadolinium are essential aids in understanding local vascular anatomy.

☐ FALX CEREBRI AND ITS ATTACHMENTS[11–15]

The *falx cerebri* is a sickle-shaped fold of dura which affixes anteriorly to the *crista galli* and blends posteriorly with the *tentorium cerebelli*. The falx separates the right and left hemispheres. The superior sagittal sinus runs in its upper margin and the inferior sagittal sinus in its lower margin. The straight sinus lies between the attachments of the falx cerebri and the tentorium cerebelli. The falx may be infiltrated by meningiomas or have enlarged collateral vascular channels with pericallosal AVMs.

The tentorium cerebelli is a crescent-shaped fold of dura which supports and separates the occipital lobes of the cerebral hemispheres from the cerebellum. Its anterior margin, the *tentorial notch,* is a gap through which the midbrain, including the third (oculomotor) and fourth (trochlear) cranial nerves, pass. It is bounded laterally by the *mesial temporal lobes (uncus).*

The tentorium has attachments to the anterior and posterior clinoid processes and petrous ridges of the temporal bones. Clinically, with temporal lobe or uncal herniation, there is compression of the ipsilateral midbrain and third nerve through the tentorial notch, leading to ipsilateral third nerve dysfunction, producing a dilated pupil, ptosis, medial rectus palsy, and contralateral hemiparesis. Because of this local anatomy, temporal lobe tumors and intracerebral hematomas may lead to varying degrees of third nerve dysfunction and hemiparesis. In "Kernohan's notch," there is uncal herniation and displacement of the brain stem, producing compression of the contralateral midbrain (cerebral peduncle) by the tentorium, which results in ipsilateral hemiparesis as well as an ipsilaterally dilated pupil, ptosis, and medial rectus palsy (ipsilateral third nerve dysfunction).

The falx cerebelli is a sickle-shaped fold of dura which separates the cerebellar hemispheres and contains the occipital sinus. The *diaphragma sellae* is a circular-shaped fold of dura which forms the roof of the *sella turcica* and through which the *pituitary stalk* passes. The diaphragma sellae may be incompetent and allow the arachnoid to develop space within the sella, leading to the "empty-sella syndrome." Visual field deficits, pituitary dysfunction, and, rarely, CSF rhinorrhea are possible results.[5–7]

☐ BRAIN TOPOGRAPHY AND LOCATION OF THE MOTOR STRIP[11–16]

The average adult male brain weighs approximately 1400 grams, of which 80 percent is water. Grossly, the brain is

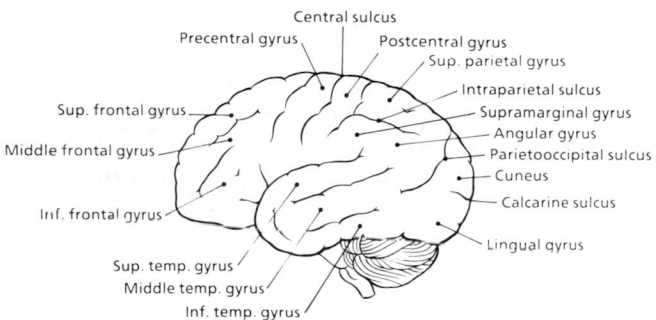

Figure 1–4 A lateral view of the cerebral cortex, illustrating the gyri and sulci.

divided into *cerebrum, cerebellum,* and *brain stem.* The cerebral surface is marked by *gyri,* or eminences, and *sulci,* or fissures (Fig. 1-4). The *major lateral sulcus,* or *sylvian fissure,* is present at the base of the brain and extends posteriorly and upward (Fig. 1-4). The *major central sulcus,* or *rolandic fissure,* extends from the hemispheric midline downward and forward until it nearly meets the sylvian fissure (Fig. 1-4). The central sulcus demarcates the key *precentral gyrus,* or *motor cortex,* and *postcentral gyrus,* or *sensory cortex.*

The *cerebral hemisphere* is divided schematically into four lobes: the *frontal, parietal, occipital,* and *temporal lobes.*

The frontal lobe occupies roughly one third of the hemisphere, beginning anteriorly and ending at the central sulcus, with lateral extension to the sylvian fissure. On the convexity it is divided into *superior, middle, inferior,* and *precentral gyri.*

The parietal lobe begins at the central sulcus and extends posteriorly to the parieto-occipital fissure; its lateral boundaries are marked by a line tangental to the sylvian fissure. It is divided into *postcentral, supramarginal,* and *angular gyri.*

The occipital lobe is situated posterior to the parieto-occipital fissure and extends inferiorly to the *preoccipital notch.*

The temporal lobe lies inferior to the sylvian fissure and extends posteriorly to the parieto-occipital fissure. The lateral surface is divided into three gyri: superior, middle, and inferior, respectively.

It is important to emphasize several *key, anatomic landmarks of skull anatomy.* The *location of the motor cortex* can be approximated by drawing a line from the pterion to a point 5 cm behind the coronal suture and at a 45-degree angle to a linear plane drawn from the *orbital plate* to the *external acoustic meatus.* The motor cortex will lie along this line. *Broca's area,* the dominant motor speech area, lies anterior to this line in the *inferior frontal gyrus.*

Further, by MRI, one can visually localize the central sulcus on the T2 axial weighted image, and relate the motor cortex to the coronal suture for safe cortical resection. By cerebral angiography, one can identify the major anastomotic *vein of Trolard,* which courses over the hemispheric convexity from the superior sagittal sinus to join the posterior aspect of the *major sylvian,* or *middle cerebral, vein,* which will localize the motor cortex. Intraoperatively, one can follow the sylvian fissure and its major middle cerebral vein posteriorly to the anastomotic vein of Trolard, thus again identifying the region of the motor cortex.

If tumors or AVMs are situated in or near the motor cortex, localization is accomplished by cortical stimulation in a patient who is awake. Alternatively, sensory evoked potentials can be used to localize important cortical structures.

☐ VISUAL SYSTEM[11–16]

OPTIC NERVE

The *optic nerve* [cranial nerve (CN) II] contains myelinated axons arising from the ganglion cell layer of the retina. The nerve fibers comprising the temporal half of the retina represent the *nasal visual field,* whereas the fibers comprising the nasal half of the retina represent the *temporal visual field.* Further, the superior half of the retina represents the inferior half of the visual field, and vice versa. Thus, the visual image is inverted and reversed left-for-right.

Structurally, the optic nerve is nearly 4 cm long and 0.5 cm wide, and it passes through the *optic canal* with the *ophthalmic artery.* The optic canal is formed by adjacent segments of *sphenoid, frontal,* and *ethmoid* bones.

Tumors such as optic gliomas, meningiomas, and cavernous hemangiomas can enlarge the optic nerve sheath, infiltrate the optic foramen, and cause decreased visual acuity.[17,18] Traumatic skull fractures may disrupt the bony optic canal and cause decreased vision in the involved eye. Complete destruction of an optic nerve leads to blindness in the denervated eye.

Idiopathic fibrous dysplasia can cause deformation of the optic canal with proptosis and decline in vision. Aneurysms at the site of the origin of the ophthalmic artery can cause decreased visual acuity in the adjacent optic nerve. In the rare *Foster Kennedy syndrome,* there may be primary optic atrophy ipsilateral to a sphenoid wing meningioma with contralateral papilledema.[17,18]

OPTIC CHIASM

Fibers from the optic nerves meet at the *optic chiasm.* There, the fibers from the nasal halves of each retina decussate, whereas fibers from the temporal halves do not cross but continue ipsilaterally with the decussated fibers as the *optic tracts.* Thus, the right optic tract will contain fibers from the right temporal retina and left nasal retina and, therefore, carry vision seen in the right nasal and left temporal visual fields.

Anatomically, the optic chiasm measures 1.2 cm wide and 0.4 cm high, and it is located above the sella turcica of the sphenoid bone. In the majority of cases (80 percent), the chiasm lies directly above the central portion of the diaphragma sellae and the pituitary gland. In the minority of cases (20 percent), the chiasm is either anteriorly situated

and overlies the *tuberculum sellae,* the so-called prefixed chiasm, or it may be posteriorly situated and overlie the *posterior clinoids, the postfixed chiasm.* As a result, the position of the optic chiasm with respect to the pituitary gland and diaphragma sellae may affect the pattern of visual field deficits seen in neurosurgical pathology.

The upper surface of the optic chiasm is attached to the *lamina terminalis* of the third ventricle, and its lower surface is separated from the pituitary gland by the diaphragma sellae, a dural leaf forming the roof of the sella. Usually a small collection of cerebrospinal fluid lies between the chiasm and the diaphragma sellae.

Pituitary tumors often compress the decussating, nasal retinal fibers from below the optic chiasm and cause a bitemporal visual field cut, beginning in the superior quadrants. Anatomically, this occurs because the lower nasal fibers, or upper temporal fields, cross low in the optic chiasm. Some loop forward into the opposite optic nerve before continuing on in the optic chiasm and tract. This loop is called "Wilbrand's knee," and is frequently damaged by lesions extending up from the pituitary fossa.

Craniopharyngiomas within the third ventricle will compress the optic chiasm from above and cause a bitemporal hemianopic visual field deficit chiefly in the inferior quadrants. Anatomically, this occurs because the upper nasal fibers, or lower temporal fields, cross high and posteriorly in the chiasm and are frequently damaged above and behind by craniopharyngiomas.

Parasellar aneurysms of the internal carotid artery and planum sphenoidale or tuberculum sellae meningiomas can cause varied chiasmal visual syndromes.[17,18] The junctional syndrome of Traquir, ipsilateral visual loss, and contralateral superior quadrantanopsia can be seen with an extrinsic tumor compressing the optic nerve near its junction with the optic chiasm. Gliomas of the chiasm may cause fusiform enlargement of the optic chiasm and often diffuse involvement of the optic nerve and tracts. Clivus chordomas arising from notochordal remnants in the dorsum sellae can extend superiorly or laterally and produce lesions in the optic chiasm or an optic tract.

OPTIC TRACTS

The *optic fibers* emerge from the posterolateral aspect of the optic chiasm as two divergent *tracts* and then pass backward along the lateral aspect of the midbrain until they reach the *left* and *right lateral geniculate bodies* of the thalamus. A smaller number of optic tract fibers subserving the pupillary and ocular reflexes bypass the lateral geniculate body and project to the pretectal area and superior colliculus, respectively.

A lesion of the optic tract disconnects fibers from one half of each retina and leads to blindness in the contralateral visual fields of both eyes, producing a homonymous hemianopsia. The field defect is also incongruous in that the visual field deficit in the half of one eye is dissimilar to that in the other eye. Homonymous hemianopsias tend to be more congruous as the lesion producing the defect is located nearer to the occipital cortex. Thus, a right mesial temporal lobe glioma may compromise the right optic tract and cause an incongruous left homonymous hemianopsia. However, primary lesions of the optic tract are rare.

LATERAL GENICULATE[11-16]

The optic tract terminates in the *lateral geniculate body,* the posterolateral portion of the thalamus, lateral to the midbrain. Each lateral geniculate body contains six layers of cells. It receives fibers from both eyes, but the fibers of the optic tract originating in the left eye terminate on only three of the six layers while those from the right eye terminate on the remaining three layers.

Lesions of the lateral geniculate body are rare and usually associated with pathology in or near the thalamus. Thalamic gliomas, metastases, and AVMs may compress the lateral geniculate body and cause an incongruous homonymous hemianopic visual field defect.

OPTIC RADIATIONS

Neurons of the lateral geniculate body give rise to fibers that form the *optic radiations,* or the *geniculocalcarine tracts,* to the *occipital cortex.* Fibers from the lateral portion of the lateral geniculate body project anteriorly and inferiorly, then bend posteriorly in a loop that passes through the temporal lobe in the lateral wall of the *temporal horn* of the lateral ventricle, sweeping posteriorly to the occipital lobe. The inferior sweep, or bundle of geniculocalcarine fibers which curves around the lateral ventricle and reaches forward into the temporal lobe, bears the eponym *Meyer's loop.* Fibers from the superomedial portion of the lateral geniculate body travel close to the inferolateral portion but take a more direct course passing through the parietal lobe to the occipital lobe.

Lesions of the optic radiations cause classic patterns of visual field defects according to their location. Temporal lobe masses will compress the inferior fibers of the optic radiations and cause a homonymous, superior quadrantanopsia, or so-called pie-in-the-sky defect. Parietal lobe masses compress the superior fibers of the optic radiations and cause a homonymous, inferior quadrantanopsia. Parietal lobe field defects are usually congruous. It should be emphasized that mass lesions in either the temporal or parietal lobe may cause a complete superior and inferior homonymous hemianopsia.

VISUAL CORTEX

Optic radiations sweep posterolaterally around the lateral ventricle and terminate in the occipital lobe. The *primary visual cortex* (area 17) is located on the medial surface of the occipital lobe above and below the calcarine fissure. The visual cortex contains six layers, and is arranged in vertical columns of ocular dominance wherein the columns receiving input from one eye alternate with columns receiving input from the other eye.

Visual cortex is known as *striate cortex* because of a horizontal stripe of white matter, called *Gennari's line,* within the gray matter of the fourth layer. This horizontal stripe is visible to the naked eye.

Within the striate cortex the *central visual fibers,* or *macular fibers,* are represented at the very tip of the occipital lobe. The *peripheral visual fibers* are represented more rostrally along the *calcarine fissure.* The most peripheral fibers, or *temporal crescent,* are situated most anteriorly in the occipital lobe at the rostral end of the calcarine fissure. The *inferior visual field fibers* (or *superior retinal*), terminate above the calcarine fissure, whereas the *superior visual field fibers* (or *inferior retinal*) are below the fissure. Each striate cortex receives the visual input from stimuli in the contralateral half of the visual field of each eye.

Lesions that destroy the entire visual area of the occipital lobe—e.g., tumors (meningiomas, gliomas, metastases) and AVMs—produce a contralateral, homonymous hemianopsia. The *hallmarks of occipital cortical lesions are congruity and macular sparing.* With small lesions in the occipital lobe, there may be macular sparing, or preservation of central vision, as there is extensive representation of macular vision at the occipital pole or tip and in the depth of the calcarine fissure. There is incomplete segregation of crossed and uncrossed fibers and double innervation of macular areas—all accounting for this macular sparing. There is also dual blood supply to the occipital lobe, the posterior cerebral artery, and middle cerebral artery.

Bilateral hemianopic lesions without any other neurologic signs or symptoms point to occipital lobe disease. Preservation or loss of the temporal crescent suggests occipital lobe disease, as a lesion rostral in the calcarine fissure may result in an isolated loss of the temporal 30 degrees of the visual field. If bilateral damage to the occipital lobe cortex occurs—e.g., trauma, vertebrobasilar ischemia—there may be bilateral homonymous hemianopsia or cortical blindness, but the pupillary reflexes, which are mediated through the colliculi, will be preserved.

Other clinical characteristics associated with cortical blindness are denial of blindness; visual hallucinations; confabulation, as in Korsakoff's psychosis; and allochiria, in which sensation from stimuli applied to one limb is localized by the patient in the opposite limb. Cortical blindness may be a complication of cerebral arteriography, but this usually has a good prognosis for return of visual function.

☐ HEARING[11-16]

AUDITORY SYSTEM

The auditory apparatus consists of the *external, middle,* and *inner ear.* Anatomically, the auditory system is contained in the petrous and tympanic portions of the temporal bone.

The external ear, or external auditory canal, is separated from the middle ear by the *tympanic membrane, or eardrum,* which receives incoming sound waves.

The middle ear is spanned by a chain of three bony ossicles: the *malleus, incus,* and *stapes.* The malleus is attached to the tympanic membrane. The incus serves as an intermediate ossicle in transmitting sound to the stapes. The stapes has a footplate which fits into an oval window between middle and inner ear cavities.

Sound transmitted to the tympanic membrane is amplified by the *ossicles* to reach the *oval window,* which represents a sealed membrane separating the air-filled middle ear from the fluid-filled inner ear. The oval window opens directly into the vestibular portion of the inner ear, which is bathed in fluid, the *perilymph.*

The inner ear is formed by the bony and membranous labyrinths. In addition, it can be divided into three distinct chambers: the *vestibule,* the *cochlea* (tube resembling the shell of a snail; from the Greek *kochlias,* meaning "snail"), and the *semicircular canals,* which are interconnected within the temporal bone to make up the *bony labyrinth.* Within this bony cavity filled with perilymph lies the *membranous labyrinth,* containing another fluid, *endolymph,* and the end organ for hearing, the *organ of Corti.* The cochlea is a spiral cavity divided into two perilymphatic chambers, the scala vestibuli and scala tympani.

The organ of Corti contains a sensory epithelium, or row of hair cells, which stretches along the length of the spiraling cochlea and rests on the basilar membrane. Sound waves transmitted to the middle ear are amplified at the stapes, the piston action of which produces an instantaneous pressure wave in the perilymph within a microsecond time scale. A traveling wave is set up on the basilar membrane, which is structurally narrower at its base than at its apex. Thus, the mechanical properties of the basilar membrane, through which the organ of Corti is stimulated, vary quite gradually from base to apex.

Pressure waves produced by sounds of specific frequency or pitch cause the basilar membrane to vibrate at specific points along its length. The organ of Corti is tonotopically organized so that the highest tones (highest, that is, in pitch and frequency) stimulate hair cells at the base of its membrane where it is most narrow, whereas tones of the lowest pitch stimulate the most apical hair cells. Sound pressure waves augmented at the oval window are ultimately dampened at the anatomical round window.

Physiologically, sound waves cause shearing forces on the hair cells, which lead to the generation of ionic fluxes in the dendrites of the spiral ganglion cells. The *spiral ganglion,* located in the cochlea, contains bipolar cells of the cochlear division of the eighth nerve. Thus, energy from sound waves is converted to physiological ionic currents, a process of sensory transduction essential for the phenomenon we call "hearing." Further, each spiral ganglion has a characteristic frequency-dependent response to sound, and hence a characteristic, specific position on the tuning curve.

Clinically, basilar skull fractures cross the *temporal bone* transversely more often than longitudinally, and they can cause hearing loss by disruption of the conduction mechanisms in the middle and inner ears. Tumors of the middle ear—e.g., schwannomas, glomus tympanicum, hemangiomas, and facial nerve neuromas—can present with conductive hearing loss, tinnitus, and facial paralysis.[4,18] The petrous portion of the temporal bone (pyramid, apex) may be eroded by a chordoma, an osteochondoma, or a squamous cell carcinoma, as well as by benign tumors. Cholesteatomas or epidermoids may erode from the tympanic membrane and cavity medially into the cerebellopontine angle. The cholesterol granuloma, an expansile accumulation of inflammatory debris, may arise from the petrous apex and likewise expand into the posterior fossa. Benign tumors may cause compression of the vestibulocochlear (CN VIII) and facial (CN VII) nerves. Often, signs and symptoms of the above cause the patient to present first to otolaryngologists. A combined surgical approach with partial or total petrosectomy is often warranted.[18]

☐ AUDITORY PATHWAYS[11-16]

BRAINSTEM

Cochlear Division of Eighth Cranial Nerve   The cochlear division of the eighth cranial nerve (CN VIII) arises from fibers of the spiral ganglion cells and enters the brainstem at the pontomedullary junction. The *cochlear nerve—first-order fibers*—passes lateral to the inferior cerebellar peduncle and restiform body and synapses in the dorsal and ventral cochlear nuclei of the medulla. The neurons that comprise these two nuclei are organized tonotopically, or from high-frequency to low-frequency sound waves. From the cochlear nuclei, nerve fibers ascend in a tract of *second-order fibers,* the *lateral lemniscus.* Also, some of these nerve fibers cross to the *contralateral lateral lemniscus* through the *trapezoid body* of the *medulla.* Thus, each lateral lemniscus carries impulses from both ears.

Three projections of axons arise from the cochlear nuclei to relay hearing centrally to the auditory cortex. The *dorsal acoustic stria* originates in the *dorsal cochlear nucleus* and crosses in the floor of the fourth ventricle to join the contralateral lateral lemniscus. The *intermediate* and *ventral acoustic stria* originate in the ventral cochlear nucleus, terminate in the ipsilateral and contralateral nuclei of the trapezoid body and superior olivary nuclei of the pons, and then ascend in both the ipsilateral and contralateral lateral lemnisci.

Some fibers in the lateral lemnisci ascend through the brain stem and synapse in the nucleus of the inferior colliculus of the midbrain, while others synapse more rostrally in the medial geniculate body of the thalamus. The *third-order fibers* project from the *medial geniculate body* ipsilaterally to the *superior temporal gyrus,* the *primary auditory cortex.*

Vestibular Division of the Eighth Cranial Nerve Of clinical importance, the *acoustic neuroma* (*schwannoma*) commonly arises from the superior vestibular portion of the eighth nerve (CN VIII) in the internal auditory meatus and causes hearing loss by compressing the cochlear nerve.

Tinnitus and symptoms of vertigo are other progressive symptoms of an expanding acoustic neuroma of this portion of the eighth nerve, known as the *vestibular nerve*. These tumors originate at the peripheral portion (PNS) of the vestibular nerve. Schwannomas are located at the porus acousticus of the temporal bone and may grow preferentially into the cerebellopontine angle cistern or laterally into the internal auditory canal. Meningiomas, cholesteatomas (epidermoids), hemangioblastomas, arachnoid cysts, metastases, and vertebrobasilar aneurysms (e.g., AICA) are cerebellopontine angle lesions which can cause ipsilateral hearing loss by compressing the eighth nerve as it enters the brain stem at the pontomedullary junction.

Hearing loss due to an intrinsic lesion of the medulla, pons, or midbrain is very rare. This is explained by the fact that the hearing pathways in the brainstem are composed of crossed and uncrossed fibers, with cross-connections between the nuclei of the trapezoid body, the superior olivary nuclei, the nuclei of the lateral lemnisci, and the nuclei of the inferior colliculi. Thus, each lateral lemniscus conducts auditory stimuli, or hearing, from both ears.

CORTEX

The third-order fibers, carrying audition, project ipsilaterally from the medial geniculate body of the thalamus, the final sensory relay station of the hearing path, to the *superior temporal gyrus,* or *transverse gyrus* of *Heschl*. This *primary auditory cortex* is located on the dorsal surface of the superior temporal convolution and is partly buried in the *lateral,* or *sylvian, fissure*. It functions to discriminate changes in the temporal patterns of sounds and recognize the location or direction of sounds. The localization of high-to-low frequency sounds is arranged tonotopically in columns.

A unilateral lesion of the primary auditory cortex in the temporal lobe does not result in marked loss of hearing. For instance, a lesion of the right temporal gyrus interrupts impulses from both ears but does not interfere with other impulses from the ears going to the left temporal gyrus. Hence, temporal lobe tumors,—gliomas, metastases, meningiomas—rarely cause noticeable hearing loss, but bilateral lesions of the transverse gyri of Heschl are known to cause deafness.

Interestingly, lesions of the nondominant (right side in right-handed patients) temporal lobe impair the appreciation of music, especially the perception of musical notes and melodies. Auditory hallucinations and agnosias may also be associated with lesions of the temporal lobe, but their origin may be in the adjacent secondary zones of the auditory cortex rather than in the primary auditory cortex, or Heschl's gyrus. Overall, these clinical entities are rare, but they are seen in neurosurgical patients having temporal lobe tumors that are epileptogenic.

☐ SMELL[11–16]

PERIPHERAL OLFACTORY APPARATUS

Olfactory receptors are found in the specialized tissue of the upper nasal mucosa, the *olfactory epithelium*. Olfactory cells are bipolar neurons organized into a pseudostratified columnar epithelium. Their axons are grouped into 10 to 15 olfactory nerves, which pass through fenestrae in the cribriform plate of the ethmoid bone and terminate in the *olfactory bulb*. These olfactory nerves convey the sense of smell to the olfactory bulb, which is an extension of the *primary olfactory cortex,* or *rhinencephalon.*

Clinically, closed or open head trauma can cause basilar skull fractures of the frontal or ethmoid bone with resultant loss of smell. This may be secondary to avulsion of the olfactory nerves at the lamina cribrosa of the cribriform plate or to interruption of the olfactory tracts. Fractures extending through the cribriform plate into the ethmoid sinus can also give rise to CSF rhinorrhea, but only if the dura is lacerated over the frontal skull base. Unilateral or bilateral anosmia is a frequent sequela of traumatic contusions of the frontal lobes.

A rare tumor of the olfactory epithelium, the esthesioneuroblastoma, can cause unilateral or bilateral anosmia. This tumor may develop in the nasal cavity near the roof of the ethmoid sinus and can frequently bridge the cribriform plate with local intracranial invasion of both frontal lobes. The tumor occurs exclusively in the anterior cranial fossa. The esthesioneuroblastoma is best managed by a combined transcranial and transnasal resection through a bicoronal scalp flap and bifrontal craniotomy with en-bloc resection of the cribriform plate and ethmoid sinuses.[8]

OLFACTORY BULBS AND CORTEX

The *olfactory bulbs* rest on the cribriform plate and project their axons into the *olfactory tracts*. Each olfactory tract lies on the orbital surface of the frontal lobe under the gyrus rectus. As the tract passes posteriorly, it divides into *lateral* and *medial olfactory striae*. The lateral stria passes laterally along the floor of the sylvian fissure near the anterior perforated substance and enters the olfactory projection area lateral to the uncus in the temporal lobe. This area includes the *pyriform cortex* (*primary olfactory cortex*), the *entorhinal cortex,* and the *amygdala*. The primary olfactory cortex enables one to discriminate one odor from another. Olfactory impulses that project to the entorhinal cortex and amygdala are believed to be implicated in the chemosensory control of social behavior and its integration with the visual, auditory, and somatosensory input from other association cortices.

The *medial stria* fibers enter the *anterior olfactory nuclei,* the *anterior commissure* for cross-connections, and the *olfactory trigone* in the *anterior perforated substance.* These fibers subserve olfactory reflex reactions. Overall, the olfactory system is anatomically uncrossed except for the anterior commissural fibers, which are axon relays from one olfactory bulb to the contralateral bulb. Because of this, the clinical presentation of anosmia can be either unilateral or bilateral.

An olfactory groove meningioma presents classically with an insidious onset of unilateral or bilateral anosmia.[17] The meningioma originates from the dura overlying the cribriform plate and often grows to considerable size before detection. A syndrome associated with this tumor has the eponym of Foster Kennedy and includes central scotoma and primary optic atrophy on the side of the meningioma, as well as papilledema in the opposite eye. Frontal lobe gliomas, metastases, and abscesses may also present with varying changes in the sense of smell. Giant aneurysms of the anterior cerebral and anterior communicating arteries can also cause anosmia, along with abulia and personality changes secondary to bilateral mesial frontal lobe dysfunction. Anosmia resulting from retraction of the frontal lobe during a craniotomy is also a frequent sequela seen in neurosurgical practice; it is attributed to the olfactory bulbs being retracted from the ethmoid bones. Lastly, pediatric patients with anterior nasal encephaloceles are anosmic—probably secondary to dysgenesis of the olfactory tract.

Temporal lobe tumors including gliomas, oligodendrogliomas and gangliogliomas can present with "uncinate fits," or bizarre olfactory sensations, as an aura for a complex partial seizure. Hamartomas, cavernous hemangiomas, or areas of mesial temporal sclerosis can also have this clinical presentation with an olfactory aura.

Cerebral Cortex

☐ SURGICAL ANATOMY OF THE CEREBRAL CORTEX[11-16]

FRONTAL LOBES: DOMINANT AND NONDOMINANT HEMISPHERES

The *frontal lobes* include the hemispheres anterior to the *central* or *rolandic sulcus* (Fig. 1-4). The *precentral sulcus* lies anterior to the *precentral gyrus,* and separates it from the three parallel gyri; the *superior, middle,* and *inferior frontal gyri.* The inferior frontal gyrus is divided into three parts by the ascending rami of the lateral sylvian sulcus: the *orbital, triangular,* and *opercular* portions (Fig. 1-4). Beneath the orbital portion in the olfactory sulcus is the *olfactory tract.* Medial to it is the *straight gyrus,* or *gyrus rectus.* Most medial is the *cingulate gyrus,* a crescentric region adjacent to and continuing along the corpus callosum.

The *key areas of neurosurgical interest* are the motor strip (precentral gyrus), supplementary motor area (superior frontal gyrus, area 6), frontal eyefields (middle frontal gyrus, area 8), and the cortical center for micturition (middle frontal gyrus). In the dominant hemisphere is the Broca's speech area (inferior frontal gyrus, area 44), which controls the motor mechanism concerned with speech articulation. It should be noted that the vast majority of right-handed patients, 99 percent, including the majority of left-handed patients, > 50 percent, have left hemispheric dominance.

The *symptoms of frontal lobe dysfunction* include personality change, new-onset focal and major-motor seizures, motor deficits, and loss of micturition control. The *signs of frontal lobe dysfunction* include decline in intellect and memory, aberrant behavior, paraparesis or hemiparesis, grasp reflexes (e.g., palmomental), abnormalities in the voluntary gaze mechanism, and Broca's or motor aphasia if the dominant frontal lobe is involved (left hemisphere in right-handed patients). Motor aphasia implies an inability to speak but with understanding of instructions.

CLINICAL EXAMPLES

Tumors, abscesses, AVMs, and giant aneurysms can cause frontal lobe dysfunction secondary to local mass effect.[3-10,17-19] Parasagittal and falx meningiomas are midline, dural-based lesions which typically cause a slowly progressive spastic weakness of the opposite leg—and later of both legs. This classical pattern underlies the fact that the motor cortex is arranged in homunculus: leg → trunk → arm → face orientation from superior to inferior.

The leg fibers project on the medial surface of the hemisphere and the face fibers project just above the sylvian fissure. Classically, destructive lesions of the motor cortex (area 4) produce a contralateral flaccid paralysis and spasticity is more apt to occur if the supplementary motor area (area 6) is ablated.

The anterior skull-base meningiomas (e.g., olfactory groove, planum sphenoidale, tuberculum sellae, anterior clinoid, and medial sphenoid wing) can attain a very large size before insidiously causing bifrontal dysfunction with personality changes, alterations in mentation, and urinary incontinence.[18]

Large and giant anterior communicating artery aneurysms can present with subtle paraparesis, abulia, or akinetic mutism, and a loss of control of micturition. These aneurysms can be approached via a pterional craniotomy through a partial cortical resection of the gyrus rectus after the standard retraction of the orbital frontal lobe.[8]

Classically, traumatic frontal lobe contusions damage the ipsilateral eye fields and cause the eyes to deviate conjugately toward the damaged side of the cortex, owing to the unopposed activity of the intact, opposite frontal lobe. Further, there is often contralateral hemiparesis associated with an ipsilateral, traumatic frontal lobe contusion, due to damage to the adjacent motor cortex. Conversely, frontal lobe tumors with epileptic foci cause "frontal adversive attacks," with the head and eyes conjugately deviated away from the side of seizure activity. Contralateral hemiparesis may be secondary to residual tumor effect. Lastly, a frontal lobe abscess can present with fever, headache, lethargy, contralateral hemiparesis, and osteomyelitis of the frontal bone originating from an infected frontal sinus.

In normal pressure hydrocephalus—or the clinical triad of gait apraxia, dementia, and sphincteric incontinence—the ventricular expansion is seen to be maximal in the frontal horns, thus explaining this hydrocephalic impairment of frontal lobe functions. The placement of a ventriculoperitoneal shunt has been quite successful in reversing the clinical symptomatology, especially the gait disturbance.[5]

INDICATIONS FOR FRONTAL LOBECTOMY[3–10]

Frontal lobe gliomas and traumatic hemorrhagic contusions may present clinically as large lesions by computerized tomography (CT) or magnetic resonance imaging (MRI) with mass effect, edema, and shift. A frontal lobectomy may be indicated. Classically, a bicoronal skin flap and ipsilateral frontal craniotomy are performed. A 7- to 8-cm resection of the frontal lobe on the dominant (left-side) or nondominant (right-side) hemisphere is considered within the safe limits of resection. This should be measured intraoperatively from the frontal lobe tip in an anterior-to-posterior direction along the length of the anterior cranial fossa. One should draw a line at a 45-degree angle to the orbital roof, and from the pterion to a point 5 cm behind the coronal suture. The motor strip will lie along this line, and Broca's area lies anterior to it in the inferior frontal gyrus. A frontal lobectomy must be designed to spare Broca's area.[5–7]

PARIETAL LOBES: DOMINANT AND NONDOMINANT HEMISPHERES[11–16]

The *parietal lobes* extend from the rolandic sulcus anteriorly to the parieto-occipital sulcus posteriorly and to the temporal lobes and sylvian fissure laterally and inferiorly (Fig. 1-4). The *postcentral sulcus* lies behind the *postcentral gyrus* (Fig. 1-4). The *intraparietal sulcus* is a horizontal groove which occasionally unites with the *postcentral gyrus,* but which separates the *superior parietal gyrus* from the *inferior parietal gyrus.* The *supramarginal gyrus* is part of the inferior parietal gyrus and arches above the ascending end of the sylvian sulcus. The *angular gyrus* is the part of the inferior parietal gyrus which caps the end of the superior temporal sulcus. These two parts of the inferior parietal gyrus have close anatomic and physiological association with the superior and middle temporal gyri.

There are *several key areas of neurosurgical interest.* The *somesthetic area,* or *sensory cortex* (postcentral gyrus, areas 3, 1, and 2), is organized the same way as the motor strip, with representation for information from the face and arm on the lateral surface and the trunk and leg areas on the top and in the parasagittal areas, respectively. The *dominant parietal lobe* (left hemisphere in right-handed patients) comprises two cortical centers for speech and writing (Fig. 1-4): the *supramarginal gyrus* (area 40) and the *angular gyrus* (area 39). These two gyri and the posterior third of the superior temporal gyrus (areas 41, 42) constitute the *Wernicke's speech area,* or *receptive speech cortex.* Lesions of Wernicke's area lead to receptive aphasia, where the patient has poor comprehension of speech with repetition of phrases characterized by spoken, but often jumbled, language along with neologisms and verbal paraphasias. The recognition and utilization of numbers, arithmetic, and calculations are also integrated through the dominant parietal lobe. Lesions of the parietal operculum lead to a conduction aphasia by disconnecting Wernicke's area from Broca's area. A patient with a focal lesion in this area has fluent aphasia with poor repetition of spoken language.

In the nondominant parietal lobe (right hemisphere in right-handed patients), the *superior* and *inferior parietal lobules* provide no sensory or motor effects but provide a region for integrating the patient's awareness of space and person. A lesion in these parietal lobules classically produces construction and dressing apraxia, geographical confusion, and inattention or neglect of the contralateral side of the body. Patients with lesions in these areas have problems in the performance of simple tasks that were previously learned skills.

It should be stressed that the parietal lobes have extensive overlap with the occipital and temporal lobe functions. Hence, there are regions which integrate visual, sensory, and auditory phenomena. As an example, the phenomenon of *opticokinetic nystagmus* (OKN) is localized to the contralateral parietal lobe and its connection with the visual association cortex in the occipital lobe (area 19). Also, the optic radiations passing through the parietal lobe *en route* to the visual cortex carry information solely from the lower visual fields; consequently, a parietal lobe lesion will produce an inferior, homonymous quadrantanopsia. More typically, a parietal lobe lesion damages both the upper and lower visual fields, as may temporal lobe lesions, and it produces a complete homonymous hemianopsia.

In summary, the *symptoms of parietal lobe dysfunction* are sensory loss, sensory inattention or even focal sensory seizures, aphasia or apraxia depending upon the dominant or nondominant hemispheres affected, visual field defects, attention hemianopsias, and visual agnosia. Other classical signs are agraphesthesia, or inability to appreciate numbers written on the skin; astereognisis, or underestimating the size of objects; and abarosthesia, or a disturbance in perception of difference in weight.

CLINICAL EXAMPLES[3–10,19]

Parietal lobe tumors, abscesses, and AVMs typically cause hemispheric dysfunction by local mass effect. Parasagittal, falx, and convexity meningiomas can present with sensory seizures or with loss of touch localization, two-point discrimination, or joint position sense on the contralateral side. Parietal AVMs may present with intracerebral hematomas or with a progressive vascular steal or shunt phenomenon, causing receptive aphasia or apraxia in the dominant or nondominant hemisphere, respectively.[19] A focal parietal tumor, such as glioma, within the angular gyrus (area 39) on the dominant hemisphere, may cause Gerstmann's syndrome, comprising four elements: agraphia, right-to-left confusion, digital agnosia, and acalculia. A parietal lobe metastasis will often evoke considerable edema around a circumscribed mass separate from the adjacent brain, which can be dissected free through an intersulcal approach advocated by Yasargil.[8]

TEMPORAL LOBES: DOMINANT AND NONDOMINANT HEMISPHERES[11–16]

The *temporal lobe* lies inferior to the lateral sylvian sulcus and extends posteriorly to the level of the parieto-occipital sulcus on the medial surface of the hemisphere (Fig. 1-4). There is no definite anatomical boundary between the temporal lobe and the occipital or posterior part of the parietal lobe. The lateral surface of the temporal lobe is divided into three parallel gyri: *superior, middle,* and *inferior.* The inferior surface includes the *fusiform, hippocampal,* and *dentate gyri,* and most medially the *uncus.*

There are *several key areas of neurosurgical interest* in the temporal lobe. The classic *Wernicke's area* (superior temporal gyrus, areas 41 and 42), a center for receptive speech, is in the dominant lobe (left hemisphere for right-handed patients). Lesions in Wernicke's area produce an aphasia wherein there is an impairment in word comprehension, but the patient has voluble speech devoid of meaning.

The *transverse gyrus* of *Heschl* (superior temporal gyrus, area 41), is the final sensory pathway for hearing in the cortex. Interestingly, the nondominant Heschl's gyrus serves a role in music appreciation, whereas the dominant Heschl's gyrus (left hemisphere in right-handed patients) is concerned with the acoustic aspects of language. The nondominant hemisphere is important for the perception of musical notes and melodies, but the naming of musical scores and all the semantic aspects of music require the integrity of the dominant temporal lobe.

The *hippocampal gyrus* is implicated in short-term memory and has extensive connections with the limbic system. Lesions affect changes in mood, personality, sexuality, and behavior. Further, there are connections to the olfactory cortex, and lesions affect the sense of smell and taste. The uncus is important in the temporal lobe herniation syndrome.

Symptoms of temporal lobe disease include temporal lobe epilepsy or complex-partial seizures, with an aura of auditory, visual, smell, taste, and visceral sensations, or psychical phenomena such as *déjà vue,* accompanied by automatisms or motor movements such as grimacing, lip-smacking, chewing, staring, or fiddling with clothes. There may be memory disturbance or personality changes. Unilateral temporal lobe lesions, specifically involving the hippocampal gyrus, rarely cause significant memory impairment, but bilateral lesions cause the syndrome of Korsakoff's psychosis—a disastrous loss of ability to learn or establish new memories—together with confabulation and psychotic behavior. Bilateral lesions can also produce the classic Kluver-Bucy syndrome, an amnestic syndrome with apathy, placidity, hypersexuality, and psychic blindness or visual agnosia.

Bilateral lesions of Heschl's gyrus are quite rare; hence, the symptom of hearing loss is quite uncommon, owing to the bilateral representation of hearing in the auditory cortex.

In summary, it appears that with symptoms learned from temporal lobe disease states, one can surmise a role for the temporal lobe in integrating sound and sight with an individual's behavior and memory.

The signs of temporal lobe disease are few and far between compared with frontal or parietal lobe lesions. The neurosurgical patient may present with new-onset complex-partial seizures or may have evidence of upper homonymous quadrantanopsia secondary to interruption of Meyer's loop, the lower arching fibers of the geniculocalcarine pathway to the occipital cortex. The patient may have subtle personality changes but neither as dramatic nor pronounced as in frontal lobe lesions. The patient with uncal herniation may present with acute third nerve dysfunction and hemiparesis due to compression of the nerve and cerebral peduncle.

CLINICAL EXAMPLES[3–10,19]

Temporal lobe tumors, abscesses, AVMs, and middle cerebral artery aneurysms may cause focal mass effect and present as a neurosurgical emergency if uncal herniation is suspected clinically or neuroradiologically. Gliomas and metastases may attain considerable size and cause edema, necessitating temporal lobectomy. These tumors often present with new-onset complex-partial seizures, with receptive dysphasia, or with a subtle upper quadrantic hemianopsia. Hemorrhage from an MCA aneurysm can present acutely as an intracerebral hematoma within the temporal lobe, requiring urgent surgical evacuation of the clot and clipping of the aneurysm at the same operation. Traumatic temporal lobe contusions and epidural and subdural hematomas present as acute emergencies requiring temporal lobe decompression to avert the consequences of uncal herniation.

Temporal lobe cavernous hemangiomas, astrocytomas, gangliogliomas, hamartomas, and oligodendrogliomas can present as intractable seizure disorders in either the pediatric or adult neurosurgical patients. The successful surgical treatment involves site-specific temporal lobectomy with intraoperative electroencephalographic (EEG) localization, a topic treated extensively in Chap. 22. Mesial temporal sclerosis is an additional pathological finding of temporal lobectomy for seizure control.

Temporal lobe abscesses can arise by direct extension from the attic or tegmen tympani of the temporal bone. The sources of infection are the ipsilateral middle ear, mastoid, or even sphenoid sinus. Abscesses of the temporal lobes often present clinically as neurosurgical emergencies requiring drainage and excision of the abscess wall.

INDICATIONS FOR TEMPORAL LOBECTOMY[3-10]

Temporal lobe tumors or hematomas may present acutely with uncal herniation, requiring urgent decompression and lobectomy. The classical "question-mark," or inverse, scalp flap is used for temporal lobectomy, and the temporal bone squama is removed inferiorly to the mastoid and temporal base as well as anteriorly to the tip of the temporal lobe. The standard temporal lobectomy should resect no more than the anterior 4 to 5 cm of the dominant temporal lobe, and it should also conserve the superior temporal gyrus for risk of producing Wernicke's aphasia. On the nondominant side the surgeon should resect no more than the anterior 5 to 6 cm of the temporal lobe. However, on nondominant temporal lobe resections the posterior extent of the cortical incision can be carried out to the supramarginal and angular gyrus.

Importantly, the posterior limit of either the dominant or nondominant resection is usually the *vein* of *Labbé,* which drains the medial, inferior, and peri-sylvian regions of the temporal lobe into the transverse sinus. (Seventy percent of cases drain into the transverse sinus while 30 percent drain into the sigmoid sinus.)[2] Interruption of this venous structure can lead to dysphasia or hemiparesis as a result of venous infarction of the temporal and/or posterior frontal lobes.

A more reliable landmark for the posterior limit of resection is the junction of the rolandic sulcus and sylvian fissure. Lastly, it should be pointed out that interruption of Meyer's loop with a resultant upper quadrantic field cut becomes a common postoperative complication if the cortical resection extends more than 6 cm from the anterior tip of the temporal lobe.

OCCIPITAL LOBES: DOMINANT AND NONDOMINANT HEMISPHERES[11-16]

The *occipital lobe* is the pyramid-shaped lobe posterior to the parieto-occipital sulcus (Fig. 1-4). This sulcus is its obvious medial boundary with the parietal lobe, but laterally it merges with the parietal and temporal lobes without definitive demarcation. The large *calcarine sulcus* courses in an anterior-posterior direction from the pole of the occipital lobe to the *splenium* of the *corpus callosum;* area 17, the *primary visual receptive cortex,* lies in its banks. The calcarine sulcus divides the medial surface of the occipital lobe into the *superior cuneus* and the *inferior lingual gyri.* The *primary visual,* or

striate, cortex is located topographically above and below the calcarine sulcus, with the posterior tip of the occipital pole concerned with macular vision and the anterior part of the calcarine cortex concerned with peripheral vision, or the so-called temporal crescent.

The key function of the occipital lobe concerns vision. The striate cortex (area 17) is the primary visual cortex, whereas the visual association areas (areas 18 and 19) are concerned with secondary phenomena, lesions of which produce visual agnosia, extinction hemianopsia, and optokinetic nystagmus.

The *symptoms* of *occipital lobe dysfunction* include seizures preceded by visual hallucinations (e.g., flashing lights and colors, visual field deficits, and visual agnosia), especially if the dominant hemisphere is involved. The signs of occipital lobe dysfunction are a classical contralateral, congruous homonymous hemianopsia, with macular sparing if the occipital tip is unaffected. Alexia, or inability to read, and visual agnosia, or inability to recognize objects, may be signs of damage to the dominant parieto-occipital lobe and the visual association areas.

CLINICAL EXAMPLES[3-10,19]

Occipital lobe gliomas and AVMs present classically with a contralateral, congruous, homonymous hemianopsia, often sparing macular vision. Tentorial meningiomas can attain large size and present with homonymous hemianopsia, papilledema, hydrocephalus, and cerebellar dysfunction, secondary to supra- and infratentorial invasion. Injury to the occiput often causes visual field deficits secondary to occipital lobe damage. Proximal and distal posterior cerebral artery aneurysms, arising from P1, P2, or P3, can also present clinically with macular sparing and congruous homonymous hemianopsia.

INDICATIONS FOR OCCIPITAL LOBECTOMY[3-10]

Large occipital gliomas and intracerebral hematomas due to rupture of an AVM can present acutely or semiacutely with marked mass effect and edema, necessitating consideration of occipital lobectomy. The neurosurgical patient can be placed in the 3/4 prone (park-bench) or sitting position, and an occipital craniotomy performed with medial access to the sagittal sinus and inferior access to the transverse sinus.

On the dominant side, the cortical incision is started 3.5 cm from the occipital tip on the superior cortical margin to avoid damage to the angular gyrus. On the nondominant side, the resection is started 7 cm from the occipital tip.

The patient will be left with a contralateral, homonymous hemianopsia. However, if there is damage to the dominant hemisphere in the area of the junction of the parietal, occipital, and temporal lobes, the patient may have dyslexia, dysgraphia, and acalculia.

Cerebellum

☐ SURGICAL ANATOMY OF THE CEREBELLUM[11-16]

The *cerebellum* is a bilaterally symmetrical structure located in the posterior fossa (Fig. 1-5). It is attached to the midbrain, pons, and medulla by the superior, middle, and inferior cerebellar peduncles, which lie at the sides of the fourth ventricle on the ventral aspect of the cerebellum. The surface of the cerebellum consists of parallel folds called *folia*. Four pairs of deep cerebellar nuclei are buried within the cerebellum. From medial to lateral they are the *fastigial, globose, emboliform,* and *dentate nuclei,* respectively.

The cerebellum can be thought of as two basic regions; the *midline structures* and the *lateral structures* (Fig. 1-5). The midline structures include the *lingula* anteriorly, the *vermis* in the middle, and the *flocculonodular lobe* posteriorly (Fig. 1-5). The lateral structures comprise the two *lateral cerebellar hemispheres,* or lobes.

The cerebellum can also be divided into functional parts that are separate and distinct embryologically. The *archicerebellum,* represented by the *flocculonodular lobe,* is phylogenetically the oldest part. The flocculonodular region is concerned with equilibrium and vestibular connections. Newer in phylogeny is the *paleocerebellum,* represented by the lingula and culmen (also the declive, uvula, and tonsil), which is concerned with the regulation of muscle tone. The lingula and culmen are also referred to as the *anterior lobe,* which is rostral to the *primary fissure* (Fig. 1-5).

Lastly, the *neocerebellum,* which is phylogenetically very new, is concerned with the coordination of fine movements. The neocerebellum is the much larger cerebellar structure and lies between the primary fissure and the *postpyramidal fissure* (Fig. 1-5). It should be pointed out that each lateral cerebellar hemisphere contains a large main nucleus, the *dentate,* through which the bulk of outflow cerebellar information is relayed.

The classical *signs and symptoms of cerebellar lesions* were well described and formulated by Gordon Holmes in his monograph, *The Cerebellum of Man,* published in 1939.[20] Lesions affecting the midline structures, particularly the vermis and flocculonodular lobe, often cause severe gait and truncal ataxia, making it impossible for the patient to stand or sit unsupported. Lesions in the lingula may extend into the superior medullary velum and cause trochlear nerve (CN

IV) dysfunction, or they may extend into the superior cerebellar peduncle ipsilaterally and cause tremor of the ipsilateral arm. Lesions in the flocculonodular lobe may also cause vertigo and vomiting in addition to the ataxia, as the lesion may damage the vestibular reflex pathways and compress the area postrema on the floor of the fourth ventricle, respectively. It should also be pointed out that midline lesions may obstruct the aqueduct, fourth ventricle, or the CSF pathways causing headache, papilledema, and vomiting from increased intracranial pressure secondary to obstructive hydrocephalus.

There are other less common but classical signs of midline lesions. Nystagmus is usually found with involvement of the flocculonodular lobe and the fastigial nucleus (vestibular connections). Opsoclonus, ocular dysmetria, and ocular flutter or oscillopsia are rapid conjugate oscillations that can be seen with midline cerebellar lesions. Titubation, a head tremor or bobbing at a rate of 3 to 4 per second in the anterior-posterior direction, can accompany midline lesions. Lastly, cerebellar speech, or scanning dysmetric speech is a thick, slow, plodding, slurred speech, "marble-mouth," a uniquely cerebellar disorder.

Lesions affecting the lateral structures (e.g., right or left cerebellar hemisphere) will cause signs of ipsilateral ataxia of the limbs. The affected limbs will have an intention tremor, past-pointing or dysmetria, decomposition of movements and fragmented or inaccurate rapid-alternating movements called dysdiadochokinesia. Other ipsilateral limb findings may be decreased muscle tone and hyporeflexia. Overall, lesions in the lateral dentate nucleus of the cerebellar hemisphere or in the superior cerebellar peduncle, the major outflow tract of the cerebellum, will produce a classical ipsilateral arm tremor.

CLINICAL EXAMPLES[11-16,19]

Tumors, AVMs, hypertensive and traumatic hemorrhages, and abscesses are the most common neurosurgical mass lesions presenting in the cerebellum. Tumors vary according to age. In the child, the medulloblastoma arises from the vermis and roof of the superior medullary velum, causes gross tunical ataxia with headache, lethargy, nausea, vomiting, and papilledema, especially if the CSF outflow pathways are obstructed (Fig. 1-5). The ependymoma arises also in the midline, but on the floor of the fourth ventricle. It can invade the adjacent brainstem, and it presents similarly with truncal ataxia and symptoms of hydrocephalus from obstruction to the CSF outflow. The cerebellar astrocytoma presents as a large, lateral hemispheric tumor with an enhancing mural nodule and consequent unilateral limb ataxia.

In the adult, cerebellar metastases are common and may present either in the vermis or laterally in the hemispheres. They may have solid or cystic components with focal enhancing areas by MRI or CT.

The hemangioblastoma is a cystic or, less commonly, solid benign, vascular tumor with a classical mural nodule, and it is found in the region of the fourth ventricle, in the vermis or hemisphere, but rarely in the substance of the medulla or

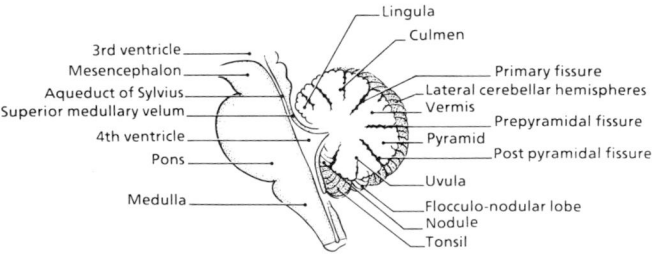

Figure 1–5 A diagram of the cerebellum and the brainstem: An oblique, midsagittal view.

pons. This tumor may be located in the inferior vermis or tonsils.

Impaction of the tumor and cerebellar tissue into the foramen magnum produces a syndrome of *tonsillar herniation*. The neurosurgical patient may have symptoms of headache, occipital pain with neck stiffness, lapses of consciousness, and intermittent "shocklike" sensations radiating into the occiput and limbs due to compression of the spinal cord (Lhermitte's sign).

Meningiomas may arise from the petrous temporal bones, occipital dura, or foramen magnum, causing ipsilateral cerebellar dysfunction. Cerebellar gliomas and the rare *Lhermitte-Duclos disease,* a glial dysplasia or gangliocytoma, may arise in the midline or laterally in the hemispheres. Other rare tumors seen in the adult, affecting the cerebellar structures, include the subependymoma, ependymoma, choroid plexus papilloma, lymphoma, epidermoid, and dermoid.

AVMs of the posterior fossa are rare, with the majority located within the substance of the cerebellum and a minority in the brainstem.[19] Nearly all infratentorial AVMs present with hemorrhages, sometimes massive and causing focal cerebellar or brainstem dysfunction, which may require emergency evacuation. Importantly, cavernous hemangiomas, venous angiomas, capillary telangiectases, and other vascular malformations can present with posterior fossa hemorrhage. Angiography and MRI are the key diagnostic procedures in these clinical situations.

Hypertensive cerebellar hemorrhages often require urgent evacuation. Spontaneous hemorrhage usually occurs laterally in the region of the dentate nucleus, but can extend into the vermis. Severe headaches in the occipital area herald the bleed. The patient is often ataxic on the side of the lesion with ipsilateral limb tremor. C. M. Fisher identified a triad seen in hypertensive cerebellar hemorrhage: ipsilateral sixth nerve dysfunction, facial palsy of peripheral type, and ipsilateral limb tremor.[21] Horizontal nystagmus is common. Lesions greater than 2.5 cm in diameter, with obliteration of the quadrigeminal cisterns by CT, require urgent surgical evacuation.

Traumatic cerebellar hemorrhages may be secondary to open, depressed skull fractures or blunt head trauma. However, blunt contusions are rare because of the lack of significant shear-strain forces in the cerebellar region. Nonetheless, large cerebellar hemorrhages can cause tonsillar herniation, in which the tonsils prolapse through the foramen magnum, obliterate the cisterna magna, and compress the medulla oblongata, with resultant apnea and death. Thus, the posterior fossa mass lesion is often a neurosurgical emergency.

In the vast majority of cases cerebellar abscesses stem from infectious otogenic disease and are usually bacterial. The recent proliferation of immunocompromised patients has led to increased cerebellar abscesses secondary to toxoplasmosis, atypical mycobacterium, cryptococcus, actinomycosis, and histoplasmosis—all rare causes of brain abscess.

REFERENCES

1. Snell RS: *Clinical Anatomy for Medical Students.* Boston, Little, Brown, 1973.
2. Osborn AG: *Introduction to Cerebral Angiography.* Philadelphia, Harper and Row, 1980.
3. Kempe LG: *Operative Neurosurgery,* vols 1 and 2. New York, Springer-Verlag, 1968.
4. Koos WT, Spetzler RF, Pendl G, et al: *Color Atlas of Microneurosurgery.* New York, Georg Thieme Verlag, Thieme-Stratton, 1985.
5. Schmidek HH, Sweet WH: *Operative Neurosurgical Techniques,* vols 1 and 2. New York, Grune and Stratton, 1982.
6. Youmans JR: *Neurological Surgery,* vols 1 to 6. Philadelphia, W. B. Saunders, 1982.
7. Wilkins RH, Rengachary SS: *Neurosurgery.* New York, McGraw-Hill, 1985.
8. Yasargil MG: *Microneurosurgery,* vols 1 and 2. New York, Georg Thieme Verlag, Thieme-Stratton, 1984.
9. Cushing H: Surgery of the head, in Keen WW (ed): *Surgery, Its Principles and Practice.* Philadelphia, W. B. Saunders, 1908.
10. Gurdjian ES, Thomas LM: *Operative Neurosurgery.* Baltimore, Williams & Wilkins, 1970.
11. Gilman S, Newman SW: *Manter's and Gatz's Essentials of Clinical Neuroanatomy and Neurophysiology.* Philadelphia, F. A. Davis, 1989.
12. DeGroot J, Chusid JG: *Correlative Neuroanatomy.* San Mateo, Calif., Appleton and Lange, 1988.
13. Patten J: *Neurological Differential Diagnosis.* New York, Springer-Verlag, 1983.
14. Carpenter MB: *Core Text of Neuroanatomy.* Baltimore, Williams and Wilkins, 1985.
15. Haymaker W: *Bing's Local Diagnosis in Neurological Diseases.* St. Louis, C.V. Mosby, 1969.
16. Adams RD, and Victor M: *Principles of Neurology.* New York, McGraw-Hill, 1981.
17. MacCarty CS: *The Surgical Treatment of Intracranial Meningiomas.* Springfield, Ill., Charles C. Thomas, 1961.
18. Al-Mefty O: *Surgery of the Cranial Base.* Boston, Kluwer, 1989.
19. Wilson CB, Stein BM: *Intracranial Arteriovenous Malformations.* Baltimore, Williams & Wilkins, 1984.
20. Holmes G: The cerebellum of man. *Brain* 62:1–30, 1939.
21. Fisher CM, Picard EH, Polak A, et al: Acute hypertensive cerebellar hemorrhage: Diagnosis and surgical treatments. *J Nerve Ment Dis* 140:38–57, 1965.

☐ APPENDIX 1: ABBREVIATIONS

ACA = anterior cerebral artery
AICA = arterior inferior cerebellar artery
Areas = cortical areas refer to Brodmann's terminology
AVM = arteriovenous malformation
CT = computerized tomography
CNS = central nervous system
CSF = cerebrospinal fluid
ECA = external carotid artery
ICA = internal carotid artery
LGB = lateral geniculate body
MRI = magnetic resonance imaging
MGB = medial geniculate body
MCA = middle cerebral artery
OKN = optokinetic nystagmus
PNS = peripheral nervous system
PCA = posterior cerebral artery
PICA = posterior inferior cerebellar artery
SS = sigmoid sinus
SSS = superior sagittal sinus
TS = transverse sinus

☐ STUDY QUESTIONS

I. A 55-year-old man is referred because of loss of vision; he is otherwise well. On examination he has a bitemporal hemianopsia that is complete in the upper outer quadrants, extends into the lower outer quadrants, but spares the lower medial segments of the inferior outer fields.

The defects are moderately asymmetrical, greater on the left than the right. Visual loss had been gradual and progressive. The patient also complains of a constant bitemporal headache. Computerized tomography (CT) reveals evidence of a tumor.

1. Where is the tumor located? **2.** What structure was most likely the source? **3.** What are possible explanations for the asymmetry of the defect? **4.** What are two other possible sources of the lesion? **5.** What changes might have been revealed on plain skull x-rays.

II. A 46-year-old woman is referred to the neurosurgeon from a psychiatric hospital because of severe headaches and progressive drowsiness during the past week. The patient has been in the psychiatric hospital for the past 2 years. She has been hospitalized because of outbreaks of unanticipated violence that the family was unable to control or tolerate.

A daughter came in with the patient and reported that the patient had begun to complain of inability to smell her food about 10 years earlier, and about 8 years earlier it was noted that the patient, who had been very careful about her dress all her life, had begun to remain in her nightclothes throughout the day. She had ceased to prepare meals on time. She would eat when food was brought to her, but for the most part, she didn't seem to care.

The outbreaks of violent behavior started about 2 years before she was admitted to the psychiatric hospital and could be triggered by almost anything. After she was admitted to the psychiatric hospital, she began to complain that she could not see and she would bump into things. She is sent for a CT scan.

1. What type of lesion would you expect to see? **2.** Where would it be located? **3.** What type of surgical incision would be appropriate to approach the lesion? **4.** How would the lesion have caused loss of the sense of smell? **5.** What might have been the cause of the violent outbreaks of behavior?

III. A 22-year-old male is brought to the emergency room with a shotgun wound to the top of his head. There is considerable bleeding from the wound, but the patient is alert enough to answer simple questions. He moves all of his extremities spontaneously and will answer simple questions with "yes" or "no," but otherwise he is somnolent.

The patient had been hunting birds with his friend. Suddenly, they came on a flock of birds which took to the air at one time. The patient, who was a few steps ahead of his friend, stood up to shoot. His friend also stood and fired, the blast striking the patient in the vertex of the head. X-rays reveal multiple bird shot in the top of the head and a large depressed fragment of bone in the midline.

1. What structures might have been damaged? **2.** How should one debride the wound? **3.** What position should the patient be placed in for the debridement? **4.** Assuming there is significant blood loss when the bone fragment is removed, what adjustments might be made in the patient's position to reduce this loss? **5.** What surgical precautions might the surgeon take to stop the bleeding?

IV. A 50-year-old lady is admitted with dizziness and loss of hearing in her right ear. Examination reveals absence of hearing in the right ear, loss of both air and bone conduction, as well as loss of corneal reflex on the right side and a slight lag of facial movement on the right. A magnetic resonance image was obtained.

1. Where is the most likely site of a lesion? **2.** What lesions might be expected to occur in the area where this lesion is most likely? **3.** What anatomical approaches might be made to remove the lesion? **4.** Assuming a posterior fossa approach is selected, what types of incision might be considered? **5.** Why might the corneal reflex be depressed?

V. A 25-year-old construction worker was working on a scaffolding when some bricks fell from the level above. Even though he was wearing his helmet, it was knocked off and he was hit by other falling objects. He fell off the scaffolding and lay unconscious for a few minutes but became alert within moments. He complained of a severe headache and then began to get more drowsy. An hour later, he was noted to have a dilated right pupil. A CT scan revealed a hematoma over the surface of the brain.

1. What is the most likely source of the bleeding? **2.** Why might the pupil be dilated? **3.** If hemiparesis is present, on which side might it have occurred? **4.** Could the hemiparesis be ipsilateral to the hematoma? How? **5.** What are the options for a surgical incision to evacuate the hemorrhage?

Neuroanatomical Basis for Surgery on the Spine

Martin Greenberg

Surgical Anatomy of the Spinal Cord

☐ EMBRYOLOGY[1-10]

The *spinal cord* develops from the ectodermal layer of the embryo during the third week of gestation. The ectodermal tissue develops folds in its dorsal edges to form a neural plate and, subsequently, a neural tube. Simultaneously, groups of cells from the ectodermal layer migrate laterally to form the dorsal roots and autonomic ganglia. By the fourth week of gestation, the spinal cord begins to segment into levels, and by the sixth week vertebrae are developing.

The *neural tube* closes at its caudal and rostral ends during the fourth week of gestation. The middle portion closes first and the ends close later. The center of the neural tube forms an ependymal cell layer around a central canal and is subsequently surrounded by circumferential zones of glial and neuronal cells. The central canal extends the length of the spinal cord during development, is lined with ependymal cells, and is filled with cerebrospinal fluid (CSF). Hence, primary tumors of the spinal cord—especially ependymomas, astrocytomas, gliomas, ganglioneuromas, and oligodendrogliomas—can be found distributed along the entire length of the spinal cord. Interestingly, ependymomas are particularly common at the level of the conus medullaris–filum terminale region, and can even present very rarely as aberrant tumors in the extraspinal lumbosacral soft tissues.

The primitive spinal cord is surrounded by a zone of tissue derived from the mesenchymal layer, which differentiates into three membranes, or *meninges:* the *dura,* the *arachnoid,* and the *pia.* Primary tumors of the meninges, *meningiomas,* can be found along the length of the spinal cord; their spinal distribution is highest in the thoracic region, which has the larger mass of spinal cord.

☐ CONGENITAL MALFORMATIONS[1-10]

The spinal cord of the human is fully formed by the first month of gestation. Of neurosurgical interest at this age are congenital malformations resulting from failure of the neural tube to form and fully close. Failure of the neural tube to close at the cranial end can result in an encephalocele, which may contain a herniated segment of neural tissue, and anencephaly, with exposed brain, which is incompatible with life. The occipital encephalocele is repaired in the postnatal period, and a ventriculoperitoneal shunt is often required to treat hydrocephalus.

Failure of the neural tube to close at the caudal end results in spina bifida aperta or cystica, which is also associated with maldevelopment of the vertebra. Most commonly, the patient has a meningomyelocele or a meningeal sac that contains dysfunctional neural tissue, and Chiari malformation. The Chiari type II syndrome is associated with a range of midline neural tube defects, which can include bulbar dysfunction secondary to malformations of cranial nerve nuclei and hydrocephalus secondary to midline obstruction of cerebrospinal fluid (CSF) pathways, e.g., aqueductal kinking. Much less common is the meningocele, a cystic lesion that contains only meninges and CSF, but no neural tissue. Both the meningomyelocele and the meningocele are surgically repaired in the early postnatal period.

Failure of the neural tube to close can also present in occult lesions. Occult spinal dysraphism includes diastematomyelia, dermal sinus tracts, dermoid cysts and lipomas, neurenteric cysts, fibrous bands, and other rare intraspinal cysts. These congenital anomalies are often associated with a visible abnormality of the overlying skin or subcutaneous tissue—e.g., dimple, nevus, and hairy patch—and they present with progressive neurological deficits. Magnetic resonance imaging

(MRI) will localize the congenital anomaly radiographically, and early surgical excision and repair will prevent further neurological deterioration.

☐ GROSS ANATOMY[1–10]

The spinal cord is a cylindrical bundle of nerve pathways that is 42 to 45 cm long and 2.5 cm wide in the normal adult. Its rostral end is continuous with the *brain stem,* whereas the distal end forms a conical tapering, the *conus medullaris,* which is usually located at the lower border of the first lumbar vertebra (L1). (See Fig. 2-1.) On occasion, it may reach only to the body of T12, or it may extend to L2 in the adult. From the conus medullaris, the lumbar and sacral nerve roots descend in a bundle known as the *cauda equina* ("horse's tail," because of their striking resemblance). Lastly, the *filum terminale* is a connective tissue filament that extends from the tip of the conus medullaris and attaches to the first segment of the *coccyx.*

The spinal cord occupies, at most, two-thirds of the spinal canal and is typically about 25 cm shorter than the vertebral column in length. In fact, the length of the spinal cord averages 45 cm in males and 43 cm in females, contrasted with a length of 70 cm for the average vertebral column. Because of this, the lower segments of the spinal cord (lumbar and sacral) are not aligned opposite their corresponding lumbosacral vertebrae. (See Fig. 2-1.)

This bears great clinical significance. As an example, a herniated cervical disk at the C5–C6 level will typically affect only the C6 nerve root, but a herniated disk at the L1–L2 level has the potential to affect *any* of the nerve roots between L2 and S5, solely because of their long course. (See Fig. 2-1.) Thus, the patient with a herniated cervical disk may have biceps weakness, whereas the patient with a herniated lumbar disk may have weakness of the iliopsoas—or even gastrocnemius with bowel and bladder incontinence. A final example might be a neurofibroma on the L2 nerve root that presents as an S1 root lesion because of the peculiar intraspinal anatomy of the cauda equina. (See Fig. 2-1.)

☐ SEGMENTAL ANATOMY[1–10]

The spinal cord is divided arbitrarily into five anatomical areas: *cervical, thoracic, lumbar, sacral,* and *coccygeal.* There are no sharp anatomical boundaries between segments within the cord. Spinal nerves exit from spinal cord segments in pairs: 8 cervical, 12 thoracic, 5 lumbar, 5 sacral, and 2 coccygeal. Each spinal nerve is formed by a dorsal root which is primarily *sensory,* and a ventral root, primarily *motor,* with some sensory fibers.

In the cervical area, the first seven nerves exit above each respective cervical vertebra, and the eighth nerve, C8, lies between the C7 and T1 vertebrae. The other spinal nerves, T1

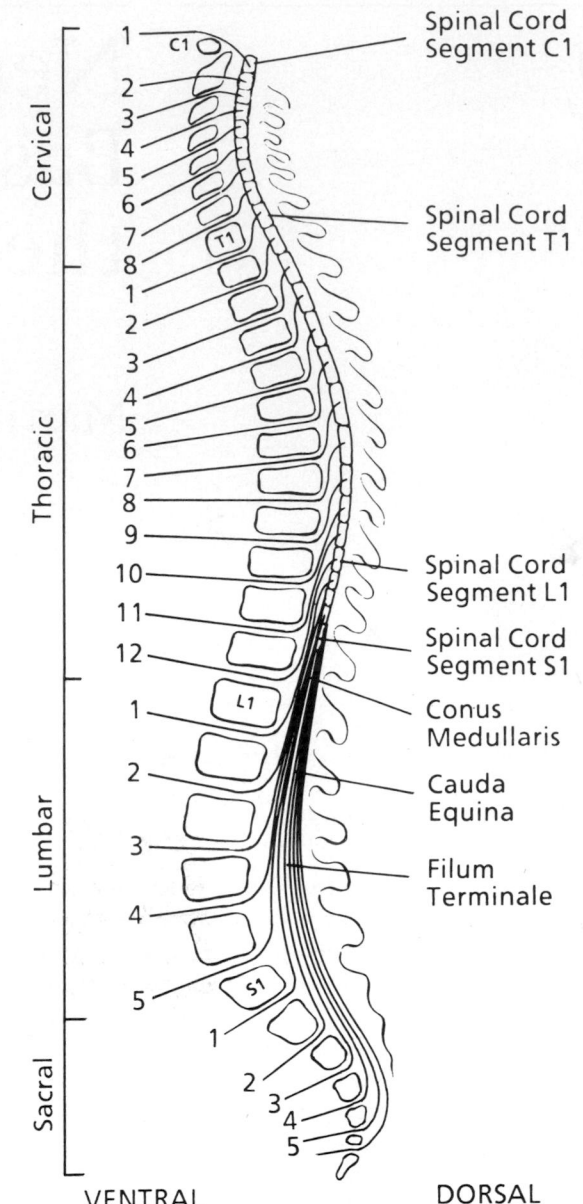

Figure 2-1 An illustration of the spinal cord and its relationship to the vertebral column, spinal segment, and nerves: a sagittal schematic.

to T12, L1 to L5, S1 to S5, and CO1 and CO2, exit below their respective corresponding vertebrae. The spinal nerves of the cauda equina are formed by dorsal and ventral roots from both sides of the lower spinal cord.

The spinal cord widens in the cervical and lumbar areas, which innervate the upper and lower extremities, respectively. In the cervical area, the spinal cord enlargement extends from the level of the third cervical vertebra, C3, to the second thoracic vertebra, T2, and it corresponds to the site of origin of the brachial plexus nerves, C5 to T1.

However, there are anatomic variations of the brachial plexus. For instance, the C4 nerve root contributes more than two-thirds of its fibers to the plexus; less than one-third of the fibers of T2 are contributed. When the contribution from C4 is large and that of T1 is negligible, the brachial plexus belongs to the *prefixed* type. Clinically, this may be significant, particularly in a neurological patient with a herniated cervical disk of the C3–C4 level who presents with weakness of the deltoid muscle. This results from compression of the C4 nerve root at the C3–C4 interspace because of its anastomotic contribution to the C5 nerve root of the brachial plexus.

In the upper cervical region, a key segment of neurosurgical interest is the *phrenic nerve,* an exclusively motor nerve that supplies the diaphragm and is derived primarily from the C4 nerve root, but which also receives smaller contributions from C3 and C5. Upper cervical cord lesions secondary to spinal trauma or tumors will cause respiratory insufficiency that results from phrenic nerve damage and interruption of reticulospinal connections from the medulla. Bilateral phrenic dysfunction usually necessitates early ventilatory assistance.

Further enlargement of the upper cervical cord can be seen with primary spinal cord tumors—especially astrocytomas, ependymomas, and, rarely, hemangioblastomas.[11–17] The holochord astrocytoma is particularly common at the cervicomedullary junction and has been described to extend the length of the spinal cord.[11–17]

The spinal cord widens laterally in the lumbar region, and its enlargement extends from the level of the T9 to the T12 vertebral body; it then tapers to form the conus medullaris. The nerves of the lumbosacral plexus arise from the lumbar enlargement and correspond to the L4 to S3 nerve roots, respectively. The lumbosacral plexus gives off one very large nerve, the *sciatic* nerve.

☐ INVESTING MEMBRANES[1–10]

The spinal cord is surrounded by three membrane layers, or meninges: dura (dura mater), arachnoid, and pia (pia mater).

DURA MATER

The *dura mater,* or *pachymeninx,* is the outermost layer of the meninges and is a tough fibrous sheath that extends from the foramen magnum to the sacral spinal vertebral body, where it ends in a cul-de-sac. Spinal dura is continuous with cranial dura, and it lines the vertebral canal around the spinal cord. An *epidural space* containing loose fatty areolar tissue and a network of venous plexuses separates the spinal dura from the vertebral canal. A potential subdural space exists between the dura and the underlying arachnoid membrane.

The dura mater is of key neurosurgical importance, posing a formidable physical barrier. Spinal cancer metastases, bacterial infection, and tuberculosis (often associated with osteomyelitis), as well as primary bone tumors, rarely penetrate the thick dura to invade the spinal canal.

On the other hand, the dura is not impregnable. A spinal meningioma, which is derived typically from the arachnoid layer where it joins the dura of the nerve root sheath, can present as a classic intradural extramedullary tumor and less commonly as a purely extradural tumor, perhaps because of the tumor's attachment to and invasion of the dura mater. Similarly, spinal neurinomas and neurofibromas can present both in the intradural *and* extradural spaces, secondary to dural invasion at the site of the dorsal root sleeve.[11–17] Lastly, epidural lipomatosis, a rare condition of overproliferation of fatty tissue in the epidural space, presents typically in the thoracic region in patients who are morbidly obese or are being administered exogenous steroids. This lesion can be treated with laminectomy and excision of epidural fat.

ARACHNOID MEMBRANE

The *arachnoid membrane layer* is a thin transparent sheath beneath the dura mater. It is separated from the underlying pia by the *subarachnoid space,* which contains cerebrospinal fluid (CSF). The arachnoid layer is rarely infiltrated by tumors or infectious processes. The subarachnoid space is readily accessible by lumbar puncture, and it serves as a diagnostic tool in determining the presence of infectious processes or subarachnoid hemorrhage.

Metastases from cancer within the central nervous system (CNS) can seed the subarachnoid space and present as "drop metastases" in the lumbosacral region. Primary brain tumors —including medulloblastomas, pinealoblastomas, germinomas, and ependymomas—are likely to disseminate here within the *leptomeninges,* or soft meninges. Magnetic resonance imaging (MRI) with gadolinium is a sensitive detector of drop metastasis. CSF cytology is also indicative.

The arachnoid membrane can present as an "outpouching" or cystic structure, which may or may not communicate with the CSF spaces—e.g., arachnoid cyst; perineural, or Tarlov's, cyst; and meningocele. These cysts can enlarge and cause progressive neurological dysfunction.

Patients with recurrent back pain secondary to postoperative spinal arachnoiditis or an inflammatory condition of the subarachnoid space develop a fibrin exudate that coats and adheres to the nerve roots and thecal sac. This clinical entity is easily diagnosed by MRI with gadolinium, which differentiates scar tissue from recurrent disk in a patient who has had multiple lumbar spine operations. Scar tissue enhances avidly and brightly with this rare earth metal cation, gadolinium, Gd^{+3}.

PIA MATER

The *pia mater,* or pial membrane layer, closely encircles the spinal cord and sends septa into the substance of the cord. The pia contributes to the formation of the *filum terminale,* a white fibrous filament extending from the conus medullaris to the tip of the dural sac and continuing extradurally to the coccyx. Also, the pia contributes to the formation of the *dentate ligament,* a long flange of whitish tissue that runs along the lateral margins of the spinal cord between the dorsal, or sensory, and ventral, or motor, roots. The ligament's medial edge is continuous with the pia at the side of the cord, and its lateral edge pierces the arachnoid to attach to the dura mater.

There are 21 pairs of dentate attachments, and they stabilize the spinal cord by cushioning it from the great motion of the dura. The most rostral dentate attachment lies at the level of the foramen magnum and serves as a useful landmark for the point at which the vertebral artery pierces the dura and enters the posterior fossa. This most superior dentate attachment lies between the vertebral artery and cranial nerve XII, the *hypoglossal nerve.* The most caudal attachment lies between T12 and L1 spinal nerves.

The dentate ligament is of primary anatomical importance. First, intraoperative visualization of the dentate ligament allows identification of the ventral, or motor, nerve root. The dentate ligament is positioned at the equator of the spinal cord and is located ventral to the corticospinal tracts and dorsal to the spinothalamic tracts. This location is important in open cordotomy performed to relieve pain.

The dentate ligament can be transected laterally, allowing the spinal cord to be rotated and enabling access to ventral tumors. This maneuver is especially helpful when foramen magnum meningiomas encroach upon the cervicomedullary junction ventrally and encase the lower cranial and upper cervical nerves, as well as the vertebral artery.[14,18]

☐ SPINAL NERVE COVERINGS

The *ventral* (or *motor*) and *dorsal* (or *sensory*) *roots* segmentally converge to become a *spinal nerve.* Thirty-one pairs of spinal nerves arise from the spinal cord. Each spinal nerve has both a ventral root and a dorsal root, and each root is made up of one to eight rootlets.

The spinal nerves are enclosed in sleeves of dura and arachnoid. Dorsal root ganglia are located close to the convergence of the roots, except they are absent in the first cervical root and the coccygeal nerves. These ganglia contain the cell bodies of afferent fibers in the dorsal root. At the dorsal root ganglion both nerve root sleeves merge to become the connective tissue sheath, or *perineurium,* of the spinal nerve. The spinal nerve exits the vertebral canal through the *intervertebral foramen.*

☐ SPINAL NERVE TUMORS

Several spinal tumors are known to develop near the spinal nerve and root sheaths.[11–18] Neurinomas and neurofibromas are located on dorsal or sensory roots, and they displace the spinal cord. They often present as dumbbell-shaped lesions from the intervertebral foramen, with both extradural and intradural extramedullary components.

Similarly, meningiomas are located near the spinal root sleeve and are often attached to the insertion of the dentate

ligament, displacing the spinal cord. Meningiomas can also present as combined extradural and intradural extramedullary lesions, although intradural presentations are more common.

Multiple neurinomas, neurofibromas, and meningiomas can be seen in the hereditary neurofibromatoses, including type I, or von Recklinghausen's disease, and type II, or bilateral acoustic neurinomas.

☐ ANATOMY OF THE SPINAL CORD PATHWAYS[1–10]

The somatotopic organization of fiber pathways in the spinal cord is illustrated schematically. (See Fig. 2-2.)

Neurons are arranged in *dorsal, lateral,* and *ventral* columns. A deep ventral median fissure divides the spinal cord into symmetrical right and left halves, and its roof, the anterior commissure, contains the crossing fibers of the spinothalamic tract, carrying sensations of pain and temperature. The ventral median fissure also contains the anterior spinal artery. This can be a useful landmark when performing the open cordotomy. A shallow dorsal median fissure also divides the spinal cord, and its floor, the gray commissure, contains motor neurons and interneurons. The central canal lies just ventral to the gray commissure.

The dorsal or sensory nerve roots are attached to the spinal cord along the shallow dorsolateral sulcus, located a few millimeters from the dorsal median fissure. (See Fig. 2-2.) The ventral nerve roots exit in the ventrolateral sulcus.

A cross section of the spinal cord reveals an H-shaped

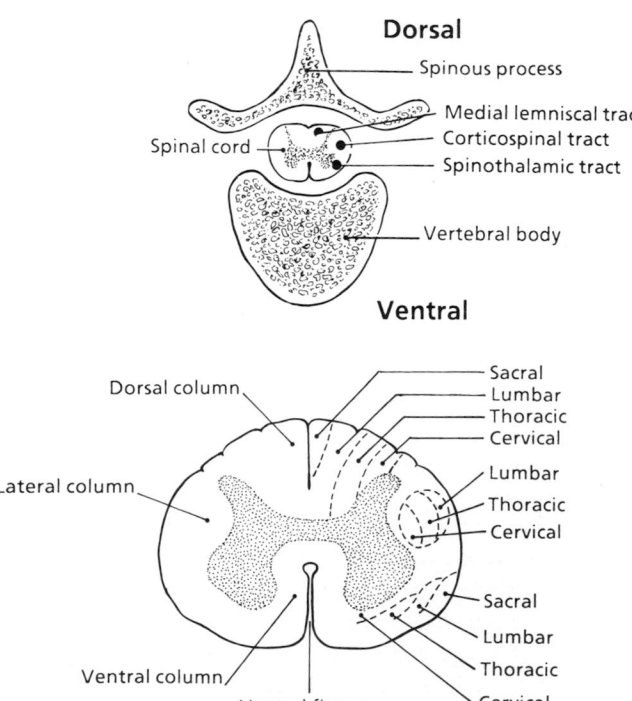

Figure 2-2 A schematic drawing of the spinal cord and its structures, including the somatotopic organization and its relationship to the spine.

mass of gray matter, containing cell bodies surrounded by white matter, the columns of nerve fiber tracts. (See Fig. 2-2.) The gray matter is arranged in 10 laminae, which are layers of neurons that subserve thermonociception, proprioception, reflex arcs, and motor function.

Functionally, each lateral half of the spinal cord is divided into dorsal, lateral, and ventral columns, which represent the medial lemniscal, corticospinal, and spinothalamic white matter tracts, respectively. (See Fig. 2-2.) Thus, the dorsal column lies between the dorsal median sulcus and the dorsolateral sulcus, and it contains axons from the ipsilateral spinal cord that convey the sensations of fine touch, vibration, two-point discrimination, and proprioception.

In the cervical and upper thoracic cord, the dorsal column is divided into a medial fasciculus gracilis from the leg and a lateral fasciculus cuneatus from the arm. These ipsilateral columns of axons are organized somatotopically with a sacral→lumbar→thoracic→cervical orientation from the dorsal median fissure to the dorsolateral sulcus. Hence, a dorsal column (proprioceptive sensory) deficit may be a sign of spinal cord compression. It can be seen with spinal cord tumors and fractures or dislocations of the vertebral column.

The lateral columns lie between the dorsolateral sulcus and the ventrolateral sulcus. (See Fig. 2-2.) The corticospinal tract, subserving ipsilateral motor function, is arranged somatotopically with a cervical→thoracic→lumbar orientation. (See Fig. 2-2.) Interestingly, an isolated lesion of the corticospinal tract often causes flaccid paralysis, whereas involvement of the adjacent rubrospinal and reticulospinal tracts can cause spastic paralysis with hyperreflexia. More typically, lesions of the corticospinal tract are characterized by clonus, Babinski and crossed reflexes, and latent reflexes, including Hoffmann's sign.

Ipsilateral lesions of the spinal cord in the corticospinal tract cause profound weakness, usually in the leg more than in the arm. Meningiomas, neurinomas, and neurofibromas develop along the course of spinal roots, mainly at cervical and thoracic levels, and compress the leg→arm fibers, producing spasticity and pathological reflexes.

In cervical spondylosis there is associated narrowing with myelopathy, causing spasticity in the lower extremities, Babinski signs, and proximal arm weakness and atrophy due to ventral motor-horn cell dropout. Focal compression by stab wounds, missile injuries, and spinal fractures—especially of the laminae and spinous processes—can cause ipsilateral leg and arm weakness due to local corticospinal tract injury. Herniated intervertebral disks at the cervical and thoracic levels can present with ipsilateral motor weakness and myelopathy.

The ventral portion of the column lies between the ventrolateral sulcus and the dentate ligament and contains the spinothalamic tracts, which convey sensations of sharp pain and temperature. (See Fig. 2-2.) The spinothalamic tract is similarly organized somatotopically: from medial to lateral is the cervical→thoracic→lumbar→sacral fiber representation, with the latter nerve fibers extending into the lateral columns. (See Fig. 2-2.) Incoming pain and temperature sensations pass to the dorsolateral funiculus, Lissauer's tract, through the anterior commissure to the opposite side of the cord, and then course upwards one to two segments before joining the spinothalamic tract. Thus, an ipsilateral lesion of the spinothalamic tract will produce a complete loss of pain and thermal sensation on the contralateral side, and the contralateral sensory loss typically extends to a level one to two segments below that of the lesion, owing to the oblique crossing of fibers. As a result, a lesion of the T8 thoracic cord segment will often produce a T9 or T10 sensory level reaction to testing with pinprick.

Intramedullary tumors—e.g., astrocytomas, ependymomas, hemangioblastomas, and syringomyelias, the Arnold-Chiari type I malformations—are characterized by a selective loss of pain and temperature sensation but retention of touch and pressure sensation, the *dissociated sensory loss*. With lesions in the cervical area, the sensory loss is usually configured in a "capelike" distribution over the neck, shoulders, and arms. A syrinx expands the gray matter and central canal, disrupting the anterior commissural fibers of the spinothalamic tracts, leading to insensitivity to pain and defective appreciation of warm or cold. Painful dysesthesias are common in intramedullary tumors, also frequently associated with syrinx formation.

Spinal Shock and Spinal Cord Syndromes of Neurosurgical Importance[1-9]

☐ SPINAL SHOCK

Acute traumatic or nontraumatic injury to the spinal cord can result in *spinal shock,* with loss of motor strength, sensation, and bowel and bladder function below the level of the lesion. If the higher cervical levels are involved, then respiratory insufficiency may ensue because of phrenic nerve paralysis (C3 to C5 roots). Following acute spinal cord transection, the paralysis is flaccid and the deep tendon reflexes are absent. Plantar stimulation gives no response, and there is often a sensory level to pinprick or touch below which the patient perceives no sensation. Occasionally, there is sensory sparing in the sacral area, which, because of its lateral and peripheral location, may be a sign of potential neurological recovery. (See Fig. 2-2.)

There may be absence of abdominal reflexes. The abdominal reflex is a superficial spinal reflex, where stroking the skin of the abdomen causes contraction of the abdominal muscles with retraction of the umbilicus to the stimulated side. The state of spinal shock often lasts several weeks and is usually followed by a state of spastic paraplegia and evidence of an upper motoneuron lesion.

Fractures of the spine, both blunt and penetrating, are the common causes of spinal cord transection and subsequent spinal shock. Treatment is aimed at decompression and stabilization. Decompression is rarely used in patients with a complete motor and sensory level from trauma.

Epidural tumors from lesions in the spine can present with spinal shock, and these are neurosurgical emergencies. Also, epidural abscesses from spinal osteomyelitis and intramedullary abscesses from hematogenous spread can present with spinal shock. Rarely, AVMs and cavernous hemangiomas of the spinal cord can present with subarachnoid hemorrhage and acute back pain, the "coup de poignard of Michon," accompanied by a catastrophic onset of paraplegia or quadriplegia. More rarely, the catastrophic onset of spinal shock without subarachnoid hemorrhage, or the syndrome of Foix-Alajouanine, is the result of spontaneous occlusion of an AVM and infarction of the spinal cord.

☐ SPINAL CORD SYNDROMES

CENTRAL CORD SYNDROME[19]

The acute *central cord syndrome* occurs most frequently in severe hyperextension injuries of the cervical spine, with simultaneous cord compression ventrally by osteophytes and dorsally by buckling of the ligamentum flavum. The syndrome is characterized by disproportionately more motor impairment in the upper extremities than in the lower extremities, bladder dysfunction (usually urinary retention), and a variable degree of sensory loss below the level of the lesion. Often, there is preservation of pinprick sensation in the sacral dermatomes, or *sacral sparing*. (See Fig. 2-2.) The motor impairment, cervical→lumbar, is considered secondary to the pattern of lamination in the spinal cord, with sacral segments most lateral in the corticospinal tract relative to cervical segments. (See Fig. 2-2.)

Pathologically, there is focal edema in the center of the spinal cord and intramedullary hemorrhage, particularly in the gray matter. As the edema subsides, the motor function returns first in the lower extremities, followed by recovery of bladder function (fibers located centrally in the intermediolateral gray columns), and, lastly, movement in the upper extremities with finger movements recovering last.

"Burning dysesthesias" in the hands and fingertips are also associated with central cord injury, and MRI can delineate the extent of central cord injury. Current neurosurgical treatment is delayed—spinal cord decompression, classically, via a posterior versus anterior approach—unless there is an acutely herniated disk, vertebral body fracture, or spinal instability associated with the initial injury. The patient with central cord syndrome will typically experience significant neurological improvement by 3 to 6 months after the injury.

SYRINGOMYELIA AND SYRINGOBULBIA[1–8,20,21]

In *syringomyelia,* there is a progressive rupture and cavitation of a dilated central canal into the gray matter of the cord, predominantly in the central region, with interruption of the spinothalamic tracts crossing through the anterior commissure and leading to a capelike sensory loss in the upper extremities. Because the spinothalamic tracts from the lumbosacral segments are lateral in the cord, pain and temperature sense are preserved in the lower extremities. (See Fig. 2-2.) Position, vibration, and touch sensation are also often preserved, as these pathways are located in the dorsal columns. (See Fig. 2-2.) The preferential loss of pain and temperature sensation with preservation of position, vibration, and touch sensation is termed *dissociative sensory loss.* Painful dysesthesias of the hands can accompany this dissociative loss, and a history of painless burns is common.

As the syrinx enlarges, there is degeneration of the ventral gray motoneurons in the cervical region and resultant amyotrophy and areflexia in the hands, the classic *main-en-griffe,* or *claw hand.* With progression and enlargement of the syrinx, there is extension into the dorsal columns and lateral columns, with very late involvement of the medial lemniscal and corticospinal tracts subserving leg function.

Overall, the neurological signs of syringomyelia are characterized by lower motoneuron (LMN) findings in the upper extremities and upper motoneuron findings (UMN) in the lower extremities. If the syrinx extends caudally to the T1 spinal segment, and particularly to T2, a Horner's syndrome can be seen. If the syrinx extends rostrally to the medulla and pons, it is termed *syringobulbia.* Many clinical signs and symptoms—including downbeat nystagmus and ataxia (cerebellum), facial hypalgesia (CN V) and weakness (CN VII), palatal and vocal cord paralysis (CN IX and X), and tongue atrophy (CN XII)—may exist. Clinically, an "onion-skin," or Balaclava helmet, pattern of facial sensory loss can be detected, as described by Dejerine, because of the laminated pattern and caudal descent of the spinal trigeminal tract as low as C2.[8,20,21] The earliest cranial nerve nuclei to be affected by syringobulbia are the hypoglossal nuclei in the floor of the canal under the obex, and this causes bilateral wasting and weakness of the tongue.

Syringomyelia and syringobulbia have a high association with such clinical entities as intramedullary cord tumors, astrocytomas, ependymomas, hemangioblastomas, and, rarely, oligodendrogliomas. Syringomyelia is also associated with the Chiari type I malformation and other congenital defects of the craniocervical junction, including platybasia, occipitalization of the atlas, basilar impression and invagination, and atlantoaxial subluxation.[22] Less common is the association with arachnoiditis and long-standing traumatic paraplegia.

The syrinx can be drained focally with a syringopleural or syringosubarachnoid shunt—or even a terminal ventriculostomy, as originally suggested by Gardner. A syrinx associated with the Chiari type I malformation is often additionally treated by posterior fossa craniectomy, cervical laminectomy, and decompression of the cerebellar tonsillar region, duraplasty, opening up the foramen of Magendie, and a controversial plugging of the central cervical canal near the obex. Resolution of the syrinx can be determined intraoperatively by ultrasonic techniques.

BROWN-SÉQUARD SYNDROME[8,20]

This classical syndrome rarely presents as a complete, clinical entity, but it will be produced by lateral hemisection of the spinal cord. (See Fig. 2-2.) Hemisection of the cord results in motor paralysis on the same side of the body below the injury, with accompanying spasticity, hyperactive reflexes, clonus, and a Babinski sign.

The dorsal column damage causes loss of position sense, vibratory sense, and tactile discrimination on the same side of the body below the injury. Damage to the ventrolateral system causes loss of pain and temperature sensation on the side opposite the lesion, typically beginning 1 to 2 dermatomal levels below the injury.

Ipsilateral symptoms may be noticeable from local damage to the dorsal and ventral nerve roots, and the neurosurgical patient may complain of radicular pain at the level of injury. For example, a patient with a neurofibroma arising from the left T6 dorsal root may complain of left-sided radicular chest pain in a girdle distribution, along with left-sided corticospinal and medial lemniscal as well as right-sided spinothalamic tract involvement below the level of the neurofibroma.

Classically, the neurofibroma, neurinoma, and meningioma arise near the spinal nerve sheath and present as a complete or incomplete Brown-Séquard syndrome; however, spinal metastases and abscesses secondary to osteomyelitis *can* present with the typical Brown-Séquard syndrome. Other presentations occur with lymphoma, sarcoidosis, and rarely infiltrating angiolipomatosis.

CONUS MEDULLARIS, OR MIDLINE, SYNDROME[8,20]

This classic syndrome rarely presents as a complete lesion but typically involves the lower sacral segments of the spinal cord, S3, S4, S5, and Coc1, in an incomplete presentation. The nerve roots are damaged at the midline from inside, i.e., S5→S4→S3→, and so on.

Clinically, there are early signs of paralytic incontinence, including urinary retention and constipation; impotence; hypalgesia or hypesthesia over the perineal and sacral dermatomas, termed "saddle anesthesia"; a lax anal sphincter with loss of anal and bulbocavernosus reflexes; and an early sign of back pain, stiffness, and muscle spasms, which are long-standing. There is an absence of motor signs in the lower limbs or a Babinski sign, as the lower limbs derive their innervation from segments of the spinal cord above the conus medullaris.

Classically, myxopapillary ependymoma arises at the conus medullaris near the filum terminale to produce the syndrome in young males. Dermoids, lipomas, teratomas, and epidermoids can also arise as congenital lesions adherent to the conus medullaris. Terminally located astrocytomas may present as the conus syndrome.

Traumatic fractures of the lower lumbar vertebrae or the sacrum have been known to cause the conus syndrome by selectively injuring the medially located roots of the cauda equina, i.e., S3 to S5. Also, a large central herniated lumbar disk at L5–S1 can present with bowel and bladder involvement merely by compression of the midline sacral nerve roots, S3 to S5, without any compromise of motor function in the lower extremities.

CAUDA EQUINA, OR EPICONUS LATERAL, SYNDROME[8,20]

This classic syndrome is characterized by considerable motor disability, in contrast to the conus syndrome, and it typically includes roots L3 to Coc1. There is a weakness of external rotation and extension of the thigh and, less commonly, abduction at the hip, flexion at the knee, and flexion and extension at the ankle. The Achilles reflex is absent, and there is commonly hypesthesia in the radicular distribution L3–Coc1, inclusive. Radicular signs are frequently predominant on one side, and bowel and bladder dysfunction are uncommon. Importantly, there are no upper motor neuron findings, nor is there a Babinski sign. Overall, the patient with cauda equina syndrome has radicular asymmetrical pain with ipsilateral radicular sensory loss.

Classically, cauda equina neurinoma or neurofibroma presents with this syndrome. Hydrocephalus might be associated with a cauda equina tumor and any intradural tumor due to the blockage of CSF protein absorption in the spinal subarachnoid spaces, as originally described by Gardner in the 1950s.[5,6,20] Less commonly, an asymmetrical ependymoma or astrocytoma arising near the conus produces the cauda equina syndrome. Metastases to the L1 or L2 vertebral body—e.g., prostate, renal, and lumbosacral chordomas—can also present similarly as either a conus medullaris or cauda equina syndrome, often a mixed presentation. CNS "drop-metastases," from medulloblastoma, ependymoma, or pinealoblastoma, may accompany either syndrome. Historically, multiple root tumors of the cauda equina are seen in patients with von Recklinghausen's disease or type I neurofibromatosis.

FORAMEN MAGNUM SYNDROME[8,18,20]

Another classic neurological syndrome, that of the foramen magnum, has protean manifestations, and its underlying cause was often overlooked until the advent of MRI. There are two presentations, craniospinal and spinocranial. Craniospinal presentation is associated with signs and symptoms referable to the lower medulla and cranial nerves, before involvement of the upper cervical cord.

The patient presents with suboccipital headache and pain in the upper cervical area and numbness and dysesthesias in the distribution of the C2 nerve root, unilaterally or bilaterally. Characteristically, this pain is aggravated by postural changes and Valsalva maneuvers.

Lhermitte's sign is occasionally reported. Cold and burning dysesthesias in the hands and astereognosis (or inability to identify an object placed in the palm) have been described, the latter due to a lesion of the nucleus cervicalis lateralis, a sensory nucleus within the medial lemniscus of the upper cervical cord.

Another classical finding is unilateral or bilateral weakness of the trapezius and sternocleidomastoid muscles, due to involvement of the eleventh cranial nerve. There is a progressive, spastic quadriparesis, first involving the upper limb on the side of the lesion. Interestingly, there is noticeable wasting of the distal upper extremity muscles, especially those of the intrinsic hand associated with compression of the upper cervical cord, although the underlying etiology appears the subject of some controversy in neurosurgical literature.

With cranial extension of the lesion there may be nystagmus, ataxia, involvement of the fifth and twelfth cranial nerves, Horner's syndrome, and ataxia. The nystagmus is classically "downbeat," or it may be horizontal, "upbeat," secondary to pressure on the sulcomarginal fibers, which are a direct extension of the medial longitudinal fasciculus in the cervicomedullary region. Papilledema is unusual unless there is a large posterior fossa component to the lesion.

Meningiomas, neurofibromas, neurinomas, ependymomas, hemangioblastomas, and large aneurysms of the posterior inferior cerebellar or vertebral arteries at the vertebral-basilar junction can cause the foramen-magnum syndrome. Much less common causes are dermoids, teratomas, lipomas, and cavernous malformations. Intramedullary tumors of the foramen magnum including astrocytomas and ependymomas—and occasionally extensions of cerebellar tumors as medulluloblastoma, choroid plexus papillomas, and hemangioblastoma—can also present similarly.

The foramen magnum meningioma is the most common cause of this clinical presentation. It is usually located predominantly anterolateral to the cervicomedullary junction. Current surgical approaches include the classic posterior route via a suboccipital craniectomy and cervical laminectomy. Recently, an anterior approach has been tried, either transoral (buccopharyngeal), transclival, or transcervical, directed through the fascial planes of the neck to the region of the foramen magnum. This tumor holds special interest for the neurosurgeon because of the problems approaching it.

Vascularity of the Spinal Cord[1–10,23–25]

☐ VASCULAR SPINAL CORD ANATOMY

ARTERIES

The *arterial supply of the spinal cord* is derived from two key sources: the *vertebral* arteries and the *radicular* arteries derived from segmental vessels, i.e., deep cervical, intercostal, lumbar, and sacral arteries. This supply is depicted schematically in Fig. 2-3. Radicular arteries course along the spinal

nerves through the intervertebral foramen and divide into smaller anterior and larger posterior radicular arteries.

The entire cervical spinal cord is supplied by branches of the paired vertebral arteries. (See Fig. 2-3.) Each vertebral artery divides into two important branches as it ascends along the ventrolateral surface of the medulla. The superior branch is the anterospinal artery, which joins with its counterpart anterior to the medullary pyramids to form a single descending *anterior spinal artery*. The inferior branch of the vertebral artery, the *posterior spinal artery,* turns dorsal to the medulla and descends on the posterior lateral surface of the spinal cord. Along its descent the posterospinal artery receives a variable number of arterial tributaries from the posterior radicular arteries arising from the vertebral artery.

The anterior spinal artery provides blood supply to the lower medulla and, caudally, gives rise to sulcal arteries that enter the ventral median fissure to supply the spinal cord on the right and left halves, respectively. The anterior spinal

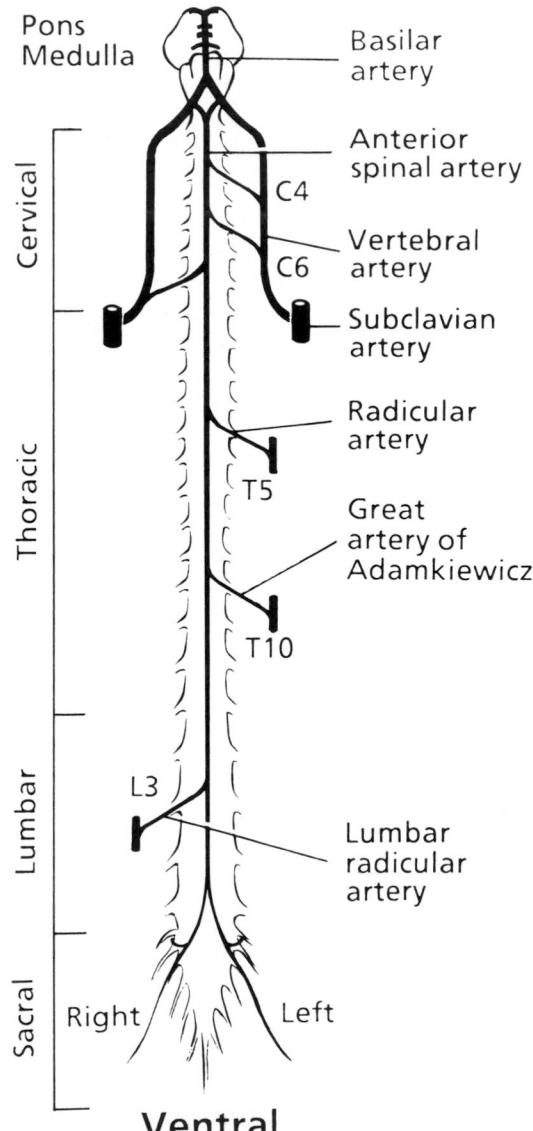

Figure 2-3 A schematic view of the vascular supply to the spinal cord, ventral view.

artery narrows below the T4 cord segment, but, nonetheless, it has rich anastomoses from radicular arteries below the spinal cord level. Anastomotic vessels unite directly with the posterior and anterior spinal arteries to form an irregular ring of arteries, the *arterial vasocorona*. Overall, the anterior spinal artery, through its sulcal branches, supplies the ventral and lateral horns, the central gray back to the dorsal horn, and the ventral and lateral columns, including the corticospinal tracts. The posterior spinal arteries supply the dorsal gray horn and the dorsal columns.

The *radicular medullary arteries* derive from segmental branches of the deep cervical, intercostal, lumbar, and sacral arteries, and they supply the spinal cord from the T2 to L2 segmental levels. The largest radicular artery, the *great artery of Adamkiewicz*, usually arises on the left but has a variable origin from the T8 to L3 cord segments. (See Fig. 2-3.) It supplies most of the arterial blood for the lower half of the thoracic and lumbar spinal cord, including the conus medullaris. Moreover, other radicular arteries derived from the lumbar, iliolumbar, and lateral sacral arteries supply the lumbosacral area, foremost of which is a major vessel usually entering the intervertebral foramen at L3 to form the lower-most portion of the anterior spinal artery, the *terminal, or ascending, artery*. (See Fig. 2-3.) This artery runs beside the filum terminale up to the conus medullaris and supplies the terminal spinal cord and the nerve roots of the cauda equina.

WATERSHED ZONES

The blood supply of the spinal cord can be compromised in transitional regions where the arterial supply is from two different sources. In the cervical cord there is very adequate supply anteriorly from the vertebral artery and anterior spinal artery and posteriorly from the ascending cervical and thyroid artery, making ischemic events rare at this level. The upper segments of the thoracic cord, T1 to T4, depend primarily on the anterior radiculomedullary branches of the intercostal arteries for their supply. T4 is considered a watershed zone.

Alternate vessels to the anterior spinal artery do not exist at the level of the upper thoracic region, probably explaining the frequency of ischemic events in the T4 region. Similarly, the L1 spinal cord segment is an equally vulnerable area, as the artery of Adamkiewicz usually originates anteriorly between T8 and T12, and the major lumbar radicular artery usually originates at L2 or L3, thus rendering L1, a midway spinal cord segment, a *watershed zone*. (See Fig. 2-3.)

Blunt trauma to the thoracolumbar region can result in damage to the artery of Adamkiewicz, resulting in an acute flaccid paraplegia with dissociated sensory loss (usually T4 to T6 sensory level), due to preservation of the dorsal columns supplied by the posterior spinal arteries. This clinical entity is known as the *anterior spinal artery syndrome*.

VEINS

Venous distribution of the spinal cord mirrors that of the arteries. There are five to ten anterior and posterior radicular veins. The posterior veins form a distinct spinal vein, as well as paired posterolateral tracts, and they drain the dorsal columns, dorsal horn, and a narrow strip of the lateral columns. Whereas the anterior veins are similarly structured and drain the ventral columns and ventral horn, a meningeal plexus of veins, the *vasocorona*, is derived from the anterior venous system and drains the anterolateral columns.

An irregular venous plexus lies in the epidural and subarachnoid spaces, and it communicates with the basivertebral veins from the vertebral column as well as the basilar plexus in the cranium. These plexuses extend the length of the spinal canal, and the spread of craniospinal metastases via Batson's plexus is explained by this route, although hematogenous-borne cancer metastases are probably a more common mode of spread.

☐ VASCULAR TUMORS[5,6,11–17,23–27]

HEMANGIOBLASTOMA[23–27]

These dense, highly vascular tumors are proliferations of endothelial cells; they can be solid or cystic, the latter type containing a classic, mural nodule that enhances radiographically with contrast agents. Hemangioblastomas are found in the upper cervical cord and cervicomedullary region, particularly in the area postrema, and they are often multiple and continuous with a syringomelic cavity.

Hemangioblastomas of the spinal cord are typically intramedullary, dorsal to the central canal, and receive their arterial supply from the anterior and posterior spinal arteries. A less common presentation is the radicular hemangioblastoma, with the tumor developing on the dorsal root and an "hourglass" extension through the neural foramen. Angiography is diagnostic and consists of intermingled vascular lakes in the form of dense multiple collections of dilated capillaries.

Spinal hemangioblastomas (10 percent) are associated with the more common cerebellar and retinal hemangioblastomas (90 percent) seen in the von Hippel-Lindau disease. Lindau's disease refers exclusively to the cerebellar hemangioblastoma. The genetics of these diseases is unclear.

Tumors in the spinal cord typically cause progressive, neurological symptoms for 1 to 2 years, and subarachnoid or intramedullary hemorrhage is rare. Tumor removal is facilitated by adjunctive use of laser with standard microneurosurgical techniques since the tumors are vascular and adherent to the medulla and spinal cord.

VERTEBRAL HEMANGIOMAS[5,6,24,25,28,29]

These benign vascular tumors usually arise from blood vessels within the vertebral body and arch, but they can also extend to the facet and lamina. They occur mainly in women, commonly in the thoracic spine, and can cause vertebral body collapse or present as an extradural mass with myelopathy. The hemangioma typically involves a single vertebral body. Classically, the hemangioma is distinctive for its thickened vertical striations, or trabeculations, which surround the dilated vascular spaces and are seen on CT scans or lateral x-rays. Angiography reveals angiomatous vertebrae with confluent vascular lacunae occupying the whole vertebra and specific tumor feeders from intercostal or lumbar arteries. Preoperative embolization of the tumor vessels is helpful before surgical decompression and stabilization to reduce the bleeding.

ANEURYSMAL BONE CYSTS[5,6,24,25]

These destructive tumors occur most frequently in children and involve the vertebral arch, with occasional extension into the spinal canal. The classical radiographic features are a thin cortical shell and honeycomb appearance. Angiography reveals an area of opacification ranging from a faint density in some cases to veritable vascular lakes.

RENAL CELL CARCINOMA[5,6,28,29]

Tumors from the kidney invading the spine include clear cell carcinomas and the hypernephromas. They are quite vascular with large feeders, destroy the vertebral body and arch, and can extend into the spinal canal. Preoperative embolization is recommended prior to surgical attack, as this tumor is very vascular and intraoperative hemorrhage sometimes leads to massive blood loss.

☐ MISCELLANEOUS TUMORS[3,5,6,24–29]

Angiosarcoma and hemangiopericytomas are rare malignant bone tumors with extreme vascularity. They metastasize and spread with dire consequences. The angiolipoma and infiltrating angiolipomatosis are very rare congenital vascular tumors commonly found in the thoracic epidural space, which may present with progressive myelopathy. They can be cured surgically.

☐ VASCULAR MALFORMATIONS[5,6,23–27]

ARTERIOVENOUS MALFORMATIONS (AVMs)

There are two distinct clinical types of spinal cord arteriovenous malformations (AVMs): the *dural* AVM and the *intradural* AVM, which includes the juvenile and glomus subtypes.

In the dural AVM, the patients are older than 40 years of age, have a gradual onset and progressive worsening of symptoms, and the lesions are midthoracic, leading to symptoms that affect the legs. The nidus of the AVM is embedded in the dural covering of the nerve root in the intervertebral foramen. This dural artery is a branch of the intercostal artery and is drained by the medullary vein, which carries blood at high pressure flowing to the meningeal plexus of veins, the vasocorona. Since there are no valves between the radicular vein and the radial veins draining the spinal cord, the high pressure and slow flow is transmitted directly to the spinal cord, leading to venous hypertension and myelopathy. Angiographically, the dural AVM is characterized as a single, tightly coiled, continuous vessel on the cord surface.

The intradural AVM is less common, constituting about 15 to 20 percent of all spinal AVMs. It presents in patients less than 30 years of age, has an acute onset of symptoms, often with paralysis, subarachnoid hemorrhage, spinal bruit, associated angioma of the back, and the site of nidus is dispersed along the axis of the cord with symptoms affecting arms as well as legs. In the intradural AVM, the nidus is within the substance of the spinal cord or pia, and it is supplied by medullary arteries from the anterior and posterior spinal arteries. In juvenile-type intradural AVM, the nidus is large, fills the spinal cord, and contains cord tissue within the interstices of the vessels of the AVM. In the glomus type of intradural AVM, there is a tightly packed nidus of blood vessels confined to a short segment of the cord, along with associated arterial or venous aneurysms.

Dural and intradural AVMs can be associated with several neurocutaneous syndromes, or *phakomatoses,* including Cobb's syndrome (cutaneous-spinal-medullary angioma), Rendu-Osler-Weber syndrome (familial telangiectasia or pulmonary-cerebral-spinal angioma), and Klippel-Trenaunay-Weber syndrome (cutaneous spinal angioma). The cutaneous hemangioma is often unilateral and follows a dermatomal pattern. The classic Wybun-Mason syndrome is a spinal or intracranial AVM associated with a truncal or facial nevus.

Selective spinal angiography defines the AVM preoperatively and is an important adjunct to microsurgical removal of these lesions. The role of preoperative embolization is still unclear in the neurosurgical literature.

CAVERNOUS HEMANGIOMAS AND MISCELLANEOUS LESIONS

The *cavernous hemangioma* is a rare cystic, intramedullary mass of thin-walled, sinusoidal spaces (arteriovenous), lined with a single layer of endothelium, containing hemosiderin (or old clot with fibrosis), gliosis, and calcification, but devoid of neural tissue. Grossly, the mass resembles a blue-brown mulberry.

The caverous hemangioma can be found anywhere in the spinal cord but characteristically occurs in the cervicothoracic region. Its clinical presentation is that of a chronic progressive paraparesis, but an acute onset with subarachnoid hemorrhage and hematomyelia has been described. MRI is diagnostic; however, selective spinal angiography will be completely normal, as cavernous hemangiomas are angiographically occult.

Venous angiomas and capillary telangiectasias are found in the spinal cord and in the brain and can cause intraspinal hemorrhage. Spontaneous epidural and intramedullary hemorrhages have been described without a clear etiology or focal pathology. Epidural hemorrhage may be associated with blunt trauma, thrombocytopenia, aspirin therapy, or it may occur spontaneously with aspirin administration.

Bone and Ligament Anatomy Supporting the Spinal Cord[1–6,9,10,28,29]

☐ VERTEBRAL COLUMN

The spinal column has 33 *vertebrae* joined by ligaments and cartilage. The cervicothoracolumbar vertebrae are mobile, but the sacral and coccygeal segments are often fused to form the sacrum and coccyx. There are 7 cervical, 12 thoracic, 5 lumbar, 5 sacral, and 4 coccygeal (Coc1 to Coc4) vertebrae. There can be sacralization of the L5 lumbar vertebra or lumbarization of the S1 sacral vertebra, congenital spinal variations with partial or complete fusion. This is important in the patient with a herniated lumbar disk, since the surgeon must identify the ruptured disk. This is determined by counting from routine thoracic and lumbosacral x-rays and correlating levels with imaging studies. Additionally, the L5 and S1 vertebrae may be identified at the time of surgery by their mobility and resonant timbre, the L5 vertebra being mobile and having a sharply resonant sound upon tapping. If levels are questionable, intraoperative x-rays will delineate them.

The vertebral column has an S-shaped curve when viewed from the side, the cervical and lumbar spine being lordotic and the thoracic spine being kyphotic. The term *normal lordotic* refers to ventral convexity. Abnormal kyphosis, or "hump back," occurs in cervicothoracic tumors, trauma, osteomyelitis, degenerating spondylosis, and in anklyosing spondylitis. Straightening of the lumbosacral spine or abnormal lordosis can be seen in discogenic disease, trauma, tumors, stenosis, and paraspinal muscle spasm. Metastases to the cervicothoracic spine cause vertebral body collapse, and kyphoscoliosis with angulation may be apparent on routine examinations.

☐ VERTEBRAE

Typical vertebrae have a body and an arch that enclose the spinal cord; the exception is the C1, which has no body. The *neural arch* comprises a *pedicle* on each side that continues posteriorly as a *lamina* behind the spinal canal. Importantly, the laminae on each side of the spinous process form shallow groves for attachment of the muscles.

Each pedicle has a *superior* and *inferior notch,* which

together with its adjacent counterpart form the *intervertebral foramen.* The spinal nerves pass through this oval-shaped foramen. Each spinous process represents the posterior midline of the neural arch and laminae. (See Fig. 2-4.) The *transverse processes* extend laterally from the junction of each pedicle, and the *superior* and *inferior articular processes* are lateral to each lamina.

Each pair of vertebral bodies is separated by an intervening fibrocartilaginous disk and is articulated on both sides by a *superior* and *inferior articular process* which is contained within a capsule. (See Fig. 2-4.) Thus the inferior articular process of L4 vertebrae relates to the superior articulate process of L5 vertebrae, surrounded by a *joint capsule.*

Each disk contains a core of gelatinous tissue with large cells, the *nucleus pulposus,* and is bound by a thick *annulus fibrosus* with radially directed attachments, *Sharpey's fibers,* to the adjacent vertebral bodies. The intervertebral disk absorbs stress and strain to the vertebral column, but progressively desiccates with age, leading to a loss of height in elderly individuals.

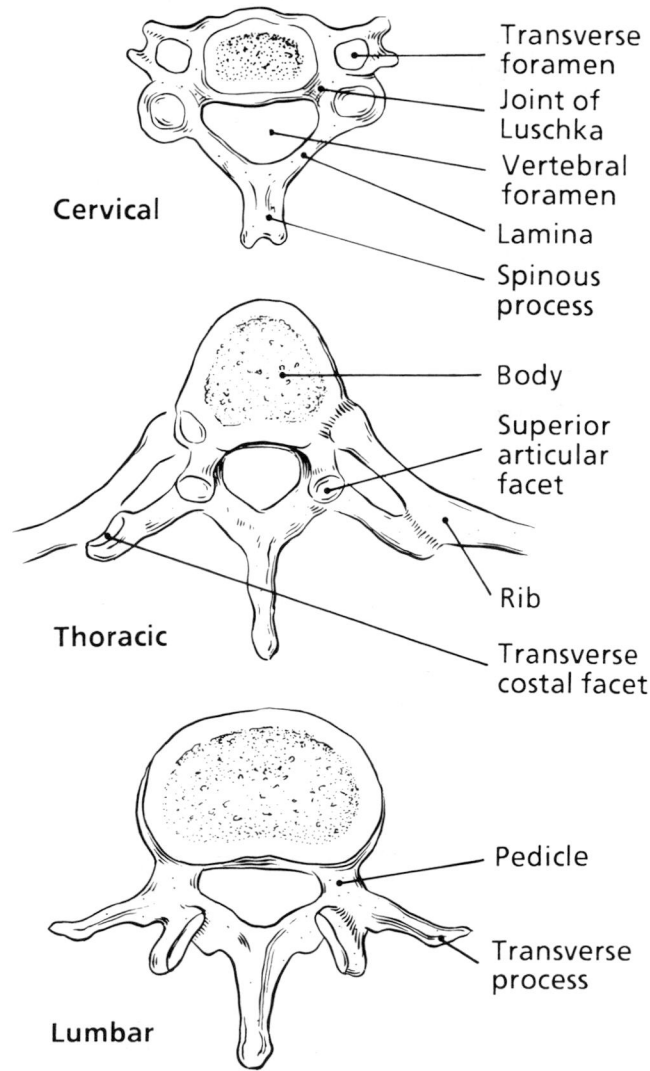

Figure 2-4   A schematic drawing of the typical cervical, thoracic, and lumbar vertebrae.

☐ SPECIAL FEATURES OF THE SPINE

CERVICAL SPINE[3-6]

There are regional differences in the vertebrae. In the cervical region the C1 to C6 vertebrae contain transverse foramina which perforate each transverse process and also contain the vertebral artery en route to the cranium. The vertebral artery enters the cervical spine through the transverse foramen of the C6 vertebral body. Trauma, tumors, osteomyelitis, and cervical spondylosis can narrow and occlude the vertebral artery within its foramen, which can cause vertebrobasilar insufficiency (VBI) with motion of the neck, depending upon flow in the contralateral vertebral artery. Classically, the cervical neurofibroma or neuroma with a dumbbell- or hourglass-shaped extension may adhere to a vertebral artery, sometimes necessitating posterior and anterolateral approaches for excision, while preserving the vertebral artery.

The *atlas,* or C1, and the *axis,* or C2, are distinctive cervical vertebrae. The C1 vertebra has neither a body nor a spinous process but consists instead of two lateral masses and two arches, anterior and posterior. Its superior facets articulate with the occipital condyles, and its inferior facets with the axis, or C2 vertebra. The atlas is prone to an axial compression fracture by trauma, the *Jefferson fracture.* It is also prone to ligamentous laxity and atlantoaxial subluxation. The atlas can be fused to the occiput, termed *occipitalization,* and is associated with a variety of craniovertebral junction anomalies, including basilar impression and invagination.[22]

The axis, C2, has a large odontoid process, the *dens,* which arises from the superior surface of the vertebral body. Large facets articulate with the atlas, and the spinous process is large. The odontoid is prone to fractures by a traumatic injury; the type II fracture through the base of the dens, is particularly unstable, perhaps because of vascular insufficiency or a "watershed" zone conjectured to be present at the base of C2. The type II fracture requires realignment and fusion. Os odontoideum, ossiculum terminate, and odontoid dysgenesis are rare congenital malformations of the odontoid which can lead to atlantoaxial subluxation and episodes of sudden quadriparesis due to ligamentous laxity.

Dimensions of the spinal canal in the cervical regions are important. As one proceeds caudally the diameter of the canal narrows. At the foramen magnum, the normal diameter is 26 to 40 mm and is acceptable with an average of 34 mm. A diameter of less than 19 mm often leads to neurological deficits. At the C5–C6 cervical level, an AP diameter less than 12 to 13 mm often is coupled with deficits and is indicative of spinal stenosis. The usual sagittal diameter at the C5–C6 level is 15 to 20 mm.

THORACIC SPINE[5,6,28,29]

The thoracic vertebrae are inherently more stable and less prone to traumatic fracture and subluxation since, in addition to the superior and inferior facets, there are two sets of facets for articulation with the *heads* and *tubercles* of the ribs. (See Fig. 2-4.) Thus, the ribs confer additional stability to the thoracic spine and as a result, traumatic thoracic fractures are uncommonly associated with movement or dislocation and are often without neurological deficits.

Importantly, the thoracic canal has an AP diameter of only 8 to 10 mm, significantly less than in the cervical or lumbar regions; hence, the thoracic canal is occupied almost completely by the spinal cord. Thoracic spinal stenosis, a degenerative, spondylitic hypertrophy of the lamina and facets, only recently recognized, leads to progressive myelopathy in the legs. Treatment is by decompressive laminectomy.

LUMBAR SPINE[5,6,28,29]

The lumbar vertebrae are uniquely massive. They provide support for bearing weight. The intervertebral disks, laminae, and pedicles are thickest in the lumbar region. The lumbar spine is subjected to much stress and strain and is frequently prone to spinal stenosis.

Importantly, the lumbar spinal canal has an average AP diameter of 15 to 25 mm. Narrowing to less than 12 to 13 mm is considered diagnostic of lumbar stenosis. Neurogenic claudication secondary to lumbar stenosis is a common and disabling disease.

Although the lumbar vertebrae are massive in size compared with other regions, traumatic fractures do occur regularly in the lumbar region, but neurologic injury is less common than in injuries at higher levels. The L1 vertebra is most prone to fractures as it lacks the rib cage support of the more rostral counterpart, the T12 vertebra.

Compromise of the AP diameter of over 50 percent is usually associated with neurologic deficit. Compression fractures require decompression and stabilization through anterior or posterior routes. The conus medullaris, or tapered end of the spinal cord, is typically near the lower border of the L1 vertebra. The L1 compression fracture needs to be decompressed and stabilized, either through an anterior or posterior route since the conus medullaris or tapered end of the spinal cord is typically near the lower border of the L1 vertebra.

☐ LIGAMENTS OF THE VERTEBRAL COLUMN[3-6,22,28,29]

Key ligaments oriented transversely and longitudinally support the spine in its normal configuration. (See Fig. 2-5.)

ANTERIOR LONGITUDINAL LIGAMENT

This ligament extends from the basion of the occipital bone caudally to the sacrum. At the C2 vertebral level it is continuous with the atlantoaxial ligament, and its rostral extent is termed the *atlantoccipital membrane.* This ligament is inti-

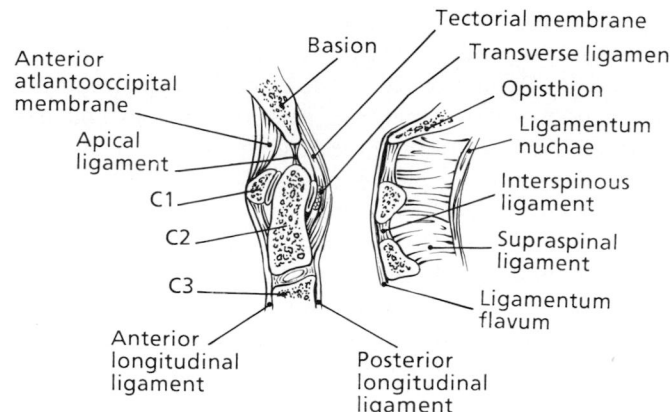

Figure 2-5 The key ligaments of the spine.

mately attached to vertebral bodies and intervertebral disks. The anterior longitudinal ligament can be torn in severe hyperextension injuries or separated from its attachment with the vertebral bodies of the neck.

POSTERIOR LONGITUDINAL LIGAMENT

This ligament extends from the basiocciput, or basion, to the sacrum, lying posterior to the vertebral bodies. Its rostral extension from the C2 vertebra to the basiocciput is termed the *tectorial membrane,* meaning "roof" or "covering." The posterior longitudinal ligament can be torn in severe hyperflexion injuries of the spine, and associated with severe vertebral fractures and instability. Ossification of the posterior longitudinal ligament (OPLL) is characterized by multisegment involvement in the spinal canal with progressive myelopathy, treated by decompression and stabilization.[5,6,28,29]

LIGAMENTUM FLAVUM

The "yellow ligament" is strong and buffers or cushions the spinal cord and cauda equina posteriorly from trauma. It attaches to the ventral surface of the lamina above, dorsal surface of the lamina below, medially to the spinous processes, and laterally to the facets. It does *not* form a continuous band posterior to the spinal cord and thecal sac dura. This is of great significance when performing a lumbar or cervical laminectomy, as great care needs to be taken not to tear the thinnest dura where the ligamentum flavum is absent or atretic. Metastatic tumors to the spine with large epidural components may replace the preexisting ligamentum flavum.

SUPRASPINOUS LIGAMENT

This ligament extends from the occiput to the sacrum and attaches to the tips of the spinous processes in the midline. In the cervical region it is termed the *ligamentum nuchae* and serves as a focal point for attachment by several fascial and muscle layers, with a most rostral attachment to the external

occipital protuberance. It is a key landmark during surgical procedures identifying the midline.

INTERSPINOUS LIGAMENT

This ligament also connects each spinous process with the adjacent level, extending from the apex to the root of each process. This becomes continuous with the supraspinous ligament dorsally and with the ligamentum flavum ventrally, adding to spinal stability.

☐ LIGAMENTS OF THE CRANIOVERTEBRAL JUNCTION[22]

There are additional key ligaments at the occiput-atlas-axis level which allow for mobility and stability at the junction of the head and neck. (See Fig. 2-6.) Ligaments between the atlas and axis allow lateral or side-to-side rotation in addition to flexion and extension.

CRUCIATE LIGAMENT

This ligament is shaped like a cross and helps stabilize the odontoid process. It extends from the odontoid process rostrally to the basion, caudally to the body of the axis, and laterally to the lateral masses of the atlas. Lateral extensions are called *transverse ligaments.* The transverse ligament forms a sling or band across the dorsal aspect of the odontoid. (See Fig. 2-6.) Thus, the transverse ligament checks the atlas from slipping forward on the odontoid (atlantoaxial subluxation).

If the transverse ligament is torn, the anterior distance between the anterior arch of the atlas and the odontoid peg is increased. Normally, in adults the predental space is 3 mm and in children 5 mm. The measurement is determined by lateral x-ray film profile. A complementary x-ray, the "open-mouth" odontoid view, may demonstrate displacement of one lateral mass of the atlas. A transverse diameter greater than 6.9 mm is indicative of atlantoaxial subluxation secondary to tear of the transverse ligament associated with fracture of the ring of the atlas.

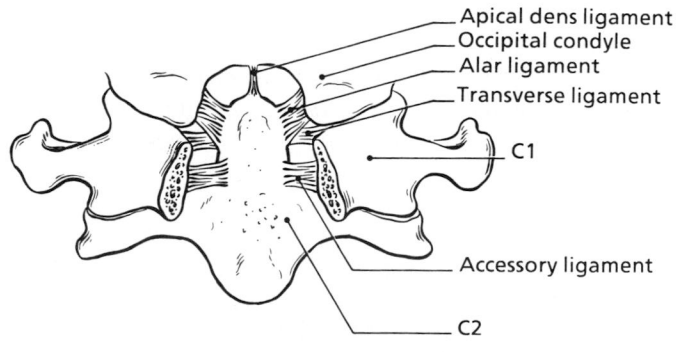

Figure 2-6 The key ligaments of the craniovertebral junction.

Other entities that tear or disrupt the transverse ligament are rheumatoid arthritis, odontoid dysgenesis, fractures, and os odontoideum. In Down's syndrome, the mucopolysaccharidoses, including Morquio's syndrome and Grisel's syndrome, acute pharyngitis, and retropharyngeal infection associated with torticollis, can be associated with atlantoaxial subluxation.

ALAR LIGAMENT

The alar ligaments have the appearance of wings. They are paired bands which attach each side of the odontoid process to the medial aspect of the occipital condyle. If the alar ligaments are torn or disrupted, the atlantoaxial space often measures 5 to 10 mm. There is a marked anterior atlantoaxial subluxation. Patients with severe rheumatoid arthritis often have atlantoaxial subluxation associated with disruption of the transverse and alar ligaments. These patients often require realignment with Gardner-Wells tongs and fusion, usually through the posterior route.

☐ MISCELLANEOUS LIGAMENTS

Other key ligaments stabilize the craniovertebral junction. The apical ligaments attach the tip of the dens to the basion or basiocciput, thus limiting rotation and flexion of the head. Also, the ligamentum nuchae, anterior and posterior atlantoccipital membranes, and atlantoaxial ligaments add to the stability of this region.

All these ligaments serve a protective role from a teleological standpoint, as the odontoid process must be stable in position. It must be prevented from compressing the cervicomedullary junction, the brainstem, and spinal cord. This duplication of ligaments in the craniovertebral junction prevents neurological deficits in cases of fractured odontoid.

☐ RELATED ANOMALIES OF THE CRANIOVERTEBRAL JUNCTION[22]

A key related group of neurosurgical diseases which are becoming more important are *basilar impression* and *invagination.* As mentioned previously, the neurosurgical patient with long-standing severe rheumatoid arthritis often has anterior atlantoaxial subluxation into the range of 10 to 20 mm, but the patient may also seem additionally predisposed to a vertical subluxation or impression of the odontoid process into the foramen magnum, a term called *cranial settling* or *basilar impression.* This descent of the skull on the eroded joints of the occipitoatlantoaxial unit will lead to ventral compression of the brainstem and accompanying neurological signs, including internuclear ophthalmoplegia, facial diplegia and hypalgesia, down-beat nystagmus, spastic

quadriparesis, and sleep apnea. The term *basilar impression* refers to a secondary or acquired form of the disease; it can be due to Paget's disease, osteomalacia, hyperparathyroidism, osteogenesis imperfecta, Hurler's syndrome, but most commonly, it is a result of rheumatoid arthritis. On the other hand this "cranial settling," or prolapse of the vertebral column into the skull base, may be a developmental defect, referred to as *basilar invagination.* It is associated with other developmental bone anomalies of the craniovertebral junction, including occipitalization of the atlas, Klippel-Feil syndrome, odontoid anomalies, and most commonly the Arnold-Chiari type I malformation associated with syringomyelia.

Several radiographic measurements are important for assessment. A line drawn along the clivus baseline, the Wackenheim line, should pass longitudinally to the posterior tip of the dens. (See Fig. 2-5.) A line connecting the posterior border of the hard palate to the opisthion should be above the tip of the dens; this is Chamberlan's line. The plane of the foramen magnum is represented by a line from the basion to the opisthion, having a normal range of 26 to 40 mm with an average of 34 mm, but it is clearly abnormal with neurological signs if it measures less than 19 mm in AP diameter.

Intervention necessitates anterior and posterior approaches in the presence of anomalies or with dislocation due to rheumatoid arthritis. Realignment may be necessary prior to transoral decompression and/or posterior stabilization. MRI delineates the abnormal ligaments and soft tissue anatomy, especially pannus or fracture anterior to the cervicomedullary junction.

☐ BONE TUMORS OF NEUROSURGICAL INTEREST[3–6,28,29]

CHORDOMA

These cartilaginous tumors arise from primitive notochord remnants at the cranial base and spine, with a predilection for the clivus (spheno-occipital) and sacrococcygeal regions, and the cervical vertebrae. The chordoma is quite destructive locally, with large soft tissue masses and calcification. Physaliparous or the "bubble" cell type have a much greater potential for metastases than the chordoid variant. The tumor is expansile and osteolytic on x-ray films of the spine and CT. Severe local pain, often nocturnal and at rest, with or without neurological deficits, is common.

Surgical approaches to the clivus include transphenoidal, transbasal via bifrontal craniotomy, transoral, transcervical, and transpalatal routes, depending upon the ventral and caudal extents of the tumor. Sacrococcygeal tumors may require anterolateral and abdominoperineal approaches in addition to a sacral laminectomy or radical sacrectomy for their removal. The chordoma is relatively radioresistant, and recent therapeutic approaches have included local interstitial brachytherapy after radical resection. Overall, it remains a therapeutic challenge for the neurosurgeon.

PLASMACYTOMA AND MULTIPLE MYELOMA

Plasmacytoma is a solitary tumor. Multiple myeloma is a malignant tumor of sites that may include vertebrae and the cranium. In the skull they are typically multiple lytic lesions, exhibiting a "moth-eaten" appearance on radiographs.

Myeloma is a B-cell lymphoma characterized by tumor cells secreting monoclonal antibodies that can be detected in the urine as Bence Jones protein by protein electrophoresis. A small percentage, 10 to 20 percent, of patients with the solitary plasmacytoma will ultimately transform to multiple myeloma. Radiographically, there is lysis and collapse of vertebral bodies, associated with local pain, often leading to paraparesis. Intervention requires anterior or anterolateral decompression and fixation.

Current medical therapy includes local radiation therapy for the solitary plasmacytoma. Medical therapy for multiple myeloma includes multiregimen chemotherapy in addition to radiation.

MISCELLANEOUS TUMORS

Rare benign bone tumors include eosinophilic granulomas, osteoblastomas, chordomyxoid fibroma, giant cell, and dermoid tumors. Localized pain is a common symptom in these, and therapeutic considerations include vertebrectomy and stabilization, with use of bone, metal, or methylmethacrylate.

Metastatic tumors to the spine are very common. Localized pain may be accompanied by pain on palpation of spinous processes, an indication of the posterior or lateral processes involvement. Neurologic deficits, including paraparesis, quadriparesis, Brown-Séquard syndrome, and bowel and bladder dysfunction, are common.

The primary lesions of breast, lung, prostate, thyroid, and colon cancer spread first to vertebral bodies, often multiple ones. They may extend posterior to the lamina and spinous processes. Pedicle erosion and vertebral body collapse are late signs of spinal metastases, and are seen on x-rays of the spine. Classically, the "ivory" vertebra is seen radiographically in prostate cancer and less commonly in lymphoma, which usually has a soft-tissue extension into the intervertebral foramen.

Because of the unique involvement of both the anterior and posterior elements of the spine in cancer metastases, current neurosurgical approaches include both anterior and posterior decompression and stabilization, tailored to each individual neurosurgical case. Unfortunately, many metastatic tumors are radioresistant. Radiation therapy is often only palliative, treating local pain.

☐ THE SPONDYLOSES OF THE SPINE[3–6,8,13,28,29]

CERVICAL SPONDYLOSIS AND MYELOPATHY[3,4]

This classical neurological problem was defined by Lord Brain in the 1950s.[8,20] Yet, its pathophysiology is still unclear. Cervical spondylosis is an accrued or congenital narrowing of the spinal canal, often slowly progressive, accompanied by formation of osteophytes, ossification of the posterior longitudinal ligament, hypertrophy of the facet joints, and ligamentum compromising the spinal cord. Elderly neurosurgical patients often develop myelopathy similar to a central cord syndrome; spastic paraparesis; upper extremity wasting, including distal atrophy and weakness; dysesthetic or hyperpathic pain in the hands; and bowel and bladder dysfunction. Although root symptoms are uncommon, the biceps (C5) and supinator (C6) reflexes may be absent, with the triceps (C7) reflex being hyperreflexic. Loss of reflexes is consistent with cord compression at the C5–C6 interspace and is classic for cervical spondylotic myelopathy (CSM). The hyperreflexia of the triceps reflex is an inverted spinal reflex, due to physiological reflex release at a lower level secondary to a block at a higher level.

Often the patient has neck pain accentuated with flexion or extension, and Lhermitte's sign upon flexion is common with severe spinal stenosis. Flexion of the neck increases the cord length by 2 cm, causing stretch and probably accounting for Lhermitte's sign. In hyperextension, there is shortening, and the cord buckles from a spondylotic bar anteriorly and the ligamentum flavum posteriorly. The cervical spinal cord is not free to allow flexion-extension movements since it is held forward by the nerve roots and prevented from moving backward by the dentate ligaments.

The presentation of a patient with cervical spondylotic myelopathy may be quite variable. Pathologically, there is demyelination of the corticospinal tracts and degeneration of gray matter, including the motor cells, which is consistent with the clinical picture of a central cord syndrome.

Radiographically, there is an average AP canal diameter of 12 to 13 mm at the C5–C6 level in patients with cervical spondylotic myelopathy. Cervical myelopathy is almost assured by a sagittal diameter of less than 10 mm. Cervical spondylotic changes are maximal at C5–C6, C6–C7, and C4–C5, as these are the points that exhibit greatest movement.

The pathophysiology of CSM is unclear. It is postulated that accentuated movement—both flexion, extension, and rotation—cause progressive spinal stenosis. A vascular mechanism of venous congestion or stasis has also been implicated.

Posterior decompression by laminectomy is the traditional treatment for spinal stenosis. Recently, there has been renewed interest in anterior decompression, including vertebrectomy and excision of the ossified hypertrophied posterior longitudinal ligament. The tested long-term benefits of posterior versus anterior surgical decompression have not been fully evaluated, but the results should be quite revealing.

LUMBAR SPONDYLOSIS AND NEUROGENIC CLAUDICATION[5,6,8,20,28,29]

Lumbar stenosis due to spondylosis is a syndrome wherein the patient complains that, while walking, he or she develops bilateral and posteriolateral leg pains with cramping or tightness and occasionally weakness with prolonged walking. Claudication of the cauda equina or neurogenic claudication is relieved with rest. Usually, when the patient is at rest, the neurological examination is normal. Nearly 25 to 50 percent of patients with lumbar stenosis have accompanying cervical stenosis, lending likely support to a common pathophysiology and pathogenesis.

Radiographically, the AP diameter of the lumbar spinal cord is 12 to 13 mm in stenosis because of bony overgrowth and compression by the ligamentum flavum. These radiographic changes are similar to those seen in cervical spondylosis. The pathophysiology is conjectured to be vascular compromise within a narrowed thecal sac which is reversed with rest, perhaps in part a result of flexion of the lumbar spinal canal.

Treatment includes wide laminectomy and partial facetectomy above and below the stenotic areas with removal of the ligamentum flavum extending into the lateral gutters. Recently, there has been an interest in bilateral hemilaminotomies as an alternative solution to this neurosurgical entity. The relief of the claudication is often dramatic postoperatively.

Congenital lumbar stenosis is quite rare, but it is seen in children with diastematomyelia and spina bifida occulta. Patients with achondroplasia have congenital stenosis with a predilection for the thoracolumbar region and the foramen magnum. This type of stenosis is exceedingly tight.

ANKLYOSING SPONDYLITIS, MARIE-STRUMPELL DISEASE[3-6,28,29]

This is a rare but fascinating spondylitic disease, linked immunologically to the HLA-B27 histocompatibility antigen complex and associated with severe kyphoscoliosis, fused or block vertebra, and a "bamboo-spine." Flexion deformity is pronounced and visible in the cervical region, and there is loss of the functional soft tissue elements to the spine.

Hence, these patients are very prone to spinal fractures and cord injury from minor trauma since their spines are fused throughout and lack the compensatory "shock-absorbing" mechanisms. Predictably, they are prone to fractures at the cervicothoracic and thoracolumbar junctions, and they can present with acute paraparesis or quadriparesis from even mild head or neck trauma, or trauma to the abdomen. The fractures may heal, but pseudoarthroses are common. An epidural hematoma can be the cause of acute neurological deterioration.

Treatment consists of immobilization, fusion often requiring instrumentation. Axial traction or a Stryker frame is contraindicated as these may dislocate the fracture further. Postoperative halo immobilization is often necessary. Anterior approaches to decompression and stabilization may be used in conjunction with the posterior decompression and fixation.

☐ DIFFUSE IDIOPATHIC SKELETAL HYPERTROPHY (DISH)[4]

This is a rare, diffuse skeletal disease that may affect the cervical spine and even simulate cervical spondylosis clinically and radiographically. First described by Forestier, this disease is characterized by extensive ligamentous calcification with formidable vertebral bridging. However, the intervertebral disk is not damaged, so the joint space may be normal in height. The posterior longitudinal ligament may also be calcified in DISH. Surgical therapy may be either anterior or posterior decompression, or both, depending on the region of cervical spine involvement. Despite the impressive bone overgrowth, myelopathy is uncommon with DISH, but radicular symptoms are common.

REFERENCES

1. Gilman S, Newman SW: *Manter and Gatz's Essentials of Clinical Neuroanatomy and Neurophysiology.* Philadelphia, Davis, 1989, pp 12–70.
2. DeGroot J, Chasid JG: *Correlative Neuroanatomy.* San Mateo, Appleton and Lange, 1988, pp 32–80.
3. Bailey RW, Sherk HH: *The Cervical Spine.* Philadelphia, The Cervical Spine Research Society, Lippincott, 1983.
4. Dunsker SB: *Cervical Spondylosis.* New York, Raven, 1981.
5. Youmans JR: *Neurological Surgery,* vols 1–6. Philadelphia, Saunders, 1982, pp 551–617, 2533–2629, 3196–3222.
6. Wilkins RH, Rengachary SS: *Neurosurgery.* New York, McGraw-Hill, 1985, vol 1, pp 927–930, 1039–1079; vol 2, pp 1694–1761; vol 3, pp 1969–1975, 2041–2081, 2219–2305, 2430–2452.
7. McLaurin RL: *Pediatric Neurosurgery; Surgery of the Developing Nervous System.* New York, Grune & Stratton, 1982, pp 1–91, 529–541.

8. Patten J: *Neurological Differential Diagnosis.* New York, Springer-Verlag, 1983, pp 139–206.

9. Truex RC, Carpenter MB: *Human Neuroanatomy.* Baltimore, Williams & Wilkins, 1973, pp 1–290.

10. Goss CM: *Gray's Anatomy.* Philadelphia, Lea & Febiger, 1971, pp 796–882.

11. Rand RW, Rand CW: *Intraspinal Tumors of Childhood.* Springfield, IL, Charles C Thomas, 1960.

12. Elsberg CA: *Tumors of the Spinal Cord and the Symptoms of Irritation and Compression of the Spinal Cord and Nerve Roots: Pathology, Symptomatology, Diagnosis, and Treatment.* New York, Paul B. Hoeber, 1925, pp 299–301.

13. Schmidek HH, Sweet WH: *Operative Neurosurgical Techniques,* vols 1 and 2. New York, Grune & Stratton, 1982, pp 1119–1977.

14. Kempe LG: *Operative Neurosurgery,* vol 2. New York, Springer-Verlag, 1968, pp 80–133.

15. Greenwood J Jr: Surgical removal of intramedullary tumors. *J Neurosurg* 26:276–282, 1967.

16. Sloof JL, Kernohan JW, McCarty CS: *Primary Intramedullary Tumors of the Spinal Cord and Flavum Terminale.* Philadelphia, Saunders, 1964.

17. Cushing H, Eisenhardt L: *Meningiomas: Their Classification, Regional Behavior, Life History, and Surgical Results.* Springfield, IL, Charles C Thomas, 1938, pp 74–133.

18. Al-Mefty O: *Meningiomas.* New York, Raven, 1991, pp 543–569, 593–621.

19. Schneider KC, Cherry G, Pantek H: The symptoms of acute central cervical cord injury. *J Neurosurg* 11:546–577, 1954.

20. Adams RD, Victor M: *Principles of Neurology.* New York, McGraw-Hill, 1981, pp 617–645.

21. Barnett HJM, Foster JB, Hudgson P: *Syringomyelia.* Philadelphia, Saunders, 1973.

22. VanGilder JC, Menzes AH, Dolan KD: *The Cranioverbral Junction and Its Abnormalities.* Mount Kisco, Futura, 1987.

23. Austin GM: *The Spinal Cord: Basic Aspects and Surgical Considerations.* Springfield, IL, Charles C Thomas, 1961.

24. Djindjian R, Hurth M, Hardart R: *Angiography of the Spinal Cord.* Baltimore, University Park Press, 1970.

25. Doppman SL, DiChiro G, Ommaya AK: *Selective Arteriography of the Spinal Cord.* St. Louis, Warren H. Green, 1969.

26. Wyburn-Mason R: *The Vascular Abnormalities and Tumors of the Spinal Cord and Its Membranes.* London, Kimpton, 1943.

27. Pia HW, Djindjian R: *Spinal Angiomas: Advances in Diagnosis and Therapy.* New York, Springer-Verlag, 1978.

28. Rothman RH, Simeone FA: *The Spine.* Philadelphia, Saunders, 1982.

29. Frymoyer JW: *The Adult Spine.* New York, Raven, 1991.

☐ STUDY QUESTIONS

I. As a resident in neurosurgery assigned to pathology, you are asked to perform an autopsy on a 75-year-old male who had died of a pulmonary embolus, having lived a normal life until he began to experience neurogenic claudication a year earlier. He had been neurologically normal with normal pulses in his lower extremities but imaging studies and myelography revealed severe stenosis at L4–L5. He had undergone laminectomy but complained of tenderness of his left calf 3 days after surgery, and he died suddenly that afternoon. You perform an autopsy.

1. What is the measured width of the spinal cord at C6? At T6? At T12? **2.** At what level might the spinal cord be expected to terminate? **3.** What would you expect to see as residual effects of the stenosis at the L4–L5 level? **4.** What is the likelihood of seeing evidence of spinal stenosis in the cervical area? Where would it most likely be located? **5.** Describe the arterial blood supply to the spinal cord.

II. A 43-year-old female is referred because of progressive weakness in the upper extremities (worse on the left than the right), weakness and atrophy of the left side of the tongue, and weakness of the left trapezius of 6 months' duration.

The patient complains of occipital headache and dizziness. Plain x-rays of the craniocervical junction are normal, but an MRI shows a large extraaxial mass lesion which appears very similar to nervous tissue in the T2-weighted image but is enhanced with gadolinium.

1. What is the most likely diagnosis? **2.** What alternative diagnoses should be considered? **3.** How can the lesion be approached surgically? **4.** What anatomical structures might be encountered? **5.** How can the spinal cord be mobilized?

III. A 40-year-old female has unrelenting pain from a sarcoma involving the left ilium. The decision is made to perform an open cordotomy on this patient.

1. At what level(s) might the procedure be accomplished? **2.** How can the spinal cord be mobilized? **3.** What quadrant of the spinal cord should be divided? **4.** What structures should one identify before making an incision in the spinal cord? **5.** What alternative surgical procedures might be considered?

IV. A 23-year-old male sustains a burst fracture of the L1 vertebra with a fragment filling 75 percent of the spinal canal.

1. What neurological deficits might be encountered? **2.** What recovery might be expected following decompression by whatever means are used? **3.** What arterial blood supply might be interrupted? **4.** What coverings of the spinal cord are present at this area? **5.** What ligaments will most likely be affected?

V. A 50-year-old male sustains a hyperextension injury of the neck with contusion of the central portion of the spinal cord. X-rays show no fracture.

1. What should be the anticipated AP diameter of the spinal canal on lateral radiographs? **2.** What neurological deficits do you expect? **3.** Explain the basis for the neurological deficits. **4.** What surgical therapy should be contemplated? **5.** When do you anticipate maximal recovery?

3

Diagnosis of Lesions Affecting the Nervous System by History and Physical Examination

Marshall B. Allen, Jr.

This chapter reviews the elements of *history taking* and *physical examination* that are important to the diagnosis and surgical therapy of persons with lesions that affect the nervous system. This review emphasizes characteristics that are peculiar to lesions of neurologic significance—both in considering a surgical procedure and in treating patients subjected to injury or disability as a result of a lesion affecting the nervous system.

Subsequent chapters will deal with diagnostic tests that confirm and, in the case of imaging, demonstrate lesions involving the nervous system, many of which might be first suspected from the patient's history and physical examination. Later chapters will apply many of the points made here that will be expanded upon as they are applied to specific cases.

History Taking

☐ PERSONAL HISTORY

A patient's *history* represents the basis on which most forms of diagnostic and therapeutic procedures are selected. It may be the only clinical clue of a major neurologic lesion, as in the case of epilepsy or transient ischemic attacks where neurological and general physical examinations may be nor-

mal. A correct diagnosis is suggested in most patients from the history alone.

The history may be difficult or impossible to obtain from the patient who is unconscious or dysphasic, and it may be misleading in a confused patient, who has lost memory function or who is subject to seizures. The history of a patient who is unconscious must be obtained from associates who accompany the patient to the examination. The history may significantly influence the order in which investigations are performed on the unconscious patient. As an example, urgency is demanded in the evaluation of a patient who has had a head injury, who was awake at the scene, but whose state of consciousness is progressively deteriorating, whereas it may be important to take a more systematic approach in the evaluation of a patient who is known to have been alert only a few minutes prior to the interview when he or she experienced a spontaneous seizure.

Details of a history will necessarily be delayed in a patient who is in respiratory difficulty or shock, immediate correction of which is necessary to sustain life. Once the life-threatening problems are corrected, however, details of the history must be sought.

Specific features of the history that are important include the patient's perception of any changes that he or she has experienced, the sequence in which these experiences have occurred, as well as their duration. Of importance in the patient with altered intellect is the perception of other people regarding length and degree of intellectual change. The family's perception of the etiology of such change may also be important.

An indication that a patient has been unconscious may be obtained by determining events which the patient recognizes as having occurred before an accident or following the event. Patients who have experienced head injuries may be unaware of loss of consciousness, but review of their recollection of details surrounding the injury may reveal evidence of *amnesia*. There can be major gaps in the memory of a patient who has experienced a recent closed head injury. Severity of the injury may be graded in part by periods of *antegrade* and *retrograde* amnesia. The period of amnesia is best determined by noting the last event that the patient remembers before the injury and the first event recalled after.

Finally, it should be recalled that the best history of an injury should be obtained shortly after the accident, since the record of events surrounding an accident may become a vital part of the medical-legal documentation.

Other points important in the history include previous infusion of blood products, types and quantities of drugs, and intimate relationships to individuals known to have evidence of disease. Intracranial mass lesions are often the result of infection and some neoplasms are related to acquired immune deficiency syndrome (AIDS).

☐ FAMILY HISTORY

A history of familial disease is important in the determination of many neurological lesions that may be neoplastic or metabolic. For instance, a family history of individuals with café-au-lait skin lesions or subcutaneous nodules may be important in a patient who evidences neurofibromatosis. A family history might indicate metabolic diseases such as diabetes. Hypertension and degenerative cardiovascular disease, as well as degenerative processes of the nervous system, are often familial. *Infectious lesions* may occur in families because of personal association. A family history of tuberculosis might draw attention in the evaluation of a patient who has a deteriorating state of consciousness or evidence of hydrocephalus. It may direct attention to evaluation of cerebrospinal fluid (CSF) for evidence of infection.

Physical Examination

☐ GENERAL EXAMINATION

A good general physical examination is an important part of the evaluation of any patient who is being considered for diagnosis and/or treatment of a lesion affecting the nervous system.

It is necessary to review cardiac and pulmonary function before any patient undergoes general anesthesia; the level of

blood pressure or evidence of organomegaly might influence the type and quantity of anesthetics administered. Evidence of oxygen deprivation may explain stupor. In infants, intracranial arteriovenous malformations exhibited first by bruits may be associated with congestive heart failure. Alterations of cardiac rhythm can account for neurological symptoms throughout life. Skin lesions, such as café-au-lait spots, cutaneous angiomata, especially in the distribution of the trigeminal nerve and adenoma sebaceum, are associated with intracranial and/or intraspinal lesions, as in the case of the midline skin defects.

Intracranial masses are often the result of metastases from lesions outside the central nervous system (CNS). Achrondroplasia is often associated with spinal stenosis, and scoliosis is often the result of neurological deficits from neoplasms or neurological disease. Severe scoliosis or acute kyphosis may be the cause of paresis below the level of deformity.

HEAD

Enlargement of the head, and especially increase in the tension and size of the anterior fontanel in infants, is a sign of hydrocephalus or some other intracranial space-occupying lesion, such as hematoma or neoplasm. Distension of veins in the scalp may be the first sign of increasing intracranial pressure. A progressively increasing circumference of the head is also an important clinical feature of inadequacy of treatment.

To the contrary, small fontanels, bony ridges, and abnormally shaped skulls represent evidence of craniosynostosis, correction of which is best accomplished at an early age.

Auscultation of heads in newborn infants is necessary since bruits may indicate the presence of intracranial vascular malformations that may be important, not only to neurological development but also for possible congestive heart failure at this early age.

Detailed evaluation of a patient with recent head injury is vital and mandatory. Lacerations may overlie fractures that are difficult to identify on plain radiographs. Depression of fragments or deformity of the skull may be apparent on direct observation or demonstrated by palpation. Subgaleal collections of fluid might represent a significant portion of the body fluids in children and can even be evidence of continuing arterial hemorrhage in adults.

Periorbital ecchymosis, a discoloration of the skin about the eye limited by the rim of the orbit or a bluish discoloration behind the ear in a patient who has recently experienced a head injury will also be apparent. (See Fig. 3-1.) *Battle's sign* suggests a fracture at the base of the skull which might not be distinguishable in plain radiographs of the skull. Blood behind a tympanic membrane is another indication of fracture to the floor of the middle cranial fossa.

Alteration of the cranium's contour is produced by metabolic lesions such as fibrous dysplasia. The contour of the cranium may also be influenced by intracranial mass lesions. In children, this can result from chronically expanding astro-

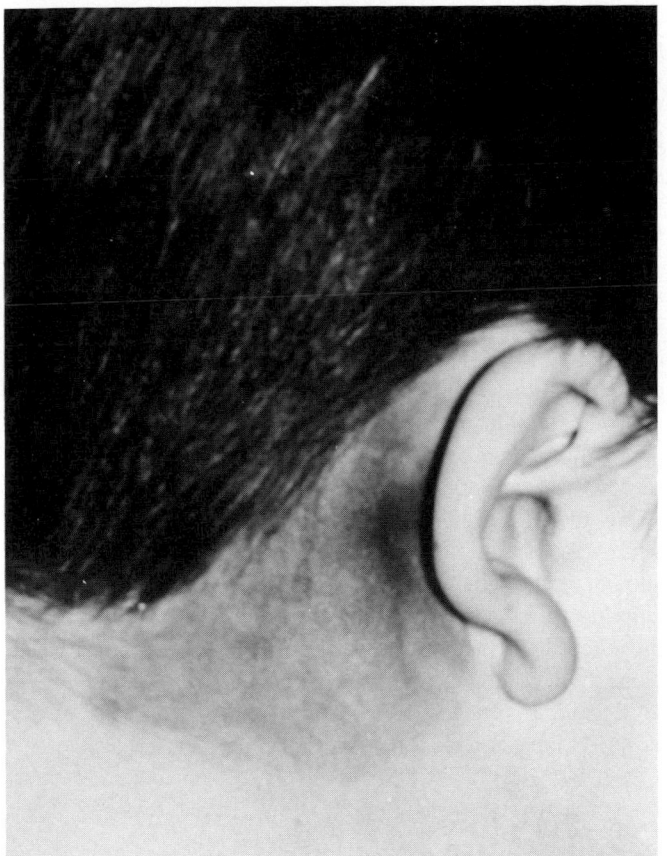

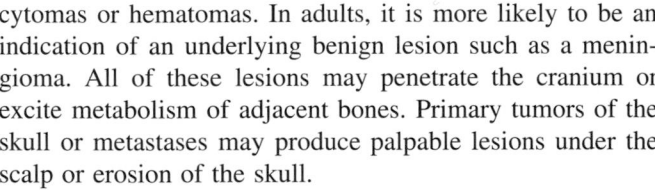

Figure 3–1 Battle's sign: Ecchymosis behind the ear indicative of a fracture at the base of the skull.

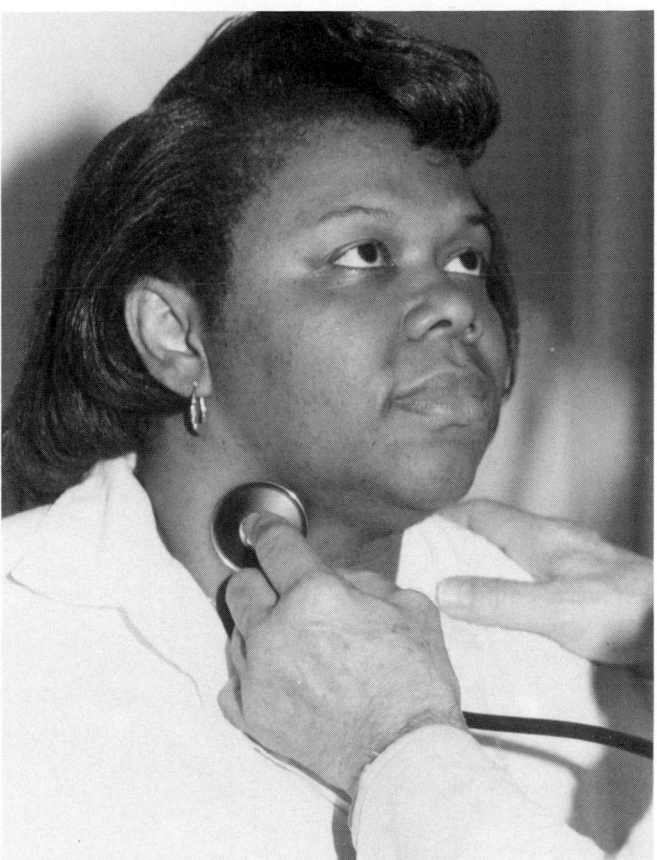

Figure 3–2 Auscultation of carotid artery in the neck.

cytomas or hematomas. In adults, it is more likely to be an indication of an underlying benign lesion such as a meningioma. All of these lesions may penetrate the cranium or excite metabolism of adjacent bones. Primary tumors of the skull or metastases may produce palpable lesions under the scalp or erosion of the skull.

Inflammatory lesions of the sinuses can produce tenderness in adjacent areas of the cranium. Extension of inflammatory processes into the subgaleal area will also at times elicit edema or fluctuation of the scalp.

Auscultation of the cranium in adults is important. Bruits are frequently associated with arteriovenous malformations. They are also associated with fistulae between arterial and venous structures. Arteriovenous fistulae may result from injury or be spontaneous. A pulsating exophthalmus is usually associated with a carotid-cavernous fistula, as is injection of the conjunctival vessels.

NECK

Examination of the neck in patients who have recently undergone severe trauma must be accomplished with caution. If consciousness is impaired, observation and palpation for deformities may provide clues to injuries. Radiographs provide more specific information. Stabilization is important

until fractures or dislocations can be ruled out. In an alert patient, pain at rest and limitation of range of motion suggest structural injury. Rigidity of the neck in the absence of trauma may indicate meningitis or subarachnoid hemorrhage. Venous distension when the head is elevated implies cardiac decompensation but may result from compression or occlusion of the superior vena cava. Auscultation is therefore very important, especially in patients with evidence of vascular disease. (See Fig. 3-2.)

BACK

The thoracic and lumbar segments of the back are examined for alignment, deformities, and limitation of motion, as well as overlying lesions of the skin and tenderness on percussion. (See Figs. 3-3A and B.) Intraspinal lesions frequently produce localized tenderness. (See Fig. 3-3C.) Pressure over nerve roots displaced or compromised by herniated discs or neoplasms may produce pain. Generalized paraspinal tenderness may represent evidence of arthritis or myositis, but rarely is associated with intraspinal pathology of surgical significance.

Examination of the back of newborn infants is especially important. Its significance is increased in children and adults

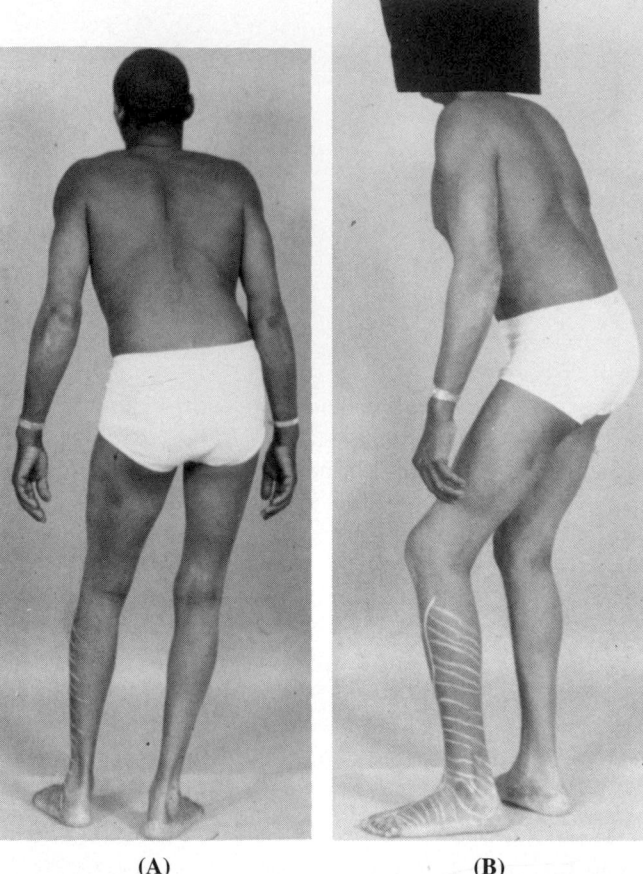

(A)   (B)

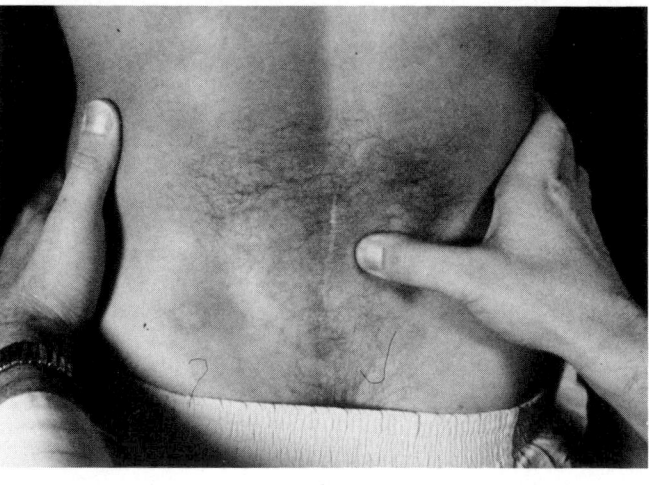

(C)

Figure 3–3 Examination of the back in patients with pain in the lumbosacral area. An acute scoliosis resulting from spasm of the paravertebral muscles in a patient with herniated intervertebral disc at the lumbosacral junction is apparent in *(A)* and *(B)*. *Note the area of hypalgesia outlined.* The paravertebral area is being palpated in a patient who had had previous surgery in *(C)*.

who have evidence of weakness, asymmetrical development of the lower extremities, or meningitis.

Dysraphic lesions such as dermal sinuses can often be visualized, as can lipomas, meningoceles, or myelomeningoceles. Each of these lesions might be associated with a tethered cord or a Chiari malformation. Other evidence of dysraphic lesions include dimples, nevi, or localized hair growth. These may be cutaneous evidence of spinal bifida, diastematomyelia, or other dysraphic processes. A dermal sinus can be the tract by which the subarachnoid space becomes contaminated.

PERIPHERAL NERVES

Evaluation of the course of peripheral nerves is important in the examination of patients with localized neurological deficits. A scar may indicate the site of an injury. Masses or tenderness along the course of the nerves may indicate sites of neoplasms, compression, or injury. Percussion along the course of a nerve which has undergone injury or repair may produce paresthesias in the distribution of the nerve (Tinel's sign). The distal point from which such a sign is elicited indicates the ends of nerve fibers, often the site of either regrowth or injury of axons. Similarly, palpation of a tender nodule under a scar can indicate the presence of a traumatic neuroma. Diffuse enlargement along the course of peripheral nerves can be a sign of hypertrophic neuropathy, neurofibromatosis or, very rarely, in the United States, leprosy.

Neurological Examination

The neurological examination is an important part of any physical examination but is most important when surgical treatment of the nervous system is being contemplated or has been performed, since it identifies specific deficits which may not be apparent to the patient but which can be important. The examination is basic to discrete diagnosis. Serial observations after treatment indicate the success of therapy or recurrence of the lesion.

☐ STATE OF CONSCIOUSNESS

A record of the patient's state of consciousness is important, especially in those with head injury or seizures, or patients with evidence of intracranial mass lesions, as well as patients who are deteriorating intellectually.

The record should indicate what the patient can and cannot do rather than make blanket statements such as "semiconscious" or "semicomatose." Even the label "comatose" has different meanings which vary with circumstances.

The record should indicate that the patient answers appropriately or does not. A patient who does not respond to verbal questions or comments may respond by flexion or extension of his extremities to painful stimulation. A patient who is less impaired may respond appropriately or be "confused."

There should be indication as to whether the patient is oriented to time, place, and person. Adult neurologic patients normally should be aware of the day of the week and most will be aware of the month and year. They should be able to identify close relatives as well. They should be able to identify their city, state, county, and country. Other aspects of the mental examination may be the ability to identify objects, to recall recent and remote events or numbers, and to perform calculations. Interpretations of proverbs becomes important in evaluation of higher functions, which will be discussed further with respect to neuropsychological evaluation.

A detailed analysis of patients with impaired states of consciousness has been published by Plum and Posner.[1] Evaluation of patients who do not respond to verbal stimuli should include a determination of whether impairment of consciousness is malingering or hysterical. The hand may be held over the face and allowed to drop. If it hits the face, the altered consciousness is most likely physiological, whereas if the hand falls away from the face, this is evidence of protection and the stupor may be nonphysiological.

In patients with physiologically impaired consciousness, there should be determination of whether bodily responses are symmetrical or asymmetrical. Except in acute trauma, symmetrical responses are suggestive of metabolic lesions, whereas asymmetrical responses suggest a structural cause for the altered state of consciousness.

Determination of pupillary size and response gives a good indication of the basis and degree of impaired consciousness. Bilaterally constricted pupils (pinpoint) indicate the presence of a drug (alkaloid) effect or a structural lesion in the region of the pons. Widely dilated pupils may be produced by drugs (atropine or similar drugs or barbiturate intoxication), anoxia, or a severe structural deficit involving the brainstem.

A unilaterally dilated pupil in a comatose patient strongly suggests an intracranial lesion and frequently represents a surgical emergency. Absence of a blink reflex to corneal stimulation in a stuporous patient suggests injury to the brainstem, although the blink reflex may be absent in the presence of intoxication with drugs, particularly barbiturates.

Eyes tend to deviate toward the side of a destructive lesion of the frontal lobe so that a gaze palsy suggests a structural lesion. Absence of "doll's eye" movements occurs in alert patients and in deeply comatose patients. (See description of determining the presence of such movements under the examination of the third, fourth, and sixth cranial nerves.) "Doll's eye" movements are usually present in patients who are drowsy, and absence suggests injury to the brainstem. The examiner should rule out a broken neck before performing this test.

The patient's response to painful stimuli (sternal pressure or pressure upon a fingernail or toenail) will determine the symmetry of response and determine whether the response is flexor (withdrawal) or extensor (decerebrate).

Cumulatively, these signs give an indication of the depth of stupor and provide a scale by which serial examinations will determine the progress of the patient.

Evaluation of Cranial Nerves

☐ I: OLFACTORY

Patients should be able to identify commonly used condiments, soap, tobacco, and coffee. Testing can be ideally accomplished by asking patients to identify odors of solutions contained in test tubes. (See Fig. 3-4.) Astringents—i.e., ammonia, ether, and formaldehyde—are not good substances to test olfaction. Even though they may have distinct odors, they are irritating to the nasal mucosa and are perceived through the trigeminal nerve. Tests of olfaction are performed through one nostril at a time. Loss of olfaction usually occurs on the side of an intracranial lesion interrupting the pathways. Loss of olfaction can result from intranasal lesions such as rhinitis or masses causing obstruction, as well as interruption of the olfactory pathways. Loss of smell may be misinterpreted as loss of taste by the patient.

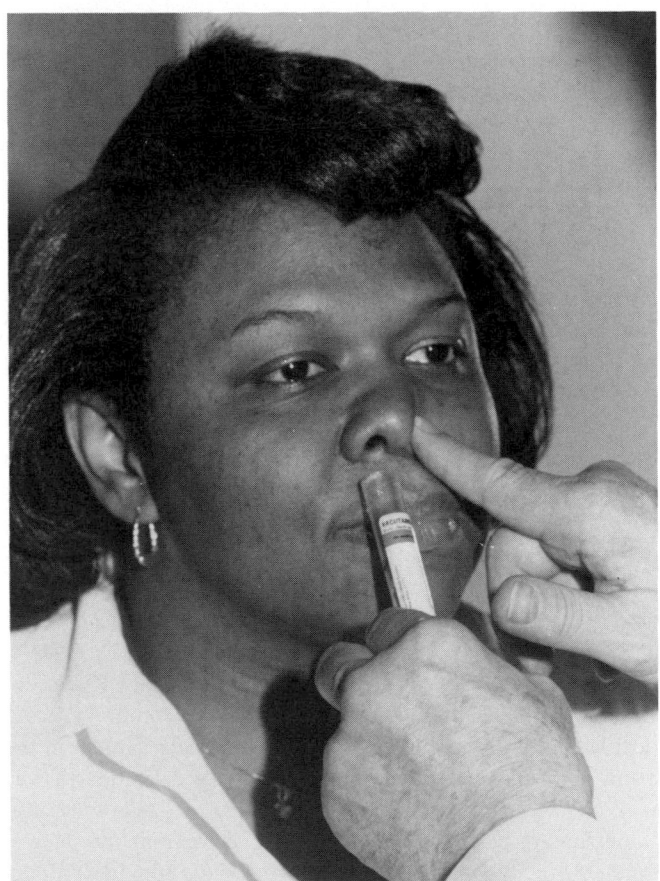

Figure 3–4 Testing olfaction. Perfumes, coffee, gum, or tobacco provide commonly identifiable odors. Astringents should be avoided.

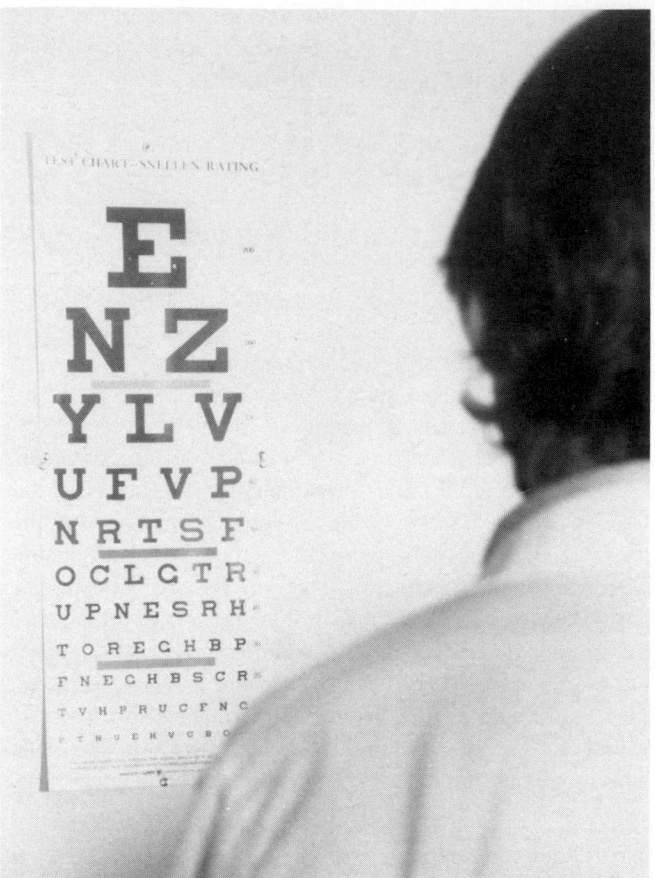

Figure 3–5 Testing visual acuity using a Snellen's chart. Acuity is most commonly altered by impairments within the eye. Visual fields are more common indications of neurological deficits.

☐ II: OPTIC

Visual acuity is tested by asking the patient to identify letters, numbers, or figures on a chart. (See Fig. 3-5.) Vision can be impaired by lesions of the cornea, lens, vitreous, retina, optic nerves, optic chiasm, and the intracranial visual pathways to the occipital cortex.

Generally, acuity is impaired by lesions or malfunction of the structures in the globe while lesions of the optic nerves and intracranial pathways are more likely to produce defects in the visual fields. Failure of accommodation or focus produces decrease in acuity which can be corrected. Increased intracranial pressure can produce papilledema, which, like optic neuritis, produces a decrease in visual acuity.

Usually, swelling of the optic disc produced by papilledema initially causes enlargement of the blind spot and decrease in the peripheral field of vision. Enlargement of the blind spot may be found in patients with optic neuritis, as well as degenerative lesions of the retina or glaucoma.[2]

Lesions that compress one optic nerve may produce a unilateral field defect which can progress to blindness in the ipsilateral eye. Pressure on an optic nerve near the optic chiasm may produce impaired acuity in the ipsilateral eye and a lateral field defect in the contralateral eye due to involvement of crossing fibers which loop into the affected optic nerve, Wilbrand's knee.[3] Lesions involving the chiasm may typically produce temporal field cuts, which usually begin in the upper outer quadrants, then progress inferiorly, later medially, and finally involve the entire field. Field defects may result from direct pressure on the optic pathways or occlusion of nutrient vessels. The field cuts may be asymmetrical. Lesions of the retrochiasmal optic pathways typically produce homonomous field defects which become more similar in the two eyes as the lesions are located more posteriorly.[2,4]

Large field defects can usually be demonstrated on confrontation by having the patient identify the presence of the examiner's moving finger when it is located in the periphery about halfway between the examiner and patient. Each eye should be tested separately. (See Fig. 3-6.) A more sensitive test of field defects is obtained by simultaneously presenting colored objects in the peripheral fields.[5] Failure to identify an object in one field suggests a deficit. Definitive examination of the visual fields is accomplished with a tangent screen usually placed 1 to 2 meters from the patient, but this may be impractical at the bedside. Automated static perimeters are often useful to determine defects in visual fields.

FUNDUSCOPIC EXAMINATION

The *funduscopic examination* is part of the general physical examination, but because of its intimate association with neurological problems, it will be given special emphasis here. (See Fig. 3-7.) Funduscopic examination will reveal opacities of the lens, swelling of the optic discs, and retinal hemorrhage. (See Fig. 3-8*A* to *D*.)

Swelling of the optic discs results from increased intracranial pressure or from inflammatory lesions of the optic nerve, i.e., optic neuritis. Frequently, differentiation can be accomplished by demonstration of venous pulsations. Pseudopapilledema can be produced by drusen (hyaline bodies derived from degenerated retinal pigment cells). Pale optic discs suggest optic atrophy which can be produced by any lesion that causes degeneration of fibers of the optic nerve.

Venous pulsations, when seen, indicate that the cerebrospinal fluid (CSF) pressure is less than the venous pressure and probably normal. Microaneurysms of the retinal arteries usually indicate *diabetes mellitus,* which may be of help in differentiation of at least one cause for coma. Arterial narrowing or occlusion and evidence of occlusion of an ophthalmic artery can be identified.

☐ III, IV, VI: OCULOMOTOR, TROCHLEAR, ABDUCENS

Determination of the function of the extraocular muscles is of vital concern in comatose patients. In the alert, coopera-

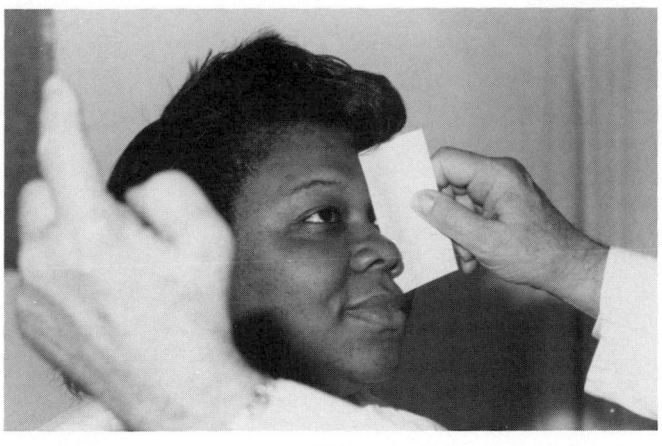

(A)

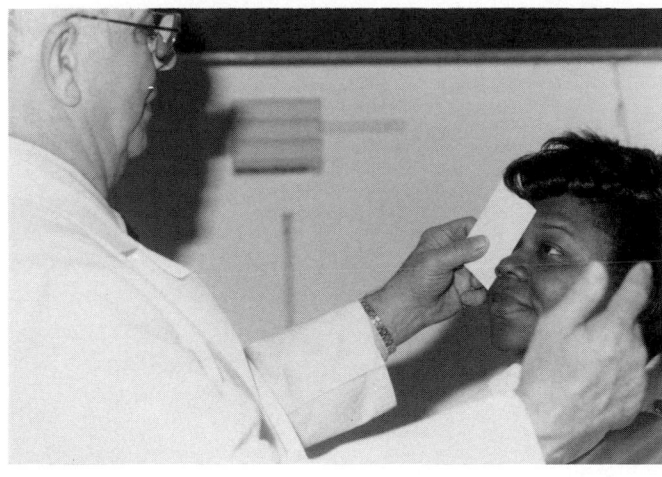

(B)

Figure 3–6 A and B Testing visual fields by confrontation, one eye at a time.

tive patient, discrete testing of the extraocular muscles is accomplished by asking the patient to follow finger movements upwards, downwards, and to either side while observing for *nystagmus* and the extent of eye movements. (See Fig. 3-9*A* to *C*.) Oblique movements should be tested as well. The patient should be questioned regarding diplopia during these maneuvers, since limitations which may be significant to the patient may not be apparent on gross examination. Viewing a light through a red glass over one eye may aid in this evaluation.

Examination of ocular movements in a patient whose consciousness is impaired may be more complex. Rotation of the head in such a patient may be used to evaluate the status of the brain stem by determining the *"doll's eye" (oculogyric) reflex.* (See Fig. 3-10.) In the normal response, eyes remain fixed—or at least relatively so—on an object when the head is turned. Consequently, they rotate away from the direction in which the head is being turned. In the abnormal response, the eyes remain fixed in the orbit and consequently move in the same direction and at the same speed as the head is turned. This response is evidence of

severe dysfunction within the brain stem in the region of the pons. The response should be described rather than called "positive" or "negative." *A loss of response only on one side indicates paralysis of ipsilateral oculomotor nerves.*

Rotation of the head should *not* be carried out to determine the presence of "doll's eyes" in a stuporous patient before ruling out concurrent neck injury. An alternative mechanism for making the same determination is the instillation of ice water against the eardrum, which normally produces nystagmus to the opposite side, after determining that the eardrum is intact.

A unilaterally dilated pupil that does not react to light indicates that the parasympathetic portion of the third nerve is not functioning. When accompanied by the acute onset of pain behind the eye, it is characteristic of pressure on a segment of the third nerve which may be produced by an aneurysm in the region of the posterior communicating artery. When seen in patients with a depressed state of consciousness, uncal herniation is implied.

A newly dilated pupil in a comatose patient with a suspected intracranial lesion constitutes a surgical emergency. Impairment of extraocular muscle action referable to the third nerve, accompanying pupillary dilation, is seen in compression of the third nerve by an aneurysm in the region of the posterior communicating artery or by herniation of the uncus through the incisura. Paralysis of muscles of the third nerve unassociated with a dilated pupil suggests intraorbital disease.

In contrast to lesions affecting the third nerve, palsies of the sixth nerve are less reliable in localizing an intracranial lesion. Sixth nerve palsies occur in association with increased intracranial pressure without shifts in the brain stem and without direct anatomical contact of the sixth nerve with known pathological lesions. Oculomotor palsies not restricted to a single nerve may be produced by lesions of the orbit, myasthenia gravis, or by myopathies which may be difficult to differentiate.

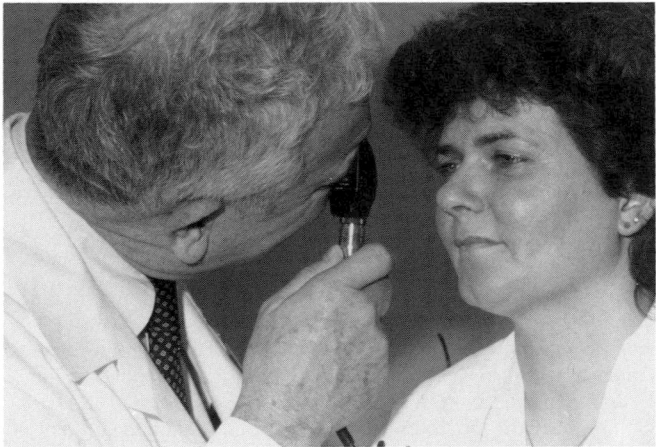

Figure 3–7 Funduscopic examination to view the lens, vitreous, and retina.

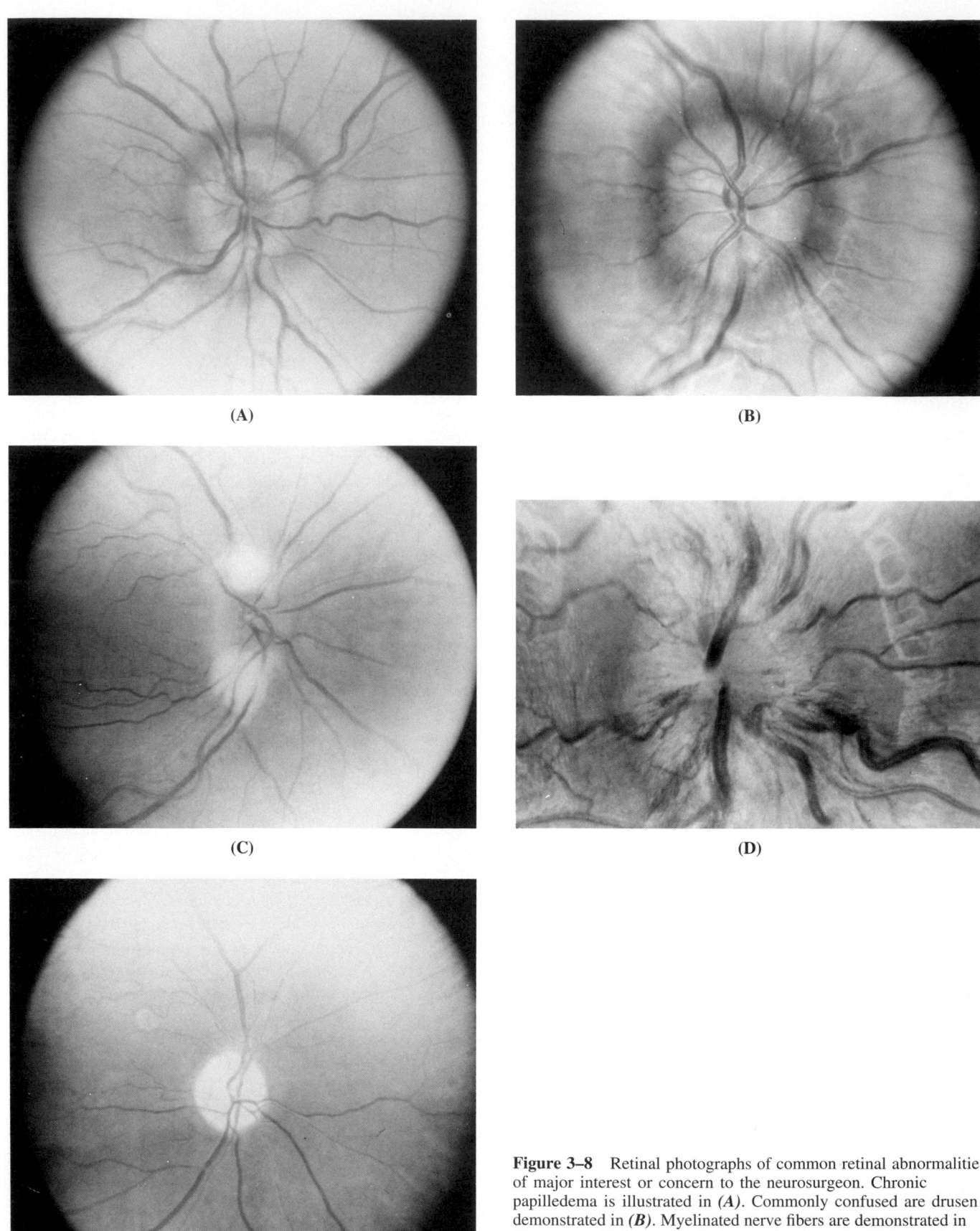

(A)

(B)

(C)

(D)

(E)

Figure 3–8 Retinal photographs of common retinal abnormalities of major interest or concern to the neurosurgeon. Chronic papilledema is illustrated in **(A)**. Commonly confused are drusen demonstrated in **(B)**. Myelinated nerve fibers are demonstrated in **(C)** and papillitis in **(D)**. Optic atrophy is demonstrated in **(E)**. (Compliments of Dr. John Kendall, Director of the Department of Ophthalmology, Allegheny General Hospital, Pittsburgh, Pennsylvania.)

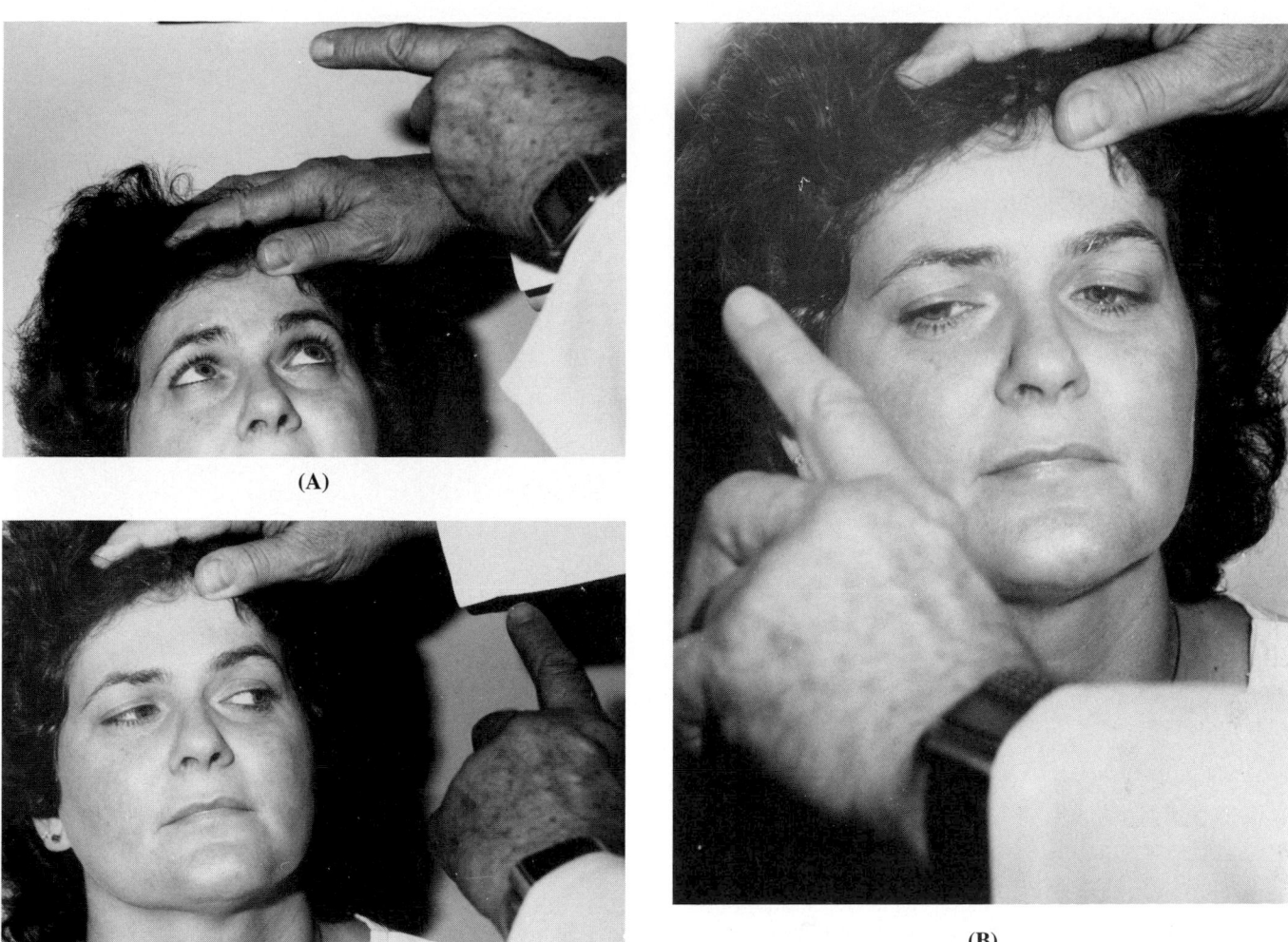

Figure 3–9 Cardinal eye movements to either side and to the left upper oblique position, obtained by asking the patient to follow the examiner's finger, are illustrated *(A–C)*. Not illustrated are verticle and other oblique movements.

☐ V: TRIGEMINAL

Both motor and sensory components of the trigeminal nerve should be tested. The *divisions of the trigeminal nerve* are the *ophthalmic, maxillary,* and *mandibular* (first, second, and third respectively). (See Fig. 3-11.) Sensation in the various divisions of the trigeminal nerve is checked by testing them individually with a pin or by light touch. Absence of the corneal reflex is a sensitive indicator of impairment of function in the first division of the trigeminal nerve in a patient with an intact seventh nerve. This is accomplished by wiping a wisp of cotton across the cornea. One should take care that the movement of the hand and cotton is not seen by the patient. In a comatose patient, the corneal reflex is used to determine the status of the brain stem in the region of the pons.

Motor fibers of the trigeminal nerve accompany the proximal portion of the mandibular division and innervate the muscles of mastication. Function may be tested by simply asking the alert patient to open his or her mouth or protrude the jaw. The jaw will deviate to the paralyzed side. Alterna-

tively, the temporalis or buccinator muscle may be palpated while the patient is gritting his teeth.

☐ VII: FACIAL

The nucleus of the facial nerve receives bilateral input from the cortex in the portion that sends fibers to the upper part of the face. Thus, a seventh nerve palsy produced by a supranuclear lesion is likely to leave function of the frontalis and corrugator muscles intact, whereas these muscles will not function when there is a lesion of the nucleus or infranuclear portion of the seventh cranial nerve. (See. Fig. 3-12*A* and *B*.)

With supranuclear lesions there may be varying degrees of involvement of the orbicularis oculi with most marked impairment of function involving the muscles about the corner of the mouth. Supranuclear lesions cause weakness of lower facial muscles on the side opposite to the lesion, whereas lesions of the facial nerve involve all facial muscles and are

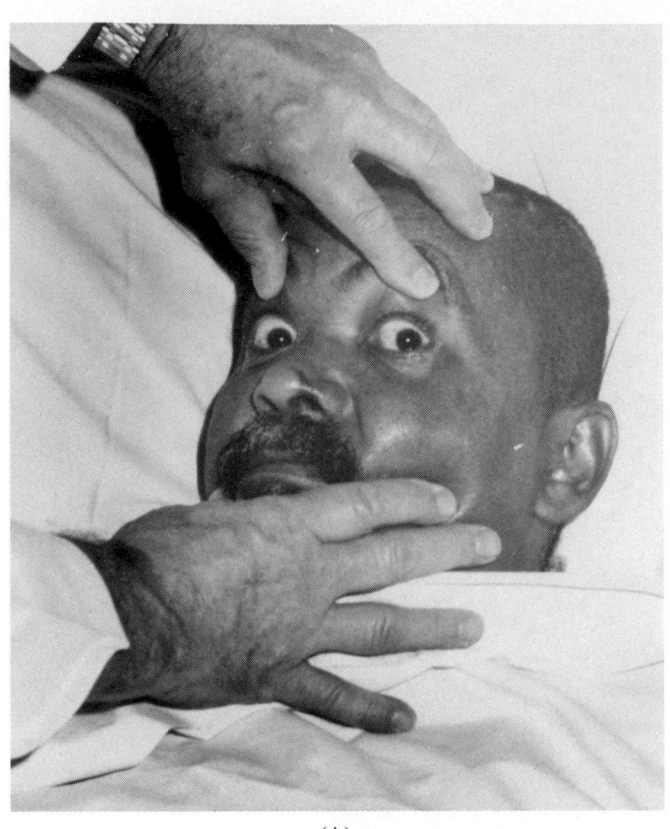
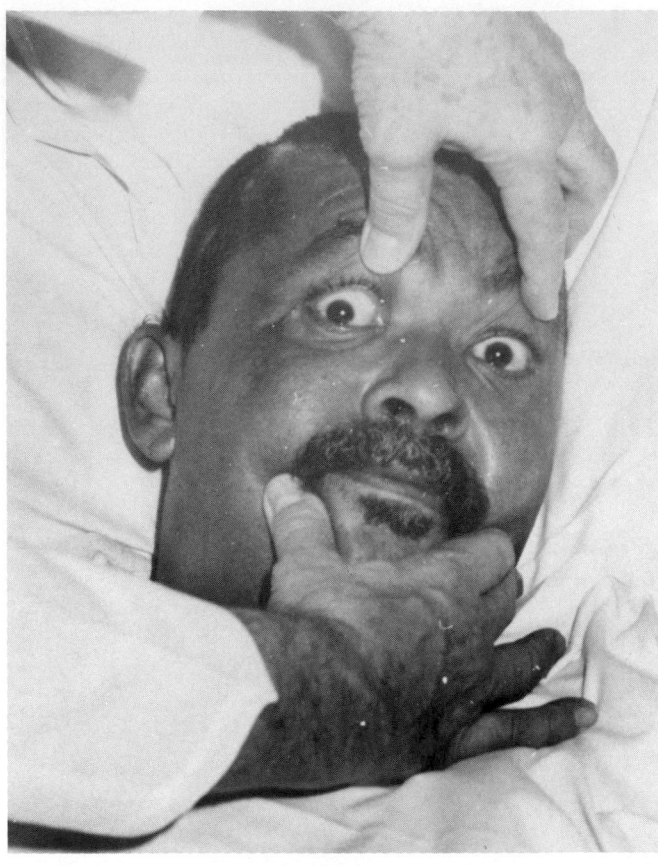

(A)   (B)

Figure 3–10   Rotation of the head to the right to illustrate "doll's eye" movements to the left, present in a stuporous patient with an intact brainstem and motor function of the eyes, illustrated in *A*. Head movement to the left is illustrated in *B*. Eye movements may be stopped by anesthesia or injury to the brainstem. Eye movements are purely volitional in an alert patient.

ipsilateral to the paresis. Minimal involvement of seventh nerve function is best recognized by observing spontaneous movements.

Fibers innervate taste buds on the anterior two-thirds of

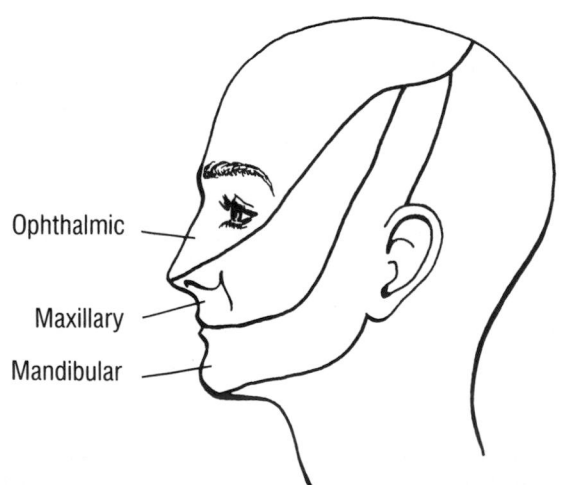

Figure 3–11   Distribution of sensation of respective divisions of trigeminal nerve.

the tongue, some fibers transmitting pain sensation from a portion of the external ear canal; motor fibers to the lacrimal gland exit from the brain stem in the nervus intermedius and travel with the facial nerve initially, before branching off in the middle ear. Loss of function of the appropriate modalities may be associated with lesions of the proximal portion of seventh nerve.

Taste is best tested on each side of the tongue separately. (See Fig. 3-13.) Solutions of salt, sugar, or bitter or sour substances (i.e., vinegar) are best used. They may be applied to the tongue by a carefully placed cotton swab. The tongue should be protruded during testing. Replacement of the tongue into the mouth causes the solutions being tested to diffuse throughout the mouth so that they may be recognized by taste buds other than those being tested.

□ VIII: ACOUSTIC

Both the auditory and vestibular divisions of the acoustic nerve can be examined. Gross testing of auditory function is initially evaluated by having the patient identify soft sounds such as a ticking watch or fingers rubbing. A more discrete determination can be made by having the patient identify a

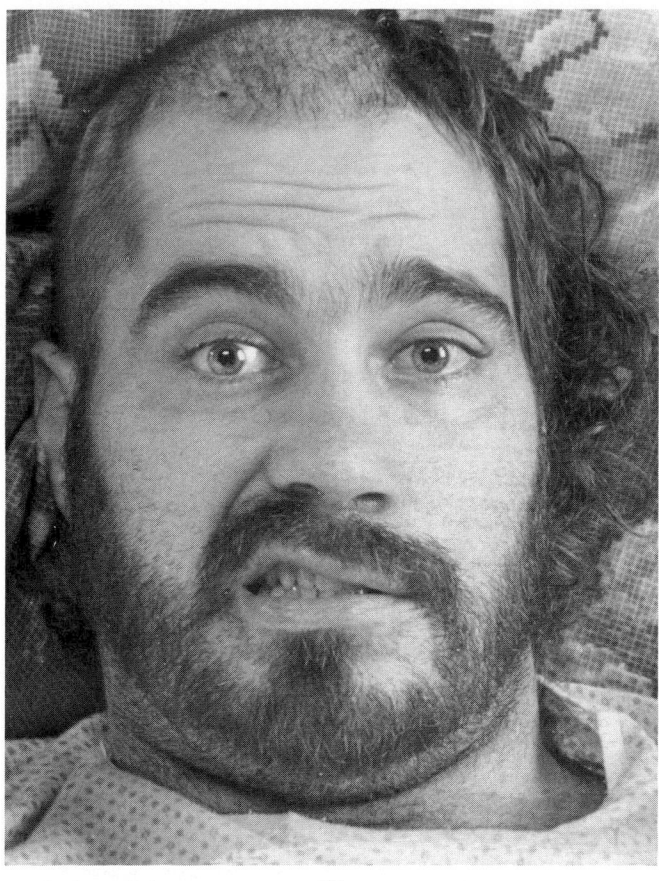

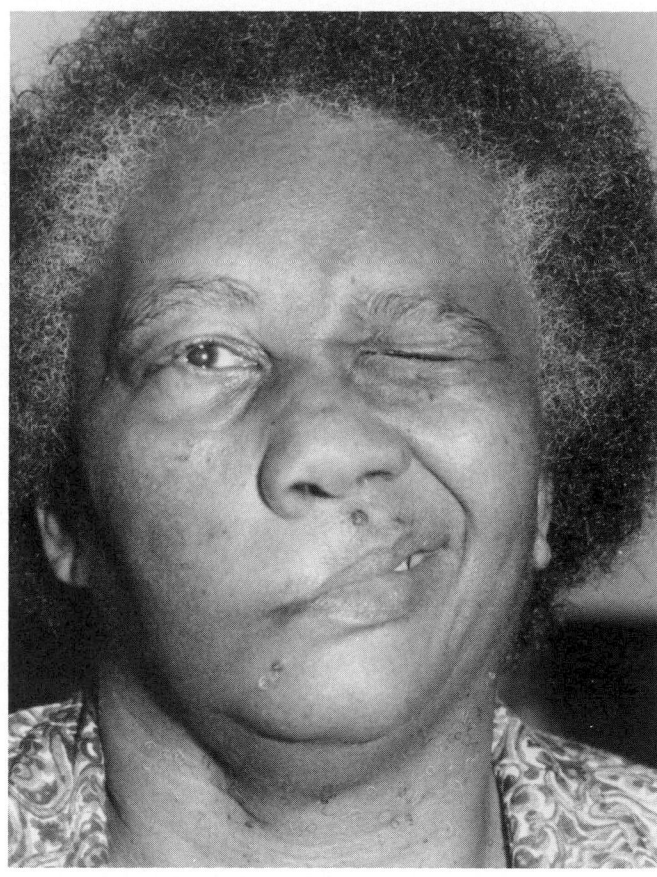

(A)   (B)

Figure 3–12   Facial palsies produced by central *A* and peripheral *B* lesions. *Note the wrinkling of the forehead of the frontalis muscle in* **A**. Although there is no wrinkling of the forehead on either side, paralysis of the entire right side of the face is apparent in **B**.

tuning fork vibration at 128 Hz, which can be used to determine both air and bone conduction.

Impairment of air conduction indicates middle ear disease, while impairment of bone conduction is caused by loss of

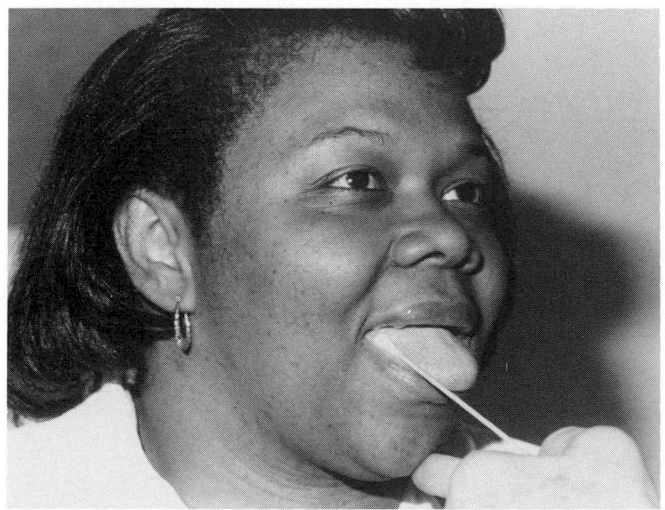

Figure 3–13   Testing taste. A swab soaked with a liquid solution of salt or sugar should be applied to the edge of the extended tongue. Taste may be identified by alternate routes when the tongue is held in the mouth.

cochlear or eighth nerve function. In the Weber test, an active tuning fork is placed on the center of the forehead or vertex. (See Fig. 3-14.) A louder sound may be heard on the side of a conductive loss, but the sound is heard less well on the side of a neurosensory loss. The Rinne test is used to help determine the defective site. The base of the vibrating tuning fork is placed on the mastoid process. When sounds are identified (bone conduction), the vibrating fork is moved to a point near the external ear (air conduction). (See Fig. 3-15.)

Air conduction is normally greater than bone conduction. Bone conduction will be equal to or greater than air conduction on the side of a conductive loss, that is on the side of involvement of the middle ear. Both air and bone conduction are decreased on the side of a lesion involving the cochlear or acoustic nerve. Air conduction will remain greater than bone conduction if the lesion is incomplete.

A more detailed evaluation of the auditory division of the eighth nerve can be obtained by an audiogram, refinements of which are used to determine the presence of small lesions involving the eighth nerve. Audiograms are important to determine the degree of functional loss. Since the advent of imaging, even small lesions of the auditory canal can be demonstrated by magnetic resonance imaging or computerized tomography before there is physiological evidence of neural loss.

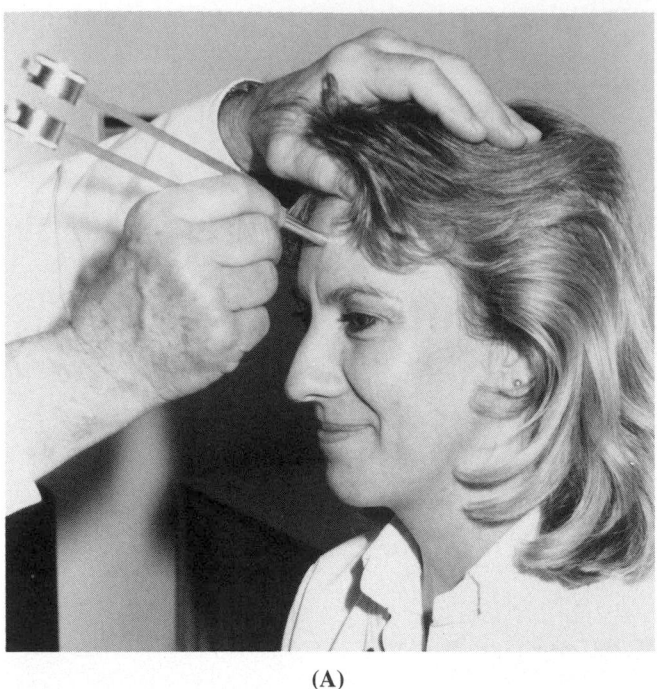

(A)

Figure 3–14 Weber's test: When the tuning fork is applied to the forehead on vertex, the sound is normally heard in both ears *(A)*. It is lateralized away from the side of loss of function of the cochlea or nerve but lateralized to the side of an occluded ear *(B)*.

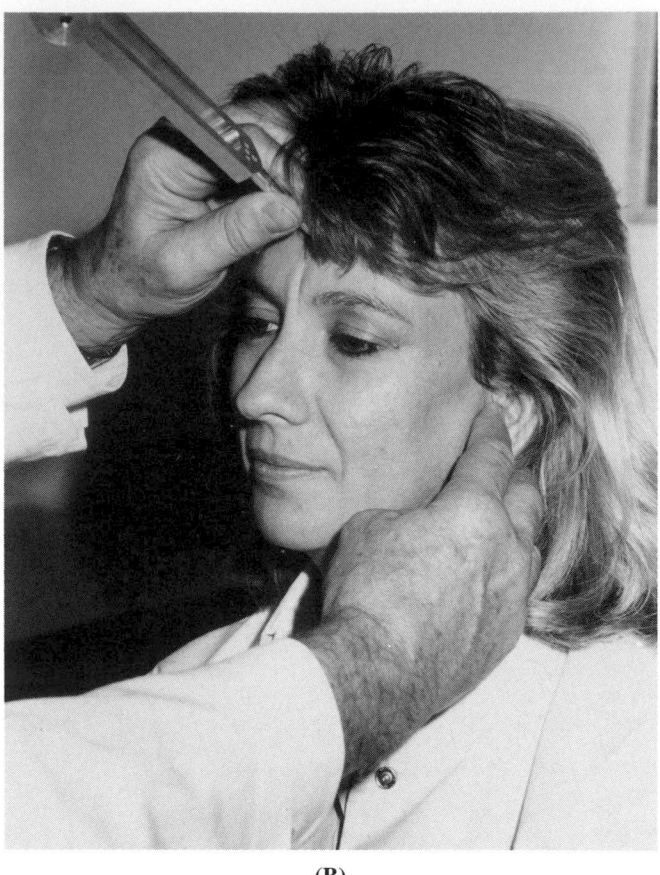

(B)

Alteration in vestibular function is suggested by the presence of an acquired nystagmus. Testing of vestibular function may be accomplished by determining the presence of "doll's eye" movements in a patient whose consciousness is impaired. (See examination of third, fourth, and sixth cranial nerves in preceding text.)

Vestibular function in an alert patient is determined by irrigating the external ear canal with 5 cm³ of ice water or warm water (44°C). The patient should be lying supine with the neck flexed 30 degrees. (See Fig. 3-16.) The intensity and length of nystagmus are observed.

Normally, the warm solution causes nystagmus with the fast component toward the side being irrigated, while cold perfusion causes the fast component to be away from the side of irrigation. The tympanic membrane should be examined before the test to determine that it is intact. In the event of a perforation, air at 2°C and 44°C may be used.

Nystagmography is a sensitive indicator of lesions involving the vestibular nerve.

☐ IX, X: GLOSSOPHARYNGEAL AND VAGUS

These two nerves are closely related, both in their function and in their sites of exit from the brain stem and cranium. Normal function of nerves IX and X is indicated by a normal gag reflex, a normally functioning soft palate (i.e., a symmetrically moving uvula), and normally functioning vocal chords, usually indicated by lack of hoarseness. The presence of hoarseness indicates the need to view the vocal cords, which requires at least indirect laryngoscopy to determine laterality of malfunction.

Although the vagus nerve includes motor and sensory fibers that are important for visceral functions, there are no good indicators to determine how they are functioning.

☐ XI: SPINAL ACCESSORY

Determination of the size and strength of the sternocleidomastoid and trapezius muscles evaluates functioning of the spinal accessory nerve. The right sternocleidomastoid muscle is tested by palpating its contraction when the patient tries to rotate the head horizontally to the left against resistance. (See Fig. 3-17A.) Elevation of a shoulder against resistance tests strength of the ipsilateral trapezius muscle and integrity of its nerve supply. (See Fig. 3-17B.)

☐ XII: HYPOGLOSSAL

Paralysis of the hypoglossal nerve is suggested when there is atrophy of the mass of the tongue or deviation of the

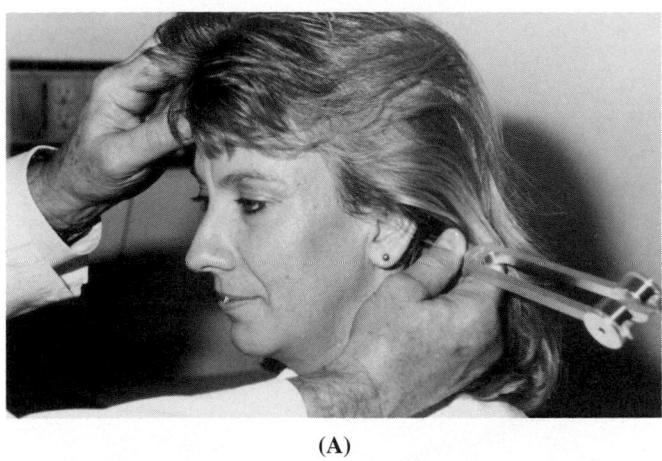

(A)

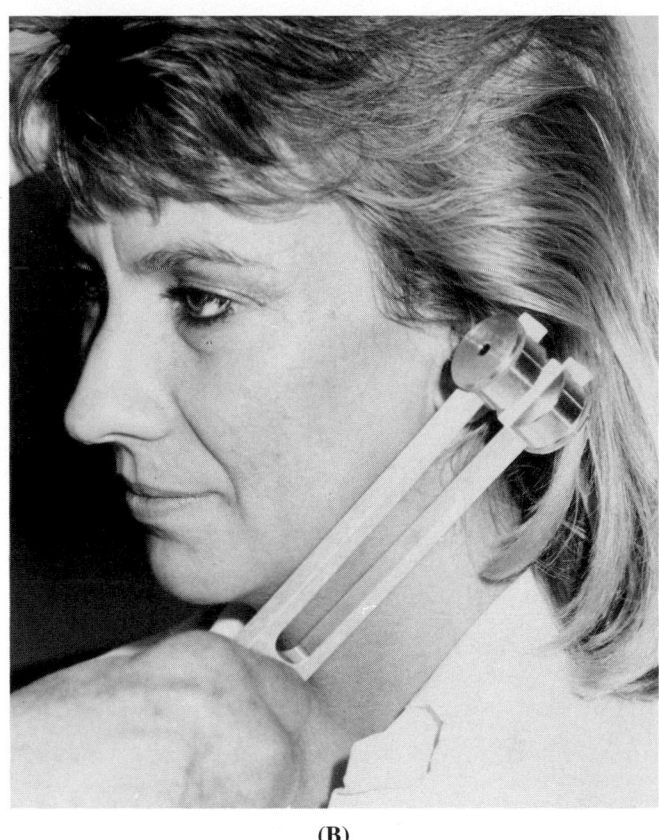

(B)

Figure 3–15   Rinne test: The sound of the tuning fork is identified when its base is applied to the mastoid process *(A)*, but it is normally perceived as much louder when the vibrating fork is placed near the ear *(B)*.

protruded tongue to the ipsilateral side. Deviation without atrophy may be seen in upper motor neuron lesions.

Fasciculations of the tongue are indicative of lesions involving the hypoglossal nerve or nucleus. Generalized diseases of the nervous system such as amyotrophic lateral sclerosis (ALS) may be implicated.

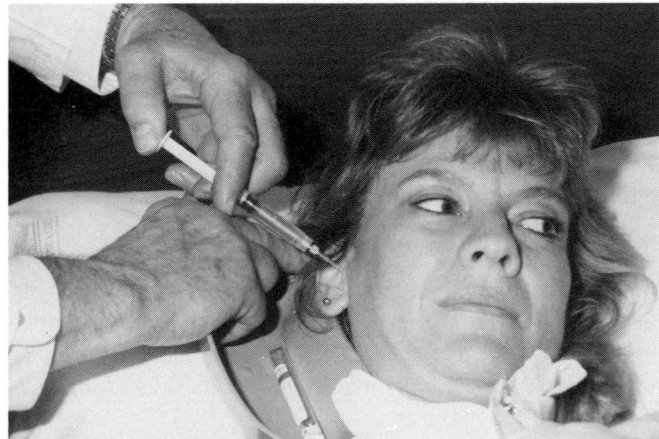

Figure 3–16   Irrigating ear canal. The head should be flexed 30°. Cold solutions normally cause the eyes to deviate toward the side of the irrigation. Irrigating with warm solution normally causes deviation of the eyes away from the side of the irrigation.

Examination of the Torso and Extremities

☐ UPPER EXTREMITIES

The type and extent of neurological examination of the extremities will depend to a large extent on the state of consciousness of the patient and location of the lesions being investigated. While it is possible and even necessary to evaluate gross movements of extremities in stuporous patients, it is necessary to have an alert, cooperative patient to evaluate individual muscles or muscle groups.

To evaluate gross movements in the extremities in a patient who is uncooperative, noncommunicative, or stuporous, simple observation will often be illuminating. Uncooperative patients will usually move about spontaneously, and paresis may be indicated by the failure to move an extremity or pair of extremities.

In the case of a mild hemiparesis, the arm and leg on one side of the body may be moved much more frequently than those of the opposite side, usually indicating an intracranial lesion contralateral to the less mobile extremities. Similarly, a patient with a lesion of the spinal cord may move his or her upper extremities much more readily than the lower extremities, even in the absence of complete paralysis. More detailed observation may reveal spontaneous purposeful movements in one pair of extremities and extensor or decerebrate movements on the opposite side.

Observation of spontaneous motor activities may be

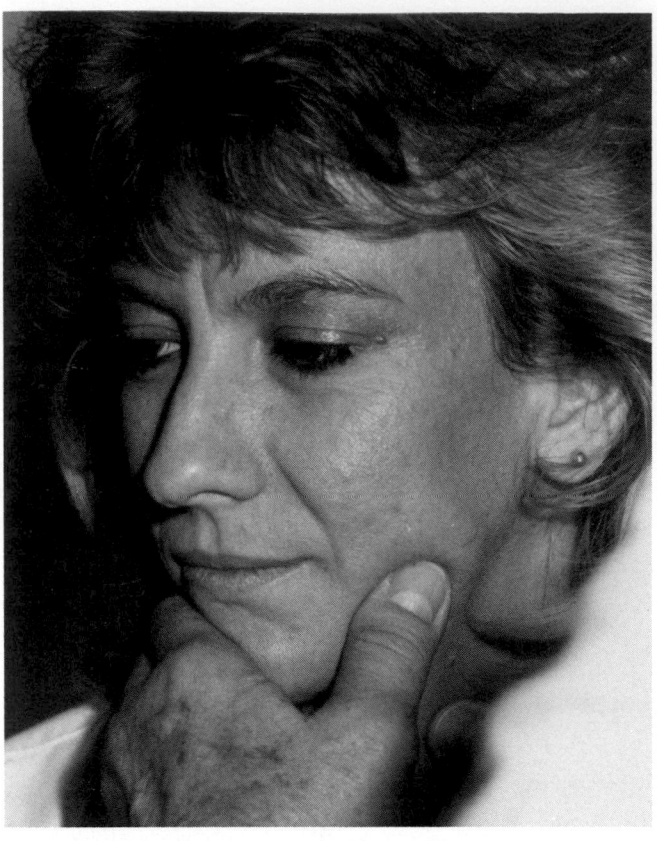

(A)

Figure 3–17 Testing function of the spinal accessory nerve. The left sternocleidomastoid is tested when the examiner pushes the head to the right *(A)*. Note the examiner's left thumb on the muscle below the chin. The latissimus dorsi is tested by pushing down on the "shrugged shoulder" *(B)*. The hand should be free so as not to resist movement of the shoulder.

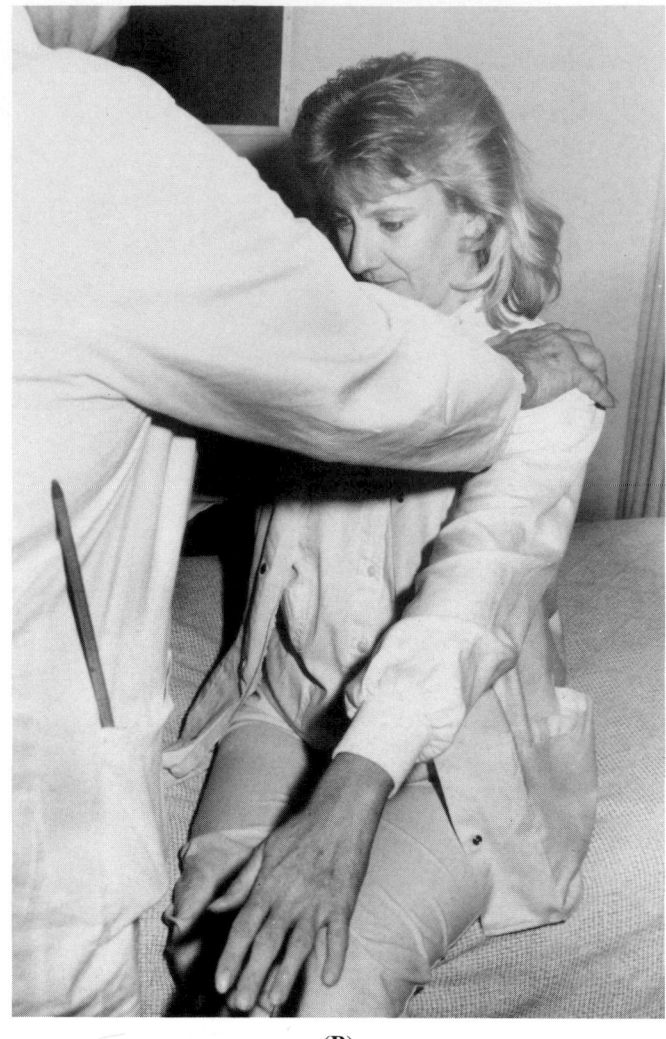

(B)

important in patients who are alert. Tremors or muscle twitching at rest are common features of certain movement disorders. Specifically, patients with Parkinson's disease may have a fine "pill-rolling" tremor of the affected hands and feet. Patients with chorea may demonstrate "squirming" movements and athetoids may have "writhing" movements, all while at rest.

Patients with hemiballismus often present with uncontrollable wildly flailing motions of an arm and leg which may cause considerable injury to their person. In addition, a much less dramatic but significant, prognostic indicator are fasciculations occurring at rest in patients undergoing degeneration of anterior horn cells. These muscular twitches or movements should be described.

In the cooperative patient, determination of subtle deficits in strength and proprioceptive sensation of upper extremities may be evaluated rapidly by asking the upright patient to extend arms and hands with palms turned upward. Weakness will be signaled by a drift downward on the affected side. Parietal lobe sensory loss may be indicated by an upward drift of the affected extremity, often with the hand rotating internally. Demonstration of weakness, in the alert patient

requires more detailed investigation to determine that the weakness is not limited to the muscles about the shoulder. The presence of pain may invalidate motor examinations.

In patients being evaluated for more peripheral lesions, discrete muscles, or muscle groups, must be evaluated. Thus, the shoulder must be evaluated for abduction, adduction, flexion and extension, and internal and external rotation. The elbow must be evaluated for flexion and extension, the forearm for internal and external rotation, and the wrist and individual digits for flexion and extension.

The thumb and fifth digit should be checked for abduction and adduction. Approximation of the thumb to the other fingers can be evaluated by asking the patient to resist the removal of a sheet of paper from the grasp. Hand grip is tested by asking the patient to squeeze the index and middle fingers of the examiner, usually on both sides simultaneously.

Evaluation of the patient's sensation of pain (pinprick) is not necessarily accomplished throughout the entire extremity when attempting to identify an intracranial lesion, but discrete testing must be accomplished for the evaluation of dermatomal lesions and for intraspinal lesions as may be

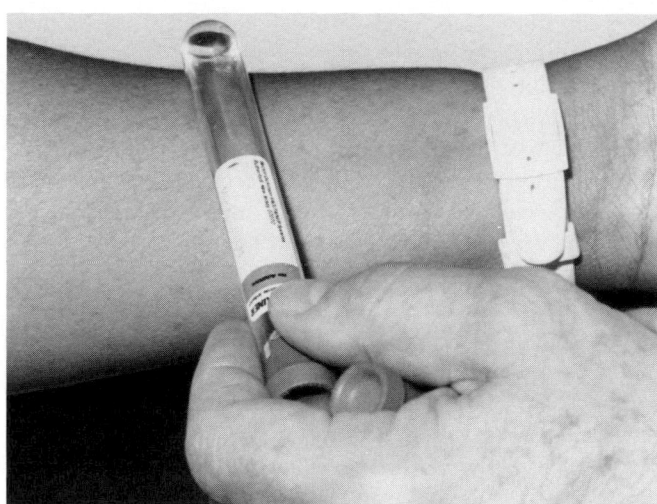

Figure 3–18 Testing sensations to temperature. Alternate test tubes filled with cold and warm water provide unmarked test objects that are easily identified.

seen with syringomyelia or injuries to the central portion of the spinal cord. Alteration in the ability to identify changes in temperature is more likely to occur in patients with intraspinal lesions than in patients with intracranial lesions. Testing is ideally accomplished by using alternate test tubes filled with warm and cold water. (See Fig. 3-18.)

Deep tendon reflexes tested in the upper extremities are the biceps, triceps, and radial periosteal. (See Fig. 3-19.) Asymmetry is most important as an indication of a neurological lesion since there may be marked variation in the response to examination in individual patients.

A Hoffman response is elicited by "clicking" the examiner's thumbnail off the end fingernail of the middle finger. (See Fig. 3-20.) An active response is indicated by flexion of the fingers. The reflex is not specific and is found in many normal individuals, but it implies decreased inhibition. In conjunction with hyperactive reflexes, it may indicate spasticity.

A "palmomental" reflex is elicited by tapping or scratching the thenar region of the hand from the base of the thumb

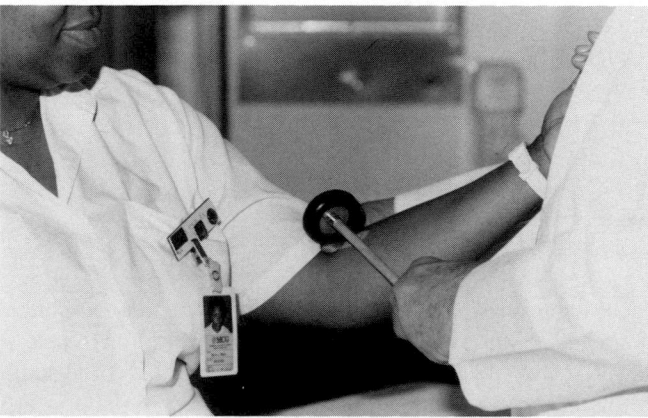

Figure 3–19 Examining the biceps reflex. The outstretched arm or hand should be resting on the examiner's arm.

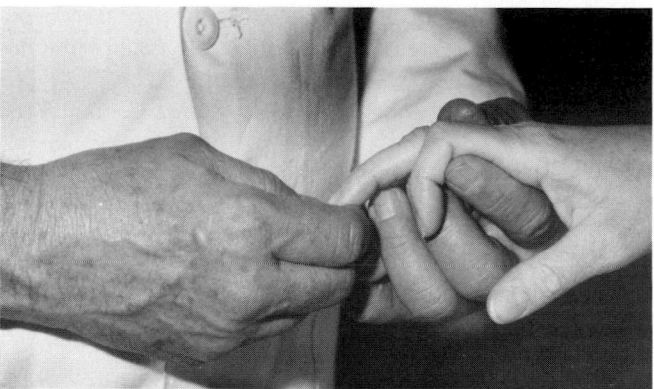

Figure 3–20 Hoffman's response obtained by "clicking" the nail of the middle finger.

to the wrist. A positive response is contraction of the muscles of the chin, slight retraction, and sometimes elevation of the angle of the mouth. The response is sometimes found in normal individuals but is more likely to be seen in disease of the pyramidal tracts or diffuse cortical disease.[6,7] This finding usually occurs in conjunction with a "snout" reflex in which there is a puckering of the lips in response to a gentle tap on the bridge of the nose. A similar response may be obtained by touching the upper and lower lips.

Evaluation of coordination is usually accomplished by simultaneously testing the upper and then lower extremities. Please note comments regarding this evaluation that will be made after the segment on examination of the lower extremities.

☐ EXAMINATION OF THE TORSO

Neurological examination of the torso usually includes determination of a sensory level in patients suspected of having injury to the spinal cord, usually accomplished with a pin. Sensory levels are determined by "walking" a pin up the body to determine where sensation is first perceived then continuing until the pinprick is perceived as "normal."

The anatomical distribution of the dermatomes should be remembered when carrying out this test. Investigation of levels of motor involvement when injury occurs between the mid and lower thoracic levels is confirmed by rectal examination to determine the strength of the sphincters and cremasteric responses as determined by stimulating the skin over the medial aspect of the upper thigh.

When the corticospinal fibers are interrupted between the eighth and tenth thoracic dermatomes, active elevation of the head of a supine patient will cause the innervated muscles of the upper but not the lower abdomen to contract, causing the umbilicus to move cephalad (Beevor's sign).[8] Such an investigation may be helpful in determining the spinal level of an injury.

Determination of rectal tone is of major importance in the case of spinal cord injury or paralysis. Paralysis of the lower extremities without loss of sphincter control suggests a peripheral lesion, whereas loss of sphincter control implies injury to the spinal cord itself.

Subtle sensory changes within the spinal cord may be documented by loss of cremasteric and/or abdominal reflexes on the side of sensory loss. Such losses may be apparent before objective sensory changes can be demonstrated.

EXAMINATION OF THE LOWER EXTREMITIES

Examination of the lower extremities mimics the examination of the upper extremities. Observation of the outstretched arms may be mimicked by turning the patient on his or her abdomen and asking the patient to hold the knees flexed.[9] Weakness of the hamstring muscles will be revealed by drifting of the feet toward the bed. Loss of proprioception may be indicated by overcompensation.

Discrete muscle testing must be accomplished by determining the strength of flexion or extension at the hips as well as abduction. The knees are examined for strength of extension and flexion, and the ankles are examined to determine the strength of dorsiflexion or plantar flexion. Since the gastrocnemius muscle is very strong, the strength of plantar flexion is usually tested by having the patients walk on the balls of their feet.

Pinprick is used to outline dermatomes if there is a suspicion of *sensory loss* in a radicular pattern or to outline loss in the pattern of a nerve. (See Fig. 3-21A and B.) *Vibratory sense* is determined with a tuning fork applied firmly over a metatarsal or malleolus. *Position sense* is tested by movement of the great toe or adjacent one up and down while asking the patient, who has his or her eyes closed, to report the way in which the toe has been moved.

Loss of posterior column function is usually more readily apparent in the lower extremities than in the upper limbs. The greater the distance between the spinal cord and the site being tested, the more likely it is that evidence of a peripheral demyelinating disease will be demonstrated by loss of sensory modalities in a stocking and glove distribution.

Sites of Destructive Lesions Affecting the Nervous System

LESIONS OF THE FRONTAL LOBES

The *frontal lobes* of the human brain primarily relate to higher levels of intellect and to motor functions. Because of close association with the olfactory nerves, chiasm, hypothalamus, and basal ganglia, lesions involving the frontal lobes are often associated with deficits which can be more specifically related to these structures.

Lesions of the prefrontal areas may be associated with behavioral changes, frequently with loss of inhibitions (which will be dealt with in Chap. 4 ("Neuropsychological Testing"). Lesions at the base of the frontal lobes may have (1) associated loss of smell due to injury to the olfactory tract, (2) loss of visual fields, and/or (3) loss of acuity due to injury to the chiasm.

The posterior extent of the frontal lobes is limited by the central sulcus. The precentral gyrus houses the primary motor cortex, destruction of which results in a contralateral hemiparesis. The premotor cortex houses supplementary motor functions which provide automatic movements and serves as a relay area for many learned skills.[10] Lesions in this area result in a grasp reflex.[11]

The frontal eye fields are located in the posterior middle frontal gyrus. Destruction of this area results in deviation of the eyes to the side of the lesion while localized seizures result in deviation of the eyes to the contralateral side.[10] Motor speech is located in Broca's area, portions of the inferior frontal gyrus bordering on the lateral fissure.

LESIONS OF THE TEMPORAL LOBES

The anatomical features of the temporal lobes include: laterally, the superior, middle, and inferior temporal gyri; and inferiorly, the hippocampal and fusiform gyri. While the anterior segments of the temporal lobe are clearly demarcated, the tempero-parietal and tempero-occipital divisions are ill-defined. The superior temporal gyrus houses the primary auditory cortex and, in the dominant hemisphere, an extension of sensory speech. Meyer's loop swings around the temporal horn of the lateral ventricle so that a lesion of the temporal lobe will produce a superior quadrantanopsia.[10]

The medial temporal lobe houses the hippocampus and amygdala, nuclei which play a major role in behavior and memory. Seizures from these structures are associated with dreamy states with altered associations with persons and places. Ablation of these nuclei in one hemisphere has limited effect on behavior, but excision of these structures bilaterally results in the Kluver-Bucy syndrome, including impaired memory, hypersexual behavior, and a hightened oral orientation toward the environment.[12]

LESIONS OF THE PARIETAL LOBES

Identifiable sensory modalities include the recognition of pain and temperature and vibratory and position sense. A lesion in one parietal lobe will result in loss of discrete localization of a stimulus, loss of position sense and in loss of the ability to differentiate minor degrees of temperature change in the opposite side of the body.

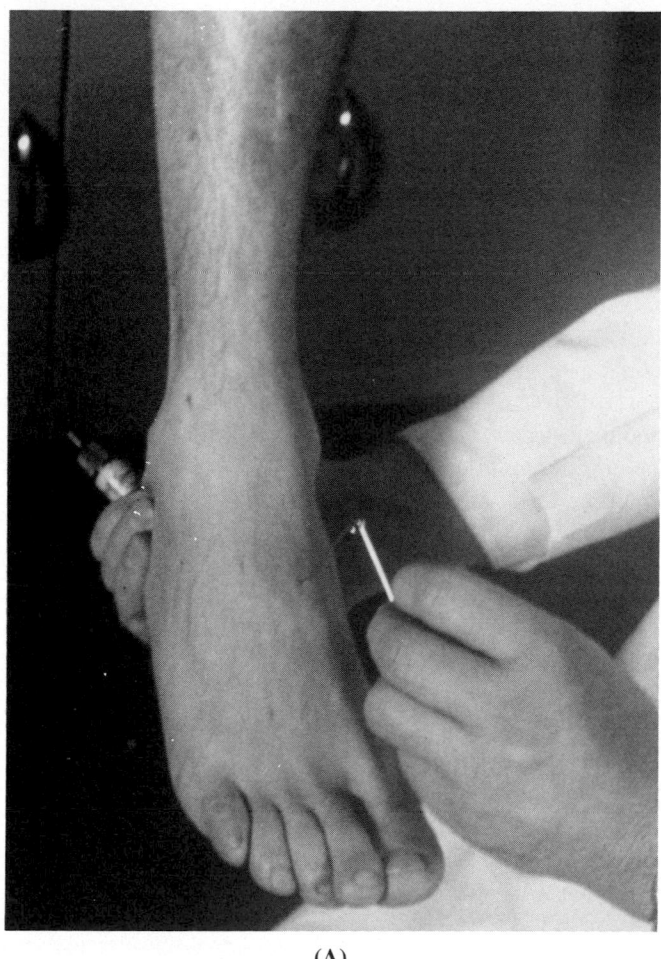

(A)

Figure 3–21 Identifying areas of hypalgesia when nerve roots are compromised. Sterilized safety pins provide good testing objects which may be discarded after each examination *(A)*. Areas of altered sensation may be mapped *(B)*.

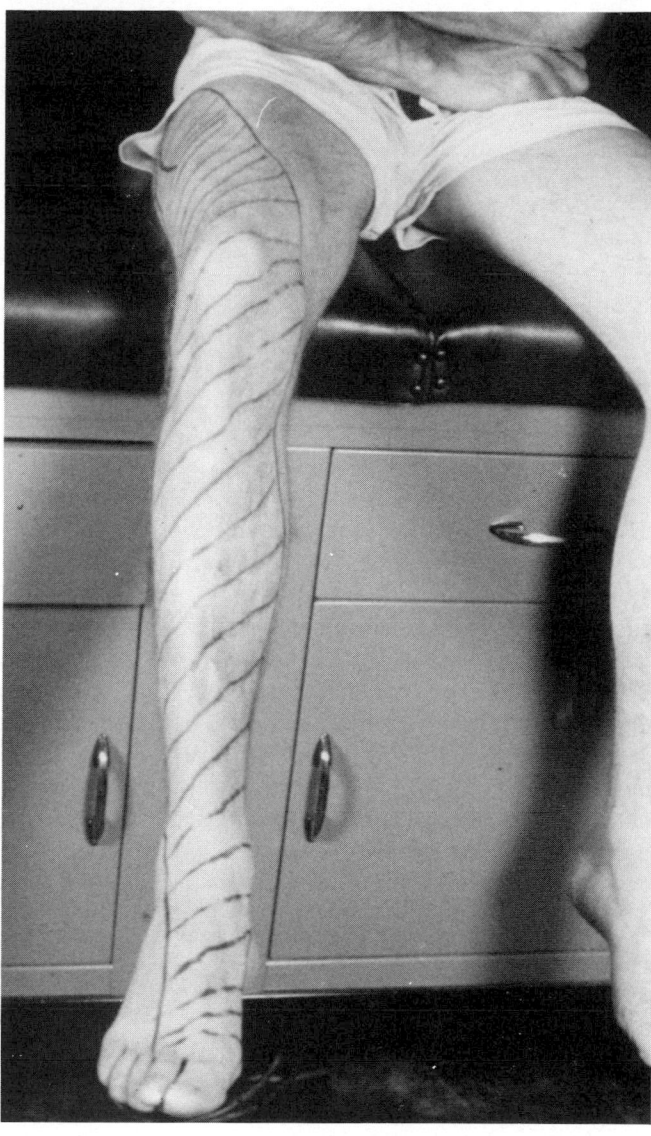

(B)

Painful stimulations and vibratory sense will still be recognized but localization of the stimulus may be impaired. Damage to the lower segments of the parietal lobe in the dominant hemisphere in adults results in varying degrees of dysphasia or aphasia, whereas lesions on the nondominant hemisphere may result in loss of spatial orientation, recognition of body parts, and inability to sketch form. The specific combination of finger agnosia, inability to perform calculations, agraphia, and alexia is known as *Gerstmann's syndrome* and signifies a lesion in the dominant parietal lobe.

Lesions in the parietal lobe will also interrupt visual pathways related to the contralateral field. More subtle lesions of the parietal lobe may result in failure to identify a contralateral stimulus when similar stimuli are applied simultaneously.

☐ LESIONS IN THE REGION OF THE OPTIC CHIASM

A majority of the lesions that affect the chiasm are neoplasms in the region of the sella. Most lesions in this area produce impairment of visual fields, or, if large enough, blindness. They may also produce hypothalamic involvement, involvement of the temporal lobes, or hydrocephalus. The physical signs of such lesions are reviewed in Chap. 12 on pituitary tumors.

☐ LESIONS OF THE POSTERIOR FOSSA

Most surgical lesions of the posterior fossa become symptomatic by involvement of the cerebellum, by obstructing the outflow of cerebrospinal fluid, by producing cranial nerve signs, or by a combination of signs and symptoms consequent to involving the cerebellum, brainstem, or cranial nerves.

Destructive lesions of the cerebellum produce *ataxia.* Hemispheric lesions cause ataxia in the ipsilateral extremities while lesions in the vermis are more prone to cause trunkal ataxia. Large mass lesions of the cerebellum or the fourth ventricle, most common in children, are likely to become apparent because of obstruction of the fourth ventricle, producing acute hydrocephalus. Ataxia may be found on examination, but complaints are more likely to be related to the hydrocephalus, producing nausea, vomiting, and unrelenting headache. Papilledema may be prominent. Malignant lesions of the fourth ventricle may cause cranial nerve deficits because of invasion of the floor of the fourth ventricle.

The most common site for extrinsic lesions of the posterior fossa is the cerebellopontine angle. Hearing may be impaired early. Vestibular function may be impaired on testing. Other cranial nerves that are likely to be involved include: the trigeminal; abducens; facial; and, less commonly, the glossopharyngeal, vagus, spinal accessory, and hypoglossal nerves. Intrinsic lesions of the brainstem may cause cranial nerve deficits, ataxia, long tract signs, and hydrocephalus as they develop.

☐ LESIONS OF THE SPINAL CORD

Tracts in the spinal cord which specifically relate to sensory deficits are in the anterolateral and posteromedial quadrants. The anterolateral quadrant of the spinal cord houses a spinothalamic tract, transmitting sensations of pain and temperature, whereas vibratory and position senses are carried in the posterior columns. Transection of the spinal cord produces anesthesia below the level of the transection. There is usually a progressive decrease in the sensation over one to two dermatomes. A unilateral lesion of the spinal cord will produce loss of pain and temperature on the contralateral side of the body, beginning one to two segments below the level of the lesion, associated with paresis below the level of the lesion on the same side (*Brown-Séquard syndrome*). If the posterior column is involved, there is loss of vibratory and position sense below the level of the lesion on the same side.

A midline lesion of the spinal cord may produce a "shawl-like" loss of pain and temperature in the area of the lesion. Sensation below the level of the lesion is variable. Such lesions are most common in the cervical area and thus affect the distal parts of the upper extremities most prominently. There is usually paresis in the same distribution. This picture is seen in patients with syringomyelia but is most prominent in patients with injury to the central portion of the spinal cord. It occurs in patients with cervical spinal stenosis, having experienced acute extension of the neck.

☐ LESIONS OF PERIPHERAL NERVES

Localized loss of pain and temperature may be related to specific lesions involving nerve roots or more peripheral nerve fibers. Traumatic injuries may involve roots, trunks, cords, or peripheral nerves or a combination of these. Disc herniations are likely to produce discrete areas of hypalgesia and paresthesias in the distribution of specific nerve roots.

Specific syndromes will be reviewed in Chap. 21. In acute lesions of the trunks, cords, or peripheral nerves, sensory deficits should be recorded by diagram. Motor deficits should also be charted. (See Table 3-1.) The neurological examination in such cases is subject to change and diagrams can be more accurate than verbal descriptions. Serial examinations reveal progressive changes.

☐ MOTOR FUNCTION

STRENGTH

Determination of the strength of individual muscles requires the cooperation of a patient and is thus impossible in a stuporous patient.

A grading system has been devised for evaluating muscle strength. In a grading of 0 to 5, the following definitions apply:

0 indicates no motor function.

1 indicates a flicker of contraction.

2 indicates ability to perform movements but not against gravity.

3 indicates that the muscle can overcome gravity.

4 indicates that muscles can work against resistance but with less than full strength.

5 indicates adequate, or "normal," strength.

A chart is advantageous for recording strength of specific muscle groups. The chart identifies nerves and roots innervating a muscle or muscle groups and indicates the function of that muscle. Using this chart, we may record serial examinations permitting comparison with accuracy and facility. Similar comparisons may be made for the reflexes.

DEEP TENDON REFLEXES

Alteration of deep tendon reflexes may result in response to lesions of the central or peripheral nervous system. Generally, an acute injury to the central nervous system (CNS) of

Table 3-1
MOTOR FUNCTION CHART

MOTOR EXAMINATION

Examiner's Initials and Date:

| | | | | | | 0–No motor function   3–Overcomes gravity
| | | | | | 1–Flicker of contraction   but quite weak
| | | | | | 2–More than flicker but   4–Slightly weak
| | | | | | can't overcome   5–Normal
| | | | | | gravity
 5 4 3 2 1 (Right)   (Left) 5 4 3 2 1

(Right) 5 4 3 2 1	Muscle	Root	(Left) 5 4 3 2 1
| | | | | |	Rhomboid	C(4),5	| | | | | |
| | | | | |	Supraspinatus	C5	| | | | | |
| | | | | |	Deltoid (circumflex)	C5(6)	| | | | | |
| | | | | |	Biceps (musculocutaneous)	C5,6	| | | | | |
| | | | | |	Supinator (radial)	C(5),6	| | | | | |
| | | | | |	Ext.carp.rad.(radial)	C6,7	| | | | | |
| | | | | |	Ext.carp.ulnaris (radial)	C7(8)	| | | | | |
| | | | | |	Ext. digitorum (radial)	C7(8)	| | | | | |
| | | | | |	Triceps (radial)	C7,8	| | | | | |
| | | | | |	Pronator teres(median)	C6(7)	| | | | | |
| | | | | |	Flex.dig.subl.(median)	C(7),8T(1)	| | | | | |
| | | | | |	Flex.dig.prof.I & II (median)	C8,T1	| | | | | |
| | | | | |	Oppenens pollicis (median)	C8,T1	| | | | | |
| | | | | |	Flex.carp.ulnarius (ulnar)	C(7),8	| | | | | |
| | | | | |	Flex.dig.prof. III & IV (ulnar)	C8,T(1)	| | | | | |
| | | | | |	Abd.dig.minimi (ulnar)	C(8),T1	| | | | | |
| | | | | |	Interossei (ulnar)	C(8),T1	| | | | | |
| | | | | |	Iliopsoas (femoral)	L(1),2,3	| | | | | |
| | | | | |	Quadriceps (femoral)	L(2),3,4	| | | | | |
| | | | | |	Thigh adductors (obturator)	L2,3,(4)	| | | | | |
| | | | | |	Thigh adductors (sup glut)	L4,5,S1	| | | | | |
| | | | | |	Gluteus maximus (inf glut)	L5,S1,2	| | | | | |
| | | | | |	Tibialis Ant. (sciatic)	L4,5	| | | | | |
| | | | | |	Toe extensors (sciatic)	L5,(S1)	| | | | | |
| | | | | |	Peronel (sciatic)	L5,S1	| | | | | |
| | | | | |	Hamstrings (sciatic)	L(4),5,S1,(2)	| | | | | |
| | | | | |	Toe flexors (sciatic)	S1,2	| | | | | |
| | | | | |	Gastroc (sciatic)	S(1),2	| | | | | |

REFLEX EXAMINATION

0–Absent 1–Hypoactive 2–Normal 3–Hyperactive 4–Very Hyperactive

	Reflex	Root	
| | | | | |	Biceps	C5,6	| | | | | |
| | | | | |	Triceps	C6,7,8	| | | | | |
| | | | | |	Abdominal	T6–L1	| | | | | |
| | | | | |	Cremasteric	L1,2	| | | | | |
| | | | | |	Patellar	L2,3,4	| | | | | |
| | | | | |	Achilles	L5,S1,2	| | | | | |
| | | | | |	Anal	S3,4	| | | | | |
| | | | | |	Bulbocavernosis	S3,4	| | | | | |
| | | | | |	Hoffmann		| | | | | |
| | | | | |	Babinski		| | | | | |
| | | | | |	Clonis		| | | | | |

Comments on: fasciculations, tone, size, spasticity or rigidity, hypotonia, tenderness or contractures. _____

_____

_____

_____

_____

major significance produces an initial decrease in deep tendon reflexes, followed within a few days by hyperactivity in the area affected by the lesion. Most chronic upper motor neuron lesions likewise result in dorsiflexion of the great toe on plantar stimulation (*Babinski sign*), although this may not be present during the period of spinal "shock" or in hypothermia.

Decrease in specific deep tendon reflexes may be the result of a lesion of a peripheral nerve or nerve root. This may result from injury in either the sensory or motor components. Alteration in deep tendon reflexes may result from specific compressive lesions of nerve roots such as are encountered with herniated disks, or from diffuse lesions, for example, peripheral neuropathy. Discrete patterns of reflex loss form part of the syndromes for specific nerve root compression, described in Chap. 20. In general, loss of reflexes associated with peripheral neuropathy is diffuse, but it is more marked distally than proximally.

☐ INVESTIGATION OF COORDINATION

Coordinated movements require good motor function, the ability to know where parts of the body are, and discrete integration of these functions. Failure on tests of coordination may be due to loss of function in any one of these modalities. For instance, injury to the premotor strip in the frontal lobe may result in spasticity. Even though muscle strength is excellent, spasticity may prohibit smooth contraction of groups of muscles, resulting in loss of finely coordinated movements. This can occur even though sites where movements are normally integrated are intact.

Proprioception is the sensibility by which one ordinarily locates parts of his extremities both in space and in relation to the rest of his body. Unless position sense is intact, coordinated movements must depend upon another method of localization. Visual signals may serve this purpose, but when proprioception is impaired, coordinated movements are lost in the dark or when one's eyes are closed.

Integration of movements is usually accomplished in the *basal ganglia* and *cerebellum*. Destructive lesions in these areas result in ataxia or inability to perform finely coordinated movements. As indicated above, adequate function of such areas requires both motor and sensory input.

Varying neurological deficits occur with lesions in different parts of these cerebral structures. Lesions in the basal ganglia are usually associated with abnormal movements in the contralateral extremities at rest. Volitional movements may be decreased or hesitant. Lesions in the cerebellum are more likely to be associated with tremors during the course of initiated movements. Likewise, lesions in the cerebellar hemispheres are frequently associated with loss of coordination of the ipsilateral extremities, while lesions in the vermis are more likely to be associated with limitation of coordinated movements of the trunk.

☐ MOVEMENT DISORDERS

Disorders of motion should be observed and described. Movements may be spontaneous and uncontrolled, as with tremor and chorea, or initiated quite slowly (hypokinetic). In certain syndromes such as Parkinson's disease, there is a combination of the two, i.e., tremor while at rest associated with difficulty initiating purposeful movements. In many cases, one feature is predominant. In other instances, patients may develop a tremor on intention or attempted movement. Intention tremors are normally associated with lesions of the region of the cerebellum.

Muscle tone must be evaluated. Decreased tone can be quite subtle and is frequently associated with lesions of the cerebellum. Increased tone or rigidity may result in a peculiar type of "gradual release" so that there is an alternate grabbing and releasing on passive motion. Examinations of coordination of movements must likewise be tested and recorded. These include finger-to-nose, finger-to-finger, heel-to-shin, and rapid alternate movements such as tapping with the toes or fingers or rapid approximation and separation of the patient's thumb and index finger of the same hand. The Romberg test is accomplished by observing the patient while having the patient stand with eyes closed and feet together. Loss of position sense or cerebellar function results in falling, which may be lateralized according to the site of the lesion. Tremors and athetoid or choreiform movements should be noted. A fall indicates the need for discrete testing of position sense and coordination.

☐ COMMENT

With completion of the bedside history and physical examination, a preliminary indication of the type and site of an anatomical lesion should be suggested. In many instances, diagnosis is indicated by the history alone. The physical examination usually indicates the site of the lesion. The history and physical examination are used to determine the need for specific ancillary examinations, which may be either physiological or imaging. Physiological investigation and imaging studies have become increasingly sophisticated in recent years. Specific tests will be described in subsequent chapters.

REFERENCES

1. Plum F, Posner JB: *The Diagnosis of Stupor and Coma,* 3d ed. Philadelphia, F.A. Davis, 1982.
2. Walsh FB, Hoyt WF: The visual sensory system: Anatomy, physiology, and topographic diagnosis, in *Clinical Ophthalmology,* 3d ed., Baltimore, Williams and Wilkins, 1969, pp 1–129.
3. Hoyt WF, Luis O: Visual fiber anatomy in the infrageniculate pathway of the primate. *Arch Ophthalmol* 68:94–106, 1962.
4. Harrington DO: Localizing value of incongruity in defects in the visual fields. *Arch Ophthal* 21:453–464, 1939.
5. Rosenberg M: Neuro-ophthalmology, in Wilkins RH, *Rengachary* SS (eds): *Neurosurgery.* New York, McGraw-Hill, 1985, pp 71–102.
6. DeJong RN: Case taking and the neurologic examination, in Baker AB, Baker LH (eds): *Clinical Neurology.* Philadelphia, Harper and Row, 1982, pp 1–87.
7. Reis DJ: The palmomental reflex: A fragment of a general nociceptive skin reflex: A physiological study in normal man. *Arch Neurol* 4:486–498, 1961.
8. Demyer W: Anatomy and clinical neurology of the spinal cord, in *Clinical Neurology.* Philadelphia, Harper and Row, 1982, vol 3, chap 31, pp 1–24.
9. Goldberg S: *The 4-minute Neurologic Exam: An Answer to the Neuro WNL problem.* Miami, Medmaster, 1984.
10. Schneider RC, Crosby EC, Calhoun HD: Surgery of convulsive seizures and allied disorders, in Kahn EA, Crosby EC, Schneider RC, Taren JA (eds): *Correlative Neurosurgery,* 2d ed. Springfield, Ill., Charles C. Thomas, 1969, chap 16, pp 279–358.
11. DeJong RN: *The Neurologic Examination,* 3d ed. New York, Hoeber, 1967.
12. Kluver H, Bucy PC: Preliminary analysis of functions of the temporal lobe in monkeys. *Arch Neurol Psychiatry* 42: 979–1000, 1939.

☐ STUDY QUESTIONS

I. A 25-year-old male suddenly screamed out with a severe headache, shortly after which he lapsed into deep stupor. He gradually awakened about 2 hours later but had a left hemiplegia that persisted. He remained quite drowsy but would answer simple questions and respond readily to deep pressure on the sternum.

A CT scan, performed without contrast, demonstrated a hemorrhage in the right frontotemporal area, clearly infiltrating the frontal and temporal lobes. There was minimal shift of the midline structures. A contrast scan revealed an aneurysm of the right middle cerebral artery from which the hemorrhage extended.

1. What would be the most likely status of the deep tendon reflexes on the day of admission? **2.** What would most likely be the status of the reflexes 2 weeks later? **3.** What is the most likely explanation for the initial loss of consciousness and why did the patient recover, at least enough to respond to pain? **4.** Which extremity would you expect to see recovery in first? Why? **5.** What changes might you expect to see in the visual fields?

II. A 35-year-old female is referred because of pain in the interscapular area and both arms. On examination the patient has marked atrophy of the hands and there is loss of sensation to pinprick and temperature throughout the upper extremities. Deep tendon reflexes in the upper extremities are absent, but they are quite active in the lower extremities and there is good strength in the lower extremities.

1. What part of the nervous system most likely has a lesion? **2.** How could the lesion be proved? **3.** What would the most likely lesion be? **4.** Could this syndrome result from trauma? **5.** Should this woman interrupt her occupation as a cook? Why?

III. A 40-year-old female was involved in an automobile accident in which she was struck by a sharp object on the left side of her head. Her cranium was penetrated in the parietal area so that she sustained contusion with considerable hemorrhage in the angular and marginal gyri of the left. The hemorrhage was controlled and the wound closed without incident.

1. What would be her expected neurological deficit? **2.** Would you expect problems with reading? With calculating? **3.** Would you expect her to verbalize? **4.** Would you expect difficulty with vision? **5.** Might there be a problem with behavior? Why?

IV. A 55-year-old male is admitted with urinary incontinence which has been progressive for a year. He has a history of a head injury 10 years earlier. A CT shows evidence of hydrocephalus.

1. What other neurological findings might one expect to see? **2.** Would headache likely be a prominent feature of this patient's problem? **3.** What is the explanation for the incontinence? **4.** Would the reflexes in the lower extremities likely be affected? **5.** What treatment might be recommended?

V. A 39-year-old male is brought in with a facial twitch. When he is examined, he is found to be demented and to have frequent choreiform movements throughout his body. His father had reportedly committed suicide and a brother was known to be hospitalized with dementia. He reportedly had some strange movements as well.

1. What is the most likely diagnosis? **2.** What are the classical neurological findings? **3.** Where are the lesions located? **4.** What would an MRI show? **5.** Will steriotaxic surgery cure this patient?

4 Neuropsychological Evaluation for Patients with Disturbances of the Nervous System

Gregory P. Lee
David W. Loring

Purposes of Neuropsychological Testing

Neuropsychological testing is an extension of the mental status examination. The goal of neuropsychological assessment is to measure possible changes of cognitive and emotional functions resulting from damage to specific regions of the brain.

In cases with known lesions and clear behavioral alterations, a complete mental status examination is frequently sufficient to answer questions regarding mental function. Although a mental status examination may be adequate to document obvious mental changes due to known brain damage, it may not identify early or mild disturbances in cognitive function. In addition, mental status examinations may also be unable to distinguish behavioral changes due to psychiatric illness from those due to neurological disorders. Because neuropsychological evaluation is more thorough and objective than the mental status examination, it offers greater sensitivity to subtle or difficult to distinguish neurobehavioral disorders such as early dementia.

In contrast to the mental status examination, neuropsychological tests are standardized procedures with groups of healthy controls or patients that comprise a comparison group. This allows for direct comparison of the patient to the standardization group's performance, and it helps to clarify the pattern of performance across different areas of cognitive function by showing areas of preserved or impaired function.

These characteristics not only help in the determination of deficit, but since the results are quantitative in nature, repeated comparisons over time, such as before and after neurosurgical intervention, may be used to evaluate improvement or deterioration in cognition. For example, serial neuropsychological testing provides information about deterioration in progressive disorders such as Alzheimer's disease or hydrocephalus. Periodic retesting also measures the degree and type of behavioral recovery following head trauma or surgery of the brain.

Lateralization between cerebral hemispheres and localization within a single hemisphere are traditional foci of neuropsychological testing. However, goals have diminished in importance as imaging techniques, such as computerized tomography (CT), magnetic imaging (MRI), and single photon emission computerized tomography (SPECT) developed and have become more widely available. Nevertheless, lateralization and localization continue to be important goals in settings such as epilepsy surgery programs where neuropsychological testing can help to document a unilateral temporal lobe seizure focus as well as provide prognostic information.

Other purposes of neuropsychological testing include determination of the cause of academic difficulties in children (such as learning disabilities or mental retardation), aiding in the design of individualized rehabilitation programs, providing data for legal purposes in patients with litigation or disability claims, and for use in research.

☐ COGNITIVE DOMAINS

The neuropsychological examination evaluates the important cognitive domains, including: attention, memory, intelligence, language, visuoperception, visuospatial judgment, and the so-called executive functions such as abstraction, complex problem solving, and concept formation. The completed neuropsychological examination should provide a comprehensive profile of cognitive abilities. Depending on the reason for referral, age of the patient, and the patient's ability to cooperate, other tests measuring sensory and motor functions, personality or psychiatric problems, and academic achievement also may provide important information.

☐ GOALS OF CHAPTER

This chapter will deal with areas of cognitive dysfunction for the major neurobehavioral syndromes, including amnesia, dementia, acute confusional states, aphasia, and pure attentional disorders. Common psychological tests used to measure each of the cognitive domains (e.g., attention, memory, intelligence) will be briefly mentioned, but describing the plethora of tests is not the purpose of the chapter. For the interested reader, an appendix is included, briefly listing common neuropsychological tests with their references. Since memory impairments are important for the differential diagnosis of many neurobehavioral disorders, it is necessary first to clarify the meaning of certain learning and memory terms before discussing the neurobehavioral syndromes.

Types of Learning and Memory

Memory refers to perceptual experiences stored in the brain that may be available to alter future thought and behavior. Learning is the process of acquiring new memories. Unfortunately, many different terms have emerged to classify functionally similar types of memory, thereby creating confusion about their precise meaning. We briefly define these terms and their equivalents in different disciplines.

☐ DEFINITION OF MEMORY IN MEDICINE

Clinical medicine categorizes memory based on the time course of learning as either *immediate, recent,* or *remote memory.* Immediate memory is the amount of information that can be recalled immediately after its presentation. Recent memory refers to learning that has taken place in the preceding days, weeks, or months. Remote memory is recall of events which occurred years earlier. The transformation of memories from recent to remote is gradual and remains imprecisely defined. This categorization of memory is not based on an understand-

ing of memory mechanisms but rather has evolved from selective disorders of memory associated with specific diseases.

☐ DEFINITION OF MEMORY IN PSYCHOLOGY

William James[1] divided memory into primary and secondary components. *Primary memory* is the immediate content of consciousness. *Secondary memory* is recalling information no longer in the consciousness.

More recently, similar distinctions have been made using the words "short-term" and "long-term memory."[2]

Short-term memory has been viewed as "working memory," in which conscious mental processes are performed, and it is analogous to immediate or primary memory. Miller[3] determined that the capacity of short-term memory is seven—plus or minus two—bits of information at any given time. Short-term memory has traditionally been measured using forward digit span.

Long-term memory is previously learned material, is considered more permanent, and encompasses both recent and remote memory concepts in clinical medical classification.

☐ DEFINITION OF MEMORY IN NEUROPSYCHOLOGY

To avoid the semantic ambiguity associated with the many different meanings of "memory," Hamsher[4] proposed substituting certain neuropsychological constructs for the immediate, recent, and remote memory concepts in clinical medicine. Immediate (primary) memory is typically measured using digit span. Because digit span loads on an attention-concentration factor in factor analytic research,[5] substituting the term attention for immediate memory will prevent misinterpretation. The equivalence of terms used in these different systems of memory classification is given in Table 4-1.

Table 4-1
SYSTEMS OF MEMORY CLASSIFICATION

Medicine	Psychology	Neuropsychology
Remote	Long-term Secondary	Intelligence
Recent	Long-term Secondary	Learning "Memory"
Immediate	Short-term Primary	Attention

Neurobehavioral Disorders

☐ AMNESIA

DEFINITION AND CLINICAL FEATURES

A generalized deficit in learning new information, when accompanied by relative sparing of intellectual and other cognitive functions, is called *amnesia* or an amnestic syndrome. Amnesic patients have difficulty learning most types of new information, except motor skill (procedural) learning, regardless of the sensory channel in which it is presented. *Immediate memory span* (also called primary or short-term memory) and remote memories are preserved. These patients are usually disoriented to time, place, and knowledge of many current personal circumstances.

ETIOLOGY

A variety of diseases and trauma may cause amnesia, including: Korsakoff's syndrome, anoxia, viral encephalitis, bilateral posterior cerebral artery infarctions, temporal lobe ablations, head trauma, and brain tumors. The common underlying neuroanatomic disruption is involvement of the limbic structures of the mesial temporal lobes, thalamus, septal forebrain, or their neural interconnections.

NEUROPSYCHOLOGICAL IMPAIRMENT

As the definition of amnesia implies, the primary neuropsychological test deficit will be seen on tests of new learning, or "memory" tests. Thus, performance on verbal memory tasks, such as word list learning (Selective Reminding Test),[6] digit supraspan (Serial Digit Learning),[7] paragraph retention (Wechsler Memory Scale),[8] and paired associate learning (Wechsler Memory Scale),[8] and tests of nonverbal, visuospatial new learning, such as complex figure recall (Rey-Osterrieth Complex Figure),[9] or learning simple geometric designs (Wechsler Memory Scale),[8] will be impaired relative to tests measuring other cognitive domains.

Tests of attentional capacity, such as digit span or mental arithmetic (subtests of the Wechsler Adult Intelligence Scale-Revised),[10] will be normal for the individual (i.e., adjusted for intellectual and socioeconomic expectations). Intelligence testing, usually measured by the Wechsler Adult Intelligence Scale-Revised,[10] will generally be preserved or only slightly below premorbid expectations.

Core linguistic functions measured by tests of visual naming, aural comprehension, sentence repetition, and verbal fluency from any common aphasia test battery[11,12,13] will be normal. Tests of visual perception[14,15] and visual spatial functions[10,16] typically will be within the normal range. Fi-

Table 4-2
PATTERN OF NEUROPSYCHOLOGICAL DEFICITS IN AMNESIA

Cognitive Domain	Performance
Attention	Normal
Memory	Impaired
Intelligence	Normal
Language	Normal
Visuospatial	Normal
"Executive"	Normal

nally, tests of "executive" or frontal lobe functions, such as those measuring abstraction, complex problem solving, reasoning, and the use of feedback to guide ongoing behavior,[17,18,19] will generally be well preserved in amnesia. The pattern of neuropsychological deficits in amnesia is given in Table 4-2.

DIFFERENTIAL DIAGNOSIS

In addition to diseases causing focal limbic lesions that result in relatively pure disorders of new learning, diseases diffusely affecting the brain may also result in severe memory disturbances. For example, patients with dementia or acute confusional states are unable to learn new information and have severe memory disorders.

The distinction between amnesia and dementia is the presence of other cognitive deficits in dementia, such as disorders of intelligence, language, and visuospatial reasoning, that are not present in amnesia. Similarly, although patients with acute confusional states are unable to form new memories, they are easily distinguished from amnesic patients by alterations in arousal, impairment in the stream of logical thought, and disruption of the sleep-wake cycle.

Psychiatric disorders may interfere with normal memory test performance as well as performance on tests of other cognitive functions. Since arousal, attention, and motivation are necessary for normal learning, psychoses may disrupt memory performance for reasons that are independent from dysfunction of important memory structures, such as the mesial temporal lobes. Consequently, psychiatric disturbances that disrupt normal memory should not be considered amnesia.

Another psychiatric disorder that should not be considered amnesia is so-called psychogenic amnesia. Psychogenic amnesia involves the sudden onset of retrograde amnesia, often with loss of remote personal memories, including knowledge of personal identity, with preservation of the ability to learn new information. These inconsistencies with established knowledge of how memory systems operate easily distinguish psychogenic amnesia from genuine amnesias.

☐ DEMENTIA

DEFINITION AND CLINICAL FEATURES

Dementia is an acquired impairment of new learning in conjunction with loss of intellectual functions of sufficient severity to interfere with the patient's social or occupational functioning. Because the brain diseases causing dementia are diffuse multifocal processes, many different cognitive functions will be impaired. Although the diseases causing dementia are different from each other, the types of cognitive deficits are generally similar regardless of etiology.

COURSE

Dementia typically begins with mild forgetfulness and slowing of mental activity. These deficits evolve to severe memory loss with multiple areas of cognitive impairment such as language and visuospatial impairment, reduced abstraction, diminished judgment, and agnosias. In addition, alterations of mood and personality are present. As intelligence continues to decline, all other cognitive domains become severely impaired and lead to a state of complete helplessness where patients are unable to feed, dress, or toilet themselves. Patients with severe dementia are vulnerable to urinary tract infections and pneumonia, and usually die of such secondary medical complications.

ETIOLOGY

Although many diseases may cause dementia, by far the most common is *Alzheimer's disease*. Adams and Victor[20] estimate that approximately 50 percent of all cases of dementia are caused by Alzheimer's disease. Vascular disease, or multiple infarcts, remains the second most common etiology of dementia, accounting for 10 to 20 percent of cases.[20,21] The remaining common dementing disorders include: Pick's, Parkinson's, and Huntington's diseases; long-standing hydrocephalus; and chronic alcohol and drug intoxication.

NEUROPSYCHOLOGICAL IMPAIRMENT

As the definition of dementia implies, the pattern of neuropsychological impairment will involve most areas of cognitive function. These are reviewed in Table 4-3 (on p. 63). The core psychological features of dementia involve impairments of memory and intelligence. Thus, tests of verbal and nonverbal learning, such as the Wechsler Memory Scale,[8] Selective Reminding Test,[6] and Rey Complex Figure-delay,[9] will be below normal levels. Further, the gold standard of psychometric intelligence, namely the Wechsler Adult Intelligence Scale-Revised (WAIS-R),[10] will show a significant

decline relative to the patient's premorbid level of intellectual functioning.

The issue of how best to estimate the premorbid IQ in the absence of previously administered intelligence tests or formal academic achievement tests is important for the behavioral diagnosis of dementia. For the majority of patients, this is not an insurmountable problem since most IQs are near the mean test scores of 100, and 68 percent are within one standard deviation (IQs between 85 and 115) of the mean.

The determination of significant IQ decline becomes more difficult with patients whose premorbid IQs were either very low (< 80) or very high (> 120). There are statistical formulas for estimating premorbid IQ,[22,23] but these also are unfortunately vulnerable to the criticism of being less accurate with extreme scores. The best method of estimating premorbid IQ is to review school, military, and employment records which frequently have some psychological test measure of intelligence. The next best method might be to use an actuarial formula. The method most open to question is the psychologist's subjective estimate based on relationships of IQs associated with various occupational and educational levels. The important point is to know which method the psychologist used to establish premorbid IQ and to understand the degree of uncertainty associated with the method employed.

In addition to impairments of memory and intelligence, there are typically deficits of visuospatial and "executive" (frontal lobe tests) functions and some aspects of language in dementia. Visuospatial difficulties include inability to properly construct two-[10] or three-dimensional[24] block designs, to draw complex geometric figures from a model,[9] or difficulties in judging the directional orientation of lines that are either presented visually[16] or drawn on the palm of the hand.

The so-called executive, or frontal lobe tests, are universally impaired in dementia. This should not, however, be interpreted as meaning there is neural damage to the frontal lobes because tests of executive functions depend upon many "lower" cognitive functions, including attention, memory, language, and visuoperception, for their successful performance.

Although patients with dementia will perform poorly on tests of executive abilities for reasons that may have nothing to do with these highest of cognitive functions, they nevertheless consistently fail executive tests due to defective subcomponent skills such as visuospatial or linguistic difficulties. Executive functions include such abilities as abstraction, complex problem solving, concept formation, planning, and the use of feedback to guide ongoing performance. Tests measuring executive functions include the Categories Test,[17] Wisconsin Card Sorting Test,[18] Porteus or WISC-R Mazes,[19,25] Stroop Test,[26] and word fluency (number of words produced beginning with a specified letter in 60 sec).[12]

In the early stages of dementia, language is typically intact. There may be slight difficulty finding appropriate words, mild problems on tests of visual naming, and a subtle paucity of ideas expressed in conversation. However, the patient is not overtly aphasic. As the dementia progresses, patients begin to show more linguistic impairment. Expressive speech

Table 4-3
PATTERN OF NEUROPSYCHOLOGICAL DEFICITS IN DEMENTIA

Cognitive Domain	Performance
Attention	Normal
Memory	Impaired
Intelligence	Impaired
Language	Normal early, impaired later
Visuospatial	Impaired
"Executive"	Impaired

becomes more empty and devoid of substantive ideas, vocabulary is reduced, and naming is impaired. Reading comprehension and written expression deteriorate more rapidly than aural comprehension and conversational speech. Grammar is usually well preserved, and paraphasic errors typically appear later in the disease. As the disease continues to take its toll, conversation is characterized by a lack of factual content, although some patients may still appear less impaired by carrying on light social conversation. In the final stages of the disease, patients become increasingly nonfluent, rarely initiate speech spontaneously, and finally become mute.

Similar to language, attention is relatively preserved in dementia, especially in the early and middle stages of progressive dementias. Patients who present with significant deficits of new learning and intellectual deterioration nevertheless are often able to repeat digits forward and backward in a normal fashion; i.e., immediate memory span is normal. However, in the later stages of the progressive dementias, attention and concentration will show impairment as well as practically all other cognitive functions. In summary, the medical classification of dementia is characterized by defects of remote memory and recent memory with normal immediate memory.

DIFFERENTIAL DIAGNOSIS

Dementia must be differentiated from several other conditions, some of which may be confused with dementia. First, dementia is not mental retardation. In retardation, low intellectual levels are developmental and present since early childhood. Dementia is an *acquired* disorder, implying that a loss of fully developed intellectual functions has taken place. *Dementia is distinguished from amnesia* by defective performances on tests of visuospatial and executive abilities, intelligence, and on tests of language.

Acute confusional states differ neuropsychologically from dementia by impaired arousal, alertness, and attention in confusion. Further, if the patient is testable, the examiner will generally be able to document normal verbal intelligence in confusion which is impaired in dementia.

Finally, dementia is distinguished from acute confusion by knowledge of the clinical history. The course of dementia is typically slow and insidious (with exceptions such as head trauma or sustained anoxia) while acute confusion often develops abruptly. The time of onset of confusional symptoms may be precisely known when questioning a relative. Because the onset of dementia is usually gradual, pinpointing the time of onset is difficult, if not impossible, for patients and relatives.

Certain psychiatric disorders, especially depression, may resemble dementia with apparent impairments of memory and general cognitive functions. In "pseudodementia," onset may be recent or abrupt, there may be a history of previous psychiatric illness, and the patient, rather than a family member, may complain of memory loss and other cognitive difficulties.[27] Psychiatric patients may highlight their deficits and give frequent "I don't know" answers to questions. Their performance on neuropsychological tests are typically more variable with areas of preserved functioning inconsistent with subjective severity of complaints.

By contrast, in dementia, the onset is gradual. Family members typically complain more about deficits than the patient himself, and performance on tests of memory, intelligence, and visuospatial functions are consistently impaired.

☐ ACUTE CONFUSIONAL STATES

DEFINITION AND CLINICAL FEATURES

The *core behavioral features of acute confusional states* are alterations in level of arousal, disturbances of attention, and impairment in the logical stream of thought. Other commonly associated features include: disturbance of the sleep-wake cycle, disorientation with respect to time and place, rambling or incoherent speech, illusions, hallucinations, and either increased or decreased psychomotor behavior.[28] Attentional capacity, speech coherence, disorientation, and tendency toward perceptual misidentification will fluctuate over the course of a day, often being worse at night. Additionally, most diagnostic criteria require that symptoms be of acute onset.

There are *two primary confusional state subtypes*. The *hyperactive type* is characterized by increased activity, overarousal, and agitation. The *hypoactive form* shows reduced arousal, underactivity, and stupor. Hyperactive confusional patients are typically restless, excitable, and distractible, and they show abnormally increased responsiveness to environmental stimuli. By contrast, in the hypoactive type, there is a reduced level of psychomotor activity and alertness. Hypoactive patients have been described as quiet and listless, speaking very little, responding slowly to stimuli, and having a tendency to drift off into sleep even when talking with others.[28]

ETIOLOGY

Toxic and metabolic disorders are among the most common etiologies of acute confusion. Metabolic diseases are systemic disorders of metabolism resulting in secondary effects on the brain. Common metabolic diseases that may cause confusion include: organ failure (liver, kidney, pancreas, and glands), systemic diseases (cancer, porphyria, Wilson's disease), deficiency of oxygen or substrates for cerebral metabolism (hypoxia, hypoglycemia), disorders of fluid, electrolyte, and acid-base balance (sodium, potassium, calcium, acidosis), vitamin deficiency or excess, and disorders of temperature regulation.[28–31]

Drug intoxication is probably the more common and important cause of acute confusional states in the elderly. In addition to prescription drugs, other common agents causing acute confusion include: alcohol, alcohol withdrawal, solvent-inhalants (glue), industrial poisons (carbon monoxide, heavy metals), and drug withdrawal (sedative-hypnotics).

NEUROPSYCHOLOGICAL IMPAIRMENT

Acute confusional states are caused by agents or processes that include almost every known drug, toxin, and acute or chronic illness that interferes with brain function. It is important to note that each toxic or metabolic cause does *not* result in a different set of behavioral symptoms. Although some metabolic disorders tend to cause hypoactive confusional states, and alcohol or sedative-hypnotic withdrawal tend to result in the hyperactive form of confusion, the essential behavioral features and neuropsychological test results seen in acute confusion remain the same despite etiology.

The pattern of neuropsychological test impairment across the major cognitive domains in acute confusional states includes deficits of attention, memory, visuospatial abilities, and executive functions. Language and verbal intellectual abilities tend to be well-preserved relative to the areas of neuropsychological impairment. This pattern is summarized in Table 4-4. Deficits of attention (digit span), concentration (mental arithmetic), vigilance (continuous performance tasks), and reaction time are among the first signs to herald the onset of acute confusion. In general, the more severe the underlying medical condition is, the greater the cognitive impairment.

Table 4-4
PATTERN OF NEUROPSYCHOLOGICAL DEFICITS IN ACUTE CONFUSIONAL STATES

Cognitive Domain	Performance
Attention	Impaired
Memory	Impaired
Intelligence	Normal
Language	Normal
Visuospatial	Impaired
"Executive"	Impaired

OUTCOME

If the medical condition causing confusion is treated promptly and successfully, neuropsychological test performance usually returns to premorbid levels. However, approximately 25 percent of confused patients develop dementia, and when treatment is unsuccessful or applied late in the course of illness, an estimated 15 to 25 percent of elderly patients die within 6 months.

DIFFERENTIAL DIAGNOSIS

Acute confusional states often require differentiation from dementia. Distinguishing acute confusion from dementia can be a difficult task since there is a global impairment of cognition in both neurobehavioral syndromes. This is further complicated by the frequent simultaneous occurrence of both disorders. However, the diagnostic distinction between confusion and dementia is important since acute confusion suggests a potentially reversible underlying medical disorder that, if not identified and treated, can progress to irreversible dementia or death. The clinical features helpful in the differential diagnosis of acute confusional state versus dementia have been detailed elsewhere[28] and are summarized in Table 4-5.

☐ APHASIA

DEFINITION AND CLINICAL FEATURES

Aphasias are acquired disorders of language not due to motor speech or articulatory disturbances. Further, aphasias are selective linguistic disorders that are not accompanied by more generalized cognitive disturbances such as those seen in dementia and acute confusional states.

Table 4-5
BEHAVIORAL DIFFERENTIAL DIAGNOSIS BETWEEN ACUTE CONFUSIONAL STATES AND DEMENTIA*

Feature	Acute Confusional State	Dementia
Onset	Acute, abrupt	Slow, insidious
Known onset time	Often, yes	No
Course	Fluctuating	Stable
Duration	Usually brief	Usually longstanding
Alertness	Abnormal	Usually normal
Awareness	Reduced	Clear

*Adapted from Lipowski.[28]

It is important to accurately diagnose aphasia since aphasia may be mistaken for acute confusion, dementia, or psychiatric illness. Accurate diagnosis is also important because various types of language disturbances have specific neuroanatomic correlates and different prognoses that may alter discussions about the patient's future. Aphasia may also be inappropriately diagnosed when language is disrupted from other causes such as dysarthria, mutism, or acute confusion.

ASSESSMENT

Aspects of language that should be assessed in patients with suspected aphasia include assessment of spontaneous speech (e.g., Is it fluent or nonfluent? Are there aphasic errors?), visual naming, sentence repetition, and aural comprehension. There are several comprehensive test batteries for the evaluation of language that have been standardized and provide data for normative comparisons.[11,12,13] In addition to assessing the core linguistic functions—namely, fluency of spontaneous speech, naming, repetition, and comprehension—most aphasia batteries also evaluate controlled word association (retrieval of words beginning with a designated letter), as well as reading and writing. Some batteries include tests for apraxia.

APHASIA SYNDROMES

The diagnosis of aphasia requires the presence of both positive and negative signs. Positive signs include such things as paraphasic errors (e.g., calling a telephone a "pookerfeld" or a "radio"), telegraphic speech (absence of connective words in ongoing speech so that "I have to go to the bathroom" becomes "Me bathroom"), or circumlocutions (When asked to name a toothbrush, the patient may say, "Oh, you know for your teeth, so you can smile."). Negative signs of aphasia include deficits in fluency of spontaneous speech, visual naming, sentence repetition, and aural comprehension. For a diagnosis of aphasia to be made, an impairment of visual naming must be present.

Table 4-6
DIFFERENTIAL DIAGNOSIS OF MAJOR APHASIA SYNDROMES

Aphasia Subtype	Fluency	Comprehension	Repetition
Nominal	Normal	Normal	Normal
Conduction	Normal	Normal	Impaired
Broca's	Impaired	Normal	Impaired
Transcortical Motor	Impaired	Normal	Normal
Wernicke's	Normal	Impaired	Impaired
Transcortical Sensory	Normal	Impaired	Normal
Global	Impaired	Impaired	Impaired
Mixed Transcortical	Impaired	Impaired	Normal

If there are both positive and negative signs of an impairment of language (and not simply impairment of articulation or speech production) in conjunction with a deficit of visual naming, the diagnosis of aphasia has been established. After it has been established that the patient is aphasic, differential diagnosis of the eight major aphasia subtypes can be made when performance on four core linguistic functions is known. Differential diagnosis of the aphasia subtypes is given in Table 4-6. There are aphasias that are atypical in that they do not conform to the classic aphasic syndromes. The *atypical aphasias,* or *subcortical aphasias,* are frequently secondary to infarctions of the thalamus or basal ganglia[32] and are not included in Table 4-6.

ETIOLOGY

Although cerebral vascular accidents involving the middle cerebral artery are probably the most common etiology of the aphasias, other focal or diffuse brain lesions—such as tumor, trauma, or end-stage Alzheimer's disease—can cause aphasia. In the overwhelming majority (approximately 98 percent) of right-handed, and in the majority of left-handed, individuals, language disturbances result from left cerebral hemisphere disease. The nonfluent aphasias are typically secondary to disease in the left frontal lobe. In *Broca's aphasia,* damage is to the posterior third of the inferior frontal convulsion (Brodmann's area 44), and in transcortical motor aphasia, the classic lesion is a crescent-shaped watershed or border-zone infarction in the superior frontal lobe between the territories of the anterior and middle cerebral arteries.

The fluent aphasias usually follow damage to the posterior regions of the left hemisphere—in *Wernicke's aphasia,* the posterior third of the superior temporal convulsion (Brodmann's area 22). In *conduction aphasia,* damage is to the supramarginal gyrus (Brodmann's area 40). In *anomic aphasia,* lesions are found in many peri-sylvian regions of the posterior left hemisphere. In transcortical sensory aphasia, the classical lesion involves a border-zone infarction of the most distal territory of anterior and middle cerebral arteries in the posterior left hemisphere.

Global aphasia results from large left hemisphere lesions that damage both anterior and posterior language areas, most commonly from occlusion of the middle cerebral artery at its origin.

Finally, *mixed transcortical aphasia,* also called isolation of the speech area, is often the result of a large borderzone, anterior-middle cerebral artery infarction extending from the frontal to the parietal lobe. Transcortical aphasias often follow cardiac arrest that in turn often occurs after prolonged hypotension or hypoxia.

OUTCOME

Prognosis of the aphasias depends on the type, size, and location of the lesion producing the disturbance. Aphasia due to cerebral vascular accidents generally have a worse prognosis than aphasia secondary to trauma. Longitudinal studies of aphasia subtypes also allows generalization about outcome. All transcortical aphasias have a favorable prognosis for return of language function. Similarly, there may be a complete return of normal language among patients with anomic and conduction aphasias. Broca's and Wernicke's aphasias have about an equal chance (fifty-fifty) for improvement to a less-severe form of aphasia, but rarely is there complete recovery. Global aphasics have the worse prognosis, and some type of significant, continuing language impairment is expected.

NEUROPSYCHOLOGICAL IMPAIRMENT

As shown in Table 4-7, the primary area of cognitive impairment in aphasia is linguistic. Because new verbal learning requires language processing, there also will be deficits of verbal, but not nonverbal (visuospatial), learning. Tests of attention, intelligence, and executive functions, not dependent on language for successful performance, will be normal. Tests of verbal intelligence, such as the WAIS-R Verbal IQ, will be defective, and they are not valid measurements of intellectual functioning in aphasia. Finally, visuospatial tests will be performed normally, provided the instructions for the test are understood.

ACQUIRED DISORDERS OF READING AND WRITING

Disturbances of reading and writing almost always parallel a patient's primary language problem. For example, patients with Broca's aphasic will read and write in a telegraphic or agrammatic manner with paraphasic errors evident when reading aloud or in writing. Although disorders of reading and writing are always present in aphasia, the reverse is not true. Acquired disorders of reading (alexia) and writing (agraphia) may be present without an accompanying aphasic disorder; that is, pure alexia or pure agraphia may exist even when the patient can speak and understand language normally.

Table 4-7
PATTERN OF NEUROPSYCHOLOGICAL DEFICITS IN APHASIA

Cognitive Domain	Performance
Attention	Normal
Memory	Impaired verbal, normal nonverbal
Intelligence	Normal
Language	Impaired
Visuospatial	Normal
"Executive"	Normal

DISORDERS OF SPEECH

Certain disorders involving the motor mechanisms of speech production may be mistaken for aphasia. *Mutism* is a disorder of speech output and is often seen in conjunction with akinesia or hypokinesia. Mutism has been associated with mesial frontal lobe lesions involving the anterior cingulate gyrus or supplementary motor area. *Aphonia,* loss of the voice, and hypophonia, diminished voice volume, may be caused by diseases of the larynx or its innervation. *Dysarthria* is a speech disorder involving the muscles of articulation. Dysarthria may occur in association with aphasia or as the sole manifestation of damage to corticobulbar tracts, cerebellum, extrapyramidal pathways, or of the cranial nerves underlying pronunciation (nerves V, VII, IX, X, and XII).

As in these pure motor disorders of speech, disturbances of prosody may also occur without compromise to linguistic processes. *Prosody* refers to the intonation or melody of speech that is produced by varying pitch and rhythm. Disorders of prosody, the *aprosodias,* are caused by lesions in the right hemisphere in most individuals and can occur in the absence of aphasia.

☐ PURE ATTENTIONAL DISORDERS

DEFINITION

Pure attentional disorders are characterized by a selective impairment in attention. This is a common, but relatively neglected, neurobehavioral syndrome primarily found among psychiatric and neurologic outpatients. The archaic term *aprosexia,* which is a Greek word meaning "attentional disturbance" or "failure to heed," has been proposed[33] as the name of this common, yet under-recognized, syndrome.

Psychometrically, aprosexia is defined as a significant impairment of attention-concentration (digit span, mental arithmetic) with preserved verbal and nonverbal (performance) intelligence. Further, aprosexic patients do not meet criteria for any of the other neurobehavioral syndromes; that is, these patients are not amnesic, demented, acutely confused, or aphasic. Psychological complaints including insomnia, loss of energy, irritability, weight loss, and depression are common, as are complaints of reduced attentional capacity, memory deficits, and diminished speed of thought.

ETIOLOGY

Aprosexia is relatively rare among neurologic patients with active central nervous system (CNS) disease. It is primarily associated with psychiatric disturbances of all types (e.g., anxiety and affective disorders, psychoses, and personality disturbances). In a neuropsychological study of 83 aprosexics,[33] despite the presence of a few cases of neurological disease which could potentially cause the selective attention deficit—such as mild head injury, seizures, metabolic diseases, and multiple sclerosis—over 90 percent of these patients obtained abnormal Minnesota Multiphasic Personality Inventory profiles. This suggests that although pure attentional disorders may be seen in patients with neurological disorders, it is chiefly associated with potentially treatable psychopathology.

PATTERN OF NEUROPSYCHOLOGICAL IMPAIRMENT

As depicted in Table 4-8, deficits on tests of attention and concentration are always present in aprosexia while impaired performance on verbal and nonverbal memory tests are common but not invariably obtained. Tests measuring visuomotor speed are also frequently impaired. Intelligence, language, visuospatial functions are always normal in aprosexia. A minority of these patients may perform in the impaired range on certain tests of executive functions that require sustained attention. However, these test failures should not be interpreted as implying defects in "frontal lobe" functioning, but rather as being due to an inability to conform to the task demands. On tests of executive abilities that do not place an undue burden on attention, aprosexics perform normally.

Table 4-8
PATTERN OF NEUROPSYCHOLOGICAL DEFICITS IN PURE ATTENTIONAL DISORDERS (APROSEXIA)

Cognitive Domain	Performance
Attention	Impaired
Memory	Variably impaired
Intelligence	Normal
Language	Normal
Visuospatial	Normal
"Executive"	Normal

DIFFERENTIAL DIAGNOSIS

Aprosexia is a common neurobehavioral disorder among neurological and psychiatric outpatients. The neurobehavioral syndromes most likely to be confused with aprosexia are amnesia and dementia (in its earliest stages). Amnesia may be distinguished from aprosexia by the knowledge that tests of attention will be normal in amnesia. In dementia, there will be a global loss of cognitive functions such as a reduction in IQ while similar losses will not be observed in aprosexia. Further, the characteristic complaints of aprosexic patients may differ from those in other neurobehavioral disorders, with common complaints being attentional disability, insomnia, energy loss, and irritability. Although aprosexia is not caused by any specific medical condition, there is a high association between aprosexia and psychological disturbances of all types.[33]

REFERENCES

1. James W: *The Principles of Psychology*. New York, Holt, Rinehart and Winston, 1890.
2. Atkinson RC, Shiffrin RM: Human memory: A proposed system and its control processes, in Spence KW, Spence JT (eds): *Advances in the Psychology of Learning and Motivation Research and Theory*, vol 2. New York, Academic Press, 1968.
3. Miller GA: The magical number seven, plus or minus two: Some limits on our capacity for processing information. *Psychol Rev* 68:81–97, 1956.
4. Hamsher KdeS: Specialized neuropsychological assessment methods, in Goldstein G, Hersen M (eds): *Handbook of Psychological Assessment*. New York, Pergamon Press, 1984, pp 235–256.
5. Mattarazzo JD: *Wechsler's Measurement and Appraisal of Adult Intelligence*, 5th ed. New York, Oxford University Press, 1972.
6. Buschke H, Fuld PA: Evaluating storage, retention, and retrieval in disordered memory and learning. *Neurology* 24:1019–1025, 1974.
7. Hamsher KdeS, Benton AL, Digre K: Serial digit learning: Normative and clinical aspects. *J Clin Neuropsychol* 2:39–50, 1980.
8. Wechsler D, Stone CP: *Wechsler Memory Scale Manual*. New York, The Psychological Corporation, 1945.
9. Osterrieth PA: Le test de copie d'une figure complexe. *Archives de Psychologie* 30:206–356, 1944.
10. Wechsler D: *Wechsler Adult Intelligence Scale Manual* (revised). New York, The Psychological Corporation, 1981.
11. Goodglass H, Kaplan E: *Assessment of Aphasia and Related Disorders*, 2d ed. Philadelphia, Lea & Febiger, 1983.

12. Benton AL, Hamsher KdeS: *Multilingual Aphasia Examination.* Iowa City, AJA & Associates, 1978.

13. Kertesz A: *Aphasia and Associated Disorders.* New York, Grune and Stratton, 1979.

14. Hamsher KdeS, Levin HS, Benton AL: Facial recognition in patients with focal brain lesions. *Arch Neurol* 36:837–839, 1979.

15. Benton AL, Hamsher KdeS, Varney NR, Spreen O: *Contributions to Neuropsychological Assessment.* New York, Oxford University Press, 1983.

16. Benton AL, Varney NR, Hamsher KdeS: Visuospatial judgment: A clinical test. *Arch Neurol* 35:364–367, 1978.

17. Boll TJ: The Halstead-Reitan neuropsychology battery, in Filskov SB, Boll TJ (eds): *Handbook of Clinical Neuropsychology.* New York, Wiley Interscience, 1981, pp 577–607.

18. Grant DA, Berg EA: A behavioral analysis of degree of reinforcement and ease of shifting to new responses in a Weigl-type card-sorting problem. *J Exp Psychol* 38:404–411, 1948.

19. Porteus SD: *The Maze Test and Clinical Psychology.* Palo Alto, Pacific Books, 1959.

20. Adams RD, Victor M: *Principles of Neurology,* 2d. ed. New York, McGraw-Hill, chap 20, 1981, p 287.

21. Joynt RJ, Shoulson I: Dementia, in Heilman KE, Valenstein E (eds): *Clinical Neuropsychology,* 2d ed. New York, Oxford University Press, chap 15, 1985, pp 453–479.

22. Wilson RS, Rosenbaum G, Brown G: The problem of premorbid intelligence in neuropsychological assessment. *J Clin Neuropsychol* 1:49–53, 1979.

23. Barona A, Reynolds CR, Chastain R: A demographically based index of premorbid intelligence for the WAIS-R. *J Consult Clin Psychol* 52:885–887, 1984.

24. Benton AL, Fogel M: Three-dimensional constructional praxis: A clinical test. *Arch Neurol* 7:347–354, 1962.

25. Wechsler D: *Wechsler Intelligence Scale for Children Manual* (revised). New York, The Psychological Corporation, 1974.

26. Perret E: The left frontal lobe of man and the suppression of habitual responses in verbal categorical behavior. *Neuropsychologia* 12:323–330, 1974.

27. Wells CE: Pseudodementia. *Am J Psychiat* 136:895–900, 1979.

28. Lipowski ZJ: *Delirium: Acute Confusional States.* New York, Oxford University Press, 1990.

29. Wells CE: Organic syndromes: Delirium, in Kaplan HI, Sadock BJ (eds): *Comprehensive Textbook of Psychiatry,* 4th ed. Baltimore, Williams & Wilkins, 1985, pp 838–851.

30. Adams RD, Victor M: *Principles of Neurology,* 4th ed. New York, McGraw-Hill, 1989, pp 323–333.

31. Levenson AJ (ed): *Neuropsychiatric Side Effects of Drugs in the Elderly.* New York, Raven Press, 1979.

32. Damasio AR, Damasio H, Rizzo M, Varney N, Gersh F: Aphasia with nonhemorrhagic lesions of the basal ganglia and internal capsule. *Arch Neurol* 39:15–20, 1982.

33. Hamsher KdeS, Lee GP: Aprosexia: An actuarial study of a nomen nudem. *J Clin Exp Neuropsychol* 8:120, 1986 (abstract).

34. Rey A: *L'examen Clinique en Psychologie.* Paris, Presses Universitaires de France, 1964.

35. Benton AL: *The Revised Visual Retention Test,* 4th ed. New York, The Psychological Corporation, 1974.

36. Terman LM, Merrill MA: *Stanford-Binet Intelligence Scale.* Boston, Houghton Mifflin, 1973.

37. Bayley N: *Bayley's Scales of Infant Development.* New York, The Psychological Corporation, 1968.

38. Gronwall D, Wrightson P: Memory and information processing capacity after closed head injury. *J Neurol Neurosurg Psychiat* 44:889–895, 1981.

39. Grant ML, Ilai D, Nussbaum NL, Bigler E: The relationship between continuous performance tasks and neuropsychological tests in children with attention-deficit hyperactivity disorder. *Percept Motor Skills* 70:435–445, 1990.

40. Weintraub S, Mesulam MM: Mental state assessment of young and elderly adults in behavioral neurology, in Mesulam MM (ed): *Principles of Behavioral Neurology.* Philadelphia, F.A. Davis, 1985, pp 71–123.

41. Matthews CG, Klove H: *Instruction Manual for the Adult Neuropsychological Test Battery.* Madison, Wisconsin, University of Wisconsin Medical School, 1964.

42. Lezak MD: *Neuropsychological Assessment,* 2d ed. New York, Oxford University Press, 1983.

43. Strub RL, Black FW: *The Mental Status Examination in Neurology,* 2d ed. Philadelphia, F.A. Davis, 1987.

☐ STUDY QUESTIONS

I. A 78-year-old female is admitted, confused, disoriented, forgetful, but with normal speech. She has slowed motor function and coordinated movements require more time than for young individuals, but discrete sensory and motor tests were normal. Reflexes were also normal.

1. What is the most likely diagnosis? **2.** What is the anticipated prognosis assuming a diagnosis of Alzheimer's disease? **3.** How might Alzheimer's disease be differentiated from an acute confusional state. **4.** How might the picture in this patient be differentiated from a described lesion of the dominant hemisphere? **5.** What are alternative causes of dementia?

II. A 30-year-old left-handed male is admitted with seizures, the focus of which are located in the medial left temporal lobe. The seizures are not controlled by medications. The patient is seeking surgical therapy.

1. How can one lateralize the dominant hemisphere? **2.** What functions might be interrupted if a large temporal lobectomy is performed on the dominant hemisphere? **3.** What type of aphasia might occur? **4.** What might be the expected effect of resection of the hippocampus unilaterally? **5.** What functional deficits might result from resection of the posterior portion of the superior temporal gyrus?

III. A 40-year-old male is admitted with confusion but no other apparent neurological deficits.

1. What are the common causes of confusion? **2.** How do confusional states affect memory? **3.** How do they affect learning? **4.** Where might cerebral lesions be located that might cause confusion? **5.** What are nonanatomical causes of acute confusion?

IV. A 20-year-old female has a head injury and is unable to carry on any meaningful conversation. She utters meaningless vocalizations.

1. What is the most likely type of aphasia? **2.** What other cognitive functions are likely to be affected? **3.** The injury is most likely lateralized to which side? **4.** Would memory likely be affected? **5.** What is the prognosis?

V. 1. What is aprosexia? **2.** Is aprosexia more likely to be associated with organic or functional disorders? **3.** How will aprosexia affect learning? **4.** How will it affect memory? **5.** What is the treatment for aprosexia?

APPENDIX A: SELECTED NEUROPSYCHOLOGICAL TESTS

Detailed descriptions of these tests may be found in Lezak[42] and Strub and Black.[43] Superscript numbers denote references.

LEARNING AND MEMORY

Wechsler Memory Scale[8]
Selective Reminding Test[6]
Serial Digit Learning[7]
Rey Auditory Verbal Learning Test[34]
Benton Visual Retention Test[35]
Rey-Osterrieth Complex Figure Test[9]

INTELLIGENCE

WAIS-R (WIPPSI, WISC-R)[10]
Stanford-Binet Intelligence Scale (4th ed)[36]
Bayley Scales for Infant Development[37]

ATTENTION AND CONCENTRATION

WAIS-R Digit Span[10]
WAIS-R Arithmetic[10]
Trailmaking Test[17]
Paced Auditory Serial Addition Task[38]
Halstead-Reitan Attention Tests (Speech-sounds & Seashore Rhythm Test)[17]
Continuous Performance Tasks[39]
Cancellation Tasks[40]

SPEECH AND LANGUAGE

Boston Diagnostic Aphasia Examination[11]
Multilingual Aphasia Examination[12]
Western Aphasia Battery[13]

VISUOPERCEPTION AND VISUOSPATIAL FUNCTIONS

Facial Recognition Test[14]
Visual Form Discrimination[15]
Judgment of Line Orientation[16]
Three-dimensional Constructional Praxis[24]

MOTOR TESTS

Finger Tapping[17]
Grooved Pegboard[41]

EXECUTIVE (FRONTAL LOBE) FUNCTIONS

Category Test[17]
Wisconsin Card Sorting Test[18]
Stroop Color and Word Test[26]
Word Fluency or F-A-S Test[12]

CHAPTER

5

Electrodiagnostic Evaluations of Patients with Lesions Involving the Nervous System

Herman F. Flanigin
Anthony M. Murro

Electrical activity of the brain is either spontaneous or event-related. *Spontaneous activity* is unrelated to transient or repetitive events occurring within the body or in the body's environment. Spontaneous activity includes *direct current (DC) potentials, alternating current (AC) potentials,* and *unit potentials* (Fig. 5-1).

DC potentials are slowly changing shifts in the brain's electrical baseline. AC potentials are more rapidly changing potentials, such as rhythmic EEG activity. Unit potentials are small intracellular or extracellular potentials of brief duration recorded by microelectrodes from individual neurons. Unit potentials depend on the spatial orientation of the neurons and their processes. In discharging, they create a dipole which may be summated by orientation, synchronization, and recruitment to reach a level that can be recorded from the scalp.

Event-related potentials (ERPs) or *event-related responses (ERRs)* occur as a result of external or internal events. The term *event-related responses* is more descriptive than evoked responses because the responses occur as a result of a transient or recurrent event.

Examples of internally generated ERPs are the prefrontal negative waves recorded while anticipating a movement and the potentials recorded from the temporal region while solving a specific problem of choice between two audible tones.

External ERPs occur following stimulation of visual, au-

ditory, and somatosensory systems. These are described as *visual evoked potentials (VEPs), auditory evoked potentials (AEPs),* and *somatosensory evoked potentials (SSEPs).*

☐ ELECTROENCEPHALOGRAPHY (EEG)

Comprehensive references covering the general topic of electroencephalography may be of assistance in understanding this subject.[1]

Scalp electroencephalography uses cup-shaped disk electrodes. The electrodes are fixed to the scalp with collodion. An electrolyte gel forms a conductive interface between the scalp and electrode. The $\frac{10}{20}$ *system*[2] has been adopted by the American EEG society as a standard system for electrode placement. The "$\frac{10}{20}$" refers to interelectrode distances expressed as percentages of anterior-posterior, transverse, and circumferential head measurements (Fig 5-2).

In addition, special electrodes inserted against the inferior surface of the greater wing of the sphenoid bone beneath the medial temporal lobe (sphenoidal electrodes) record from the basilar and medial temporal lobe regions (Fig. 5-3).

The electroencephalograph amplifies minute scalp potentials as low as 2 to 3 microvolts (μV) and provides a record of the scalp voltage over time. Differential amplifiers

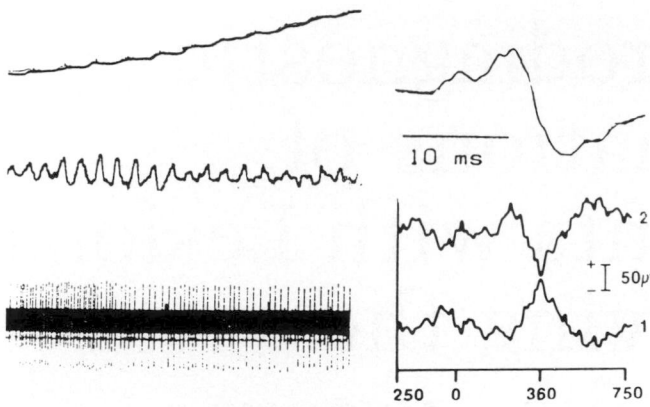

Figure 5–1 Spontaneous brain electrical activity (left): DC current (top), alternating current (middle), unit potentials (bottom). Event-related responses (right): somatosensory evoked response recorded over the sensory cortex (top), cognitive related response showing phase reversal (bottom), recorded from limbic structures.

amplify the difference in potentials between two input leads but are insensitive to the potentials common to both input leads *(common mode rejection)*.

The EEG amplifier's bandwidth is usually between 0.5 and 70 hertz (Hz). The low and high filter settings are adjusted to accentuate low or high EEG frequencies for interpretation. Notch filters exclude a 60-Hz artifact from external power sources. Although DC currents occur in the brain, special DC amplifiers are required to record signals below 0.5 Hz. At a typical sensitivity of 7 μV per millimeter, a 50-μV calibration signal produces a 7-mm deflection.

The time constant of the EEG filter is the time for a sustained calibrated input signal to decay or fall to 37 percent of its initial deflection. This decay of pen deflection to a sustained voltage input explains why DC voltages require special recording equipment. Amplifier sensitivity and paper speed may be adjusted to enhance EEG interpretation.

EEG amplifiers have two inputs, designated as "input 1" and "input 2." By convention, when the potential of input 1 is more negative than input 2, the EEG produces an upward pen deflection. Multiple matched calibrated amplifiers,

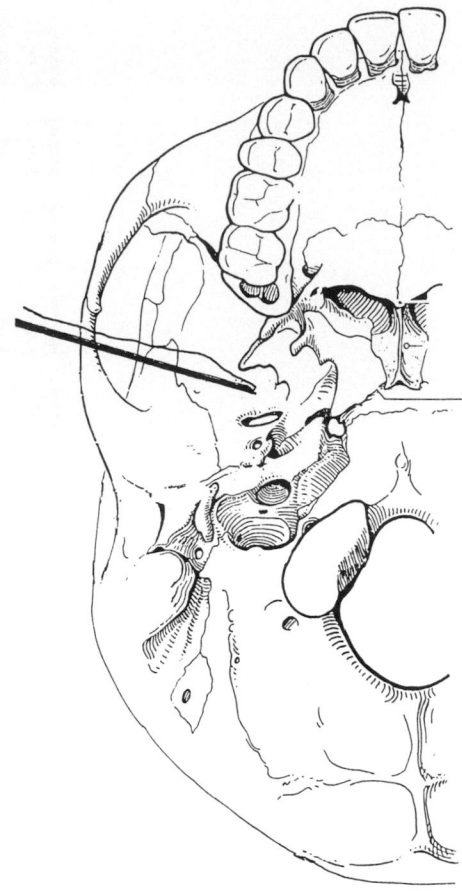

Figure 5–3 Schematic drawing of introducer placing sphenoidal electrode on the inferior surface of the greater wing of the sphenoid bone near the foramen ovale.

called "channels," simultaneously record from sixteen or more scalp areas. The filter and sensitivity settings are usually the same for all channels. The recording montage is the list of recording sites used for inputs 1 and 2 of each channel. A recording is made between an active site and a single inactive site *(referential, or monopolar, montage)* or between successive adjacent recording sites *(sequential, or bipolar, montage)*.

With a specific localized electrical discharge in the brain, in a referential montage, the maximum pen deflection occurs in the channel recording from the most-active scalp site. In a sequential, or bipolar, montage, a reversal in polarity between two adjacent channels *(phase reversal)* determines the most-active recording site (Fig. 5-4).

EEG interpretation depends on the duration, topography, and form of EEG waves. *Waveforms* may be described as rhythmic, sinusoidal, transient, spike, sharp, sharply contoured, truncated, biphasic, polyphasic, spike and wave, multiple spike and wave, amorphous, or polymorphous.

EEG ACTIVITY IN THE NORMAL BRAIN

Normal electrical brain activity depends on the recording site, the subject's age, and the state of alertness (alert,

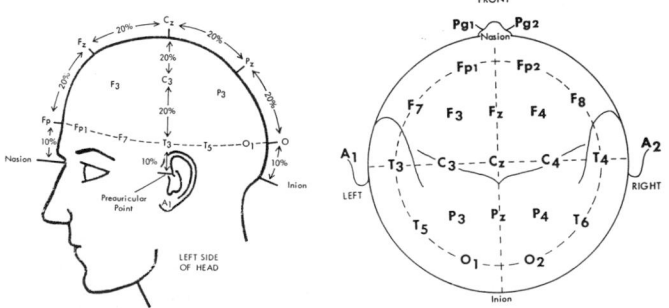

Figure 5–2 Standard 10-20 international system of electrode placement. Position and measurements for electrode placement, viewed from the left side (left). Electrode positions viewed from the vertex (right).

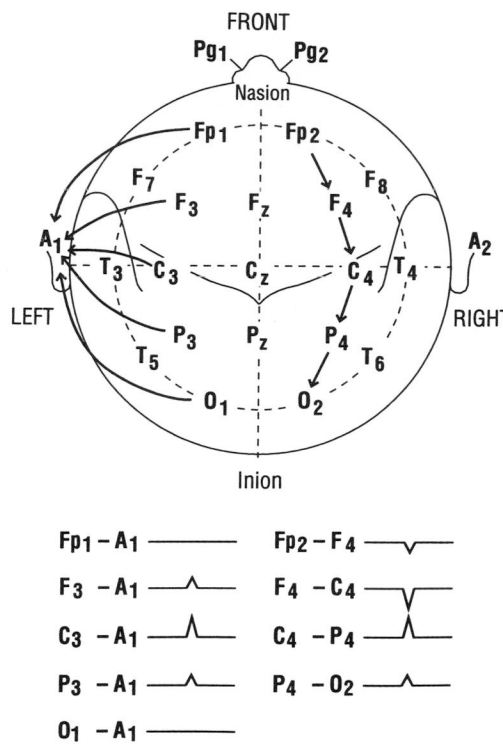

Figure 5–4 The montage for a referential montage is illustrated on the left side of the head and a sequential montage on the right (top). Stylized tracings on the left illustrate an assumed spike focus at the C3 electrode recorded with a referential montage and on the right an assumed spike focus at F4 recorded with a sequential montage (bottom).

drowsy, or asleep). In general, however, the activity recorded in an individual should be fairly symmetrical.

Frequency is designated in cycles per second, or Hertz (Hz), and is divided into four *bands*. The bands are *delta* (0.5–4 Hz), *theta* (4–8 Hz), *alpha* (8–13 Hz), and *beta* (13 Hz and above) (Fig. 5-5).

Amplitude varies markedly from one individual to another, from one location to another, and with frequency.

ADULT EEG ACTIVITY

Alpha activity is best seen in the awake, resting subject with the eyes closed. The amplitude is generally about 20 to 50 μV and the frequency ranges from 8 to 12 Hz. It is recorded maximally over the parietal and occipital regions but may appear to a lesser degree over other areas. Alpha activity often attenuates or modulates with eye opening or with mental activities. The amplitude often waxes and wanes over periods of 1 to 2 s, a phenomenon called "spindling." Alpha activity is absent during sleep.

Beta activity is usually less than 20 μV in amplitude. It is often maximal over the frontal and central regions. Under careful observation, it may diminish with voluntary motor tasks. Some intermingling occurs over other head regions.

Theta activity intermingles with other frequencies. Its usual location is in the temporal and central regions.

NORMAL SLEEP ACTIVITY

Decreased axial muscle tone, phasic eye movements, irregular cardiac and respiratory activity, penile erections, vivid dreaming, EEG sawtooth waves, and EEG low-voltage theta and delta activity occur during *rapid eye movement (REM)* sleep.

Non-REM sleep is divided into stages I to IV. The occurrence of sleep transients (sleep spindles and K complexes) and the amount of sleep delta determines the non-REM sleep stage. Sleep delta is less than 2 Hz and greater than 75 μV.

Stage I sleep contains no sleep transients, and the EEG consists of low-voltage 2- to 7-Hz activity. Sleep transients occur during the remaining non-REM sleep stages. *Stage II sleep* contains less than 20 percent sleep delta. *Stage III sleep* contains 20 to 50 percent sleep delta. *Stage IV sleep* contains greater than 50 percent sleep delta.

NORMAL INFANTS AND CHILDREN

There are major differences between EEGs recorded from infants and children of different ages and the adult. In the premature infant with a conceptual age of less than 30 weeks, a discontinuous EEG pattern of prolonged low-voltage periods alternating with brief slow-wave bursts occurs. Continuous EEG patterns develop between 30 and 34 weeks conceptual age. Distinct EEG patterns that distinguish sleep from wakefulness develop between 35 and 37 weeks of conceptual age. Fully developed neonatal sleep patterns of quiet and active sleep occur after 37 weeks of conceptual age.

During infancy, a posterior rhythmic 3- to 4-Hz activity occurs by 3 months of age. This background frequency increases to 5 Hz at 6 months, 6 to 7 Hz at 1 year, 7 to 8 Hz at 18 months, and 9 to 11 Hz during young adulthood. Theta and delta activity is commonly seen in the posterior scalp regions during childhood and young adulthood (posterior slow waves of youth).

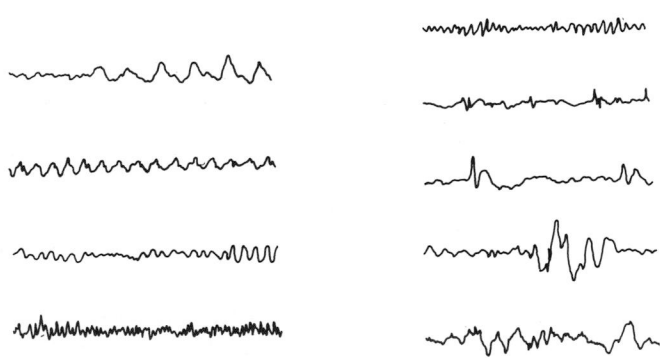

Figure 5–5 Frequency bands top to bottom (left): delta, theta, alpha, and beta. Typical waveforms top to bottom (right): rhythmic sinusoidal, rhythmic low-voltage spikes, spike and slow wave, polyspike and slow wave, and polymorphous waves.

ABNORMAL WAVE FORMS

Spikes are sharply contoured waves, less than 80 ms in duration. They occur repetitively and have an amplitude significantly greater than the background. Spikes occur alone or followed by a slow wave (spike and wave). Multiple spikes followed by a slow wave *(polyspike and wave)* are associated with generalized seizures. Spike and wave discharges can be regular (rhythmic) or irregular.

Sharp waves are similar to spikes but have a duration between 80 to 200 ms. Spikes and sharp waves are epileptiform discharges and are associated with epilepsy.

Persistent polymorphic focal delta activity is associated with focal structural brain lesions such as stroke, tumor, abscess, or contusions. The location of this EEG abnormality corresponds closely to the site of the structural brain lesion.

Intermittent bilateral synchronous rhythmic delta is associated with diffuse metabolic, degenerative, or toxic disease. The location of this EEG abnormality is usually frontal or occipital and does not correspond to the site of the underlying brain abnormality.

ACTIVATION PROCEDURES

Activation procedures have been developed to precipitate abnormal EEG activity.

Hyperventilation over 3 min reduces arterial CO_2, produces cerebral vasoconstriction, and results in bilateral rhythmic EEG slowing in normal patients. In patients with absence seizures, hyperventilation will produce paroxysmal rhythmic spike and wave discharges.

Photic stimulation often produces rhythmic synchronous posterior activity in normal patients *(photic driving response)*. In some patients, photic stimulation produces synchronous myoclonic jerks *(photomyoclonic response)*. In patients with generalized epilepsy, photic stimulation may produce seizure activity *(photoconvulsive response)*.

Sleep deprivation, on the evening prior to the EEG recording, increases the diagnostic sensitivity of the EEG for patients with epilepsy. Epileptiform discharges occur more frequently during non-REM sleep. In some patients, sleep deprivation will induce seizures.

Hydration, alcohol, metrazol, amytal, and brevital have all been used to precipitate epileptiform discharges, but this will not be discussed further here (Fig. 5-6).

PROLONGED MONITORING

Prolonged EEG-video monitoring is used to evaluate episodic events such as seizures. Multiple EEG channels are encoded (multiplexed) as a single channel that is stored on an audio channel of a videotape. A video camera simultaneously records the patient's behavior onto the same videotape. Radio or cable telemetry EEG recordings allow the patient to remain mobile during the recording.[3] A technologist may communicate with the patient and record significant behavioral observations for correlation with the EEG.

ELECTROENCEPHALOGRAPHIC INVESTIGATION

While imaging studies reveal structural brain abnormalities, the EEG reveals functional brain abnormalities. The EEG will reveal abnormalities associated with clinically latent disease in patients with epilepsy and in metabolic, toxic, and traumatic disease.

The site of seizure onset *(seizure focus)* is determined by the location of epileptiform discharges in the initial stages of electrographic seizure activity. Focal slow-wave activity may occur in association with epileptiform discharges at the same site.

Diffuse polymorphic activity is associated with diffuse brain disease such as results from inflammatory, toxic, vascular, anoxic, and degenerative disorders.

Diffuse rhythmic 10-Hz sinusoidal activity is seen at times in coma states *(alpha coma)*. The frontal predominance, absence of spindles, and lack of modulation distinguish this from true alpha as seen in the normal subject.

Acute hemispheric brain lesions and acute exacerbations of partial seizures are associated with periodic lateralized epileptiform discharges (PLEDS). Periodic bisynchronous 0.5- to 2-Hz discharges are associated with Jakob-Creutzfeld (JC) disease. Periodic discharges on a flat background are associated with anoxic coma and myoclonus. In patients with subacute sclerosing panencephalitis (SSPE), periodic 100- to 1000-μV, 0.5- to 3-s, slow-wave bursts occur with 4- to 15-s interburst intervals.

CORTICAL MAPPING

Cortical mapping includes the recording of spontaneous electrical activity, stimulation of the cortex for localizing cortical representation of function, and evoked potential recording for localization of sensory primary projection cortex. The latter will be described later in this chapter. The use of mapping techniques is not confined to epilepsy surgery. The preservation of functional cortex during resection of intracerebral tumors and vascular malformations is aided by accurate identification of speech and sensorimotor cortex, and, at times, of visual cortex.

STIMULATION STUDIES

When stimulation mapping is required for identification of speech and sensorimotor cortex, it is necessary to perform the studies under local anesthesia, as described in Chap. 22. Electrocorticography may be indicated for seizure activity associated with the lesion to be resected. Following acquisition of spontaneous electrographic activity, stimulation studies are performed as described in Chap. 22.

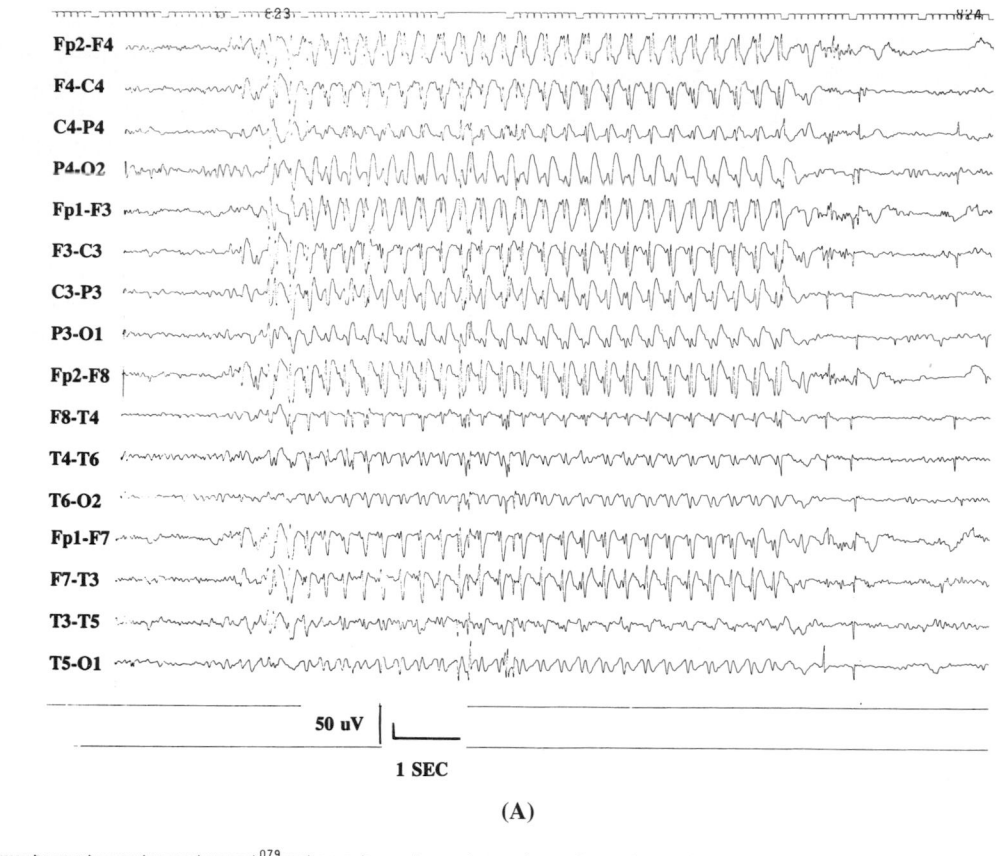

50 uV

1 SEC

(A)

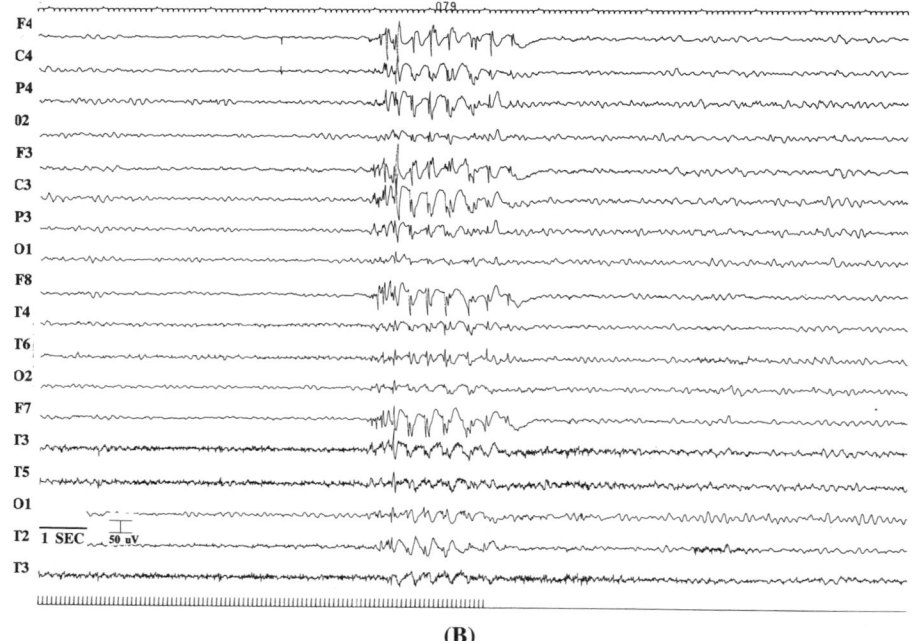

(B)

Figure 5–6 Activation by hyperventilation (*A*) and photic stimulation (*B*). (Note photic stimulation artifact in last channel.)

Cortical threshold for stimulation parameters is determined by responses in the lower sensorimotor strip, after which motor and speech areas are identified by stimulation. A response cannot be considered negative unless the threshold for stimulation parameters has been established by positive responses reproducible elsewhere in the cortex in the same patient. Cortical response positions are indicated with numbered tickets and recorded photographically.

☐ EVENT-RELATED RESPONSES (EVOKED POTENTIALS): SENSORY

A flash visual evoked response sometimes occurs in the occipital region during photic stimulation on the routine EEG; however, low-amplitude electrical response to a stimulus is usually obscured by ongoing spontaneous electrical brain activity. The appearance of the event-related response is improved by

76   CHAPTER 5

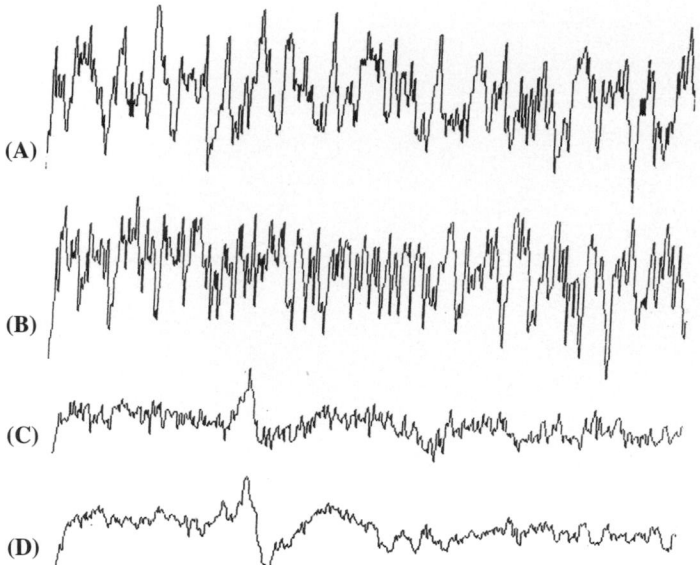

Figure 5–7 Effect of averaging on recorded signals. *A.* Single sweep. *B.* Averaging of 10 sweeps. *C.* Averaging of 100 sweeps. *D.* Averaging of 1000 sweeps.

averaging multiple responses that are time-locked to the stimulus. These responses are summated and averaged so that with a sufficient number of epochs the background activity is canceled and the response can be identified (Fig. 5-7).

INSTRUMENTATION

Stimulating Device The stimulating device must produce an appropriate stimulus type and signal the onset of the stimulus to the computer that performs the signal averaging. Stimulus intensity and frequency are programmable.

Visual stimulation for visual evoked responses (VERs) includes flash, pattern reversal (PR), and light-emitting diode (LED) array stimuli. All VERs are performed with monocular testing. During a pattern reversal VER, the patient maintains fixation on a screen of alternating bright and dark squares. Stimulation occurs when the dark squares become bright and the bright squares simultaneously become dark.

Retrochiasmatic lesions of the visual pathways are evaluated using monocular hemifield stimulation. The pattern reversal VER is more sensitive than the other VERs for detecting conduction defects of the visual pathways. The pattern reversal study, however, requires greater patient cooperation and concentration, which are not necessary with flash or LED VERs.

Auditory stimulation is obtained from broad-spectrum clicks, or single-frequency tone pips. Stimulus intensity is measured in decibels (dB) above a reference level. The commonly used reference levels are the normal hearing level (NHL) and the sensation level (SL). NHL is the average auditory threshold from a normal population. SL is the auditory threshold of the subject's ear. Each ear is tested separately while the opposite ear is masked with white (broad-spectrum, multifrequency) noise.

Auditory stimuli are also used to obtain the P300 cognitive evoked potentials. For this study the auditory stimulus is either a low- or high-pitched tone. One of the tones is presented rarely, and the sequence of rare and frequent tones is random. The patient is asked to identify and count the number of rare tones. The average evoked response to rare tones will contain a positive potential with an average latency of 300 ms (P300).

Audiometry may also be obtained by AEPs using tone pips. The threshold for hearing successive frequencies is charted for each ear while the opposite ear is masked. These studies may be obtained for both air and bone conduction.

Somatosensory evoked potentials (SSEPs) are obtained from mechanical or electrical stimuli applied to the upper extremities (median nerve SSEP) or lower extremities (posterior tibial or peroneal nerve SSEP). Stimulus duration, intensity, and frequency are adjustable.

Recording Instrumentation Each channel amplifies up to 500,000 times. The low filter settings are typically 1, 5, 10, 25, 50, 100, and 300 Hz, and the high filter settings are 100, 250, 500, 1000, and 3000 Hz, providing for cutoff of high frequencies. The rate of signal attenuation (rolloff) is greater for digital than analogue filters. Phase-free digital filters, unlike analogue filters, do not change evoked potential peak latencies. A 60-Hz notch filter reduces artifact from external power sources.

Averaging Equipment Averaging is accomplished by computer. The analogue-to-digital converter (ADC) transforms the analogue signal to a digital form. An 8-bit ADC has a resolution of 1/256 of the full ADC voltage range. A 12-bit ADC has a finer resolution of 1/4096 of the full ADC voltage range. Signals with an amplitude beyond the ADC voltage range are rejected for averaging *(artifact rejection).*

The computer averages serial-recorded samples *(epochs)* triggered by the stimulator. The evoked response is enhanced because it is time-locked to the stimulus; however, spontaneous activity unrelated to the stimulus is nullified by averaging. The *intersample interval (ISI)* is the time between successive ADC voltage measurements. The reciprocal of the ISI is the ADC's *sampling frequency.* The sampling frequency must exceed twice the fastest frequency component of the recorded data *(Nyquist frequency).* A sampling frequency below the Nyquist frequency causes an aliasing *(harmonic error).* Sweep time is the duration of the entire recorded epoch. Usually 4 to 8 channels are used to record progressive transmission of neural activity from multiple sites of the nervous system.

A record of the average baseline prior to stimulation is obtained by a triggered average for a fixed period prior to stimulation. Recorded stimulus artifact is reduced by beginning the triggered averaging a fixed interval after stimulation. Using a cursor, the amplitude and latencies of evoked responses are measured on a screen. This information is stored on a computer disk and printed by the computer. The convention on the direction of pen deflection and signal polarity varies among manufacturers and laboratories.

The distance between the active recording electrode and the neural generator of an evoked potential peak varies. If this distance is small, the response is termed a *near field potential*. If this distance is large, the response is termed a *far field potential*. The short latency brainstem auditory evoked responses (BAERs) are examples of far field potentials. Physiological transmission must be distinguished from electrical conduction.

☐ AUDITORY EVOKED RESPONSES

The *brainstem auditory evoked responses (BAERs)* or *brainstem auditory evoked potentials (BAEPs)* are also referred to as *auditory brainstem responses (ABRs)*. These short latency responses arise from cranial nerve VIII and the brainstem. Auditory stimuli are also used to elicit the long latency P300 cognitive evoked response.

Waves I to VIII may be present, but only waves I to V are of significant clinical value.

The auditory nerve generates waves I and II. The auditory nerve produces a positive wave II recorded from the vertex. The auditory nerve near the porus acusticus produces the second negative peak recorded from the earlobe. The interval between these positive and negative waves measures the *intracranial auditory nerve transmission time*. This travel time is abnormal in neurovascular compression syndromes.[4]

Wave III is generated in the lower pons by the cochlear nucleus.[5] Wave IV may receive input from several sources, including the lateral lemniscus and the superior olivary nucleus.[5] This is also the earliest wave that receives contributions from contralateral structures. Wave V appears to be derived from the lateral lemniscus and the inferior colliculus. Waves IV and V tend to fuse on the ipsilateral side and become more discrete on the contralateral side. Waves VI and VII may be generated in the inferior colliculus (Fig. 5-8).

☐ SHORT LATENCY SOMATOSENSORY EVOKED RESPONSES

These responses are most frequently used for study of the sensory pathways from the median nerve in the upper extremity or the tibial nerve in the lower extremity. Stimulating electrodes are placed over the median nerve at the wrist or over the tibial nerve at the ankle.

Direct somesthetic pathway recordings suggest that the P13 cervical cord neurons generate the P13 wave and that the rostral brainstem medial lemniscus or ventral posterior lateral thalamic neurons generate the P14 wave.[6]

Height and age correlate with median nerve peak latencies but not with median nerve interpeak latencies. Men have longer N13 and N19 peak latencies than women.[7]

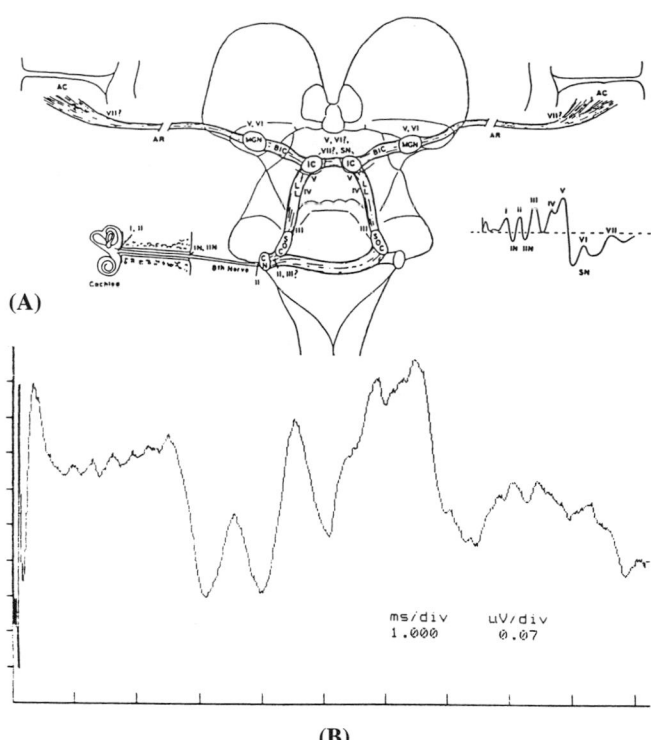

(A)

(B)

Figure 5–8 *A.* Schematic for stylized auditory evoked response and its anatomical generators. (*Legatt AD, Arezzo JC, Vaughn HG Jr: The Anatomic and physiologic bases of brain stem auditory evoked potentials. Neurol Clin 6:681–704, 1988. Reproduced with permission.*) *B.* Normal auditory evoked response, showing clearly defined waves I to IV. Vertex positive is up.

Depth electrode studies suggest that a positive 15.5-ms wave originates from postsynaptic activity of the nucleus ventrocaudalis. A much-lower-voltage, positive-negative-positive triphasic response with peak latencies of positive 13.3 and negative 16.0 ms maximum in the nucleus intermedius represents a presynaptic axonal potential generated in the rostral part of the lemniscal pathway and recorded by volume conduction (Fig. 5-9).[8]

TRIGEMINAL EVOKED RESPONSES

In addition to involvement in trigeminal neuralgia, the trigeminal nerve may be compressed by tumors of the skull base at several sites.

Stimulation is by a Teflon-coated electrode with bared tip inserted into the infraorbital foramen. The depth of insertion is critical for latency, and symmetrical placement is necessary. Square-wave stimulation parameters of 0.05 ms duration, with a frequency of 2 per second and intensity of 3 times the sensory threshold are satisfactory.

Recording electrodes are placed at Cz with reference to the C7 vertebral spinous process (Cv7).

Bilateral studies provide the opportunity for evaluation of a control and determination of symmetry.

With negative deflection upward, waves 1, 2, and 3 have latencies of 0.88, 1.80, and 2.44 ms, respectively. Interwave

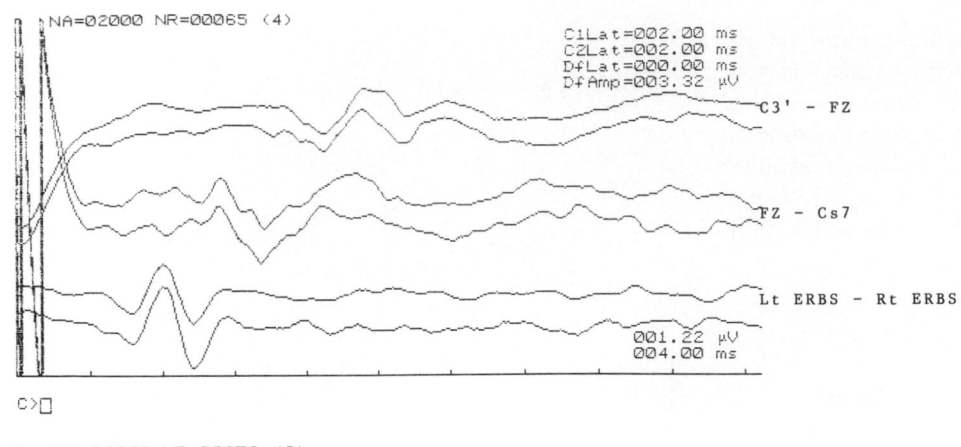

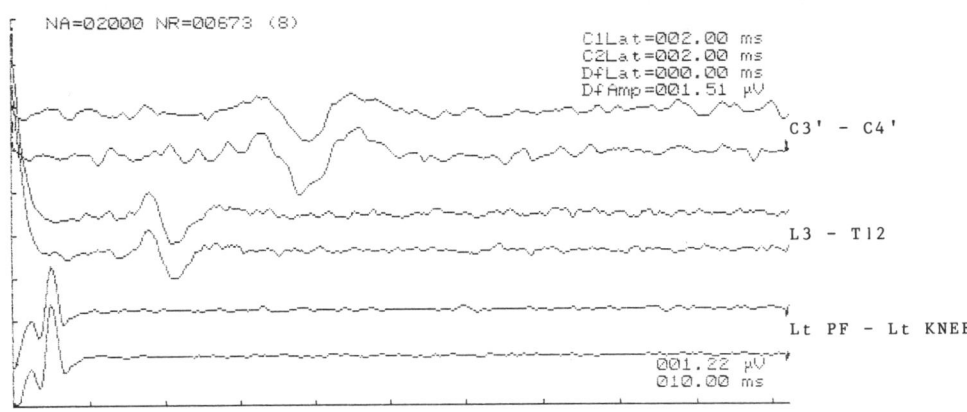

(B)

Figure 5–9 Normal SSERs obtained by stimulation of median nerve (*A*) and posterior tibial nerve (*B*). Negative is up.

latencies of 1 to 2 and 2 to 3 are 0.90 and 1.55 ms, respectively. An increase in the latency of wave 1 of more than 0.32 ms when compared to the normal side is considered abnormal. Wave 1 originates at the entrance of the maxillary division into the gasserian ganglion. Wave 2 originates from the root entry zone into the pons. The origin of wave 3 is at the presynaptic portion of the trigeminal tract within the pons.

Delay or absence of wave 2 and/or 3 on the affected side is seen in tumors of the skull base and in trigeminal neuralgia. This may be demonstrated even in patients with subclinical involvement of the nerve.

Anteriorly placed lesions along the trigeminal pathways are characterized by similar delays of waves 2 and 3. Lesions of the cerebellopontine angle produce greater changes in wave 3 than in wave 2. Wave 1 is altered only with anteriorly placed peripheral lesions. Absence of waves 2 and 3 may be demonstrated in patients successfully treated by surgery for trigeminal neuralgia.[9]

Evoked responses may also be obtained from stimulation of the supraorbital nerve. These are harder to obtain because of the difficulty involved in stabilization of the stimulating electrode and the need to anesthetize the scalp around the stimulating electrode to avoid motor responses. The amplitude of these responses is lower than those obtained by stimulating the maxillary division. While not identical to the responses from infraorbital stimulation, there are similarities in waveforms, latencies, and probably generators (Fig. 5-10).

☐ ELECTRORETINOGRAMS

Electroretinograms (ERGs) are responses in the retinae evoked by visual stimulation. Waves at less than 50 ms latency are thought to originate in the eye. Recording from stimulation of both eyes permits comparison of the responses, since only slight contralateral response to unilateral stimulation occurs. Stimulation by pattern reversal is preferred but flash may be used. The alpha (α) wave appearing at about 26 ms is mediated by the receptors, and the beta (β) wave appearing at about 45 ms is mediated by the ganglion cells. Rapid stimulation may result in overlapping responses [fast frequency following (FFF) or steady state]. Retinal disease may impair this response.[11]

Recording is accomplished, preferably from gold-foil electrodes inserted beneath the lower lid or from cup electrodes on the lower lid. For ERG recording, the reference electrode is placed on the ipsilateral temporal region, since VER contamination is reduced. Simultaneous recording of the VER using occipital electrodes permits correlation of the responses.[12] The ERG may persist in the absence of intracranial response in brain death (Fig. 5-11).

☐ VISUAL EVOKED RESPONSES

For usual clinical study, *pattern shift* (or *reversal*) *visual evoked responses* (PSVERs, PRVERs) are used. These have

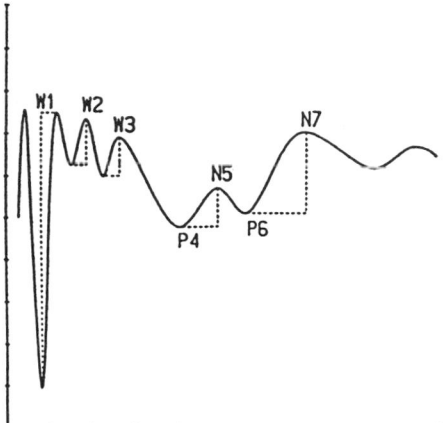
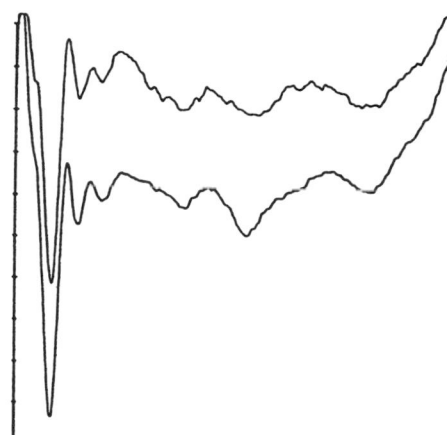

Figure 5–10 Stylized and actual normal trigeminal evoked responses. Negative is up. (*Leandri M, Parodi CI, Favale E: Normative data on scalp responses evoked by infraorbital nerve stimulation.* Electroencephalogr Clin Neurophysiol *71:415–421, 1988. Reproduced with permission.*)

less variability than strobe light studies and are more sensitive to abnormalities. For infants and uncooperative or unconscious patients, strobe light or LED studies are necessary.

PSVERs are obtained using a video screen placed 1 m from the patient, who may wear appropriate corrective lenses. A point of fixation is situated in the center of the screen. The screen is illuminated in a checkerboard pattern that alternately reverses the illuminated squares. The size of the squares and the frequency of reversal are controlled by computer. Control of half and quarter fields is also programmable. Sensitivity to detection of abnormalities is increased with smaller squares.

Depth electrode studies reveal both flash VERs and PRVER responses, as recorded from the scalp, and they appear to be generated entirely in the visual cortical structures. The initial negativity has a more-superficial generator than the large positive peak at 80 to 100 ms.[14] The response is dipole-oriented to the visual cortex, and placement of the recording electrode is critical to the response. Of note is the maximal response in the occipital region on the side of an absent occipital lobe (Fig. 5-12).

☐ OLFACTORY EVOKED POTENTIALS

Special techniques have been designed to record evoked potentials from the olfactory system. Stimulation is deliv-

ered unilaterally to the olfactory mucosa by switching cleaned filtered air, flowing at 20 ml per second, to similar air-containing odoriferous substances. The continuous flow prevents somatosensory response from a puff of air on the nonolfactory nasal mucosa.

The switching mechanism serves as the sweep trigger with a sweep time of 2048 ms. Recording is from Cz referred to A1. Waves designated as N1 may be obtained at 306 to 484 ms and P1 at 349 to 455 ms. Anosmic subjects are unable to generate evoked responses to vanillin.[15]

☐ INTRAOPERATIVE MONITORING

PRINCIPLES

The use of intraoperative evoked potential monitoring, particularly VERs, has been criticized for its inability to predict the outcome of a surgical procedure.[16] The expectation that intraoperative monitoring can predict the outcome of an operation is doomed to disappointment, although a high degree of correlation has been reported. Current evaluation of the use of intraoperative monitoring has been published by the American Academy of Neurology.[17]

The concept of "false negatives" and "false positives" as an evaluator of intraoperative monitoring is subordinated by whether neural damage is reduced by monitoring. The likelihood of prevention of a major neurological deficit by recognition and reversal of lost evoked potentials is so high that a

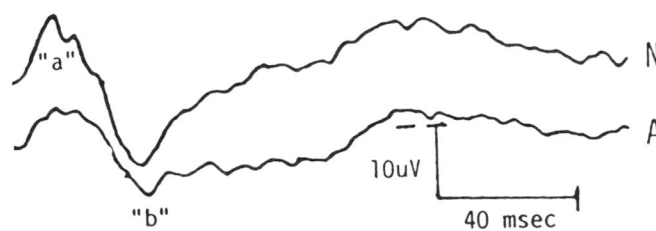

Figure 5–11 Electroretinograms. Normal eye (N). Abnormal eye (A) with optic neuritis associated with multiple sclerosis. Negative is up. (*Papakostopoulos D, Fotiou F, Hart JC, Banerji NK. The electroretinogram in multiple sclerosis and demyelinating optic neuritis.* Electroencephalogr Clin Neurophysiol *74:1–10, 1989. Reproduced with permission.*)

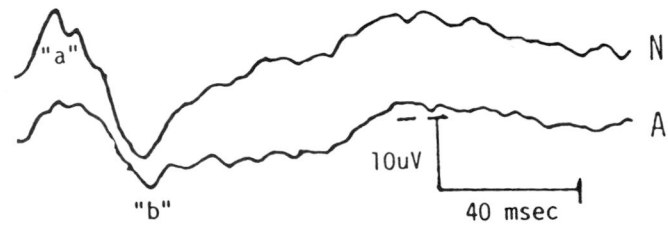

Figure 5–12 Visual evoked response. Sweep time, 200 ms. Positive is down.

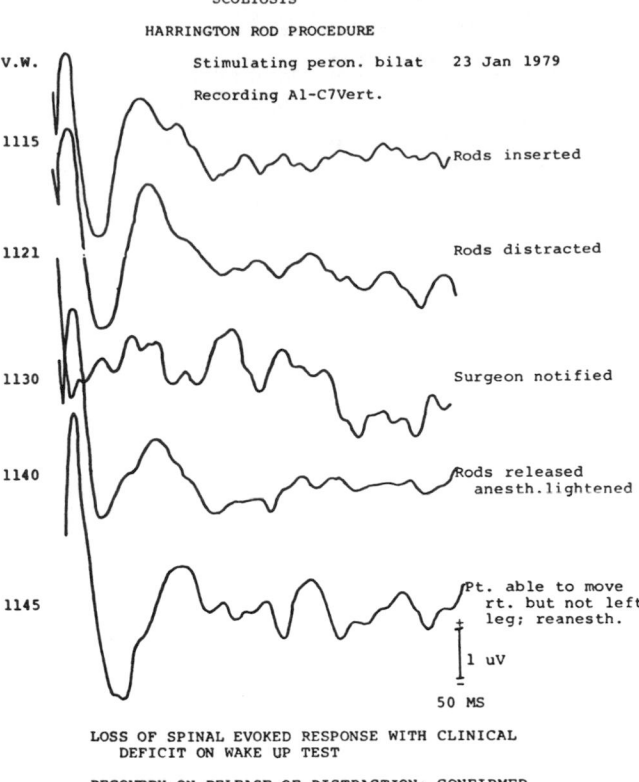

SCOLIOSIS

HARRINGTON ROD PROCEDURE

V.W.   Stimulating peron. bilat   23 Jan 1979

Recording Al-C7Vert.

1115   Rods inserted

1121   Rods distracted

1130   Surgeon notified

1140   Rods released
                                                               anesth.lightened

1145   Pt. able to move
                                                               rt. but not left
                                                               leg; reanesth.

                                                               1 uV

                                                        50 MS

LOSS OF SPINAL EVOKED RESPONSE WITH CLINICAL
DEFICIT ON WAKE UP TEST

RECOVERY ON RELEASE OF DISTRACTION: CONFIRMED
POST OPERATIVELY

Figure 5–14   IORSER during insertion of Harrington rods.

increase in latency is also a potential warning sign, but the delay in conduction with decrease in body or extremity temperature must be considered. Frequent dialogue with the surgeon permits meaningful correlation between steps in the surgery and the observed evoked responses (Fig. 5-14).

Patients operated on in the sitting position may accumulate intracranial subdural air. This alters conduction of the electrical response from the cortex to the conventional recording electrodes. This may be detected by a decrease in amplitude without an increase in latency in the response, and in the absence of alteration in anesthesia or vital signs. It may be confirmed by preservation of the response using a different montage recording from T3 to T4, as well as the bimodal use of concurrent IOAERs.[31]

☐ INTRAOPERATIVE VERs (IORVERs)

Several authors have found that intraoperative VERs are useful,[29,32–39] but others have denied their significance.[30,40,41] Of the modes of intraoperative monitoring in use, VERs are the most susceptible to instability. As noted above, the waves with longer latencies represent those with a greater number of synaptic passages and are, therefore, most sus-

ceptible to systemic changes due to anesthesia or alterations in blood pressure, oxygenation, and electrolytes.

Stimulation may be by LED arrays mounted in goggles, but more satisfactory are LED arrays mounted in scleral cups placed beneath the eyelids. A local anesthetic is applied to the conjunctiva prior to placement. It may be necessary to use a short-acting mydriatic to produce pupillary dilation.[4,29,42–46]

The stimulation controllers illuminate the arrays in flashes of 5 ms duration at variable frequencies. Because of the sweep duration for averaging, a frequency of <5 Hz is required. With pathological delay of the visual pathway conduction, a range of 1 to 2 Hz may be desirable. The flashes may be given to either eye, bilaterally, or to alternate eyes. The last technique may permit the ongoing averaging of potentials from each eye separately during a single sweep, but sweep time must be doubled to prevent superimposition of responses.

Recording electrodes are Oz electrodes referred to Cz electrodes, but in some instances 01 and 02 are added.

Low filter settings of 1 to 30 Hz and high filter settings of 100 to 250 Hz have proved satisfactory for intraoperative VERs. This may vary with individual patients, and it should be set for the optimal response that is replicable. Amplification may vary from 10K to 100K, depending on the individual case. The preoperative baseline may help in the selection of recording parameters. Once an optimal and stable setting is reached in the initial phases of the operation, it is desirable to retain the same settings during the critical part of the procedure.

The latency of the P100 wave in patients with impaired conduction of the anterior visual pathways is frequently increased significantly. Selection of an appropriate sweep time should be increased sufficiently to permit identification of this wave not only at the beginning of the operation, but also during periods of monitoring when the latency may be increased. Sweep times of 300 to 400 ms may therefore be appropriate. This may require an appropriate adjustment in the stimulation frequency to avoid superimposition. The number of sweeps required varies with replicability. Where reliable responses are obtained, 100 to 200 sweeps will suffice. The number of required sweeps together with the stimulation frequency determines the recycling time per average. During critical times in the procedure the shortest stable recycling time is desirable.

A decrease in amplitude of 50 percent, an increase in latency of 5 ms, or a change in morphology are indications for notifying the surgeon. At that time, information as to the manipulation being done should be obtained and documented. It is important to recognize that each patient serves as his or her own control, and the thrust of the entire monitoring procedure is to record deviations from the baseline responses since they may be affected by the surgical procedure. The informed surgeon may then alter the manipulations, if possible, and reduce the threat of increased visual deficit. An improvement in responses with release of visual pathway compression is gratifying (Fig. 5-15).

MOTOR EVENT RELATED RESPONSES (MERs), MOTOR EVENT RELATED POTENTIALS (MEPs)

The development of somatosensory evoked responses has by far preceded that of motor evoked responses. The importance of the motor system in volitional activities has prompted the development of techniques for clinical assessment of the function of the motor system in the laboratory and in the operating room.[47] The history of the observation that stimulation of the motor cortex resulted in movement is well-documented and will not be repeated. Assessment of the function of the motor pathways, however, has required development of replicable quantitative techniques comparable to those used for sensory studies but equally noninvasive. Motor response to electrical stimulation through the intact scalp has been observed, and techniques have been developed for stimulation of the motor cortex through the intact skull. This involves placement of a large electrode (anode) over the motor strip and another against the palate or other distant site (cathode).

The impedance to stimulating currents in ohm-cm is scalp, 300 to 1000; skull, 5000 to 15,000; CSF, 65; gray matter, 250; and white matter, 750.[48] The attenuation of the stimulating current by high tissue resistance requires relatively large voltages—up to 700 V—and currents of up to 1 A. The resistance and current dispersion results in discomfort or pain in alert patients.

The development of stimulating electromagnetic coils provides a more-acceptable method of transcranial cortical stimulation and is now the preferred method.[49] Large electrical fields are not created at the surface of the scalp, and little discomfort is produced. The stimulating coil does not require contact with the scalp.[50] Transcranial electrical stimu-

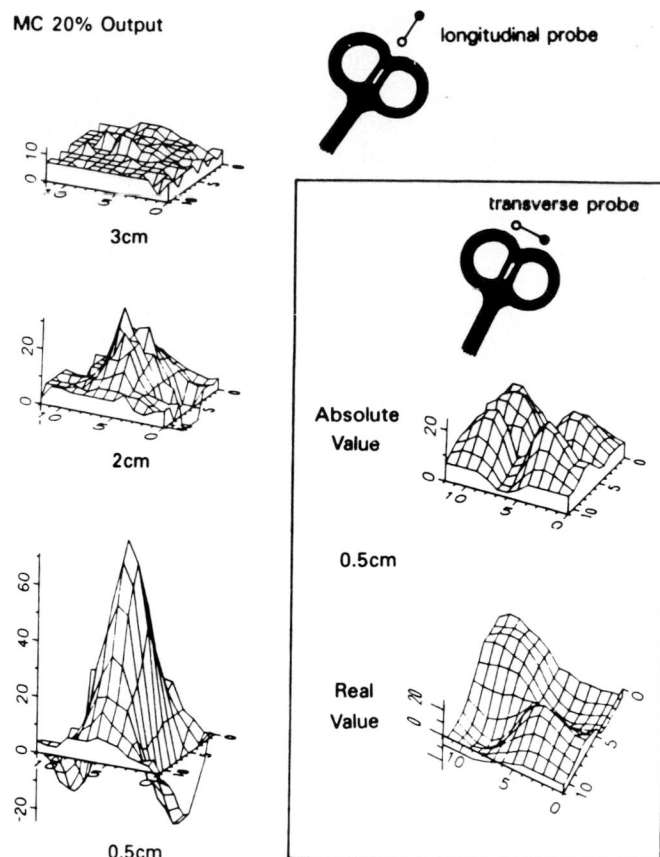

Figure 5–16 Magnetic stimulating coil showing field strength at 0.5, 2, and 3 cm from the center of the figure-8 coil with the center of the coil oriented longitudinally to the recording probe. The insert shows the field strength with the coil oriented transverse to the recording probe. (*Maccabee PJ, Eberle L, Amassian VE, et al: Spatial distribution of the electric field induced in volume by round and figure '8' magnetic coils: Relevance to activation of sensory nerve fibers.* Electroencephalogr Clin Neurophysiol 76:131–141, 1990. Reproduced with permission.)

lation may still be preferable for intraoperative monitoring where the patient is anesthetized and paralyzed, since the equipment is less complicated to organize in the operating room environment (Fig. 5-16).

Recording may be from surface electrodes over peripheral muscles as performed with EMG or over nerves as is used for recording of action potentials. Intraoperative recording is more reliable from needle electrodes inserted in peripheral nerves or along the spinal axis. As in SSEPs, the responses referable to the upper extremities are more easily elicited than those of the lower extremities.

In electromagnetic stimulation, it is the changing magnetic field that produces the stimulation. The field strength is determined by the number of ampere turns. To achieve a high rate of change in current, a capacitor is discharged into the excitation coil. The current induced in tissue is proportional to the rate of change of the magnetic field, which is proportional to the current in the coil. Living tissue is freely permeable to magnetic fields without attenuation. Because of the high current required in the coil, the discharge from the

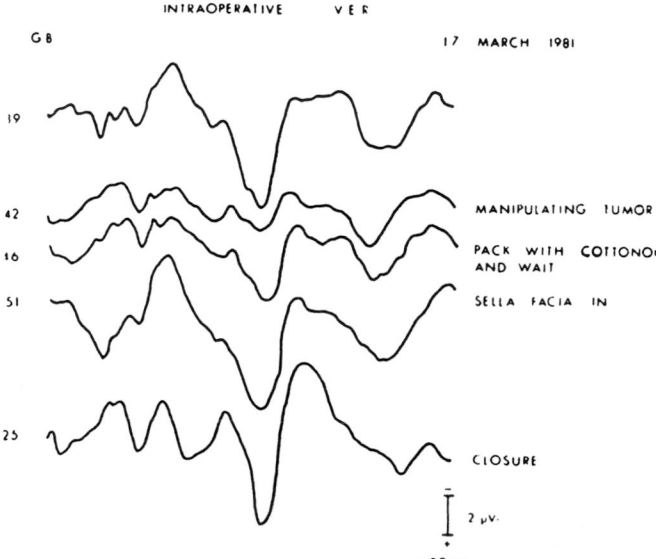

Figure 5–15 IOVER during transsphenoidal removal of pituitary tumor. Note marked decrease in response during tumor manipulation with subsequent recovery after surgeon was alerted.

capacitor from which the current originates is very brief, while recharging the capacitor requires more time. This limits the repetition rate of the stimulus. Rates more rapid than 0.3 per second require a cooling coil for heat dissipation. A stimulus duration of 100 μs has been found to be satisfactory.[48]

The magnetic field produced is 1 to 2.5 tesla in the center of the coil. An electrical field is generated at right angles to the magnetic field, parallel to the plane of the coil, and it is proportional to the time rate change of the magnetic field. The direction of current flow determines the orientation of the field.[51] Action potentials are produced in excitable cells lying in the electrical field.

The geometry of the coil determines the 3-dimensional power of the induced electrical field. Coils formed in a single loop produce maximal electrical fields near the margin of the loop decreasing to the center, with reversal of the field outside the margins of the loop. Smaller coils and more tightly wound coils produce more focalized electrical fields.[52]

Adjacent coils forming a butterfly or figure-8 shape with current flowing in opposite directions in the two loops produce electrical fields maximal under the center of the butterfly, and they are considered best-suited for localized transcranial cortical stimulation and mapping. The magnitude of the electrical field decreases with the square of the distance from the plane of the coil, so that at 2, 3, and 4 cm the value is 50 percent, 27 percent, and 16 percent of the value 1 cm below the plane.[52]

In addition to transcranial stimulation of the brain, electromagnetic stimulation may also be used on peripheral nerves for SSEPs and nerve conduction studies. This produces less discomfort than electrical stimulation. For nerve conduction studies, the exact position of the stimulation field may be difficult to define. The butterfly coil also appears superior in this application. The orientation of the junction of the two loops should be parallel to the nerve for maximal stimulation.[53]

Motor responses following electrical and magnetic stimulation of the cerebral cortex are very similar, although latencies are about 2 ms shorter with electrical stimulation. Differences are also observed in response to active contraction of the stimulated muscle, with only a small decrease in latency observed with magnetic stimulation, while latencies with electrical stimulation were decreased 2 to 6 ms.[49,54]

Although the motor strip is the area of principle interest for stimulation, the cells of origin of the fibers in the pyramidal tract are not exclusively located in the precentral gyrus. In the primate only 31 percent arise in area 4, 20 percent from area 6, and 40 percent from the parietal lobe.[55] The direct response from the Betz cells is, therefore, supplemented by an indirect delayed response from collateral pathways of other origins. In general, the direct response pathways are required for fine motor activity of the distal limbs and digits, and the slower indirect responses are associated with more proximal structures involved in posturing and locomotion. An increased intensity of the stimulus may increase the distribution of pathways involved by including collateral structures.[56]

The safety of transcranial magnetic stimulation remains unproven, but the maximal charge of 50 μC per pulse appears to be acceptable. Thermal effect on the tissues at maximal stimulus of 3 per second is only 1/300 the limits suggested by international standards.[57] A study of 58 epileptic patients on medication who received an average of 25 *transcranial magnetic stimuli (TMS)* revealed no statistical change in seizure frequency on follow-up.[58]

Rapid rate TMS (rTMS) is possible with a stimulation coil which is cooled to prevent overheating. Stimulation rates of up to 25 Hz in trains of 10 s have permitted identification of language lateralization in preoperative studies. Stimulation of both left and right hemispheres induced speech arrest and counting errors during stimulation on the left, but not on the right. Subsequent intracarotid amytal studies confirmed speech lateralization on the left. One of the six patients studied had an after-discharge following an initial train of stimuli, as well as a partial motor seizure compatible with the area stimulated following a second train. This was different from the patient's habitual seizures. EEG monitoring is indicated for such an application, and an after-discharge is a contraindication to continuing stimulation at that intensity.[59]

Significant increases in motor latencies have been demonstrated in subjects with multiple sclerosis. This is also seen in cervical myelopathy, cervical spondylosis, spinal cord trauma, hemiplegia, and hereditary spastic paraparesis.[49,50,57] On the other hand, motor latencies are reported as normal in Parkinson's disease, essential tremor, Huntington's disease, and torsion dystonia.[50,54]

Intraoperative monitoring using MEPs provides assessment of the potential threat to motor pathways not demonstrated by SSEPs. Recording is from the peripheral nerves, using needle electrodes. This avoids displacement and alteration of EMG response by muscle-relaxing agents used during surgery. To avoid the enhancing effect of muscle contraction, drip titration rather than bolus administration of muscle relaxants should be used. A combination of SSEP and MEP monitoring is desirable since the integrity of both motor and sensory systems can be assessed. In addition, the SSEP has an enhancing effect on the MEP. When loss of MEP does not occur or is transient, no permanent motor deficit is present, but when a weakened MEP does not resolve, a resulting permanent or slowly resolving deficit is observed. An optimal monitoring system should provide feedback to the surgeon approximately every 30 s for maximal safety (Fig. 5-17).[47]

☐ MAGNETOENCEPHALOGRAPHY (MEG)

Electroencephalography is handicapped by the high impedance of tissues through which a signal from an electrical generator must pass before being recorded. Tissue imped-

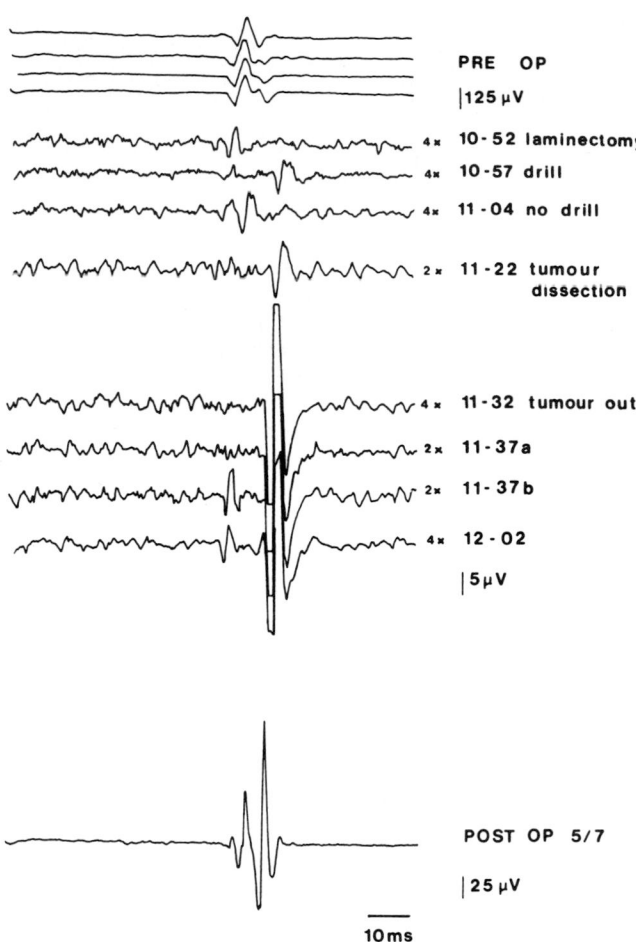

PRE OP

|125 μV

4× 10-52 laminectomy

4× 10-57 drill

4× 11-04 no drill

2× 11-22 tumour dissection

4× 11-32 tumour out

2× 11-37a

2× 11-37b

4× 12-02

|5μV

POST OP 5/7

|25 μV

10ms

Figure 5–17 Intraoperative monitoring of spinal tumor removal using MEP. (*Jellinek D, Jewkes D, Symon L: Noninvasive intraoperative monitoring of evoked potentials under propofol anesthesia: Effects of spinal surgery on the amplitude and latency of motor evoked potentials.* Neurosurgery 29:551–557, 1991. *Reproduced with permission.*)

ance measures 250 ohm/cm in gray matter, 750 ohm/cm in white matter, 65 ohm/cm in CSF, 5000 to 15,000 ohm/cm in skull, and 300 to 1000 ohm/cm in scalp.[48]

Magnetoencephalography is emerging as a method not only for detection of epileptic foci but also for studying the physiology, pharmacology, and psychology of the CNS. The electrical currents created by neuronal activity follow the right-hand rule of current flow in physics. Thus electrical currents produced by neurons create electromagnetic fields of 10^{-15} to 10^{-12} tesla (1 femtotesla to 1 picotesla), compared with ambient magnetic field strengths of 5×10^{10} ftesla. These fields in the brain are recorded by arrays of detectors [Superconducting Quantum Interference Devices (SQUIDS)] placed over the scalp. The superconducting state is achieved by cooling the device with liquid helium in a dewar flask. The maneuverability of the system is limited to an angulation of 45° or less to avoid spilling the helium. This requires that the study be made with the patient in the lateral position, and simultaneous recording from both sides cannot be done with currently available instruments.[60]

The data acquired are digitized and may be displaced in a manner similar to EEG recordings, or as graphic displays of the dipole.[61,62] Using stereotactic references, magnetic spike activity may be localized in 3-dimensional stereotactic space and then onlayed over multiplaner MRI views to display anatomical location. The potential advantage over EEG is that the signals are detected directly rather than after volume conduction, and are not attenuated by bone or altered by conflicting electrical signals. Therefore MEG may have better potential for localizing foci from deep structures. Unfortunately, the strength of the signal diminishes with the square to cube of the distance,[60] so that a signal 3 cm deep is attenuated by 80 percent. Like EEG, MEG detects signals in relation to the orientation of the recording sites, but magnetic dipoles are at right angles to their electrical dipoles. Also, like EEG, a large number of recording points are necessary for localization. The signals recorded by EEG are of voltage differences, whereas MEG records the magnetic fields produced by current flow. MEG records signals that are parallel to the plane of the recording device, or the surface of the scalp. Thus superficial currents tangential to the surface are recorded, while radial currents are only detected as distant deep signals when parallel to the detectors.

As in the study of EEG activity, attention is directed at dipole generators. The dipole localization method (DLM) based on the equivalent current dipole (ECD) has proved extremely accurate in the localization of high-amplitude and event-related responses, particularly in superficial locations. Demonstration of tonotopic auditory responses in the relatively superficial auditory cortex of the first temporal convolution has been correlated with MRI imaging and displayed with a resolution of less than 1 mm.[63] An ECD at a deeper site involves decreased signal-to-noise ratio (SNR), and computation of spatial orientation is required for identification.[64]

With the development of 37-channel MEG and improved data processing, the capability has been developed to process acquired information to focus on the activity in a specific region of the brain. After simultaneous acquisition of data from the contour-placed detectors, the stored data is computer processed in a manner similar to that used in the astronomically applied radiotelescope. With this algorithm of space-filtered imaging (SFI), it is possible to reconstitute the electrical currents in deep brain structures. Figure 5-18 shows evoked spike activity in a 7×7 cm grid reformatted in a plane 5 cm lateral to the midsagittal plane. Signals arising in deep brain structures have lower SNRs, and those of spontaneous normal activity have lower SNRs than pathological spikes or evoked responses. In comparative studies with ECD, in the presence of multiple dipole sources or low SNR a localization advantage was displayed by SFI.[65] This method appears to enhance the potential for study of slow wave foci and for the determination of the sites of action of pharmacological agents used in neurology and psychiatry (Fig. 5-18).

In clinical applications, SFI has shown neuronal activity

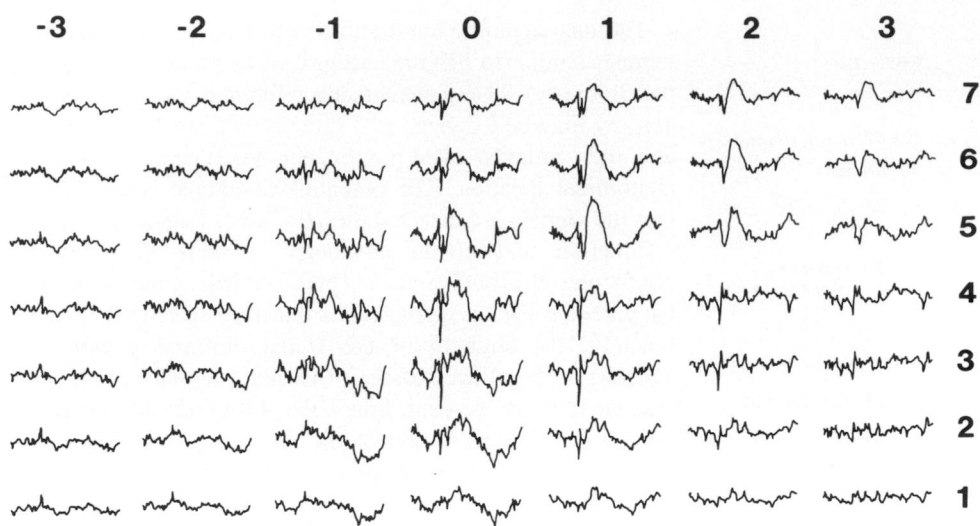

Figure 5–18 MEG study of SERs showing evoked spike activity in a 7 × 7 cm grid reformatted in a plane 5 cm lateral from the midsagittal plane. Recording sites are separated 1 cm. Numbers at top represent distances posterior and anterior to the preauricular point; numbers at right represent distance above the basal plane. (*Reproduced courtesy of Robinson SE.*)

at the onset of interictal discharge, with 3-dimensional spread away from the onset location and resolution of multiple areas of excitation that are separated 1 to 2 cm and have different time amplitude patterns.[66] MEG has the capability of determining latency differences and propagation distances of spikes consistent with the conduction velocity of corticocortical fibers.[61] Noninvasive derivation of the cortical surface area of spikes agrees with localization obtained by electrocorticography over temporal neocortex.

Using replicated preoperative MEG studies with dipole electrical signals inserted through depth electrodes, spatial correlation has been found to be within 1 cm. These were localized within the area subsequently resected. The MEG localization was also in close agreement with intraoperative cortical recordings.[67]

At present the role of MEG may be to provide information complementary to EEG.[68] It has added a more realistic approach to quantification of the interictal spike zone in the study of epilepsy.[69] Its potential for both research and clinical application seems to be on the threshold of significant contribution.[70]

REFERENCES

1. Kooi KA: *Fundamentals of Electroencephalography.* 2d ed. New York, Harper & Row, 1978.
2. Jasper HH: The ten-twenty electrode system of the International Federation. *Electroencephalogr Clin Neurophysiol* 10:371–375, 1958.
3. Binnie CD: Telemetric EEG monitoring in epilepsy, in Pedley TA, Meldrum BS (eds): *Recent Advances in Epilepsy, I.* Edinburgh, Churchill Livingstone, 1983, pp 155–178.
4. Møller AR: *Evoked Potentials in Intraoperative Monitoring.* Baltimore, Williams & Wilkins, 1988, pp 50–60.
5. Møller AR, Jannetta PJ, Sekhar LN: Contributions from the auditory nerve to the brain-stem auditory evoked potentials (BAEPs): Results of intracranial recording in man. *Electroencephalogr Clin Neurophysiol* 71:198–211, 1988.
6. Jacobson GB, Tew JM: The origin of the scalp recorded P14 following electrical stimulation of the median nerve: Intraoperative observations. *Electroencephalogr Clin Neurophysiol* 71:73–76, 1988.
7. Mervaala E, Paakkonen A, Partanen JV: The influence of height, age and gender on the interpretation of median nerve SEPs. *Electroencephalogr Clin Neurophysiol* 71:109–113, 1988.
8. Morioka T, Shima F, Kato M, Fukui M: Origin and distribution of thalamic somatosensory evoked potentials in humans. *Electroencephalogr Clin Neurophysiol* 74:186–193, 1989.
9. Leandri M, Parodi CI, Favale E: Early trigeminal evoked potentials in tumors of the base of the skull and trigeminal neuralgia. *Electroencephalogr Clin Neurophysiol* 71:114–124, 1988.
10. Leandri M, Parodi C, Favale E: Early scalp responses evoked by stimulation of the supraorbital nerve in man. *Electroencephalogr Clin Neurophysiol* 74:367–377, 1989.
11. Kaufman D, Celesia GG. Simultaneous recording of pattern electroretinogram and visual evoked responses in neuro-ophthalmological disorders. *Neurology* 35:644–651, 1985.
12. Tan CB, King PJL, Chiappa KH: Pattern ERG: Effects of reference electrode site, stimulus mode and check size. *Electroencephalogr Clin Neurophysiol* 74:11–18, 1988.
13. Chiappa KH: *Evoked Potentials in Clinical Practice,* 2d ed. New York, Raven, 1990.
14. Ducati A, Favi E, Motti EDF: Neuronal generators of the visual evoked potentials: Intracerebral recording in awake humans. *Electroencephalogr Clin Neurophysiol* 71:89–99, 1988.

15. Kobal G, Hummel C: Cerebral chemosensory evoked potentials elicited by chemical stimulation of the human olfactory and respiratory nasal mucosa. *Electroencephalogr Clin Neurophysiol* 71:241–250, 1988.

16. Aminoff MJ: Intraoperative monitoring by evoked potentials for spinal cord surgery: The cons. *Electroencephalogr Clin Neurophysiol* 73:378–380, 1989.

17. American Academy of Neurology: Report of the therapeutics and technology assessment subcommittee of the American Academy of Neurology. Assessment: Intraoperative neurophysiology. *Neurology* 40:1644–1645, 1991.

18. Daube JR: Intraoperative monitoring by evoked potentials for spinal cord surgery: The pros. *Electroencephalogr Clin Neurophysiol* 73:374–377, 1989.

19. Grundy BA. Monitoring of sensory evoked potentials during neurosurgical operations: Methods and applications. *Neurosurgery* 11:556–575, 1982.

20. Hargadine JR: Intraoperative monitoring of sensory evoked potentials, in Rand RW (ed): *Microneurosurgery,* 3rd ed. St. Louis, Mosby, 1985, pp 91–110.

21. John R, Prichep LS, Ransohoff J, Epstein F: Real-time intraoperative monitoring of evoked potentials using optimized digital filtering. *Electroencephalogr Clin Neurophysiol* 61:20P, 1985.

22. Prichep LS, John ER, Ransohoff J, et al: Real-time intraoperative monitoring of cranial nerves VII and VIII during posterior fossa surgery, in Morocutti C, Rizzo PA (eds): *Evoked Potentials: Neurophysiological and Clinical Aspects.* Amsterdam, Elsevier, 1985.

23. Clark DL, Rosner BS: Neurophysiologic effects of general anesthetics. *Anesthesiology* 38:564–582, 1973.

24. Drummond JC, Todd MM, Sang H: The effect of high dose sodium pentothal on brain stem auditory and median nerve somatosensory evoked responses in humans. *Anesthesiology* 63:249–254, 1985.

25. McPherson RW, Mahla M, Johnson R, Traystman R: Effects of enflurane, isoflurane, and nitrous oxide on somatosensory evoked potentials during fentanyl anesthesia. *Anesthesiology* 62:626–633, 1985.

26. Uhl RR, Squires KC, Bruce DL, Starr A: Effect of halothane anesthesia on the human cortical visual evoked response. *Anesthesiology* 53:273–276, 1980.

27. Radtke RA, Erwin W, Wilkins RH: Intraoperative brainstem auditory evoked potentials: Significant decrease in postoperative morbidity. *Neurology* 39:187–191, 1989.

28. Allen A, Starr A, Nudleman K: Assessment of sensory function in the operating room utilizing cerebral evoked potentials: A study of fifty-six surgically anesthetized patients. *Clin Neurosurg* 28:457–481, 1981.

29. Nuwer MR. Evoked potential monitoring in the operating room. New York, Raven, 1986, pp 49–101, 172–187.

30. Raudzens PA. Sensory potentials: An outline for surgical monitoring. *Barrow Neurological Institute Quarterly* 1:40–48, 1985.

31. Watanabe E, Schramm J, Schneider W: Effect of a subdural air collection on the sensory evoked potential during surgery in the sitting position. *Electroencephalogr Clin Neurophysiol* 74:194–201, 1989.

32. Harding GFA, Bland JDP, Smith VH: Visual evoked potential monitoring of optic nerve function during surgery. *J Neurol Neurosurg Psychiatry* 53:890–895, 1990.

33. Feinsod M, Selhorst JB, Hoyt WF, Wilson CB: Monitoring optic nerve function during craniotomy. *J Neurosurg* 44:29–31, 1976.

34. Flanigin HF, Allen MBJ. Reducing risk of pituitary surgery by intraoperative visual evoked response monitoring. *Proceedings of the Second International Evoked Potentials Symposium.* Cleveland, 1982.

35. Wilson WB, Kirsch WM, Neville H, et al: Monitoring of visual function during parasellar surgery. *Surg Neurol* 5:323–329, 1976.

36. Wright JE, Arden G, Jones BR: Continuous monitoring of the visually evoked response during intraorbital surgery. *Transactions Ophthalmol Soc (London)* 93:311–314, 1973.

37. Koshino K, Kuroda R, Mogami H: Flashing diode evoked potentials and optic nerve function during surgery. *Electroencephalogr Clin Neurophysiol* 43:449, 1977.

38. Groswasser Z, Kriss A, Halliday AM, McDonald WI: Visual evoked potentials in optic nerve gliomas. *Electroencephalogr Clin Neurophysiol* 60:20P, 1985.

39. Costa I, Silva E, Wang AD, Symon L: The application of flash visual evoked potentials during operation on the visual pathways. *J Neurol Neurosurg Psychiatry* 47:1144–1145, 1984.

40. Cedzich C, Schramm J, Mengedoht CF, Fahlbusch R: Factors that limit the use of flash visual evoked potentials for surgical monitoring. *Electroencephalogr Clin Neurophysiol* 71:142–145, 1988.

41. Celesia GG: Visual evoked responses, in *Evoked Potential Testing.* San Diego, Grune & Stratton, 1985, pp 1–54.

42. Feinsod M, Madey JMJ, Susal A: A new photostimulator for continuous recording of the visual evoked potential. *Electroencephalogr Clin Neurophysiol* 38:29–31, 1975.

43. Kramer KK, Przybyla VAJ, LaPiana FG: A light emitting diode array globe protector photostimulator. *J Clin Neuroophthalmol* 4:53–55, 1984.

44. Lesser RP, Luders H, Klem G: LED evoked potentials: Characteristics and clinical correlations. *Electroencephalogr Clin Neurophysiol* 54:63–64P, 1982.

45. Norcross K: Comparison of VEPs elicited with pattern reversal and light emitting diode stimulation. *Electroencephalogr Clin Neurophysiol* 58:49P, 1984.

46. Skuse NF, Burke D, McKeon B: Reproducibility of the visual evoked potential using a light-emitting diode stimulator. *J Neurol Neurosurg Psychiatry* 47:623–629, 1984.

47. Levy WJ: Clinical experience with motor and cerebellar evoked potential monitoring. *Neurosurgery* 20:169–182, 1987.

48. Geddes LA: Optimal stimulus duration for extracranial cortical stimulation. *Neurosurgery* 20:94–99, 1987.

49. Mills KR, Murray NMF, Hess CW: Magnetic and electrical transcranial brain stimulation: Physiological mechanisms and clinical applications. *Neurosurgery* 20:164–168, 1987.

50. Cracco RQ: Evaluation of conduction in centralmotor pathways: Techniques, pathophysiology, and clinical interpretation. *Neurosurgery* 20:199–203, 1987.

51. Chiappa KH, Cros D, Cohen D: Magnetic stimulation: Determination of coil current flow. *Neurology* 41:1154–1155, 1991.

52. Cohen LG, Roth BJ, Nilsson J, et al: Effects of coil design on focal magnetic stimulation: Technical considerations. *Electroencephalogr Clin Neurophysiol* 75:350–357, 1990.

53. Maccabee PJ, Eberle L, Amassian VE, et al: Spatial distribution of the electrical field induced in volume by round and figure '8' magnetic coils: Revelance to activation of sensory nerve fibers. *Electroencephalogr Clin Neurophysiol* 76:131–141, 1990.

54. Rothwell JC, Day BL, Thompson PD, et al: Some experiences of techniques for stimulation of the human cerebral motor cortex through the scalp. *Neurosurgery* 20:156–163, 1987.

55. York DH: Review of descending motor pathways involved with transcranial stimulation. *Neurosurgery* 20:70–73, 1987.

56. Amassian VE, Stewart M, Quirk GJ, Rosenthal JL: Physiological basis of motor effects of a transient stimulus to cerebral cortex. *Neurosurgery* 20:74–93, 1987.

57. Barker AT, Freeston IL, Jalinous R, Jarratt JA: Magnetic stimulation of the human brain and peripheral nervous system: An introduction and the results of an initial clinical evaluation. *Neurosurgery* 20:100–109, 1987.

58. Tassinari CA, Michelucci R, Forti A, et al: Transcranial magnetic stimulation in epileptic patients: Usefulness and safety. *Neurology* 40:1132–1133, 1990.

59. Pascual-Leone A, Gates JR, Dhuna A: Induction of speech arrest and counting errors with rapid rate transcranial magnetic stimulation. *Neurology* 41:697–702, 1991.

60. Sato S, Ballish MS: Principles of magnetoencephalography, in Luders H (ed) *Epilepsy Surgery.* New York, Raven, 1992, pp 415–421.

61. Sutherling WW, Barth DS: Neocortical propagation in temporal lobe spike foci on magnetoencephalography and electroencephalography. *Ann Neurol* 25:373–381, 1989.

62. Barth DA, Sutherline W, Engel J Jr, Beatty J: Neuromagnetic localization of epileptiform spike activity in the human brain. *Science* 218:891–894, 1968.

63. Pantev C, Hoke M, Lehnertz K, et al: Identification of sources of brain neuronal activity with high spatiotemporal resolution through combination of neuromagnetic source localization (NMSL) and magnetic resonance imaging (NMI). *Electroencephalogr Clin Neurophysiol* 75:173–184, 1990.

64. Kaufman L, Kaufman JH, Wang JZ: On cortical folds and neuromagnetic fields. *Electroencephalogr Clin Neurophysiol* 79:211–226, 1991.

65. Robinson SE, Rose DF: Current source estimation by spatially filtered MEG (abstract). Eighth International Conference on Biomagnetism, 1991, pp 337–338.

66. Rose DF, Robinson SE, Ebersole JS, Karnaze D: 3D current imaging of interictal spikes in spatially filtered MEG (abstract). Eighth International Conference on Biomagnetism, 1991, pp 39–40.

67. Eisenberg HM, Papanicolaou AC, Baumann SB, et al: Magnetoencephalographic localization of interictal spike sources. (case report). *J Neurosurg* 74:660–667, 1991.

68. Cohen D, Cuffin BN, Yunokuchi K, et al: MEG versus EEG localization test using implanted sources in the human brain. *Ann Neurol* 28:811–817, 1990.

69. Sutherling WW, Levesque MF, Crandall PH, Barth DS: A complete physical description of the dynamic electric currents of human partial epilepsy and essential cortex using MEG, EEG, chronic ECoG grid recordings, and direct cortical stimulation, in Luders H (ed) *Epilepsy Surgery.* New York, Raven, 1992, pp 429–450.

70. Stefan H: Multichannel magnetoencephalography: Recordings of epileptiform discharges, in Luders H (ed) *Epilepsy Surgery.* New York, Raven, 1992, pp 423–428.

☐ STUDY QUESTIONS

I. A 25-year-old male, having recently had a series of generalized seizures beginning in the left arm, is sent for an EEG. The report indicates alpha activity throughout except for the right frontal area where there is a focal area of delta activity with intermittent spikes.

   1. What is the size and frequency of the alpha activity? **2.** When is it most likely to appear? **3.** What is the implication of delta activity? **4.** What is its rate? **5.** What is the interpretation of the spike activity?

II. An 18-year-old girl has an EEG after being kept awake all night the night before. She falls asleep during the examination, progressing through the various levels of sleep to REM sleep.

   1. What was the most likely rhythm when the individual being examined was awake? **2.** Describe the expected EEG recordings during non-REM sleep. **3.** What is the appearance of the EEG during REM sleep? **4.** What is the explanation of this later category? **5.** What is the purpose of depriving a patient of sleep before an EEG?

III. A 36-year-old female is being monitored with auditory evoked responses while undergoing a surgical procedure in the posterior fossa.

   1. What anesthesia should be used? **2.** What are the most important waves to be observed? **3.** What are the sources of these waves? **4.** How are the response waves differentiated from the routine electrical activity of the brain? **5.** Initial recordings show prolongation between the waves recorded from the vertex and that recorded from the earlobe. What is the significance of this increase in conduction time?

IV. Intraoperative evoked responses are being recorded during the course of resection of a vascular malformation at the cervicomedullary junction.

   1. Where should the recording electrodes be placed? **2.** What are the normally recorded responses? **3.** Of what significance is an increase in the latency of responses? **4.** What is the significance of loss of the later responses during the administration of anesthesia? **5.** How should the head be held during the recordings?

V. A 40-year-old male is undergoing laminectomy for an extraaxial mass of the mid-cervical area.

   1. What form of evoked potentials (sensory or motor) would be most predictive of future function? **2.** Where might stimulations for each of these forms of monitoring be performed? **3.** Where would recording electrodes be placed? **4.** What are the advantages and disadvantages of magnetic stimulation as compared to electrical stimulation? **5.** What indications on the recordings would lead one to recommend an alteration of the conduct of the procedure?

Radiographic Examinations and Imaging of Patients with Lesions Affecting the Nervous System

Edward K. Mark, Jr.
Ramón E. Figueroa
Alexis Norelle

The technological evolution which has occurred in neuroradiology over the past 20 years is without parallel in clinical medicine and is a major factor in the development of neuroradiology as a distinct discipline within radiology.

This rapid acceleration of imaging technology was spawned by the development of computer-assisted imaging techniques such as computerized tomography (CT), magnetic resonance imaging (MRI), and ultrasonography (US). These techniques employ powerful computers and complex computer programs to collect, analyze, and reconstruct enormous amounts of data into digitized images.

From a clinical perspective, computer-assisted imaging techniques have greatly enhanced diagnostic sensitivity and specificity, with minimal risks to the patient. They have practically replaced certain traditional imaging methods such as pneumoencephalography and significantly limited the indications for others such as arteriography, myclography, and radioisotope scanning.

In this chapter we will attempt to convey what we believe are the essentials of contemporary neuroradiology as it is practiced at our institution. Emphasis has been placed on the computer-assisted imaging techniques—CT, MRI, and US —since these comprise the mainstay of our diagnostic imaging. Arteriography, myelography, and ultrasonography have been reviewed disproportionately to their relative application in contemporary neuroradiology; however, we feel this was necessary to clearly convey their essentials. Other techniques, such as pneumoencephalography, radioisotope scanning, positron emission tomography (PET) scanning, and diskography have received quite summary discussion, which is indicative of their limited use at our institution. This should not be interpreted as a condemnation.

Applications of the various imaging modalities to intracranial pathology are presented first, followed by their application to spinal pathology. Neurosonology is presented separately from other imaging techniques, primarily to limit the confusion that can occur when describing the physical and technical principles involved in different imaging modalities. Throughout this discussion, we have included numerous illustrations to support the text. Most of these describe normal anatomy or its variations. We have deferred presentation of images describing pathology to their respective chapters elsewhere in this book.

The conclusion provides a modest list of suggested review texts that give a more in-depth treatment of specific aspects of neuroradiology.

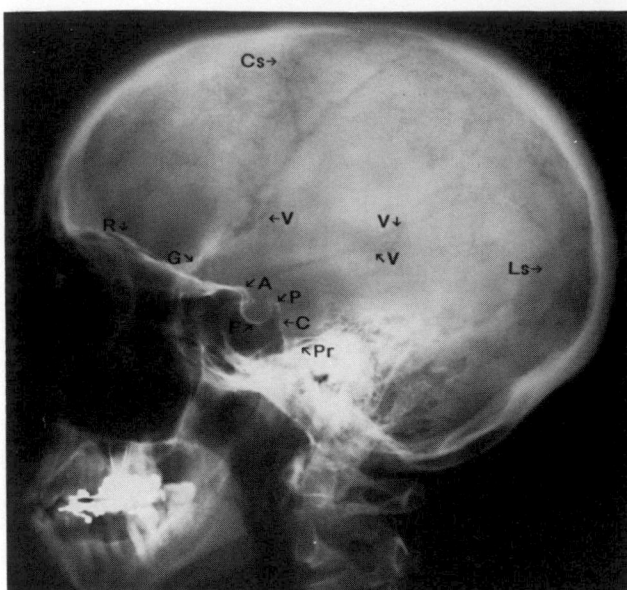

Figure 6–1   Lateral skull x-rays. A = anterior clinoid; C = clivus; Cs = coronal suture; E = ethmoid air cells; F = floor of sella; Fs = frontal sinus; G = greater wing of the sphenoid; I = internal auditory canal; L = lesser wing of sphenoid; Ms = mastoid air cells; Mx = maxillary sinus; N = nasal septum; P = posterior clinoid; Pr = petrous ridge; R = orbital roof; S = superior orbital fissure; Ss = sphenoid sinus; V = vascular grooves of meningeal vessels.

☐ NEURORADIOLOGY OF THE HEAD

PLAIN SKULL RADIOGRAPHY

Traditionally, the radiographic investigation of suspected calvarial and intracranial lesions begins with a series of plain skull radiographs. A variety of projections and techniques for plain radiographs relate radiographic features to specific intracranial lesions as well as some systemic disease.[1] The major handicap of radiography of the skull arises from its inability to image intracranial lesions directly.

Direct imaging of intracranial lesions is best achieved by the use of computer-assisted imaging techniques, computerized tomography (CT), and magnetic resonance imaging (MRI). These provide the capability of obtaining high-resolution images and specific localization of intracranial lesions.

As a result, interest in plain skull radiographs has declined. Its principal application today is as a screening or adjunctive imaging technique in the evaluation of suspected calvarial lesions, such as bony metastatic disease, reactive or inflammatory bone disease, congenital skull deformities, and skull trauma. For the astute clinician, plain radiographs of the skull also reveal evidence of elevated intracranial pressure or space-occupying lesions, such as thinning of the cortical floor of the sella, displacement of the normally midline pineal gland, widening of the bony sutures in children, and enlargement of the vascular grooves. The most useful views for accomplishing these objectives include the following:

Lateral projection. Most useful for observation of patterns of intracranial and craniovertebral junction pathology (Fig. 6-1).
20° Anteroposterior (AP). Demonstrates the position of the calcified pineal gland.

In addition to the lateral and AP views, the standard skull series typically includes:

25° Posteroanterior (Cauldwell) view. Useful in demonstration of fractures and lesions of the midfacial sinuses.
30° Anteroposterior (Townes) view. Useful in the demonstration of lesions involving the mastoid and petrous bones.
Submental vertex (Hirtz) view. May demonstrate abnormalities of the skull base foramina.

Additional applications of the skull x-ray to the neurosurgeon include the evaluation of ventricular or cisternal shunts for continuity and placement and the intraoperative localization of foreign bodies or outlining adjacent structures as is required in pituitary surgery. Figure 6-1 provides the essential anatomy of normal lateral skull x-rays.

INTRACRANIAL COMPUTERIZED TOMOGRAPHY

The introduction of CT in 1972 initiated a major evolution in the field of diagnostic neuroimaging with its ability to

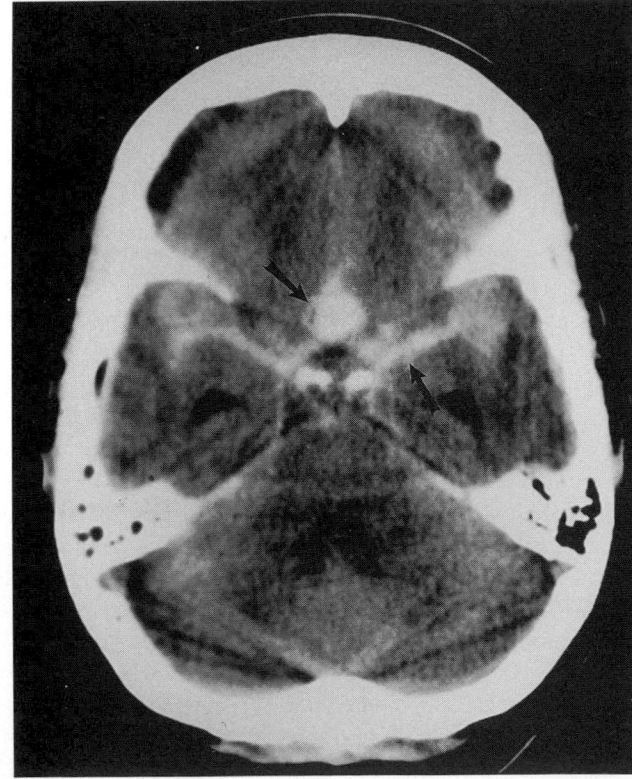

Figure 6–2   CT of head without contrast showing a subarachnoid hemorrhage.

analyze the absorption of x-rays by all tissues to produce an image of high resolution in the transaxial (horizontal) plane.[2,3] At the present time, CT is readily available in most major hospitals, making it the most widely used neurodiagnostic modality. CT is accurate, fast, and well tolerated by patients—even those who have difficulty remaining motionless or who require life support systems.

The physical principle underlying the CT image is the same as in all radiography—the selective absorption of x-rays (photons) by tissues of different densities.[4] Tissues with greater density—for example, bone—will exhibit more absorption of the x-ray beam and will be displayed on the CT image as areas of high density (white). Tissues with less absorption (attenuation) of x-ray beams will be displayed as areas of lower density (varying shades of gray to black). Routine examinations of the brain with CT are performed with axial 10-mm slices through the entire brain and the base of the skull. Some specific anatomic regions—such as the posterior fossa, sella, orbits, temporal bone, or paranasal sinuses—can be evaluated with thinner sections in axial, axial oblique, and/or coronal imaging planes.

It is vital to recognize the advantages and limitations of CT relative to other imaging techniques such as MRI in the evaluation of intracranial pathology. Selection of the study of choice depends on multiple factors, such as history of acute or chronic trauma, the presence of cardiac pacemakers or metallic implants, the monitoring needs of the patients, or the presence of bone pathology versus soft tissue pathology. Generally, CT will be the initial study in patients presenting suspected intracranial hemorrhage that might be the result of head trauma, hypertension, or rupture of an aneurysm or infarction, as well as suspicion of intracranial tumors, either primary or metastatic.[5] CT of the head is the study of choice as well for evaluation of craniofacial trauma to include facial and skull base fractures.

Thus, a nonenhanced CT of the head is recommended for evaluation of acute head trauma, subarachnoid hemorrhage (Fig. 6-2), acute stroke, follow-up of hydrocephalus or shunt malfunction, and for general evaluation of patients with dementia. A CT of the head should be obtained with intravenous contrast enhancement as a screening study for possible metastases, headaches of unknown etiology without neurological deficit, suspected aneurysms or vascular malformations, intracranial infections or abscess, or primary and metastatic brain tumors. CT supplemented by intrathecal contrast is excellent in evaluating CSF fistulas. CT of the head with 3-dimensional reconstruction is the study of choice preoperatively and postoperatively for evaluation of facial anomalies and craniosynostosis prior to surgery as well as for postsurgical evaluation.

Nevertheless, there are certain limitations of CT. Routine CT is suboptimal for evaluation of the prepontine and cerebellopontine angle cisterns unless special angulation is used and thin sections are obtained. This is due to the absorption of the x-ray beam by the thick petrous bones ("Hounsfield artifact"). The evaluation of the sellar region by CT should be performed in the coronal plane with intravenous contrast;

however, the patient's position for the study may be awkward and uncomfortable, resulting in inconsistent image quality. Therefore, MRI is the study of choice for suspected lesions in the region of the sella.

INTRACRANIAL MAGNETIC RESONANCE IMAGING

The next major evolution in neuroimaging following CT in 1972 occurred with the clinical application of magnetic resonance imaging (MRI) in 1982.[6] MRI is a noninvasive computer-assisted imaging technique that differs from CT in the type of energy used. The MRI is based on measuring the phenomenon of *nuclear magnetic resonance* of the hydrogen atom in various tissues. Magnetic resonance imaging uses a strong magnetic field and the application of radiofrequency pulses to generate 2-dimensional or 3-dimensional images.

Nuclei of certain atoms, particularly hydrogen, respond to a strong magnetic field by aligning with or against the longitudinal axis of that magnetic field. This process is called *magnetization*. The number of hydrogen atoms aligned in the direction of the magnetic field is slightly greater than the number aligned against it, producing a net magnetization in the direction of the magnetic field. The magnitude of this net magnetization is related to the number of hydrogen nuclei in each volume of tissue (*proton density*). The direction of the net magnetization may be altered by the addition of energy in the form of a radiofrequency (RF) pulse of appropriate frequency.[7] This extra energy flips the magnetization vector away from its alignment with the primary magnetic field.

When the RF pulse is terminated, the hydrogen protons will begin to realign in the direction of the external magnetic field, releasing the excess energy initially used to deflect them from alignment. The rate at which this realignment occurs depends on the rate that the added energy is released to the surrounding environment. This process is called *longitudinal relaxation*. The time required for 63 percent of the magnetization vector to return to alignment with the external magnetic field is designated *T1*, or *longitudinal relaxation time*.

A second component of relaxation occurs in the transverse plane around the axis of the magnetic field. The magnetization vector in the transverse plane is the sum of many nuclei rotating at slightly different frequencies, which are forced together by the application of the external RF pulse (*coherence*). The net magnitude of the transverse vector and its signal strength diminishes as the nuclei fan out within the transverse plane (*loose coherence*). The time required for 63 percent loss of the transverse coherence is designated *T2*, or *transverse relaxation time*. Different tissues will exhibit different T1 and T2 relaxation patterns, making their magnetic behavior different enough to be recognized as separate entities in the MR image.

The excess energy released by the protons as they realign with the magnetic field is radiated to the environment as a

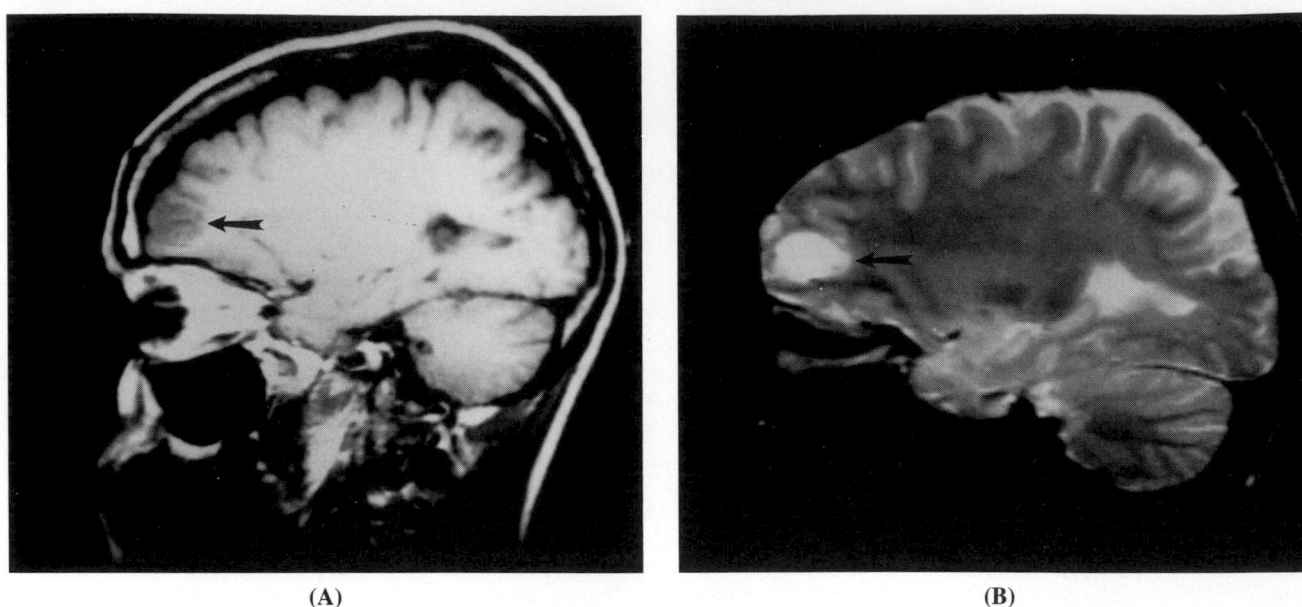

(A)   (B)

Figure 6–3 MRI of cranium of a patient with astrocytoma. Sagittal T1 image to show MRI anatomic detail *(A)*. Sagittal T2 image enhances visualization of lesion *(B)*.

radio frequency "signal." The amount of signal (*signal intensity*) emitted per unit of volume will be correlated to a gray scale, where high signal intensity will be white and absence of signal will be black. The signal intensity of a tissue is related to its T1 and T2 relaxation times and its proton density.

MR images can be obtained in such a way as to favor the demonstration of structures with predominant T1 or with T2 characteristics. T1-weighted images produce a strong MRI signal that results in anatomic images. In a T1-weighted image, cerebrospinal fluid (CSF), cortical bone, air, and rapidly flowing blood will have negligible signals, appearing dark. The gray matter and white matter will show different shades of gray, with the gray matter appearing slightly darker. Fat is intensely bright on T1-weighted images, which is an advantage when outlining orbital fat or the epidural space or marrow in the spinal column. Subacute and chronic hematomas are seen as high signal intensity. The abundant signal of the T1-weighted image is ideal for demonstrating detailed intracranial or spinal anatomy, for example, in evaluating the cerebellopontine angle cistern or the pituitary fossa. This is due to its high contrast between normal structures and the adjacent darker CSF. T1-weighted images, however, are relatively insensitive to small changes in the water content of tissue. Therefore, small brain lesions that do not cause anatomic distortion are often invisible (Fig. 6-3).[8]

T2-weighted images are much more sensitive in the detection of small changes in the water content of the tissue examined.[9] Regions of increased water content (*edema*) are imaged as regions of high signal intensity superimposed on a darker background. Because of the lack of a strong background tissue signal, T2-weighted images do not display the anatomy as sharply as the T1-weighted image does. Nevertheless, the high sensitivity of T2-weighted images for the detection of changes in tissue water content is the primary reason for the increased sensitivity of MRI over CT in the detection of brain and spinal cord pathology. In T2-weighted images, the dominant tissue producing the highest signal intensity will be bulk water, making CSF the dominant bright signal factor in comparison to gray and white matter. Cortical bone, air, and rapidly flowing blood still present negligible signals (black). Fat in T2-weighted images presents lower signal intensity than in T1-weighted images. Areas of demyelination, edema, infarction, or tumor infiltration will have higher water content (more hydrogen atoms) and will produce higher signal intensities than the surrounding tissues.

A definite advantage of MRI over all other imaging modalities is its ability to image multiple direct planes (axial, sagittal, coronal, or any degree of oblique projections) without a change in the patient's supine position. The absence of signal from surrounding bone allows excellent anatomic detail of structures adjacent to bone, both intracranially and throughout the spinal canal. Most MRI examinations of the brain include sagittal, coronal, and axial projections. The axial images are most commonly obtained to evaluate the brain. The coronal images are most useful in evaluating sellar and parasellar regions. With both, the axial or the coronal images, side-to-side comparison is possible. Direct sagittal images are extremely useful when evaluating midline pathology of the brain, such as sellar tumors, pineal masses, brainstem tumors, vermian atrophy, obstructive hydrocephalus, or congenital malformations. They are also helpful in visualizing the location of other internal pathology in the lateral view (Fig. 6-4).

Gadolinium (Gd), a heavy rare-earth element, is being used in special solutions as the intravenous contrast agent for MRI of the central nervous system (CNS).[10] Although free Gd is toxic, its compound chelated to diethylenetriamine

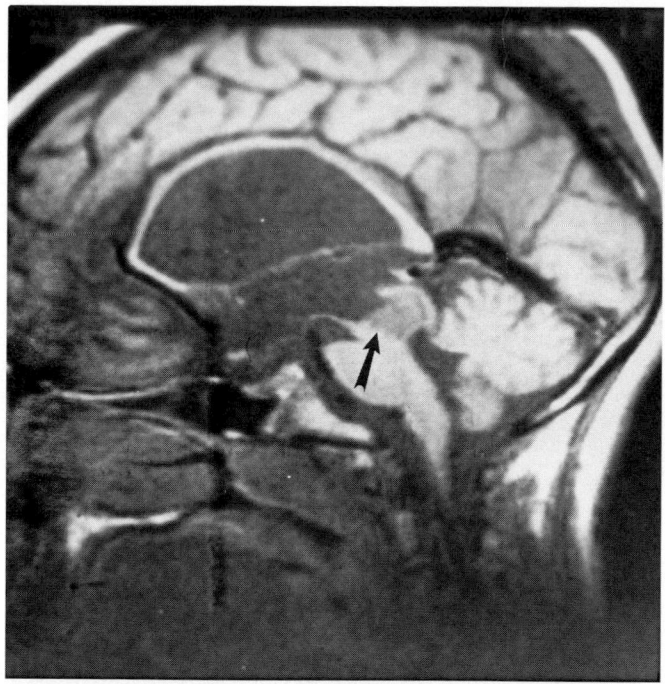

(A)

(B)

Figure 6–4 MRI of cranium showing midbrain tumor and hydrocephalus. Sagittal T1 image shows aqueductal obstruction by tumor *(A)*. Axial T2 image shows tumor involvement *(B)*.

pentaacetic acid (DTPA) or other chelating agents exhibits "paramagnetic behavior." When deposited within tissue, this compound greatly decreases the T1 relaxation time of the surrounding tissue, resulting in a high signal intensity on T1-weighted images. Because of the nature of the blood-brain barrier, Gd will only move outside of the intravascular space in areas of absence or breakdown of the blood-brain barrier. Damage to the blood-brain barrier is a nonspecific

alteration that occurs with pathology within the brain, as seen with tumors, infection, and infarction. Gadolinium-DTPA, the current agent employed for contrast MRI, has been shown to be safe, with very few reported allergic reactions in over 5 million administered doses. The use of paramagnetic contrast increases the sensitivity of MRI for detection of specific disease processes, particularly small tumors. The pattern of contrast enhancement in MRI allows for better tissue characterization of the visualized lesions. Pituitary gland, infundibulum, choroid plexus, pineal gland, and dural reflections lack a blood-brain barrier and will normally enhance with Gd. Slowly flowing blood within the cavernous sinus or in the cortical veins will also exhibit normal enhancement (Fig. 6-5).

Contraindications to MRI include the presence of ferromagnetic materials in soft tissues of the body, such as old intracranial aneurysm clips or intraocular metallic foreign bodies that could move in the fluctuating magnetic field and damage structures on which they are located.[11] Contraindications also include such devices as cardiac pacemakers that could malfunction in the magnetic field or large metallic implants that may become heated by magnetic induction.[12] Since the effect of high magnetic fields and radiofrequency energy on fetuses has not been determined, pregnant patients are generally excluded at the present time. Patients with claustrophobia may not be able to remain in the MR unit for the required time. Quality MRIs require patients to remain motionless for 10 to 15 min. The magnetic environment restricts the use of conventional electronic monitoring devices. Therefore, critical or unstable patients are difficult to monitor and require special attention or equipment while undergoing MRI.

MRI is most sensitive in detection of pathology in the CNS, except for evaluation of acute intracranial hemorrhage or parenchymal calcifications.[13] MRI is rapidly becoming the study of choice in many other conditions that affect the brain, the reason being the absence of artifacts from bony structures surrounding the brain, especially in the posterior fossa (Fig. 6-6). Also, MRI has the capability of acquiring multiplanar images without the need for manipulation of position of the patient, which is especially useful for evaluation within or around the pituitary fossa. Nonenhanced MRI of the brain is useful for screening demyelinating diseases like multiple sclerosis (Fig. 6-7), ischemic brain disease, dementia, and for primary evaluation of the etiology and site of obstruction in hydrocephalus. MRI of the brain is also routinely used to diagnose tumors in pediatric patients. It is the study of choice in the evaluation of congenital anomalies of the CNS, such as agenesis of the corpus collosum (Fig. 6-8), Chiari malformations, migrational anomalies, schizencephaly, problems of brain maturation, or pediatric vascular accidents and vascular malformations.

Recent advances in MRI include magnetic resonance angiography (MRA) and magnetic resonance spectroscopy. MRA has the potential to replace routine angiography for screening of disease at the carotid bifurcation (Fig. 6-9). Its potential in the evaluation of intracranial vascular

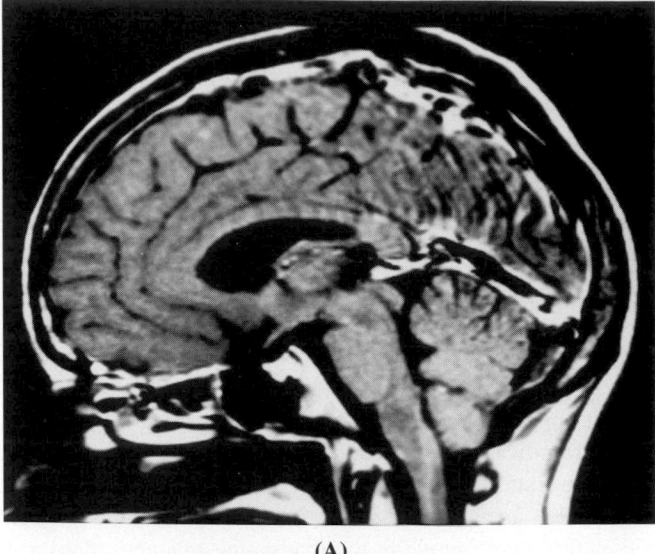

(A)

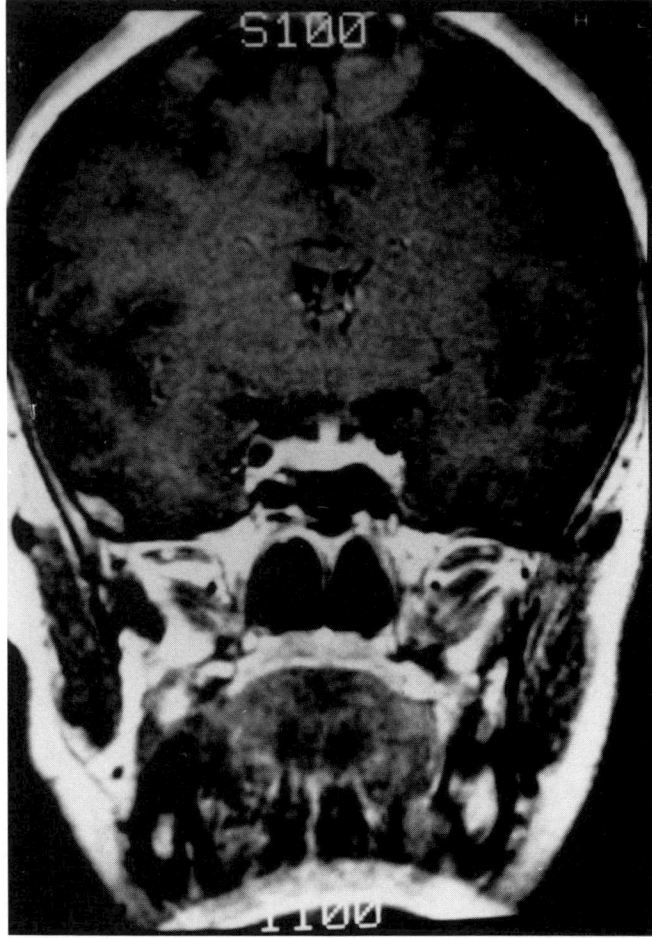

(B)

Figure 6–5 MRI of normal cranium after administration of gadolinium. Midline sagittal enhancement *(A)*. Coronal sella enhancement *(B)*.

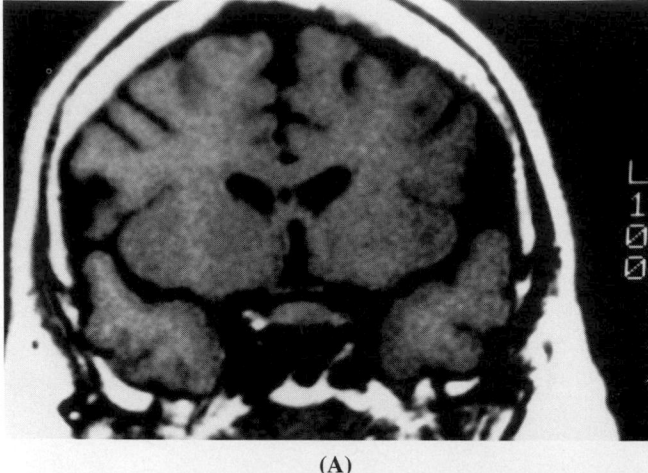

(A)

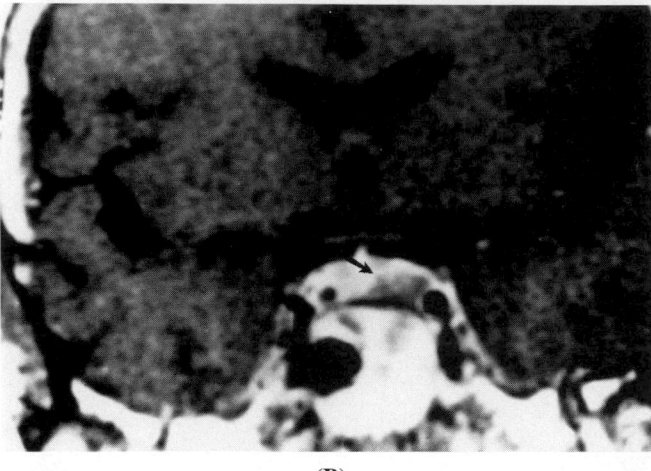

(B)

Figure 6–6 MRI of cranium demonstrating pituitary microadenoma. Coronal T1 image without Gd *(A)*. Coronal T1 image with Gd, showing lesion *(B)*.

of patients with temporal lobe epilepsy, Alzheimer's disease, brain tumors, and determination of brain death.[15] The selection of MRI, CT, or a combination of these examinations depends on the kind of information sought and the time needed to acquire that information.

CEREBRAL ANGIOGRAPHY

The radiographic demonstration of the vasculature of the head and neck using an intraarterial contrast media was first described by Moniz in 1927.[16] Initially, the morbidity associated with this procedure was high, owing to the techniques employed and the toxicity of the contrast media. In 1944, Engeset reported 100 cases using a carotid cannulation technique with relatively low morbidity.[17] Less-toxic contrast media were developed and the technique gained widespread acceptance by the late 1940s. In 1953, Seldinger described a technique for femoral artery cannulation and selective arterial injection, further enhancing the diagnostic capabilities and relative safety of cerebral angiography.[18]

From the early 1950s until the early 1970s, cerebral

malformations and occlusive vascular disease (for example, moyamoya disease) is being explored.[14] MR spectroscopy may provide information on the metabolic status of different areas within the brain and may be helpful in the evaluation

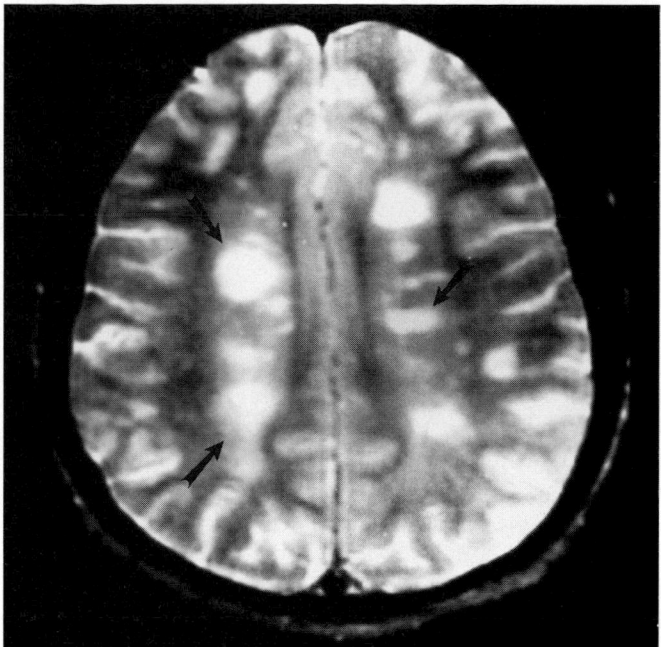

Figure 6–7 MRI of cranium of patient with multiple sclerosis. Axial T2 image showing paraventricular lesions.

angiography in tandem with pneumoencephalography was the mainstay of diagnostic cranial neuroradiology. With the advent of CT scanning in the early 1970s, the use of angiography was significantly curtailed, particularly for evaluating trauma.[5] The evolution of third- and fourth-generation CT scanners and the incorporation of MRI into the diagnostic armamentarium have resulted in the elimination of many of the diagnostic applications of cerebral arteriography.

At facilities where high-quality CT imaging and MRI are available, indications for cerebral angiography are usually limited to the following:

1. Demonstration of the vascular supply of tumors or demonstration of the relationships of major arteries or veins to tumors.

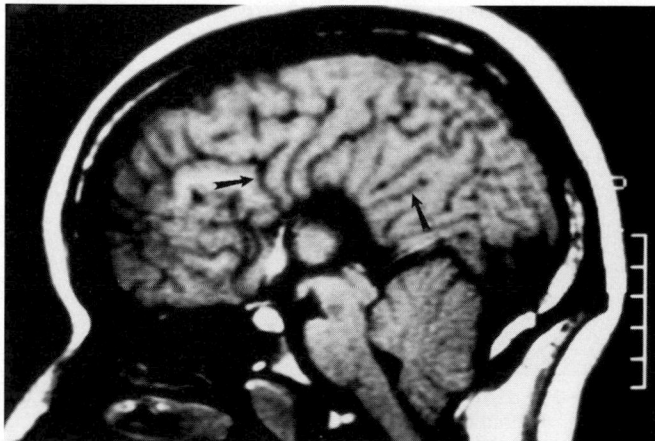

Figure 6–8 MRI of cranium demonstrating agenesis of corpus callosum. Sagittal T1 image.

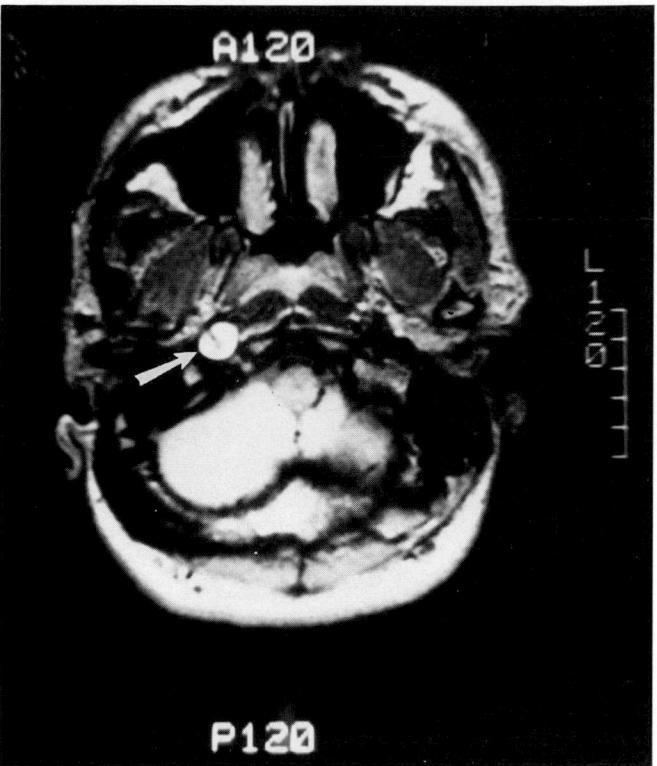

Figure 6–9 MRI/angiogram demonstrating carotid dissection. Magnetic resonance angiography.

2. Evaluation of cerebrovascular lesions such as arteriovenous malformations (AVM), aneurysms, arteriosclerosis, or arteritis.
3. Specialized studies such as Wada testing for hemispheric dominance.
4. Endovascular embolization procedures.

Contemporary cerebral angiography employs electronic digital imaging with computerized subtraction and/or biplanar arteriography and fluoroscopy, an automatic contrast injector, and automatic film changers. The Seldinger technique, or a modification thereof, in most cases provides the safest means of selective arterial injection; however, on rare occasions a retrograde brachial or direct carotid injection may be necessary to obtain a complete study.[18]

Physicians requesting or performing cerebral angiography should be familiar with the normal cerebrovascular anatomy, commonly occurring anatomical variations, and typical angiographic patterns, as well as appearance of various lesions.

Aortic Arch The *aortic arch* study is traditionally part of the standard cerebral angiogram. Currently, many institutions perform this study using digital subtraction angiography (DSA) in an effort to reduce the total amount of contrast media. The study is usually obtained in right posterior oblique (RPO) and left posterior oblique (LPO) projections. These views are important in the evaluation of ischemic cerebrovascular disease, since lesions or anomalous vascular origins in the region of the aortic arch may have an impact on treatment planning (Fig. 6-10).

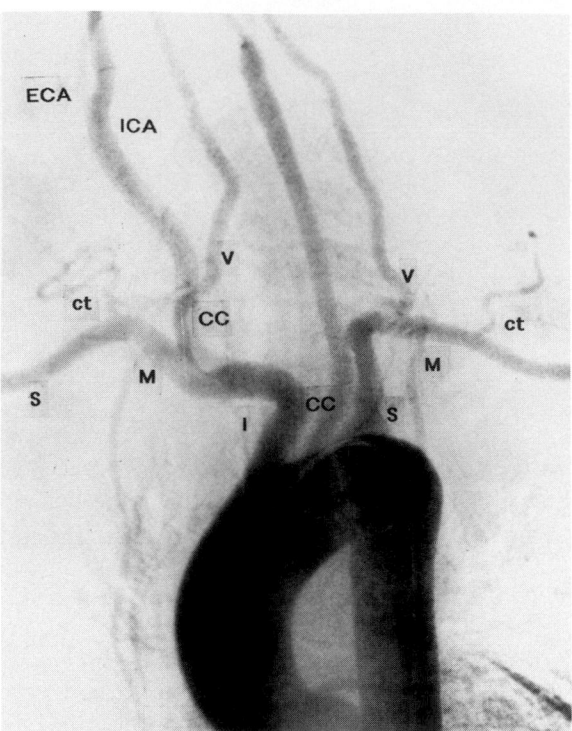

Figure 6–10 Angiogram of the aortic arch. I = innominate; M = mammary; S = subclavian; CC = common carotid; V = vertebral; ECA = external carotid artery; ct = thyrocervical trunk; ICA = internal carotid artery.

external carotid arteries for varying distances, creating turbulence and obstruction to blood flow (Fig. 6-11).

External Carotid Artery The *external carotid artery* is most often found anteromedial to the internal carotid artery and is normally the smaller of the two vessels. Of the seven to eight branches that arise from the external carotid artery, the internal maxillary, the major terminal branch, is of principal importance in neuroradiology. This artery gives rise to the middle meningeal artery, which enters the base of the skull via the foramen spinosum and provides blood supply to the dura over the sphenoid wing and over the frontal and parietal lobes. The meningeal arteries and their branches enlarge to supply meningeal tumors or dural arteriovenous malformations in this region. Terminal branches of the internal maxillary artery anastomose with distal branches of the ophthalmic artery, thus providing an important avenue of collateral blood flow to the intracranial arterial circulation. This is most commonly demonstrated after complete occlusion of the internal carotid artery proximal to

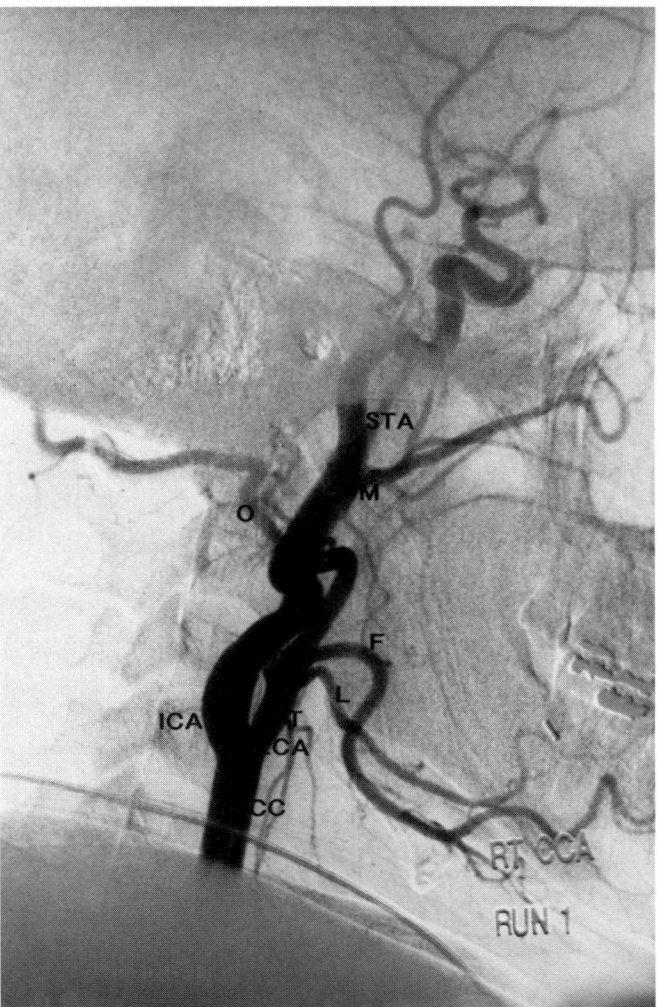

Figure 6–11 Arteriogram. Lateral views of extracranial carotid artery. CC = common carotid; ICA = internal carotid artery; ECA = external carotid artery; T = superior thyroid; L = lingual; F = facial; O = occipital; M = maxillary; STA = superficial temporal; arrow = catheter tip.

The innominate artery is the most proximal major branch of the aortic arch. This vessel divides into the right subclavian and right common carotid arteries. The right vertebral artery typically arises from the right subclavian artery within a couple of centimeters of its origin. On rare occasions an aberrant right subclavian artery may arise from the posterior wall of the aortic arch at or just distal to the origin of the left subclavian artery.

The left common carotid artery usually arises as a separate branch of the aortic arch just distal to the origin of the innominate artery, although these arteries may share a common origin. The left subclavian artery consistently arises from the anterosuperior surface of the aortic arch distal to the left common carotid origin and almost immediately gives rise to the left vertebral artery. Occasionally, the left vertebral artery will originate directly from the aortic arch between the origin of the left common carotid artery and the left subclavian artery. The left vertebral artery is typically the dominant vertebral artery and is therefore the preferred vessel for injection in the performance of posterior fossa angiography.

Carotid Artery The *common carotid artery* arises from the innominate artery or the aortic arch and usually has no major branches until its bifurcation into internal and external carotid arteries in the midcervical region. The bulbous-shaped bifurcation is the most common site of origin of atherosclerotic plaques that extend into the internal and

the supraclinoid segment. These vessels may also enlarge to supply meningeal tumors in the region of the sphenoid planum or olfactory groove. In cases of arteritis, the terminal branches of the external carotid artery frequently demonstrate typical angiographic patterns of this disease.

Internal Carotid Artery The *internal carotid artery* may be divided into four anatomical segments: cervical, petrous, cavernous, and supraclinoid. The cervical segment has few angiographically demonstrable branches except when there is persistence of a primitive hypoglossal artery. When present, this vessel arises from the cervical segment and ascends through the hypoglossal canal to anastomose with the basilar artery in the posterior fossa. Similarly, the petrous segment has few branches of angiographic significance save for the rare occurrence of a persistent primitive acoustic artery anastomosing with the basilar artery of the posterior circulation. Occasionally, a caroticotympanic branch feeds a glomus tumor in this region.

The cavernous segment of the internal carotid artery sometimes gives rise to a persistent trigeminal (mesencephalic) artery connecting the anterior and posterior circulations. This anomaly may be associated with an atretic posterior communicating artery, an atretic anterior cerebral artery, or an intracranial aneurysm. The cavernous segment also gives rise to a meningohypophyseal artery, which divides into the meningeal artery, supplying the tentorium and the inferior hypophyseal arteries. The meningeal artery, the artery of Bernasconi and Casanori, is rarely apparent except in association with a meningioma of the clivus or the tentorium or with a local dural arteriovenus malformation (AVM).

The supraclinoid segment gives rise to three major branches, the ophthalmic, the posterior communicating, and the anterior choroidal arteries, prior to its terminal bifurcation into the anterior and middle cerebral arteries (Fig. 6-12). The ophthalmic artery arises from the ventral surface of the internal carotid artery as it exits the cavernous sinus. From the initial segment of the ophthalmic artery originate a number of small arteries (ethmoidals), which supply the ethmoid sinuses and the dura overlying the sphenoid planum and floor of the frontal fossa. These arteries become prominent in the presence of meningeal tumors of the region. A recurrent meningeal artery may arise from the ophthalmic artery, and rarely this vessel gives rise to the middle meningeal artery. The terminal branch of the ophthalmic artery is the retinal artery. Angiograms outlining the retinal artery often demonstrate a choroidal blush of the posterior globe.

The posterior communicating cerebral artery (PComA) arises from the posterior wall of the supraclinoid internal carotid artery and courses posteromedially to join the posterior cerebral artery (PCA). The branch point of the PComA from the internal carotid artery is one of the most common sites of occurrence of a saccular (berry) aneurysm. The artery may be atretic. Rarely, there may be "fetal origin" of the PCA, where it arises directly from the supraclinoid ICA without an intervening PComA, in which case there is no communication with the basilar artery.

The anterior choroidal artery arises from the intracranial carotid artery just distal to the PComA. This point of branching is another common site for a saccular aneurysm. The anterior choroidal artery initially courses posteromedially and ultimately turns superolateral to enter the choroidal fissure and supply the choroid plexus of the temporal lobe.

The intracranial carotid artery terminates by bifurcating into the anterior and middle cerebral arteries.

The initial segment of the anterior cerebral artery (ACA) complex courses anteromedially from the bifurcation, beneath the orbital portion of the frontal lobe and turns superiorly in the cistern of the lamina terminalis. Here, it gives rise to a short segment, the anterior communicating artery (AComA), which anastomoses with the opposite anterior cerebral artery. The segment from the bifurcation of the intracranial carotid artery to the anterior communicating artery is often referred to as the *A-1 segment.* The segment of anterior cerebral artery beyond the origin of the anterior communicating artery is referred to as the *A-2 segment* and gives rise to one or two small lenticular branches, the larger of which is usually called the "recurrent artery of Huebner." The region around the AComA is where most saccular aneurysms of the ACA occur. Beyond this point, the distal anterior cerebral artery, which is also known as the "pericallosal artery," gives rise to the frontopolar branch and proceeds superiorly and posteriorly above the genu and over the superior surface of the corpus callosum. The artery terminates in a number of callossomarginal branches and the artery of the pericallosal sulcus.

The middle cerebral artery, as it originates from the bifurcation of the intracranial carotid artery, courses slightly anteriorly and superiorly and then becomes almost horizontal as it courses laterally toward the sylvian fissure. This horizontal segment gives rise to a number of small lenticulostriate vessels, which are barely demonstrable on angiography, followed by major branches to supply the frontal and/or anterior temporal lobes. The segment of the middle cerebral artery proximal to its turn (genu) into the sylvian fissure is referred to as the *M-1 segment.* From the genu, the artery courses posteriorly and superiorly in the sylvian fissure, typically giving rise to two or three major branches, referred to as the *bifurcation* or *trifurcation.* Any of these branch points may be the sites of saccular aneurysms; the trifurcation is the most common site for aneurysms of the middle cerebral artery. Distally, branches of the middle cerebral artery extend over the surface of the frontal, temporal, and parietal lobes. Other major branches, deep in the sylvian fissure loop over the insular cortex, the island of Reil. Viewing the angiogram made in the AP projection, the terminal loop of middle cerebral artery most posterior and medial is referred to as the *sylvian point.* Viewing the lateral projection, the sylvian point is again identified as the most distal point of the terminal loop of the middle cerebral artery. A triangle may be constructed by drawing a line from the sylvian point to the genu of the middle cerebral artery, and another line from the sylvian point tangential to the

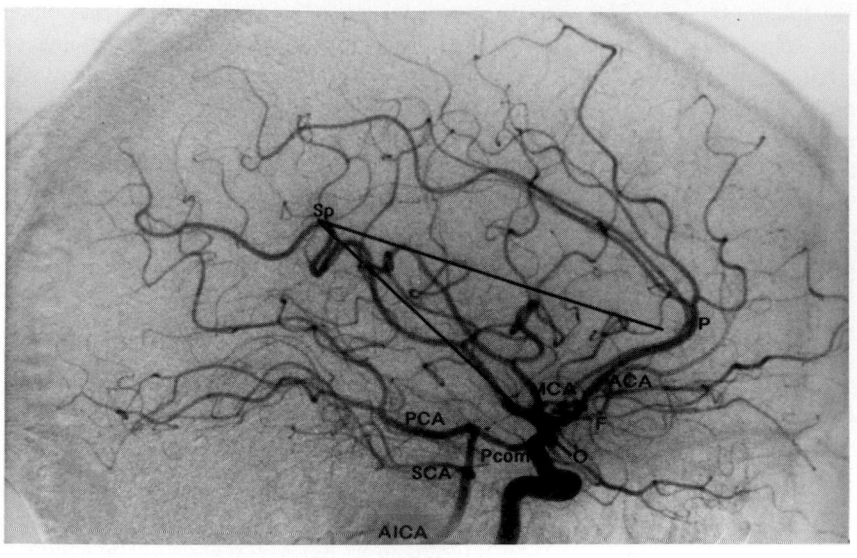

(A)

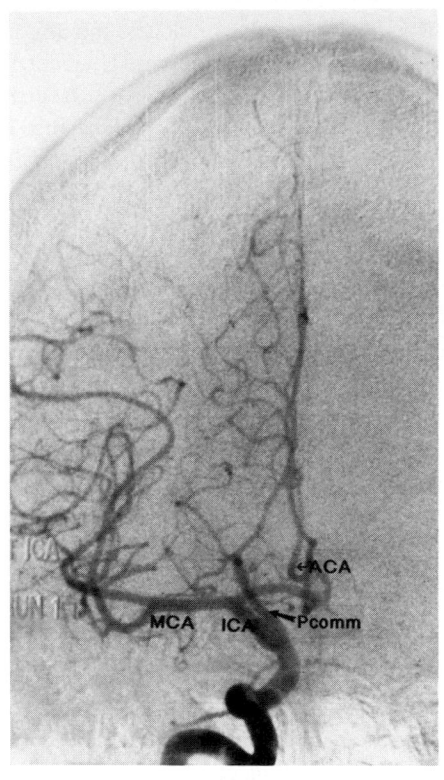

(B)

Figure 6–12 Normal carotid angiogram demonstrating primitive-type posterior communicating artery (Pcom) with filling of the right anterior and entire posterior circulation. Note also the well-defined sylvian point (Sp) and outline of the sylvian triangle. Lateral projection carotid angiogram *(A)*. AP projection carotid angiogram *(B)*. MCA = middle cerebral artery; ACA = anterior cerebral artery; O = ophthalmic; PCA = posterior cerebral artery; F = frontopolar; P = pericallosal; SCA = superior cerebellar artery; AICA = anterior inferior cerebellar artery.

middle cerebral artery loops over the insular cortex to the level of the carotid bifurcation (Fig. 6-12). These two landmarks, the sylvian point and the sylvian triangle, are useful in locating intracranial masses by cerebral angiography.

Posterior Circulation Other than the exceptions of aberrant circulation previously noted, the posterior cerebral circulation is supplied principally by the vertebral arteries and a variable contribution from the posterior communicating arteries. The vertebral arteries enter the skull through the foramen magnum posterolateral to the brainstem. At approx-

imately the level of the caudal pons, they course ventromedially and join in the midline to form the basilar artery. Prior to this junction, each vertebral artery gives rise to a posterior inferior cerebellar artery (PICA). Aneurysms of the posterior circulation commonly occur where the PICAs branch from the vertebral arteries. Each PICA has two major branches: a tonsillohemispheric branch with a caudal loop which passes around the lowest extent of the cerebellar tonsils prior to terminating over the posteroinferior aspect of the cerebellar hemisphere and a terminal vermian branch which approaches the midline (Fig. 6-13). The caudal drop of the tonsillo-

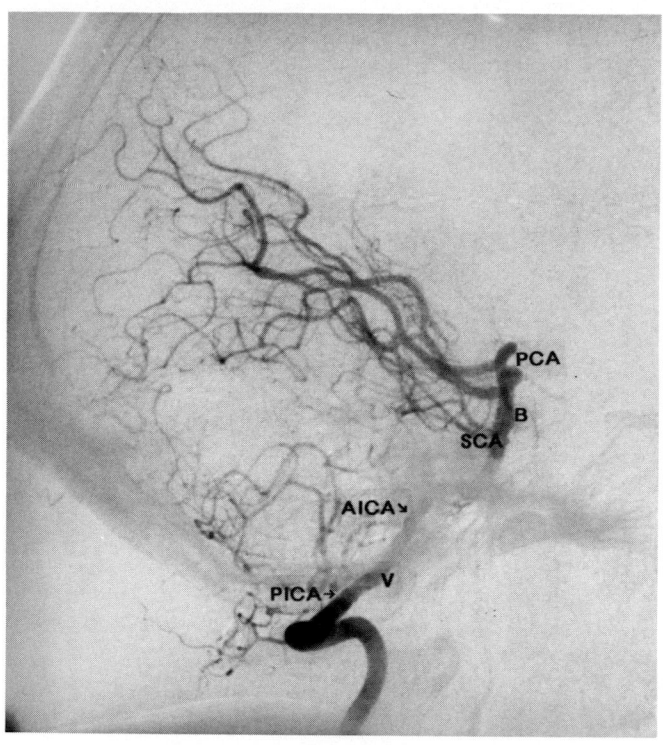

(A)

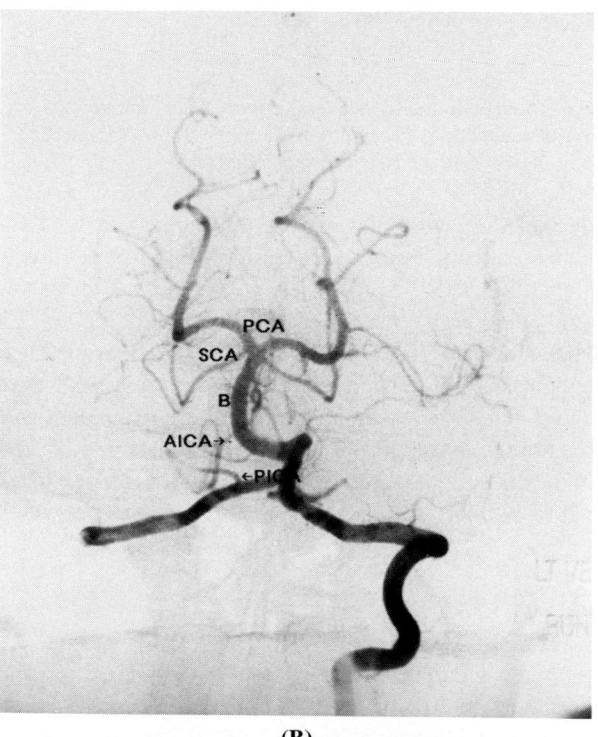

(B)

Figure 6–13 Normal vertebral angiogram. Lateral *(A)* and AP projection *(B)*. V = vertebral; PICA = posterior inferior cerebellar artery; AICA = anterior inferior cerebellar artery; B = basilar artery; SCA = superior cerebellar artery; PCA = posterior cerebral artery.

hemispheric artery is useful in identifying caudal descent of the cerebellar tonsils through the foramen magnum, as may be seen in tonsillar herniation and Chiari malformations. The

vermian branch may be helpful in lateralizing intraaxial posterior fossa tumors.

The first major branch of the basilar artery is the anterior inferior cerebellar artery (AICA), which courses laterally around the pons to become adjacent to the seventh and eighth cranial nerves. It then continues laterally over the ventrolateral surface of the cerebellar hemisphere. This vessel is frequently elevated by tumors in the region of the cerebellopontine angle; it is occasionally the site of aneurysms or may supply arteriovenous malformations.

The superior cerebellar arteries arise as paired branches from the distal basilar artery and course laterally around the brainstem in the ambient cistern and then superiorly over the surface of the cerebellum beneath the tentorium. The origin of these vessels is infrequently the site of aneurysms. The vessels may supply AVMs or tumors. Their initial segments may be displaced upward or downward by transtentorial herniation.

The large paired posterior cerebral arteries are the terminal branches of the basilar artery. Basilar tip aneurysms occur at the branching point. The posterior cerebral artery courses around the midbrain above cranial nerve III and becomes supratentorial. The artery then divides and gives off branches posteriorly, superomedially, and laterally.

Cerebral Veins The cerebral venous drainage may be divided into superficial and deep venous systems. The superficial venous system is primarily composed of veins that overlie the gyral surfaces and drain into major venous sinuses. The deep venous system, for angiographic purposes, includes the paired internal cerebral veins and the deep medullary veins, which ultimately drain into the vein of Galen and the straight sinus (Fig. 6-14).

Lesions overlying the surface of the brain, such as subdural or epidural hematomas, visibly displace the superficial cerebral veins away from the inner table of the skull. Deeper lesions, within the brain substance, displace the deep veins with reference to the midline. Other lesions demonstrated by venous angiography include the early draining veins of a neoplasm or vascular malformation or venous sinus occlusion. The sequence and timing of venous drainage may also be helpful in identifying such signs as the early draining vein of a neoplasm or vascular malformation or a venous sinus occlusion or thrombosis.

ENCEPHALOGRAPHY

Encephalography, which encompasses pneumoencephalography and ventriculography, was described by Walter Dandy in 1918 and is one of the oldest neuroradiological imaging techniques.[19] By convention, encephalography combines the use of plain skull x-rays or polytomograms with the use of air or other radiographic contrast media injected into the ventricular or subarachnoid spaces of the brain.[20] In pneumoencephalography, air is injected into the subarachnoid space via a lumbar or cisternal puncture and subsequently

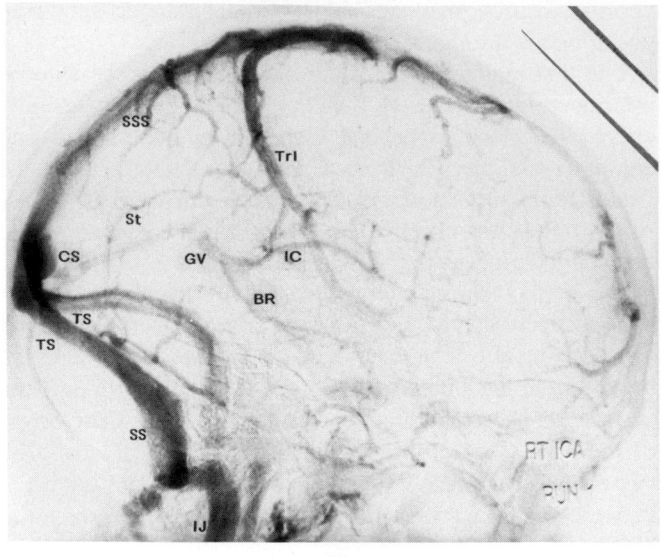

(A)

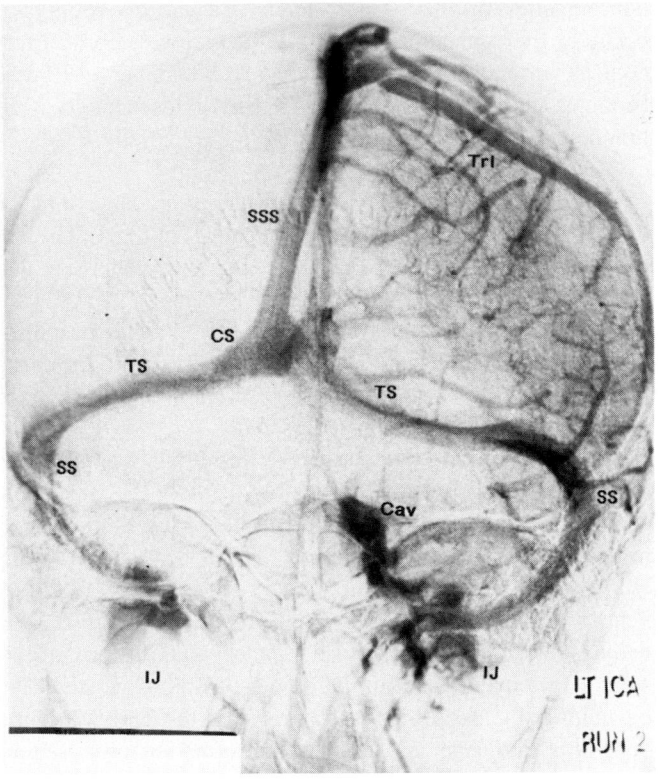

(B)

Figure 6–14 Normal venous phase of carotid angiogram. Lateral *(A)* and AP *(B)* projection of venous phase.
IJ = internal jugular; SS = sigmoid sinus; SSS = superior sagittal sinus; St = straight sinus; TS = transverse sinus; Trl = trolardi vein; CS = confluence of sinuses; Cav = cavernous sinus; GV = great vein of Galen; BR = basal vein of Rosenthal; IC = internal cerebral vein.

skull x-rays or polytomograms obtained in various projections, while manipulating the position of the patient to accomplish movement of the air throughout the ventricular and cisternal systems.

In ventriculography, air or other contrast media is injected

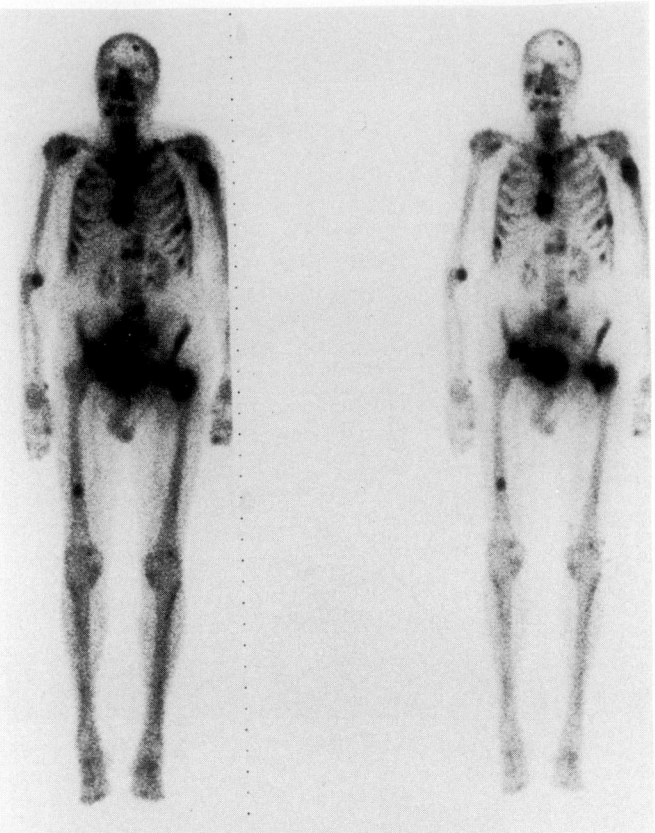

Figure 6–15 Radionuclide skeletal survey after intravenous injection of technetium (Tc) demonstrating multiple metastatic lesions in patient with primary cervical cancer.

directly into the ventricular system through a burr hole and ventricular catheter and, again, skull x-rays or polytomograms are obtained.[21]

In contemporary neuroradiology, the availability of CT and MRI has supplanted the general applications of encephalography and eliminated the attendant morbidity of these procedures. The specific application of these techniques may be expeditious, as in the intraoperative assessment of ventricular or cisternal catheter position or the assessment and removal of pituitary tumors.

RADIONUCLIDE SCANS

Radionuclide scanning involves the injection of a small amount of radioactive isotope, usually technetium (Tc) into the blood or cerebrospinal fluid (CSF).[22] The location and relative activity of the isotope is subsequently detected at various time intervals by a scintillation camera or a series of scintillation detectors. CT scanning and MRI have replaced radionuclide scanning for many applications. Remaining applications include: (1) skeletal surveys for metastatic disease or infection (Fig. 6-15); (2) cranial surveys (cisternography) for CSF fistulae (Fig. 6-16); (3) radionuclide angiography, which provides physiological information related to cerebral blood flow and compensated collateral flow (Fig. 6-17); and

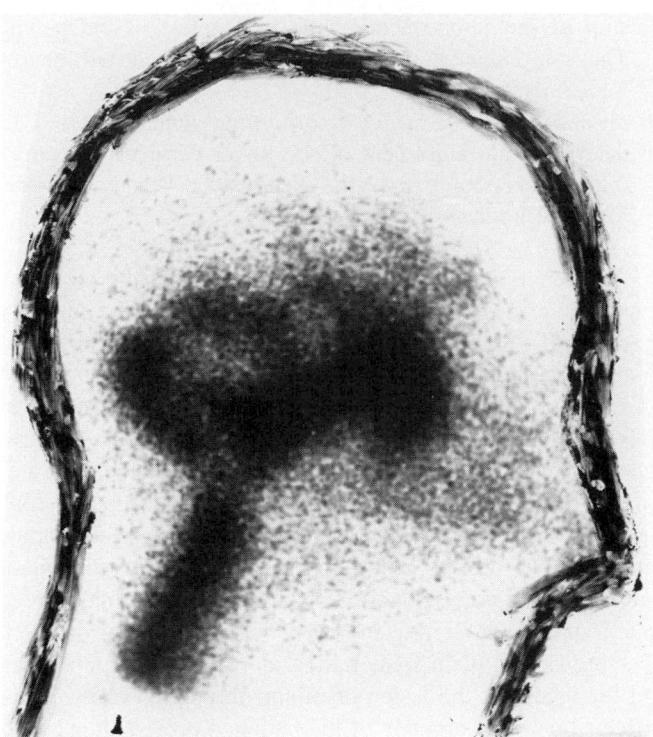

Figure 6–16 Radionuclide cisternogram using indium to demonstrate anterior fossa CSF fistula.

(4) radionuclide investigation of shunts ("shunt-o-grams") which may demonstrate the existence of obstruction to CSF flow between the ventricles or subarachnoid spaces and the recipient cavity. Examples of these studies are provided below.

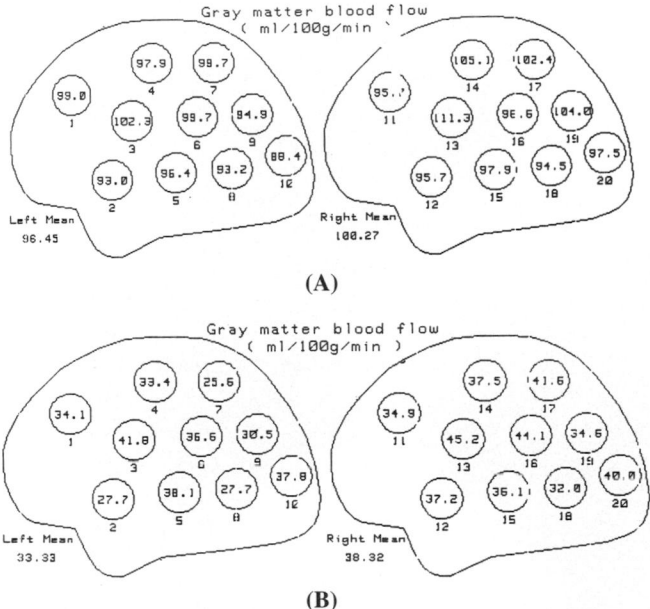

(A)

(B)

Figure 6–17 Regional cerebral blood flow scans. Computer-generated scintigraphs of normal xenon (Xe) uptake over various brain regions *(A)*. Computer-generated scintigraph demonstrating diffuse cerebral hypoperfusion *(B)*.

POSITRON EMISSION COMPUTED TOMOGRAPHY (PET)

PET employs the use of positron emission radionuclides attached to metabolites, typically glucose. After intravenous administration, these radionuclides are detected by specialized scanning devices, similar to the scintillation detectors used in traditional radionuclide scanning. The major advantage of this technique is that it provides images that reflect physiological information, specifically the relative increase or decrease in the activity of the positron-tagged metabolite in the brain.[23] The major disadvantages are the enormous expense of acquiring and maintaining a cyclotron to generate the positrons and the rather limited clinical applications.

☐ NEURORADIOLOGY OF THE SPINE

PLAIN SPINE RADIOGRAPHY

Plain radiographs of the spine are still the first imaging studies obtained in the evaluation of patients with suspected spinal disease or injury. Portable radiographs of the spine may be performed on site, with a minimum of patient manipulation. More extensive protocols involving multiple views and patient manipulation may be employed in an effort to define more clearly the anatomy of bones and joints. The major failing of plain spine radiography is its inability to image adequately noncalcified tissue intimately related to the spine, such as the spinal cord, intervertebral disks, and adjacent soft tissues. The most important observations made from plain spine radiographs relate to the structural integrity of the spinal column and the adequacy of the spinal canal. The most useful views for this purpose are the following:

Lateral projection. Demonstrates the anterior-posterior diameter of the canal, the alignment and regional contour of the spine, the height and shape of the vertebral bodies and disk spaces, the joint spacing and continuity of the posterior elements, and the relationship of the atlas and axis at the craniovertebral junction (Fig. 6-18).
Lateral views. May also be obtained with the patient in flexion and extension to aid in the assessment of structural integrity (Fig. 6-19).
Anteroposterior projections. Demonstrate the interpedicular distance or coronal diameter of the spinal canal, the shape and thickness of the pedicles, and the presence of dysraphic lesions or soft tissue masses (Fig. 6-20).

Additional projections may include the following:

Open mouth views of the odontoid. Used to assess the integrity and continuity of the dens and its relationship to the lateral masses of the atlas (Fig. 6-21).

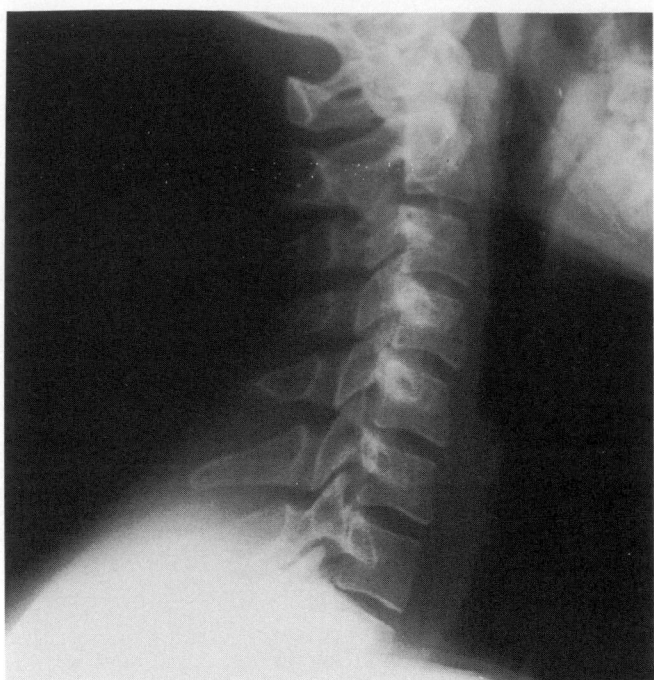

Figure 6–18 Normal lateral projection of cervical spine.

Oblique views. Used to assess the pedicles, neural foramina, lamina, and articular pillars and joint spaces.
Anteroposterior pelvic views. Demonstrate the relation-ship of the lumbosacral spine to the rest of the pelvis. They may identify pelvic fractures associated with neurological dysfunction.

Swimmers' views of cervicothoracic junction. Used to determine the alignment of the lower cervical and upper thoracic vertebrae and the height and shape of these vertebral bodies.

In practice, a complete spinal survey employing all of the views described above in each region of the spine is rarely required. The extent and direction of the radiographic examination is usually determined from the information obtained through the history and physical examination, with historical information often being the major determinant. Consequently, the judgment of what constitutes an adequate examination varies. In the situation presented by an unconscious trauma victim with an apparent paraparesis, the radiographic examination may be extensive, whereas the evaluation of subacute neck pain with a discrete radiculopathy may forego plain spine radiography in favor of myelography or MRI. The efficacy of plain spine radiography will vary, depending on the nature of the lesion or injury, the region of the spine affected, and the urgency of the patient's presentation.

In general, nonskeletal lesions and lesions with extraskeletal extension—such as neoplasms, infectious processes, vascular malformations, herniated intervertebral disks, and some congenital malformations—are rarely adequately iden-

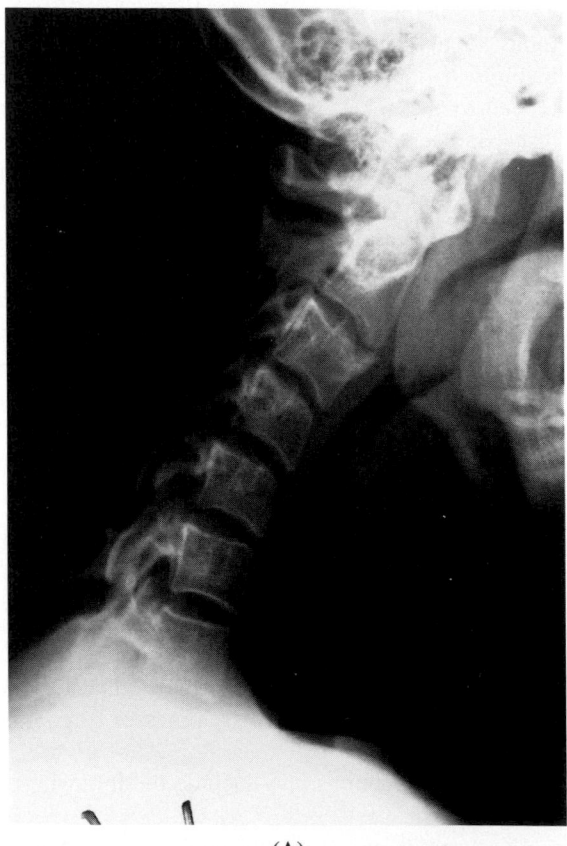

(A)

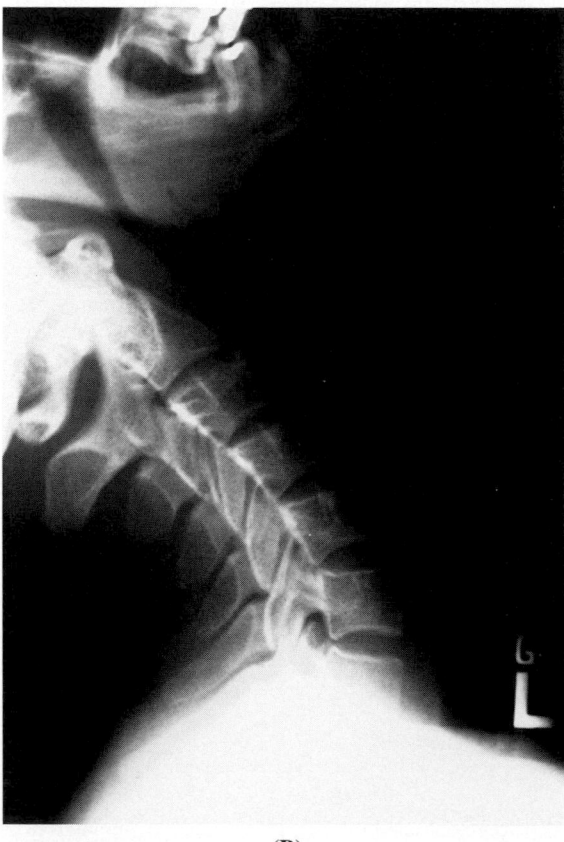

(B)

Figure 6–19 X-ray of cervical spine in extreme flexion and extension. Note the even distribution of movement over all motion segments. Lateral cervical spine in extreme flexion *(A)*. Lateral cervical spine in extreme extension *(B)*.

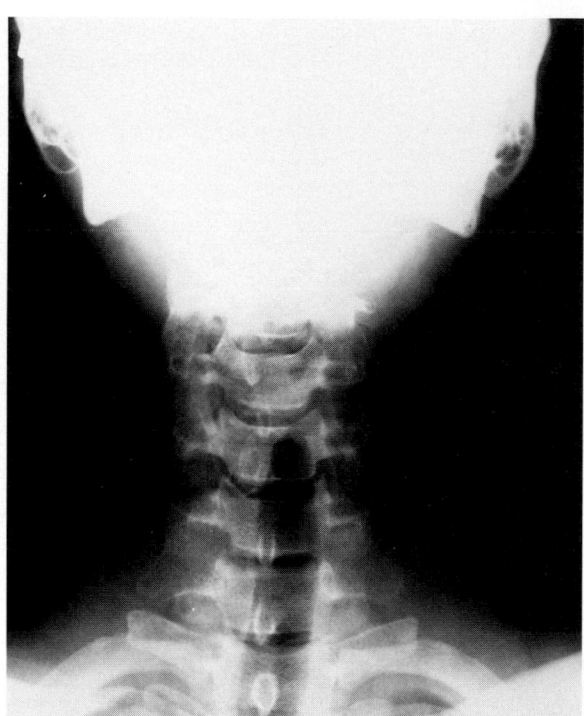

Figure 6–20 Normal AP projection cervical spine.

tified by plain radiography, and they require specialized imaging techniques, such as myelography, CT scan, and MRI, for appropriate evaluation and planning of treatment.[24]

In the region of the CV junction, skeletal lesions such as rheumatoid pannus, os odontoideum, odontoid fracture, platybasia, basilar impression, achondroplasia, and Paget's disease, which may have an impact on CNS function, can be rapidly and reliably identified by lateral and open mouth radiographs.[25] More specialized imaging techniques may not be indicated.

In the cervical, thoracic, and lumbar regions, plain radiographs may effectively identify degenerative and destructive

lesions of the spine and demonstrate the effect of these lesions on the structural integrity of the spinal column; however, plain radiographs do not illustrate the impact of such lesions on the nervous system. Consequently, specialized imaging techniques are often employed prior to surgical intervention.

In the evaluation of vertebral trauma, plain radiography is normally the initial imaging technique. Lateral views are usually the most revealing, especially in the cervical and lumbar areas, and coupled with an AP view, these images may provide sufficient information to determine the need for stabilization or surgical intervention, particularly in the event of neurological deficits. A complete spine series may be required in symptomatic cases prior to concluding a normal examination or negative evaluation. In the event of positive physical or neurological findings and a negative plain radiographic examination, more specialized studies are often necessary. Table 6-1 details the suggested views for a complete series for each region of the spine.

COMPUTER ASSISTED IMAGING OF THE SPINE

Magnetic resonance imaging is the study of choice for the evaluation of abnormalities of the spinal canal, spinal cord, vertebral body marrow spaces, and intervertebral disk disease.[26] This is due to the absence of mobile protons in the cortical bone of the vertebral bodies and the neural arches, as well as the excellent soft tissue discrimination of MRI. MRI outlines the spinal cord within the CSF, allowing the differentiation of intramedullary and extramedullary lesions. It provides for the noninvasive diagnosis of primary spinal cord tumors (Fig. 6-22), syringohydromyelia, spinal cord demyelination or infarcts, and congenital malformations of the spinal cord or the spinal column. MRI is also ideal for the evaluation of pediatric spinal anomalies, i.e., meningoceles, myelomeningoceles, lipomyelomeningoceles, diaste-

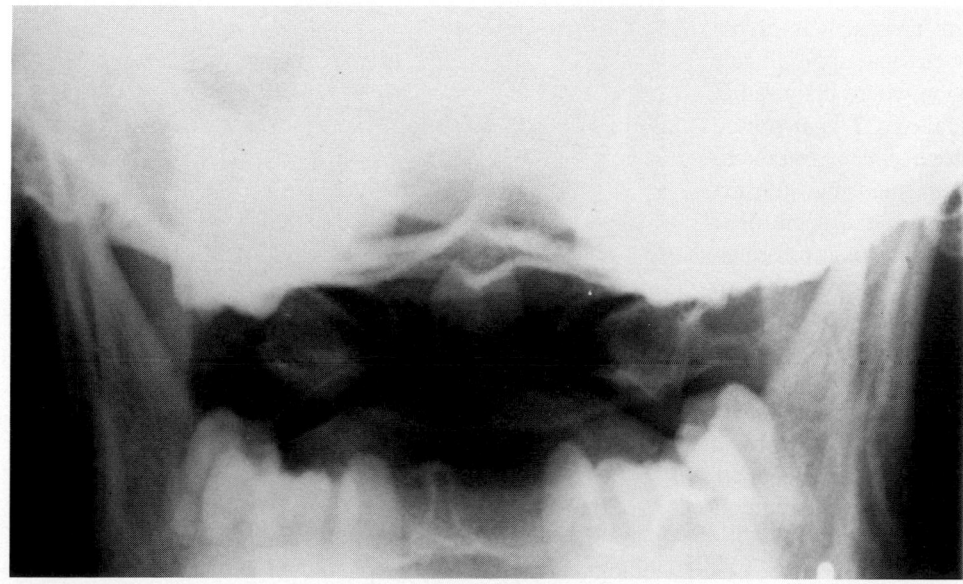

Figure 6–21 Open mouth view of odontoid. Note the symmetry of space between right and left lateral masses of CT and the odontoid process.

Table 6-1
SUGGESTED PLAIN RADIOGRAPHS IN THE EVALUATION OF SUSPECTED VERTEBRAL INJURY

Cervical Spine
1. Lateral
2. Anteroposterior
3. 30° Obliques
4. Upright weight bearing lateral
5. Flexion and extension laterals
6. Open mouth odontoid view of atlas and axis
7. Swimmers view of cervical thoracic junction

Thoracic Spine
1. Lateral
2. Anteroposterior

Lumbar Spine and Sacrum
1. Lateral
2. Anteroposterior lumbosacral spine
3. Anteroposterior pelvis

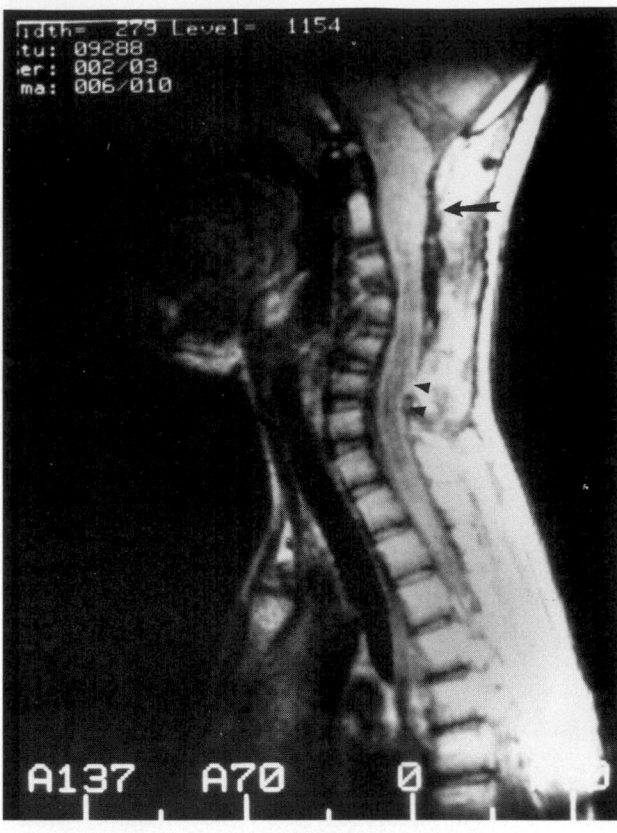

(A)

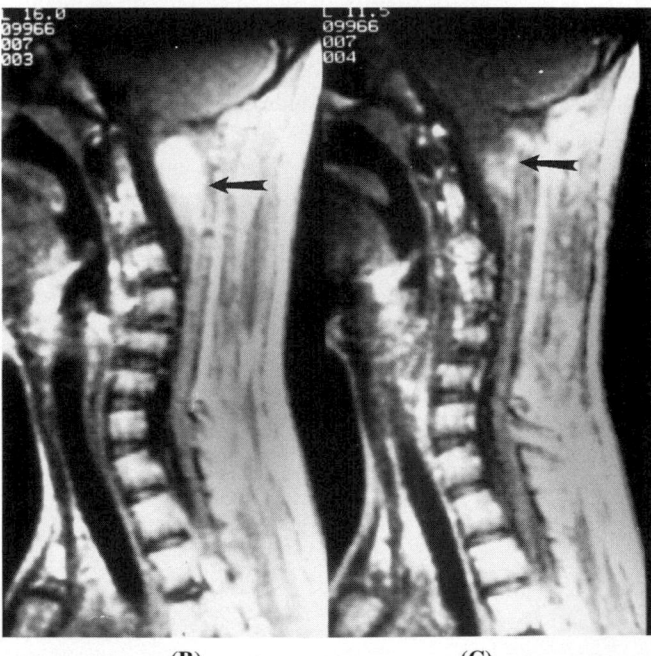

(B)   (C)

Figure 6–22 Sagittal T1 image *(A)*; sagittal T2 image *(B)*, sagittal T1 image after administration of Gd *(C)*.

matomyelia, or tethered cord (Fig. 6-23). MRI with gadolinium-DTPA is recommended for investigation of neoplasms, both primary and metastatic, of the spinal canal.[27] Additionally, in patients with failed back syndrome, it can differentiate scar tissue from recurrent disk herniations (Fig. 6-24).

Limitations of MRI include the significant artifacts surrounding metallic hardware (Harrington rods, Halifax clamps, or metallic plates). Signal loss is also seen in areas of spinal surgery where metal deposition from use of surgical drills occurs, as in anterior cervical diskectomies. For this reason we routinely use diamond bits, but burrs are becoming available that do not leave behind materials that cause artifacts.

The use of MRI for evaluation of spinal lesions has changed the role of CT in recent years. At the present time, CT is the study of choice for evaluation of spinal trauma, especially when considering the presence of fractures or dislocations of the facets and/or neural arches. It is highly desirable to obtain a CT of the lower cervical spine to rule out lesions at the cervical-dorsal junction where plain radiographs of this region are of limited quality. CT is also used in evaluating burst fractures with retropulsion of fragments into the spinal canal, trauma to the spine by gunshot wounds, and abnormalities in alignment of the spine after deceleration injuries. Two- and three-dimensional reformatted CT images may also be helpful in the evaluation of complex injuries, developmental abnormalities, and degenerative changes of the spine (Fig. 6-25). There has been a continuous decline in the use of CT for the evaluation of routine lumbar spine diskogenic disease in favor of MRI. In cases where the MRI findings are equivocal, myelography in combination with CT (CT-myelogram) is recommended. The role of myelography and CT-myelogram is still important in the evaluation of abnormalities of alignment of the spine, including scoliosis and spondylolisthesis.

MYELOGRAPHY

Myelography combines the use of contrast media injected into the subarachnoid space with spinal radiographs or polytomograms to outline the spinal cord and nerve roots. Walter

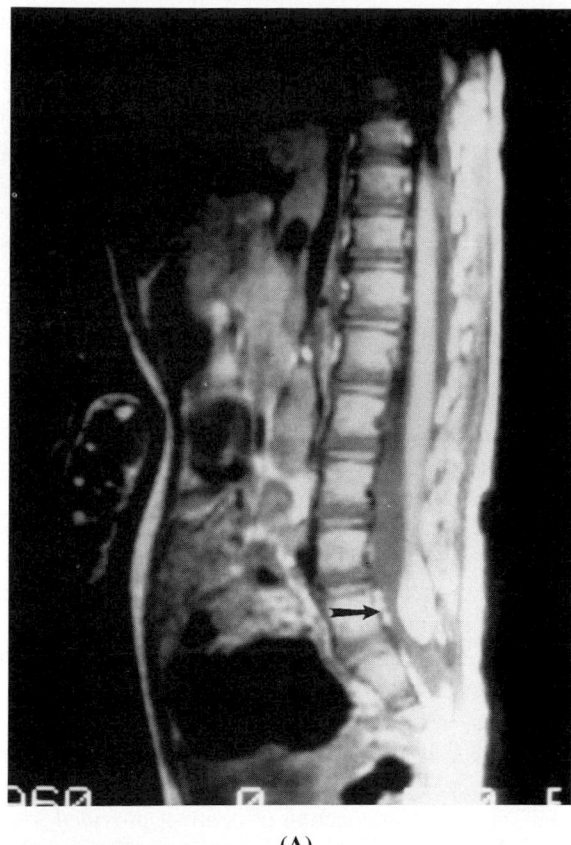

(A)

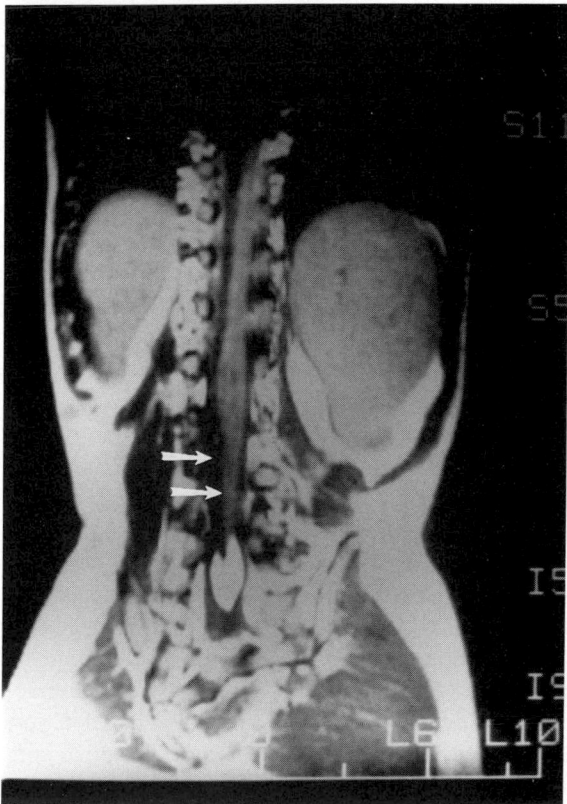

(B)

Figure 6–23 MRI of lumbar spinal region demonstrating lipoma with cord tethering. Sagittal T1 *(A)*. Coronal T1 *(B)*.

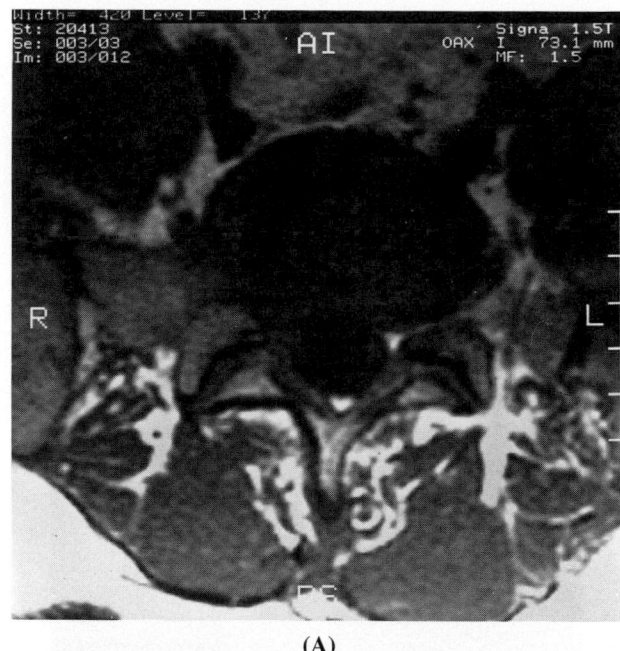

(A)

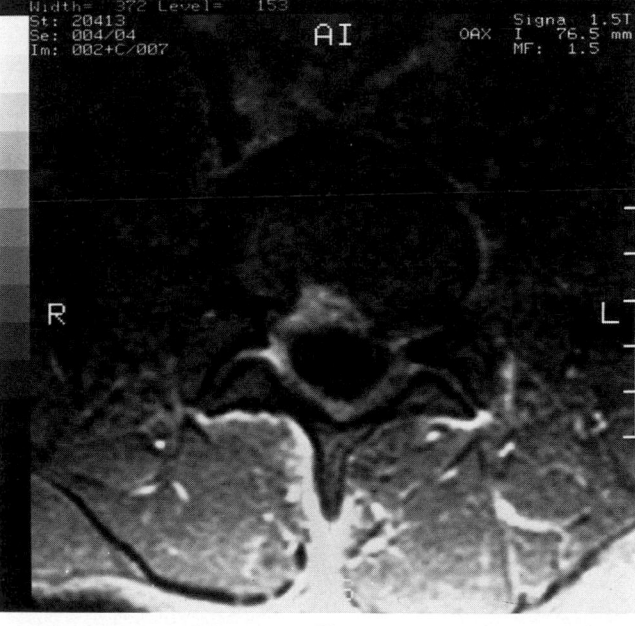

(B)

Figure 6–24 MRI of postsurgical lumbar spine *(A)*. Axial T1 image with poor definition of dura/scar interface *(B)*. Axial T1 image after Gd demonstrating dura/scar interface.

Dandy, in his 1919 paper on pneumoencephalography, advocated the use of air to contrast the subarachnoid space of the spinal column.[28] By 1921, Jacobeus in Sweden and Forestier and Sicard in Paris, using air and lipiodol, respectively, described the use of subarachnoid contrast media in the diagnosis of spinal cord tumors.[29] During the early 1940s, a less-viscous and less-toxic contrast medium was introduced, and myelography gained widespread use. With the availability of water-soluble contrast media by the mid-1970s came the capability for full volume opacification of the subarach-

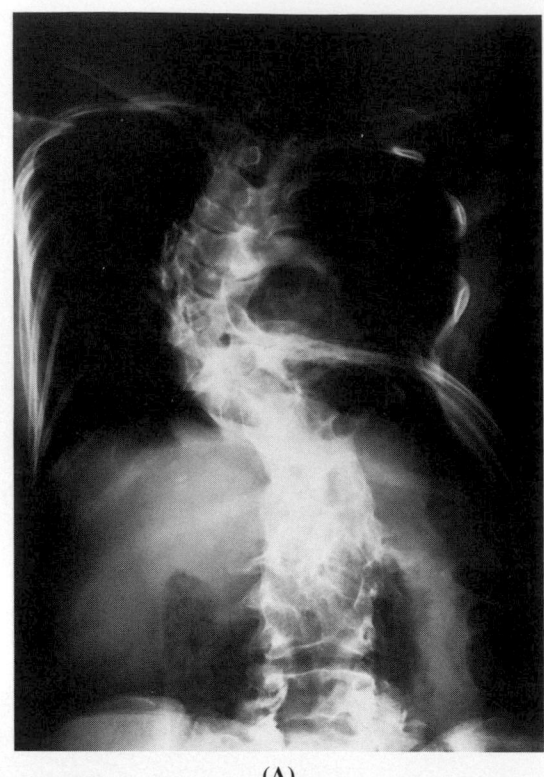

(A)

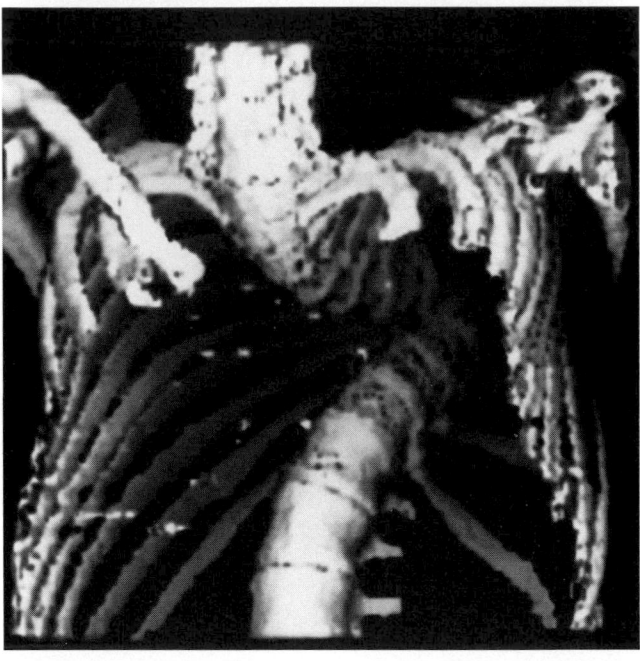

(B)

Figure 6–25 Scoliosis of thoracic and upper lumbar spine. *(A)* AP projection plain spine film. CT 3-dimensional reconstruction *(B)*.

noid space, thus enhancing the diagnostic sensitivity and accuracy of myelography.[30]

The tandem combination of myelography and the postmyelogram CT were the mainstay in neuroradiology of the spine by the mid-1980s.[31] This combination affords multiple orientations from which to view the spinal canal and its contents. Myelography affords the versatility to focus on a specific region of the spine or a survey of the entire spinal axis. The patient may be repositioned during the study to simulate symptomatic postures or to facilitate the flow of contrast. Nerve root lesions and traumatic nerve root avulsions are often best demonstrated by myelography. Obstruction of the subarachnoid space (myelographic block) and cavitary spinal cord lesions, such as syringomyelia, may also be indicated by myelography; however, in general, the postmyelogram CT scan is more sensitive and more specific in the demonstration of spinal cord and spinal column lesions and may also identify lesions beyond the level of a complete myelographic block.

While a detailed discussion of the technique of myelography is beyond the scope of this text, some familiarity with the procedure will provide the insight necessary for selecting the appropriate imaging techniques.

The patient is placed on a radiolucent myelography table in the prone or a lateral decubitus (fetal) position in order to achieve separation of the spinous processes to provide easy access to the spinal canal. Mild sedation is frequently required; however, an awake, cooperative patient is preferred, and general anesthesia is seldom indicated.

The lumbar puncture is usually attempted at the L2–L3 level unless this is the area of particular interest. Adequate studies of the cervical, thoracic, and lumbar regions may be obtained via a lumbar injection of contrast provided meticulous attention to technique is maintained. Occasionally a cervical (C1–2) puncture and injection are necessary to obtain adequate opacification in the cervical region or to image the spinal canal above the level of a myelographic block. Once the needle enters the subarachnoid space and there is prompt return of CSF, the patient is positioned prone and the contrast medium is allowed to drip into the subarachnoid space. This aspect of the procedure should be observed under fluoroscopy to avoid a subdural or epidural injection. After the radiopaque contrast has been manipulated into the appropriate region, a series of lateral, anteroposterior, and oblique films is obtained. The protocol varies slightly between institutions. Depending on the diffusion of the contrast media and the extent of the study, a postmyelogram CT scan may be performed immediately or within 4 hours after the myelogram.

The indications for myelography are fairly broad—in essence, whenever there is a need to image the spinal cord or nerve roots. The most common application is in the evaluation of patients with neck pain, low back pain, and radicular pain; however, any complex of symptoms or signs which implicates spinal cord or nerve root involvement may be considered an appropriate indication for myelography. There are few, if any, contraindications to the use of water-soluble contrast myelography; however, neurological deterioration of patients with inflammatory diseases of the spinal cord has been reported after the use of some water-soluble contrast agents. In many institutions, myelography has been supplanted by MRI as the initial study of choice in the evaluation of the spine, particularly in an emergency.

In the normal myelogram, the radiopaque column that

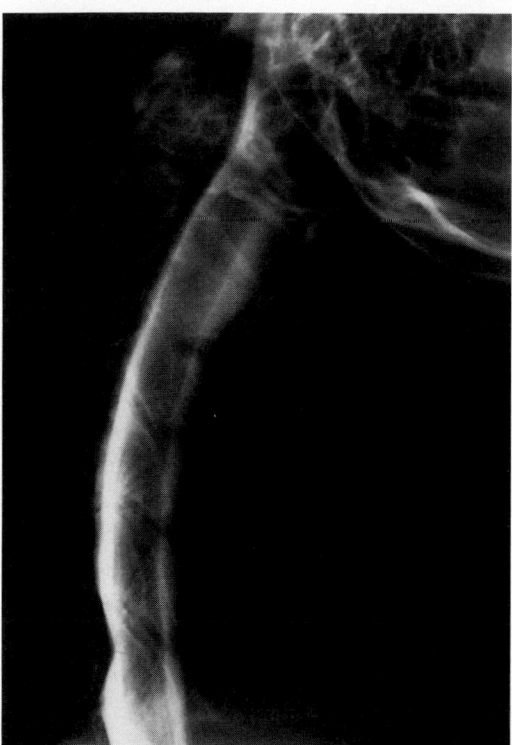

Figure 6–26 Lateral projection of cervical myelogram. Note the dark shadow of the spinal cord outlined by the radiopaque water-soluble contrast. There is a slight disk bulge at the C5–6 level encroaching on the anterior meningeal space.

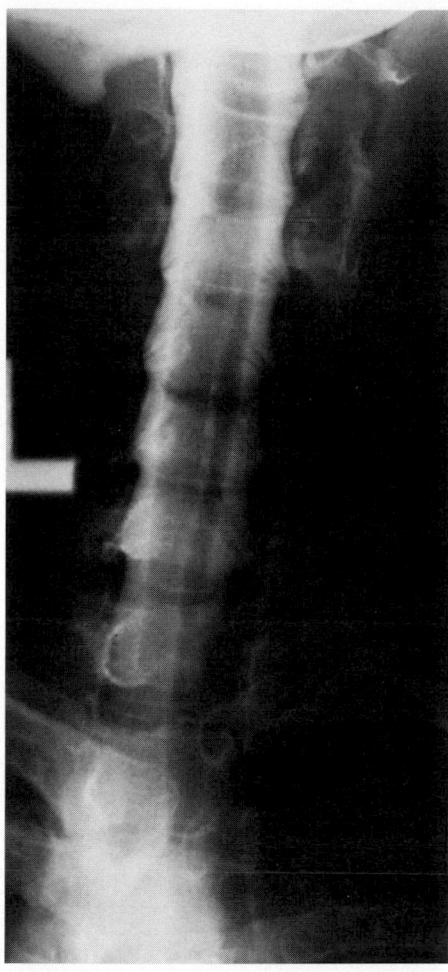

Figure 6–27 AP projection of cervical myelogram. The dark shadow of the spinal cord is centrally located within the canal and the nerve roots are demonstrated coursing inferolaterally from the spinal cord to the neural foramina.

results from water-soluble contrast media filling the sub-arachnoid space will exhibit regional variations due to the changes in the size of the vertebral canal, the size and trajectory of exiting nerve roots, and the cross-sectional diameter of the spinal cord. Nevertheless, there should be a uniform and symmetrical outline of the centrally positioned spinal cord from the upper cervical region to the level of the conus.

In the cervical region, the lateral projection usually demonstrates a relatively wide subarachnoid space ventral to the spinal cord and a narrower subarachnoid space posteriorly (Fig. 6-26). This is, in part, due to the moderate degree of extension in which the patient is positioned for cervical myelography. The anteroposterior diameter of the spinal cord viewed from the lateral projection remains rather uniform throughout the cervical region (Fig. 6-27). The anteroposterior projections should demonstrate uniform radiopaque margins bordering a central radiolucent shadow of the spinal cord, which may exhibit a slight increase in the cross-sectional diameter in the middle and lower cervical region. The fine linear radiolucencies of nerve rootlets are commonly outlined by the contrast within the subarachnoid space as they pass from the spinal cord and exit the neural foramina. Their appearance should be symmetrical at each segment. One common exception is presented by the occasional demonstration of perineural cysts, which fill with subarachnoid contrast material and give the nerve root

sheath a bulbous appearance (Fig. 6-28). Usually, these cysts are not pathological.

In the thoracic region, the lateral projection outlines a spinal cord that adheres closely to the normal thoracic kyphotic curvature and demonstrates a constant anteroposterior diameter throughout the region (Fig. 6-29). The ventral subarachnoid space is usually defined by a fine radiopaque line separating the posterior aspect of the vertebral bodies from the radiolucent shadow of the spinal cord. The posterior subarachnoid space is much wider and remains uniform in its contour throughout the region. In the anteroposterior projections, the cross-sectional diameter of the spinal cord remains constant throughout the region; however, the subarachnoid space is narrowest in the midthoracic region and widens in the upper and lower thoracic regions (Fig. 6-30). The linear radiolucencies of the thoracic nerve rootlets, although not prominent, should be symmetrical. Thoracic myelography is frequently supplemented with polytomography or CT scan in a region of primary interest. A swimmer's view may be obtained if the cervicothoracic junction is suspect.

In the lumbar region, the subarachnoid space is usually

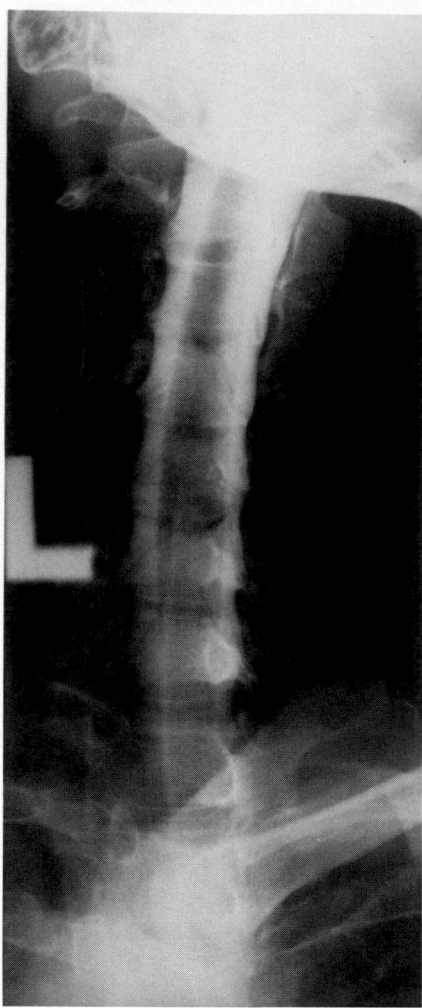

Figure 6–28 Oblique view cervical myelogram demonstrating perineural cysts of lower cervical roots.

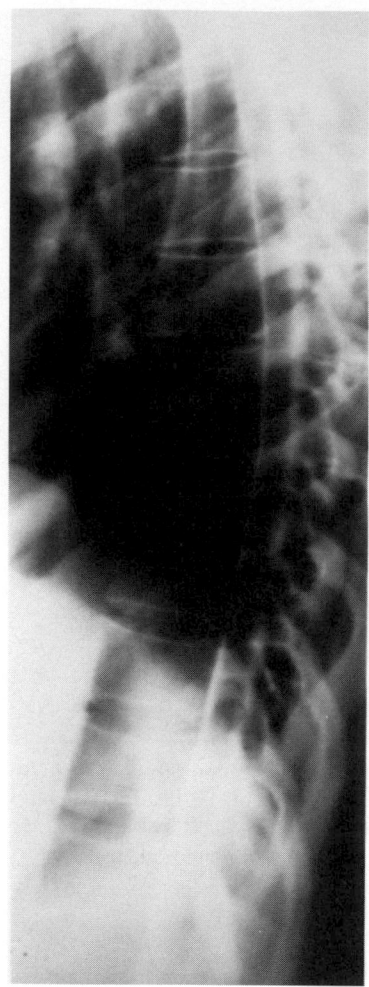

Figure 6–29 Lateral projection thoracic myelogram.

uniform in both the AP and lateral projections, down to the level of the lumbosacral junction. The caudal extent of the subarachnoid space may exhibit considerable variability but most often occurs below the S1 spinal level. The radiolucent shadow of the terminal segment of the spinal cord, the conus medullaris, should taper to a blunted point not lower than the L2 spinal level. In the lateral projection the collected radiolucencies of the cauda equina are usually observed in the posterior third of the lumbar subarachnoid space, with the fine linear radiolucencies of individual nerve roots coursing ventrally and caudally. In the AP projections, the paired nerve roots course caudally and laterally, ultimately turning lateral as they enter the neural foramina (Figs. 6-31 and 6-32). Occasionally, two nerve roots will share a common sheath as they exit the thecal sac (*conjoined nerve roots*), thus giving an asymmetrical appearance. This is a normal anatomical variant.

The myelographic appearance of lesions involving the spinal cord may be placed into one of three categories: (1) extradural, (2) intradural extramedullary, and (3) intramedullary—each with a distinct myelographic pattern. Extradural lesions tend to displace the dura and the spinal cord to the opposite side, thus resulting in narrowing of the subarachnoid space between the lesion and the spinal cord and of the subarachnoid space between the spinal cord and the opposite side of the spinal canal. Depending on the size and orientation of the lesion and the projections being viewed, the contrast should outline a gentle curve around the lesion. Intradural-extramedullary lesions tend to displace the spinal cord and dura in opposite directions, thus widening the subarachnoid spaces, above and below and ipsilateral to the lesion. The contrast will outline the lesion, demonstrating a meniscus at its rostral and caudal poles. A myelographic block may result in the ability to visualize only one pole of the lesion. Intradural lesions in the lumbosacral region fill the subarachnoid space before they cause significant symptoms or signs. If they have not resulted in a complete myelographic block, the subarachnoid contrast will usually outline menisci at the rostral and caudal poles. Intramedullary lesions enlarge the radiolucent shadow of the spinal cord, thus narrowing the subarachnoid space on both sides of the cord. In most instances, lesions must be viewed from at least two projections in order to make the above distinctions, and some lesions may provide appearances not distinctive of one particular category. In these instances, a postmyelographic CT scan may be helpful.

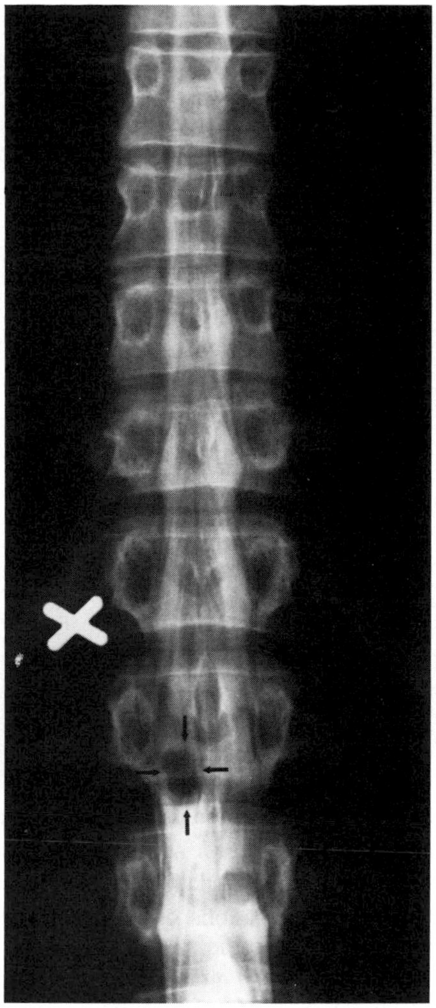

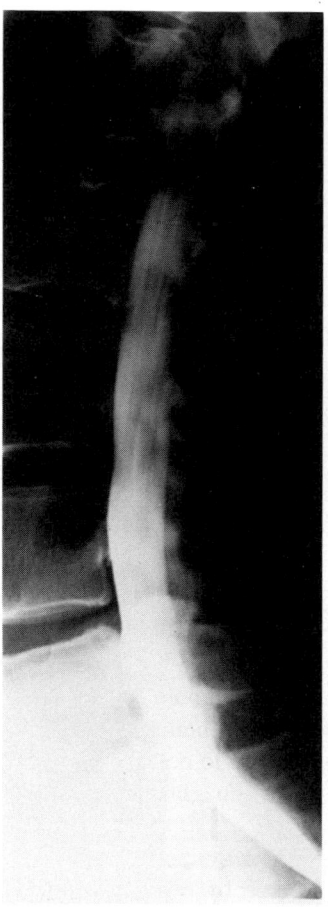

Figure 6–31 Lateral projection lumbar myelogram.

Figure 6–30 AP projection of lower thoracic and upper lumbar region. Note the symmetrical tapering of the conus at L1–L2 and the intradural-extramedullary lesion *(arrows).*

Lesions that affect the filling of nerve root sheaths, producing filling defects, are usually described in the cervical and lumbosacral regions. The majority of these lesions are extradural defects resulting from herniations of intervertebral disks and degenerative diseases of the spinal column. The typical myelographic findings include defects of the ventral subarachnoid space on lateral projections and root sleeve effacements or filling defects at the same spinal level on the AP and oblique projections.

DISKOGRAPHY

Diskography involves the injection of small quantities of water-soluble contrast media into the nucleus palposis.[32] The placement of the needle and the injection of contrast media are performed with the aid of fluoroscopy, and subsequently plain radiographs of the region of interest are obtained. More than one disk space may be contrasted during the same study. The normal spinal disk will accept between 0.25 cc and 0.5 cc (cervical vs. lumbar, respectively) of contrast

media, and they will distribute the contrast media in a smooth centrally positioned ellipsoid pattern. Injection of contrast material into a degenerated disk typically outlines a flattened disk space with an irregular contour. Tears in the annulus or fissures in the cartilaginous end plates may allow seepage of contrast to define a plane of separation between the degenerated disk and the adjacent vertebral bodies or the anterior and posterior longitudinal ligaments and over adjacent vertebrae (Fig. 6-33). During the injection, the patient's symptoms may be reproduced or exacerbated, thus suggesting a symptomatic degenerative disk.[33]

Diskography was popularized in the mid-1940s as a means of assessing the integrity of cervical and lumbar spinal disks. The information provided by this technique is limited to the intervertebral disk space and surrounding ligaments. Although an abnormal diskogram may be associated with reproduction of pain or other symptoms, many still question the validity of the technique in establishing a true cause-and-effect relationship. The general acceptance and usefulness of this imaging technique in contemporary neuroradiology has declined since, under usual circumstances, MRI or myelography and CT scan provide sufficient information for clinical assessment and treatment planning. Diskography may be employed when there is need for intraoperative identification of the disk space or when the MRI

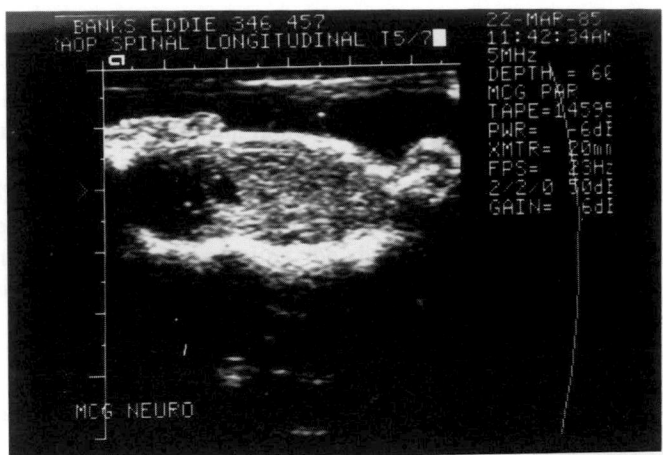

Figure 6–38 Longitudinal intraoperative sonogram of spinal cord tumor. Cyst can be visualized within the spinal cord.

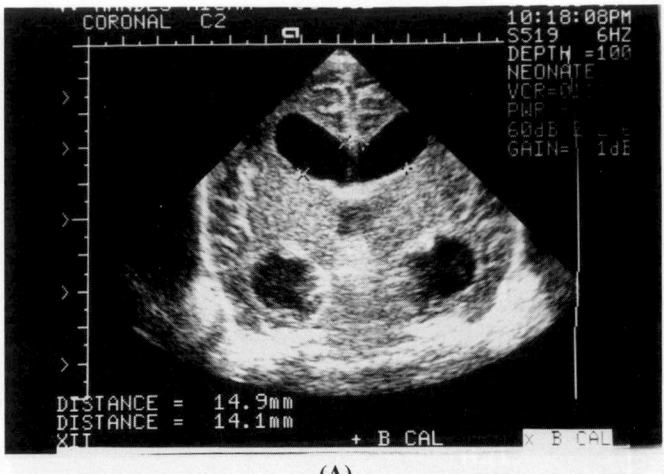

(A)

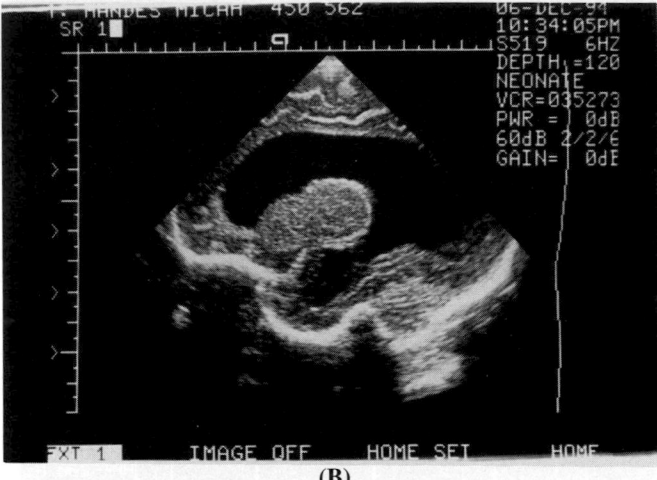

(B)

Figure 6–39 Coronal sonogram through dilated lateral ventricles and third ventricle with large temporal horns (*A*). Parasagittal sonogram shows dilatation of one lateral ventricle, trigone, and temporal horns (*B*). No atrophy of parenchyma is seen.

on sonography.[53] Calcification within tumors causes acoustic shadowing. Areas of edema surrounding tumors can be differentiated on ultrasound from actual infiltration by the tumor.[59,63,64] Feeding vessels or major cerebral vessels located near tumors can be identified.[57] By ultrasonic imaging, intracerebral abscesses have a well-defined hyperechoic rim with a hypoechoic center. Septations within an abscess cavity can be visualized.[55,58,64]

Arteriovenous malformations are echogenic, and most can be localized by standard gray scale real-time ultrasonography.[56] More useful is the color-flow Doppler sonography of vascular malformations. This produces an image in which the color red is encoded for flow in one direction and the color blue for flow in the opposite direction. Thus, a malformation and its feeding arteries and draining veins can be quickly and easily located. Prior to closure of the craniotomy, the area can be scanned to detect any residual malformation or complicating hematoma. Intraoperative sonography can also be used to locate small mycotic aneurysms and to help determine the patency of cerebral vessels after placement of aneurysm clips.[42]

Intraoperative sonography is used to locate missiles, bone, and other debris embedded within the cerebrum after trauma. It has been found helpful in the placement of ventricular catheters for shunts or Ommaya reservoirs, especially in patients who have very small ventricles. Imaging is performed through open fontanelles in infants and through small trephines in adults. Malposition of ventricular catheters can be accurately determined and immediately corrected.[54,58,59,62,63,67]

INTRAOPERATIVE SPINAL SONOGRAPHY

Ultrasonography has been utilized in the management of a variety of spinal lesions, including resection of intramedullary and extramedullary tumors, placement of shunts into syringes, decompression of traumatic fractures, location of

herniated disks, and in the management of congenital anomalies such as Chiari malformations.[68–74]

Intraoperative sonography can be performed with the pa-

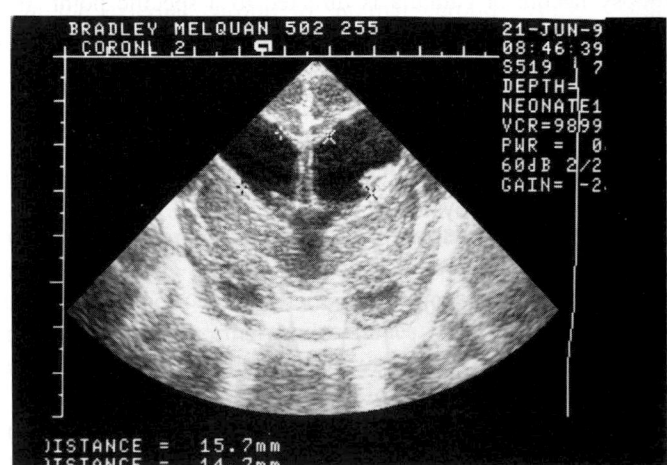

Figure 6–40 Grade III intraventricular hemorrhage. Note hyperechoic areas that represent hemorrhage in the lateral ventricle. Ventricles are markedly dilated.

tient in the supine or prone position but not in the lateral position. After the laminectomy is performed, the wound is filled with sterile saline to prevent near-field artifact and to avoid direct contact of the probe with the spinal cord and nerve roots. Usually a 7.5 MHz transducer is used for visualization, although it may be desirable to use 10 MHz. The spinal cord, nerve roots, dentate ligaments, intervertebral disks, and vertebral bodies can be imaged without opening the dura. The area is examined systematically in the transverse and sagittal planes. An initial examination is performed to establish the landmarks and to locate lesions. Sonography can then be performed during the course of surgery to monitor progress and, at the termination of the case, to document the extent of resection or decompression.[68,72–75]

Intraoperative sonography can identify tumors and delineate the margins for biopsy or resection. Intramedullary tumors are typically isoechoic or hyperechoic when compared to the normal spinal cord. Cystic and solid portions of a tumor may be clearly identified (Fig. 6-38). Sonography shows expansion of the cord and concomitant narrowing of the subarachnoid space. The normal central echo of the cord is absent and is thought to represent the transition zone from normal cord into tumor.[70–73,75,76]

Sonography can differentiate intramedullary from extramedullary masses. Extramedullary masses—i.e., meningiomas, neurofibromas and lipomas—are usually homogeneous and hyperechoic as compared to normal spinal cord. They have well-defined borders. Sonography reveals compression of the spinal cord and enlarged subarachnoid spaces above and below the lesions.[68,71,73–75]

Extradural lesions such as metastases or herniated disks are imaged as hyperechogenic masses which narrow the subarachnoid space. If large, the mass may compress the spinal cord and obliterate the central echo in the cord. Stretching of nerve roots can also be imaged. Scar tissue, however, can mimic disk protrusion or metastases.[68,73,75]

Intraoperative sonography is useful in monitoring the degree of reduction of a fracture without manipulating the spinal cord.[69,77,78] A laminotomy no larger than 1 square centimeter will permit introduction of an ultrasonic probe to visualize the area.

Intraoperative sonography can be used to localize bone and missile fragments within the canal and is particularly useful when these fragments are mobile. The image generally conforms to the shape of the fragment. Sonography can also detect syringomyelia, myelomalacia, pseudomeningocele, dural tears, tethered cord, and arachnoiditis.[54,69,73,75]

A syrinx within the spinal cord is imaged as an anechoic space with well-defined borders. It is typically surrounded by abnormal spinal cord. The size and number of cystic cavities and the presence of septations are all easily demonstrated. Sonography can direct placement of the catheter into the syrinx and monitor the amount of reduction. If decompression is inadequate, immediate surgical maneuvers, such as catheter manipulation, can be performed.[63,70,73,75]

Intraoperative sonography can be used to image the poste-

rior fossa after bony decompression of a Chiari malformation. If sonography shows that the decompression is inadequate, a patch graft and plugging of the obex can be performed when the surgical management involves decompression of the fourth ventricle and dissection of the vermian peg from the medulla.[71,75,79,80,81]

TRANSCRANIAL DOPPLER SONOGRAPHY

Transcranial doppler (TCD) sonography was introduced in 1982 by Aaslid.[82] It is a noninvasive, easily reproducible technique for determining blood flow velocities in the major intracranial arteries. A special transducer is used to insonate the basal cerebral arteries directly through the squamous portion of the temporal bone, the orbit, and the foramen magnum. The most common application of TCD sonography has been in the evaluation of cerebral vasospasm. TCD sonography can also be used intraoperatively to monitor cerebral blood flow.[83] The physical principles of TCD sonography are essentially the same as Doppler sonography of carotids except that a lower frequency is used.

The internal carotid, anterior cerebral, anterior communicating, posterior cerebral, and posterior communicating arteries are insonated through the squamous portion of the temporal bone. The carotid and ophthalmic arteries, carotid siphon, and, occasionally, the anterior cerebral artery are insonated through the orbit. A low-power setting must be used to reduce the ultrasonic exposure to the eye. Through the suboccipital approach, the vertebral and basilar artery signals are obtained.[82,83]

Descriptions of the methods for localizing each of the basal arteries can be found in detail elsewhere.[84] Normal values of the velocities for the various cerebral vessels are available for comparison.

In contrast to arteriography, TCD sonography is noninvasive, easily reproducible, and can be performed at the bedside. It has been used clinically in the evaluation of cerebral vasospasm.[35,85,86] It is a sensitive measure of the development as well as resolution of vasospasm. Flow velocity is inversely related to vessel diameter. With vasospasm, the vessel diameter decreases, and TCD sonography records the increased velocity in the artery. This is used as a guide for treatment of the patient.

TCD sonography is used intraoperatively to identify pathological flow patterns during carotid endarterectomy or open heart surgery. EEG or other electrophysiologic monitoring is indirect and often shows changes only after tissue injury has occurred. TCD sonography detects a disruption of flow before any ischemic injury has developed.[34,83] TCD sonography has also been used intraoperatively to localize AVMs and their feeder vessels.[87] The utility of TCD sonography is being assessed in the evaluation of increased intracranial pressure, in monitoring cerebral flow in seizure patients, in the evaluation of ventriculomegaly and hydrocephalus, and in intraoperative monitoring for cerebral emboli, as well as confirmation of brain death.[83]

EXAMINATION OF THE NEONATE WITH ULTRASOUND

Ultrasonography is used to screen neonates for intraventricular hemorrhage, congenital malformations, and tumors (Fig. 6-39). Testing is often performed in the nursery, minimizing stress to the infant. Since the examination is noninvasive and involves no radiation, scans can be repeated frequently. For most infants, a 5- or 7.5-MHz probe is used to insonate through the anterior or posterior fontanelle for visualization of the intracranial structures.[88,89]

Premature infants are screened for intraventricular hemorrhage within the first 3 days of life (Fig. 6-40). Ultrasonography has a sensitivity of 96 percent and specificity of 94 percent for diagnosing intraventricular hemorrhage.[84] If indicated, follow-up scans can be easily obtained. Over a period of weeks, the hematoma changes to a hypoechoic area surrounded by an echogenic rim. With time, the area develops into a porencephalic cyst which appears anechoic.[38,89–91]

Ultrasonography of the craniocervical junction via the posterior cervical approach provides good visualization of the medulla, tonsils, vermis, and cervical cord in infants because the posterior arches of the cervical spine are minimally ossified. This allows evaluation of the infants for a Chiari malformation and for evidence of intracranial hemorrhage.[92,93] Other congenital malformations that can be evaluated by ultrasonography include the Dandy-Walker syndrome, agenesis of the corpus callosum, holoprosencephaly, lissencephaly, and schizencephaly, among others.[91,93]

In summary, tumors have a greater echogenicity than normal brain. Ultrasound is also used to evaluate tumors in infants. Cysts, necrosis, and calcifications can be identified, but the specific pathology cannot be determined by ultrasound alone. It may also be difficult to differentiate infarctions or hemorrhage from tumor. CT scan or MRI scan is required for further evaluation.[38]

SUGGESTED READING

Ramsey RG: *Neuroradiology.* 2d ed. Philadelphia, Saunders, 1987.
Burrows EH, Leeds NE: *Neuroradiology.* New York, Churchill Livingstone, 1981.
Kirkwood JR: *Essentials of Neuroimaging.* New York, Churchill Livingstone, 1990.
Daffner RH: *Imaging of Vertebral Trauma.* Rockville, Md, Aspen, 1988.

Gehweiler JA Jr, Osborne RL Jr, Becker RF: *The Radiology of Vertebral Trauma.* Philadelphia, Saunders, 1980.
Petersen HO, Kieffer: Neuroradiology, in Baker AB, Baker LH (eds): *Clinical Neurology.* Philadelphia, Harper & Row, 1987.

REFERENCES

1. Pendergast EP, Schaeffer JP, Hodes PJ: *The Head and Neck in Roentgen Diagnosis,* 2d ed. Springfield, Ill, Charles C. Thomas, 1956.
2. Hoursfield N: A method of and apparatus for examination of a body part by radiation such as x-ray or gamma radiation. British Patent 1283915, 1972.
3. Ambrose J: Computerized transverse axial scanning (tomography): II. Clinical application. *Br J Radiol* 41:1023–1047, 1973.
4. Villafana T: Physics and instrumentation, in Lee SH, Rao KCVG (eds): *Cranial Computed Tomography.* New York, McGraw-Hill, 1985, chap 1, pp 1–46.
5. Williams AL: Trauma, in Williams AI, Haughton VM (eds): *Cranial Computed Tomography.* St. Louis, Mosby, 1985, pp 37–87.
6. Smith FW: NMR—Historical aspects, in Newton TH, Potts DG (eds): *Modern Neuroradiology,* vol 2: *Advanced Imaging Techniques.* San Francisco, Clavadel Press, 1983, pp 7–14.

7. Bradley WG, Crooks LE, Newton TH: Physical principles of NMR, in Newton TH, Potts DG (eds): *Modern Neuroradiology,* vol 2: *Advanced Imaging Techniques.* San Francisco, Clavadel Press, 1983, pp 15–61.
8. Bradley WG: Effect of magnetic relaxation times on magnetic resonance image interpretation. *Noninvasive Med Imaging* 1:195–204, 1984.
9. Wehrli FW, MacFall Jr, Newton TH: Parameters determining the appearance of NMR images, in Newton TH, Potts DG (eds): *Modern Neuroradiology,* vol 2: *Advanced Imaging Techniques.* San Francisco, Clavadel Press, 1983, pp 81–117.
10. Weinman HJ, Gries H, Speck U: Gd-DTPA and low osmolar Gd chelates, in Runge V (ed): *Enhanced Magnetic Resonance Imaging.* St. Louis, Mosby, 1989, pp 74–86.
11. New PFJ, Rosen BR, Brady TJ, et al: Potential hazards and artifacts of ferromagnetic and nonferromagnetic surgical and

dental materials and devices in nuclear magnetic resonance imaging. *Radiology* 147:139–148, 1983.

12. Kelly WM: Image artifacts and technical limitations, in Branelt-Zawadzki M, Norman D (eds): *Magnetic Resonance Imaging of the Central Nervous System.* New York, Raven, 1986, chap 1, pp 43–82.

13. Brooks RA, DiChiro G, Patroras N: Magnetic resonance imaging of cerebral hematomas at different field strengths: Theory and applications. *J Comput Assist Tomogr* 13(2):194–206, 1989.

14. Litt AW, Eidelman EM, Pinta RS, et al: Diagnosis of carotid artery stenosis: Comparison of 2 DFT time-of-flight MR angiography with contrast angiography in 50 patients. *AJNR* 12:149–154, 1991.

15. Watson GB, Weimer MW: MR spectroscopy in vivo: Principles, animal studies and clinical applications, in Stark DD, Bradley WG (eds): *Magnetic Resonance Imaging.* St. Louis, Mosby, 1988, pp 201–228.

16. Moniz E: L'encephalographic arterielle, sou impertance dans la localization des tumeurs cerebrales. *Rev Neurol* 342:72–90, 1927.

17. Engeset A: Cerebral angiography with Per-Abrodil. *Acta Radiol,* suppl 56, 1944.

18. Seldinger SI: Catheter replacement of the needle in percutaneous angiography: A new technique. *Acta Radiol* 39:368–376, 1953.

19. Dandy W: Ventriculography following the injection of air into the cerebral ventricles. *Ann Surg* 68:5, 1918.

20. Ruggiero G: Encephalography today. *Acta Radiol* 5:715, 1966.

21. Corrales M: The chain guide technique for selective ventriculography. *Neuroradiology* 9(5):243–246, 1975.

22. Webber MM: Normal brain scanning. *Am J Roentgen* 94:815–818, 1965.

23. Hayman LA, Taber KA, Jhingran SG, et al: Cerebral infarction: Diagnosis and assessment of prognosis by using [123]IMR-SPECT and CT. *AJNR* 10:557, 1989.

24. McRae DL: The significance of abnormalities of the cervical spine. Caldwell Lecture, 1959. *Am J Roentgen* 34:3–25, 1960.

25. Hinck VC, Hopkins CE, Savara BS: Diagnostic criteria of basilar impression. *Radiology* 76:572, 1961.

26. Norman D: MRI of the spine, in Brandt-Zowadski M, Norman D (eds): *Magnetic Resonance of the Central Nervous System.* New York, Raven, 1987, pp 289–328.

27. Ross JS, Hueftle MG: Postoperative spine, in Modic MT, Masaryk TJ, Ross JS (eds): *Magnetic Resonance Imaging of the Spine.* Chicago, Year Book, 1989, pp 120–148.

28. Dandy W: Roentgenography of the brain after injection of air into the spinal canal. *Ann Surg* 70:397, 1919.

29. Sicard JA, Forestier J: Methode generale d'exploration radiologique par l'hoils iodee (Lipiodol). *Bell Mem Soc Med Hosp,* Paris, 46:463, 1922.

30. Orvell S: Myelography with water soluable contrast. *Acta Radiol,* suppl 75, 1988.

31. Anand AK, Lee BCP: Plain and metrizamide CT of lumbar disk disease: Comparison with myelography. *AJNR* 3:567–571, 1982.

32. Feinberg SB: The place of discography in radiology as based on 20 cases. *AJR* 92:1275, 1964.

33. Wilson DH, McCarly WC: Discography: Its role in the diagnosis of lumbar disc protrusions. *J Neurosurg* 31:520, 1969.

34. Smith R, Brown R, Martin J, Wilson R: Noninvasive carotid artery testing—an expanding science, in Wood JH (ed): *Carotid Artery Surgery in Stroke: Neurosurgery State of the Art Reviews,* 1989, chap 4, pp 27–42.

35. Kremkau JFW: *Diagnostic Ultrasound: Principles, Instrumentation and Exercises.* New York, Grune and Stratton, 1984.

36. Wicks JD, Harve KS: *Fundamentals of Ultrasonographic Technique.* Chicago, Year Book, 1983.

37. Bartrum RJ, Crow HC: *Real-Time Ultrasound: A Manual for Physicians and Technical Personnel.* Philadelphia, Saunders, 1983.

38. McGahan JP, Lindfors KK, Carroll BA: Diagnostic ultrasound in neurologic surgery, in Youmans JR (ed): *Neurologic Surgery.* Philadelphia, Saunders, 1990, chap 8, pp 187–204.

39. Kremkau FW: Technical considerations, equipment, and physics of duplex sonography, in Grant EG, White EM (eds): *Duplex Sonography.* New York, Springer-Verlag, 1988, chap 1, pp 1–6.

40. Grant EG: Duplex sonography of the cerebrovascular system, in Grant EG, White EM (eds): *Duplex Sonography.* New York, Springer-Verlag, 1988, chap 2, pp 7–68.

41. Baker DW: Applications of pulsed Doppler techniques. *Radiol Clin North Am* 18:79–103, 1980.

42. Black KL, Rubin JM, Chandler WF, McGillicuddy JE: Intraoperative color flow Doppler imaging of AVMs and aneurysms. *J Neurosurg* 68:635–639, 1988.

43. Zwiebel WJ, Austin CW, Sackett JF, Strother CM: Correlation of high-resolution B-mode and continuous-wave Doppler sonography with arteriography in the diagnosis of carotid stenosis. *Radiology* 149:523–632, 1983.

44. James EM, Earnest F, Forbes GS, et al: High-resolution dynamic ultrasound imaging of the carotid bifurcation: A prospective evaluation. *Radiology* 144:853–858, 1982.

45. Blackshear WM Jr, Phillips DJ, Thiele BL, et al: Detection of carotid occlusive disease by ultrasonic imaging and pulsed Doppler spectrum analysis. *Surgery* 86:698–706, 1979.

46. Barnes RW, Russell HE, Bone GE, Slaymaker EE: Doppler cerebrovascular examination: Improved results with refinements in technique. *Stroke* 8:468–471, 1977.

47. Wolverson MK, Heiberg E, Sundaram M, et al: Carotid atherosclerosis: High-resolution real-time sonography correlated with angiography. *AJR* 40:355–361, 1983.

48. Fell G, Phillips DJ, Chikos PM, et al: Ultrasonic duplex scanning for disease of the carotid artery. *Circulation* 64:1191–1195, 1981.

49. Croft RJ, Ellam LD, Harrison MJG: Accuracy of carotid angiography in the assessment of atheroma of the internal carotid artery. *Lancet* 1:997–1000, 1980.

50. Eikelboom BC, Riles TR, Mintzer R, et al: Inaccuracy of angiography in the diagnosis of carotid ulceration. *Stroke* 6:882–885, 1983.

51. Cooperberg PL, Robertson WD, Fry P, Sweeney V: High resolution real time ultrasound of the carotid bifurcation. *J Clin Ultrasound* 7:13–17, 1979.

52. Knot RA, Phillips DJ, Breslau PJ, et al: Empirical findings relating sample volume size to diagnostic accuracy in pulsed Doppler cerebrovascular studies. *J Clin Ultrasound* 10:227–232, 1982.

53. Chandler WF, Knake JE: Intraoperative use of ultrasound in neurosurgery. *Clin Neurosurg* 30:550–563, 1984.

54. Knake JE, Bowerman RA, Silver TM, McCracken S: Neurosurgical applications of intraoperative ultrasound. *Radiol Clin North Am* 23:73–90, 1985.

55. McGahan JP, Boggan JE, Gooding GAW: Intraoperative use of ultrasound, in Youmans JR (ed): *Neurologic Surgery,* vol 2. Philadelphia, Saunders, 1990, chap 36, pp 1033–1046.

56. Rubin JM, Dohrmann GT: Efficacy of intraoperative US for evaluating intracranial masses. *Radiology* 157:509–511, 1985.

57. Gooding GAW, Boggan JE, Powers SK, et al: Neurosurgical sonography: Intraoperative and postoperative imaging of the brain. *AJNR* 5:521–525, 1984.

58. Dohrmann GJ, Rubin JM: Intraoperative real-time ultrasonography: Localization, characterization and instrumentation of lesions of brain and spinal cord, in Fasano VA (ed): *Advanced Intraoperative Technologies in Neurosurgery.* New York, Springer-Verlag, 1986, chap 1, pp 3–19.

59. Quencer RM, Montalvo BM: Intraoperative cranial sonography, in Naidich TP, Quencer RM (eds): *Clinical Neurosonography: Ultrasound of the Central Nervous System*. New York, Springer-Verlag, 1987, pp 162–184.

60. Chaunge S, Harwood-Nash D: Tumors and cysts, in Naidich TP, Quencer JRM (eds): *Clinical Neurosonography: Ultrasound of the Central Nervous System*. New York, Springer-Verlag, 1987, pp 97–109.

61. Rubin JM, Dohrmann GJ: A canulla for use in ultrasonically guided biopsies of the brain. *J Neurosurg* 59:905–907, 1983.

62. Rubin JM, Dohrmann GJ: Use of ultrasonically guided probes and catheters in neurosurgery. *Surg Neurol* 18:143–148, 1982.

63. Chandler WF, Knake JE, McGillicuddy JE, et al: Intraoperative use of real-time ultrasonography in neurosurgery. *J Neurosurg* 57:157–163, 1982.

64. Chandler WF: Use of ultrasound imaging during intracranial operations, in Rubin JE, Chandler WF (eds): *Ultrasound in Neurosurgery*. New York, Raven, 1990, chap 2, pp 67–106.

65. Lange SC, Captain, Harve JF, et al: Intraoperative ultrasound detection of metastatic tumors in the central cortex. *Neurosurgery* 11:219–221, 1982.

66. Gooding GAW, Boggan JE, Bank WO, et al: Sonography of the adult brain through surgical defects. *AJNR* 2:449–452, 1981.

67. Shkolnik A, McLone D: Intraoperative real-time ultrasonic guidance of ventricular shunt placement in infants. *Radiology* 141:515–517, 1981.

68. Knake JE, Gabrielsen TO, Chandler WF, et al: Real-time sonography during spinal surgery. *Radiology* 151:461–465, 1984.

69. Montalvo BM, Quencer RM, Green BA, et al: Intraoperative sonography in spinal trauma. *Radiology* 153:125–134, 1984.

70. Platt JF, Rubin JM, Chandler WF, et al: Intraoperative spinal sonography in the evaluation of intramedullary tumors. *J Ultrasound Med* 7:317–325, 1988.

71. Quencer RM, Montalvo BM, Green BA, Eismont FJ: Intraoperative spinal sonography of soft-tissue masses of the spinal cord and spinal canal. *AJR* 143:1307–1315, 1984.

72. Rubin JM: Ultrasonography in spinal cord surgery, in Rubin JM, Chandler WF (eds): *Ultrasound in Neurosurgery*. New York, Raven, 1990, chap 3, pp 107–182.

73. Rubin JM, Dohrmann GJ: The spine and spinal cord during neurosurgical operations: Real-time ultrasonography. *Radiology* 155:197–200, 1985.

74. Rubin JM, Dohrmann GJ: Work in progress: Intraoperative ultrasonography of the spine. *Radiology* 146:173–175, 1983.

75. Montalvo BM, Quencer RM: Intraoperative sonography in spinal surgery: Current state of the art, in Naidich TP, Quencer RM (eds): *Clinical Neurosonography: Ultrasound of the Central Nervous System*. New York, Springer-Verlag, 1987, pp 185–224.

76. Braun IF, Raghavendra BN, Kricheff II: Spinal cord imaging using real-time high-resolution ultrasound. *Radiology* 147:459–465, 1983.

77. McGahan JP, Benson D, Chehrazi B, et al: Intraoperative sonographic monitoring of reduction of thoracolumbar burst fractures. *AJR* 145:1229–1232, 1985.

78. Quencer RM, Montalvo BM, Eisomont FJ, Green BA: Intraoperative spinal sonography in thoracic and lumbar fractures: Evaluation of Harrington rod instrumentation. *AJR* 145:343–349, 1985.

79. Di Pietro MA, Venes JL, Rubin JM: Arnold-Chiari II malformation: Intraoperative real-time ultrasound. *Radiology* 164:799–804, 1987.

80. DiPietro MA, Venes JL: Intraoperative sonography of the Arnold-Chiari malformations, in Rubin JE, Chandler WF (eds): *Ultrasound in Neurosurgery*. New York, Raven, 1990, chap 4, pp 183–199.

81. Venes JL, Black KL, Latack JT: Preoperative evaluation and surgical management of the Arnold-Chiari II malformation. *J Neurosurg* 64:363–370, 1986.

82. Aaslid R, Markwalder TM, Nornes H: Noninvasive transcranial Doppler ultrasound recording of flow velocity in basal cerebral arteries. *J Neurosurg* 57:769–774, 1982.

83. Ringelstein EB: Transcranial Doppler monitoring, in Aaslid R (ed): *Transcranial Doppler Sonography*. New York, Springer-Verlag, 1992, chap 10, pp 147–163.

84. Aaslid R: Transcranial Doppler examination techniques, in Aaslid R (ed): *Transcranial Doppler Sonography*. New York, Springer-Verlag, 1992, chap 4, pp 39–59.

85. Aaslid R, Huber P, Nornes H: Evaluation of cerebrovascular spasm with transcranial Doppler ultrasound. *J Neurosurg* 60:37–41, 1984.

86. Seiler RW, Aaslid R: Transcranial Doppler for evaluation of cerebral vasospasm, in Aaslid R (ed): *Transcranial Doppler Sonography*. New York, Springer-Verlag, 1992, chap 8, pp 118–131.

87. Lindegaard KF, Aaslid R, Nornes H: Cerebral arteriovenous malformations, in Aaslid R (ed): *Transcranial Doppler Sonography*. New York, Springer-Verlag, 1992, chap 6, pp 86–105.

88. Donn SM, Goldstein VW, Silver TM: Real-time ultrasonography: Its use in the evaluation of neonatal intracranial hemorrhage and post-hemorrhagic hydrocephalus. *Am J Dis Child* 135:319–321, 1981.

89. Grant EG, Borts FT, Schellinger D, et al: Real-time ultrasonography of neonatal intraventricular hemorrhage and comparison with computed tomography. *Radiology* 139:687–691, 1981.

90. Sauerbrei EE, Digney M, Harrison PB, Cooperberg PL: Ultrasonic evaluation of neonatal intracranial hemorrhage and its complications. *Radiology* 139:677–685, 1981.

91. Grant EG: Sonography of the premature brain: Intracranial hemorrhage and periventricular leukomalacia, in Naidich TP, Quencer JRM (eds): *Clinical Neurosonography: Ultrasound of the Central Nervous System*. New York, Springer-Verlag, 1984, pp 110–124.

92. Cramer BC, Jequier S, Gorman AM: Ultrasound of the neonatal craniocervical junction. *AJNR* 7:449–455, 1986.

93. Rumak CM, Johnson ML: Congenital brain malformations, in Rumak CM, Johnson ML (eds): *Perinatal and Infant Brain Imaging: Role of Ultrasound and Computed Tomography*. Chicago, Year Book, 1984, chap 5, pp 91–115.

☐ STUDY QUESTIONS

I. A 28-year-old male was involved in an automobile accident in which he was thrown from the car. He sustained multiple abrasions of the head and body but no gross deformities. Over the next 2 days he become progressively more alert but complained of neck pain.

1. What imaging and/or radiographic study(ies) might be recommended upon admission to the emergency room? Why? **2.** Which imaging study might be most likely to show evidence of subarachnoid hemorrhage within the first 24 hours? **3.** What imaging study might best demonstrate evidence of cerebral contusion after 6 days? Why? **4.** What imaging study might best demonstrate evidence of a fractured odontoid process? **5.** What imaging study would most likely show evidence of a basilar skull fracture?

II. A 60-year-old male who had known carcinoma of the prostate began complaining of midthoracic back pain and gradually developed weakness, first in his left lower extremity, then the right. A plain x-ray of the thoracic and lumbar spine showed multiple areas of increased density and other areas of erosion.

1. What initial imaging study might best demonstrate the extent of bony involvement with metastases? **2.** What imaging study might best demonstrate a specific site of involvement of the spinal canal which could account for the paresis? **3.** What is the classic study that would have been used to demonstrate evidence of a spinal block? **4.** What would be the expected appearance of a partial spinal block by myelography? **5.** What imaging study would most likely demonstrate evidence of a fracture?

III. A 60-year-old diabetic hypertensive Caucasian lady is admitted with a sudden onset of left hemiparesis and right monocular blindness, each of which lasted for a half-hour. Both cleared. The patient had a bruit over the right carotid artery.

1. What scanning study should be used to indicate evidence of disease of the carotid artery? **2.** What study would most likely demonstrate evidence of cerebral damage initially? 48 hours later? **3.** What would Doppler flow studies of the carotid artery show if the carotid artery were 60 percent occluded? 80 percent occluded? **4.** Under what conditions might a direct arteriogram be required? **5.** What might an MRI of the head show?

IV. An infant was born at 30 weeks of gestation. Within the day he developed a full fontanel and persistent drowsiness.

1. What diagnostic evaluations might be considered? **2.** Assuming an intracerebral hemorrhage, what forms of imaging might be used to follow the progress of the hemorrhage? **3.** What form of imaging might be used to follow the progress of hydrocephalus? **4.** What imaging study might demonstrate the sight of aqueductal stenosis? **5.** How might a subependymal hemorrhage be differentiated from a subarachnoid hemorrhage on CT?

V. A 25-year-old male suddenly complained of the "worst headache I've ever had in my life" and then lost consciousness. He was also nauseated, vomited twice, and had a stiff neck.

1. What imaging study would most likely indicate the cause of the headache? **2.** Assuming evidence of subarachnoid hemorrhage, how might the source be first identified? **3.** How might an aneurysm be identified noninvasively? **4.** What is the best imaging examination to outline discretely the aneurysm? **5.** How might one determine evidence of chronic vasospasm noninvasively?

Diagnosis and Surgical Treatment of Congenital Lesions of the Nervous System

Ann Marie Flannery

Neurosurgical disorders of infants and children may be classified into three categories. The first group includes disorders generally unique to the age group, including most congenital anomalies, such as myelomeningocele, and associated dysraphic states, congenital hydrocephalus, encephaloceles, and craniofacial anomalies. The second group includes conditions not necessarily unique to the young but more likely to be seen in infancy and childhood, such as acquired hydrocephalus and some brain tumors. (Pediatric tumors will be discussed separately.) The third and final group of disorders includes those commonly seen at any age but which have an altered presentation and prognosis in the young due to ongoing development of the nervous system. Cranial trauma is the most common member of this group.

Comments on the special effects and treatment of cranial trauma that relate to infants and children are included in Chap. 18. Chapters 7 and 8 will concentrate on the anatomic descriptions and the most common therapeutic interventions for developmental disorders and congenital anomalies.

☐ DEVELOPMENTAL ANATOMY

DEVELOPMENT

Of the three embryonic layers, endoderm, mesoderm, and ectoderm, *ectoderm* gives rise to the principal neural struc-

tures in the developing human. An important developmental milestone includes the period of time between 21 and 25 days of fetal development. At that time, the neural placode forms the neural tube. (See Fig. 7-1.) Failure of tubulation results in *neural tube defects*, including anencephaly, and myelomeningocele, with its complex of associated congenital anomalies to be discussed below.[1] At about the same time in neural development, failure to close the anterior neuropore may result in *encephaloceles*.[2] Further along in development, between 6 and 20 weeks of gestation, complex cellular migration and hemispheral separations and cortical infoldings result in the organization of the human brain.[3]

SPINAL DYSRAPHISM

The most common manifestation of the spinal dysraphic state is a *myelomeningocele*, sometimes referred to as *spina bifida aperta*. Other forms of *spinal dysraphism* include diastematomyelia, spinal lipomas, lipomyelomeningoceles, and dural sinuses. These anomalies are classified as *spina bifida occulta*. The terms *aperta* and *occulta*, to modify spina bifida, are used to imply that the lesion is either covered by skin (occulta) or open, uncovered (aperta). In most populations, myelomeningocele is far more common than the varied manifestations of spina bifida occulta.

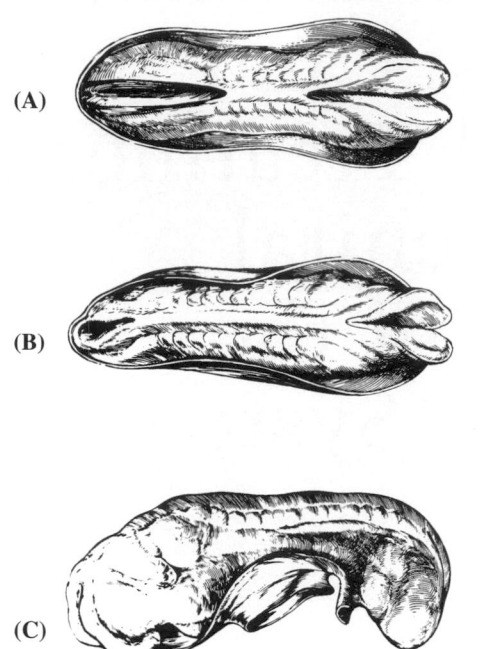

Figure 7–1 Normal closure of the neural tube. *A.* Early closure, approximately day 22 of embryologic development. *B.* Day 23, showing continued fusion of neural folds. *C.* Sagittal view, day 25, neural tube is nearly closed.

MYELOMENINGOCELE

Myelomeningoceles develop very early in gestation, generally long before most women are aware of their state of pregnancy. The etiology of the disorder is understood descriptively; the actual cause is related to folate. Currently, either a lack of exogenous folate or an inability to maintain adequate endogenous levels is implicated. Current recommendations are that all women of childbearing potential should consume 0.4 mg of folate daily.[4,4a,4b]

It is known that certain populations are more prone to have myelomeningocele. The best-studied of these are from England, Ireland, Scotland, and Wales, where the overall incidence is between 3 and 4 per 1000. The general occurrence rate for this complex congenital anomaly is 1 per 1000 live births.[5] Those who move from an endemic area to an area where the background rate exists tend to have an intermediate rate of occurrence.[6] Subsequent pregnancies of the mother of a dysraphic child have an increased risk of about tenfold as do other first-degree relatives.

Prenatal Diagnosis Myelomeningocele and other neural tube defects, where central nervous system tissue is exposed to amniotic fluid, such as *anencephaly,* may be detected by *serum alpha-fetaprotein screening* between the 15th and 18th week of fetal gestation. If the alpha-fetaprotein is elevated, further studies including amniocentesis with amniotic fluid sent for alpha-fetaprotein and acetylcholinesterase, as well as ultrasonagraphic imaging with attention to the spine and brain, are recommended. Fetal age and fetal number must also be determined. The most common causes of an

elevated maternal serum alpha-fetaprotein are incorrect dating of pregnancy or multiple gestation.[7,8] These situations may be determined by the use of ultrasound and be differentiated from a neural tube defect.[9]

Postnatal Diagnosis Following birth, the most notable defect is the myelomeningocele on the back. (See Fig. 7.2.) Myelomeningocele, however, is associated with two other major central nervous system (CNS) anomalies, *hydrocephalus* and the *Chiari II malformation.* Affected children have a 90 to 95 percent risk of hydrocephalus.[10] Those with myelomeningocele will frequently, but not invariably, have radiographic evidence of the Chiari II malformation.

The myelomeningocele may occur at any level, from cervical to sacral. The most common level is the lumbosacral region.[11] Often, but not always, the motor and sensory function below the level of the lesion is lost. The repair of a myelomeningocele should occur as soon as feasible, usually within the first 24 h of life. Failure to close the myelomeningocele defect results in a high risk of CNS infection, including meningitis and ventriculitis. The surgical closure is aimed at creating a watertight barrier between the open neural tube and the external environment. The second goal of surgical correction is to prevent, as much as possible, tethering of the neural tube in the surgical scar.

Surgical Repair (Fig. 7-3) The anatomy of the myelomeningocele can be thought of as concentric circles of normal tissues in abnormal locations. The innermost circle, or *placode,* is composed of neural elements that under normal circumstances would have fused to create the neural tube and then the spinal cord. This center circle is usually fused to the surrounding epithelium. In the process of the surgical correction, the connections between the placode and the epithelium are gently incised. The placode is mobilized and a tube is created and secured using a fine suture, creating a surface most of which is covered in pia arachnoid, except in the area of actual suturing. This pial surface is less prone to be tethered in scar tissue. The next concentric circle of the myelomeningocele is the dura. This tissue is generally mobilized from the dysplastic bone elements which are present. Dissected free and occasionally reinforced with muscle and fascia, the dura is brought to the midline and closed in a watertight fashion. Appropriate flaps of skin and fascia are brought to the midline and closed. Occasionally, it is necessary to close very large defects with rotated flaps of skin and other soft tissues or by the use of relaxing incisions. Plastic surgical consultation is appropriate in these situations.[12,13]

☐ PROBLEMS ASSOCIATED WITH MYELOMENINGOCELE

Hydrocephalus, which occurs in 90 to 95 percent of cases, will be discussed in Chap. 8.

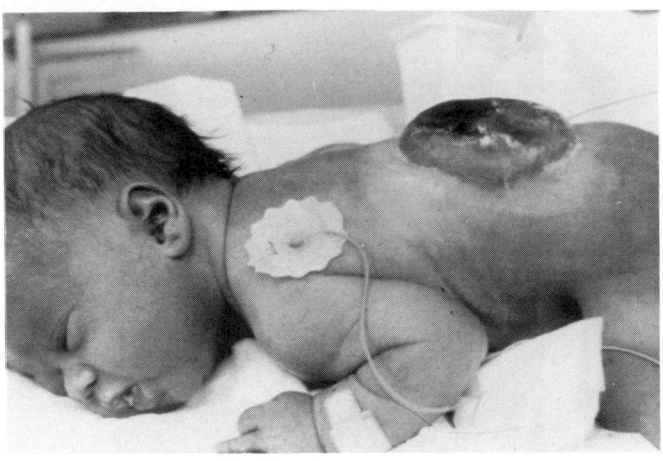

(A)

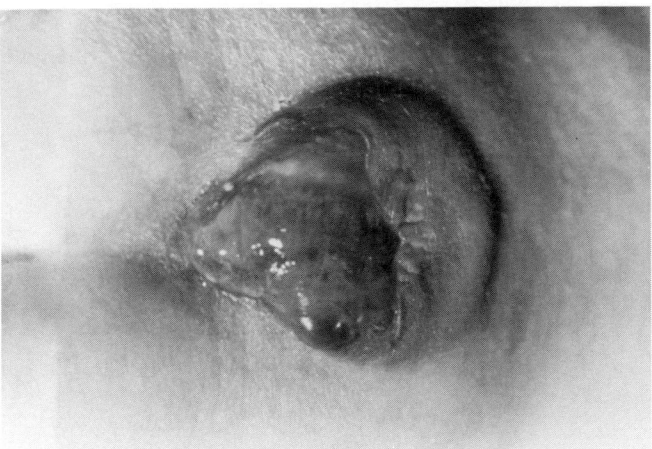

(B)

Figure 7–2 *A.* Infants with moderately large myelomeningocele sacs. Note normal size head and relatively normal size and configuration of legs and feet. *B.* A smaller myelomeningocele located just above the gluteal crease.

THE CHIARI II MALFORMATION

The complex hindbrain anomaly, the *Chiari II malformation,* is found by imaging studies. Only approximately 5 to 10 percent of individuals who have a myelomeningocele become symptomatic from the Chiari II malformation.[14] The malformation consists of beaking of the tectum, kinking and elongation of the brainstem below the foramen magnum, and herniation of the cerebellar vermis, the vermian peg, below the foramen magnum. (See Fig. 7-4.) The bony posterior fossa is usually small.[15] Symptoms of this problem include respiratory distress, cranial nerve palsies—particularly palsies of cranial nerves VI, VII, IX, and X—hypotonia, spasticity, and quadriparesis.[16] If symptoms develop during infancy, the prognosis is fair with aggressive management. Up to 30 percent of infants will die of respiratory complications.[17] Individuals who become symptomatic in childhood or adolescence generally do well.[16]

Magnetic resonance imaging (MRI) is the best examination to demonstrate the Chiari II malformation. Severity of the disorder seen by imaging does not correlate well with the clinical presentation. Treatment usually includes laminectomy of the upper levels of the cervical spine and in some cases removal of the posterior rim of the foramen magnum to decompress the contents of the posterior fossa which have herniated. The dura must be opened and a dural patch graft implanted. Some authors advocate dissection of the arachnoid around the vermian peg.[15] *Hydromyelia* may occur. Often the hydromyelia resolves after the Chiari II malformation is decompressed, but some experts advocate plugging the obex of the medulla with muscle.

MENINGOCELE

Much less common than myelomeningocele, the *meningocele* is a variant of spina bifida aperta in which the meninges are distended, often resulting in distension or ballooning of the skin and subjacent tissue. The spinal cord and nerves are usually not involved. Affected individuals are usually neurologically normal.

SPINA BIFIDA OCCULTA OR (OCCULT SPINAL DYSRAPHISM)

The embryology of myelomeningocele is well understood. That of spina bifida occulta is diverse and continues to be obscure. As with spina bifida aperta, in normal spina bifida occulta normal elements are present but are found in abnormal locations. The simplest form of spina bifida occulta is probably that of the thickened, *fatty filum terminale.* More complex anomalies include spinal cord *lipomyelomeningoceles* and *diastematomyelia.*

DERMAL SINUS

A tract extending from the epidermis through deeper layers, the *dermal sinuses* often penetrate the dura into the subarachnoid space. Externally, the sinus has the appearance of a pit or dimple, often with a tuft of hair on or near the midline. (See Fig. 7-5.) Dermal sinuses are most common in the lumbosacral region but can appear in association with any midline structure, including the underside of the tip of the nose, the occipital bone, and the cervical spine.[18] The dermal sinus is often asymptomatic, but when it extends through the dura, it may be associated with recurrent meningitis. The therapy for dermal sinus is excision. Preoperative MRI may aid in the detection of associated congenital anomalies, which can include a thickened or fatty filum terminale, lipomas, or epidermoid tumors. The planned excision should be complete. The dermal sinus must be followed to its full extent. This may include laminectomy and opening of the dura, as well as surgical correction of the associated soft tissue anomalies.

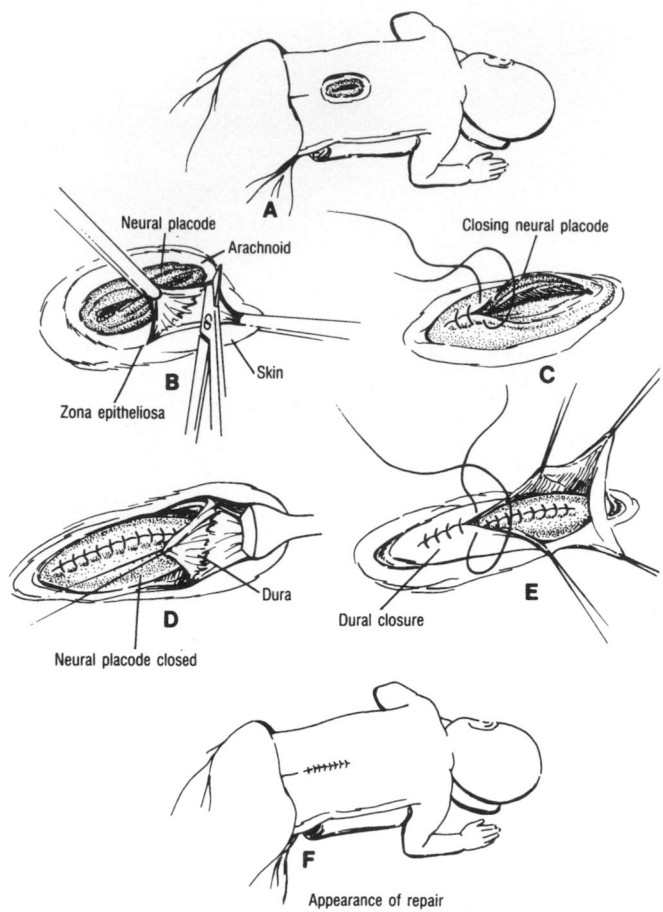

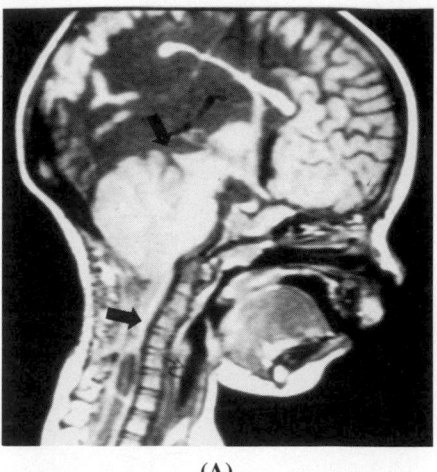

(A)

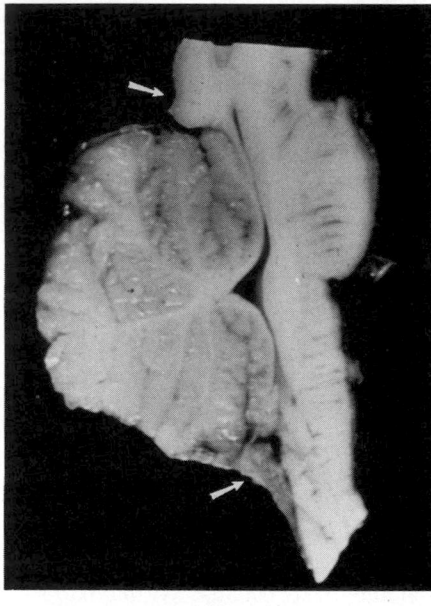

(B)

Figure 7–3 Repair of myelomeningocele. *A.* Positioning of patient. Note the rolls supporting and suspending the chest and abdomen and the "doughnut" under the head for support, without compression of the external ear. *B.* The initial repair dissection of the neural placode. *C.* Repair of placode by formation of a tube. *D.* Mobilization of dura. *E.* Dural repair with formation of watertight sleeve. *F.* Appearance of final repair.

Figure 7–4 Chiari II malformation. *A.* MRI image. *B.* Autopsy specimen. Note the beaked tectum *(arrow)* and the position of the cerebellar vermis extending to about C3 *(arrow).*

TETHERED SPINAL CORD

Although often initially asymptomatic, any lesion that tethers the spinal cord puts the individual at risk for eventual neurological dysfunction, which may occur during periods of axial growth, or during periods of adipose deposition, which in the case of tethering, may cause lipomatous structures to enlarge. Although the signs and symptoms may include pain, most often, they include loss of control of bowel or bladder, loss of sensation in the feet or motor dysfunction in the sacral and lower lumbar segments. Surgical therapy of any of the lesions which cause spinal cord tethering is directed at release of the tethering.

THICKENED FILUM TERMINALE

The most elementary form of tethering of the spinal cord occurs when the filum terminale is excessively thickened. In these cases, the filum terminale is often infiltrated with fatty tissue. Normally, the filum is a fibrous structure, a continua-

tion of the arachnoid which invests the conus medullaris.[11] Tethering of the spinal cord is indicated when imaging studies show that the conus is located below L2 in the older child or below L3 in the infant. Surgical therapy of the thickened filum terminale includes a laminectomy, opening of the dura, and sectioning of the thickened filum. When a thickened filum terminale is detected early, neurological dysfunction may be prevented, or, in some cases, reversed.[19]

LIPOMA (Fig. 7-6)

The embryological development of lipoma of the spinal cord is not well-understood. As in other forms of spinal dysraphism, normal elements are present, but are found in abnormal locations. One hypothesis is that during embryological development after the neural tube is formed, disrup-

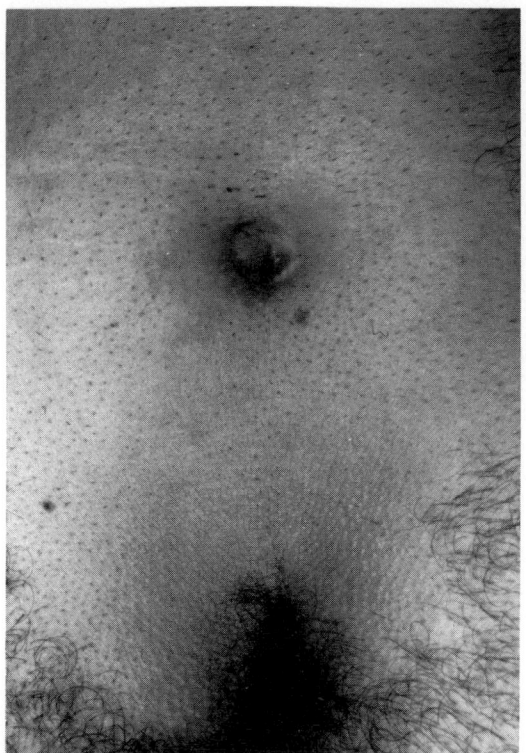

Figure 7–5 Dermal sinus indicated by a large dimple.

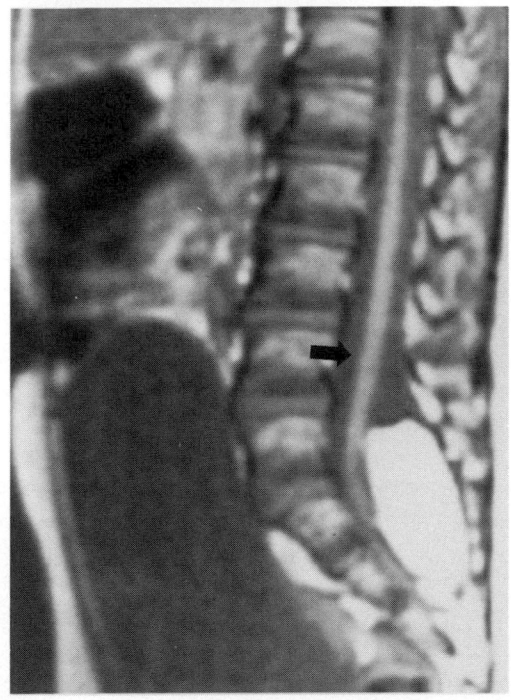

Figure 7–6 Lipoma, tethering the spinal cord. The cord *(arrow)* continues beyond its normal termination into the fatty mass located in the sacral spinal canal.

tion occurs and subcutaneous fat is allowed to herniate into the region of the neural tube.[20,21] The lipomatous tissue fuses with the neural tissue, and the resulting lipoma tethers the spinal cord. Tethering may result in neurological dysfunction.

The therapy of this disorder is resection of the fatty tissue. Laminectomy, opening of the dura, and resection of the lipomatous tissue will effectively release the spinal cord. The surgical carbon dioxide laser is very useful in removing fatty tissue without disturbing neural structures. "Lasering" allows decompression and release without damage to the spinal cord and nerve roots.[19]

LIPOMYELOMENINGOCELE

The lipomyelomeningocele is often detected as a fatty lump in the back, usually in the lumbosacral region. (See Fig. 7-7.) Often dismissed as a cosmetic deformity, the lipomyelomeningocele is, in reality, a complex congenital anomaly which demonstrates not only lipomatous elements and infiltration of neural tissues by fat as in the lipoma but also a large associated meningocele or myelomeningocele. The entire anomaly may be covered with skin.

Surgical correction of this disorder includes release of the tethering, removal of the lipomatous tissue, and reconstruction of the dural sheath around the spinal cord. As with all lesions which tether the spinal cord, the risks of failure to diagnose and correct a lipomyelomeningocele include loss of neurological function of the lower extremities and urinary and rectal sphincters.[19,20]

DIASTEMATOMYELIA

A relatively rare manifestation of spinal dysraphism is diastematomyelia, a disorder that includes the following components:

1. The spinal cord is split, usually asymmetrically, into two hemicords. The dura may or may not be split to surround each hemicord separately.
2. A spike protruding from the vertebral body, consisting of bone or cartilage, may further separate the two hemicords.
3. Diastematomyelia usually occurs at thoracic or thoracolumbar levels, and the associated vertebral body is usually congenitally abnormal, often a hemivertebrae.
4. The interposed bone or cartilaginous spike will tether the cord, and surgical excision is indicated. Careful retraction of the hemicords and resection of the spike and dural septum will release the cord.

A cutaneous hallmark of this disorder is a hairy patch on the back at the level of the diastematomyelia. It has been hypothesized that in ancient times, when the neurological dysfunction resulted in an equinovarus deformity of the feet, individuals with diastematomyelia and a hairy patch may have been the human basis for the mythological centaur—half human, half horse.

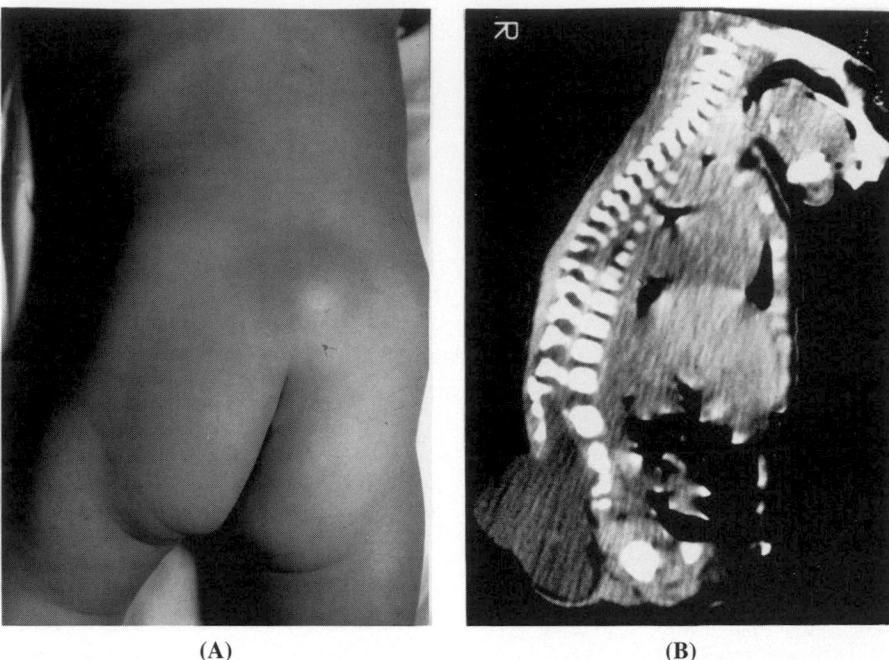

(A)   (B)

Figure 7–7 *A.* Lipoma of the back. Note midline position and physical appearance of scoliosis. *B.* CT scan cross section through lipomyelomeningocele. The skin covered lesion is apparent, and there is a large CSF-filled meningeal sac. The spinal cord is not seen because no subarachnoid contrast has been given.

ENCEPHALOCELE

Encephaloceles are congenital CNS anomalies in which disruption of the developing cranium allows herniation of tissues normally located within the cranium. Encephaloceles and variants of encephaloceles result from defective closure of the rostial neuropore during the fourth week of fetal development. The spectrum of this disorder is variable and depends on the timing and severity of intrauterine disruption.

The most basic variation is *cranium bifidum,* in which only the calvarium fails to form; meninges and neuroectoderm are not involved. A cranial meningocele will include herniation of meninges through the calvarial defect. Encephalocele is broadly defined to include herniation of the encephalon (brain), meninges, and CSF-filled ventricles. One variation is *encephalocystocele,* in which the brain, meninges, and ventricles with choroid plexus are herniated through the calvarial defect. An *encephalomeningocele* involves only meninges and brain.[21]

Encephaloceles may occur in any area of the cranium from the anterior skull base to the occipital bone. Anterior encephaloceles predominate in Asia; occipital encephaloceles are more common in the West.[23] The reason for this distribution is unknown.[21] The anatomical and neurological alterations of affected individuals depend on the amount and organization of the brain tissue remaining intracranially. Hydrocephalus may coexist and require shunting of cerebrospinal fluid (CSF).

Clinical Presentation Many encephaloceles are detected prenatally or at birth. (See Fig. 7-8.) Although the entire mass is usually covered with skin, some areas of the encephalocele may be covered only by meninges and may leak CSF. Encephaloceles which involve the anterior skull and skull base, including the nasal, ethmoidal, sphenoidal, and orbital regions, may not be detected until later in life, when they cause airway obstruction, and then they may be mistaken for nasal polyps. Meningitis may result from communication between the airways and the meninges.[21] Exophthalmos may also occur.

Preoperative evaluation should include computerized tomography (CT) scanning, which will provide images of both the neural structures and the bony defects,[21] or mag-

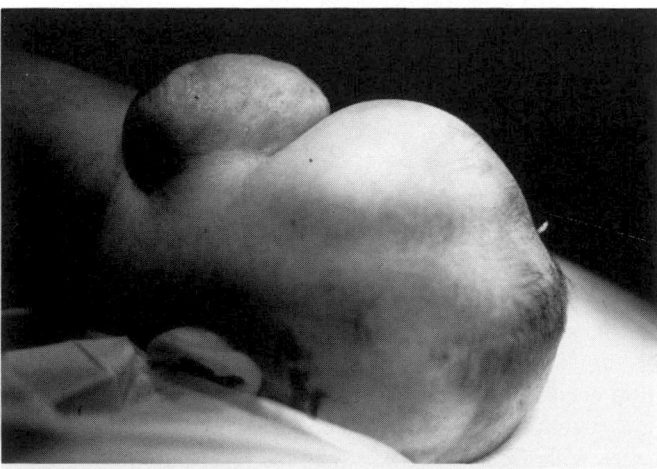

Figure 7–8 Large occipital encephalocele. The child's forehead is right; the encephalocele protrudes to the left.

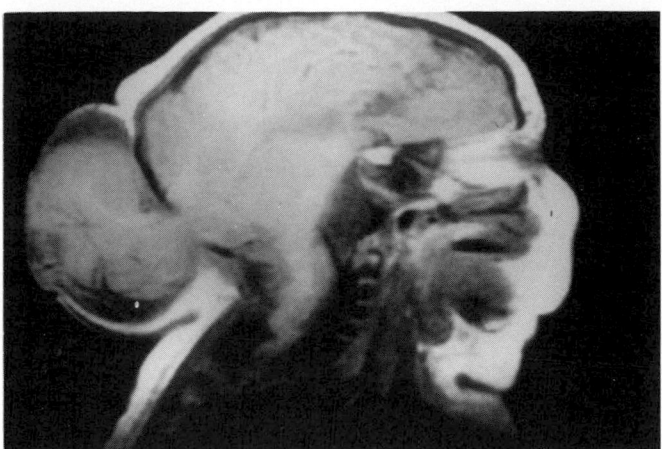

Figure 7–9 Magnetic resonance image (MRI) showing occipital lobe in the encephalocele sac.

netic resonance imaging (MRI) may be very helpful in showing fine details of involved neural structures. (See Fig. 7-9.)

Surgical Therapy The time for repair of encephaloceles should be based on the clinical presentations. A defect with a CSF leak should be repaired within a short period of time (12–24 h) to decrease the risk of infection.[21,22,23] Surgical correction of all encephaloceles should occur as early as the clinical conditions of the patient permits.

The goal of surgery is to repair the defect and preserve neural tissue. Skin and dura should be mobilized. A watertight dural closure is necessary.[24] No attempt is made to repair the calvarial defect, initially. Later, surgery may include calvarial reconstruction, which will be similar to complex calvarial reconstructions described for severe craniofacial anomalies.[25] Occipital, parietal, and temporal defects are approached directly. Anterior and basicranial encephaloceles are approached intracranially through a bicoronal incision. This approach protects neural tissue and minimizes cosmetic deformities.

CHIARI I MALFORMATION

Chiari I malformation is a congenital anomaly consisting of caudal migration of the cerebellar tonsils. (See Fig. 7-10.) Often, affected individuals have associated hydrosyringomyelia and hydrocephalus.

Although the Chiari I malformation may remain asymptomatic, clinical symptoms may occur at any age but most commonly in adolescence or young childhood.

Clinical Manifestations Clinical manifestations of the Chiari I malformation are variable. Headache and cervical pain are common.[26] Motor weakness, especially of the upper extremities, is frequent. A central cord syndrome with upper extremity weakness and hypotonia is frequently associated with hydrosyringomyelia. Other clinical manifestations in-

clude sensory loss, lower cranial nerve weakness, scoliosis, ataxia, sleep apnea, and diplopia.

Nystagmus on lateral gaze and downbeat nystagmus, characteristic of lesions at the foramen magnum, are seen. The Klippel-Feil syndrome, characterized by limited neck movement, web neck, and low hairline, has been associated with Chiari I malformation.[27]

Treatment Symptomatic Chiari I malformations are treated by surgery. CT scans and MRI show the bony and CNS anomalies well. Preoperative CT demonstrates the size of the foramen magnum. Pathology also occurs below the

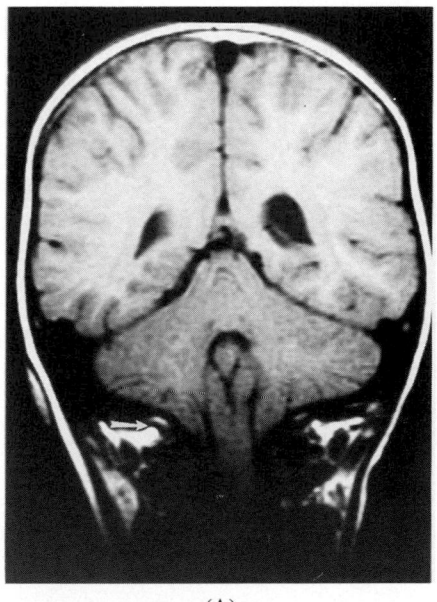

(A)

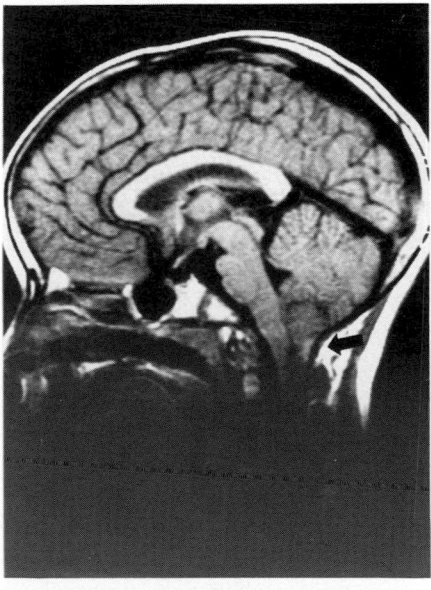

(B)

Figure 7–10 Chiari I malformation. *A.* Coronal view. *B.* Sagittal view. Note tonsils herniating below foramen magnum. (Compare with Fig. 7-4.)

foramen magnum as the upper cervical cord is crowded by the low-lying cerebellar tonsils.

Surgical corrections consist of a posterior fossa decompression by removing the occipital bone to decompress the foramen magnum. The cervical spine is decompressed by removing laminae to a level below the herniated tonsils as seen on the preoperative examinations and visualized at surgery.[28,29]

After the bone is removed, the dura is opened. Usually, the arachnoid is densely adherent to the anomalous structures. Under high-power magnification, dissection of these adhesions and plugging of the obex with muscle and the fourth ventricle to subarachnoid shunt may be undertaken, depending on surgical judgment and severity of the congenital anomaly.

Outcome As with other congenital anomalies, the goal of surgery is to prevent worsening. Some patients, especially those who present with weakness or pain, improve, In younger patients, the outlook is generally more favorable. Overall, Menzes et al. report that 85 percent of patients improved with surgery.[30]

DEVIATIONS FROM THE NORMAL IN CRANIAL GROWTH

Head circumference measurement [occipital-frontal circumference (OFC)] is a routine part of the physical assessment of infants. Children whose measurements are above the 98th percentile or below the 5th percentile, as well as those who cross percentiles rather than growing along a curve, require evaluation.

MACROCEPHALY (CRANIAL ENLARGEMENT)

Macrocephaly may be due to hydrocephalus. Commonly, however, the child is macrosomic. Macrocephaly is often a benign familial variant. Careful inquiry into the maternal and paternal history should reveal a pattern of benign enlargement. The dolicephalic head of the child with sagittal synostosis will also have an increased OFC and will, therefore, appear macrocephalic. Other diagnoses associated with macrocephaly include chronic subdural hematomas, Sotos's syndrome, spongy degeneration of infancy (Canavan Van Bogaert-Bertrand disease) neurofibromatosis, and achondroplasia.[31]

MICROCEPHALY

Children who are microcephalic are often evaluated because of the possibility of closure of sutures (craniosynostosis). Like macrocephaly, microcephaly can be a benign familial variation. The cranium may also fail to increase in size because the brain is not growing normally as a result of central nervous system damage or malformation. This damage results in secondary craniosynostosis. Secondary craniosynostosis is not amenable to surgical correction.

CRANIOFACIAL ANOMALIES

CRANIOSYNOSTOSIS

The human cranium accommodates the rapid brain growth which occurs postnatally in human infants. At birth, the cranial sutures are normally open, but, occasionally, sutures fuse prematurely or in utero. The affected child may be detected early in life. Involved sutures are usually palpably ridged. The pattern of early fusion of cranial sutures results in pathonomonic cranial appearances as described below.

SURGICAL CORRECTION

Surgical correction for most of the single suture craniosynostoses varies with the age of the child and the severity of the deformity. For premature fusion of the sagittal or lambdoid sutures noted prior to the age of 6 mo, simple strip craniectomy along the affected suture is probably sufficient. When children are older than 6 mo, when the coronal suture is involved, or when there is severe distortion of the cranium, complex cranial reconstructions are necessary.[32]

Evaluation of patients should include a history, physical examination, and developmental assessment. Radiographs of the skull will often reveal suture closure and abnormal configuration. Computerized tomography of the brain and bones will give additional information related to the status of the sutures, as well as revealing congenital or cerebral malformations which may influence cranial development.

Sagittal Suture (Fig. 7-11) Premature fusion of the sagittal suture is the most common of single suture craniosynostoses. Males are affected more often than females.[33] Compensation and growth may only occur at the coronal and lambdoid sutures. The head shape, characteristically elongated, is described as *dolicephalic.* If the deformity is allowed to progress beyond the fourth to sixth month, significant prominence of the forehead and occiput will occur. As there is significant deformity and the possibility of increased pressure on the developing brain, surgical correction is advocated.[33]

Coronal Suture (Fig. 7-12) Premature fusion of one or both coronal sutures is referred to as *plagiocephaly.* Affected children have a shallow anterior fossa, flattened forehead, shallow orbit, and elevated brow ridge on the affected side. The cosmetic deformity is significant and may be progres-

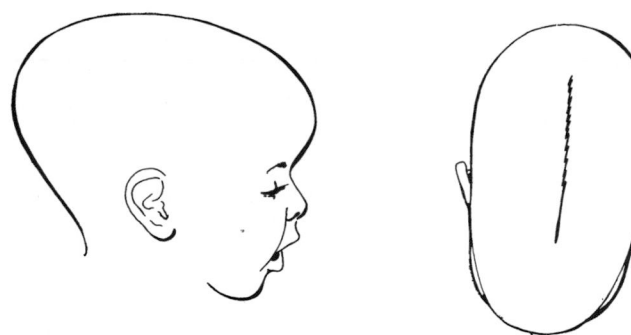

Figure 7–11 Sagittal synostosis. The calvaria is long and narrow with a prominent forehead and occiput.

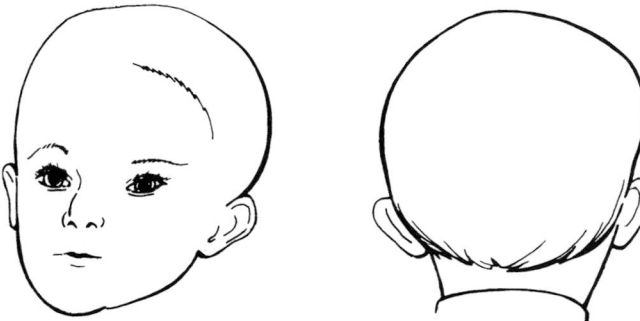

Figure 7–12 Unilateral coronal synostosis. The entire calvaria is asymmetrical with flattening of the forehead on the effected side.

sive. If left uncorrected, not only is there compression of the developing brain, but also the excessively shallow orbit allows inadequate space for the developing globe of the eye. The surgical correction includes not only the release of the coronal suture, but also advancement of the forehead and realignment of the orbits and browridge.[34] This complex surgery is best accomplished by a craniofacial team, including a neurosurgeon and a plastic surgeon.

Lambdoid Suture (Figs. 7-13 and 7-14) Premature fusion of the lambdoid suture shows a characteristic flattening of the occipital region. This may be unilateral or bilateral, the former being more frequent. In its most severe manifestation, there is a compensatory bulge at the contralateral parietal eminence. In the most serious cases, the ear of the affected side may also be displaced forward and out; milder cases, however, are much less deforming. Surgical correction which includes resection of the lambdoid suture in those less than 6 months of age is usually employed only in the most severely affected children.[33]

Metopic Suture Premature fusion of the metopic suture results in a triangular-shaped forehead, *trigoencephaly*. Although less threatening to the developing brain than plagiocephaly, the cosmetic deformity may be significant. The neurosurgeon and plastic surgeon work together to resect the suture and reshape the forehead to achieve a more normal contour. In its most severe form, trigonocephaly may be associated with *hypotelorism*, abnormally small space be-

tween the two orbits. In this case, the orbits should be moved outward during reconstruction.[34]

Occasionally, a child will be born with all cranial sutures prematurely fused. The calvarial bone between sutures is expanded by the developing brain but held at the area of the sutures. The resulting cloverleaf–shaped skull is referred to as *kleebatschadel*. This disorder is uncommon. When detected, urgent surgical correction is indicated to release the compression on the brain. All sutures are resected. The skull is morcellized. Bone fragments may be replaced and sutured loosely to the dura.[34] An alternative surgical approach removes all bone.

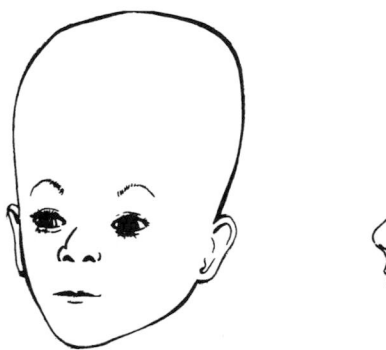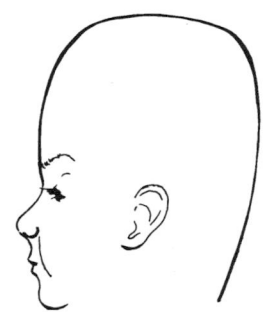

Figure 7–13 Brachycephaly. This vertically elongated head may occur with bilateral lambdoidal fusion.

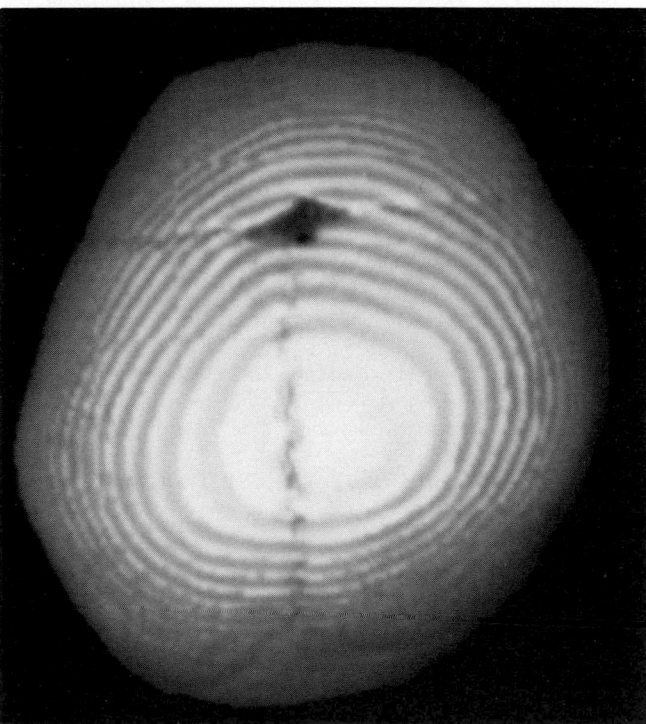

Figure 7–14 A 3-dimensional CT reconstruction of a skull, demonstrating unilateral lambdoidal synostosis. Note the flattening of the skull on the right with the loss of the lambdoidal suture, as well as the compensatory bulge of the skull on the left.

REFERENCES

1. Wasrkany J: Morphogenesis of spina bifida, in McLaurin (ed): *Myelomeningocele.* New York, Grune & Stratton, 1977, pp 31–35.
2. Campbell JB: Congenital anomalies of the neural axis. *Am J Surg* 75:231, 1948.
3. Moore KL: *The Developing Human,* 4th ed. Philadelphia, Saunders, 1988, chap 18, pp 364–401.
4. Czeizel AE, Dud'as I: Prevention of the first occurrence of neural-tube defects by periconceptional vitamin supplementation [see comments]. *N Engl J Med* 327(26):1832–1835, 1992.
4a. Recommendations for the use of folic acid to reduce the number of cases of spina bifida and other neural defects. *MMWR Morb Mortal Wkly Rep* 41(RR-14), 1–7, 1992.
4b. From the Centers for Disease Control and Prevention: Recommendations for use of folic acid to reduce number of spina bifida cases and other neural tube defects. *JAMA* 269(10): a1233, 1236–1238, 1993.
5. Knoury MJ, Erikson JD, James LM: Etiologic heterogeneity of neural tube defects: Clues from epidemiology. *Am J Epidemiol* 115:538, 1982.
6. Elwood JH: Major central nervous system malformations notified in Northern Ireland, 1964–1968. *Den Med Child Neurology* 26:177, 1984.
7. Lorberg J, Ward AM: Spina bifida—A vanishing nightmare? *Arch Dis Child* 60:1086, 1985.
8. Report of the UK collaborative study on alpha-feta-protein in relation to neural tube defects. *Lancet* 1:1323, 1977.
9. Filly R: The fetus with a CNS malformation: Ultrasound evaluation, in Harrison M, Galbus M, Filly R (eds): *The Unborn Patient.* Philadelphia, Saunders, 1990, chap 34, pp 304–436.
10. McLone DG, Dias L, Kaplan WE, et al: Concepts in the management of spina bifida, in Hemphreys RP (ed): *Concepts in Pediatric Neurosurgery.* Basel, S Karger, 1985, pp 97–106.
11. French BL: Midline fusion defects and defects of formation, in Youmans J (ed): *Neurological Surgery,* 3d ed. Philadelphia, Saunders, 1990, chap 39, pp 1081–1235.
12. Reigel D: Spina bifida, in McLauren RL, Schut L, Venes JA, Epstein F (eds): *Pediatric Neurosurgery,* 2d ed. Philadelphia, Saunders, 1989, chap 3, pp 35–53.
13. McLone DG: Technique for closure of myelomeningocele. *Child's Brain* 6:65, 1980.
14. Hoffman HJ, Hendrick EB, Humphrey RP: Manifestations and management of Arnold-Chiari malformations in patients with myelomeningocele. *Child's Brain,* 1:255, 1975.
15. Park TS, Hoffman HJ, Hendrick EB, et al: Experience with surgical decompression of the Arnold-Chiari malformation in young infants with myelomeningocele. *Neurosurgery* 13:147, 1983.
16. Nardich TP, McLone DG, Fulling KH: The Chiari II malformation: IV. The hind brain deformity. *Neuroradiology* 25:179, 1983.
17. McLone DG, Nardich TP: Myelomeningocele outcome and late complications, in McLaurin RL, Schut L, Venes JA, Epstein F (eds): *Pediatric Neurosurgery,* 2d ed. Philadelphia, Saunders, 1989, chap 4, pp 53–70.
18. French BN: Abnormal development of the central nervous system, in McLaurin RL, Schut L, Venes JA, Epstein F (eds): *Pediatric Neurosurgery,* 2d ed. Philadelphia, Saunders, 1989, chap 2, pp 9–34.
19. McLone DG, Nardich TP: Laser resection of fifty spinal lipomas. *Neurosurgery* 18:611, 1986.
20. Hoffman HJ, Hendrick EB, Humphrey RP: The tethered spinal cord: Its protein manifestations, diagnosis and surgical correction. *Child's Brain* 2:145, 1976.
21. James HE: Encephalocele, dermoid, sinus, and arachnoid cyst, in McLaurin RL, Schut L, Venes JA, Epstein F (eds): *Pediatric Neurosurgery,* 2d ed. Philadelphia, Saunders, 1989, chap 6, pp 97–106.
22. Luyendijk W: Intranasal encephaloceles: A survey of 8 neurosurgically treated cases. *Psych Neurol Neurochir* 72:77, 1969.
23. Matson DD: *Neurosurgery of Infancy and Childhood.* Springfield, IL, Charles C. Thomas, 1969.
24. Yokota A, Kajiwara H, Kohchi M, Fuwa I, et al: Parietal cephalocele: Clinical importance of its atretic form and associated malformations. *J Neurosurg* 69:545–551, 1988.
25. Berman DE, Persing JA: Total cranial vault reconstruction for parietal encephalocele. *Plast Reconstr Surg* 86(3):554–557, 1990.
26. Saez et al: Experience with Arnold-Chiari malformation, 1960–1970. *J Neurosurg* 45:416–422, 1976.
27. Sherk HH, Dawoud S: Congenital os odontoideum with Klippel-Feil anomaly and fatal atlantoaxial instability: Report of a case. *Spine* 6:42–45, 1981.
28. Garcia-Uria J, Leunda G, Carillo R, Bravo G: Syringomyelia: Long-term results after posterior fossa decompression. *J Neurosurg* 54:380–383, 1981.
29. Levy WJ, Mason L, Hahn JF: Chiari malformation presenting in adults: A surgical experience in 127 cases. *Neurosurgery* 12:377–390, 1983.
30. Menezes AH, Smoker WR, Dyste GN: Syringomyelia, Chiari malformations, and hydromyelia, in Youmans JR (ed): *Neurological Surgery,* 3d ed. Philadelphia, Saunders, 1990, chap 46, pp 1421–1459.
31. Adams RD, Victor M: *Principles of Neurology,* 3d ed. New York, McGraw-Hill, 1985, chap 43, p 904.
32. Laurent JP, Cheek WR: Craniosynostosis, in McLaurin RL, Schut L, Venes JA, Epstein F (eds): *Pediatric Neurosurgery,* 2d ed. Philadelphia, Saunders, 1989, chap 7, pp 107–119.
33. Hoffman HJ, Raffel C: Craniofacial surgery, in McLaurin RL, Schut L, Venes JA, Epstein F (eds): *Pediatric Neurosurgery,* 2d ed. Philadelphia, Saunders, 1989, chap 8, pp 120–141.

☐ STUDY QUESTIONS

I. A newborn female is referred because of a mass on the back, located at the lumbosacral junction, measuring 4 cm in diameter and paresis of the lower extremities. Epidermis is missing from the central $1\frac{1}{2}$ cm of the mass which is fluctulant.

1. What is the most likely diagnosis? **2.** What therapy should be administered? When? **3.** What is the purpose of early surgery? **4.** What are the chances of hydrocephalus? **5.** What is the most likely relationship between the spinal cord and the skin?

II. An infant is referred because of a peculiar-looking head. The forehead is flattened on the right and the orbit is "raised," with the globe of the eye appearing to be protruding. A ridge is palpated over the usual site of the coronal suture.

1. What is the most likely diagnosis? **2.** What surgical therapy should be administered? When? **3.** How can the orbit be reshaped? **4.** What is the explanation for the ridge over the coronal suture? **5.** What would radiographs show?

III. An infant, 6 mo of age, is brought into the emergency department with fever and seizures. The fontanel is bulging and there is a dimple over the upper sacrum in the midline, surrounded by a small tuft of hair. The neck is stiff and the temperature is 40°C.

1. What is the most likely acute diagnosis? **2.** What is the most likely origin of the infection? **3.** How should the dimple be treated? When? **4.** How could the infection have been prevented? **5.** What organisms are most likely to be the cause of the infection?

IV. A 28-year-old female is complaining of intermittent "dizziness," headaches, and weakness in her hands. Examination showed bilateral lateral nystagmus and decreased sensation to pinprick and temperature in the distribution of the hands. Neurological examination was otherwise normal.

1. What is the most likely diagnosis? **2.** How can the diagnosis(es) be proved? **3.** What forms of therapy might be considered? **4.** What are the chances for hydrocephalus in this patient? Why? **5.** What is the explanation for the altered sensation in the hands?

V. A newborn is referred because of a mass on the back of the head, the base of which is located near the junction of the parietal and occipital bones. The mass is fluctulant.

1. What is the most likely diagnosis? **2.** What determines the degree of neurological deficit? **3.** What type of surgical therapy might be administered? **4.** What other alterations in the anatomy of the head might be anticipated. **5.** Is there a chance of hydrocephalus?

Diagnosis and Surgical Treatment of Patients with Hydrocephalus or Pseudotumor

Ann Marie Flannery

☐ HYDROCEPHALUS

CEREBROSPINAL FLUID PHYSIOLOGY

Cerebrospinal fluid (CSF) surrounds the brain and fills the ventricles within it. Normally, CSF is produced at a rate of 0.3 mm per minute, or approximately 500 cm³ per day. Approximately 50 to 70 percent of the CSF is secreted by the choroid plexus; the remainder is a venous transudate. At the time of production, CSF reflects its origin, containing approximately the same amount of sodium, chloride, and potassium as plasma. Other normal constituents of cerebrospinal fluid include: glucose, approximately two-thirds of the amount being found in plasma; small amounts of protein, mainly albumin; and a few white cells—all lymphocytes.[1]

Most CSF is produced in the lateral ventricles. From there, it moves by bulk flow, propelled by the pulsation of the cardiac output and by respiration. Propelled CSF exits from the lateral ventricles through the paired foramina of Monro, into the third ventricle, exiting through the aqueduct of Sylvius, a narrow channel of 1 to 2 mm, in the midbrain. From the aqueduct, CSF flows into the fourth ventricle, then into the subarachnoid space through the paired lateral foramina of Luschka and medial foramen of Magendie to enter the basal cisterns. Once in the basal cisterns, some fluid flows along the spinal cord, while the remainder is pumped slowly over the convexity of the brain to the arachnoid granulations and villi, where most is reabsorbed.[1]

This simple, yet effective, system may be disrupted at many points. Disturbances in flow may result in hydrocephalus, which has numerous causes. The pathophysiology usually occurs in one of three ways. First, excessive quantities of CSF may be produced. This cause of hydrocephalus is the least common. It is, most likely, the result of a tumor, the choroid plexus papilloma, which secretes excessive amounts of CSF. Second, CSF production may be normal in amounts, but its circulation may be blocked—most commonly where the pathway is narrowest, at the aqueduct of Sylvius, but also at the foramen of Monro, the third or fourth ventricles, or in the subarachnoid spaces. Finally, the pathways may be open, but the reabsorptive mechanism may malfunction, usually the result of hemorrhage or an inflammatory process. The result of any of these pathological events is hydrocephalus. Imaging ultrasound, computerized tomography (CT), or magnetic resonance imaging (MRI) reveal enlarged ventricles.

☐ SIGNS AND SYMPTOMS OF HYDROCEPHALUS

The diagnosis of hydrocephalus may be made when ventriculomegaly is noted in association with signs or symptoms consistent with increased intracranial pressure. Table 8-1 lists the symptoms and signs of hydrocephalus.

☐ CLASSIFICATION OF HYDROCEPHALUS

Hydrocephalus may be classified by its pathophysiology or etiology. The pathophysiology, as listed previously, may include excessive production, obstruction, or failure of reabsorption. Excess production is seen only from an uncommon tumor, the choroid plexus papilloma. Hydrocephalus caused

Table 8-1
HYDROCEPHALUS IN CHILDREN AND ADULTS

Symptoms	Signs
	In Adults
Emesis	VIth nerve palsy
Neck pain	Ataxia
Developmental delay	Gait disturbance
Developmental regression	Dementia
Personality changes	Incontinence
Intellectual decline	Paresis of upward gaze
Irritability	(Parinaud's syndrome)
Lethargy	Hypertension
Headache	Bradycardia
	Apnea
	Coma
	In Infants
	Increasing head circumference
	Full fontanel
	Split sutures

by obstruction above the spinal cord is called *noncommunicating hydrocephalus*. Obstruction may be due to tumors, blood clots, congenital malformations, or arachnoiditis. When the CSF pathways are open, but reabsorption fails, *communicating hydrocephalus* results. Causes of communicating hydrocephalus include intraventricular hemorrhage, subarachnoid hemorrhage, and meningitis. Details will be given in the following sections.

When hydrocephalus is classified by etiology, a division is made between congenital hydrocephalus and acquired hydrocephalus. *Congenital hydrocephalus* is present from birth and is the result of a central nervous system malformation. *Acquired hydrocephalus,* secondary to a postnatal occurrence, is caused by infection, trauma, or tumor.

CONGENITAL HYDROCEPHALUS

The majority of cases of congenital hydrocephalus are categorized as idiopathic; that is, no known cause can be found. Some are diagnosed prenatally. Although prenatal therapy has been advocated, intrauterine CSF shunts are rarely performed at present. Children with idiopathic hydrocephalus may have a good prognosis. Normal intelligence is possible, and it is likely if anomalies are minimized and the hydrocephalus is not severe.[2] Congenital hydrocephalus is usually noncommunicating. This anomaly in many cases includes obstruction to CSF flow at some point in the pathway. Aqueductal stenosis is accompanied by enlargement of the lateral and third ventricles and a normal-sized fourth ventricle. (See Fig. 8-1.) Some, but not all, cases of aqueductal stenosis are X-linked disorders. Hydrocephalus associated with a myelomeningocele is usually noncommunicating. The hypothesized obstruction to flow is in or around the fourth

ventricle; however, the absorptive mechanisms may also be developmentally abnormal. Hydrocephalus occurs in up to 95 percent of children with myelomeningoceles. With adequate treatment, 80 percent of these children will have an intelligence quotient (IQ) above 80.[3]

A unique variant of congenital hydrocephalus is the Dandy-Walker syndrome. Characterized by a large posterior fossa cyst, with or without dilitation of the lateral ventricles, the Dandy-Walker syndrome is thought to be a congenital atresia of the outflow of the fourth ventricle, the foramina of Luschka and Magendie. Midline cerebellar hypoplasia is characteristically seen. (See Fig. 8-2.) Seizures, developmental delay, and agenesis of the corpus callosum are often associated.[4,5]

ACQUIRED HYDROCEPHALUS

While most cases of congenital hydrocephalus are due to obstruction, acquired hydrocephalus may be communicating or noncommunicating. Increased survival of premature infants has resulted in a number of infants with intraventricular hemorrhage. Neonates, born between 28 and 32 weeks of gestation, have a layer of subependymal tissue, the germinal matrix, which is richly supplied with blood vessels. It has been hypothesized that, as a result of respiratory distress from immature lungs along with episodes of hypoxemia, vessels in the germinal matrix of these infants have a tendency to rupture and hemorrhage into the ventricles.[6] Most of the hemorrhages are asymptomatic and resolve without therapy. A small number of the most severe type (grades III to IV) cause communicating hydrocephalus, probably because of the effects of the red blood cells on the immature arachnoid villi. Many of these children can be managed by maneuvers which temporarily drain CSF, such as serial lumbar punctures. Although some children require a ventriculoperitoneal shunt, the overall outlook for these infants is relatively good, but up to 25 percent will be more severely affected with major motor dysfunction and/or developmental delay.[7,8] (See Fig. 8-3.)

Any event resulting in red blood cells in the CSF, such as head trauma, subarachnoid hemorrhage from a ruptured aneurysm, or arteriovenous malformation may result in communicating hydrocephalus. The mechanism is similar to that postulated as causing hydrocephalus secondary to intraventricular hemorrhage. Occasionally, this hydrocephalus is temporary and resolves spontaneously or with temporary drainage. Intracranial pressure may be controlled by drainage of the CSF by lumbar puncture or by an external ventricular drainage system. Permanent shunting will be necessary if the hydrocephalus persists.

The inflammatory responses incited by meningitis may also affect the ability of the arachnoid villi and granulations to absorb CSF. Communicating hydrocephalus is most commonly seen after bacterial meningitis.[9] Tuberculous meningitis has a unique tendency to cause dense inflammatory adhesions of the basilar meninges.[10] (See Fig. 8-4.) This

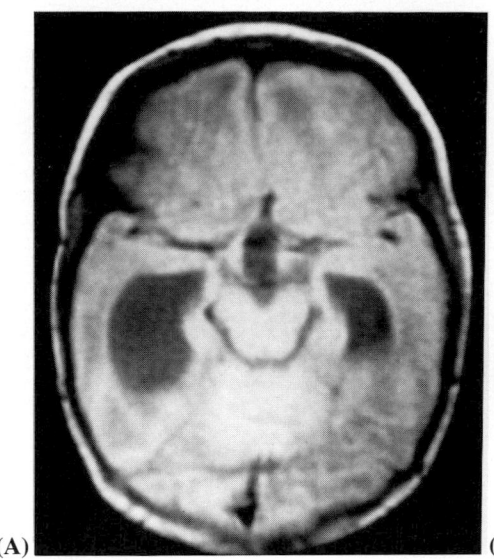

(A)

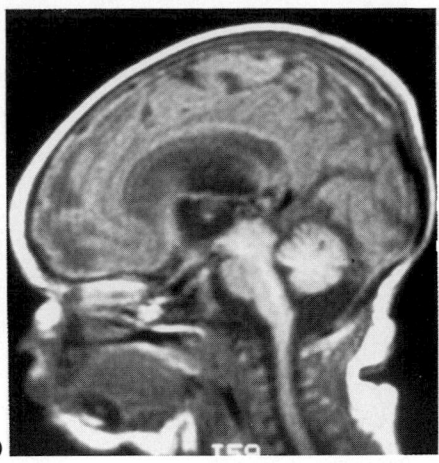

(B)

Figure 8–1   Aqueductal stenosis. *A.* Axial MRI. *B.* Sagittal MRI. Note the lack of signal flow void in the aqueduct of Sylvius.

intense inflammatory response may bring about obstructive hydrocephalus, which can be treated temporarily by external ventricular drainage or permanently by placement of a ventriculoperitoneal (VP) shunt. Intraventricular brain tumors—especially those in or around the aqueduct of Sylvius and the fourth ventricle—may also cause acquired hydrocephalus.

☐ TREATMENT OF HYDROCEPHALUS

The treatment goals of hydrocephalus include control of increased intracranial pressure and avoidance of infection. Achieving these allows the preservation of maximal intellec-

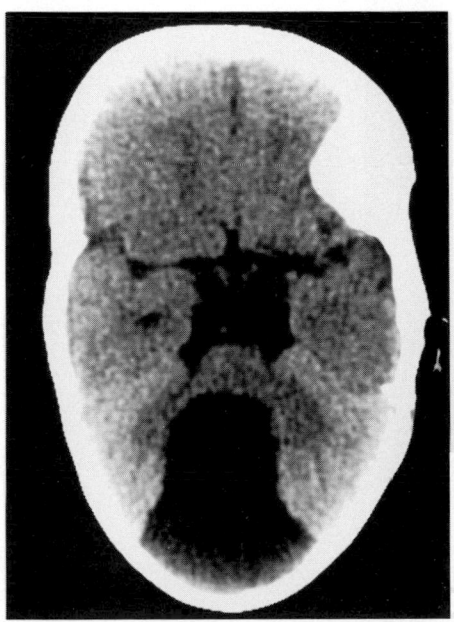

Figure 8–2   The Dandy-Walker syndrome. Characteristic features include a large posterior fossa cyst.

tual function and minimizes neurological deficits. Many of the congenital forms of hydrocephalus are associated with an overall good outcome. The definitive therapy for hydrocephalus is shunting the CSF from the lateral ventricles to another region where it can be absorbed. The VP shunt, first available in the 1950s, but improved after silastic tubing became available, is now the standard of therapy. Cerebrospinal fluid may be shunted to other locations, including the right atrium and pleura. Historically, CSF has been diverted to other areas, including the gall bladder, stomach, fallopian tube, and ureter.

Placement of the VP shunt, under general anesthesia, is usually well-tolerated, even in the youngest individuals. Risks of the ventriculoperitoneal shunt do include infection, malfunction, and hemorrhage into the brain or ventricles, but these complications are uncommon. The expected rate of infection is 3 to 5 percent.[11]

SURGERY

A VP shunt is placed by making a cranial incision and an abdominal incision and tunneling a valve and silastic tube between the two incisions.

The ventricular catheter is introduced frontally, anterior to the coronal suture in the midpupillary line. The alternative standard introduction is posterior parietal-occipital, inferior and posterior to the parietal boss and well away from the sensorimotor cortex, with the tip being directed toward the frontal horn. After shaving, the patient is placed with the neck extended and the head turned away from the side to be shunted. Shunts are usually placed on the right side to avoid the dominant hemisphere areas.

The scalp incision is made through skin and galea and a C-shaped flap is centered on the chosen burr hole site. The scalp is held open by a self-retaining retractor.

The abdominal incision may be located below the costal edge, below the xyphoid, or along the lateral border of the

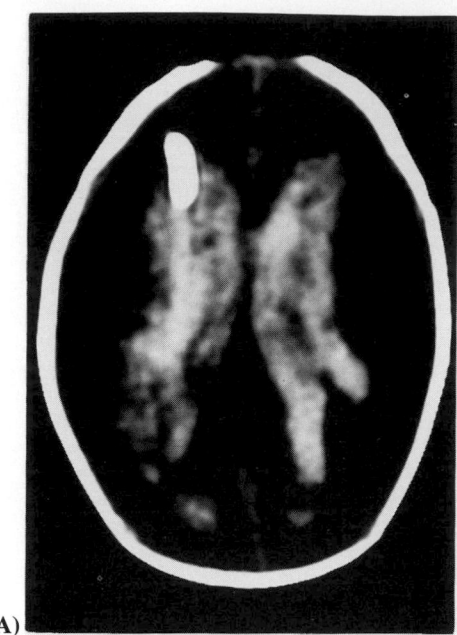

(A)

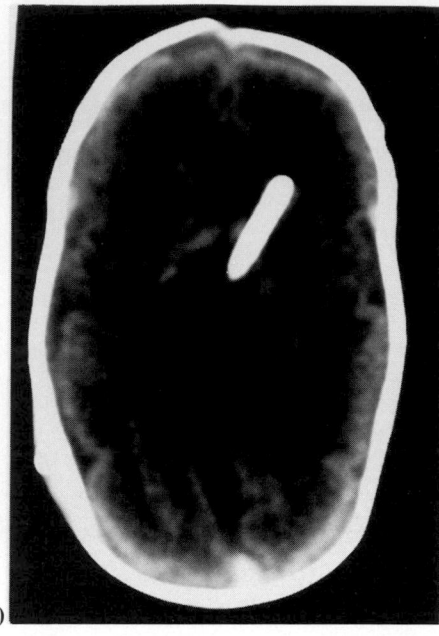

(B)

Figure 8–3 *A.* Grade IV intraventricular hemorrhage seen in a 26-week infant. *B.* Same patient as *A,* following placement of a ventriculoperitoneal shunt.

rectus sheath near the level of umbilicus. The skin is incised and sharp and blunt dissection divides the subcutaneous fat to the external oblique fascia. A tunneling device is used to create a subcutaneous tunnel between the cranial and abdominal incisions. (See Fig. 8-5A.) The chosen shunt is passed into the subcutaneous tunnel and the tunneler is removed.

At the cranial incision, the pericranium is incised. A small burr hole, 3 to 8 mm in diameter, penetrates the skull. The dura is incised. A ventricular catheter is passed into the lateral ventricle. Catheters which start from a posterior burr hole are directed into the frontal horn of the ventricle by aiming toward the medial canthus of the eye on the ipsila-

teral side. This landmark may vary with the configuration of the lateral ventricles.

Good flow of CSF confirms appropriate placement. CSF pressure is checked by a manometer connected to the ventricular catheter. CSF is collected for cell count, Gram's stain, protein, and glucose. The ventricular catheter is cut to an appropriate length and connected to the distal valve and tubing. CSF flow is checked at the distal end.

The layers of the abdominal wall are opened by muscle splitting or penetrated by a blunt trocar. If a trocar is used, the bladder must be emptied by preoperative catheterization. During passage of the catheter through the abdominal wall, the anesthesiologist should increase the intra-abdominal

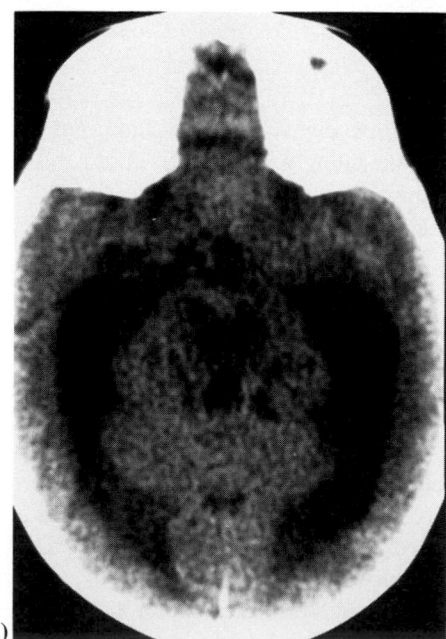

(A)

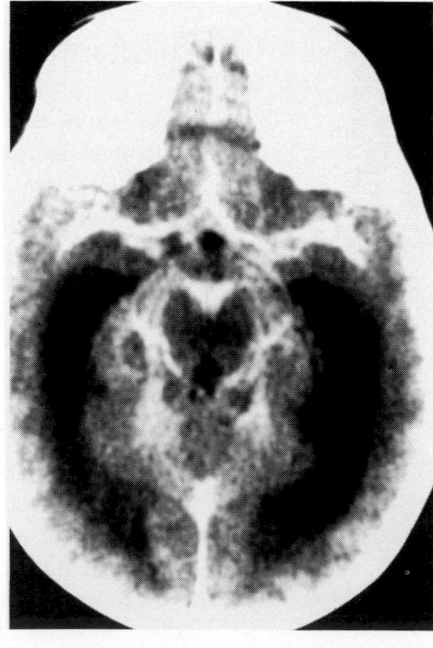

(B)

Figure 8–4 *A.* Hydrocephalus secondary to tuberculosis. *B.* Note enhancing basilar meninges.

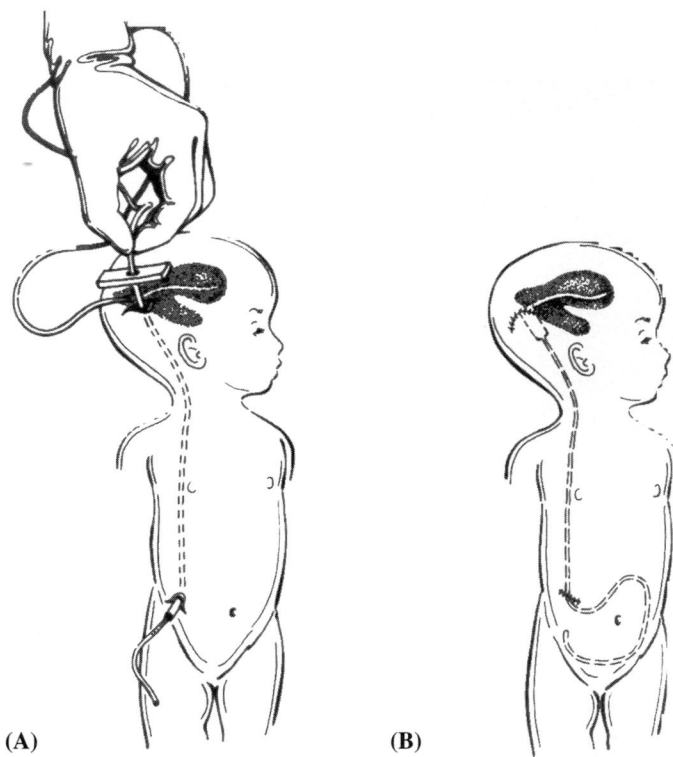

(A)   **(B)**

Figure 8–5 *A.* Placement of the ventriculoperitoneal shunt. Note incisions and the placement of subcutaneous tunneling device. *B.* Ventriculoperitoneal shunt. Ventricular subcutaneous and peritoneal catheters in final position. This figure illustrates the parietal occipital approach.

pressure of the patient by inflating the patient's lungs and delaying expiration (Valsalva's maneuver). Each incision is then closed. (See Fig. 8-5*B*.)

VENTRICULOPERITONEAL (VP) SHUNT INFECTIONS

The VP shunt may become infected, with shunt infection manifesting as acute or chronic. Although the treatment is similar for both presentations, the clinical presentation is different for each and is important to discuss.

Acute shunt infection occurs days to weeks after the placement of the shunt. The patient is usually febrile. The wound often, but not always, demonstrates erythema and may have a purulent drainage. The subcutaneous tract of the shunt can also become erythematous. The peripheral blood count will demonstrate an elevated white count with a left shift. If the shunt is percutaneously tapped, the CSF will generally have an increased number of white cells and positive cultures. The CSF Gram's stain may also be positive. An infected shunt will usually malfunction, and the resultant increased intracranial pressure combined with the infection will cause the patient to appear very ill.

Chronic shunt infections occur weeks to months after the shunt has been placed. The most common presentation for a chronic shunt infection is that of repeated malfunctions. Systemic signs such as fever and elevated peripheral white count may or may not be present. If the shunt is tapped, the CSF white count may be only slightly elevated, the Gram's stain may be negative, but the culture will usually be posi-

tive. Occasionally, infection can be diagnosed only when the shunt device is cultured.

Treatment of a shunt infection, whether acute or chronic, is accomplished by removing the entire system. Particular attention must be paid to extracting all foreign bodies from the ventricular system. An external ventricular drain is then placed to control CSF flow. Appropriate antibiotics are started after cultures of CSF and removal of the shunt hardware. Duration and dosage of antibiotics are determined by the organism infecting the shunt. The draining CSF should be cultured daily to monitor the effectiveness of the chosen antibiotic and to detect suprainfections, which may occur. When the culture shows that the infection has been eradicated, a new shunt system is installed.

Alternative therapeutic plans to treat shunt infections may be effective. The treatment should include high-dose intravenous antibiotics, plus installation of antibiotics into the shunt via percutaneous puncture, with or without preplacement of the system. Other plans use the externalization of the existing system via an incision at the cervical, thoracic, or abdominal tract of the shunt, draining the CSF and antibiotic administrations. The system is then replaced after an appropriate period of antibiotic therapy.

Organisms which commonly infect the shunt include *Staphylococcus epidermidis* (SE) and *Staphylococcus aureus*. SE is the most common infecting organism. Less-common infections are caused by anaerobic diphtheroids, *Escherichia coli* (seen most commonly in premature and term infants), as well as organisms known to cause meningitis. Treatment duration is usually 10 to 14 days after the culture becomes negative. The treatment for virulent or highly resistant organisms may be longer.

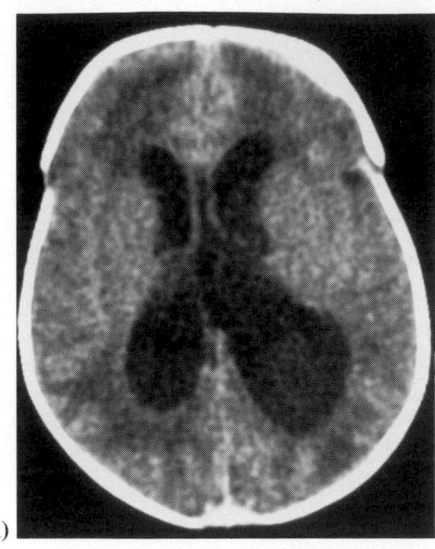
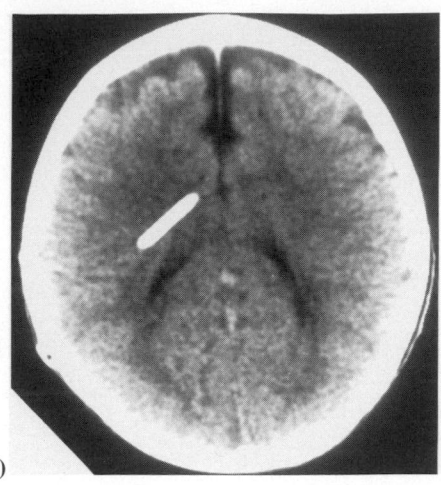

(A)   (B)

Figure 8–6 *A.* Idiopathic hydrocephalus with marked ventriculomegaly prior to placement of a shunt. *B.* Same child, age 3, with excellent ventricular decompression. Development is so far normal.

If treated promptly and vigorously, shunt infections usually resolve without sequelae. Complications, however, can include cerebritis with cortical damage, polycystic ventricles, brain abscess, and peritoneal CSF malabsorption. Developmental delay has been associated with severe shunt infections with *E. coli* occurring in the neonatal period.

PSEUDOTUMOR CEREBRI

Intracranial pressure may be increased without ventricular enlargement. This disorder is termed *benign intracranial hypertension,* or *pseudotumor cerebri.* Affected individuals present with papilledema, or, in infants, bulging fontanels. The primary symptom is headache. Other symptoms include dizziness, nausea, vomiting, paresthesia, diplopia, tinnitus, and blurred vision. Signs include abducens and facial nerve palsy, especially in children.[13] The most serious symptom is visual loss, which can be abrupt and irreversible.[14] Affected individuals may demonstrate hemianopia, quadrantanopia, and, following prolonged visual loss, optic atrophy.[13]

Imaging studies will usually include a CT to screen for overt hydrocephalus. An MRI with gadolinium enhancement should be performed to evaluate the patient for tumor and vascular occlusions. Lumbar puncture will demonstrate intracranial pressure, which is significantly above normal (greater than 200 mm of water.)[14]

Multiple etiologies have been proposed as the cause of pseudotumor. The most commonly affected individual is an obese young woman, often with menstrual irregularities. Usually, no clear anatomical or endocrinological abnormality is found in this group of patients who have idiopathic pseudotumor.

Pseudotumor cerebri has been found in association with numerous lesions or agents. The leading cause in the preantibiotic era was mastoiditis. Other proposed etiologies include: antibiotics, especially tetracycline; steroids; oral contraceptives; excesses and deficiencies of vitamin A; hypothyroidism; anemia; polycythemia vera; head injury; and infection, including Lyme disease; as well as autoimmune disorders, including discoid lupus erythematosis.[13]

Treatment of pseudotumor includes detecting and correcting the underlying problem. For idiopathic pseudotumor, medical management may include exogenous corticosteroids and diuretics, such as furosemide (Lasix) or acetazolamide. If symptoms continue or visual acuity worsens, lumbar puncture, sometimes once or serially, is often effective. If the need for serial lumbar punctures persists and the symptoms persist or worsen despite therapy, a permanent diversion of CSF via shunt, usually lumbar subarachnoid-peritoneal, is indicated.

NORMAL PRESSURE HYDROCEPHALUS

Normal pressure hydrocephalus is one of the few treatable causes of dementia. First described by Hakim and then by Adams in 1965, this disorder is characterized by the clinical triad of dementia, gait ataxia, and urinary incontinence. Additional features include usually normal intracranial pressure and enlarged ventricles.[15]

Some patients who present with normal pressure hydrocephalus have a known or probable cause, including trauma, meningitis, subarachnoid hemorrhage, or tumors. The decision to treat is often straightforward, and the outcome is usually quite satisfactory in this group.

Idiopathic normal pressure hydrocephalus can be difficult to treat. Those patients who are most likely to benefit have a significant gait disturbance and a limited degree of dementia. A radionuclide cisternogram may provide useful objective data of altered CSF dynamics. Some reports favor the use of lumbar puncture to assess improvement and pressure prior to shunting.[16] (See Fig. 8-6.)

Placement of a shunt in these patients is similar to the procedure described above. Technical difficulties include the selection of the correct valve pressure to achieve maximum benefit with minimum risk. The most significant risk is that of extra-axial fluid collections of CSF or blood due to overshunting. These collections may be asymptomatic, but often the patient presents with headache, a diminished level of consciousness, or new neurological deficits. When the clinical situation warrants, additional surgery to drain the subdural collection, adjust the shunt pressure, or remove the shunt completely may be necessary.

REFERENCES

1. Rowland LP: Blood brain barrier, cerebrospinal fluid, brain edema, and hydrocephalus, in Kandel ER, Schwartz JH (eds): *Principles of Neural Science,* 2d ed. Amsterdam, Elsevier, 1985, pp 837–844.

2. Hudgins R et al: History of fetal ventriculomegaly. *Pediatrics* 82:692–697, 1988.

3. McLone DG, Nardic TP: Myelomeningocele: Outcome and late complications, in McLaurin RL et al (eds): *Pediatric Neurosurgery.* Philadelphia, Saunders, 1989, chap 4, pp 53–70.

4. Raimondi AJ, Sato K, Shimoji T: *The Dandy Walker Syndrome.* Basel, S Karger, 1984.

5. Pasueal-Castroviejo I et al: Dandy Walker malformation: Analysis of 38 cases. *Child's Nervous System.* 7:88–97, 1991.

6. Hill A, Shackelford GD, Volpe JJ: A potential mechanism of pathogenesis for early post-hemorrhagic hydrocephalus in the premature newborn. *Pediatrics* 73:19–21, 1984.

7. Palmer P, Dobowitz LMS, Levene MI, et al: Developmental and neurological progress of preterm infants with intraventricular hemorrhage and ventricular dilation. *Arch Dis Child* 57:748–753, 1982.

8. Paplie LA, Munsick Bruno G, Schaefer A: Relationship of cerebral intraventricular hemorrhage and early childhood: Neurological handicaps. *J Pediatr* 103:273–276, 1983.

9. Handler LC, Wright MGE: Post meningitis hydrocephalus in infancy. *Neuroradiology* 16:31–35, 1978.

10. Adams RD, Victor M: *Principles of Neurology,* 3d ed. New York, McGraw-Hill, 1985, chap 31, pp 510–544.

11. McLaurin RL: Ventricular shunts: Complications and results, in McLaurin RL et al (eds): *Pediatric Neurosurgery.* Philadelphia, Saunders, 1989, chap 15, p 223.

12. Chutorian AM, Gold AP, Braum CW: Benign intracranial hypertension and Bell's palsy. *N Engl J Med* 296:1214–1215, 1977.

13. Gree M: Pseudotumor cerebri, in Youmans J (ed): *Neurological Surgery.* Philadelphia, Saunders, chap 122, pp 3514–3530.

14. Jefferson A, Clark J: Treatment of benign intracranial hypertension by dehydrating agents with particular reference to measuring the blend spot area as a means of recording improvement. *J Neurol Neurosurg Psychiatry* 39:627–639, 1976.

15. Adams RD et al: Symptomatic occult hydrocephalus with "normal" cerebrospinal fluid pressure. A treatable syndrome. *N Engl J Med* 273:117–126, 1965.

16. Wood JH et al: Normal pressure hydrocephalus: Diagnosis and patient selection for shunt surgery. *Neurology* 24:517–526, 1974.

☐ STUDY QUESTIONS

I. A newborn was referred because of a large head. Delivery had been by C section because the head did not engage. Pregnancy had been normal.

1. What diagnoses might be entertained? **2.** How could they be differentiated? **3.** What respective treatments might be instituted? **4.** What accompanying conditions might influence the intellectual outcome? **5.** What might be the anatomical causes of hydrocephalus?

II. The patient described in question I above has hydrocephalus and is treated by a ventriculoperitoneal shunt. Four days later the patient begins running a fever, vomiting, and developing a tight fontanel. There is erythema about the incision over the cranium.

1. What is the most likely complication of the shunt?

2. How should it be treated? **3.** What is the most likely offending organism? **4.** For how long should the shunt be externalized? **5.** How might this complication influence the eventual outcome?

III. A 45-year-old male with a previous history of a ruptured aneurysm treated successfully 10 years earlier is referred because of an increasingly ataxic gait and deteriorating intellect. Detailed history reveals that the patient has also been experiencing urinary incontinence in recent months. The patient denies headaches. A CT scan reveals enlarged ventricles and the sulci are almost completely obliterated.

1. What is the most likely diagnosis in this patient? **2.** What therapies might be considered? **3.** What is the likelihood of recovery of the described deficits? **4.** What is

year of age. Newborns have approximately 80 cc per kilo-gram. Premature infants may have up to 105 cc per kilo-gram. The circulating blood volume is relatively small; therefore, meticulous hemostasis is an essential part of pediatric neurosurgery.[5]

Children have a larger surface-to-volume ratio than adults. They have tendency to decrease their core temperature in a cold operating room. Hypothermia can lead to complications including cardiac arrhythmias and hypotension. As a result, preservation of normal core temperature is very important during the preoperative positioning, operation, and postoperative periods.

Positioning of children for surgery is generally similar to that used for adults. Surgical judgment is called for in balancing the risks of pin fixation versus the benefits of immobilization. Most pediatric neurosurgeons avoid the use of the pin head holders in children less than 4 years of age because of the relative fragility of the infant skull. Skull fractures and epidural hematomas are known complications of the use of the pin fixation in children. Often in a child, a horseshoe head holder can be substituted.

A preponderance of posterior fossa tumors in the pediatric age group dictates that posterior fossa craniotomy is among the most common procedures performed for tumors in children by pediatric neurosurgeons. Although the sitting position has been employed for children, the risk of air embolism and the effects of excessive loss of CSF have led to the adoption of the prone position for most posterior fossa operations in children.

The surgical approach—following prone positioning on chest roles for most posterior fossa brain tumors in pediatric patients, especially cerebellar astrocytomas, medulloblastomas, and ependymomas as described below—includes a midline incision from approximately the external occipital protuberance (inion) to the upper or midcervical levels, usually about C2–C3. Following retraction of skin and muscles, the occipital bone is removed, by craniotomy, which we prefer, or a craniectomy; the dura is visualized and incised by a Y-shaped incision; and the cerebellum is exposed. This approach allows adequate access to the cerebellar midline, fourth ventricle, and hemispheres.

Approaches to the cerebellar-pontine angles are similar to those described for adults. However, the surgical position is likely to be the "park bench" or lateral decubitus position to avoid the risks of the sitting position in this population.

CEREBELLAR ASTROCYTOMA

The most common pediatric brain tumor is among the benign and treatable. The cerebellar astrocytoma may occur at any age from infancy to adulthood; however, the classic presentation is in the school-age child at about 5 to 10 years of age. A slowly growing tumor, astrocytoma, frequently presents as described in the clinical section, with signs and symptoms of increased intracranial pressure including head-

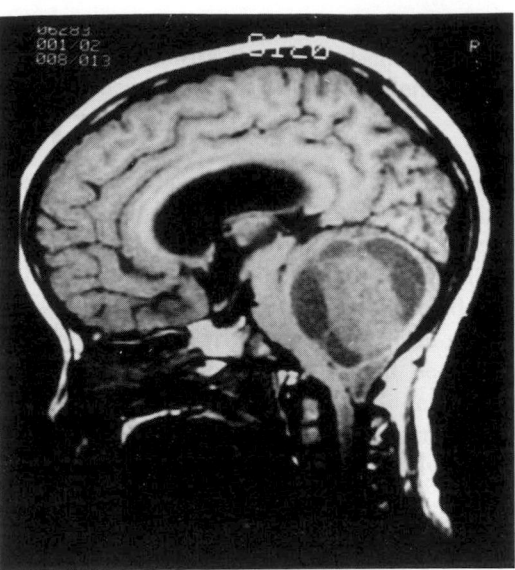

Figure 9-1   Cerebellar astrocytoma, MRI. The low-signal cysts outline the more dense tumor. The cerebellar tonsil has herniated below the foramen magnum.

ache and vomiting, but the tumor is frequently not diagnosed until ataxia and sixth nerve palsies herald the intracranial location of the pathology.

Cerebellar astrocytomas are usually located in a hemisphere, although they may be midline (Fig. 9-1). These tumors may be either solid or cystic with an enhancing nodule (Figs. 9-2 and 9-3). The most common histologic pattern is pilocytic (Fig. 9-4).

Following the surgical approach through the midline, efforts are made to resect the entire lesion. Complete resection is usually possible and results in cures. Many patients with cerebellar astrocytomas have been followed for periods of over 25 years. Follow-up has shown that, although late recurrences are possible, surgical cure may be expected.[7]

Additional therapy is rarely indicated in the treatment of cerebellar astrocytomas, although when tumors with anaplastic histologic features are found, adjuvant therapy is indicated.[8]

MEDULLOBLASTOMAS

The most common malignant brain tumor of childhood is the medulloblastoma, sometimes referred to as the posterior fossa primitive neuroectodermal tumor (PNET). As cerebellar astrocytomas, medulloblastomas may present at any age but are commonly seen in children of preschool and early school years. They present with clinical signs and symptoms, reflecting the tendency of these midline posterior fossa tumors to cause hydrocephalus, usually including headache, lethargy, vomiting, papilledema, sixth nerve cranial palsies, and ataxia.

Medulloblastomas are highly cellular tumors composed of relatively undifferentiated cells. Theoretically, this tumor is

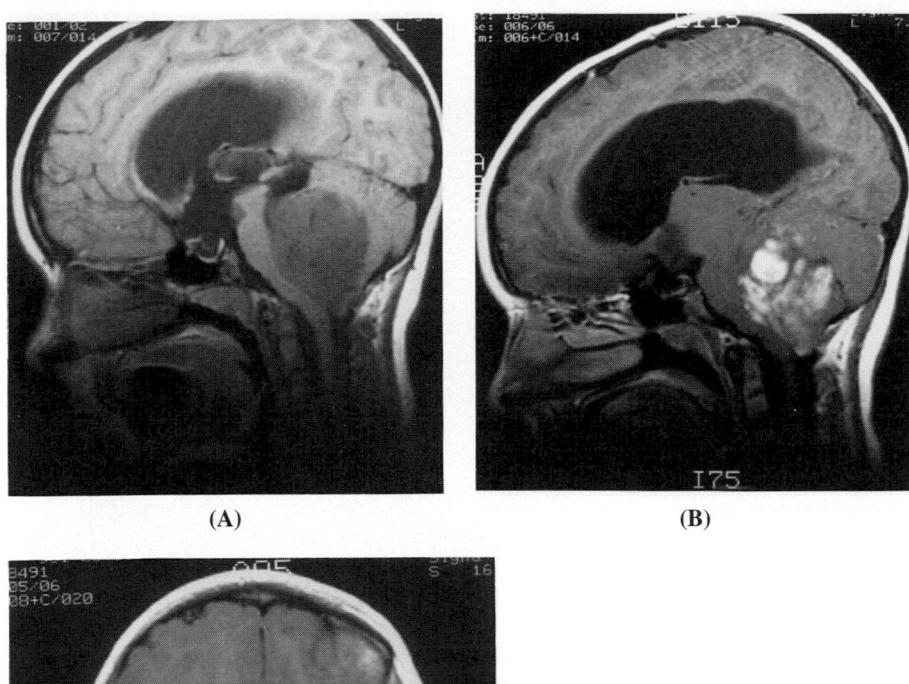

(A)

(B)

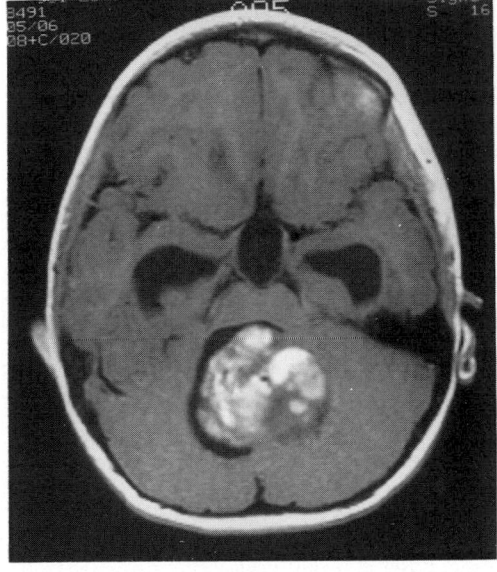

(C)

Figure 9-2 Cerebellar astrocytoma. *A.* MRI, sagittal section. This tumor is lower signal than the brain. *B.* MRI, following gadolinium enhancement. The tumor enhances inhomogeneously. *C.* MRI, same patient, cross section. The fourth ventricle is present but displaced by the tumor, which arises from the cerebellum.

derived from the granular cell layer in the cerebellar vermis (Fig. 9-5). These tumors tend to be midline (Figs. 9-6 and 9-7).

Patients who undergo total or near-total resection of the tumor have an overall better outcome than similar patients who receive biopsy only or very limited resection.[9] Medulloblastoma has a tendency to have spread by the time of diagnosis. Cells are frequently transported along cerebrospinal fluid (CSF) pathways.[10]

Following surgical resection, patients with medulloblastomas are staged clinically. Staging depends on the size of the primary tumor and the extent of its spread. Important factors include the preoperative size of the tumor and whether or not hydrocephalus is present, intraoperative findings including involvement of the brainstem, and extent of resection (Fig. 9-8). Postoperatively, CSF is examined for tumor cells. Evidence of spread of disease is sought by examining bone marrow and by looking for "drop" metastases along the spinal subarachnoid space. Myelography has been used to detect metastatic disease; however, in many medical centers, magnetic resonance imag-

ing (MRI) of the spine with gadolinium enhancement has been found to be more sensitive and less invasive.

Since the period 1965–1970, survival with medulloblastoma has improved significantly.[11–13] Supplementation of surgery by radiation therapy to the posterior fossa and craniospinal axis provided the first improvement. The addition of adjuvant chemotherapy has resulted in further prolongation of survival without significant morbidity.[12–14] A variety of chemotherapeutic regimens has shown some success, including: CCNU, vincristine, and prednisone; CCNU, procarbazine, and prednisone (MOPP); and cisplatin and vincristine.[12,13,15,16]

☐ BRAINSTEM GLIOMAS

Brainstem gliomas frequently present in school-aged children (6–12 years). Unlike many of the tumors discussed in this chapter, brainstem gliomas do not usually present with

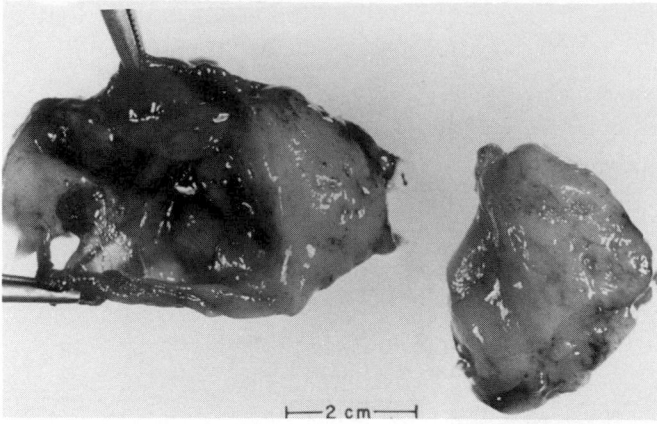

Figure 9-3 Cystic juvenile cerebellar astrocytoma. In this unfixed surgical specimen, a large, cystic, thin-walled cavity (held at the edges with surgical clamps) forms the main bulk of the tumor. The cyst was filled with 15 ml of amber fluid that coagulated in a tube at room temperature. The active parts of the tumor are two "mural nodules" seen as the solid parts at the right (larger), and the left (smaller) sides of the cystic cavity. The freestanding solid tumor tissue is part of the larger mural nodule.

signs or symptoms of increased intracranial pressure. The classic presentation includes cranial nerve palsies, especially of the sixth and seventh nerves, often combined with signs of cerebellar dysfunction such as ataxia and nystagmus. The tumor usually infiltrates the pons; thus pontine cranial nerve palsies are usually seen before signs of increased intracranial pressure caused by obstruction of the fourth ventricle by the expanding tumor mass (Fig. 9-9*B*).

On computerized tomography (CT), brainstem gliomas are hypodense lesions usually in the region of the pons, and enhancement by contrast media is variable. MRI demonstrates the tumor clearly and is the preferred technique for imaging. While the most common type of brainstem glioma

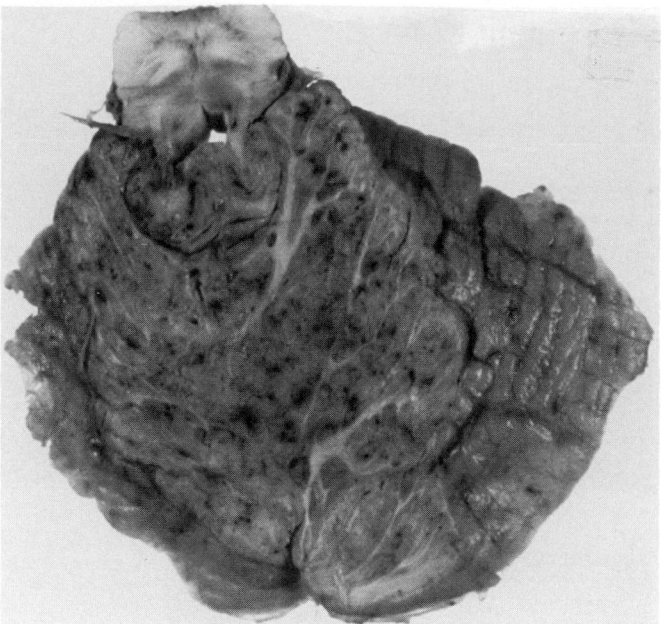

Figure 9-5 Medulloblastoma. This is a transverse section of cerebellum and brainstem at the midpons level. Notice the infiltrating tumor that has greatly enlarged the surface area of cerebellum. In the central parts of the cut surface of cerebellum, bulk of pure tumor is seen, whereas in the periphery, infiltration of cerebellar folia and the subarachnoid space is noticeable.

involves the pons, any part of the brainstem may be involved. Others are radiographically classified exophytic, focally cystic, or at the cervicomedullary junction.[17] MRI outlines these variations (Fig. 9-9*A* and *B*).

TREATMENT

Brainstem gliomas have a highly variable prognosis, depending on location and tumor type. Improvements need to

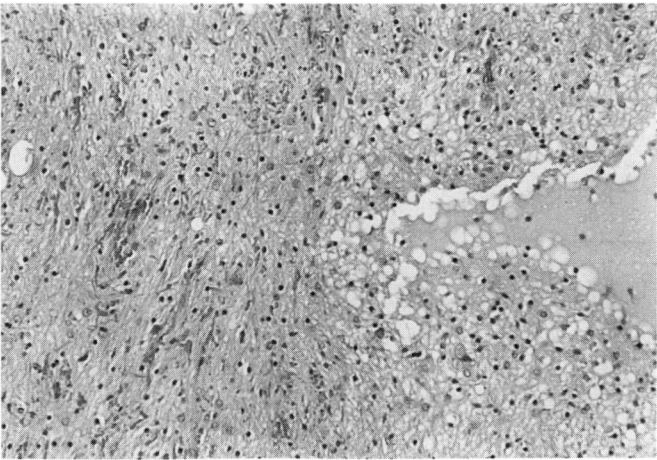

Figure 9-4 Juvenile (pilocytic) astrocytoma of cerebellum. This tumor is one of the most benign gliomas. Many examples have a cystic component. In this photomicrograph, a microcystic area is seen to one side. The surrounding astrocytes have round and ovoid small nuclei. The other part of the tumor shows a denser architecture with more prominent pilocytic elements. Minimal surgical hemorrhage is noted. H&E ×100.

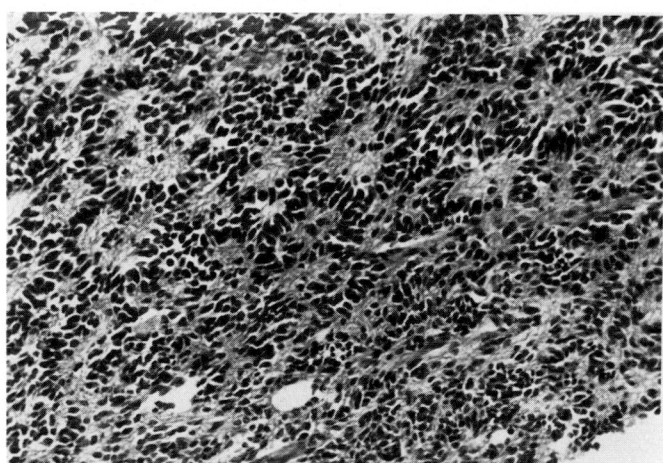

Figure 9-6 Medulloblastoma. In this example, the potential of tumor for neuroblastic differentiation is noticeable. There is an abundance of Homer-Wright rosettes. These are round and off-round formations of tumor cells surrounding a fibrillar zone without a lumen or vessel. H&E ×200.

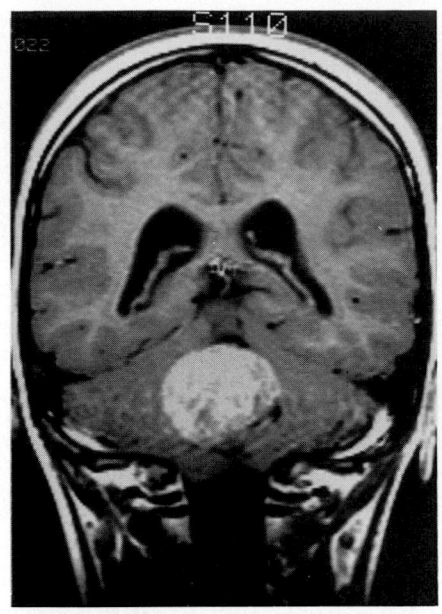

(A)

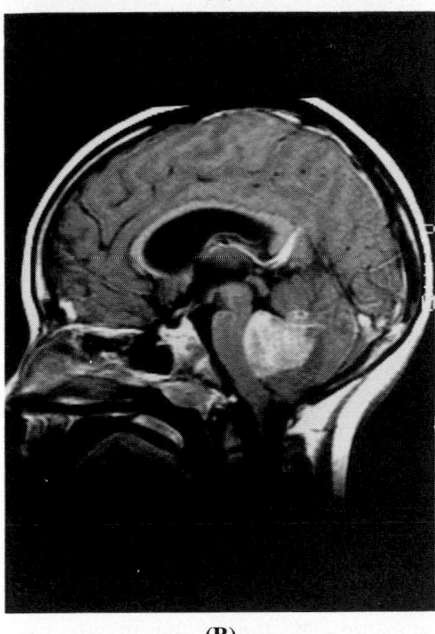

(B)

Figure 9-7 Medulloblastoma. *A*. MRI, coronal section. This densely enhancing posterior fossa lesion is a medulloblastoma. The midline position is a characteristic. *B*. MRI, sagittal section, same patient. This tumor arises from the cerebellar vermis.

be sought in the measurement of the diffuse pontine and malignant types.

Localization of brainstem gliomas and identification of histology directs treatment plans and prognosis. Patients with gliomas located outside the pons—including focal cystic, exophytic, and cervicomedullary tumors—frequently benefit from debulking. Prolonged survival is reported.[18–20]

Patients with diffuse gliomas which involve the pons and other portions of the brainstem are not surgical candidates. Stereotaxic biopsy may be indicated. Imaging by MRI, how-

ever, is usually diagnostic. Therapy usually includes conventional radiation to the tumor. Experimental protocols include twice-daily radiation therapy treatments to increase the tolerance without increasing toxicity. The outlook for diffuse pontine gliomas, however, is poor, even with radiation therapy. Only 30 percent of treated children survive for 1 year and 5-year survival is less than 10 percent.[21] Chemotherapy has improved survival in small trials.[22] If a brainstem glioma has a malignant pathological picture on biopsy, survival will be zero percent at 12 months, despite therapy.

□ PRIMITIVE NEUROECTODERMAL TUMORS (PNET)

PNETs of children are supratentorial lesions which tend to grow rapidly. Like other pediatric brain tumors, these lesions often present with signs of increased intracranial pressure, including: increasing head circumference; emesis; lethargy; and, most commonly in the older child, headache. Focal neurological deficits and seizures may also occur.

The diagnosis is usually made by CT, MRI, or ultrasound (Fig. 9-10). The hemispheral mass is often quite large by the time of diagnosis. PNETs are usually enhanced with contrast although the pattern of enhancement may not be homogenous (Fig. 9-11).[23]

PNETs are poorly differentiated tumors that occur in the cerebral hemispheres but appear histologically similar to medulloblastomas. Medulloblastomas are sometimes referred to as PNETs of the posterior fossa.

TREATMENT

When possible, a gross total resection is attempted in these large cerebral lesions. Occasionally, involvement of deep structures or functional areas precludes total excision. Postoperatively, an evaluation similar to that in medulloblastomas should search for metastatic lesions. Spread may be by CSF pathways and evaluation includes a myelogram or MRI of the spine with gadolinium. The CSF is sampled for tumor cells postoperatively. The bone marrow is aspirated and examined for tumor cells.

Following surgery and tumor staging, additional therapy is probably beneficial. Radiation therapy has been useful in the treatment of some PNET patients.[24] Radiation in young children frequently causes developmental delay and is therefore avoided. Younger patients, especially those less than 3 years, may have prolonged survival when given chemotherapy. Chemotherapy has also been used efficiently with radiation therapy in children more than 36 months. The drugs and dosages employed are similar to those utilized for medulloblastomas. Data on the effectiveness of these approaches is currently under evaluation.

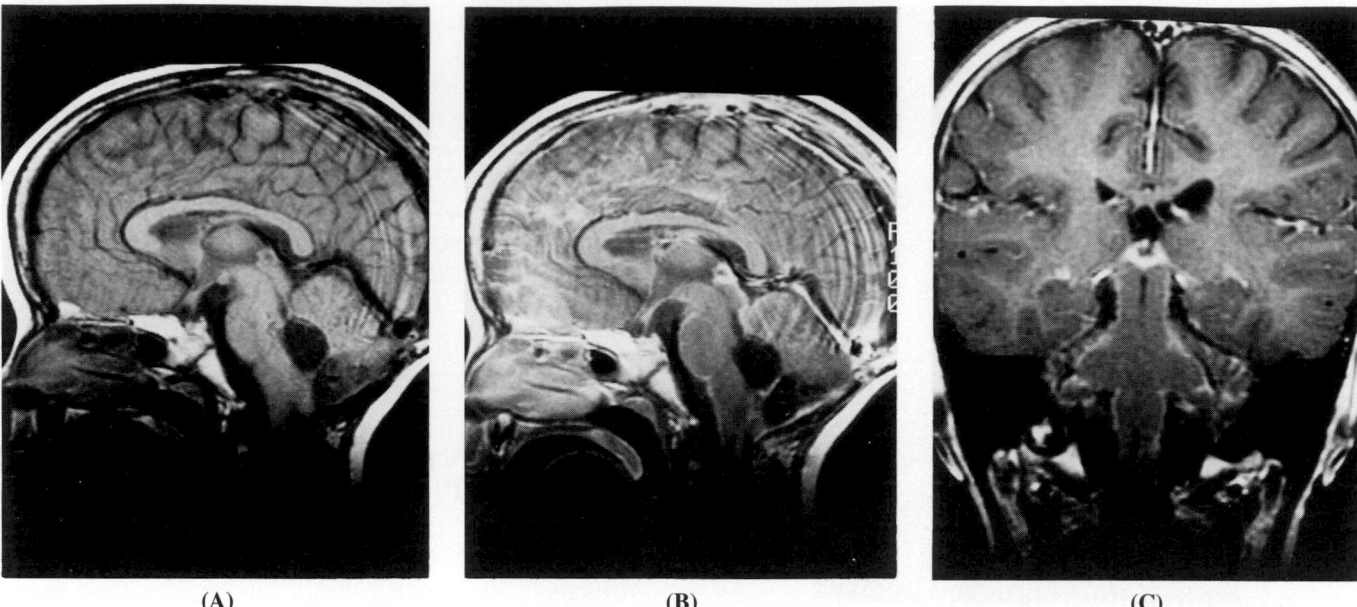

(A)   (B)   (C)

Figure 9-8 Postoperative medulloblastoma. *A*. MRI, sagittal section. Removal leaves an enlarged fourth ventricle. *B*. MRI, sagittal section following gadolinium. The enhancement in the subarachnoid space outlines posterior fossae structures, especially the pons. This enhancement is seen with metastatic spread of medulloblastoma. *C*. Coronal section, MRI, with gadolinium enhancement. The subarachnoid spread of tumor outlines the medulla, brachium pontins, cerebellar folia, and midbrain.

☐ GLIOMAS OF THE OPTIC PATHWAYS

Gliomas of the optic pathways may involve optic nerves, the optic chiasm, or the optic tracts. Often they extend onto the hypothalamus. These anatomic involvements cause the clinical presentation to include visual loss and endocrinological dysfunction in addition to the classic findings of pediatric brain tumors.

When such tumors occur in the first year of life, the chiasm and structures posterior to it are often involved. Affected infants have macrocephaly, irritability, and ocular findings, including spasmus nutans. Older children may have visual loss, and visual field defects can be documented. Endocrinological dysfunction may include the diencephalic syndrome and precocious puberty.[25] Tumors that are confined to the orbit are often stable or very slowly growing lesions which occasionally cause proptosis.

Both MRI and CT may show these tumors, but the resolution of involvement seen with an MRI scan is superior. The MRI may show no contrast enhancement, variable enhancement, or intense uniform enhancement. The contrast pattern does not correlate with the pathological grade of the tumors (Fig. 9-12).

The differential diagnosis of lesions for optic pathways varies with the clinical situation. These tumors are frequently associated with neurofibromatosis. In children without neurofibromatosis (NF), the differential includes germinomas, craniopharyngiomas, and pituitary tumors. Children with masses of the optic pathways, who do not have NF, may need surgery for diagnostic purposes prior to starting other therapy.[27]

TREATMENT

Treatment options may include surgical debulking for large lesions.[26] Radiation therapy has been useful in slowing growth in tumors with proven histology that are very likely to be gliomas such as those with progressive growth in patients with NF. Chemotherapy has also shown promise in small numbers of patients.[27]

☐ EPENDYMOMAS

Ependymomas are CNS tumors that may be found supratentorially and infratentorially. In children, the posterior fossa location predominates. These tumors usually arise from the fourth ventricle and spread directly by CSF metastasis through the CSF pathways. The clinical presentation is very similar to that of other midline posterior fossa tumors with early nonspecific signs and symptoms, including headache, irritability, emesis, and failure to thrive. Later developments may include ataxia, papilledema, and cranial nerve palsies, especially of the sixth cranial nerve (Fig. 9-13).

The age of onset of symptoms tends to be younger than other posterior fossa tumors. The peak age of occurrence in children is 1 year, the mean age at diagnosis is 5 years, averaging just over 3 years.[26] Ependymomas also occur in the adult population, where 23 years is the mean age of presentation.[29] The overall mean age of presentation is about 16 years.[30]

The relationship between histopathological appearance

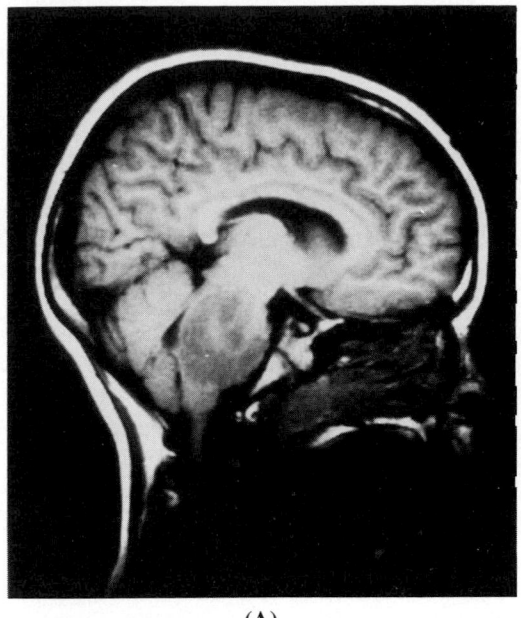
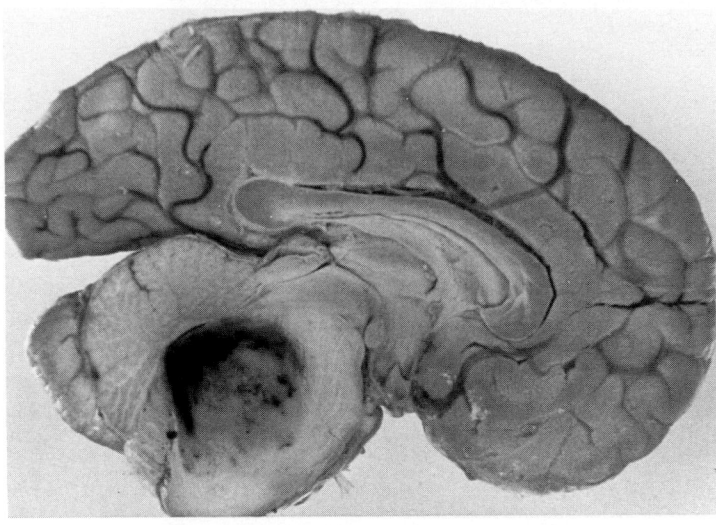

(A)   (B)

Figure 9-9 Pontine glioma. *A*. T1-weighted sagittal MRI. This low-grade glioma has diffusely enlarged the brainstem from diencephalon to lower pons. The medulla and cervical cord are spared. Brainstem glioma. *B*. This is a midsagittal section of brain at autopsy at approximately 8 months after the MRI in Fig. 9*A*, showing the left cerebral hemisphere. Notice that the infiltrating tumor has markedly enlarged the volume of pons and medulla. The tumor in its anterior and inferior parts blends into the structure of pons and medulla. In its central and posterior parts, it has formed a rather pure tumor mass with variegated texture (hemorrhage, necrosis) and has evolved into a markedly anaplastic glioma (glioblastoma multiforme). Notice the slit-like fourth ventricle.

and outcome has caused significant discussion. Evaluation of the prognostic importance of histological features such as anaplasia and the number of mitoses favors the use of the latter rather than the former to predict survival.[31]

Anaplastic ependymomas usually have a poor prognosis, however. Even tumors with a more benign pathological appearance may behave malignantly.

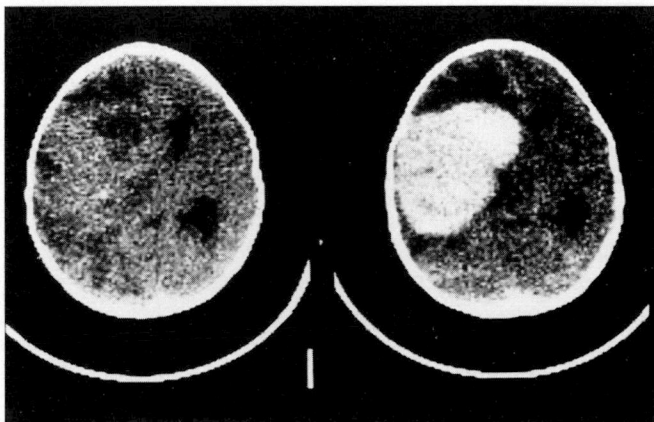

Figure 9-10 Right cerebral PNET. CT scan with and without contrast. This tumor is isointense with brain before contrast but enhances brilliantly and uniformly.

TREATMENT

The surgical approach to posterior fossa ependymomas is similar to that for medulloblastomas and other midline posterior fossa tumors. If possible, the tumor should be completely removed. The outlook for this tumor is not as favorable as for medulloblastoma, even with gross total resection.[32]

Postoperatively, residual or metastatic tumor is sought by checking CSF cytology, screening bone marrow aspirates, and biopsy for tumor cells, as well as by use of MRI of the spine with gadolinium or a myelogram to look for metastatic deposits along the spinal subarachnoid space.

Treatment includes radiation therapy and may include chemotherapy. A variety of radiation doses and protocols has been used, as well as a number of chemotherapeutic agents. To date, however, no therapy has been found to be very effective. The 5-year survival rate is approximately 20 percent.[33]

☐ TERATOMAS

Teratomas are seen most commonly in neonates and young infants.[34,35] They are frequently found in the pineal region, supratentorially, and in the sacrococcygeal region.[35] The clinical signs and symptoms of the intracranial tumor reflect

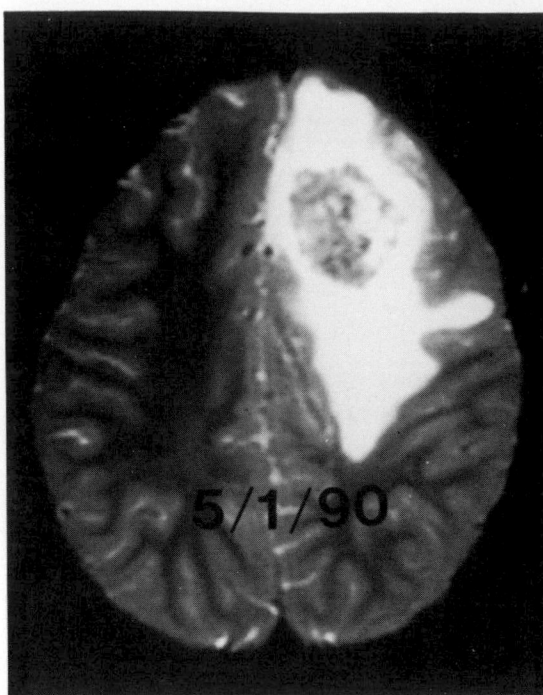

Figure 9-11 PNET, MRI, transaxial, T-2 weighted. This left frontoparietal PNET is surrounded by a large area of peritumoral vasogenic edema.

the increased intracranial pressure and include macrocephaly, a full fontanel, irritability, and lethargy. Teratomas include tissue from all three germ cell layers.[35]

Teratomas are usually debulked and are completely resected if possible. Benign teratomas have a favorable prognosis after complete excision.[36,37] Malignant teratomas or

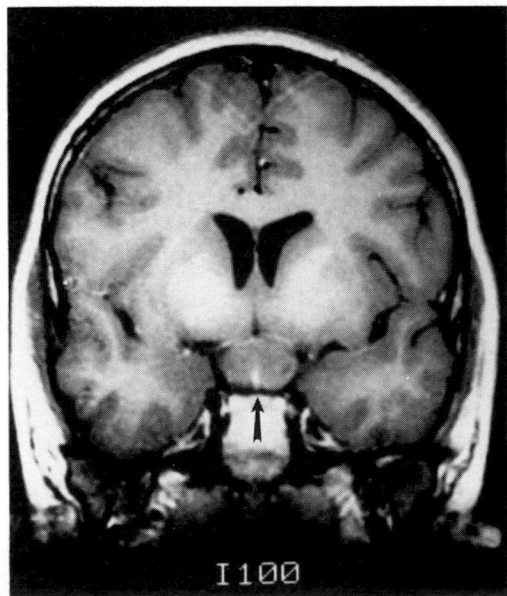

Figure 9-12 Optic chiasm glioma. T-1 weighted, coronal MRI. The optic chiasm (arrow) is diffusely enlarged by a chiasmatic glioma.

teratocarcinomas are less favorable, but, occasionally, infants with malignant teratomas survive.

☐ EPIDERMOID TUMORS

Epidermoids are frequently called "pearly tumors." The glistening white appearance is due to the capsule of stratified squamous epithelium. Derived from a single germ cell layer of the developing embryo, epidermoid tumors grow slowly and are located along the cisterns in the cerebellopontine angle or in the parasellar area, but they may occur at other locations including the fourth ventricle, lateral ventricles, cerebrum, cerebellum, and brainstem (Fig. 9-14).[39–41]

The CT appearance of epidermoids is that of a low-density lesion that does not enhance with contrast. The MRI appearance is hypointense compared to brain in the T1-weighted image and hyperintense in the T2-weighted image (Fig. 9-15).[42]

The clinical presentation reflects the slowly growing nature of these tumors and their anatomical location. Symptoms are often gradual in onset and may include signs of increased intracranial pressure, cranial nerve dysfunction, endocrine dysfunction, aseptic meningitis, and seizures.[40]

Treatment of epidermoid tumors is excision. The lesions should be removed in toto whenever possible. The capsule may be densely adherent to other structures, and viable portions of capsule that are not removed reform tumors. Residual epidermoid cells, however, grow slowly, and the patient may remain asymptomatic for prolonged periods.[40,43]

☐ DERMOID TUMORS

Dermoid tumors are composed of epidermoid cells plus dermal elements which may include hair. The tumors enlarge slightly more rapidly than epidermoid tumors and thus commonly present in the first two decades of life. Dermoids are characteristically midline tumors. They are also often associated with sinus tracts that extend from the skin deep to the tumor.

Symptoms of these tumors reflect their tendency to be midline lesions and the resultant hydrocephalus. If a dermal sinus is present, bouts of bacterial meningitis may occur. Occasionally, the tumors cause chemical meningitis.

Imaging reflects the midline location and the high fat content of these lesions. CT shows a hypodense lesion. The signals on MRI reflect a higher fat content than that of the brain.

Surgery for dermoids is similar to that for epidermoids. Problems include the adherence of the capsule to intracranial structures and the risk of spilling of the tumor contents.

Both inclusion tumors are benign, and the overall outlook is generally good but dependent on the risks of, and outcome from, the surgical resection.[39,43]

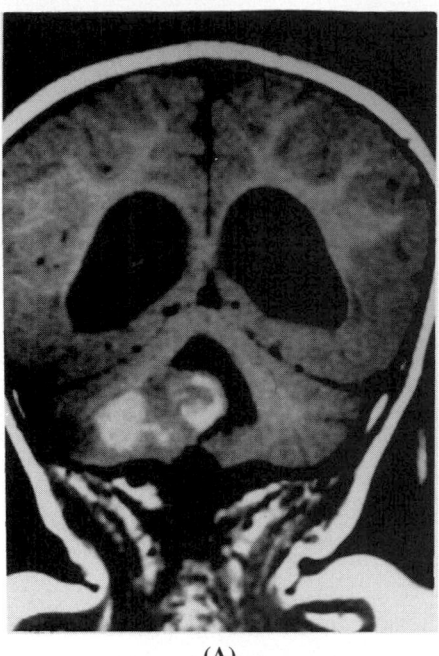
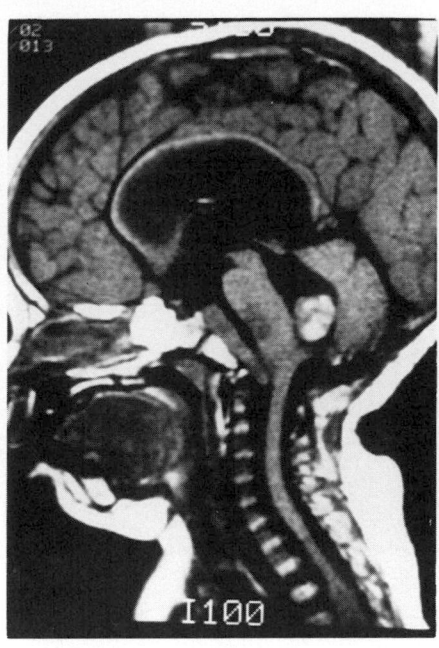

(A)   (B)

Figure 9-13 Ependymoma. T-1 weighted sagittal *(A)* and coronal *(B)* MRI. The tumor mass enhances inhomogeneously with contrast and extends into the fourth ventricle.

☐ TUMORS OF THE PINEAL REGION

Tumors in the pineal region include tumors found in other parts of the brain, such as gliomas, epidermoids, dermoids, and meningiomas, all of which are described elsewhere. Tumors that are unique to the pineal region are grouped into two categories: (1) *germ cell tumors,* derived from nests of primitive, totipotential germ cells that occur in midline structures, and (2) *pinealomas,* including pineocytomas and

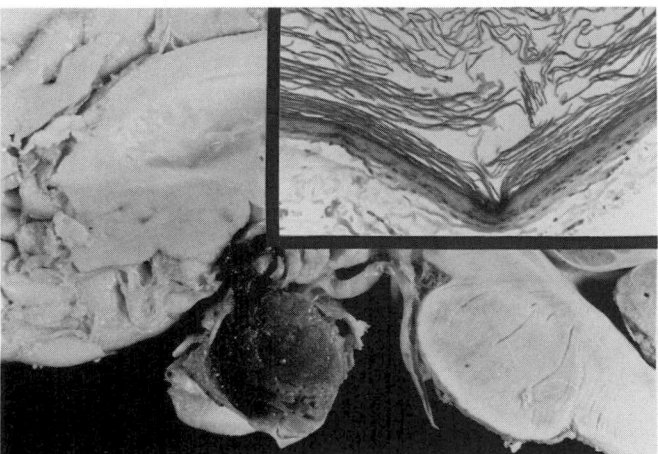

Figure 9-14 Epidermoid cyst of suprasellar region. In this sagittal hemisection of brain, a large, round, thin-walled epidermoid cyst is seen. The contents are friable keratinous material. This cyst was an incidental autopsy finding in a middle-aged woman, retrospectively with some hypothalamic-pituitary dysfunction. The inset shows the typical wall structure of an epidermoid cyst. H&E ×63. There is an external fibrous matrix on which sits a thin, compressed layer of squamous epithelium, slowly producing the keratinous matter, filling the interior of the cyst. In contrast with dermoid cysts, no skin appendages are found within the wall of the cyst.

pinealoblastomas, which are believed to be derived from parenchymal pineal cells.[44]

Nonneoplastic pineal region cysts are common at autopsy.[45] MRI has also revealed that asymptomatic cysts occur frequently (Fig. 9-16).[46,47] Occasionally a benign cyst, because of size and location, can become large enough to cause symptoms (Fig. 9-17). Symptoms will include headache and gaze paresis, with or without hydrocephalus and papilledema and pineal apoplexy with acute hydrocephalus. Surgical excision of the cyst will usually result in improvement.[48]

CLINICAL PRESENTATION

Obstruction to CSF flow results in hydrocephalus, making the clinical presentation of tumors of the pineal region similar to that of other tumors that present with increased intracranial pressure. Pineal region tumors are associated with Parinaud's syndrome, which includes "nystagmus retractorius," paresis of upward gaze, inability to converge, and midposition, unreactive pupils. Nystagmus retractorius is the appearance of the globe being withdrawn into orbit when an attempt is made to converge. These findings are thought to be due to compression of the quadrigeminal plate.[49]

Pineal tumors may invade adjacent structures, including the basal ganglia, hypothalamus, thalamus, internal capsule, inferior collicular plate, and adjacent midbrain structures and fornixes.

DIAGNOSIS

Computerized tomography and magnetic resonance imaging show ventricular enlargement and the pineal region mass.

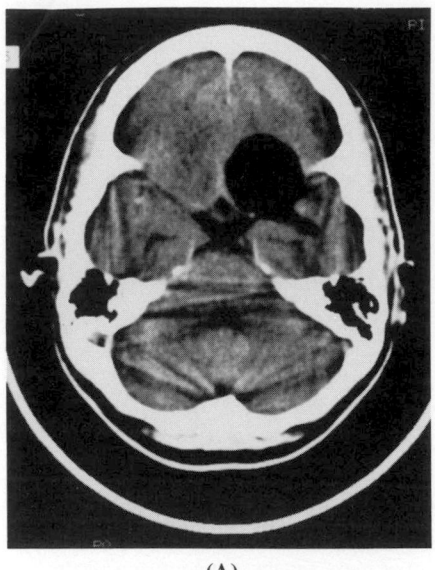
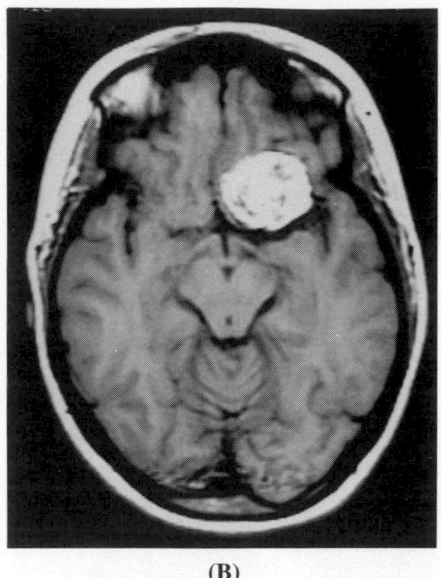

(A)   (B)

Figure 9-15 Epidermoid tumor. *A.* CT scan. The low-density (black) mass on the sphenoid wing is an epidermoid tumor. *B.* MRI, same patient. The T1-weighted MRI reveals the fat density of the epidermoid tumor and allows differentiation from a CSF collection.

Characteristic findings include a lesion that is hypointense or isointense compared with brain prior to contrast. Contrast enhancement usually shows a uniform uptake (Fig. 9-18).

THERAPY

In the past, the therapy of tumors of the pineal region was limited because of the risks of surgery. Therapy advocated at that time included only ventricular shunting and radiotherapy.[35] Currently, recommended therapy includes resection under direct vision. Resection is beneficial because there are multiple types of tumors in this region, and improvements in surgical technique, especially the use of the microscope, has greatly enhanced the outcome. Tumors in the pineal region may be totally removed.

The pineal region is approached by one of three ways. The occipital transtentorial approach elevates the occipital lobe and divides the tentorium to reach the pineal region.[50] The infratentorial, supracerebellar approach achieves access by retracting the cerebellum down and working in the space between the tentorium and the cerebellum.[51] Both of these approaches were initially described with patients in the sitting position. A modification of positioning, the "Concorde position," may be more suitable for pediatric patients as they can be operated on in a prone position, with a decreased incidence of air embolism.[52] This modification is described with the infratentorial approach.

A transcallosal approach has also been utilized in a pediatric population with excellent results. The mortality, in the period of CT and the operating microscope, is about 4.3 percent. This approach is similar to most transcallosal procedures. The patient is positioned supine with the head elevated and flexed.[53]

The choice of approach to tumors of the pineal region depends on the preference and the experience of the surgeon.

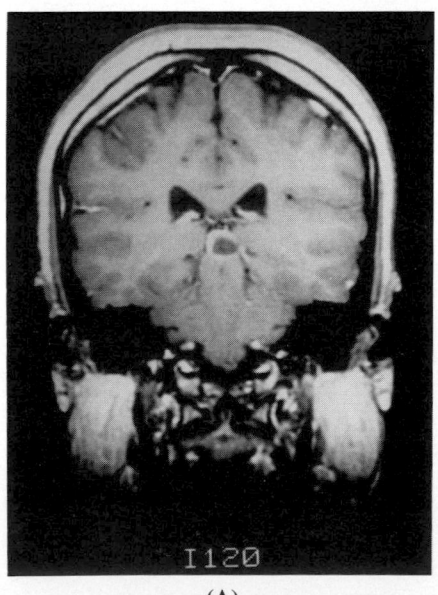
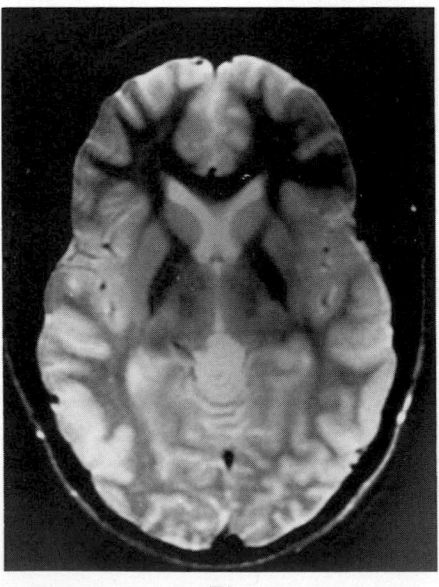

(A)   (B)

Figure 9-16 Pineal region cyst. T1-weighted coronal MRI. *A.* The thickened, enhancing rim of this pineal region cyst contrasts with its nonenhancing, low signal center. The cyst has no mass effect or edema. The T-2 weighted image is presented in *B.*

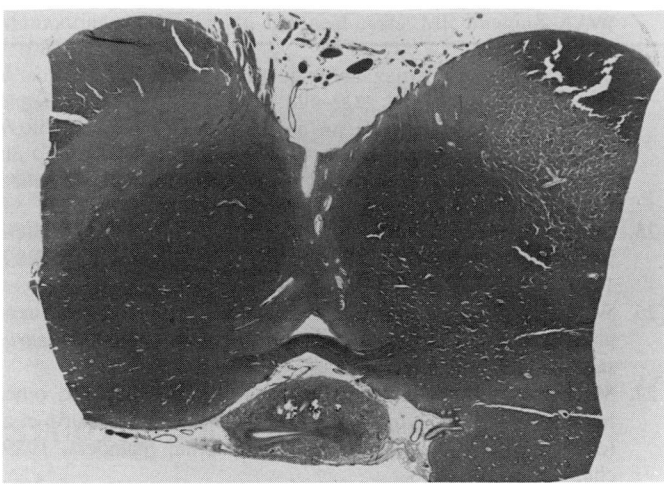

Figure 9-17 Cyst of pineal body. In this horizontal cut of the region of midbrain, an incidental pineal body cyst is seen in the lower midportion of this very low power pictomicrograph. A cyst of this size is a common autopsy finding. Cysts of dimensions to be demonstrable by imaging are seen in about 3–4 percent of population; larger cysts should not be mistaken for genuine neoplastic lesions.

Pineal tumors are very deep and surrounded by structures that cannot be sacrificed or imperiled such as the vein of Galen, the internal cerebral veins, and the basilar veins of Rosenthal. The occipital transtentorial approach may give better visualization of tumors straddling the tentorial notch and extending above the tentorium. The infratentorial, supra-cerebellar approach is probably best for tumors that extend primarily below the tentorial notch,[54] avoiding the risk of postoperative hemianopsia.[51] The transcallosal approach allows excellent access to tumors that may have expanded into the third ventricle.

Surgical therapy of pineal tumors improves the outcome by decompressing large or malignant lesions, permitting total excision of benign lesions, and establishing the pathological identity of the tumor to allow for the safest, most-effective postoperative therapy.

Additional therapy will be dictated by the pathological identification of the tumor. Radiation therapy is particularly important in the treatment of pineal germinomas, which are very sensitive to relatively low doses of radiation therapy (2000 cGy). Other tumors may be treatable by a combination of radiation and chemotherapy.

CONCLUSION

The role of the neurosurgeon in the treatment of pediatric brain tumors has become increasingly important and parallels the improved outlook for children with brain tumors. Although some tumors, such as intrinsic brainstem gliomas, continue to have a poor prognosis, with others such as cerebellar astrocytomas, medulloblastomas, and tumors of the pineal region, surgery can be curative or provide the basis for a multidisciplinary effort including radiation therapy and chemotherapy, which is likely to lead to a cure or at least long-term survival.

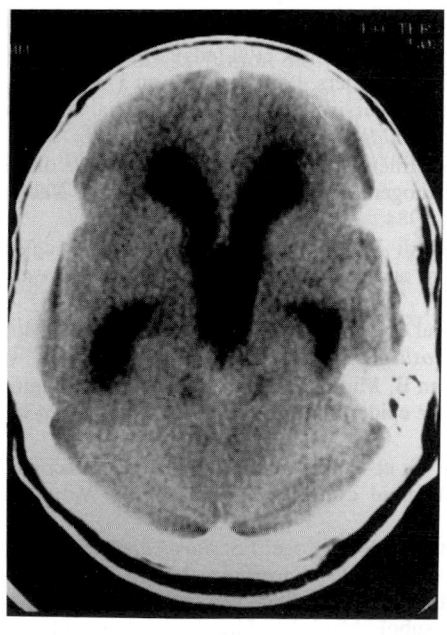
(A)

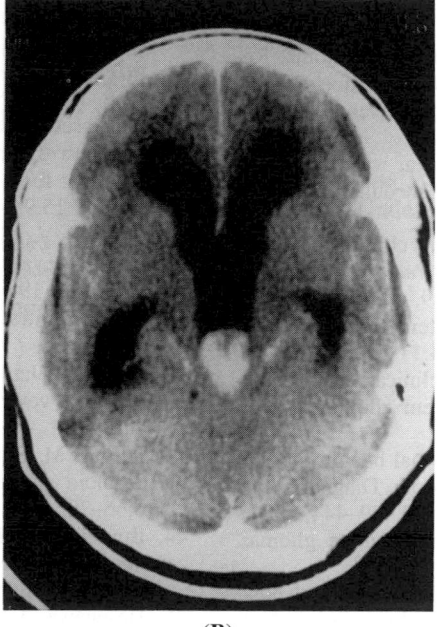
(B)

Figure 9-18 Pineal tumor. CT scan with and without contrast. *A*. The pineal region tumor is located posterior to the third ventricle and is isointense with the brain. It obstructs CSF flow from the third ventricle and causes hydrocephalus, as demonstrated by the enlarged ventricle. *B*. When iodinated contrast is given, the tumor enhances and becomes much more apparent.

CLASSIFICATION OF CNS TUMORS

Following is the 1993 classification of CNS tumors by the World Health Organization. Classifications vary and are based on cell origin, histology, and biological behavior. For the utility of the student of neurosurgery, we present in Table 10-2 the latest available classification of the World Health Organization. It is not necessary to utilize this classification routinely. There are varieties of rare tumors that are not listed in the WHO classification. One such example is the "Primitive Neuroectodermal" tumor. It does not contain a modernized version of pituitary tumors. (See Table 10-2).

Table 10-2
HISTOLOGICAL TYPING OF TUMORS OF THE CNS

I. **Tumors of Neuroepithelial Tissue**
   A. **Astrocytic tumors**
      1. Astrocytoma
         Variants:
         a. Fibrillary
         b. Protoplasmic
         c. Gemistocytic
      2. Anaplastic (malignant) astrocytoma
      3. Glioblastoma
         Variants:
         a. Giant cell glioblastoma
         b. Gliosarcoma
      4. Pilocytic astrocytoma
      5. Pleomorphic xanthoastrocytoma
      6. Subependymal giant cell astrocytoma (Tuberous sclerosis)
   B. **Oligodendroglial tumors**
      1. Oligodendroglioma
      2. Anaplastic (malignant) oligodendroglioma
   C. **Ependymal tumors**
      1. Ependymoma
         Variants:
         a. Cellular
         b. Papillary
         c. Clear cell
      2. Anaplastic (malignant) ependymoma
      3. Myxopapillary ependymoma
      4. Subependymoma
   D. **Mixed gliomas**
      1. Oligo-astrocytoma
      2. Anaplastic (malignant) oligo-astrocytoma
      3. Others
   E. **Choroid plexus tumors**
      1. Choroid plexus papilloma
      2. Choroid plexus carcinoma
   F. **Neuroepithelial tumors of uncertain origin**
      1. Astroblastoma
      2. Polar spongioblastoma
      3. Gliomatosis cerebri
   G. **Neuronal and mixed neuronal-glial tumors**
      1. Gangliocytoma
      2. Dysplastic gangliocytoma of cerebellum (Lhermitte-Duclos)
      3. Desmoplastic infantile ganglioglioma
      4. Dysembryoplastic neuroepithelial tumor
      5. Ganglioglioma
      6. Anaplastic (malignant) ganglioglioma
      7. Central neurocytoma
      8. Paraganglioma of the filum terminale
      9. Olfactory neuroblastoma (Esthestoneuroblastoma)
         Variant:
         a. Olfactory neuroepithelioma

   H. **Pineal parenchymal tumors**
      1. Pineocytoma
      2. Pineoblastoma
      3. Mixed/transitional pineal tumors
   I. **Embryonal tumors**
      1. Medulloepithelioma
      2. Neuroblastoma
         Variant:
         a. Ganglioneuroblastoma
      3. Ependymoblastoma
      4. Primitive neuroectodermal tumors (PNETs)
      5. Medulloblastoma
         Variants:
         a. Desmoplastic medulloblastoma
         b. Medullomyoblastoma
         c. Melanocytic medulloblastoma
II. **Tumors of Cranial and Spinal Nerves**
   A. **Schwannoma (Neurilemoma, Neurinoma)**
         Variants:
         a. Cellular
         b. Plexiform
         c. Melanotic
   B. **Neurofibroma**
      1. Circumscribed (solitary)
      2. Plexiform
   C. **Malignant peripheral nerve sheath tumor (MPNST) (Neurogenic sarcoma, Anaplastic neurofibroma, "Malignant schwannoma")**
         Variants:
         a. Epithelioid
         b. MPNST with divergent mesenchymal and/or epithelial differentiation
         c. Melanotic
III. **Tumors of the Meninges**
   A. **Tumors of meningothelial cells**
      1. Meningioma
         Variants:
         a. Meningothelial
         b. Fibrous (fibroblastic)
         c. Transitional (mixed)
         d. Psammomatous
         e. Angiomatous
         f. Microcystic
         g. Secretory
         h. Clear cell
         i. Chordoid
         j. Lymphoplasmacyte-rich
         k. Metaplastic
      2. Atypical meningioma
      3. Papillary meningioma
      4. Anaplastic (malignant) meningioma

Table 10-2
(Continued)

B. Mesenchymal, nonmeningothelial tumors
1. Benign neoplasms
   a. Osteocartilaginous tumors
   b. Lipoma
   c. Fibrous histiocytoma
   d. Others
2. Malignant neoplasms
   a. Hemangiopericytoma
   b. Chondrosarcoma
      Variant:
         Mesenchymal chondrosarcoma
   c. Malignant fibrous histiocytoma
   d. Rhabdomyosarcoma
   e. Meningeal sacromatosis
   f. Others
C. Primary melanocytic lesions
   a. Diffuse melanosis
   b. Melanocytoma
   c. Malignant melanoma
      Variant:
         Meningeal melanomatosis
D. Tumors of uncertain histogenesis
1. Hemangioblastoma (Capillary hemangioblastoma)
IV. Lymphomas and Hemopoietic Neoplasms
1. Malignant lymphomas
2. Plasmacytoma
3. Granulocytic sarcoma
4. Others
V. Germ Cell Tumors
1. Germinoma
2. Embryonal carcinoma
3. Yolk sac tumor (Endodermal sinus tumor)

4. Choriocarcinoma
5. Teratoma
   a. Immature
   b. Mature
   c. Teratoma with malignant transformation
6. Mixed germ cell tumors
VI. Cysts and Tumor-like Lesions
1. Rathke cleft cyst
2. Epidermoid cyst
3. Dermoid cyst
4. Colloid cyst of the third ventricle
5. Enterogenous cyst
6. Neuroglial cyst
7. Granular cell tumor (Choristoma, Pituicytoma)
8. Hypothalamic neuronal hamartoma
9. Nasal glial heterotopia
10. Plasma cell granuloma
VII. Tumors of the Sellar Region
1. Pituitary adenoma
2. Pituitary carcinoma
3. Craniopharyngioma
   Variants:
   a. Adamantinomatous
   b. Papillary
VIII. Local Extensions from Regional Tumors
1. Paraganglioma
2. Chordoma
3. Chondroma
4. Chondrosarcoma
5. Carcinoma
IX. Metastatic Tumors
X. Unclassified Tumors

Source: Kleihues P, Burger PC, Scheithauer BW: *Histological Typing of Tumors of the Central Nervous System,* 2d ed. Geneva, World Health Organization, 1993. This classification is in collaboration with L.H. Sobin and pathologists in fourteen countries, and was obtained by personal communication from Dr. P.C. Burger. The classification will soon be published by Springer-Verlag, Berlin, Heidelberg, New York, London, Paris, Tokyo, Barcelona. Reprinted with permission.

extensively that complete removal is impossible, but long-term survival can be achieved.

In this tumor group, there may be an indication for physiological mapping. Mapping procedures for identification and preservation of function are described in detail in Chaps. 5 and 22.

Slow indolent growth and high seizure incidence make it desirable to excise the tumor as thoroughly as possible, while preserving functions of speech, memory, movement, sensation, and vision. Unfortunately, incompletely removed tumors eventually progress. Repeat surgical resection may be accomplished when preservation of function is possible.[19,20] Recurrent tumors may have more aggressive behavior, which is reflected histologically by more anaplasia.

Postoperative radiation therapy for astrocytomas is controversial. Most surgeons advocate extensive resection, the extent of removal being the most important factor in long-term survival.[21] Others believe that postoperative irradiation is more significant than the extent of surgical removal. This distinction becomes trivial after 3 years, with radiation showing no statistical difference in the survival rate for

patients with grade I tumors.[22] Younger age correlates best with duration of survival.

Pilocytic astrocytomas generally follow a more benign course and can be removed without recurrence. They are more common in younger patients but also occur in adults. When the tumor is grossly removed, the survival rate is reported to be 83 percent at 10 years and 70 percent at 20 years. With incomplete resection and having 40 Gy postoperative radiation, 74 percent of patients survived 10 years and 41 percent 20 years. This series also included 22 out of 36 cases that are cerebellar and therefore much more benign. Histological changes in tumors of the nonsurvivors showed progression to anaplastic astrocytoma.[23]

Oligodendroglioma *Oligodendrogliomas* comprise 2 to 5 percent of gliomas. The oligodendroglia appear on microscopy as uniform, small round cells with clear cytoplasm. Oligodendrogliomas usually grow slowly. Seizures frequently initiate symptoms. Microhemorrhages give rise to calcifications within the tumor, which may be identified on plain x-ray and CT. (See Fig. 10-2.)

Although mostly indolent, malignant changes do show

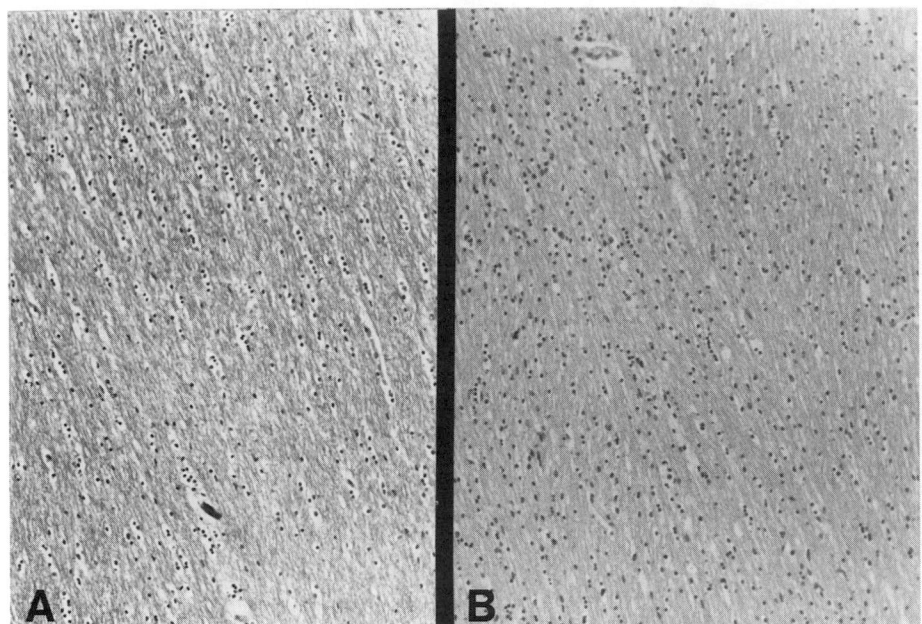

Figure 10–6 *Astrocytoma.* **A.** The *left* photomicrograph shows normal cerebral white matter. Notice the short single files of oligodendroglial cells as the predominant cell type. They are recognized by their round, small, dark nuclei and clear perinuclear halo (cytoplasm). The astrocytes are inconspicuous and occasionally seen with slightly more irregular nuclei (H&E ×63). **B.** The *right* photomicrograph is a field of an astrocytoma. Notice increased number of astrocytes and mild disturbance of the architecture of the infiltrated white matter. This tumor may also be considered a grade I, or benign, astrocytoma in different nomenclatures (H&E ×63).

surrounding the growth zone into which tumor cells infiltrate. These cells have an affinity to infiltrate along fiber tracts. Extensions along major fiber pathways account for neoplastic progression deep in the cerebrum near such structures as the corpus callosum, anterior commissure, fornix, and internal capsule. These regions are especially prone to rapid recurrence following local therapy.[34]

The extent of tumor involvement as defined by imaging studies is a critical parameter for planning surgical and radiation treatment. It has been proposed that a margin of 2 cm beyond the visualized tumor margins usually includes the invaded tissue. Tumor cells may extend beyond the enhanced margin into the surrounding low-density zone and beyond, especially in the corpus callosum and other fiber tracts. Thus a margin of resection of 2 or even 3 cm beyond

the enhancing lesion may not include all tumor.[34] (See Fig. 10-10.)

There are significant differences between anaplastic gliomas and glioblastomas, but in many respects their management is similar. Accurate histological classification is important in correlating survival rate with treatment results. Median survival time reported for glioblastoma multiforme is 32 weeks and for anaplastic astrocytoma is 63 weeks.[35]

Several factors affect the clinical course of malignant astrocytomas and glioblastomas. Factors that influence prognosis are (1) location of tumor, (2) extent of resection, (3) age of the patient, and (4) neurological functional level.

Preserving neurological function requires that tumors in eloquent brain areas be treated by partial resection or biopsy. Lesions in noneloquent brain areas may be resected more

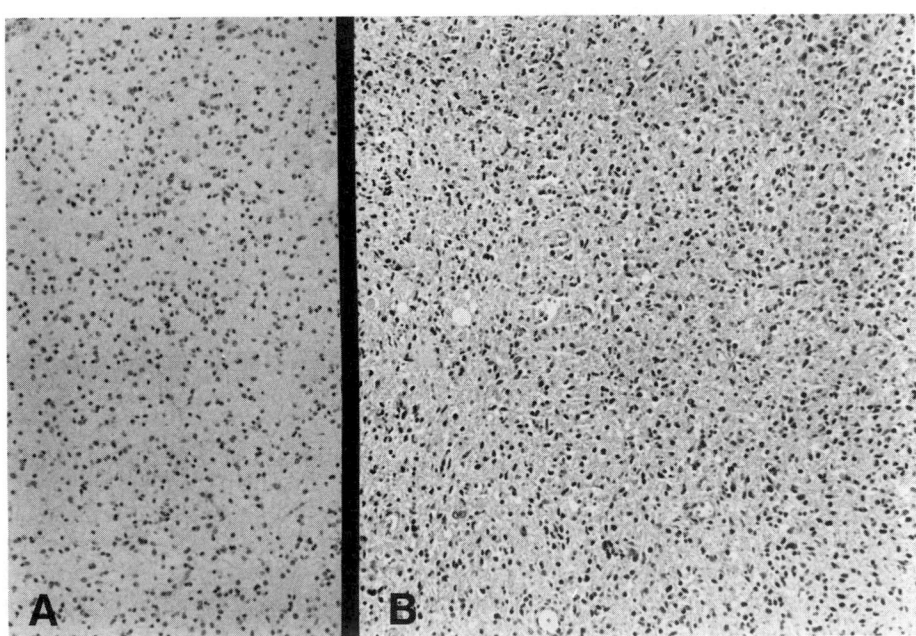

Figure 10–7 *Astrocytoma.* **A.** The *left* photomicrograph is a field of astrocytoma with more cellularity. The background white matter has lost its architecture, and the myelinated fibers have been extensively displaced by the processes of astrocytes. This is considered grade II or benign (H&E ×63). **B.** The *right* photomicrograph shows an anaplastic, or malignant, astrocytoma. The background tissue is almost replaced by the tumor cells. The nuclei are larger, hyperchromatic, and, to some degree, vary in shape and chromatin density. Mitoses are rare (H&E ×63).

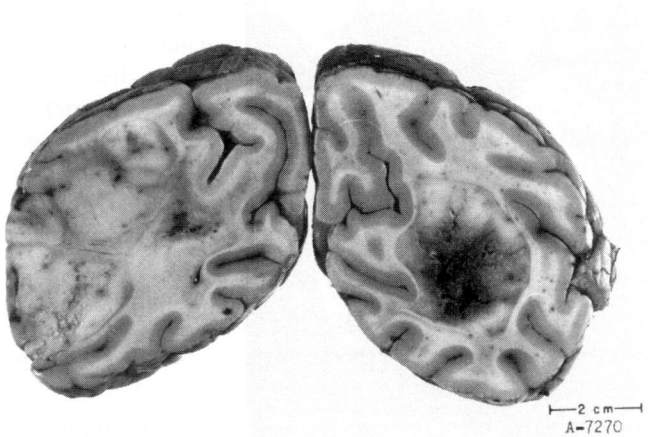

Figure 10–8 *Glioblastoma multiforme*. This is a coronal section of brain at the posterior parietal-occipital level. This tumor is seen extensively and bilaterally. The tumor in the left hemisphere is seen at the convexity and the deep white matter, with ill-defined borders. The tumor was traceable through the corpus callosum (not shown here) to the right hemisphere, where it has maintained a usually well circumscribed contour. Areas of hemorrhage and necrosis (with moth-eaten appearance) are seen.

extensively. Tumors in lobar or noncentral locations can be resected regionally with less risk of increased functional impairment and consequently have better palliation with surgical resection.[32,36]

Tumors in functionally indispensable locations such the thalamus and basal ganglia are generally not amenable to surgical intervention.[27] However, stereotactic laser resection techniques have resulted in longer postoperative survival than biopsy alone in patients with thalamic lesions.[37] Bihemispheric tumors have a poor prognosis.[35]

There is lack of consensus concerning the effect of cytoreductive surgery. Evidence suggests that patients with gross total resection live longer than those with partial resection and patients with any degree of resection live longer than those who have biopsy only.[27,38] One study of patients with just biopsy showed only a median 19-week survival time.[35]

Resection documentation merits consideration. Contrast-enhanced CT scanning is performed during the first 24 to 48 h after surgery, before a misleading vascular response is fully developed. Absence of abnormal enhancement on the postoperative CT scan indicates gross total resection. A partial resection is indicated when more than 10 percent of the enhancing lesion persists. Gross total removal results in 97 percent improved stable postoperative neurological status compared to 40 percent postoperative neurological morbidity following partial resection. Residual tumor and necrotic tissue have an effect similar to that of a foreign body in the brain, promoting cerebral edema and its sequelae.[31]

Patients having total tumor removal showed a higher 5-year survival, whereas no patient with partial removal survived more than 5 years. Biopsy in recurring astrocytomas has revealed a 79 percent incidence of anaplastic transformation.[21]

There is a strong correlation between younger age and longer survival in adults with supratentorial intermediate or high-grade astrocytomas.[31] Median survival time from diagnosis has been reported to be 107 weeks, for patients aged 18 to 44 years, 42 weeks for those aged 45 to 65 years, and 23 weeks for those above the age of 65.[35]

The Karnofsky performance scale 3 weeks after surgery is an independent prognostic factor. Patients with better function live longer. Patients with scores of 20 to 40 survived 15 weeks, those with scores 50 to 70 survived 36 weeks, and those with scores of 80 to 100 survived 76 weeks.[35]

Ganglioglioma Gangliogliomas are tumors containing a mixture of glial and neuronal cells, both of which are neoplastic. When there is a predominance of neurons, the term

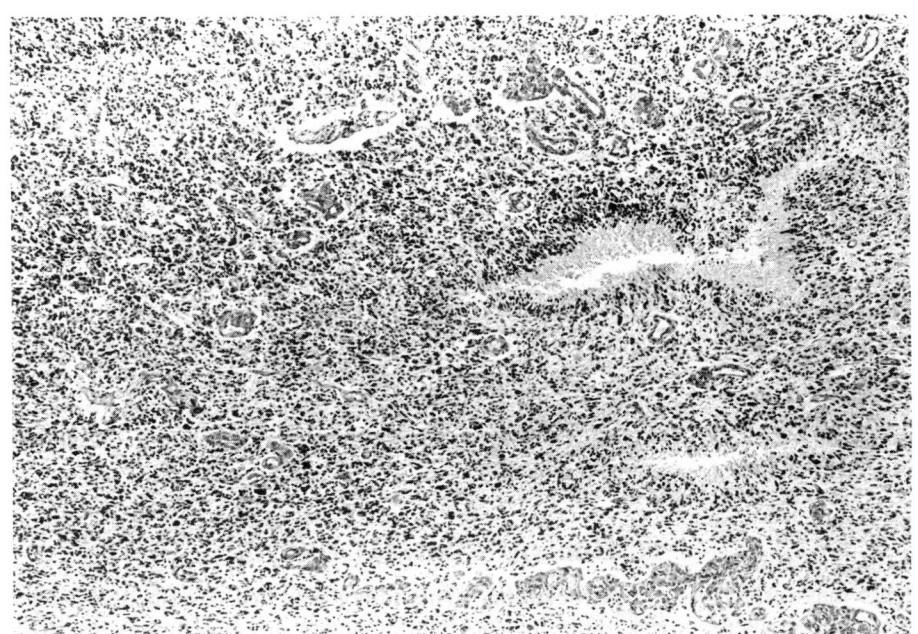

Figure 10–9 *Glioblastoma multiforme*: Microscopically is signified by marked cellularity, pleomorphism of the tumor cells, occasional tumor giant cells, vascular prominence, and pseudopalisading. Pseudopalisading (two areas are seen in the right side of the photo) is signified by a curving arrangement of several layers of condensed tumor cells around a zone of necrosis. Vascular prominence is mainly in the form of proliferated endothelial lining of small vessels, compiling in round-to-irregular structures (seen at the lower part of photomicrograph, obstructing the lumen). Mitoses were seen at higher powers (H&E ×40).

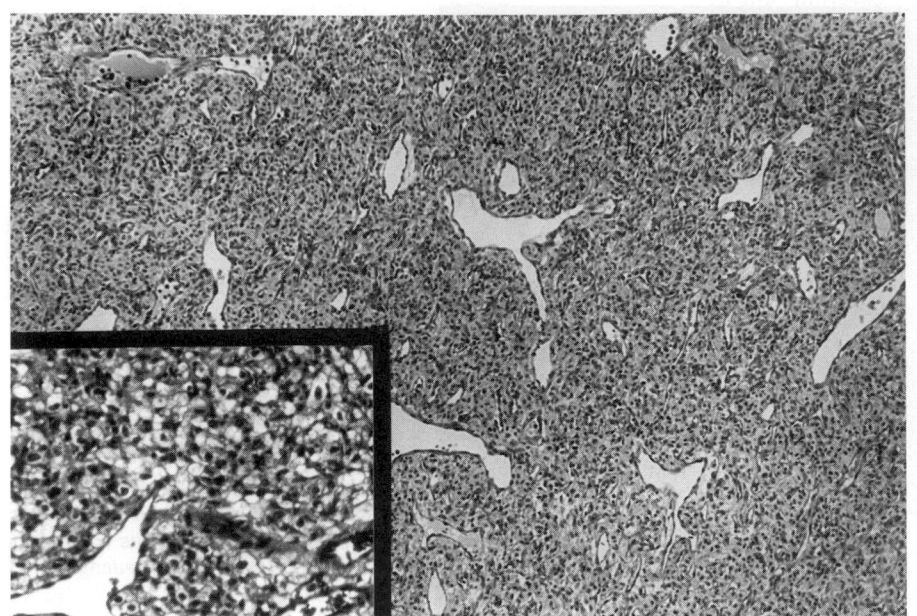

Figure 10–18 *Hemangioblastoma.* This microphotograph represents the mural nodule, which is the solid part of an example of cerebellar hemangioblastoma. Besides the obvious vessels with open lumen, many capillaries exist with slitlike contours. The cell population consists of an intermixture of endothelial-perithelial cells and the stromal cell (H&E ×63). The inset (H&E ×160) shows more details of the round "foamy cells," which have clear cytoplasm due to the high content of glycogen.

HEMANGIOENDOTHELIOMA

Benign hemangioendotheliomas are more familiar as capillary hemangiomas or "strawberry nevi," and they are very rare tumors within the CNS; however, they can occur anywhere in the neuraxis. They consist of aggregates of capillary channels in a reticulin background with endothelial proliferation. These can become adherent to the dura, which increases their vascularity. They should be biopsied with caution, as bleeding tends to be profuse. Unlike hemangioblastomas, these lesions have not been demonstrated in the cerebellum, and they are histologically and biologically unique.[71] Surgical resection of hemangioendothelioma may be difficult because of tumor vascularity; but it may respond to radiotherapy.[72]

☐ METASTATIC CARCINOMA

Metastasis to the brain occurs in about 25 percent of patients with systemic cancer, and it is the most common type of intracranial tumor at autopsy. Carcinoma of the lung is the origin of over half of all cerebral metastases in the United States. The prognosis for patients with such lesions is poor. Response to treatment is closely related to the aggression of the tumor, the host response, and treatment modality.[73]

A cerebral metastasis is the result of a complicated series of conditions and events. An individual or group of cells separates from the primary tumor and enters the vascular system, resulting in dissemination. The explant may arrest in the cerebral microvasculature, adhering to the endothelium and causing retraction of the endothelial cells as well as exposure of the subendothelial collagen membrane. The tumor cells traverse this basement membrane to become an intraparenchymal metastatic colony. The tumor cells must

alter local cerebral tissues to become an established self-propagating tumor. Cerebral metastases usually originate at the more vascular grey and hypovascular white matter junction.[74] (See Fig. 10-20.)

The three steps of metastatic invasion are: (1) tumor cell adherence to the basement membrane (laminar receptor on cell wall binds to type IV collagen), (2) proteolytic breakdown of the basement membrane (tumor cell–generated type IV collagenase), and (3) tumor cell migration through the defect (autocrine cytokine stimulation of psuedopodal motility). These tumor-active gene components are potential sites for a therapeutic attack on metastatic cancer.[74]

The anatomic compartments involved in brain metastasis are the skull, dura, leptomeninges, and cerebral parenchyma. Frequency of involvement correlates with regional brain mass and blood flow. Eighty percent of metastases occur in the supratentorial compartment. Parenchymal tumors expand in the white matter and precipitate vasogenic edema that exaggerates local mass effect and tissue distortion.[75]

The CNS is a site preferentially involved by certain cancers. In men the most common primaries are lung, gastrointestinal tract, and urinary tract cancers. In women the most common primaries are breast, lung, gastrointestinal tract tumors, and melanoma. Carcinoma of the lung is the most common origin of cerebral metastatic tumor; however, melanoma and choriocarcinoma are the most likely tumors to metastasize to the brain. Sixty-five percent of melanomas metastasize to the brain.

Brain metastasis clinically presents in a time frame related to the primary tumor: *precocious* (undetected primary); *synchronous* (simultaneous primary); and *metachronous* (antecedent primary)—the most common.[75]

Contrast-enhanced CT demonstrates many lesions and gives good bone detail to the skull base and calvarium. Gadolinium-DPTA–enhanced MRI is the most sensitive study for detecting metastatic lesions. Typical metastatic

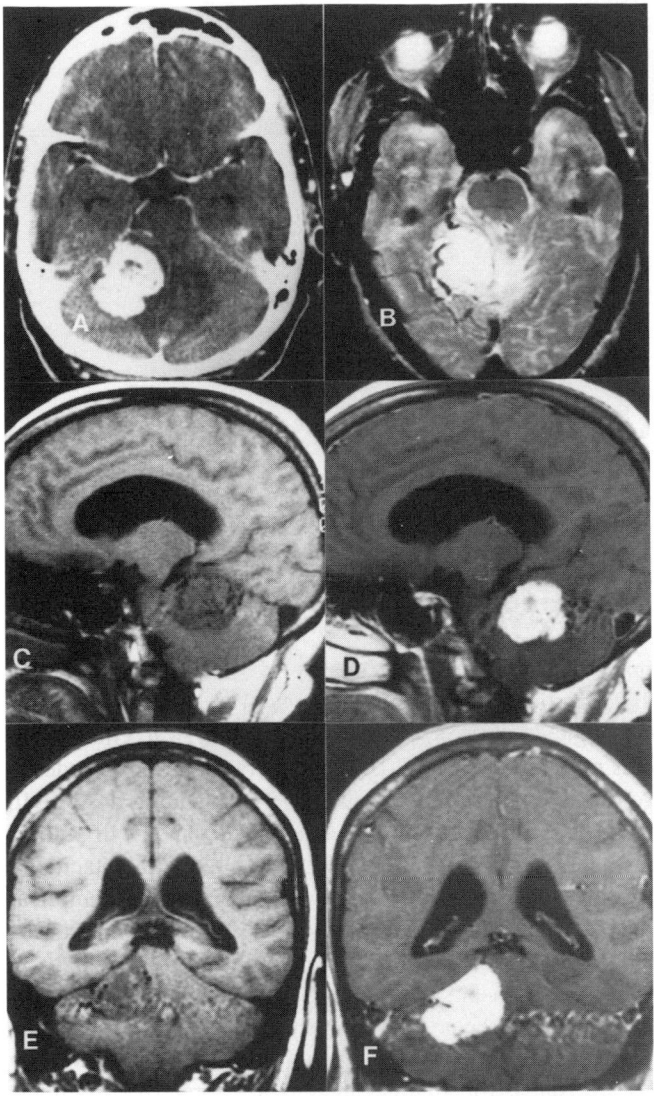

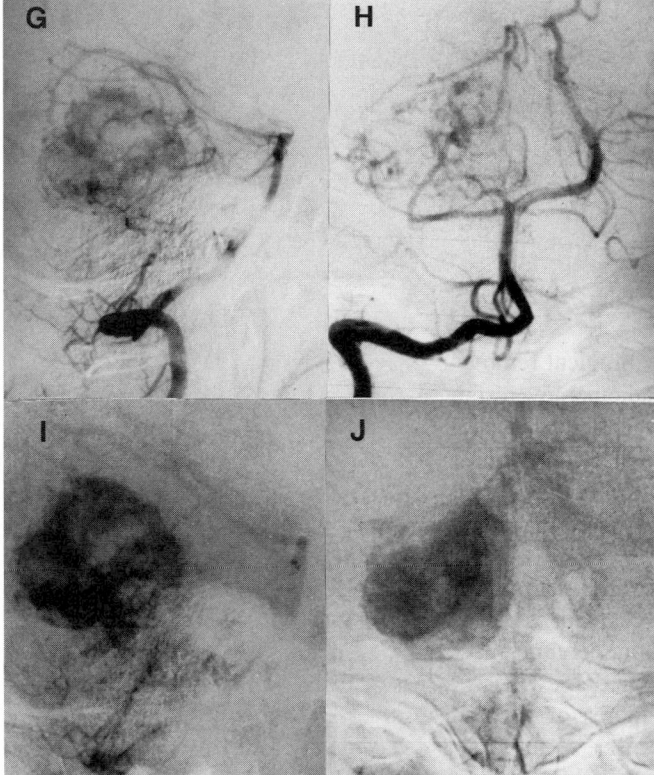

Figure 10–19 J.P., woman aged 57 years with progressive headache and morning vomiting over 3 months associated with recent falls and confusion while driving an automobile. An ataxic wide-based gait with falling backward and to the right on Romberg along with nystagmus and papilledema were noted on exam. *A.* Enhanced CT scan shows a large enhancing mass in the right superior cerebellum. *B.* Transverse MR scan with gadolinium enhancement brainstem compression and closing of the aqueduct by the cerebellar mass effect and edema. Also note curvilinear flow void, suggesting adjacent vascularity. *C.* Sagittal MR scan with right superior cerebellar mass and early hydrocephalus. *D.* Sagittal MR scan with gadolinium enhancement shows the enhancing mass in the superior cerebellum. *E.* Coronal MR shows the lesion to be in the superior cerebellar position predicted by the CT. *F.* Coronal MR with gadolinium enhancement shows mass abutting the tentorial undersurface, a solid type hemangioblastoma.

Figure 10–19 *(Continued) G.* Vertebral angiogram, lateral view, shows a highly vascular cerebellar mass supplied by branches of the posterior cerebral, superior cerebellar, and anterior inferior cerebellar arteries. *H.* Anterior-posterior view of the vertebrobasilar system shows the multiple sources of supply to this highly vascular tumor. *I.* Lateral view late arterial phase shows highly vascular mass homogeneously filled with contrast medium. *J.* Anterior-posterior view in capillary phase abutting the tentorium, a hemangioblastoma.

lesions are spheroid, surrounded by a zone of edema. Imaging studies not only assist in the initial diagnosis but also can be used serially to follow the progress of treatment. They detect complications of cerebral metastases such as hydrocephalus, hemorrhage, infection, edema, and occurrence of new lesions. (See Fig. 10-21.)

Cerebral lesions from radiosensitive primary tumors are best managed by establishing diagnosis through stereotactic biopsy and starting treatment with chemotherapy, radiotherapy, or a combination of both. Examples of such lesions are small cell carcinomas of the lung, germ cell tumors, lymphomas, leukemias, and myeloma. Some germ cell tumors are best treated by chemotherapy (cisplatin, vinblastin, and bleomycin) and surgical resection in selected patients.[76]

Table 10-3
MANAGEMENT ALGORITHM FOR
CEREBRAL METASTATIC NEOPLASM

Symptoms	Headache, 50%; focal weakness, 40%; mental change, 30%; seizures, 15%
Signs	Impaired cognition,75%; hemiparesis, 60%; ataxia, 25%; papilledema, 25%
Study	CT without + with contrast, MRI without + with gadolinium enhancement

KNOWN PRIMARY, NONLYMPHOMATOUS

Single metastasis and no systemic metastases	Steroid + surgical excision + radiation
Single or multiple metastasis and systemic metastases	Mass or no mass: steroid + radiation + chemotherapy
Multiple metastases and no systemic metastases	No hydrocephalus: steroid + radiation Hydrocephalus: steroid + VP shunt + radiation
Single life-threatening tumor	Steroid + surgical excision + radiation

UNKNOWN PRIMARY

Single metastasis	Steroid + surgical excision + radiation
Multiple metastases	Steroid + stereotaxic biopsy + radiation
Multiple metastases with a single life-threatening tumor	Steroid + surgical excision + radiation

Nonlocalized headache is a common complaint. Alteration of mental status with confusion, loss of memory, and lethargy are dysfunctional complaints which occur, but cognitive impairment is more commonly evident on examination.[81,82]

The diagnosis is suggested by gadolinium-enhanced MRI scanning.[83] CSF studied cytologically may demonstrate malignant cells. Humoral tumor markers within CSF in the absence of specific cytology may also verify the diagnosis.[84,85]

Treatment involves intrathecal methotrexate via a subcutaneous ventricular reservoir usually combined with radiation therapy directed to a specific cranial location or to the whole brain. Recently, immune therapy trials using intraventricular recombinant interleukin-2 and lymphokine-activated killer (LAK) cells have been used experimentally.[86]

Principals of Surgical Management

Cerebral neoplasms require surgical intervention for establishing tissue diagnosis and for relieving intracranial mass effect; these two indications are accepted and well-estab-

lished for effective management.[87] The effects of aggressive resection of tumor and cytoreductive surgery on longevity and outcome are less clear and more controversial.[35]

Evaluation of the general status of a patient with an intracranial mass using the Karnofsky scale will help to establish the urgency of the need for intervention. The use of steroids for transient relief of increased intracranial pressure has reduced the incidence of emergency craniotomies for tumor, although decompression on an urgent basis is still required on occasion. Examples may be the case of ventricular obstruction or the case of threatened herniation of brain structures through the incisura, under the falx, or through the foramen magnum. Even in these emergency situations, imaging investigations are mandatory to develop a plan of management.

The most readily available diagnostic imaging is computerized tomography (CT). CT is most useful when images are obtained both with and without contrast, for comparison. The examination provides visualization of the lesion as well as the ventricular system, which may provide evidence of obstruction, distortion, displacement, or brainstem compression. Magnetic resonance imaging (MRI) may provide greater resolution and better delineation of the margins and extent of the neoplasm, leading to a better-planned procedure, but a stable, cooperative, or immobile patient is necessary. In the event of threatened herniation due to ventricular obstruction, ventricular puncture and drainage may be guided by the study and provide time for a definitive operation. The operator must be cautioned about the possibility of a reverse herniation from the compartment of the tumor, particularly when associated with a mass in the posterior fossa.

The patient should be prepared from a cardiopulmonary standpoint to undergo the operation. Nutrition and fluids and electrolytes should be within acceptable limits. The patient and/or responsible relatives should be appropriately informed of the procedure to be done and apprised of realistic expectations.

Actual planning of the operation begins with imaging studies. Parenchymal tumors usually extend well beyond the demonstrable margins of the imaged lesion, while extraparenchymal lesions may have infiltrative attachments to the dura, bone, or skull base. Tumors located in functionally eloquent areas might best be managed by stereotactic biopsy to verify diagnosis, followed by adjunctive therapy.[88] Longer preservation of neurologic function affords better quality of life without change in overall longevity.[35]

The surgeon must have a definite approach in mind before the patient reaches the operating room. This includes a plan for the scalp flap designed to preserve circulation regardless of the approach.

The dura may be densely adherent to overlying bone, requiring that it be stripped by dissection before the bone flap can be elevated. This may be very difficult—in the elderly, in the case of hyperostosis frontalis interna, and in neoplasms involving bone and dura.

The craniotomy flap should adequately expose the region

of brain containing the tumor. If the lesion is superficial, a resection margin on all sides is desirable. If the lesion is subcortical, eloquent areas are to be avoided in the approach in order to preserve speech, movement, and visual functions. This may necessitate approaching the lesion obliquely. Microsurgical dissection through a sulcus and corticotomy might be preferable to cortical entry through the gyral crown in order to gain access to deep lesions or for en bloc resection of cerebral-lobar tumors.[89] Structural appearance is not a reliable assurance of function, and cortical mapping may be necessary to delineate and preserve eloquent cortex. Stereotactic implantation of catheters around the periphery of the tumor as demonstrated on MRI has been proposed as a guide to the surgeon during resection.[90]

Preservation of cerebrovascular supply and drainage is essential. This may require alteration of the approach. If both arterial and venous supplies of a structure are to be sacrificed, the arterial supply should be interrupted first to avoid congestion, bleeding, and swelling in the field.

Positioning of the patient is important. Once the plan for an approach has been made, the position of the patient is considered. Principles include the following:

1. The position must permit access by the surgeon and assistants, as well as equipment such as microscope, laser, and aspirator.
2. The surgical team must be able to operate in comfort throughout the procedure.
3. The head must be stable and secure but capable of being repositioned.
4. The anesthesiologist must have adequate access to the patient.
5. Pressure areas and the eyes must be adequately protected.

Elevation of the head above the heart augments venous drainage, reducing intracranial pressure and bleeding. Rotation or flexion of the neck that might compress jugular veins or kink the endotracheal tube should be limited. Fixation of the head provides stability and allows attachment of retractors.

If the operation is to be performed under local anesthesia for cortical mapping, the patient should be positioned for maximum possible comfort.

It is also desirable to plan positioning so that retraction of the brain is aided by gravity wherever possible. This may prevent retractor pressure from producing ischemic and necrotic changes in the brain. Care must also be exerted to avoid compression of major vessels by retractors.

☐ OPERATION

Once the brain has been exposed, resection of neoplasms varies according to their type and location. Resection of tumors of moderate and high malignancy may require physi-

ological mapping using techniques discussed for lower-grade tumors in order to preserve function. Distortion of structures by an expanding mass makes topographic identification of functional areas questionable.

Having outlined the areas to be preserved, a corticotomy may be made in an adjacent gyrus and extended into the circumscribed area to be removed. Blood vessels supplying normal brain must be carefully preserved. Before entering the brain substance, the overlying blood vessels must be controlled by displacement or by coagulation and division.

The pia-arachnoid is opened using bipolar coagulation along the line of incision which is made by sharp dissection. It is usually safe to make a subpial dissection to the adjacent sulcus, continuing into the white matter and seeking a plane between the tumor and edematous brain. Some tumors present with a false capsule, but such lines of demarcation are usually delimited. Generally, brain substance is divided by suction or blunt dissection. Division of low-grade gliomas or sclerotic areas may require sharp dissection or ultrasonic aspiration. Dissection around the base of the tumor continues until the tumor is isolated. If a ventricle is opened, it should be walled off to prevent blood from collecting within it. If cortex is reached opposite the entry site, the cortical vessels must be individually occluded and divided by sharp dissection. The plane of dissection can be preserved by the use of cottonoid strips to protect the brain.

Planes of demarcation can usually be developed between metastatic lesions and the surrounding brain, aided by strips of cottonoid to wall off the brain. Bridging vessels are divided, and separation along lines of cleavage is continued until the tumor is surrounded.

Many infiltrating lesions have pseudocapsules that may be well-demarcated, but usually such lines of delineation fade out so that separation must continue along areas of infiltration. In other cases where the infiltrating lesion is limited to a lobe, a standard lobectomy may be selected, dividing the pia and pial vessels, and transecting lobar structures so as to include the neoplasm. If cortex is reached opposite the entry site, the cortical vessels must be individually occluded and divided by sharp dissection. Ultrasonic aspiration may supplement suction and coagulation.

Resection of infiltrating lesions requires debulking of the mass—usually by aspiration and often with ultrasonic aspiration. Generally, blood loss from highly vascular neoplasms will be less by working at the edge of the tumor. When this is impossible, aspiration must begin within the tumor.

Care must be taken against undermining or even excessive retraction of functional cortex to be preserved. Hemostasis during the dissection aids visualization of structures and identification of vessels. When the bulk of the tumor has been removed, further search for additional tumor is carried out and such fragments are removed. The ultrasonic aspirator is helpful in this maneuver.

The tumor cavity is then examined for bleeding points, and meticulous hemostasis is secured prior to closure. Persistent bleeding may be due to residual tumor, and it will require direct bipolar cauterization or topical gelatin foam,

10. Westphal M, Herrmann HD: Growth factor biology and oncogene activation in human gliomas and their implications for specific therapeutic concepts. *Neurosurgery* 25:681–694, 1989.

11. Maruno M, Kovach JS, Kelly PJ, Yanagihara T: Transforming growth factor-a, epidermal growth factor receptor, and potential in benign and malignant gliomas. *J Neurosurg* 75:97–102, 1991.

12. Samuels V, Barrett JM, Bockman S, et al: Immunocytochemical study of transforming growth factor expression in benign and malignant gliomas. *Am J Pathol* 134:895–902, 1989.

13. Hoshino T, Wilson CB: Cell kinetic analysis of human malignant brain tumors (gliomas). *Cancer* 44:956–962, 1979.

14. Hoshino T: A commentary on the biology and growth kinetics of low-grade and high-grade gliomas. *J Neurosurg* 61:895–900, 1984.

15. Kriecbergs A, Tribukait B, Williams J, Bauer HC: DNA flow analysis of soft tissue tumors. *Cancer* 59:128–133, 1987.

16. Salcman M: Survival in glioblastoma: Historical perspective. *Neurosurgery* 7:435–439, 1980.

17. Piepmeier JM: Observations on the current treatment of low-grade astrocytic tumors of the cerebral hemispheres. *J Neurosurg* 67:177–181, 1987.

18. Hylton PD, Reichman OH: Clinical manifestation of glioma before computed tomographic appearance: The dilemma of a negative scan. *Neurosurgery* 21:27–32, 1987.

19. Salcman M, Kaplan RS, Ducker TB, et al: Effect of age in reoperation on survival in the combined modality treatment of malignant astrocytoma. *Neurosurgery* 10:454–463, 1982.

20. Harsh GR IV, Levin VA, Gutin PH, et al: Reoperation for recurrent glioblastoma and anaplastic astrocytoma. *Neurosurgery* 21:615–621, 1987.

21. Sofietti R, Chio A, Giordano MT, et al: Prognostic factors in well-differentiated cerebral astrocytomas in the adult. *Neurosurgery* 24:686–692, 1989.

22. Weir B, Grace M: The relative significance of factors affecting postoperative survival in astrocytomas, grades one and two. *Can J Neurol Sci* 47–50, 1976.

23. Wallner KE, Gonzales MF, Edwards MSB, et al: Treatment results of juvenile pilocytic astrocytoma. *J Neurosurg* 69:171–176, 1988.

24. Sun ZM, Genka S, Shitara N, et al: Factors possibly influencing the prognosis of oligodendroglioma. *Neurosurgery* 22:886–891, 1988.

25. Ludwig CL, Smith MT, Godfrey AD, Armbrustmacher VW: A clinicopathologic study of 323 patients with oligodendrogliomas. *Ann Neurol* 19:15–21, 1986.

26. Wallner KE, Gonzales MF, Sheline GE: Treatment of oligodendrogliomas with or without postoperative irradiation. *J Neurosurg* 68:684–688, 1988.

27. Winger MJ, Macdonald DR, Cairncross JG: Supratentorial anaplastic gliomas in adults. The prognostic importance of extent of resection and prior low grade glioma. *J Neurosurg* 71:487–493.

28. Schiffer D, Chio A, Cravioito H, et al: Ependymoma: Internal correlations among pathologic signs: The anaplastic variant. *Neurosurgery* 29:206–210, 1991.

29. Rawlings CE III, Giangaspero F, Burger PC, Bullard DE: Ependymomas: A clinicopathologic study. *Surg Neurol* 29:271–281, 1988.

30. Barone BM, Elvidge AR: Ependymomas: A clinical survey. *J Neurosurg* 33:428, 1970.

31. Ciric I, Ammirati M, Vick N, Mikhael M: Supratentorial gliomas, surgical considerations and immediate post operative results. *Neurosurgery* 21:21–26, 1987.

32. Jelsma R, Bucy PC: The treatment of glioblastoma multiforme of the brain. *J Neurosurg* 27:388–400, 1967.

33. Jelsma R, Bucy PC: Glioblastoma multiformi: Its treatment

34. Burger PC, Heinz ER, Shibata T, Kleihues P: Topographic anatomy and CT correlations in the untreated glioblastoma multiforme. *J Neurosurg* 68:698–704, 1988.

35. Nazzaro JM, Neuwelt EA: The role of surgery in the management of supratentorial intermediate and high-grade astrocytomas in adults. *J Neurosurg* 73:331–344, 1990.

36. Lieberman AN, Foo SH, Ransahoff J, et al. Long term survival among patients with malignant brain tumors. *Neurosurgery* 10:450–453, 1982.

37. Kelly P: Stereotactic biopsy and resection of thalamic astrocytomas. *Neurosurgery* 25:185–195, 1989.

38. Coffey RJ, Lunsford LD, Taylor FH: Survival after stereotactic biopsy of malignant gliomas. *Neurosurgery* 22:465–473, 1988.

39. Kalyan-Raman UP, Olivero WC: Ganglioglioma: A correlative clinicopathological and radiological study of ten surgically treated cases with follow-up. *Neurosurgery* 20:428–433, 1987.

40. Katz MC, Kier EL, Schechter MM: The radiology of gangliogliomas and ganglioneuromas of the central nervous system. *Neuroradiology* 4:69–73, 1972.

41. Bowles AP, Pantazis CG, Allen MB Jr, et al: Ganglioglioma, a malignant tumor? Correlation with flow deoxyribonucleic acid cytometric analysis. *Neurosurgery* 23:376–381, 1988.

42. Nishio S, Tashima T, Takeshita I, Fukui M: Intraventricular neurocytoma: Clinicopathological features of six cases. *J Neurosurg* 68:665–670, 1988.

43. Goldstein JD, Zeifer B, Chao C, et al: CT appearance of primary CNS lymphoma in patients with acquired immune deficiency syndrome. *J Comput Assist Tomogr* 15:39–44, 1991.

44. Correale JD, Montverde DA, Bueri JA, et al: Craniocerebral involvement in lymphoma. *Arq Neuropsiquiatr* 48:306–314, 1990.

45. Kanavaros P, Mikol J, Nemeth J, et al: Stereotactic biopsy diagnosis of primary non-Hodgkin lymphoma of the central nervous system. A histological and immunohistochemical study. *Pathol Res Pract* 86:459–466, 1990.

46. Goldstein JD, Dickson DW, Moser FG, et al: Primary central nervous system lymphoma in acquired immune deficiency syndrome. A clinical and pathological study with results of treatment with radiation. *Cancer* 67:2756–2765, 1991.

47. Rubinstein LJ: *Tumors of the Central Nervous System.* Washington, D.C., Armed Forces Institute of Pathology, 1970, pp 300–311.

48. Riikonen R, Simell O: Tuberous sclerosis and infantile spasms. *Dev Med Child Neurol* 32:203–209, 1990.

49. Shepherd CW, Scheithauer BW, Gomez MR, et al: Subependymal giant cell astrocytoma: A clinical, pathological, and flow cytometric study. *Neurosurgery* 28:864–868, 1991.

50. Nixon JR, Houser OW, Gomez MR, Okazaki H: Cerebral tuberous sclerosis: MR imaging. *Radiology* 170:869–873, 1989.

51. Costantino PD, Friedman CD, Pelzer JH: Neurofibromatosis type II of the head and neck. *Arch Otolaryngol Head Neck Surg* 115:380-383, 1989.

52. Mulvihill JJ, Parry DM, Sherman JL, et al: NIH conference. Neurofibromatosis 1 (Recklinghausen's disease) and neurofibromatosis 2 (bilateral acoustic neurofibromatosis): An update. *Ann Intern Med* 113:39–52, 1990.

53. Brill CB: Neurofibromatosis. Clinical overview. *Clin Orthop* 245:10–15, 1989.

54. Samuelsson B, Riccardi VM: Neurofibromatosis in Gothenburg, Sweden: III. Psychiatric and social aspects. *Neurofibromatosis* 2:84–106, 1989.

55. Senveli E, Altinors N, Kars Z, et al: Association of von

Recklinghausen's neurofibromatosis and aqueduct stenosis. *Neurosurgery* 24:99–101, 1989.

56. Senveli E: Association of von Recklinghausen's neurofibromatosis and aqueduct stenosis. (Correspondence.) *Neurosurgery* 25:318–319, 1989.

57. Pou-Serradell A, Ugarte-Elola AC: Hydrocephalus in neurofibromatosis contribution of magnetic resonance imaging to its diagnosis, control, and treatment. *Neurofibromatosis* 2:218–226, 1989.

58. Mirowitz SA, Sartor K, Gado M: High-intensity basal ganglia lesions on T1-weighted MR images in neurofibromatosis. *AJR Am J Roentgenol* 154:369–373, 1990.

59. Glasscock ME III, Woods CI, Jackson CG, Welling DB: Management of bilateral acoustic tumors. *Laryngoscope* 99:475–484, 1989.

60. Linskey ME, Lunsford LD, Flickinger JC: Radiosurgery for acoustic neurinomas: Early experience. *Neurosurgery* 26:736–744, 1990.

61. Maher ER, Yates JR, Harries R, et al: Clinical features and natural history of von Hippel-Lindau disease. (See comments.) *Q J Med* 77:1099–1100, 1990.

62. Filling-Katz MR, Choyke PL, Patronas NJ, et al: Radiologic screening for von Hippel-Lindau disease: The role of Gd-DTPA enhanced MR imaging of the CNS. *J Comput Assist Tomogr* 13:743–755, 1989.

63. Filling-Katz MR, Choyke PL, Oldfield E, et al: Central nervous system involvement in von Hippel-Lindau disease. *Neurology* 41:41–46, 1991.

64. Smalley SR, Schomberg PJ, Earle JD, et al: Radiotherapeutic considerations in the treatment of hemangioblastomas of the central nervous system. *Int J Radiat Onc Biol Phys* 18:1165–1171, 1990.

65. Sperner J, Schmauser I, Bittner R, et al: MR-imaging findings in children with Sturge-Weber syndrome. *Neuropediatrics* 21:146–152, 1990.

66. Hoffman HJ, Freeman A: Primary malignant leptomeningeal melanoma in association with giant hairy nevi. Report of two cases. *J Neurosurg* 26:62–71, 1967.

67. Kasarskis EJ, Tibbs PA, Lee C: Cerebellar hemangioblastoma symptomatic during pregnancy. *Neurosurgery* 22:770–772, 1988.

68. Kruse FK Jr: Hemangiopericytoma of the meninges (angioblastic meningioma of Cushing and Eisenhardt): Clinicopathologic aspects and follow-up studies in 8 cases. *Neurology* 11:771–777, 1961.

69. Dardick I, Hammar SP, Scheithauer BW: Ultrastructural spectrum of hemangiopericytoma: A comparative study of fetal, adult, and neoplastic pericytes. *Ultrastruct Pathol* 13:111–154, 1989.

70. Mena H, Ribas JL, Pezeshkpour GH, et al: Hemangiopericytoma of the central nervous system: A review of 94 cases. *Hum Pathol* 22:84–91, 1991.

71. Pearl GS, Takei Y, Tindall GT, et al: Benign hemangioendothelioma involving the central nervous system: "Strawberry nevus" of the neuraxis. *Neurosurgery* 7:249–256, 1980.

72. Chedid MK, Maroon JC: Radiation therapy of hemangioendotheliomas. *Neurosurgery* 20:995–996, 1987.

73. Patchell RA, Posner JB: Neurologic complications of systemic cancer. *Neurol Clin* 3:729–750, 1985.

74. Liotta LA, Kohn E: Cancer invasion and metastases. *JAMA* 263:1123–1126, 1990.

75. Wright DC, DeLaney TF: Treatment of metastatic cancer to the brain, in De Vita VT, Hellman S, Rosenberg SA (eds): *Cancer: Principles and Practice of Oncology*. Philadelphia, JB Lippincott, 1989, pp 2245–2645.

76. Jelsma RK, Carroll M: Brain metastasis from nonseminomatous germ cell tumors of the testis: Case report and review of the role of surgery. *Neurosurgery* 25:814–819, 1989.

77. Patchell RA, Tibbs PA, Walsh JW, et al: A randomized trial of surgery in the treatment of single metastases to the brain. *N Engl J Med* 322:494–500, 1990.

78. White KT, Fleming TR, Laws ER Jr: Single metastasis to the brain: Surgical treatment in 122 consecutive patients. *Mayo Clin Proc* 56:424–428, 1981.

79. Posner JB: Management of central nervous system metastases. *Semin Oncol* 4:81–91, 1977.

80. Black P: Brain metastasis: Current status and recommended guidelines for management. *Neurosurgery* 5:617–631, 1979.

81. Olson ME, Chernik NL, Posner JB: Infiltration of the leptomeninges by systemic cancer: A clinical and pathologic study. *Arch Neurol* 30:122–137, 1974.

82. Little JR, Dale AJD, Okazaki H. Meningeal carcinomatosis: Clinical manifestations. *Arch Neurol* 30:138–143, 1974.

83. Sze G, Soletsky S, Bronen R, Krol G: MR imaging of the cranial meninges with emphasis on contrast enhancement and meningeal carcinomatosis. *AJNR Am J Neuroradiol* 5:965–975, 1989.

84. Bach F, Soletormos G, Bach FW, Pedersen AG: TPA and CK-BB: New tumor markers in leptomeningeal carcinomatosis secondary to breast cancer. *J Natl Cancer Inst* 82:320–322, 1990.

85. Bach F, Bach FW, Pedersen AG, et al: Creatin kinase-BB in the cerebrospinal fluid as a marker of CSF metastases and leptomeningeal carcinomatosis in patients with breast cancer. *Eur J Cancer Clin Oncol* 25:1703–1709, 1989.

86. Heimans JJ, Wagstaff J, Schreuder WO, et al: Treatment of leptomeningeal carcinomatosis with continuous intraventricular infusion of recombinant interleukin-2. *Surg Neurol* 35:244–247, 1991.

87. Ammitrati M, Vick N, Liao Y, et al: Effect of the extent of surgical resection on survival and quality of life in patients with supratentorial glioblastomas and anaplastic astrocytomas. *Neurosurgery* 21:201–206, 1987.

88. Green GM, Hitchon PW, Schelper RL, et al: Diagnostic yield in CT-guided stereotactic biopsy of gliomas. *J Neurosurg* 71:494–497, 1989.

89. Harkey HL, Al-Mefty O, Haines DE, Smith RR: The surgical anatomy of the cerebral sulci. *Neurosurgery* 24:651–654, 1989.

90. Kelly PJ: Stereotactic technology in tumor surgery. *Clin Neurosurg* 35:215–253, 1987.

91. Salcman M: Resection and reoperation in neuro-oncology: Rationale and approach. *Neurol Clin* 3:831–842, 1985.

92. Rostomily RC, Berger MS, Ojemann GA, Lettich E: Postoperative deficits and functional recovery following removal of tumors involving the dominant hemisphere supplementary motor area. *J Neurosurg* 75:62–68, 1991.

93. Shapiro WR, Green SB, Burger PC, et al: Randomized trial of three chemotherapy regimens and two radiotherapy regimens in postoperative treatment of malignant glioma. Brain Tumor Cooperative Group Trial 8001. *J Neurosurg* 71:1–9, 1989.

94. Liang BC, Thornton AF Jr, Sandler HM, Greenberg HS: Malignant astrocytomas: Focal tumor recurrence after focal external beam radiation therapy. *J Neurosurg* 75:559–563, 1991.

95. EORTC Brain Tumor Group: Evaluation of CCNU, VM-26 plus CCNU and procarbazine in supratentorial brain gliomas: Final evaluation of a randomized study. *J Neurosurg* 55:27–31, 1981.

96. Walker MD, Green SB, Byar DP, et al: Randomized comparisons of radiotherapy and nitrosureas for the treatment of malignant glioma after surgery. *N Engl J Med* 303:1323–1329, 1980.

97. Green SB, Byar DP, Walker MD, et al: Comparison of carmustine, procarbazine and high dose methylprednisolone

Table 11–1
THE KARNOFSKY SCALE

100	Normal—no evidence of disease
90	Able to carry on normal activity—minor symptoms
80	Normal activity with effort—some symptoms
70	Cares for self—unable to carry on normal activity
60	Requires occasional assistance—care for most needs
50	Requires considerable assistance
40	Disabled
30	Severely disabled
20	Very sick—active supportive treatment needed
10	Moribund

☐ NEOPLASMS OF THE BRAIN COVERINGS

MENINGIOMAS

The early history of treatment of these tumors is interesting.[2,3] Meningiomas comprise 15 to 20 percent of primary intracranial tumors.[4] Although they may occur at any age, they peak about 45 years of age, with a predominance of women over men in a ratio of approximately 2:1. Meningiomas are derived from arachnoid cap cells with which tumor cells share many features. Microscopic classification of five types includes syncytial, transitional, fibrous, angioblastic, and malignant.[4,5] *Syncytial* tumors are characterized by homogenous cytoplasm with poorly defined margins surrounding round nuclei. A vascular trabeculation with collagen and reticulin fibers is present. *Transitional* tumors have a swirling pattern of cells around central areas of hyalinization (Fig. 11-1). Calcified psammoma bodies are common. Syncytial and transitional types account for most meningiomas. *Fibrous* or *fibroblastic* types are composed of fibrocytic cells with increased collagen and reticulin. *Angioblastic* meningiomas are highly cellular tumors with prominent vascular channels. Mitoses are frequent. Malignant meningiomas are locally invasive and have many mitoses and atypical histopathological changes, including anaplasia. Sarcomatous changes occur.

Cerebral edema adjacent to meningiomas is frequently encountered. This is partly due to the breaching of the leptomeninges and cortex separating the tumor from the white matter. This allows the extracellular fluid from the tumor to accumulate in the adjacent white matter. It may also be the effect of a direct secretory substance from the tumor. The degree of edema correlates with the size of the tumor and is more marked in transitional and meningiotheliomatous tumors. There is no correlation with location.[5,6] Edema may present a problem in management postoperatively. This is seen in Fig. 11-3.

There are multiple clinical features supporting concepts that meningiomas may be related to sex hormones. Sixty-six percent of intracranial and 80 percent of intraspinal tumors are in women. The majority of meningiomas contain high-affinity receptors for progesterone, and a few contain estrogen receptors. Some of the receptors appear to be functional. Tumor growth may be hormonally affected, increasing during pregnancy and in the luteal, but not in the proliferative, phase of the menstrual cycle. Nuclear binding assays indicate functional receptors of both hormones.[7–10]

Most meningiomas appear globular with a smooth or nodular surface, but flat *en plaque* growth occurs at times. Tumors locally invade the dura, dural sinuses, and overlying bone, depending on the duration and type. When meningiomas are small, they may indent the brain, which accommodates to their presence, but with enlargement, the growth may expand beneath the cerebral cortex. The tumor then assumes the shape of a doorknob.

Approximately 20 percent of meningiomas are on the convexities, with the remainder occurring at the base and other locations described in the text following. Symptoms are related to the structures being compressed or activated, with seizures being prominent in almost one third of the patients. Therapy of seizures may be part of the therapeutic surgical procedure.

Special features of meningiomas in specific locations require individual attention.

Olfactory Groove About one-fifth of intracranial meningiomas are located in the olfactory groove. They arise from the lamina cribrosa. Because of their position beneath the frontal lobes, they may be very large when diagnosed. Symptoms referable to the frontal lobes may be quite subtle and escape detection until well advanced. Visual impairment may be among the first reported symptoms. Loss of olfactory function often escapes notice until other symptoms lead to investigation.

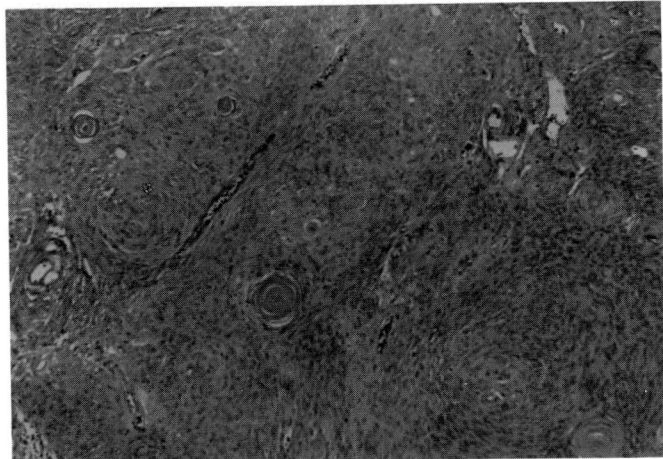

Figure 11–1 Meningioma. These tumors have many histologic forms. This is an example of *transitional meningioma*. A major part has a syncytial pattern, being formed of round uniform tumor cell nuclei distributed within a cytoplasmic mass with indistinct cell membranes in light microscopy. Small groups of cells swirling in small circles (*whorls*) and small hyalinized concentric structures (*psammoma bodies*), which are typical of meningiomas, are seen (H & E × 63).

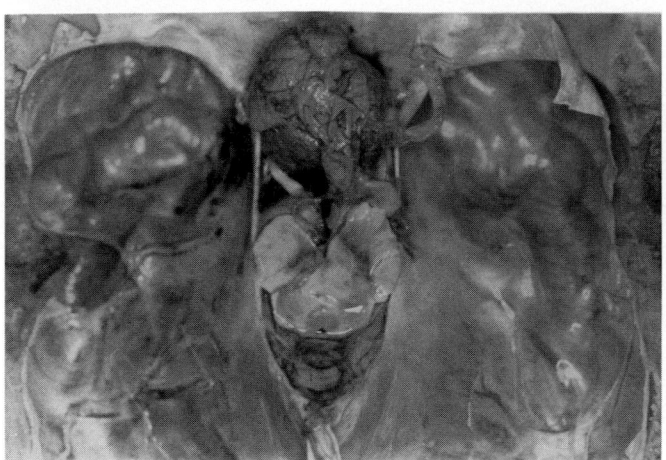

Figure 11–2 Meningioma of tuberculum sellae. This autopsy view of the skull cavity shows a transverse cut of the midbrain and the cerebellar tentorium intact. Notice the round lobulated tumor overlying the region of the sella turcica, which had caused marked visual deficits in this patient.

Tuberculum Sellae Ten percent of meningiomas may arise from the region of the tuberculum sellae. Visual symptoms are usually the first experienced. Visual field defects assume patterns dependent on the optic fibers involved. Extension of the tumor anteriorly mimics the symptoms of tumors of the olfactory groove. More posterior and superior extension may produce symptoms related to the hypothalamus (Fig. 11-2).

Sphenoid Wing Less than one in five meningiomas arises from the sphenoid ridge, but meningiomas produce a variety of neurological symptoms and related signs, according to location.

Lateral Wing Meningiomas at the lateral end of the sphenoid wing may reach a moderate size before seizures or headache lead to a diagnosis. If the tumor is *en plaque* rather than globular, the growth pattern along the dura toward the cavernous sinus and superior orbital fissure produces symptoms similar to the more medially placed tumors (Fig. 11-3).

Medial Wing Meningiomas of the medial sphenoid ridge frequently encroach on the optic nerve and carotid artery and may surround these structures. With infiltration of the sphenoid sinus, involvement of third, fourth, and fifth cranial nerves may be apparent. Invasion of the superior orbital fissure and even the orbit results in proptosis. Venous congestion of the cavernous sinus may produce proptosis as well (Fig. 11-4).

Parasagittal Convexity The most common site for meningiomas is in the convexity parasagittal region, about one fourth occurring here. This may be due to the high concentration of pacchionian granulations in this location. Tumors are more common in the central region and may extend laterally over the convexity or deep along the falx. Seizures are common, often focal, beginning in the foot.

Superior Sagittal Sinus Early invasion of the dura, including the sagittal sinus, is characteristic. With progressive occlusion of the sinus, collateral pathways of venous drainage develop. The location of such occlusion in relationship to the rolandic veins is of critical importance in planning surgical intervention. If occlusion is anterior to the central (rolandic) veins, the sagittal sinus may be resected. If the occlusion is more posterior in the sagittal sinus and is complete, it too may be resected, but if the sinus is incompletely occluded, resection may result in disastrous venous obstruction and edema. Angiography and magnetic resonance imaging (MRI) studies may aid in this determination of blood flow in the sinus (Fig. 11-5).

Falx Meningiomas arising below the sagittal sinus and growing along the falx are usually located in the anterior part of the falx and may infiltrate or grow through defects in the falx to become bilateral. They are frequently large. Their anterior location frequently makes it possible to resect the sinus, falx, and tumor completely.

Tentorium Tentorial meningiomas may arise from the superior or inferior surface or the tentorial margin. Symptoms depend on whether there is compression of the contents of the middle or posterior fossa or both. At the tentorial edge, the fourth cranial nerve may be involved. Tumor invasion may extend into the straight, lateral, or sigmoid sinuses or the torcular Herophili. Precautions regarding acute occlusion or resection of a sinus prevail; otherwise, extensive resection should be done wherever possible. Adequate demonstrable patency of the opposite lateral or sigmoid sinus may permit resection of the involved sinus. The size of the sinus, however, at times may permit reconstruction of the sinus after removal of one wall from which the tumor extends into the lumen.

Foramen Magnum Meningiomas of the foramen magnum have often gone unrecognized. Their location produces symptoms of slowly progressive long pathway involvement, often with suboccipital headaches. Various lower cranial nerves may be involved. Differential diagnoses include intramedullary tumors, cysts, and syringes as well as demyelinating and degenerative diseases. Current imaging methods of computed tomography (CT) and MRI have made possible early and accurate diagnoses, resulting in preservation of function (Fig. 11-6).

Orbit Meningiomas of the sphenoid wing may extend into the orbit. Of particular interest are those which arise within the optic sheath or the orbit.

Optic Sheath Meningiomas within the optic sheath characteristically produce slowly progressive loss of vision, beginning in the macular region. Optic atrophy occurs before loss of vision is complete. A patient presenting such symptoms must be suspected of this diagnosis until proven otherwise. Imaging with contrast is the most accurate method of diagnosis. Rarely, bilateral lesions occur.

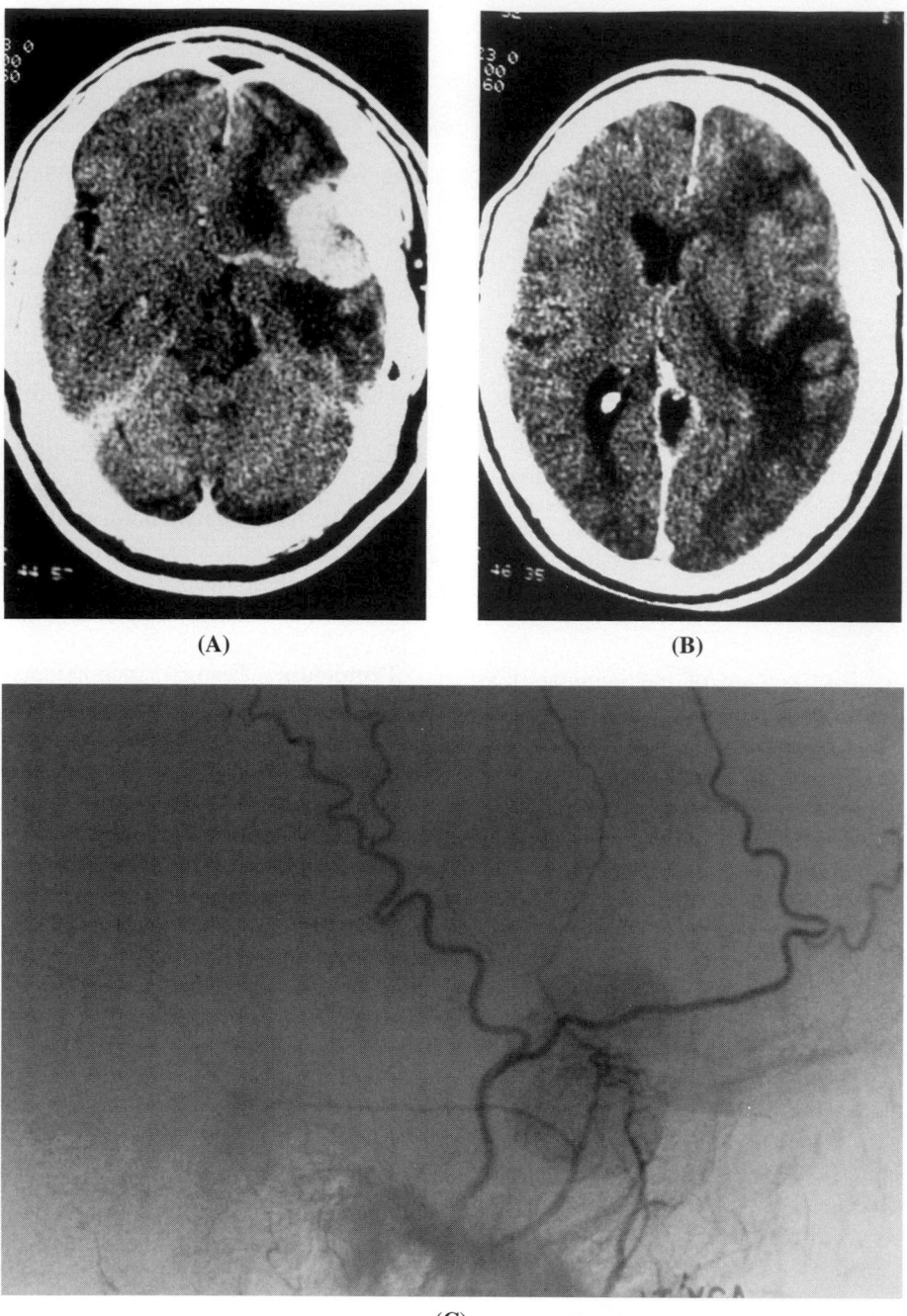

(A)   (B)

(C)

Figure 11–3 Lateral sphenoid wing meningioma. A 56-year-old male with a 3-week history of progressive frontal headache that was worse in the morning and would awaken him from his sleep. He also complained of recurrent dizziness, frequent falls, and syncope. He was neurologically intact. He could *not* tolerate undergoing an MRI scan. *A.* Contrast-enhanced CT shows a lateral sphenoid wing tumor with a wide surrounding zone of decreased attenuation, as evidence of reactive white matter edema. *B.* The CT cut through the anterior and temporal horns of the ventricles shows extensive edema beyond the immediate vicinity of the tumor, extending into the frontal and temporal lobes and causing effacement of the ipsilateral ventricle and shift of the septum pellucidum as well as collapsed third ventricle contralateral to the midline. *C.* Selective external carotid angiogram shows branches of the middle meningeal artery and accessory dural branches from the internal maxillary artery, supplying the tumor as demonstrated by the homogeneous vascular blush—typical for meningioma.

Large Orbit Large intraorbital meningiomas originate from the roof of the orbit or extend into the orbit through the superior orbital fissure.

Clinoidal Meningioma Meningiomas arising from the anterior clinoid process present special problems because of involvement of both the optic nerve and the internal carotid artery. The resectability of these tumors relates to the presence of interfacing arachnoid membranes between the tumor and adjacent neural and vascular structures, and this depends on the precise origin of the tumor. Such tumors can then be grouped according to origin: (1) proximal to end of carotid cistern, (2) superior and/or lateral aspect of anterior clinoid

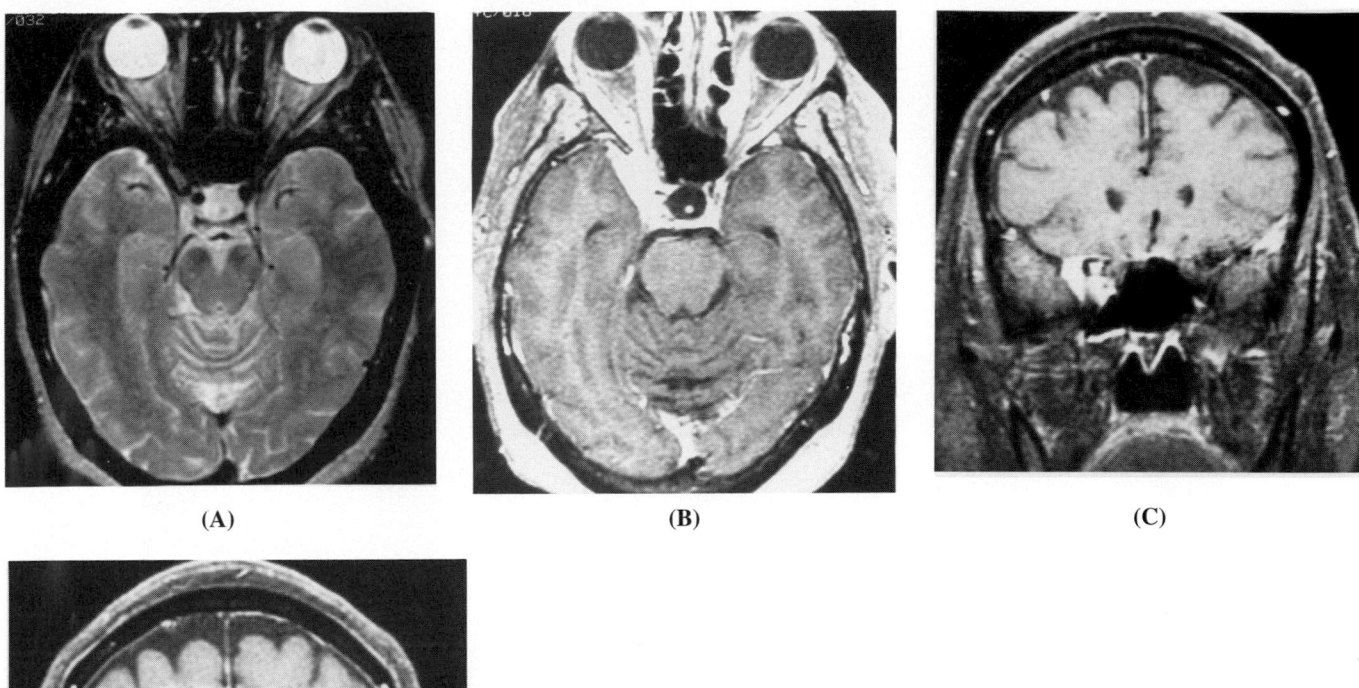

Figure 11–4   Medial sphenoid wing meningioma. A 60-year-old female with severe constant pain in the right eye of 6 months duration. She had a constant burning pain in the "eyeball" and was no longer relieved by narcotic analgesics. Diplopia was present in lateral and right upward gaze. The corneal reflex was diminished in the right eye and the right pupillary response to light was slightly diminished. She was otherwise neurologically intact. *A.* Plain MRI transverse cut suggests subtle thickening in the region of the right cavernous sinus. *B.* Contrasted MRI clearly shows an enhanced mass in the cavernous sinus with *en plaque* extension along the anterior medial middle fossa and orbital apex. *C.* Contrasted MRI coronal view through the sphenoid wing shows enhanced tumor mass in the right sphenoid wing and superior orbital fissure. *D.* Same study cut through the cavernous sinus shows involvement of the cavernous carotid artery.

above the segment of carotid invested in carotid cistern, and (3) at the optic foramen, extending into the optic canal. The adjacent structure becomes encased if there is no arachnoid interface.[11] The surgical dissection of a neural or arterial structure encased by meningioma is under extreme risk of damage with resultant functional morbidity or mortality. Mortality for surgical removal of meningiomas in this location is as high as 42 percent.[12]

Clivus   Tumors arising from the clivus extend superiorly and posteriorly compressing long pathways and encompassing cranial nerves and blood vessels. In addition to symptoms due to involvement of local structures, obstruction of the incisura results in increased intracranial pressure.

Petrous Ridge   Meningiomas along the superior surface of the petrous ridge encroach on the gasserian ganglion, causing symptoms of trigeminal neuralgia. Encroachment on the inferior mesial temporal lobe may produce seizures of the complex partial type. Tumors arising from the posterior surface may mimic acoustic nerve tumors with involvement

of the fifth, seventh, and eighth cranial nerves. Hearing loss, vertigo, facial palsy, and facial pain may be experienced.

☐ SURGERY OF MENINGIOMAS

The surgical treatment of meningiomas requires special consideration. Since bone is frequently invaded as well as the dura, it may be necessary to remove involved bone while protecting the brain, cranial nerves, and blood vessels. For example, in dealing with a convexity tumor invading the dura and cranium, the elevation of a bone flap in the usual manner may damage the underlying brain. One plan is to form a free flap of bone immediately adjacent to the tumor, separated from a larger second flap that encompasses the entire area. The second flap may be elevated to expose the dura surrounding the tumor and invaded dura and bone. The tumor may be separated from the brain by careful dissection of the arachnoid and separation of the tumor from the brain, preferably using magnification.[13] The brain should be protected by cottonoid or telfa strips.

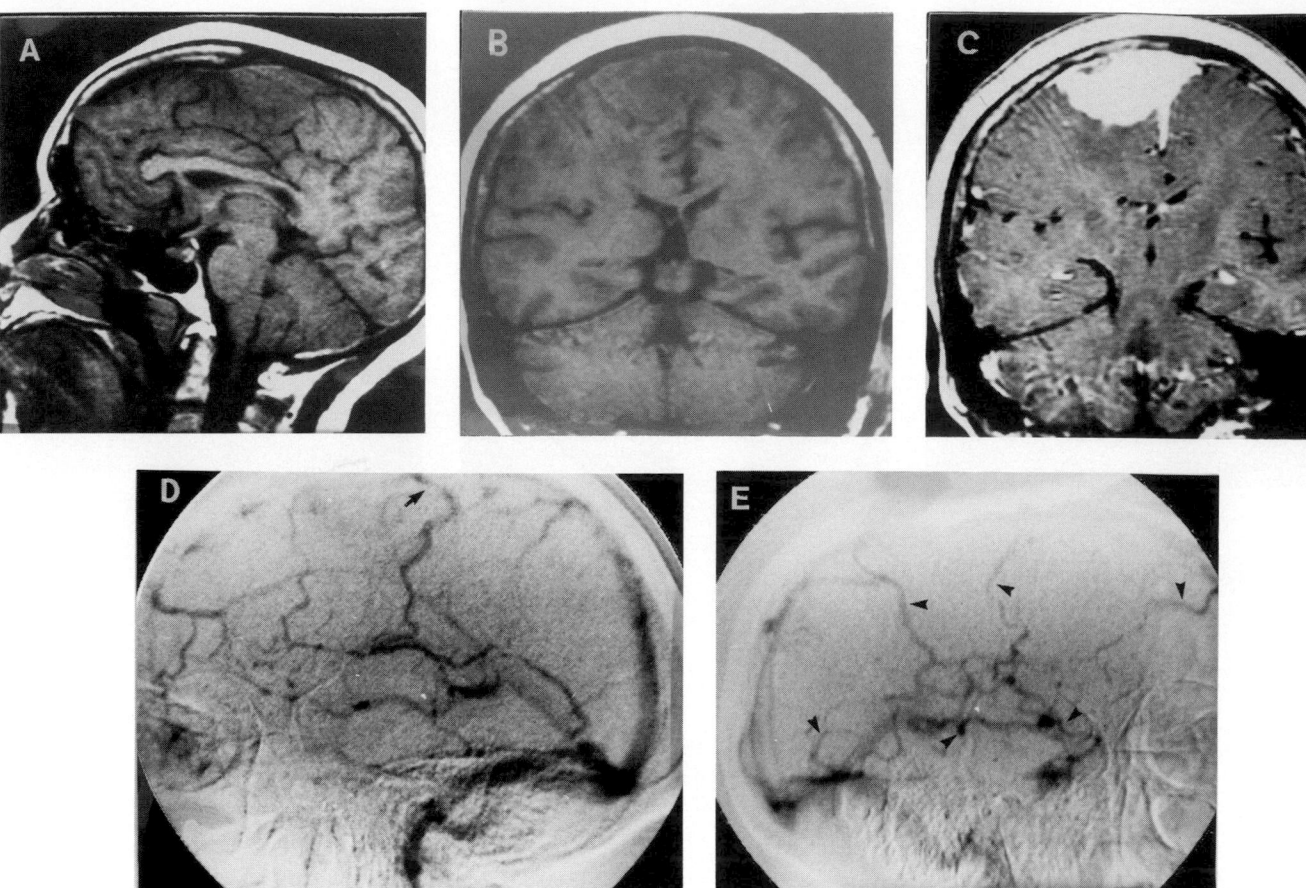

Figure 11–5 Parasagittal meningioma involving superior sagittal sinus. A 49-year-old female with nagging constant dull headache across the forehead and right temporal region. Headache had been present for over 5 years and became "unbearable" over the preceding 3 weeks. She was neurologically intact. *A.* MRI midsagittal view shows tumor mass posterior to the bregma with downward compression of the corpus callosum. There is attenuation of the high fat signal in the adjacent calvarium. *B.* MRI coronal view shows the mass extending from the midline to the right parasagittal convexity. The triangular profile of the superior sagittal sinus is faintly outlined and filled with tumor. *C.* Gadolinium enhancement verifies obliteration of the sinus and more clearly delineates the extent of the tumor mass. *D.* Venous phase left carotid angiogram shows segmental nonfilling of the superior sagittal sinus, with a prominent vein of Trolard filling along the posterior limit of the tumor into superior sagittal sinus (*arrow*). *E.* Venous phase of the right carotid angiogram shows collateral venous drainage (*arrowheads*) that has compensated for occlusion of the superior sagittal sinus.

In incising the dura, it may be helpful to surround the tumor attachment completely in order to control bleeding and to have a site of traction while dissecting the tumor. If an enlargement of the tumor extends below the cortex, debulking by suction, ultrasonic aspiration, laser, or cautery-cutting loop may be necessary.

Dural defects remaining after tumor removal should be repaired by a graft. Living tissue is always preferable to preserved tissue. Pericranium or fascia lata provide satisfactory grafts, although there is some evidence that there may be fewer complications with pericranium than with fascia lata. Inorganic prosthetics should be the last choice. Connective tissue proliferation simulating recurrence has been reported as a complication of the use of prosthetic dural substitutes.[14]

Invaded bone may be discarded. If the invasion involves the inner table only, this may be removed by burring. If removal is more extensive, the bone flap may be autoclaved and replaced. A defect left by a discarded flap may be corrected by an acrylic prosthesis at the same, or at a later, operation.

Recent developments in surgery of the skull base have provided aggressive new approaches to meningiomas attached to the orbital roof, sphenoid wing, and posterior fossa. Such approaches permit resection of the skull base directed at eradication of the entire tumor.

In dealing with basilar meningiomas, preservation of blood vessels and cranial nerves becomes paramount, and use of the operating microscope is necessary. Microdissection of the nerves and blood vessels at the base of the brain, using appropriate instrumentation and lasers, decreases postoperative deficits and morbidity.

The pterional or anterior temporal approach to the region of the clivus or tuberculum sellae is enhanced by careful dissection of the arachnoid and vessels between the temporal and frontal lobes.

Displaced but noninvaded brain tissue should be preserved. Mannitol, hyperventilation, aspiration of cerebral

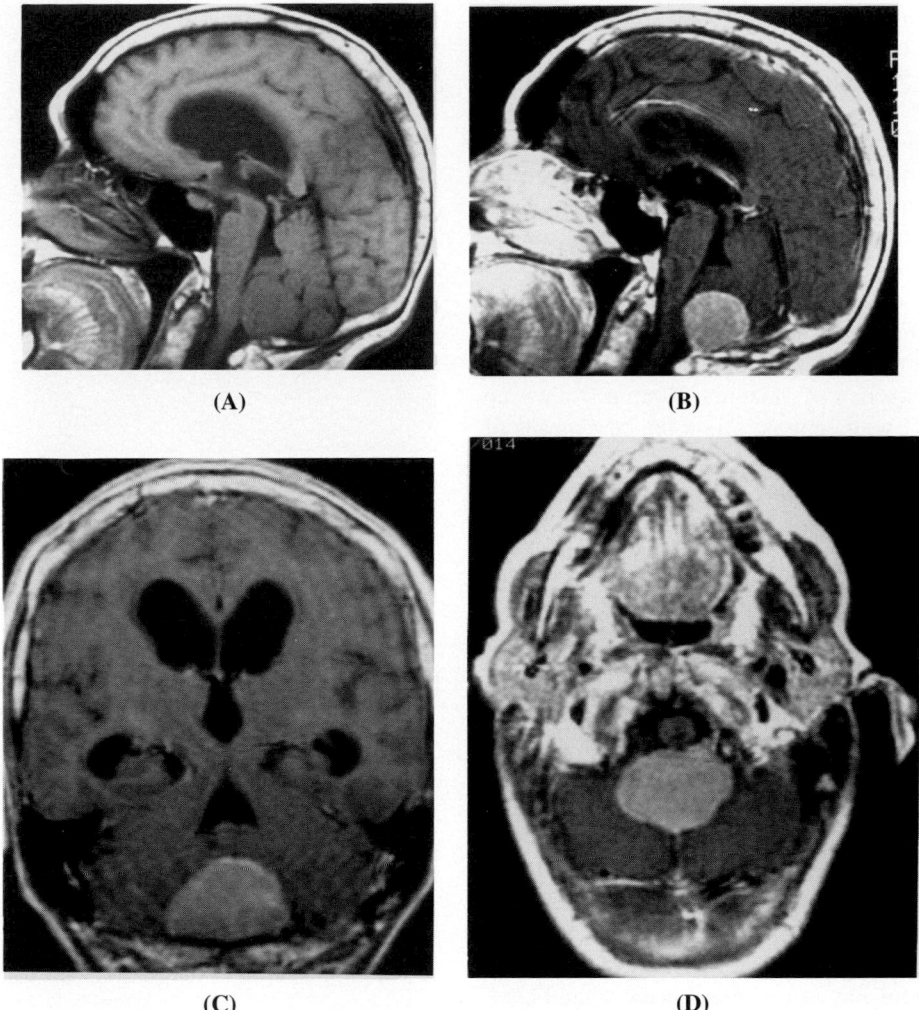

(A)

(B)

(C)

(D)

Figure 11–6 Foramen magnum meningioma. A 70-year-old female with progressive loss of cognitive function and impaired ambulation along with high blood pressure over 18 months. She had headache, dizziness, vomiting, and urge incontinence. Because of repeated falling she was not walking and in a wheelchair for the past 3 months. There was hyperreflexia but no clonus or Babinski response evident. *A.* Plain midsagittal MRI shows hydrocephalus and suggestion of an isodense inferior cerebellar mass. *B.* Contrast-enhanced MRI clearly shows the spheroid tumor mass with posterior compression of the medulla. *C.* Contrasted MRI coronal section shows the midline mass caudal to the fourth ventricle and hydrocephalus. *D.* Contrasted MRI transverse section through the arch of C1 shows homogeneous enhancement and extent of the mass with proximity to the medulla.

spinal fluid (CSF) from cisternae, and the use of gentle, broadly contoured, padded, mechanical retractors aided by gravity will help in the preservation of function.

Pressure from a meningioma can produce marked atrophy of the compressed and devitalized cortex; epilepsy may result. Removal of the atrophic cortex using techniques ordinarily applied to seizure surgery should be considered (Penfield, personal communication).[13a]

The goal of surgery for meningiomas is total removal. A wide dural margin along with all hyperostotic bone and adjacent pericranium in *en bloc* resection has been shown to eliminate recurrence, at least for convexity meningiomas.[13] When this is not possible in a single stage, a second stage may be necessary. Despite benign tissue predominance, recurrence is frequent.

In a review of over 600 patients with apparent complete tumor removal, a recurrence rate of 19 percent at 20 years was reported.[15] Tumors with anaplasia were excluded. Risk factors subjected to multivariate analysis were coagulation rather than removal of the dura, bone invasion, and soft consistency of the tumor. The 20-year recurrence rate was estimated at 11 percent with no risk factors, 15 to 24 percent with one, and 34 to 56 percent with two risk factors.

In a review of 235 patients operated in the Oxford series, Simpson[16] graded the extent of removal. Where removal was complete including the dura, the recurrence rate was 9 percent, while if the dura could only be coagulated, the rate was 19 percent. Infiltration of the venous sinuses was found in 15 percent of the cases, of bone in 20 percent, and of the brain in 3.7 percent. Of interest is the absence of recurrence in the 12 angioblastic meningiomas. Recurrent tumor merits reoperation in most cases.

The proliferative potential of meningiomas may be predicted by labeling with bromodeoxyuridine (BrdUrd). Preoperative infusion of BrdUrd is followed by indirect immunoperoxidase staining of the excised specimen to determine the BrdUrd index. Recurrence rate was 100 percent in patients with indices greater than 5 percent, 44 percent with indices of 1 to 5 percent, and 6.1 percent with indices less than 1 percent.[17]

Flow cytometry has predictive value for recurrence. DNA analysis has a significantly higher proliferative index in a group of recurrent tumors than in a nonrecurrent group, even though the histological subtyping of the two groups is similar.[18]

Clinical evidence of recurrent meningioma can be obscured by the space remaining after initial removal. Alerting symptoms include progressive neurological deficits and altered patterns or frequency of seizures. Routine follow-up evaluation using MRI with contrast offers the best means of detecting recurrence.

Where the quality of life permits, reoperation for recurrent meningiomas should be considered. The opportunity for a more complete removal may present at reoperation, as when the sagittal sinus becomes completely occluded.

MALIGNANT MENINGIOMA

The distinction between benign and malignant meningioma may at times be equivocal when there is persistent recurrence, multiple new occurrence, and even metastasis. Malignant meningiomas display nonrandom karyotypic aberrations, particularly in chromosome 22.[19] Men seem to be more commonly afflicted. Suspicion is raised when there is rapid progression of the tumor with recurrences that frequently become inoperable. Ominous histologic features are anaplasia and numerous mitosis, whereas necrosis and cerebral invasion may not always indicate malignancy.[20] This is to be distinguished from *primary leptomeningeal sarcomatosis,* which is a rare malignant neoplasm that arises from and diffusely infiltrates the leptomeninges without forming large or discrete tumor masses. This condition is often confused with chronic meningitis, metastatic carcinoma, and sarcoidosis.[21]

□ RADIATION THERAPY OF MENINGIOMAS

The role of radiation therapy in the management of meningiomas remains controversial. Postoperative irradiation following total removal of a meningioma is not indicated. Incomplete removal, particularly in angioblastic tumors and in tumors of the medial sphenoid wing, suggests the need for postoperative radiation. Its use is indicated in recurrent tumors involving the cavernous sinus or orbit, or where reoperation is not considered feasible. In vascular tumors, radiation has been proposed to reduce the size and vascularity, followed by resection about 6 months later. Using this protocol, 8 of 12 meningiomas, initially considered unresectable because of vascularity, were resected at reoperation,

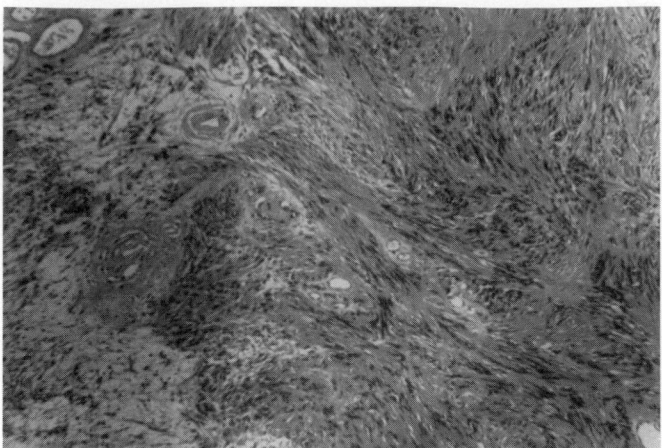

Figure 11–7   Schwannoma. The tumor is formed mainly of the densely cellular areas, which are referred to as "Antoni type A" areas. These are composed of parallel rows of elongated nuclei and intermittent bands of pink cytoplasm. A small area of round, loose, sparsely arranged cells, "Antoni type B" area, is seen at the lower left part of the picture (H & E × 63).

with 7 remaining free of recurrence up to 13 years following irradiation.[22]

Radiation therapy ranging from 4800 to 6080 rad (median, 5490 rad) is given over a 6-week period. The use of radiation therapy in case of incomplete removal is particularly indicated in medial sphenoid wing lesions and may provide a prolongation of the interval before recurrence.[23] There may be special application of stereotactic interstitial radiation (brachytherapy) using ^{125}I seed implants in selected small meningiomas around the petrous apex and cavernous sinus.[24]

□ CRANIAL NERVE NEOPLASMS

ACOUSTIC SCHWANNOMA

Schwannomas of the eighth nerve account for approximately 8 percent of intracranial tumors. They arise from Schwann cells of the vestibular nerve within the internal auditory canal. There are both dense (Antoni, type A) and loose (Antoni, type B) tumor cells, with the more-dense regions showing the typical palisading of the elongated nuclei. Collagen may be present (Fig. 11-7).

As the tumor grows, it encroaches on the acoustic nerve and then the facial nerve. While the tumor is still within the internal auditory canal, bony erosion of the canal wall occurs so that x-rays or CT studies show a columnar or bell-shaped enlargement of the canal. As the tumor grows beyond the limits of the canal, it encroaches on the pons, the trigeminal nerve, and the cerebellum. While still small and within the canal, the tumor attached to the superior vestibular nerve is frequently easily separated from the acoustic, the facial, and even, at times, from the inferior vestibular nerves. With an increase in the size of the tumor, however, both vestibular nerves and the acoustic nerve become incorporated. The facial nerve is usually displaced anteriorly and inferiorly and incorporated in the tumor capsule where it may remain as a single strand, but it is usually splayed into several fiber bundles, which may be identified at surgery. Larger tumors produce impressions in the cerebellum and pons and may incorporate the basilar artery and its branches.

Acoustic schwannomas are characteristically unilateral, but bilateral acoustic neuromas occur in von Recklinghausen's disease. Bilateral tumors exhibit a tendency for the facial and acoustic nerves to be incorporated into the tumor, even in the early stages. The opportunity to preserve these structures is reduced.

The earliest symptoms of eighth nerve tumors are usually referable to the acoustic nerve in the form of tinnitus and hearing loss in the higher frequencies, which is typically retrocochlear. Audiological studies reveal decreased discrimination, decay, and reduced recruitment. Auditory evoked responses show retrocochlear changes. Decreased or absent caloric responses are seen. Facial nerve involvement produces numbness of the posterior surface of the external auditory canal and facial paresis, with delayed blink and EMG changes. Increasing tumor size and encroachment on the pons and cerebellum result in impairment of balance and gait. Encroachment on the fifth nerve produces paresthesias or pain and eventually numbness, with decreased corneal sensation and reflex. The diagnosis of acoustic neuroma is made by CT or MRI, supported by clinical findings. Consequently surgical treatment may be planned for maximal preservation of function (Fig. 11-8).

The neurosurgical approach to these tumors is through the posterior fossa, usually with a vertical incision between the inion and the mastoid process. While the sitting position is preferred by some, many surgeons use the lateral or park bench position, with a few using the prone or semiprone position. Use of the microscope and microsurgical techniques is imperative. With proper positioning, dehydration, and retraction, it is usually possible to expose the small and medium-sized tumors without resecting any cerebellum as may be required with large lesions. Intracanalicular tumors and intracanalicular portions of larger tumors can be exposed by burring off the posterior wall of the internal auditory canal after turning a small dural flap to expose the bone directly. Small tumors, thus exposed, may be separated from the facial and sometimes from the acoustic nerve. Preservation of the facial nerve is frequently possible, and preservation of hearing occasionally occurs, but preservation of useful hearing is rare. Attempts should be made to preserve hearing whenever possible. The suboccipital retrosigmoid approach is used in such cases.

Surgical removal of larger tumors is more difficult. A total removal should be the goal, but an aggressive threat to the brainstem should be avoided. Identification of the facial nerve by stimulation and meticulous dissection make preservation of facial function possible. The same care should be exerted in dealing with the blood vessels, trigeminal and glossopharyngeal nerves, and brainstem.

Hemostasis should be secure, and the dural closure should be watertight. Opened mastoid cells require occlusion with bone wax. Large bone and dural defects, such as with a translabyrinthine approach are closed by an autogenous free fat graft.

FIFTH NERVE NEUROMA

Schwannomas of the trigeminal nerve are rare. Histopathological characteristics are the same as those of the eighth nerve. Malignant changes are extremely rare and show increased mitoses and invasion of adjacent tissues.[25] Symptoms are isolated ipsilateral abducens nerve palsy, with trigeminal nerve dysfunction several years later.[26] Other symptoms are dependent on the direction of growth. Extension into the cavernous sinus produces symptoms referable to its contents, while posterior extension produces symptoms related to the cerebellopontine angle.[27] Anterior extension through the optic canal and superior orbital fissure produces painless proptosis.[28]

The site of origin of the tumor presents problems in imaging while it is still small. With an increase in symptoms MRI reveals its presence. With an increase in the size of the tumor, it becomes more easily imaged.

The surgical treatment should be directed at complete removal if possible. The approach is dependent on the location. Subtemporal, frontal, and suboccipital approaches have been described, some resulting in total removal[29] (Fig. 11-9).

☐ CAVERNOUS SINUS TUMORS

Tumors in the cavernous sinus are extensions of meningiomas above, pituitary adenomas below, and schwannomas within. They present with focal periorbital pain and visual impairment, usually with decreased ocular motility due to third, fourth, and/or sixth cranial nerve compression. The optic nerve can be impaired when larger lesions compress the optic nerve or chiasm.[29] Neuromas of the ocular cranial nerves uncommonly occur; usually they are associated with sensory nerves, such as the vestibular and trigeminal nerves, but they can involve the sheaths of other cranial nerves.[30]

☐ GLOMUS JUGULARE

Tumors of the glomus jugulare, paragangliomas, or chemodectomas are rare tumors arising from extra-adrenal paraganglia. In addition to a jugular origin, tympanic and vagal origins occur. They are histologically similar to carotid body tumors. Familial occurrence from alternate locations has been reported.[31] They secrete neuropeptides such as chole-

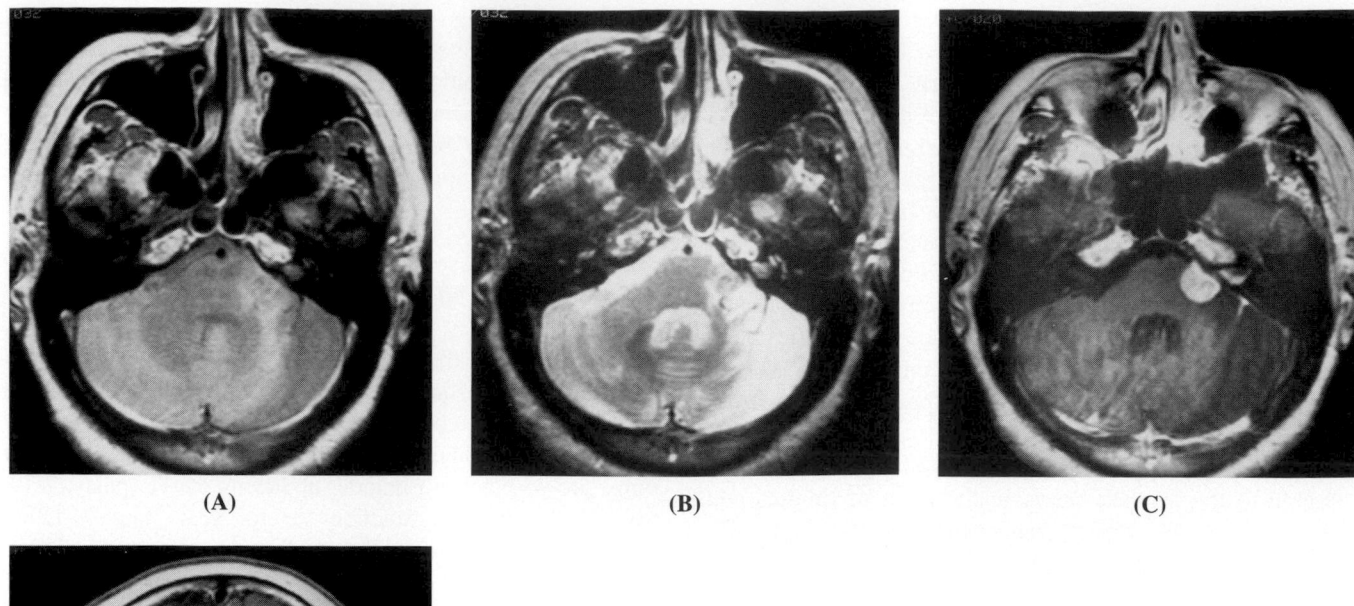

(A)   (B)   (C)

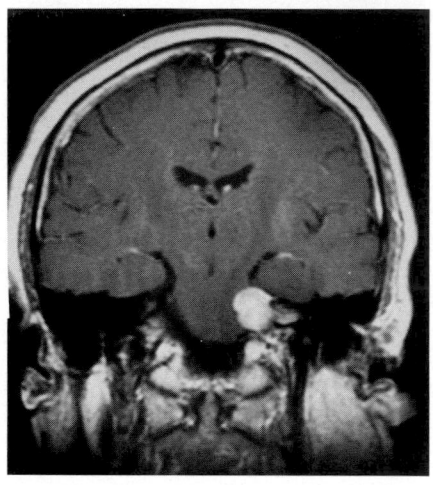

(D)

Figure 11–8   Recurrent acoustic schwannoma. A 52-year-old female had undergone subtotal surgical resection of a left acoustic tumor via a suboccipital craniectomy 5 years previously. She had loss of hearing and headache at that time. A complete left facial nerve palsy had persisted since the surgery. She presented with increasing headache and right eye blinking. She was deaf in the left ear; there was a left peripheral facial paralysis and diminished pin stick in the left face. The left corneal reflex was decreased. T1 MRI (*A*) and T2 MRI (*B*) show postoperative atrophy of the left cerebellar hemisphere and suggest recurrent tumor. *C.* Enhanced MRI (transverse cut) shows globoid brightly enhancing tumor. *D.* Coronal MRI shows the mass arising from the internal acoustic canal and bulging into the lateral wall of the pons.

cystokinin in addition to catecholamines.[32] Malignant characteristics and metastases are rare.[33] The tumors are very vascular, a trait that aids in angiographic diagnosis, but that presents surgical risk. Biopsy of these tumors is likely to cause significant hemorrhage.

Diagnosis is suggested by deficits of the tympanic, jugular, or vagal nerves. Hearing loss and tinnitus are common, but initial vocal cord paralysis points to a vagal origin. Catecholamine secretion results in hypertension and tachycardia. Tomography and MRI with gadolinium enhancement have become the imaging studies for paragangliomas. Angiography is required for preoperative embolization or in preoperative determination of the extent of the tumor and its blood supply.[34]

Surgery and radiation are used in treatment. The local control rates for surgery alone, surgery with pre- or postoperative radiation, and radiation alone are similar: 86, 90, and 93 percent.[35] Preoperative embolization of the glomus jugulare tumors significantly reduces blood loss and operative time.[36] The surgical approach may be subtemporal, transtemporal, or suboccipital.

Complications of surgery include increased cranial nerve deficits. Continuous intraoperative facial nerve monitoring

provides warnings that may reduce postoperative facial paresis.[37]

☐ PHACOMATOSIS

NEUROFIBROMATOSIS

Neurofibromatoses are manifestations of two autosomal dominant disorders. Neurofibromatosis 1 (NF-1, von Recklinghausen's disease) and neurofibromatosis 2 (NF-2) result in neurofibromas, but they are distinct disorders resulting from defective genes on chromosome 17 in NF-1 and chromosome 22 in NF-2.[38] Acoustic neuromas occur in NF-2 but have rarely been documented in NF-1. Iris hamartomas, or Lisch bodies, in NF-1 cause no problem with vision, whereas posterior lens opacity in NF-2 may produce a handicap in addition to the potential for auditory loss.[39]

Essentially, all organ systems can be affected either directly or through neural or vascular involvement. Clinical manifestations include mental retardation, learning and be-

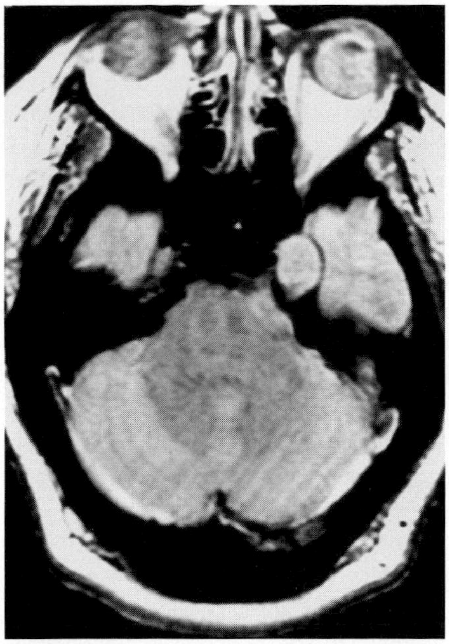

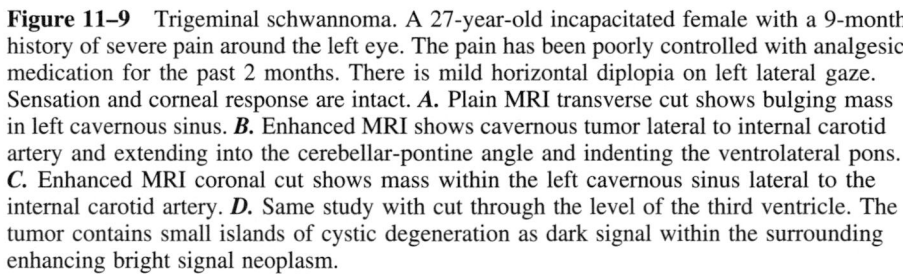

(A) 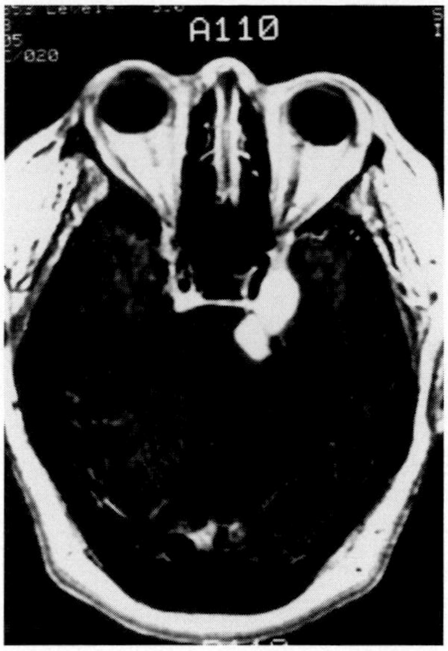   (B) 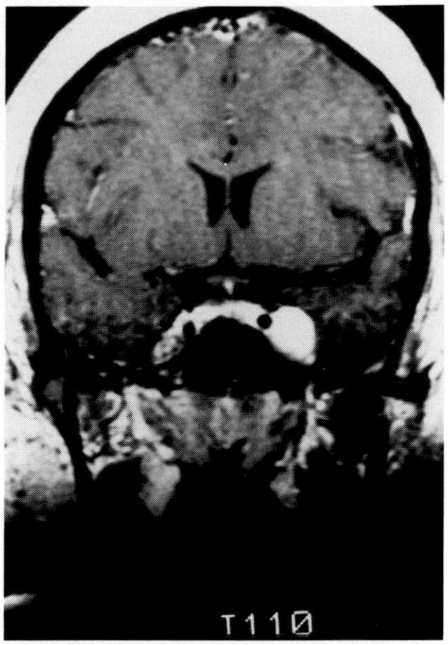   (C)

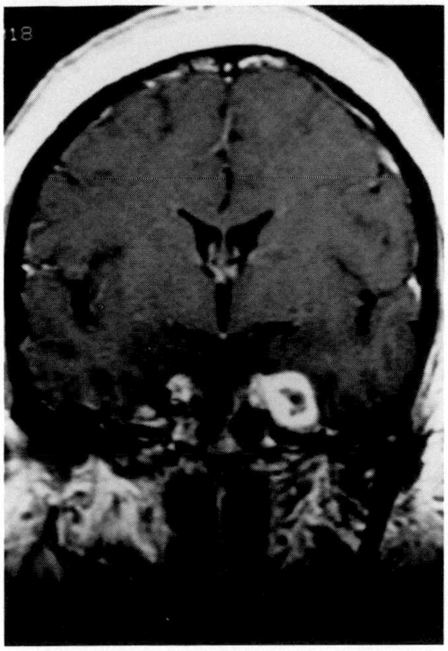

Figure 11–9   Trigeminal schwannoma. A 27-year-old incapacitated female with a 9-month history of severe pain around the left eye. The pain has been poorly controlled with analgesic medication for the past 2 months. There is mild horizontal diplopia on left lateral gaze. Sensation and corneal response are intact. *A.* Plain MRI transverse cut shows bulging mass in left cavernous sinus. *B.* Enhanced MRI shows cavernous tumor lateral to internal carotid artery and extending into the cerebellar-pontine angle and indenting the ventrolateral pons. *C.* Enhanced MRI coronal cut shows mass within the left cavernous sinus lateral to the internal carotid artery. *D.* Same study with cut through the level of the third ventricle. The tumor contains small islands of cystic degeneration as dark signal within the surrounding enhancing bright signal neoplasm.

(D)

havioral disorders, seizures, and intracranial or intraspinal tumors. They may be meningiomas or gliomas in addition to neurofibromas.[40] Mental disorders in the form of depression, anxiety, or organic brain syndrome have been reported in as much as one-third of patients with NF-1.[41] Hydrocephalus due to obstruction of the aqueduct of Sylvius or the foramina of Lushka and Magendie may occur in over one fifth of the patients and may require surgical treatment.[42,43] Café-au-lait skin lesions are frequently seen and suggest the diagnosis. Diagnosis is by MRI. Early studies are emphasized. Small acoustic tumors within the internal auditory meatus may be removed with preservation of hearing and facial nerve function. Lesions in the globus pallidus and internal capsule,

bilaterally, may appear on T1-weighted studies, while smaller foci appear on T2-weighted studies. They may represent heterotopias of neural crest origin.[44]

Treatment of the NF-1 neurofibromas is directed primarily at removal of those that, by position, produce pain or disfigurement. Malignant changes may necessitate an aggressive form of approach.

Treatment of NF-2 neurofibromas is more challenging. Threatening meningiomas or gliomas must be dealt with individually. Diagnosis of bilateral acoustic neuromas at the earliest possible time offers the greatest possibility for preservation of hearing.[45] Preservation of hearing has been reported in 8 out of 20 patients when it was attempted at surgical removal.[46] Stereotactic radiosurgery offers an alternative to conventional operation. Preservation of facial nerve and hearing functions is frequently possible.[47]

☐ CRANIAL BASE TUMORS

CHORDOMA

Chordoma is a unique and rare neoplasm originating from embryonic remnants of the notochord. It rarely presents clinically until middle age. It involves midline structures and usually has a benign histological architecture. It is indolent, relentless, and locally aggressive. It can metastasize and even change histologically late in its course. Chordomas present from the cranial base to the coccyx and at intervening spinal segments. Chordomas are rare among the spinal tumors of children. They have a tendency to recur locally after subtotal resection. They are relatively resistant to radiation treatment.

In his 1857 monograph on the development of the skull base, Virchow described and illustrated these clival excrescences and their large vacuolated cells, which he termed *physaliphorous* (Gk., "bubble-bearing").[48] He considered these tumors to contain mucous-filled cells of cartilaginous origin, and he named them *ecchondrosis physaliphora*. In 1858, Muller noted the resemblance of these excrescences to the notochord and called them *chordoid tumors*. Muller noted persistent notochordal remnants in the skull base, odontoid process, and coccyx.[49]

Notochordal rests are seen occasionally in adults along the spinal axis and within the nucleus pulposus. Notochordal tissue appears to have potential for cellular proliferation.[50] Similar locations and cell types of the notochordal rests, nucleus pulposus, ecchordosis, and chordoma occur at different levels along the original tract of the notochord, suggesting a relationship in these structures.[51-54]

Approximately 50 percent of chordomas originate in the sacrum, 35 percent at the skull base and upper cervical region, and 15 percent in the intervening vertebrae.[55-59] The mean age of onset is older for the sacrococcygeal tumors (63 years) than for tumors of other locations (35 years).[60-62] They are resistant to treatment and tend to recur locally and metastasize. Eventually they are lethal; the 5-year overall survival rate for cranial base tumors is 35 percent and for the sacrococcygeal group 66 percent.[59,63]

CT gives precise information about chordomas, demonstrating bone destruction in 90 percent; it directly images the soft tissue mass. Calcific debris is noted in 87 percent, compared with only 44 percent seen on plain films.[64,65]

MRI provides superior contrast of chordoma with surrounding soft tissues because of its prolonged T1 and T2 times. The direct sagittal images of MRI indicate extent.[66] It images spinal canal invasion, with dural displacement or occlusion.[67,68]

Chordomas are lobulated, pseudoencapsulated, gray, semitranslucent, soft, and mucinous. Hemorrhage can convert the translucent lobules into "currant-jelly" masses. The involved bone is expanded and destroyed by the tumor, infiltrating between the bony trabeculae. The pseudocapsule is not evident within the bone.[69] Adjacent bony invasion is present but obscured. There may be extension into the spinal canal. Focal calcification is seen frequently.[70,71]

Microscopic septations provided by the fibrovascular connective pseudocapsule render a lobular pattern within which tumor cells are seen. Three types of tumor cells are recognized: (1) Physaliphorous cells, seen consistently, are large and distended by abundant vacuolated (mucin) cytoplasm. The nuclei of these cells are small, dark, and eccentric. Physaliphorous cells can become quite large, with distended and stringy cytoplasmic extensions. The cells may occur in groups or cords with an epithelioid pattern or in lobules and clusters. The vacuoles are within a faintly eosinophilic cytoplasm. The cells are separated by a similar frothy vacuolated mucinous matrix.[72,73] These features are similar to the histological appearance of the notochord and ecchordosis. (2) Other cells are smaller, polygonal or spherical, and arranged in trabeculae, cords, or clusters. They show few cytoplasmic vacuoles. (3) More sparsely found cells are close to the rim of the lobules, compactly arranged with smaller cell size of "collapsed" fusiform and stellate shape.

Histological evidence of malignancy is not rare in chordomas, at least in parts of the tumor. Features include anaplasia, mitotic divisions, nuclear hyperchromasia, and irregularity.[72]

Initially, chordoma was considered a tumor of local invasion.[72] It is now recognized that the spinal and sacral chordomas eventually disseminate.[59,74,75] Cranial chordomas are being reported to disseminate more often as improved local treatment lengthens survival.[64] Histological anaplasia seems to be a factor, but microscopic criteria cannot predict metastatic potential with any certainty.

Radiation may be a factor in survival. Sixty-seven percent of cases with reported metastasis had been irradiated. Death frequently follows complications of local recurrence[60] (Fig. 11-10).

Sarcomatous metaplasia is frequently reported in chordoma. The metastatic lesions and biologic behavior are those of the sarcomatous component.[76]

Radiation Therapy   Chordoma is relatively radioresistant and is rarely destroyed by radiation alone (using standard megavoltage beams) at tolerable doses. The median relapse time was 3.5 years.[77] There is no difference in survival rate between the various sites, nor is there any difference whether they received palliative doses of radiotherapy (up to 4500 rad) or not.[78] Response to high-dose radiation therapy is slow, with pain resolving over 1 to 2 months and tumor regression continuing 4 to 5 months after completion of treatment.[79,80]

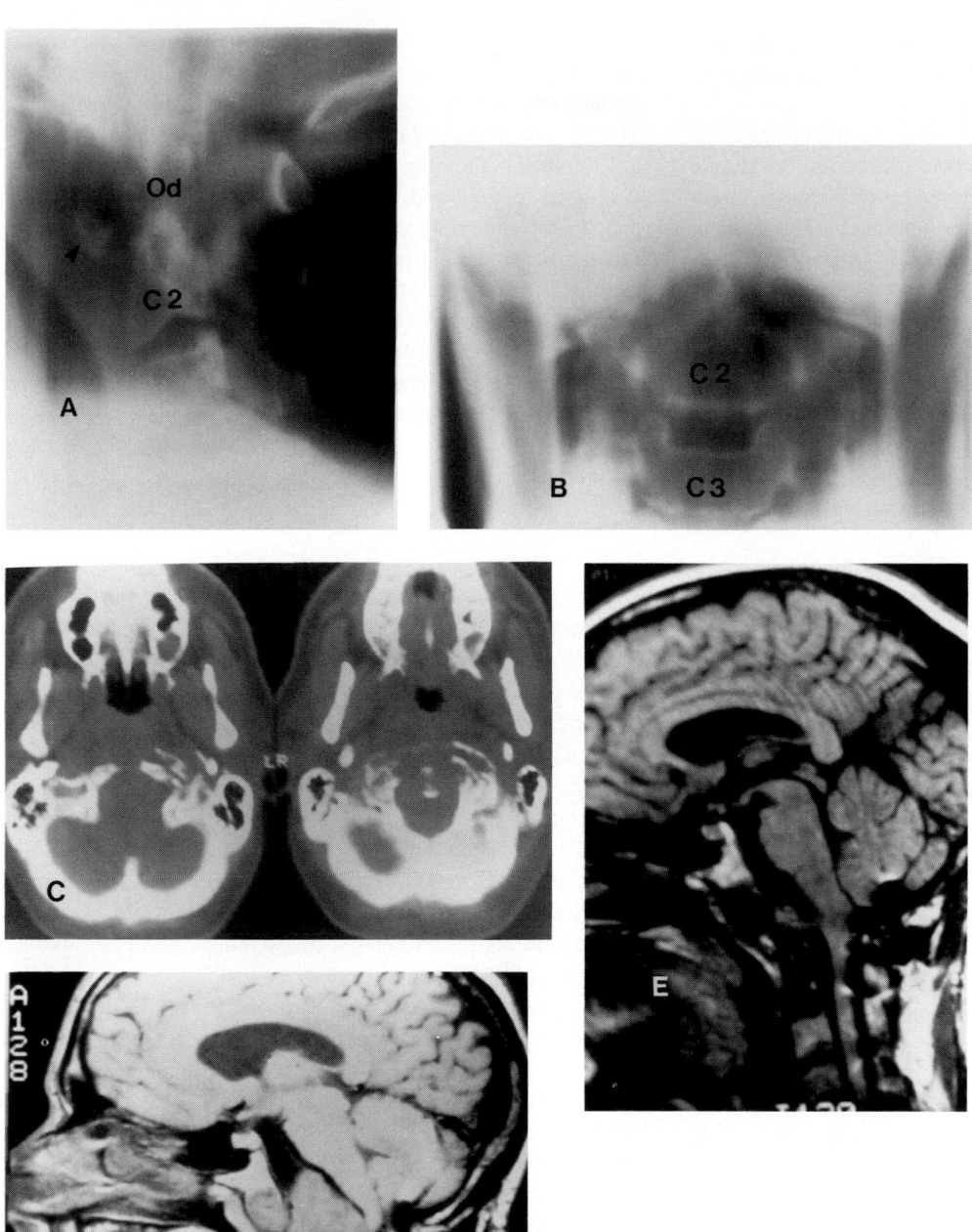

Figure 11–10 Craniovertebral chordoma. A 35-year-old male with persistent intractable neck pain after doing calisthenics. He was neurologically intact initially. *A.* Polytomogram of occiput, C1–C2 lateral view shows settling and anterior subluxation of C1 on C2 (Od = odontoid; *arrowhead* = C1 anterior arch). *B.* Anterior-posterior view shows erosion of the odontoid and splaying of the C1 lateral masses. *C.* CT cuts through the foramen magnum, and occipital condyles shows irregular destruction of these bony structures. The patient underwent transcervical subtotal resection of chordoma, followed by posterior resection of C1 and occipital cervical fusion and then 60 Gy cobalt 60 radiation. He presented $2^1/_2$ years later with clumsiness and unilateral numbness with dystaxia and dysmetria. *D.* Midsagittal MRI shows recurrant chordoma at C1–C2 with clival extension and ventral compression of the medulla. *E.* Midsagittal MRI after suboccipital far-lateral tumor resection and fascial graft to clival base.

Principals of Surgical Management

Many patients with extra-axial tumors do not have increased intracranial pressure and many extra-axial tumors are slowly growing, accommodating neural structures to the mass. Rating the patient using the Karnofsky scale helps to establish the degree of urgency for intervention. The use of steroids for transient relief of increased intracranial pressure has reduced the incidence of emergency craniotomies for tumors, although some emergencies still occur. Steroids may reduce symptoms of cranial nerve compression.

Diagnostic imaging by CT, without and with contrast, provides adequate identification of lesions of the calvarium. Lesions at the base are likely to be obscured by bone. MRI provides greater resolution of the margins and extent of the neoplasm and also affords optimal imaging of lesions about the skull base. Patients must be stable and cooperative.

Patients should be medically prepared for surgery. Nutrition and fluids and electrolytes should be within acceptable limits. The patient and/or responsible relatives should be appropriately informed of the procedure and of the realistic expectations thereof.

Planning for surgery begins with imaging. Extraparenchymal lesions may have infiltrative attachments to overlying bone or the skull base.

The surgeon must have a definitive approach planned before the patient reaches the operating room. It should include a plan for the scalp flap designed to preserve circulation of the scalp regardless of the approach. The base of the flap should be toward the base of the skull unless other priorities such as a previous scar prevail (see Chap. 1).

The sequence of the burr holes and saw cuts is planned. For example, in turning a flap near the pterion the burr hole closest to the position of the middle meningeal artery as well as the saw cuts in this area should be last. Likewise, in turning a flap near or across the vertex, the burr holes and saw cuts nearest the superior sagittal sinus should be last. The same applies to the region of the transverse sinus and the torcular Herophili.

The dura may be densely adherent to the overlying bone, requiring that it be stripped before the bone flap can be elevated. This may present a problem in the elderly and in the case of hyperostosis frontalis interna, as well as with some neoplasms.

Preservation of the vascular supply and drainage is also stressed. This may require alteration of the approach. If arterial and venous supplies of a structure are to be sacrificed, it is desirable to interrupt the arterial supply first.

Once the plan for a surgical approach has been made, proper positioning of the patient is required. Principals include the following: (1) The position must permit the surgeon and assistants access for a planned approach. (2) Access to special instrumentation such as the microscope, ultrasonic aspirator, laser, and so forth must be provided. (3) The surgical team must be able to operate in comfort over the period of the procedure. (4) The head must be stabilized and secured but capable of being repositioned. (5) The anesthesiologist must have adequate access to the patient. (6) Pressure areas and structures, including the eyes, must be adequately protected.

Elevation of the head above the rest of the body optimizes venous drainage and aids in controlling intracranial pressure and bleeding. Undue rotation or flexion of the neck that may produce jugular compression or kinking of the endotracheal tube should be avoided. Generally headpin fixation is desirable for stability and for retractor fixation. The head is positioned so that retraction of the brain is aided by gravity where possible. This may reduce the need for retractor pressure which can produce ischemic and necrotic changes. Compression of major vessels by retractors should be avoided.

☐ SURGICAL APPROACHES ORIENTED TOWARD THE SKULL CONVEXITIES

FRONTAL

The patient is supine. A unilateral frontal craniotomy posterior to the forehead may utilize a horseshoe or L-shaped scalp incision. If the craniotomy is low, an L-shaped flap may still be used, but a midline scar through the forehead is undesirable unless combined with a transfacial approach. The bicoronal scalp flap is preferred. The bicoronal incision has the advantage of greater relaxation of the reflected scalp. It is used for bilateral frontal approaches, such as for olfactory groove meningiomas. The head may be flexed for a more-superior lesion or extended for inferior or subfrontal lesions to utilize gravity as an aid in retraction. At least one olfactory bulb and tract should be preserved. Inclusion of the supraorbital ridge with the frontal bone flap greatly improves exposure of the anterior fossa and considerably reduces frontal lobe retraction.[81,82]

TEMPORAL

Two approaches to the temporal lobe may be utilized. The "question mark" incision swings from the lateral frontal hairline to a point above the pinna of the ear, then down toward the ear, curving just above and anterior to the ear to descend vertically anterior to the tragus to the zygomatic arch. The temporal artery and the branches of the facial nerve to the frontalis muscle should be preserved. The size and extent of the flap may vary. The scalp flap is retracted forward exposing the temporalis muscle, which is incised with the pericranium to permit reflection of a free flap or, preferably, an osteoplastic flap with the muscle used as a hinge. The lateral extent of the sphenoid bone is removed and the middle meningeal artery controlled.

An "inverted U" flap may also be used, with the anterior limb in front of the ear and anterior to the temporalis artery, while preserving the branches of the facial nerve to the frontalis muscle. The posterior limb of the incision is located behind the ear. The flap is reflected inferiorly, and the temporalis muscle and bone flap may be reflected as in the question mark flap.

In both incisions it is advantageous to have the patient on the side or semisupine with the midline nearly horizontal, the face slightly superior to the occiput, and the base of the skull more elevated than the vertex. This permits direct vision of the mesial temporal structures with minimal retraction.

CENTRAL

The approach to the temporal lobe may be used for an approach to low central structures. A horseshoe-shaped incision extending to or across the midline is suitable for the exposure of superior central structures near the midline. Dimensions may be adjusted appropriately. Working in the region of the superior sagittal sinus requires specific precautions. Bridging cortical veins should be preserved, using microdissection of the vessels and arachnoid if necessary.

PARIETAL

The approach to the parietal lobe may be a more posteriorly placed flap of the central type or a more anteriorly placed occipital flap, described below.

OCCIPITAL

The occipital flap must be closely coordinated with the positioning of the patient. An L-shaped flap with a midline incision extending from the inion to the parietal region and turning laterally and inferiorly preserves the blood supply and permits a bone flap to expose the sagittal and lateral sinuses and the underlying occipital lobe. The larger size of the venous sinuses posteriorly requires caution to avoid their laceration.

☐ SURGICAL APPROACHES ORIENTED TOWARD THE SKULL BASE

Current interest in the skull base is an evolution of knowledge and techniques that have progressed since the introduction of the operating microscope to clinical surgery. The dexterity of the surgeons is limited only by what can be visualized. The "keyhole" stereoscopic view presents the surgeon with a panorama of the CNS. Microsurgical techniques imply gentle handling of tissues, with improved overall results and reduced morbidity. The successes enjoyed by adhering to microsurgical principles along with improved diagnostic imaging by CT and MRI have encouraged more aggressive interventions to previously "inoperable" lesions of the basal segments of the brain, skull, and craniovertebral junction. Skull base neoplasms are being excised with significant alteration of palliative or curative outcome. Skull base principles have application to reconstruction of congenital craniofacial malformations, excision of neoplasms, treatment of vascular lesions, debridement of infection, and restoration of trauma.

☐ COMPLICATIONS OF CONCERN TO SURGICAL THERAPY

Impaired healing due to poorly vascularized resurfaced cranial floor will lead to CSF rhinorrhea and resultant meningitis. Ischemia and contusion of underlying brain can result from excessive retraction. Use of the microscope for intracranial stages of surgery improves visualization while minimizing brain retraction. Pneumocephalus and CSF rhinorrhea can be controlled with judicial use of lumbar subarachnoid drainage.[83,84] This will reduce intracranial hydrostatic pressure and avoid CSF rhinorrhea and its inherent risk of postoperative meningitis. It will facilitate the soft tissue "seal" of the frontal cranial base. This is best initiated before the patient leaves the operating room. The authors prefer to establish the lumbar CSF drain prior to the procedure. Nutritional support with enteric or intravenous alimentation helps reduce the incidence of infection and facilitate recovery.

☐ THE ANTERIOR CRANIAL BASE

The anterior cranial base is most frequently involved by extracranial neoplasms from the paranasal sinuses, nasopharynx, or orbits. Such lesions of the pericranial sites that involve the intracranial base must be approached primarily as intracranial lesions. Therefore, craniotomy and intracranial manipulation of the lesion are parts of the definitive procedure, since adequate visualization of cerebral structures along with dural reconstruction are required for safe and adequate tumor removal. The ethmoid sinuses are the most-common site of origin for tumors of the anterior extracranial base. The most-common malignant tumor arising in the pericranial sinuses is the squamous cell carcinoma. Esthesioneuroblastoma occurs more commonly in young adults, and rhabdomyosarcoma occurs in children. Sepsis of pericranial sinuses may complicate intracranial structures, leading to epidural and subdural empyema as well as frontal and temporal lobe abscesses.

The patient's overall prognosis for treatment of neoplasms is related to histological type. For example, anaplastic carcinoma is a separate entity from poorly differentiated squamous cell carcinoma. It is more common in women. The 5-year survival rate is only 15 percent if the lesion arises from the sinuses. Wide excision of more locally infiltrative lesions such as basal cell or squamous cell carcinoma may be curative. The intimate relationship of the sinuses and nasal cavity potentiates spread of tumor through compartments. Ethmoidal tumors often involve the orbit and orbital exenteration may be required for ultimate tumor control.

☐ APPROACHES IN SKULL BASE SURGERY

For greater clarity the approaches in skull surgery are described in the following text by steps in detail. The craniofacial and subfrontal approaches comprise features in common regardless of pathology.

GOALS OF SURGICAL TREATMENT OF FRONTAL BASAL LESIONS

There should be an attempt to excise the lesion completely. The dural enclosure is reconstructed. Hydrostatic pressure of CSF requires reduction at the repair site. A vascularized barrier between the intracranial contents and paranasal spaces is reestablished. Frontal-orbital cosmetic contours are rebuilt. Denuded paranasal and nasal walls are epithelialized with skin grafts. The palatal mechanism for phonation and deglutition is reestablished with prosthetics.[85–88]

1. *Bicoronal scalp incision.* A bicoronal incision is based on the supraorbital and supratrochlear vessels inferiorly and the superficial temporal vessels laterally. It can include the pericranial membrane or be separated at the areolar subgaleal space. It is reflected inferiorly on its base over the orbital ridges to expose the superior orbital cavities, nasion and medial orbit, and zygoma and lateral orbit.

2. *Bifrontal craniotomy.* Low supraorbital, or including the orbital ridge: An osteoplastic flap can be left attached to the temporalis fascia to preserve blood supply to the flap. Commonly, a free bone flap is raised.

3. *Cranialization of frontal sinus.* The posterior wall of the frontal sinus is removed from the bone flap and cranial base. The interior of the remaining sinus wall is drilled to remove all remnants of sinus mucosa. The nasofrontal ducts are obliterated to avoid delayed mucocele formation and CSF leaks.

4. *Extradural delineation of pathology.* The dura is striped from the anterior fossa, avoiding tears of the dura, which may be thin and adherent. Tumors can be devascularized or delineated.

5. *Resection of orbital plates or skull base bone as needed.* Care is taken to dissect and preserve the periorbital membrane.

6. *Transverse opening of supraorbital dura.* This step gains entrance to the subdural space. The frontal lobes are gently elevated. The olfactory bulbs and tracts are preserved unless the lesion renders this inappropriate.

7. *Ligation and transection sagittal venous sinus.* This gains control of the rostral sagittal sinus.

8. *Transection of the falx at crista galli.* This exposes the expanse of the anterior fossa and interhemispheric fissure. It accesses midline lesions at the basal anterior fossa.

9. *Gentle elevation of frontal lobes and retraction of orbital gyri.* This should expose the lesion for resection, debridement, and repair.

☐ TUMOR: INCISIONAL PIECEMEAL EXCISION VERSUS EN BLOC RESECTION

INCISIONAL PIECEMEAL EXCISION

This procedure is applicable where *en bloc* resection is unnecessary or impossible. It is used for histologically benign tumors that are confined to the frontal cranial base with

dural and/or bony invasion such as meningiomas or epidermoids.

10. The tumor mass is debulked using an ultrasonic aspirator or laser. Precise tumor resection is best visualized and facilitated by illumination and magnification.

11. Transection of olfactory tracts avoids inadvertent avulsion of the olfactory bulbs that sometimes results in delayed CSF rhinorrhea.

12. Excision of involved dura, bone, and paranasal sinuses prevents delayed local recurrence of the neoplasm. A high-speed drill is advantageous in the bony resection.

EN BLOC RESECTION

This procedure is applicable in tumors arising from paranasal sinuses or nasopharynx with invasion of the intracranial frontal base. It is used for those tumors that are histologically or biologically benign and are circumscribed and amenable to en bloc removal with margins free of tumor. This is a resection directed by natural anatomical boundaries such as the medial orbital walls, cribriform plate, nasal septum, sphenoid wing, and hard palate.[89–99]

Steps 1 through 9 are the same as previously described.

10. Bicoronal scalp flap is repositioned for viscerocranial access. This frees the face, nasal cavity, and maxilla for surgical resection.

11. Bone cuts are circumferential around the lesion, visualized directly. This disconnects the intracranial portion of the tumor and frees it to be delivered from below. Posterior cuts across the optic canal and orbital apex are made if the orbit and contents are to be included with the resected specimen. Bone cuts are planned so that tumor margins are not transgressed.

12. Facial incisions are unilateral rhinotomy or gingivolabial.

    a. Unilateral rhinotomy incision may be extended to split the upper lip. This "lateral rhinotomy" allows reflection of facial soft tissues for bone exposure of the nasal cavity, medial orbital wall, maxilla, and orbital floor.

    b. Gingivolabial sulcus incision may permit elevation of all tissues. This "degloving" avoids external facial incisions and affords bony exposure for osteotomies to communicate with superior cuts and allow mobilization and removal from below.

13. The base of the nasal bone is separated, and the contralateral nasal bone then scored and fractured, allowing the nose to be folded to contralateral side. This opens the entire nasal cavity and gives access to the hard palate and nasopharynx.

14. Soft tissue flaps are elevated by separating mucoperiosteum, exposing the osseous visceral cranium and providing bone cuts with tumor-free margins.

15. Bony cuts are made into the maxillary, ethmoid, and sphenoid sinuses. This frees the specimen from below.

16. The specimen is mobilized and soft tissue attachments cut. The tumor mass and entire resection specimen is thus loosened.

17. The specimen is delivered from below in the rhino-antral direction. The tumor is resected *en bloc* with wide tumor-free margins. Preoperative CT and MRI will visualize gross tumor margins and adjacent cranial structures so that resection is preplanned with close multidisciplinary collaboration among otolaryngology, plastic surgery, oncology, radiotherapy, and neurosurgery.

☐ RECONSTRUCTION AND CLOSURE

PIECEMEAL INCISIONAL EXCISION AND TRAUMA (LIMITED TO THE CRANIAL PROCEDURE)

The following steps are applicable if the surgical procedure has been limited to the intracranial vault and rostral portion of the frontal, ethmoid, and sphenoid sinuses. This would occur in most cases, including trauma, meningioma, empyema, or abscess. Local tissues often can be used to reconstruct the anterior fossa.[100,101]

1. Dural replacements are sutured circumferentially. Autologous fascia, pericranium, or allograft dura is used to reconstruct dural covering of the frontal base.

2. Autologous bone grafts are positioned at the opened cranial base. This can be obtained from the inner table of the bone flap. It is usually unnecessary unless there is a very large bone defect (> 9 cm^3) or there is inadequate soft tissue for local reconstruction of the base.

3. The vascularized cranial periostium is draped over the frontal base. This isolates the intracranial contents from the external environment with a viable vascularized membrane and barrier. The galeofrontalis flap supplied by the superficial temporal arteries is another suitable vascularized flap. It is stronger than the pericranial flap, but its use devascularizes the scalp, which severely limits this flap's utility.

4. Suturing the periosteal flap to the intact dura proximally to any dural graft ensures that a vascularized barrier will remain covering the desired position. It also bolsters the primary dural repair. The P-2 semicircular needle with 5-0 Dexon helps this maneuver since its small 5-mm girth allows easier manipulation in the narrow crevice formed by the frontal base epidural space.

5. Autogenous fat grafts from the abdominal wall or lateral thigh can be used to fill in dead space formed by the cranialized frontal sinus. This step is necessary only if the frontal sinuses are the very large "wrap-around" type, which leave a large intracranial dead space that should be filled by the graft.

6. Temporalis muscle and fascia are a source of vascularized graft. These can be used to supplement frontal base reconstruction if necessary and can also be employed instead of a free bone graft in the frontal base bony defect.

7. The frontal bone flap is reconstructed from the inner table. Bony defects are reconstructed for optimal cosmetic results. The outer table from the intact calvarium is a source of compact bone for cranial reconstruction.

8. The reconstructed bone flap is secured. Fragments can be secured with multiple wires or mini screw plates. Wire (No. 28) twisted at bone bridges and inverted into the drill holes secures the calvarial replacement. Drill holes can be filled with bone dust to enhance the final cosmetic result. Titanium miniplates and screws are an alternative method for fixation and drill hole occlusion.

9. Scalp edges are secured with double-layer closure. A tight galea closure with interrupted absorbable suture, supplemented by superficial wound edge approximation, gives optimal closure and minimizes CSF leakage.

10. Systemic antibiotic and irrigation with Bacitracin, 1g/500 ml, reduces the incidence of postoperative infection.

11. CSF diversion by lumbar subarachnoid external drain reduces intracranial hydrostatic pressure and avoids CSF rhinorrhea as well as its inherent risk of postoperative meningitis. It facilitates the soft tissue "seal" of the frontal cranial base. This should be done before leaving the operating room. It is preferable to establish the lumbar CSF drain prior to starting the procedure.

12. Beware of tension pneumocephalus and meningitis in the early postoperative period. Excessive drainage of CSF can lead to intracranial hypotension and tension pneumocephalus if there is a "flap valve" effect formed by the soft tissue flaps used to reconstruct the frontal base.

EN BLOC RESECTION

Procedures may include the visceral skull. They create wide communication between the cranial cavity and the contaminated environment of the nasopharynx and pericranial sinuses. For effective isolation of intracranial contents, the guiding principles of closure should include vascularity, simplicity, and cosmetic result. Protracted malignant tumors such as esthesioneuroblastoma are often best managed by en bloc resection; they are also somewhat sensitive to radiation treatment.[102]

1. The dura is closed with repositioning of the pericranial flap along the floor. This gives a vascularized barrier from the nasal cavity and opened sinuses as previously described.

2. A split-thickness skin graft is positioned over the denuded nasal cavity. This supplies coverage of exposed bony surfaces of the nasal cavity and sinuses to avoid chronic osteitis and sequestration.
3. The nasal cavity is packed and stented, ensuring skin graft contact with bone surface and blood supply to improve graft viability. It forms a base to support cosmetic and functional prosthetics.
4. The maxillary obturator is placed to assist deglutition and phonation. Consultation with the prosthetic service prior to surgery will optimize design and fit of any prosthetic insert to assist in glossopharyngeal function required following resection.

RECONSTRUCTION ALTERNATIVES

Methods of closure are dependent on the extent to which original tissues are resected and residual viable tissues made available for closure. All methods require temporary lumbar drainage of CSF. Floating facial bones require securing and bone graft struts are used to reform contours. The medial canthal ligaments must be stabilized. The following lists tissues used for closure in ascending complexity.

Tissues that are vascularized locally are the following:

1. A broad bipedicle scalp flap is used.
2. The dural replacement is circumferentially sutured.
3. An attached pericranial flap is sutured to the dural base.
4. A bone flap is reconstructed and replaced.
5. A double-layered scalp closure without tension is used.
6. A split-thickness skin graft is onlayed to pericranial spaces.

Myocutaneous flaps are repositioned with vascular supply maintained through a remote pedicle. This is required when the orbital contents are excised with the specimen.

1. Trapezius myocutaneous flap is dissected on a vascular pedicle.
2. The flap is rotated and positioned by a tunneled pull-through on its pedicle.
3. The skin surface is deepithelialized for sinus obliteration.
4. The flap is sutured securely in place.

A free myocutaneous flap or greater omentum flap requires microvascular anastomosis of arteries and veins to local vessels. It is an alternative when local tissues are inadequate for effective closure[103,104] (Fig. 11-11).

ANTEROLATERAL CRANIAL BASE

The approach to the cranial base by way of the pterion is one of the most familiar and versatile approaches used for intracranial surgery, particularly for parasellar lesions and carotid system aneurysms.[105,106] The pterional approach can be expanded to excise tumors located in the orbit, cavernous sinus, greater wing of the sphenoid, maxillary sinus, pterygoid space, and infratemporal fossa. Specific structures requiring preservation and control are the internal carotid artery and the facial, optic, extraocular, and trigeminal nerves as they course in their various compartments. Wide bony resection and "exposure osteotomies" of the superior orbital ridge, zygoma, and sphenoid wing give access to deep cranial structures with minimal brain retraction, and most bony resection is accomplished extradurally.[107] Incisional and piecemeal excision techniques are used for most intracranial and orbital tumors, i.e., meningiomas, teratomas, chordomas, and chondrosarcomas.[108] Meningiomas frequently produce hyperostosis and bony infiltration so that involved bone and dura have to be excised to avoid local recurrence. Bone resection assists in exposure of deep structures. Preoperative planning, using imaging with CT, MRI, and angiography, is important.

If the carotid artery is involved, a carotid occlusion test is helpful in determining whether carotid repair or bypass will be needed. This is necessary with lesions of the cavernous sinus. Management of the carotid artery determines incisions, bony removal, and facial nerve relocation.

PTERIONAL ORBITAL ZYGOMATIC APPROACHES

EXPOSURE

The pterion is the junction of the greater wing of the sphenoid with the frontal and temporal bones. There are numerous variations in pterional approaches. Essential steps and principles are presented in a generic fashion, and they can be modified to anatomic specifics for individual lesions.[109]

1. The "hidden Dandy" incision extends from behind the hairline to below the tragus. This is cosmetically acceptable and may be extended as a coronal incision contralaterally, allowing forward reflection of the scalp flap when the orbital ridge and zygoma are to be exposed and removed. The frontalis branch of the facial nerve is avoided by keeping the incision close to the tragus. An attempt is made to preserve the superficial temporal artery.
2. A keyhole is drilled behind the zygomatic process of frontal bone to gain access to both the orbit and the anterior fossa without altering the superior orbital ridge. Resection of the orbital plate through this hole forms the inferior bony cut for inclusion of the orbital ridge with the bone flap.
3. A free frontotemporal bone flap with orbital ridge allows protection of the periorbital membrane by dissecting it from the orbital walls when the scalp flap is

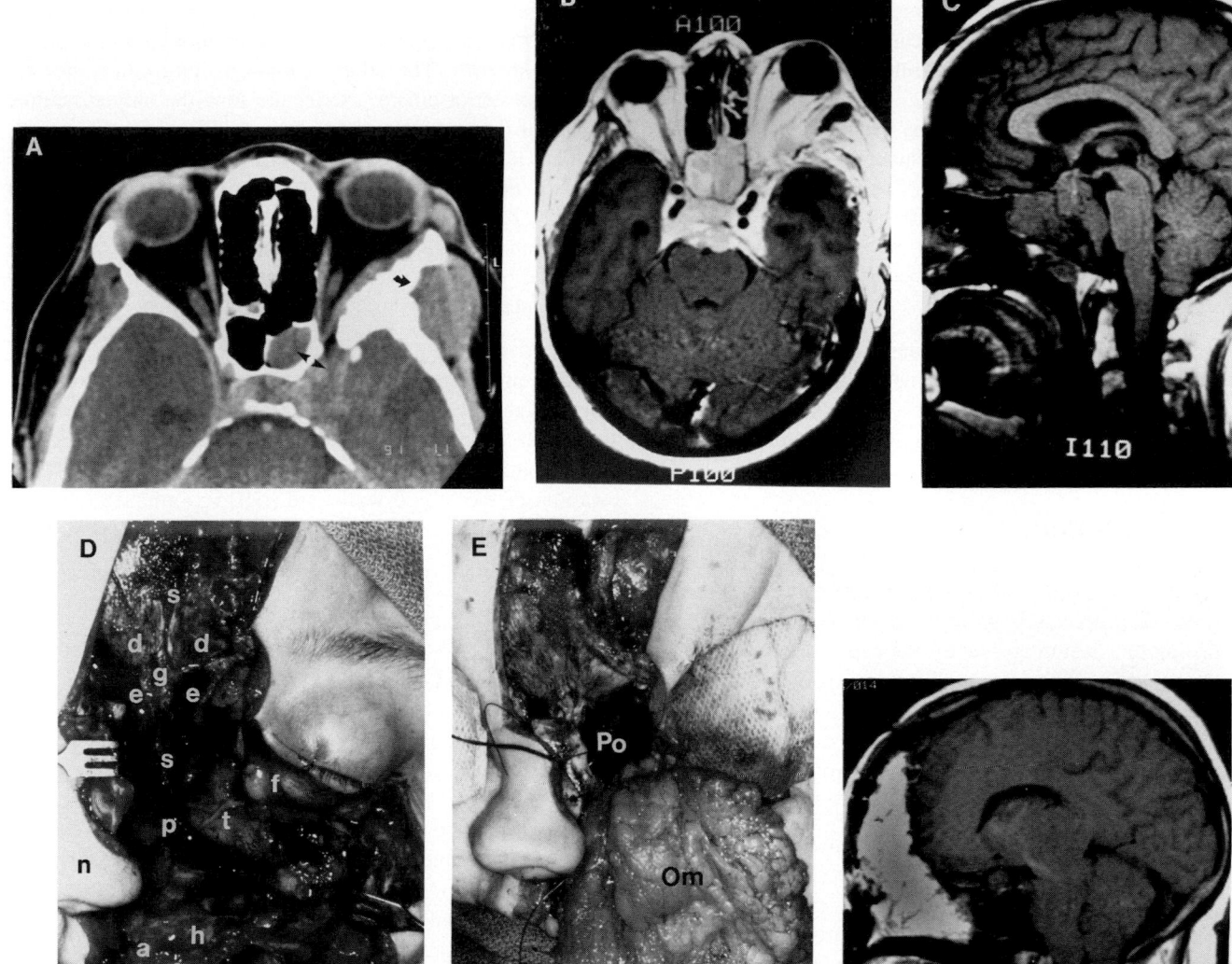

Figure 11–11 Basisphenoid invasive meningioma. A 29-year-old female with 3 months of left orbital pain and temporal headache, left ocular proptosis, and temporal swelling. **A.** CT shows thick lateral wall of orbit with bulged mass in temporalis muscle (*arrow*), small mass in sphenoid sinus, and thick medial dura (*opposing arrowheads*). *She underwent left frontal-orbital-temporal-zygomatic resection of the sphenoid wing.* She returned 1 year later with left ophthalmoplegia and recurrent proptosis. **B.** Enhanced MRI transverse cut now shows progression of tumor through the clivus into the prepontine cistern and filling the sphenoid sinus. **C.** MRI midsagittal cut shows tumor extension through the basisphenoid into the posterior fossa and nasopharynx. *Combined bifrontal orbital craniotomy and LeForte I left transmaxillo-* *orbital resection of the clival and pharyngeal tumor.* **D.** Operative photograph shows view of approach via a left paranasal midline incision (Weber-Ferguson) to the nasopharynx (s = sagittal sinus, d = frontal dura, g = crista galli, e = ethmoid sinuses, s = sphenoid sinus removed, f = orbital fat, p = nasopharynx, t = inferior turbinate, n = nose retracted, h = hard palate, a = superior alveolar ridge). **E.** Vascularized free omental graft (Om) anastomosed to the external carotid artery and external jugular vein after being tunneled over the mandible and through the maxilla to close off the gap between exposed pons (Po) and pharynx after resection of clivus. **F.** MRI midsagittal cut shows omental graft filling the sphenoid resection site.

reflected inferiorly. A Gigli saw and high-speed pneumatic drill are used to disconnect the flap at the frontal sinus medially and at the zygomatic process laterally.

4. The zygoma is separated at the maxilla and root of the arch and is removed. This exposure complements removal of the superior orbital ridge to gain exposure from the superior lateral orbit to the floor of the middle fossa with minimal retraction. The temporalis muscle is

reflected inferiorly. Alternatively, the temporalis-coronoid insertion is reflected superiorly, being attached at its origin along the superior temporal line for blood supply.

5. The sphenoid ridge is resected to the orbital fissure and anterior clinoid process. This removes the lesser wing of sphenoid and expands access to the anterior and rostral middle fossa. Since drilling of the medial portion is extradural, the position of the carotid artery and optic

nerve is heralded by the medial clinoid, a thin bony strut from the anterior clinoid, forming the lateral optic canal and medial boundary of the carotid at its emergence from the cavernous sinus, 20 mm beyond the superior orbital fissure.

6. The orbital plate is excised after separation of the periorbita. This opens the entire superior orbital expanse. Gentle orbital retraction offers further exposure of the medial anterior fossa. The orbital plate can be removed as a single piece to be later replaced, avoiding the pulsating ophthalmus that can occur if there is no intervening orbital roof.

This completes the extradural exposure ostectomies of the anterior lateral skull base. Lesions of the orbit, pterygoid space, optic canal, anterior cavernous sinus, parasellar, and sylvian fissure are visually accessible for surgical management.

ORBITAL PROCEDURES

The majority of orbital masses present with painless proptosis. When the proptosis is painful, an inflammatory, malignant, or vascular lesion is usually the cause. Loss of vision without proptosis suggests a small lesion involving the optic nerve at the orbital apex. CT, MRI, and ultrasonographic images are diagnostic. Location of the lesion determines the surgical approach. Access is planned to avoid injury to the cranial nerves by using the most direct route to the lesion.[110]

1. Completion of the optic canal and superior orbital fissure exposure is accomplished to preserve the optic nerve, which can be mobilized slightly after it has been freed from its bony confines. The periorbita is a continuation of the dura at the supraorbital ridge and superior orbital fissure.
2. The superior periorbita is opened longitudinally from the apex. Laterally, the trochlear and frontal nerves are vulnerable, coursing beneath the periorbita through the superior orbital fissure outside the relative protection of the annulus of Zinn and muscle cone. The levator superior rectus muscle complex is medial to these nerves and acts as a guide to intraorbital structures.
3. The levator and superior rectus muscles are retracted with sutures opposite to the direction of concern. The oculomotor innervation is on the ventral surface. This opens the muscle cone to lesions located in the superior orbital compartment. The superior and inferior divisions of the oculomotor nerve, the abducens, and nasociliary nerves enter through the oculomotor foramen made by the inferolateral annular ligament. These are identified and protected upon opening the annular ligament of Zinn.
4. The periorbital fat is retracted using self-retaining blade devices. This exposes deeper structures, allowing visualization of the lesion.
5. The ophthalmic artery is exposed as it crosses the optic nerve. This landmark identifies the midpoint of the or-

bital course of the optic nerve. It crosses lateral to medial, over the nerve in 70 percent and under the nerve in 30 percent of cases, forming ethmoidal and supraorbital arteries. The ciliary ganglion, long ciliary nerves, and posterior ciliary arteries are now the only structures obscuring the optic nerve.

6. The lesion is managed microsurgically according to individual requirements. Adjunctive measures such as CO_2, KPT/532, or Argon laser along with bipolar coagulation and microinstrumentation allow total excision while reducing morbidity of visual and extraocular impairment.

Orbital edema and paresis of the ocular muscles often result in ptosis and impaired ocular motility that may persist for several weeks. Neural paresis can persist for several months but also frequently recovers with time. Pulsatile ophthalmus and enophthalmus can be avoided by replacement or reconstruction of the orbital walls and roof. Extradural dissection reduces cerebral complications and avoids a CSF orbital fistula.

☐ CAVERNOUS SINUS

The cavernous sinus is no longer considered a surgical "no-man's-land," and is often approached with safety and effectiveness. Neoplastic (meningioma + neuroma) and vascular lesions (aneurysm + arteriovenous fistula) can be treated directly. Insight into the anatomical relationships of cranial nerves to the dural and venous compartments and the contained internal carotid artery (ICA) is critical for safety.[111,112] The course of the cranial nerves is an anatomical guide through this region. Masses tend to compress venous channels so that venous bleeding is minimal and controlled by local hemostatic tamponade. The key to this region is proximal and distal control of the ICA.

PREOPERATIVE PLANNING

Surgical procedures within the cavernous sinus should be planned with MRI and CT imaging. Carotid angiography with assessment of toleration of ICA occlusion determines the need for carotid bypass or reconstruction if carotid occlusion is necessary. Balloon occlusion is performed under protection of heparin anticoagulation and with cerebral blood flow and transcranial Doppler flow studies correlated with clinical assessment. Approximately 30 percent of patients will not tolerate ICA occlusion.

Alternative measures such as radiosurgery for residual tumor or stereotaxic interstitial radiation may be preferable to risks of morbidity involved with intracavernous surgery. Trap or bypass may be preferred to direct clipping for some intracavernous aneurysms.

1. The head is rotated 30° and elevated with the neck

extended. This facilitates venous drainage and assists hemostasis.

2. Bone is removed extradurally from the orbital roof, superior orbital fissure, optic canal, anterior clinoid, and the foramina rotundum-spinosum-ovale. This step is as described for the orbital exposure. A diamond drill avoids inadvertent neural and vascular injury. The more extensive resection of the sphenoid greater wing includes the foramen rotundum, foramen spinosum, and foramen ovale, and it allows access to the rostral cavernous sinus. The middle meningeal artery is occluded and transected. The second and third trigeminal divisions are exposed within their dural sheath.

3. Removal of Glasscock's triangle exposes the petrous carotid. Glasscock's triangle is a line from the foramen spinosum to the arcuate eminence laterally, the groove for the greater superficial petrosal nerve (GPN) medially, and the third trigeminal division at the base. Cutting the GPN here avoids transmitting traction to the geniculate ganglion and facial paresis. This unroofs the lateral loop of the petrous carotid artery. Avoid drilling posterior to the carotid canal at the vertical carotid, which risks injury to the cochlea. This gives proximal control of the cavernous carotid artery as well as access to the caudal cavernous sinus.

4. A frontotemporal transverse dural opening exposes the carotid cistern; the intracranial ICA is fully dissected to the carotid bifurcation. A wide dissection of the arachnoidal compartments of the carotid and chiasmatic cisterns ensures distal carotid control and mobility.

5. The two fibrous rings anchoring the emerging ICA are dissected. The segment of ICA beneath the clinoid is between the fibrous ring of emergence from the cavernous sinus and the fibrous ring of intracranial emergence from the basal dura. Separation of the ICA from the adjacent attachments of these two rings frees the ICA for entry into the anterior cavernous sinus.

6. The dura is incised rostrally along the course just medial to the oculomotor nerve. This opens the superior lateral cavernous sinus and exposes the anterior loop of ICA, which is crossed laterally by the oculomotor nerve. Care is taken to avoid injury to the trochlear nerve.

7. The trochlear nerve is dissected along its course to the orbital fissure. This extends the exposure of the lateral wall of the cavernous sinus. The trochlear nerve crosses over the oculomotor nerve as they both enter the superior orbital fissure, and both are vulnerable to injury here.

8. The ophthalmic division of the trigeminal nerve (V_1) is dissected. The second trigeminal division (V_2), previously identified at the foramen rotundum and dissected proximally toward Meckel's cave, assists in exposing V_1. Exposure of the V_1 course identifies the lower border of Parkinson's triangle and frees the entire lateral wall.

9. Interface of a lesion with the wall of the ICA is established. This completes the goal of exposure of the cavernous sinus. Contingencies for management of the ICA and lesion must be preplanned.

CAROTID RECONSTRUCTION AND WOUND CLOSURE

1. Temporary clips are applied to the intracranial ICA proximal and distal to the posterior communicating artery, ophthalmic artery, and proximal ICA. This isolates carotid flow for management. The common carotid is released to allow ongoing external carotid flow.

2. The ICA is bypassed or reconstituted using a saphenous vein graft. As much as 2 h of carotid occlusion may be necessary. Protection of the brain is accomplished with parenteral dexamethasone, 20 mg q 4 h, with pentothal given to produce burst suppression on the electroencephalogram (EEG). Profound hypothermia with cardiac bypass is an alternative.

3. The saphenous vein is harvested from the groin. The saphenous vein from the groin matches the ICA for size. It is oriented for direction of flow. The distal end of the graft to be joined to the supraclinoid ICA is beveled to prevent kinking or twisting. It is flushed with cold heparinized saline. Interrupted sutures of 7-0 proline on B-V1 needle are used for anastomosis of the posterior lateral wall of supraclinoid to the proximal ICA. The proximal ICA anastomosis is performed prior to the distal.

4. The temporary clips are released to reestablish carotid flow. The ophthalmic artery trial release will show leaks in anastomosis. Next the proximal supraclinoid ICA releases posterior communicating artery flow through the ophthalmic artery and anastomosis. The distal ICA is released and collateral carotid flow is reestablished. Leaks at the anastomosis are bolstered with topical microfibrillar collagen.

5. The eustachian tube is plugged proximally with cottonoid and muscle. The eustachian tube is always opened when the petrous ICA is exposed. Plugging it prevents CSF rhinorrhea via this route.

6. The dura is closed using fascia or dural allograft along the base. A temporal myofascial flap inversion can close a large defect along the cranial floor.

7. Exposed ostectomy grafts are replaced and secured by wire twists or miniplates. Replacement of supraorbital ridge and zygomatic arch preserves the contours needed for a satisfactory cosmetic result.

☐ LATERAL APPROACH TO THE SKULL BASE

Tumors located at the petrous apex, pterygoid fossa, infralabyrinthine, and jugular foraminal region require extensive extracranial and intracranial dissection. Anterolateral and posterior approaches do not allow sufficient visualization of structures to excise the muscles. The expertise of otolaryngology is needed to manage this approach. Large paraganglioma or glomus jugulare tumors require this approach: Fisch class C tumors arising in the dome of the jugular bulb and extending through adjacent bone to involve the extracranial skull base and class D tumors that have intracranial extension (both extradural and intradural).[113–116]

INFRATEMPORAL PETROSAL APPROACH TO PARASELLAR CLIVUS

1a. A retroauricular incision is carried to the anterior cervical triangle. This incision is used when the lesion involves retrojugular and posterior fossa structures requiring suboccipital craniectomy, the external ear canal is sutured closed to reduce bacterial contamination.

1b. A coronal and preauricular incision is extended to the anterior cervical region. This incision is used when the posterior fossa is not involved.

2. A scalp-skin flap is reflected forward and the external ear canal transected.

3. The extracranial facial nerve is dissected from the foramen through the parotid gland. This is the initial phase for anterior relocation of the facial nerve.

4. The sternocleidomastoid and digastric muscles are transected at the mastoid tip. This initiates the exposure of the cranial nerves and major vessels.

5. The hypoglossal, spinal accessory, and vagus nerves are dissected.

6. The jugular vein at jugular foramen and the ICA are dissected.

7. The ECA, pharyngeal, and occipital arteries are exposed and transected. This interrupts some blood supply to the tumor.

8. The zygomatic arch is removed and the temporalis muscle is reflected forward. This prepares the field for temporal and mastoid bone removal.

9. The sigmoid sinus and facial nerve are exposed, using microsurgical drilling.

10. The external ear canal along with the tympanic membrane and middle ear are removed.

11. A mastoidectomy is performed, exposing, ligating, and transecting the sigmoid sinus. This frees the tumor extent posteriorly and initiates entrance to the jugular bulb. Venous drainage is previously assessed.

12. The facial nerve is freed from the mastoid canal. The labyrinth is preserved. Care is taken along the tympanic portion of the nerve to avoid injury to the lateral semicircular canal. The facial nerve can now be moved anteriorly, thus displacing it away from the carotid canal. The eustachian tube identifies the medial border of the carotid canal.

13. The ICA is exposed in the petrous carotid canal lateral to the eustachian tube. The carotid canal is drilled laterally to the carotid foramen. This gains proximal control of the ICA and completes the posterior subtemporal middle fossa exposure. The foregoing can be added to anterolateral approaches when proximal control of ICA is needed intracranially rather than at the cervical carotid level.

14. The corticotympanic artery is identified and transected. This is the major ICA blood supply to a paraganglioma tumor mass.

15. The styloid process is removed and the cervical jugular vein ligated. The bone overlying the jugular bulb is drilled away, exposing it.

16. The jugular bulb is opened, exposing the tumor, and the inferior petrosal sinus is plugged. Removal of the tumor mass completes the exposure-resection using the Fisch Type A infratemporal approach to the jugular foramen. A temporal muscle flap is rotated into the defect before closure.

The Fisch Type B infratemporal approach to the clivus involves a medial extension of the procedure described. It is extracranial and requires disarticulation or removal of the mandibular condyle.

The Fisch Type C infratemporal approach to the parasellar region involves extension of the procedure rostrally along the subtemporal region. This is a variation of the anterolateral exposure previously described, but this is from an extracranial perspective.[113]

1. The temporal muscle and coronoid process attachment are reflected upward. This exposes the pterygoid fossa.

2. The base of the pterygoid process is resected by drilling. This allows rostral exposure of the petrous carotid coursing toward the cavernous sinus.

3. The mandibular and maxillary divisions of the trigeminal nerve are exposed. These may even be electively transected to facilitate ICA exposure and translocation, for tumor removal from the medial pterygoid fossa.

☐ COMBINED SUBTEMPORAL SUBOCCIPITAL TRANSTENTORIAL APPROACH

The wide translabyrinthine or retrolabyrinthine lateral temporal bone resection combined with a low subtemporal craniotomy affords access to the brainstem, superior cerebellum, and cerebellopontine angle. Care is taken to dissect the vein of Labbé so as to avoid tearing it and causing a venous infarct. This is a quite useful and widely accepted approach for tumors along the petrous apex and posterior cavernous sinus. Dissection of the posterior petrous wall and complete tentorial transection are critical to adequate exposure. The superior petrosal sinus is a guide.[117–119]

FAR LATERAL TRANSCONDYLAR APPROACH TO CLIVUS

Extensive bone resection of the squamous suboccipital bone, along with the posterior arch of C1 and superior edge of the C2, combined with resection of the posterior and medial thirds of the occipital condyle gives access to the basi-occiput of the clivus and ventral brainstem with minimal cerebellar retraction. The vertebral artery is "skeletonized" and can be moved from its position if needed. This is the preferred approach for meningioma on the anterior lip of the foramen magnum. A disadvantage is that the dissection must deal with the perivertebral artery venous plexus. Also the lower cranial nerves, draped over the posterior tumor surface, are vulnerable to surgical trauma.[120,121]

CLOSURE AND RECONSTRUCTION

Large defects require myofascial flap rotations or free composite grafts with microvascular anastomosis to cover dural exposure to the pharynx or pericranial sinuses. The eustachian tube is occluded to prevent a CSF fistula and pneumocephalus.

SUMMARY

The anterior, orbital, and lateral skull base approaches have been detailed in a stepwise fashion, with anatomical and technical notations cited.

RADIONEUROSURGERY

This is a therapeutic alternative to open surgical procedures for selected extra-axial neoplasms.

DEFINITION

It is essentially destruction or interruption of a precisely defined and stereotactically determined three-dimensional intracranial target using a multidirectional controlled beam of high-energy radiation stereotactically centered to the target, delivered in a single dose.

HISTORY

Lars Leksell of Sweden was the first to conceive, design, and produce instrumentation that allowed stereotactically directed radiosurgery to be accomplished. The method destroys tissue within the brain without mechanically entering it. He used several modes of radiation energy including x-ray, positrons, and gamma rays. He worked with the radiation physicist and therapist Bjorn Larsson and finally settled on gamma radiation from cobalt 60 in the form of multiple sources housed in a fixed shield. The sources are angled and columnated so that the multiple narrow beams intersect in an isocenter. The shield housing is integrated with the Leksell stereotactic instrument. The size of the lesion can be varied by using different sized columnators in the steel helmet that integrates the Leksell frame to the cobalt 60 shield housing. He named it the "gamma knife," emphasizing the surgical aspects of this device.[122]

This method has been used clinically at the Karolinska hospital in Stockholm since 1956. Initially lesions were accomplished in deep-brain structures for treatment of physiologic abnormalities. This required small $5 \times 8 \times 5$ mm lesions precisely targeted in the thalamus or brainstem. When the surgical treatment of Parkinson's disease gave way to medical treatment with dopamine, stereotactic surgery declined. Leksell then adapted the gamma knife for treatment of anatomical lesions such as AVMs and selected tumors. The lesion produced was enlarged to a maximum of 25 mm in diameter. The Leksell instrument can be adapted for stereotactic angiography. Using orthogonally centered radiography with the patient mounted in the stereotactic frame, the dimensions of the AVM can be determined in three dimensions relative to reference points on the frame. If the size of the AVM is within 50 percent isodose limit of the radiosurgical beam, the AVM can be irradiated with a tissue-destructive dose of radiation 25 Gy (2500 rad). The tissue absorption falloff is sharp so that normal cerebral tissues beyond the 50-percent isodose line are not significantly affected by the radiation. This results in gradual obliteration of the AVM over 1 to 2 years. Similar results are noted when this procedure is applied to small localized tumors such as acoustic neuromas.[123,124]

Development of improved imaging technology with CT in the 1970s and MRI in the 1980s allowed noninvasive imaging of intracranial structures. Stereotactic instrumentation was soon adapted to these imaging techniques. This had led to a resurgence of stereotactic surgery. Emphasis has been on anatomical structures since these are displayed. Deep-seated intracranial lesions are now commonly approached stereotactically for biopsy, aspiration, and implantation of treatment modalities, i.e., radioisotopes.[24,125]

Adaptation of linear accelerators (LINACs) to radiosurgery technique evolved in the 1970s. This requires precise mechanical coordination between the moving gantry, the patient support system (couch or chair), and columnation of the exiting proton beam. Isocentering and calibration require computerized control. Most centers have developed computer programs for control of the system as well as isodose curves of tissue absorption of radiation energy and three-dimensional construction of the target in reference to the stereotactic instrumentation. Computerized systems have proved to be effective, precise, and reliable. The advantage of these techniques was in the employment of linear accelerators already in use for conventional radiotherapy. By adapting them for stereotactic radiosurgery the major capital expense of a new radiation source hardware was avoided.[126–129]

TECHNIQUE

The technical aspects of stereotactic surgery are described in Chap. 23.

RADIATION SOURCES

1. Cyclotron.
2. Proton beam from a linear accelerator on a fixed center rotational gantry aimed through variably sized columnators.
3. Gamma radiation from multiple sources of Cobalt[60]

housed, shielded, fixed, and directed by variably sized calumniators aimed to a fixed isocenter.

NEOPLASMS AMENABLE FOR TREATMENT

1. Meningiomas
2. Acoustic or trigeminal neuromas
3. Recurrent pituitary adenomas
4. Solid residuals of craniopharyngiomas
5. Hemangioblastomas
6. Glomus jugulare chemodectomas (small)
7. Histologically malignant, sharply localized tumors
8. Metastatic carcinomas (single or multiple)
9. Selected gliomas (thalamus or brainstem)

Radioneurosurgery may also be used to create anatomical physiological lesions for pain and movement disorders (see Chaps. 24 and 25).

REFERENCES

1. Karnofsky DA, Burchendl JH, Armstead GC, et al: Triethylene melamine in the treatment of neoplastic disease. *Arch Intern Med* 87:477–516, 1951.
2. Al-Rodhan NRF, Laws ER, Jr: Meningioma: A historical study of the tumor and its surgical management. *Neurosurgery* 26:832–847, 1990.
3. Bakay L: Cruveilhier on meningiomas (1829–1842). *Surg Neurol* 32:159–164, 1989.
4. Rohringer M, Sutherland GR, Louw DF, Sima AF: Incidence and clinicopathological features of meningiomas. *J Neurosurg* 71:665–672, 1989.
5. Russell DS, Rubinstein LJ: *Pathology of Tumors of the Nervous System,* 4th ed. Baltimore, Williams & Wilkins, 1977, chap 3, pp 48–73.
6. Go KG, Wilmink JT, Molenaar WM: Peritumoral brain edema associated with meningiomas. *Neurosurgery* 23:175–179, 1988.
7. Benzel EC, Gelder FB: Correlation between sex hormone binding and peritumoral edema in intracranial meningiomas. *Neurosurgery* 22:169–174, 1988.
8. Halper J, Colvard DS, Scheithauer BW, et al: Estrogen and progesterone receptors in meningiomas: Comparison of nuclear binding, dextran-coated charcoal and immunoperoxidase staining assays. *Neurosurgery* 25:546–553, 1989.
9. Waelti ER, Markwalder TM: Immunocytochemical evidence of progesterone receptors in human meningiomas. *Surg Neurol* 31:172–176, 1989.
10. Schrell UMH, Adams EF, Fahlbusch R, et al: Hormonal dependency of cerebral meningiomas. I. Female sex steroid receptors and their significance as specific markers for adjuvant medical therapy. *J Neurosurg* 73:743–749, 1990.
11. Al-Mefty O: Clinoidal meningiomas. *J Neurosurg* 73:840–849, 1990.
12. Bonnal J, Thibaut A, Brotchi J, et al: Invading meningiomas of the sphenoid ridge. *J Neurosurg* 53:587–599, 1980.
13. Kinjo T, Al-Mefty O, Kanaan I: Grade zero removal of supratentorial convexity meningiomas. *Neurosurgery* 33:394–399, 1993.
13a. Penfield W: Personal communication.
14. Ng TH, Chan KH, Leung SY, et al: An unusual complication of silastic dural substitute: Case report. *Neurosurgery* 27:491–493, 1990.
15. Jaaskelainen J, Haltia M, Servo A: Atypical anaplastic meningiomas: Radiology, surgery, and outcome. *Surg Neurol* 25:233–242, 1986.
16. Simpson D: The recurrence of intracranial meningiomas after surgical treatment. *J Neurol Neurosurg Psychiatry* 20:22–39, 1957.
17. Lee KS, Hoshino T, Rodriguez LA, et al: Bromodeoxyuridine labeling study of intracranial meningiomas: Proliferative potential and recurrence. *Acta Neuropathol* 80:311–317, 1990.
18. May PL, Broome JC, Lawry J, et al: The prediction of recurrence in meningiomas. A flow cytometric study of paraffin-embedded archival material. *J Neurosurg* 71:347–351, 1989.
19. Benedict WF, Porter IH, Brown CD, et al. Cytogenic diagnosis of malignancy in recurrent meningioma. *Lancet* 1:971–973, 1970.
20. Thomas HG, Dolman CL, Berry K: Malignant meningioma: Clinical and pathological features. *J Neurosurg* 55:929–934, 1981.
21. Thibodeau LL, Ariza A, Piepmeier JM: Primary leptomeningeal sarcomatosis. *J Neurosurg* 68:802–805, 1988.
22. Wara WM, Sheline GE, Newman H, et al: Radiation therapy of meningiomas. *AJR* 123:453–458, 1975.
23. Petty AM, Kun LE, Meyer GA: Radiation therapy for incom-

pletely resected meningiomas. *J Neurosurg* 62:502–507, 1985.

24. Kumar PP, Patil AA, Leibrock LG, et al: Brachytherapy: A viable alternative in the management of basal meningiomas. *Neurosurgery* 29:676–680, 1991.

25. Horie Y, Akagi S, Taguchi K, et al: Malignant schwannoma arising in the intracranial trigeminal nerve. A report of an autopsy case and a review of the literature. *Acta Path Jpn* 40:219–225, 1990.

26. Del Priore LV, Miller NR: Trigeminal schwannoma as a cause of chronic, isolated sixth nerve palsy. *Am J Ophthalmol* 108:726–729, 1989.

27. Bordi L, Compton J, Symon L: Trigeminal neuroma. A report of eleven cases. *Surg Neurol* 31:272–276, 1989.

28. Faucett DC, Dutton JJ, Bullard DE: Gasserian ganglion schwannoma with orbital extension. *Ophthal Plast Reconstr Surg* 5:235–238, 1989.

29. Al-Mefty O, Smith RR: Surgery of tumors invading the cavernous sinus. *Surg Neurol* 30:370–381, 1988.

30. Celli P, Ferrants L, Acqui M, et al: Neurinoma of the third, fourth, and sixth cranial nerves: A survey and report of a new fourth nerve case. *Surg Neurol* 38:216–224, 1992.

31. Geysens P, D'Haenens P, Van Steenberge R, et al: Familial occurrence of paragangliomas. *J Belge Radiol* 72:95–99, 1989.

32. Jackson CG, Gulya AJ, Knox GW, et al: A paraneoplastic syndrome associated with glomus tumors of the skull base? Early observations. *Otolaryngol Head Neck Surg* 100:583–587, 1989.

33. Johnstone PA, Foss RD, Desilets DJ: Malignant jugulotympanic paraganglioma. *Arch Pathol Lab Med* 114:976–979, 1990.

34. Phelps PD, Cheesman AD: Imaging jugulotympanic glomus tumors. *Arch Otolaryngol Head Neck Surg* 116:940–945, 1990.

35. Springate SC, Weichselbaum RR: Radiation or surgery for chemodectoma of the temporal bone: A review of local control and complications. *Head Neck* 12:303–307, 1990.

36. Murphy TP; Brackmann DE: Effects of preoperative embolization on glomus jugulare tumors. *Laryngoscope* 99:1244–1247, 1989.

37. Leonetti JP, Brackmann DE, Prass RL: Improved preservation of facial nerve function in the infratemporal approach to the skull base. *Otolaryngol Head Neck Surg* 101:74–78, 1989.

38. Costantino PD, Friedman CD, Pelzer HJ: Neurofibromatosis type II of the head and neck. *Arch Otolaryngol Head Neck Surg* 115:380–383, 1989.

39. Mulvihill JJ, Parry DM, Sherman JL, et al: NIH conference. Neurofibromatosis 1 (Recklinghausen's disease) and neurofibromatosis 2 (bilateral acoustic neurofibromatosis). An update. *Ann Intern Med* 113:39–52, 1990.

40. Brill CB: Neurofibromatosis. Clinical overview. *Clin Orthop* 245:10–15, 1989.

41. Samuelsson B, Riccardi VM: Neurofibromatosis in Gothenburg, Sweden. III. Psychiatric and social aspects. *Neurofibromatosis* 2:84–106, 1989.

42. Senveli E, Altinors N, Kars Z, et al: Associations of von Recklinghausen's neurofibromatosis and aqueduct stenosis (see comments): *Neurosurgery* 25:318–319, 1989.

43. Pou-Serradell A, Ugarte-Elola AC: Hydrocephalus in neurofibromatosis. Contribution of magnetic resonance imaging to its diagnosis, control and treatment. *Neurofibromatosis* 2:218–226, 1989.

44. Mirowitz SA, Sartor K, Gado M: High-intensity basal ganglia lesions on T1-weighted MR images in neurofibromatosis. *Am J Roentgenol* 154:369–373, 1990.

45. Baldwin D, King TT, Chevertton E, et al: Bilateral cerebello-

pontine angle tumors in neurofibromatosis type 2. *J Neurosurg* 74:910–915, 1991.

46. Glasscock ME III, Woods CI, Jackson CG, et al: Management of bilateral acoustic tumors. *Laryngoscope* 99:475–484, 1989.

47. Linskey ME, Lunsford LD, Flickinger JC: Radiosurgery for acoustic neurinomas: Early experience. *Neurosurgery* 26:736–744, 1990.

48. Virchow R: Die Entwicklung des Schadelgrundes. Berlin, G. Zeimer, 1857, pp 57, 127.

49. Muller H. Ueber das Vorkommen von Resten der Chorda dorsalis bei Menschen nach der Geburt und uber ihr Verhaltniss zu den Gallertgeschwulsten am Clivus. *Zischr f Rationelle Med* 2:202–227, 1858.

50. Heaton JM, Turner DR: Reflections on notochord differentiation arising from a study of chordomas. *Histopathology* 9:543–550, 1985.

51. Congdon CC: Benign and malignant chordomas: A clinicoanatomical study of 22 cases. *Am J Pathol* 28:793–821, 1952.

52. Horowitz T: *Human notochord: A study of its development and regression, variation, and pathologic derivative, chordoma.* Indianapolis, private printing, 1977.

53. Beaugie JM, Mann CV, Butler ECB: Sacrococcygeal chordoma. *Brit J Surg* 56:586–588, 1969.

54. Wright D: Nasopharyngeal and cervical chordoma. Some aspects of their development and treatment. *J Laryngol Otol* 81:1337–1355, 1967.

55. Mirra J, Picci P, Gold H: *Bone Tumors: Clinical, Radiologic, and Pathologic Correlations.* Lea & Febiger, 1989, vol 2, pp 648–672.

56. MacCarty CS, Waugh JM, Coventry MB, et al: Sacrococcygeal chordomas. *Surg Gynecol Obstet* 113:551–554, 1961.

57. Sundaresan N, Galicich JH, Chu FCH, et al: Spinal chordomas. *J Neurosurg* 50:312–319, 1979.

58. Sundaresan N: Chordomas. *Clin Orthop Related Res* 204:135–142, 1986.

59. Sen CN, Sekhar LN, Schramm VL, et al: Chordoma and chondrosarcoma of the cranial base: An 8 year experience. *Neurosurgery* 25:931–941, 1989.

60. Azzarelli A, Quagliuolo V, Cerasoli S, et al: Chordoma: Natural history and treatment results in 33 cases. *J Surg Oncol* 37:185–191, 1988.

61. Hansen PH, Rasmussen LB: Chordoma. *Spine* 8:802–803, 1983.

62. Kamrin RP, Potanos JN, Pool JL: An evaluation of the diagnosis and treatment of chordoma. *J Neurol Neurosurg Psychiatry* 27:157–165, 1964.

63. Paavolainen P, Teppo L: Chordoma in Finland. *Acta Orthop Scand* 47:46–51, 1976.

64. Smith J, Ludwig RL, Marcove RC: Sacrococcygeal chordoma: A clinicoradiological study of 60 patients. *Skeletal Radiol* 16:37–44, 1987.

65. Bouropoulou V, Bosse A, Roessner A, et al: Immunohistochemical investigation of chordomas: Histologic and differential diagnostic aspects. *Current Topics Pathol* 80:183–203, 1989.

66. Rosenthal DI, Scott JA, Mankin HJ, et al: Sacrococcygeal chordoma: Magnetic resonance imaging and computed tomography. *Am J Roentgenol* 145:143–147, 1985.

67. Pettersson H, Hudon T, Hamlin D, et al: Magnetic resonance imaging of sacrococcygeal tumors. *Acta Radiol Diagn (Stockholm)* 26:161–165, 1985.

68. Yuh WTC, Lozano RL, Flickinger FW, et al: Lumbar epidural chordoma: MR findings. *J Comput Assist Tomogr* 13:508–510, 1989.

69. Sundaresan N, Rosenthal DI, Schiller AL, et al: Chordomas, in Sundaresan N, Schmidek HH, Schiller AL, Rosenthal DI

(eds): *Tumors of the Spine, Diagnosis and Clinical Management.* Philadelphia, Saunders, 1990, pp 192–213.

70. Dahlin DC, MacCarty CS: Chordoma a study of fifty-nine cases. *Cancer* 5:1170–1178, 1952.

71. Turner ML, Mulheren CB, Dalinka MK: Lesions of the sacrum. Differential diagnosis and radiological evaluation. *JAMA* 245:275–277, 1981.

72. Crawford T: The staining reactions of chordoma. *J Clin Pathol* 11:110–113, 1958.

73. Erlandson RA, Tandler B, Lieberman PH, et al: Ultrastructure of human chordoma. *Cancer Research* 28:2115–2125, 1968.

74. Chambers PW, Schwinn CP: Chordoma: A clinicopathologic study of metastasis. *Am J Clin Pathol* 72:765–776, 1979.

75. Kasantikul V, Shuangshoti S: Positivity to glial fibrillary acidic protein in bone, cartilage, and chordoma. *J Surg Oncol* 41:22–26, 1989.

76. Knechtges TC: Sacrococcygeal chordoma with sarcomatous features (spindle cell metaplasia). *Am J Clin Pathol* 53:612–616, 1970.

77. Cummings BJ, Hodson DI, Bush RS: Chordoma: The results of megavoltage radiation therapy. *Int J Radiation Oncol Biol Phys* 9:633–642, 1983.

78. Chetiyawardana AD: Chordoma: Results of treatment. *Clin Radiol* 35:159–161, 1984.

79. Tewfix HH, McGinnis WL, Nordstrum DG, et al: Chordoma. Evaluation of clinical behavior and treatment modalities. *Int J Radiat Oncol Biol Phys* 2:959–962, 1977.

80. Fuller DB, Bloom JG: Radiotherapy for chordoma. *Int J Radiation Oncol Biol Phys* 15:331–339, 1988.

81. Jane JA, Park TS, Pobereskin LH, et al: The supraorbital approach: Technical note. *Neurosurgery* 11:537–542, 1982.

82. Al-Mefty O: Supraorbital-pterional approach to skull base lesions. *Neurosurgery* 21:474–477, 1987.

83. Ketcham AS, Hoye RC, Van Buren JM, et al: Complications of intracranial facial resection for tumors of the paracranial sinuses. *Am J Surg* 112:591–596, 1966.

84. McCallum J, Maroon JC, Jannetta PJ: Treatment of postoperative cerebralspinal fluid fistulas by subarachnoid drainage. *J Neurosurg* 42:434–437, 1975.

85. Schramm VL Jr: Craniofacial resection, in Sasaki CT, McCabe BF, Kirchner JA (eds): *Surgery of the Skull Base.* Philadelphia, Lippincott, 1984, pp 43–61.

86. Blacklock JB, Weber RS, Lee YY, et al: Transcranial resection of tumors of the paranasal sinuses and nasal cavity. *J Neurosurg* 71:10–15, 1989.

87. Persing JA, Jane JA, Levine PA, et al: The versatile frontal sinus approach to the floor of the anterior cranial fossa. Technical note. *J Neurosurg* 72:513–516, 1990.

88. Lalwani AK, Kaplan MJ, Gutin PH: The transphenoethmoid approach to the sphenoid sinus and clivus. *Neurosurgery* 31:1008–1014, 1992.

89. Tessier P, Guiot G, Rougerie J, et al: Osteotomies, cranio-naso-orbitofasciales pour hypertelorism. *Ann Chir Plast* 12:103, 1967.

90. Belmont JR: The Le Fort I osteotomy approach for nasopharyngeal and nasal fossa tumors. *Arch Otolaryngol Head Neck Surg* 114:571–574, 1988.

91. Utley D, Moore A, Archer DJ: Surgical management of midline skull-base tumors: a new approach. *J Neurosurg* 71:705–710, 1989.

92. Sandor GK, Charles DA, Lawson VG, et al: Transoral approach to the nasopharynx and clivus using the Le Fort I osteotomy with mid palatal split. *Int J Oral Maxillofac Surg* 19:352–355, 1990.

93. Fujitsu K, Saijoh M, Aoki F, et al: Telecanthal approach for meningiomas in the ethmoid and sphenoid sinuses. *Neurosurgery* 28:714–720, 1991.

94. Kawakami K, Yamanouchi Y, Kubota C, et al: An extensive transbasal approach to frontal skull-base tumors. Technical note. *J Neurosurg* 74:1011–1013, 1991.

95. Spetzler RF, Pappas CTE: Management of anterior skull base tumors. *Clin Neurosurg* 37:490–501, 1991.

96. Arriaga MA, Janecka IP: Facial translocation approach to the cranial base: The anatomic basis. *Skull Base Surg* 1:26–33, 1991.

97. Anand VK, Harkey HL, Al-Mefty O: Open-door maxillotomy approach for lesions of the clivus. *Skull Base Surg* 1:217–225, 1991.

98. Rabadan A, Conesa H: Transmaxillary-transnasal approach to the anterior clivus: A microsurgical anatomical model. *Neurosurgery* 30:473–482, 1992.

99. Origitano TC, Al-Mefty O, Leonetti JP, et al: *En bloc* resection of an ethmoid carcinoma involving the orbit and medial wall of the cavernous sinus. *Neurosurgery* 31:1126–1131, 1992.

100. Johns ME, Winn R, McLean WC, et al: Pericranial flap for closure of defects of craniofacial resections. *Laryngoscope* 91:952–958, 1981.

101. Arita N, Mori S, Sano M, et al: Surgical treatment of tumors in the anterior skull base using the transbasal approach. *Neurosurgery* 24:379–384, 1989.

102. Elkon D, Hightower SI, Lim ML, et al: Esthesioneuroblastoma. *Cancer* 44:1087–1094, 1979.

103. Barrow DL, Nahia F, Tindall GT: The use of the greater omentum vascularized free flaps for neurosurgical disorders requiring reconstruction. *J Neurosurg* 60:305–311, 1984.

104. Yamaki T, Uede T, Tano-oka A, et al: Vascularized omentum graft for the reconstruction of the skull base after removal of a nasoethmoidal tumor with intracranial extension: Case report. *Neurosurgery* 28:877–880, 1991.

105. Yasargil MG, Antic J, Laciga R, et al: Microsurgical pterional approach to aneurysms of the basilar bifurcation. *Surg Neurol* 6:83–91, 1976.

106. Long DM, Rhoton AL: The pterional approach in aneurysm surgery (part II), in Hopkins LN, Long DM (eds): *Clinical Management of Intracranial Aneurysms.* New York, Raven Press, 1982, pp 245–262.

107. Hakuba A, Liu SS, Nishimura S: The orbitozygomatic infratemporal approach: A new surgical technique. *Surg Neurol* 26:271–276, 1986.

108. Hassler W, Zentner J: Pterional approach for surgical treatment of olfactory groove meningiomas. *Neurosurgery* 25:942–947, 1989.

109. Close LG, Mickey BE, Samson DS, et al: Resection of upper aerodigestive tract tumors involving the middle cranial fossa. *Laryngoscope* 95:908–914, 1985.

110. Housepian EM: Microsurgical anatomy of the orbital apex and principles of transcranialorbital exploration. *Clin Neurosurg* 25:556–573, 1978.

111. Parkinson D: A surgical approach to the cavernous portion of the carotid artery. Anatomical studies and case report. *J Neurosurg* 23:474–487, 1965.

112. Harris FS, Rhoton AL Jr: Anatomy of the cavernous sinus: A microsurgical study. *J Neurosurg* 45:169–180, 1976.

113. Fisch U: Classification of glomus temporale tumors, in Fisch U, Mattox D (eds): *Microsurgery of the Skull Base.* New York, Thieme, 1988, pp 149–152.

114. Fisch U, Oldring DJ, Senning A: Surgical therapy of internal carotid artery lesion of the skull base and temporal bone. *Otolaryngol Head Neck Surg* 88:548–554, 1980.

115. Goldenberg RA: Surgeon's view of the skull base from the lateral approach. *Laryngoscope Suppl 36* 94:1–21, 1984.

116. Pellet W, Cannoni M, Pech A: The widened transcochlear approach to jugular foramen. *J Neurosurg* 69:887–894, 1988.

117. Kawase T, Shiobara R, Toya S: Anterior transpetrosal-transtentorial approach for sphenopetroclival meningiomas:

Surgical method and results in 10 patients. *Neurosurgery* 28:869–876, 1991.

118. Spetzler RF, Daspit CP, Pappas CTE: The combined supra- and infratentorial approach for lesions of the petrous and clivus regions: Experience with 46 cases. *J Neurosurg* 76:588–599, 1992.

119. Ammirati M, Ma J, Cheatham ML, et al: Drilling the posterior wall of the petrous pyramid: a microneurosurgical anatomical study. *J Neurosurg* 78:452–455, 1993.

120. Heros RC: Lateral suboccipital approach for vertebral and vertebrobasilar artery lesions. *J Neurosurg* 64:559–562, 1986.

121. Spetzler RF, Grahm TW: The far-lateral approach to the inferior clivus and the upper cervical region: Technical note. *BNI Quarterly* 6:35–38, 1990.

122. Leksell L: Stereotactic radiosurgery. *J Neurol Neurosurg Psychiatry* 46:797–803, 1983.

123. Steiner L: Stereotactic radiosurgery with the ^{60}Cobalt gamma in the surgical treatment of intracranial tumors and arteriovenous malformations, in Schmidek HH, Sweet WH (eds): *Operative Neurosurgical Techniques.* Orlando, Grune and Stratton, 1988, pp 515–530.

124. Lunsford LD, Flickinger J, Linder G, et al: Stereotactic radiosurgery of the brain using the first United States 201 cobalt-60 source gamma knife. *Neurosurgery* 24:151–159, 1989.

125. Mundinger F, Ostertag C, Birg W, et al: Stereotactic treatment of brain lesions; biopsy, interstitial radiotherapy (iridium 192 and iodine-125) and drainage procedures. *Appl Neurophysiol* 43:1988–204, 1980.

126. Winston KR, Lutz W: Linear accelerator as a neurosurgical tool for stereotactic radiosurgery. *Neurosurgery* 22:454–464, 1988.

127. Friedman WA, Bova FJ: The University of Florida radiosurgery system. *Surg Neurol* 32:334–342, 1989.

128. Luxton G, Petrovich Z, Jozef G, et al: Stereotactic radiosurgery: Principles and comparison of treatment methods. *Neurosurgery* 32:241–259, 1993.

129. Duma CM, Lunsford LD, Kondziolka D, et al: Stereotactic radiosurgery of cavernous sinus meningiomas as an addition or alternative to microsurgery. *Neurosurgery* 32:699–705, 1993.

☐ STUDY QUESTIONS

I. A 46-year-old female is referred because of pain in the right forehead, blindness, proptosis, and paresis of movements of the right eye for one year. A CT scan shows a large mass in the medial third of the sphenoid wing, involving the anterior cavernous sinus and posterior orbit.

1. What is the most likely diagnosis? **2.** How should the lesion be approached? **3.** What is the explanation for pain in the forehead? **4.** What is the most dangerous part of a therapeutic operation for this patient? **5.** What therapeutic procedures other than surgery might be considered?

II. A 33-year-old female has noted loss of hearing in her right ear for about 6 months. She is now experiencing pain in the right occipital area. Examination reveals loss of hearing and a diminished corneal reflex on the right. An MRI shows a mass 2½ cm in diameter in the right cerebellopontine angle.

1. What is the likely diagnosis? **2.** What other lesion could be considered? **3.** What would tomograms of the petrous ridges likely show? **4.** How should the lesion be approached? **5.** Where is the seventh nerve likely to be located in relation to the mass?

III. A 58-year-old male is referred to a psychiatrist because of a developing difficulty in relating to his colleagues. The patient has made many poor business decisions in recent years. He would become quite hostile with almost any provocation. Skills that he had developed years earlier were now recognized as being lost. He now was noticing loss of vision in the right eye. A CT scan reveals a large mass lesion at the base of the frontal fossa slightly to the right of the midline.

1. What is the most likely diagnosis? **2.** What alternative diagnosis should be considered? **3.** What are the most likely sources of blood supply for this lesion? **4.** How should this lesion be approached surgically? **5.** How can the floor of the frontal fossa be repaired, assuming that the mass is totally removed?

IV. A 40-year-old male begins to complain of difficulty swallowing. Examination of the throat reveals a bulging mass behind the pharynx on the right with intact overlying mucosa. The patient is hoarse with a paralyzed right vocal cord. The gag reflex is decreased on the right. A CT scan shows the mass to involve the basiocciput of the skull base and to extend into the upper cervical spine. A needle biopsy shows large cells filled with mucous-appearing cytoplasm, but the cells appear benign.

1. What is the differential diagnosis? **2.** What might the origin of the cells composing this tumor be? **3.** Where else in the body might such lesions be found? **4.** How should this lesion be surgically attacked? **5.** How might radiation therapy affect this lesion?

V. A 60-year-old female is admitted to the hospital complaining of occipital headaches, primarily on the left. She notes pain on rotating her head. She has numbness of the left face. The left side of her tongue is paralyzed. She is ataxic in her gait and paretic in her left arm and leg. The MRI shows a mass in the anterior foramen magnum, primarily on the left side.

1. What is the most likely diagnosis? **2.** What other lesions might be considered? **3.** How might this lesion be approached? **4.** What alternative approaches might be considered? **5.** What stabilizing procedures should be considered assuming that the anterior portions of C1 and C2 as well as part of the clivus are removed?

12

Diagnosis and Treatment of Pituitary Tumors and Craniopharyngiomas

Marshall B. Allen, Jr.
Farivar Yaghmai

Pituitary Tumors

The *pituitary* is the seat of a number of neoplasms for which optimal treatment may require surgery alone or in combination with pharmacological manipulation and/or irradiation.[1] The pituitary rests in the sella turcica, or "Turkish saddle." (See Fig. 12-1.) It is surrounded by the dura mater, which separates it from the sphenoid bone, the cavernous sinuses, and the suprasellar cistern. The diaphragma, which attaches to the clinoids, has a defect of variable size, allowing passage of the pituitary stalk and the surrounding arachnoid. The stalk connects the hypothalamus with the posterior pituitary. Thus, the subarachnoid space extends into the pituitary fossa.

The normal pituitary of an adult weighs less than a gram, measuring up to 1.5 cm at greatest width and about 8.2 mm in height.[2] The normal gland reaches its maximum size in adolescents and is slightly larger in adult women than in men.

The pituitary is made up of two *lobes*: the *anterior* lobe, or *adenohypophysis,* derived from the primitive stomadeum of the oropharynx; and the *posterior* lobe, derived from a downward extension of the diencephalon. These join early in embryonic life.

The anterior lobe is composed of: the pars distalis, the largest segment of the adenohypophysis; the pars intermedia; and the pars tuberalis—the latter being intimately attached to the pituitary stalk.

The adenohypophysis consists of glandular cells interposed among numerous vascular channels. (See Fig. 12-2.) These cells provide hormones that influence body growth, metabolism, lactation, response to stress, body pigment, levels of sex hormones, and ovulation.

The *neurohypophysis* persists as a downward extension of the hypothalamus, being made up primarily of axons and their processes, the cell bodies of which are located in the paraventricular and supraoptic nuclei. Its hormones influence water balance and the contraction of selective smooth muscles under varying conditions.

There are no neuronal connections between the brain and the anterior pituitary. Hypothalamic influences on the adenohypophysis are mediated through hormones transported from the hypothalamus by the portal veins, which are intimately attached to the pituitary stalk and neurohypophysis.

Blood is supplied to these structures through the superior and inferior *hypophyseal arteries,* branches of the internal carotid artery given off above and within the cavernous sinus, respectively. These vessels divide into arterioles and eventually capillaries, blood from which is collected in the portal veins and transported to the anterior pituitary, from where it eventually returns to systemic circulation. Some venous blood, after passing through the adenohypophysis, passes back up the portal system to the hypothalamus.[3]

The pituitary is located directly under the optic chiasm in the majority of cases. The chiasm is fixed anteriorly in about 9 percent of cases and behind the pituitary in 11 percent. (See Fig. 12-3.) Thus, symptoms of visual impairment are the most common complaints related to mass lesions in the region of the pituitary. Microadenomas (less than 10 mm) are usually asymptomatic or produce symptoms due to endocrinological abnormalities. (See Fig. 12-4.)

Dura mater separates the pituitary from the cavernous sinuses, which house the internal carotid arteries on either side. Lateral to the carotid arteries, but still within the cavernous sinuses, are the third, fourth, sixth, and first two divisions of the fifth cranial nerves. The medial parts of the temporal lobes are adjacent to the cavernous sinuses.

The *sella turcica* is located in the midline in the body of

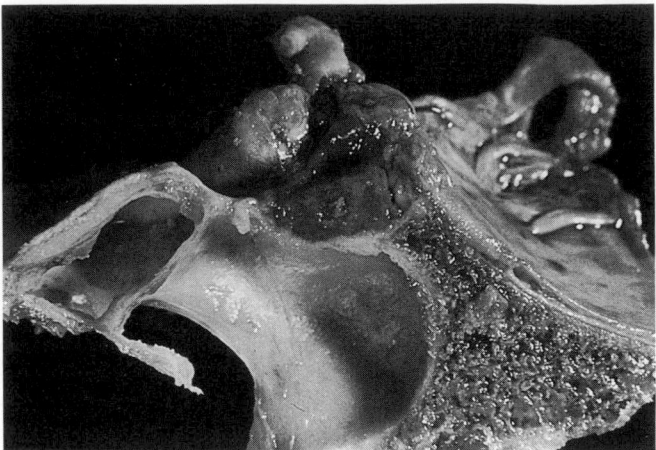

Figure 12–1 Midsagittal section of base of the skull showing the correlation of sella turcica, diaphragm sellae, pituitary (partially autolyzed), the right optic nerve, the sphenoid sinus, and clivus.

the sphenoid bone. The sphenoid sinus is located anterior and inferior to the sella in 88 percent of adults.[1] The sinus is located adjacent to the anterior surface of the sella in most other adults. Cortical bone separating the sella and the sphenoid sinus is quite thin in normal individuals, and it is often eroded by intrasellar masses.

In a very small group of cases—most of whom are children or young adults—the sphenoid sinus is poorly developed or absent, leaving cancellous bone between the sella and the posterior nasopharynx. Extending laterally from the body of the sphenoid on either side are the lesser and greater wings of the sphenoid, which mark the site of junction of the frontal and temporal lobes and represent the anterior floor of the middle fossa, respectively,

MASS LESIONS IN OR ADJACENT TO THE PITUITARY

Tumors in the region of the pituitary include: (1) neoplasms of the parenchyma of the adenohypophysis, which exhibit varying degrees of cellular growth; (2) neoplasms of adjacent structures, including the optic nerves and chiasm and the hypothalamus; (3) congenital neoplasms; (4) metastatic neoplasms; (5) aneurysms; (6) cysts; and (7) miscellaneous disorders, including infections and sarcoidosis.

In the authors' experience, craniopharyngiomas, aneurysms, meningiomas, gliomas, and sarcoidosis are the more common lesions—aside from neoplasms of pituitary parenchyma.

Of the hormonally active tumors, prolactinomas are the most common, followed in order of frequency by tumors secreting growth hormone, tumors secreting more than one hormone (mixed), mammosomatotrophic lesions, and tumors secreting adrenocorticotropic hormone.[4]

Tumors which produce gonadotropic and thyrotrophic hormones are rare; the authors have not recognized them in their series. Hormonally inactive neoplasms of the adenohypophysis include null cell adenomas, which produce inactive hormones and chromaphobic tumors.

CLINICAL PRESENTATIONS OF NEOPLASTIC LESIONS IN THE REGION OF THE PITUITARY

Indications of neoplastic lesions of the pituitary gland or those adjacent to it are usually neurological or endocrinolog-

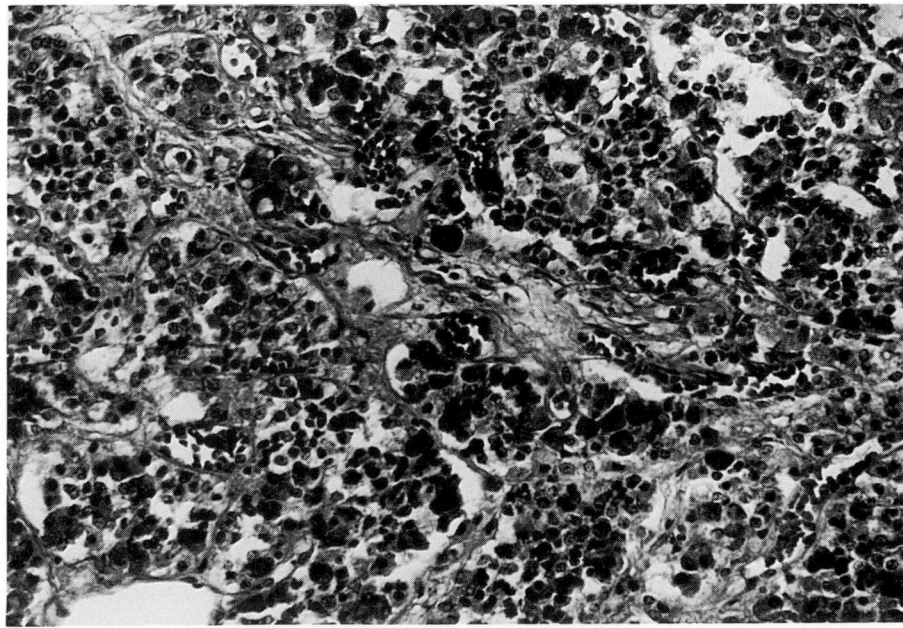

Figure 12–2 Microscopic section of normal anterior pituitary. Note the admixture of different types of adenohypophyseal cells with varying amounts of hormonal collections in the cytoplasm. Also note capillaries coursing through the normal anterior pituitary. H&E × 160.

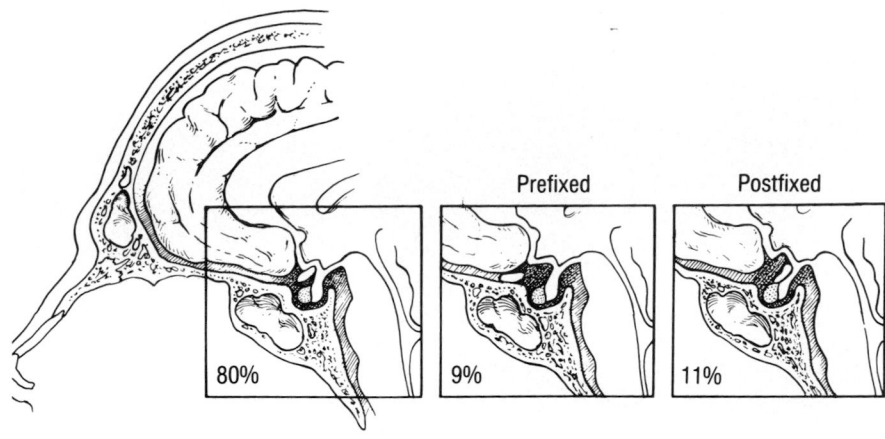

Figure 12–3 Schematic illustration of pituitary showing usual relationship, compared with the prefixed and postfixed chiasm.

ical. Since the pituitary lies directly beneath the optic chiasm in most cases, *alteration of vision is the most common initial evidence of a mass lesion in the region of the pituitary gland.*

Visual field deficits may be produced by direct pressure on the optic chiasm or by interruption of flow in nutrient vessels supplying the optic pathways. Direct pressure on the optic chiasm from an underlying lesion initially produces defects in the fields of vision in the upper outer quadrants that extend to the lower outer quadrants as the lesion progresses. These defects subsequently extend to the lower inner quadrants as a result of further expansion of the mass.

Deficits produced by mass lesions pressing directly on the midportion of the chiasm are likely to be more symmetrical than lesions resulting from ischemia produced by occlusion of nutrient vessels. A unilateral mass located anterior to a postfixed chiasm may produce a central scotoma in one eye with a defect in the upper outer quadrant of the contralateral eye—due to the looping of crossing fibers in the proximal segment of the optic nerve opposite the side of their retinal origin (von Willebrand's knee).

The optic tracts may be affected by laterally located mass lesions situated behind a prefixed chiasm. Masses from the region of the sella may involve the frontal lobes or hypothalamus, causing behavioral problems. Impingement on the hypothalamus may cause alterations in the state of consciousness, memory, thirst, appetite, and the intake of food and water. Obstruction of the third ventricle or foramina of Monro may produce hydrocephalus.

Mass lesions extending laterally from the sella may displace or invade the cavernous sinuses, stretching the cranial nerves which innervate the muscles of ocular motility and the first two divisions of the trigeminal nerve, producing pain in the face. The sudden occurrence of headache followed by altered consciousness and paralysis of two or more of the extraocular muscles is the classical clinical picture of pituitary apoplexy.

Occlusion of the carotid arteries by an expanded intrasellar mass due to pituitary apoplexy precipitated by a "triple bolus test," involving the intravenous injection of luteinizing hormone–releasing hormone, thyrotropin-releasing hormone, and insulin—has recently been reported.[5] Extension of a mass into the middle fossa may lead to temporal lobe seizures. Headaches, associated with an intrasellar expanding mass, are thought to result from stretching the dura and/or vessels in the area. Headaches are usually localized to the distribution of the ophthalmic division of the trigeminal nerve.

SIGNS AND SYMPTOMS OF SUPPRESSED PITUITARY ACTIVITY

Hypopituitarism may be the result of injury to the pituitary stalk or gland by tumors or other lesions—or in some instances by pituitary apoplexy, which usually occurs in a neoplasm.[1]

When the hormonal deficiency is severe, patients develop pale, waxy appearances with fine wrinkles about the eyes and mouth. There is a loss of axillary and pubic hair and a slowing of beard growth, in males.

Diminished bone marrow function is often indicated by moderate anemia. Nausea and vomiting may be prominent, as may be postural hypotension and hypothermia. Loss of adrenal function may result in collapse, whereas loss of thyroid function may result in cold intolerance, sluggishness, dryness of the skin, and myxedema.

Loss of activation of the gonads results in amenorrhea and sterility in females and testicular atrophy with loss of libido and potency in males. Marked diminution of vasopressin results in diabetes insipidus. Urinary output is increased and the specific gravity is reduced, usually below 1.004.

The alert patient without severe damage to the hypothalamus usually complains of thirst and with unrestricted access to water will control fluid balance; but if consciousness is impaired and there is damage to the hypothalamus, or if water is restricted, severe water loss may result, and concentrations of electrolytes and osmolarity of the blood will rise. Osmolarity of the urine remains low. Shock and eventual mortality can result.

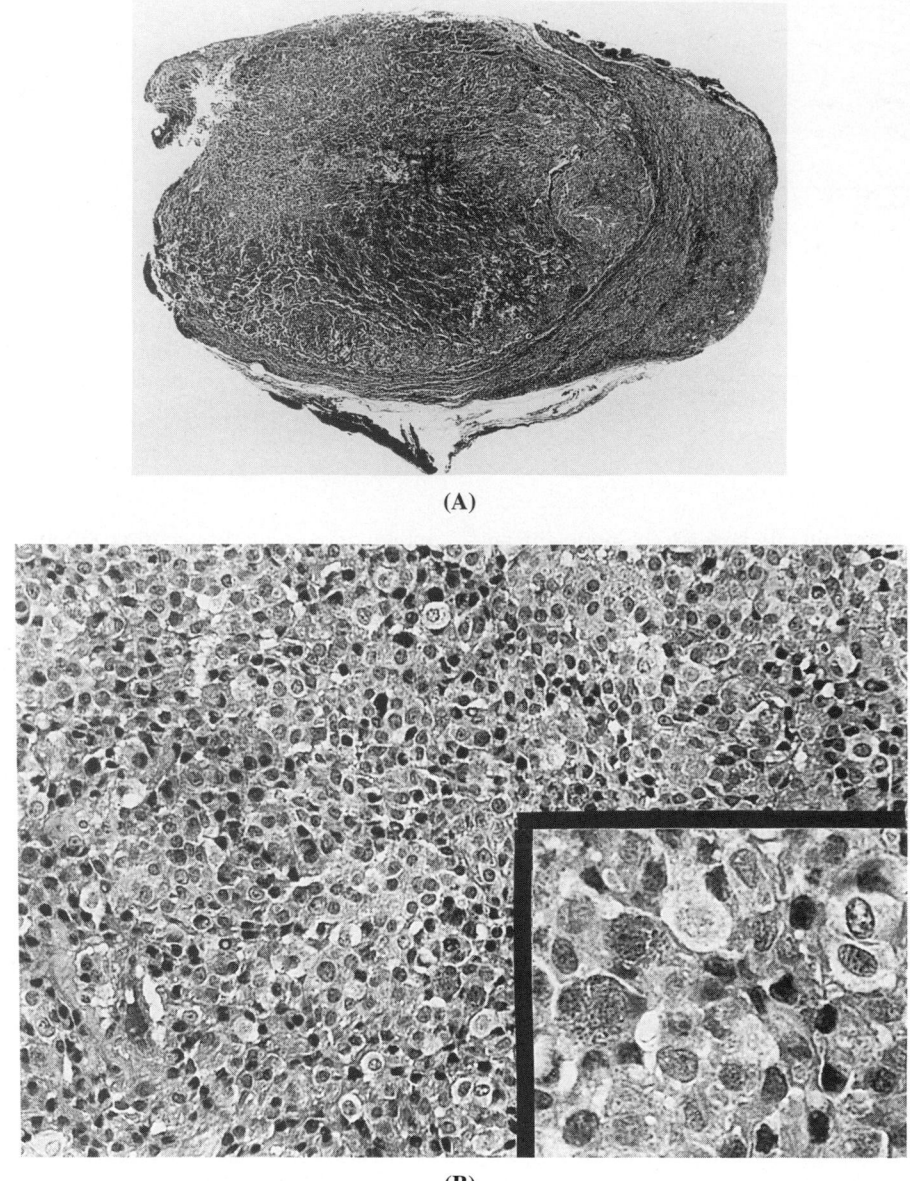

(A)

(B)

Figure 12–4 *A.* Photograph of microadenoma of adenohypophysis. This adenoma, which measures 0.9 cm in largest diameter, is an incidental null cell adenoma found at postmortem. The tumor is well delineated and has compressed the residual still functional adenohypophysis to a crescent shape. H&E × 15. Microscopic sections are in *B.* H&E × 160, inset H&E × 400.

☐ SIGNS AND SYMPTOMS OF HORMONALLY ACTIVE PITUITARY TUMORS

Prolactinomas are the most common endocrinologically active pituitary tumors. The most common symptoms are amenorrhea and galactorrhea in females. These may present primarily—the women never experiencing normal menstrual periods—or the symptoms may interrupt cyclic menses. Menses may not return after a delivery, or patients who are utilizing oral contraceptives may experience interruption of menses. Offending lesions range from microadenomas (less than 10 mm diameter) to macroadenomas that produce signs of mass lesions as well as symptoms of excessive prolactin production.

The normal level of prolactin in a nonpregnant female who is not in the early postpartum period is less than 20 nanograms per mililiter. A level above 200 ng/ml almost uniformly indicates a prolactinoma. Levels between these figures may be open to question.

The production of prolactin is controlled by inhibitory influences from the hypothalamus. Division of the pituitary stalk results in a rise in the level of prolactin. There is evidence that these inhibitory influences, normally passing from the hypothalamus to the anterior pituitary, may be interrupted by mass lesions such as craniopharyngiomas or aneurysms, resulting in a rise in the level of prolactin.[6,7]

Clearly, the use of medications such as thyrotropin-releasing hormone, antidepressants, phenothiazenes, estro-

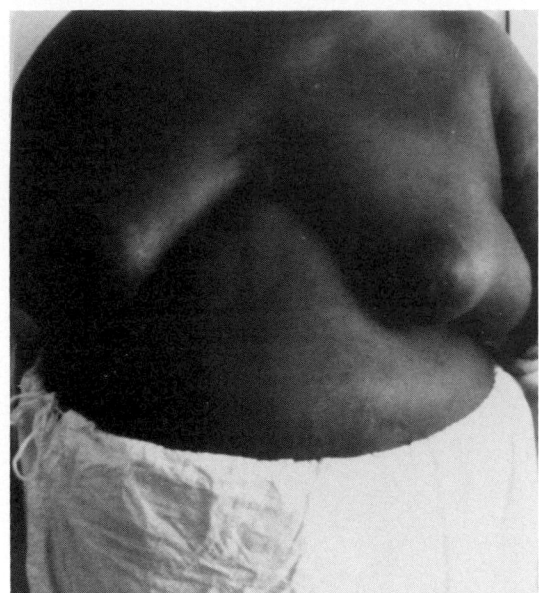

Figure 12–5 Photograph of breasts of 57-year-old obese male with large prolactinoma.

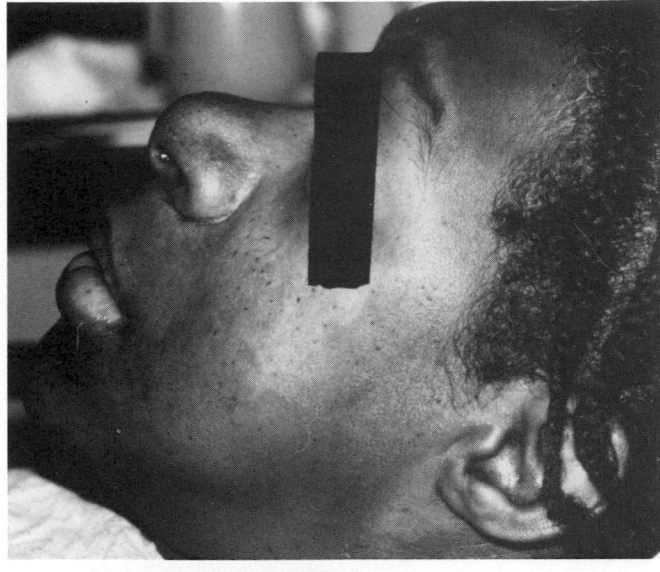

(A)

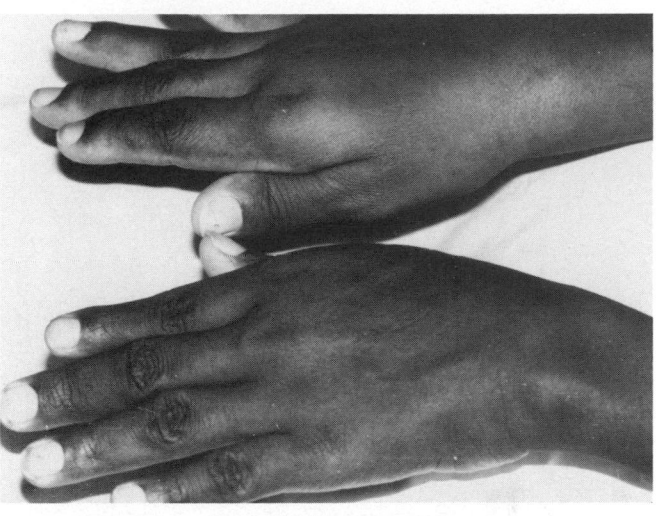

(B)

Figure 12–6 Photographs of 37-year-old female with growth hormone secreting pituitary adenoma. *Note enlarged soft tissues of face (A) and hands (B).*

gen-containing oral contraceptives, and certain antihypertensives is associated with elevated prolactin levels.[8] How high the level of prolactin might reach is not clear. Amenorrhea, ovulatory defects, menstrual disorders, and hirsutism are common complaints in females with elevated prolactin levels.[9]

Prolactinomas are less frequently diagnosed in males than in females. Hyperprolactinemia in males is associated with loss of libido and impotency; testicular atrophy; oligospermia; and, rarely, galactorrhea.[9] Levels of prolactin in males have generally been much higher at the time of diagnosis of a prolactinoma than in females.[1] The tumors are often much larger when diagnosed in males. (See Fig. 12-5.)

Obesity is common to both men and women with prolactinomas, and there is the suggestion that the obesity may respond to less-vigorous therapy when the tumor is adequately treated.

Adenomas that produce excessive quantities of growth hormone in mature adults produce signs and symptoms of *acromegaly.* These are overgrowth of soft tissues, including the tongue, lips, and scalp. In addition, there is growth of the bones of the nose, jaw, and hands and feet. (See Fig. 12-6.)

Facial features become "coarse." (See Fig. 12-7.) There is general organomegaly. Frequently, there are pains in joints due to degenerating joint disease, and there may be intolerance to glucose. Spinal stenosis has been reported.[10] One of the severest consequences of acromegaly is progressive arteriosclerotic cardiovascular disease.

The life expectancy for uncontrolled acromegalics is significantly reduced, in large measure, as a result of cardiovascular and respiratory disease.[1] The mortality rate is almost twice that of the normal population.[11]

When pituitary adenomas produce excessive growth hormone becomes apparent before the epiphyses have closed,

and the features are those of *gigantism.* The individual continues to grow at excessive rates.

The normal level of growth hormone in adults beyond 25 years is less than 5 ng/ml. An exact correlation between the level of growth hormone and signs and symptoms of acromegaly is not possible. The effects of growth hormone are mediated through somatocedin C, and one of the best indications of success in the treatment of acromegaly is determination of the level of somatocedin C.[12,13] Normal levels of 0.4 to 2.2 units per milliliter should be achieved.

Pituitary adenomas that produce excessive quantities of adrenocorticotrophic hormone (ACTH) lead to the clinical features of Cushing's syndrome, including: truncal obesity, hypertension, hirsutism, bruising, mental disturbances, alteration of menstrual cycles and libido, striae about the abdomen and breasts, myopathy, diabetes mellitus, acne, osteoporosis, and fatigue.[14] (See Figs. 12-8 and 12-9.)

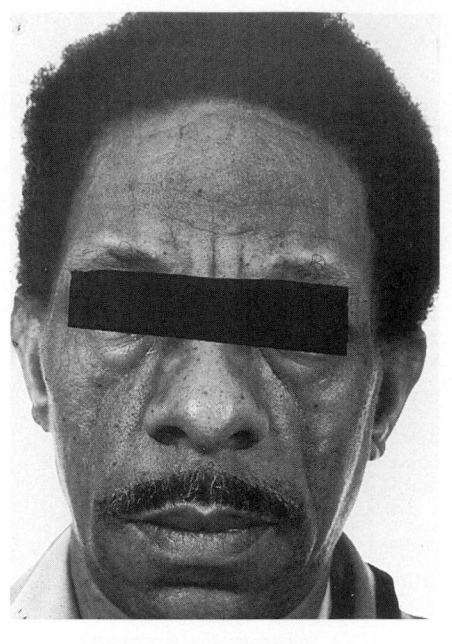

(A)

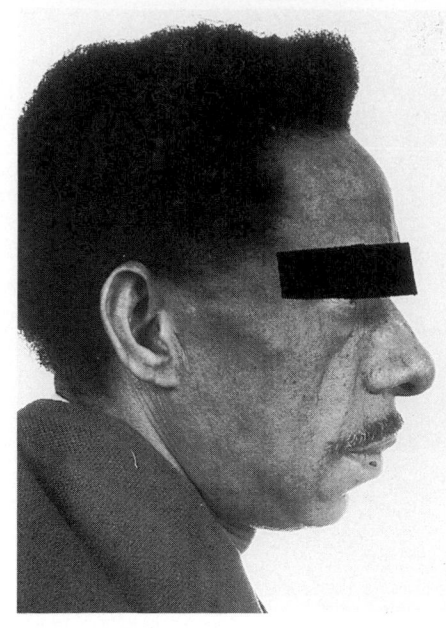

(B)

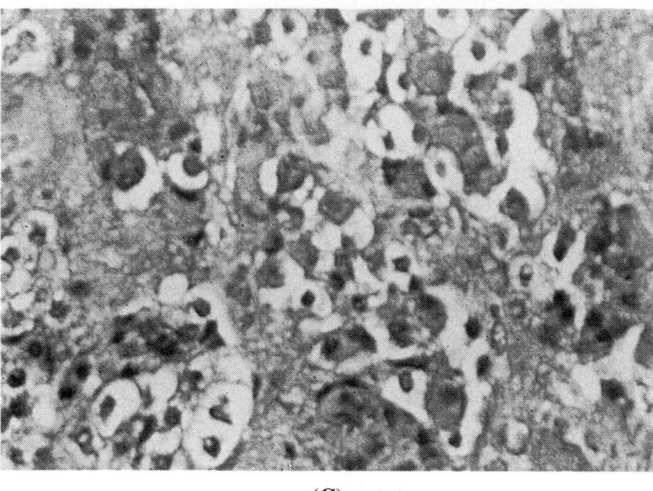

(C)

Figure 12–7 Frontal *(A)* and lateral *(B)* photographs of the head of a 45-year-old male with acromegaly who had had previous irradiation of the pituitary with limited effect on the level of growth hormones. Note the coarse facial features and receding hairline and a photomicrographing of the actively growing tumor with an acellular area between clumps of adenomatous cells *(C)*.

The most common cause of Cushing's syndrome is a pituitary adenoma, explaining 60 to 80 percent of cases. Neoplastic lesions of the adrenal cortex cause 15 to 25 percent of cases, and ectopic foci of hormonal production explain the remainder.[1,15]

Ectopic foci occur in malignant tumors of the lung, carcinoids, thymomas, islet cell tumors of the pancreas, carcinomas of the thyroid, and pheochromocytomas. Differentiation among these lesions requires determination of levels of ACTH—especially in conjunction with corticotropin-releasing hormones, via the dexamethasone suppression test and the metyrapone test. (See Tables 12-1, 12-2, and 12-3.)

Other adenomas of the pituitary may produce excessive quantities of thyroid-stimulating hormone or gonadotrophins.

☐ THYROID-STIMULATING HORMONES (TSH)[19,20]

Adenomas secreting TSH are rare but well-documented. Diagnosis is based upon the following criteria:

1. Elevated level of thyroxine.
2. Inappropriately high TSH determined by RIA's specific for human TSH.
3. Finding of pituitary tumor with typical thyrotrophs.
4. Absence of infiltrative ophthalmopathy or acropathy.
5. Undetectable thyroid-stimulating immunoglobulins.
6. The disappearance of hyperthyroidism after removal of the pituitary adenoma.

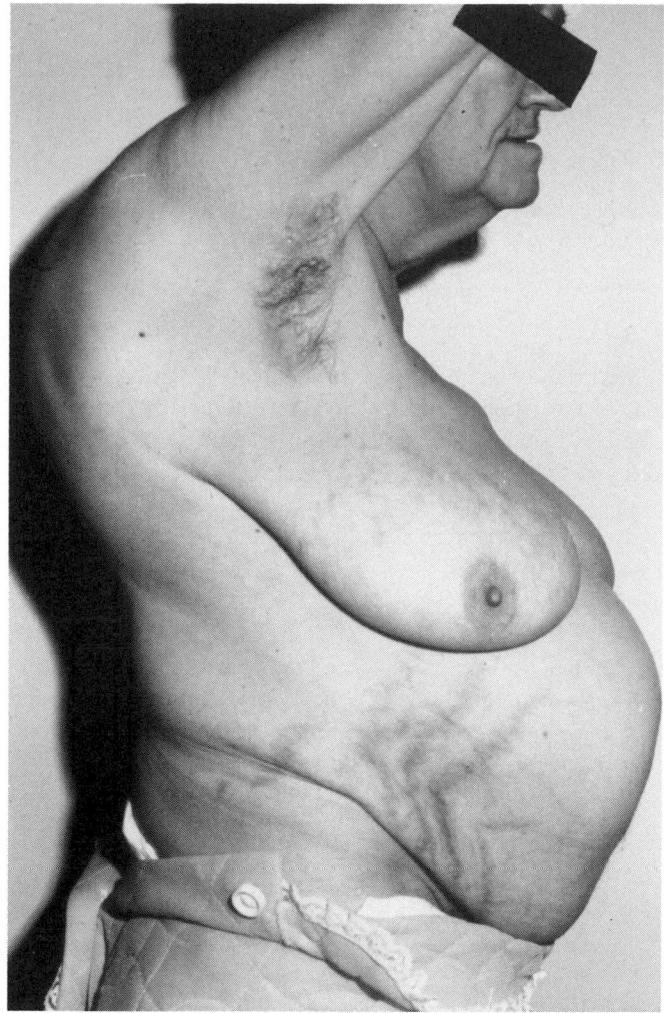

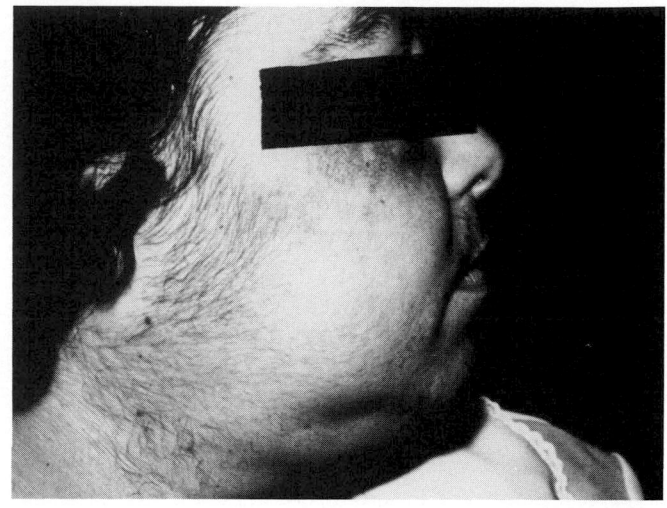

(A)

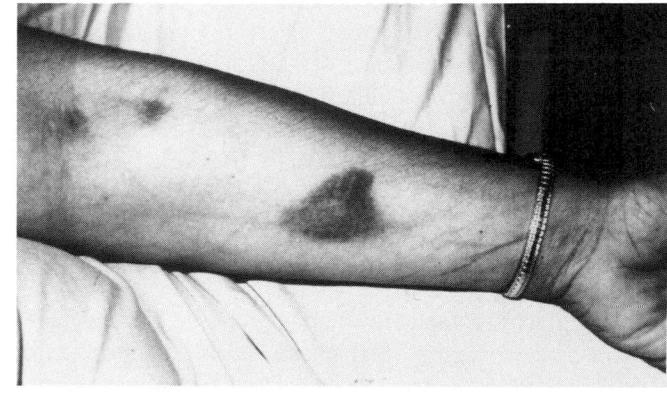

(B)

Figure 12–8 Photograph of Cushing's disease in middle-aged female, showing marked obesity, thoracic kyphosis, and striae of the abdomen and breasts.

☐ ADENOMAS SECRETING GONADOTROPHINS

These are rare lesions, usually found in patients with primary hypogonadism.[21,22,23] Even more rarely have cases been documented without hypogonadism.[24,25] Most secrete follicle-stimulating hormone (FSH). Rarely have tumors secreting both FSH and luteinizing hormone (LH) been documented.[1]

Investigation of hormones produced by the pituitary has indicated that TSH, FSH, and LH are glycoproteins composed of two subunits, *alpha* and *beta.* Alpha units are similar for all three hormones, but neither the alpha or beta units demonstrate biological activity unless both units are present.[26] Tumors producing only alpha subunits have been described. Since they are biologically inactive, they usually are recognized because of their neurological deficits. It is now apparent that many tumors formerly thought to be "nonfunctioning" are producing hormones.[27,28]

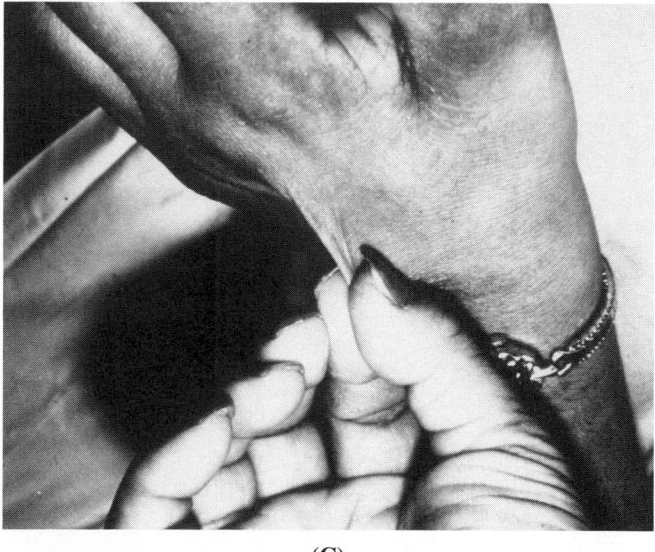

(C)

Figure 12–9 A facial photograph *(A)* of a young adult female with Cushing's disease, showing hirsutism and hyperpigmentation. Ecchymoses from bruising are seen in *(B)*, and poor skin turgor of the dorsum of the hand is seen in *(C)*.

Table 12-1
NORMAL VALUES OF CORTISOL AND ACTH

Cortisol: 6.5–20.5 μg/dl with diurnal variation.
            AM twice afternoon levels.
ACTH: 41–68 pg/ml

☐ DIAGNOSTIC IMAGING IN THE EVALUATION OF PATIENTS WITH LESIONS IN THE REGION OF THE PITUITARY

We routinely obtain plain radiographs of the skull in patients being considered for lesions in the region of the pituitary. These radiographs outline the sella and paranasal sinuses. They may show evidence of calcification in patients with craniopharyngiomas. They may also show clouding in the paranasal sinuses or evidence of mass lesions which represent (1) invasions of the sella from lesions in the region of the oropharynx or (2) extension of intrasellar lesions into the sphenoid sinus.

Absence of/or distortion of the sphenoid sinus or clouding indicates the need for additional evaluation of the paranasal sinuses if a lesion of the pituitary is to be attacked by the transsphenoidal route.

Imaging with computerized tomography (CT) and magnetic resonance imaging (MRI) have become the most definitive diagnostic procedures for lesions of the pituitary parenchyma or surrounding structures.

CT findings which suggest pituitary adenomas include: (1) increase in tissue contents of the sella, (2) abnormal configuration of the pituitary gland, (3) hypodensity within the gland on a nonenhanced or contrast-enhanced scan, (4) hyperdensity on a nonenhanced scan, (5) concentration of contrast medium on enhanced CT scan, and (6) enhancement and displacement of the secondary hypophyseal capillary bed.[29] Adenomas frequently are enhanced before the remainder of the pituitary, and the stalk is usually deviated away from an adenoma. Within a few minutes, the adenoma may become isodense.[30]

Table 12-2
DEXAMETHASONE SUPPRESSION TEST[16,17]

Dexamethasone suppression (6-day test)

First 2 days: Basal urine. Over 7 mg/gm (cortisol).
Second 2 days: Give decadron: 2.0 mg q 6 h. Should reduce urine cortisol to 50%.
Third 2 days: Give decadron: 8.0 mg q 6 h. The urinary excretion of cortisol is not suppressed in patients with Cushing's disease on 2.0 mgm, but it is with 8.0 mgm of decadron.

The cortisol output of patients with Cushing's syndrome of extra pituitary origin is not suppressed.

Table 12-3
METYRAPONE TEST[18]

Metyrapone

(750 mg q 4 h × 24 h. Check urine 17-hydroxycorticoids.)
First 24 hours: Basal urine.
Second 24 hours: Cushing's disease gives positive response (2× rise). Cushing's syndrome of extrapituitary origin: No increase in 17-hydroxycorticoids.

MRI has assumed a major role in the evaluation of adenomas of the pituitary; it clearly delineates enlargement of the gland and outlines the relationships between the adenomas and parasella structures. MRI locates and demonstrates deformations of the optic tracts, chiasm, and optic nerves, and it demonstrates invasion of the cavernous sinuses by neoplasms. It will also show neoplasms in surrounding structures.[29,31]

MRI frequently outlines the adenoma more discretely than CT. Enhancement can be accomplished with gadolinium. MRIs are particularly helpful in outlining blood vessels and ruling out aneurysms. Angiography is rarely necessary except for lesions with parasellar extensions.

☐ PATHOLOGY OF PITUITARY ADENOMAS

A discussion of the pathology of tumors in the region of the pituitary will be limited to a discussion of *pituitary adenomas;* other lesions in the area will be discussed under their appropriate headings.

Adenomas of the pituitary are classified according to size of *microadenomas* (less than 10 mm in diameter) and *macroadenomas* (see text previous). The neoplasms are usually clearly identifiable by their greyish red appearance, which is usually gelatinous, although they may be quite fibrous. Macroadenomas usually begin within the sella but may extend well above the sella or into the sphenoid sinus, laterally into the adjacent cavernous sinuses, or over the sinuses into the region of the temporal fossa.

Microscopically, the normal pituitary is made up of glandular cells which usually appear cuboidal, with capillary channels interspersed among small clumps of cells. (See Fig. 12-4B.) There is usually considerable variation in the amount of acidophilic and basophilic dye taken up in the cytoplasm of cells so that there is much variation of cells, from one to another in the normal pituitary. Adenomas take on a monotonous appearance. Vascular channels are scarce and the cytoplasm of the cells stains similarly. Cells appear in "sheets." (See Fig. 12-10.)

Pituitary adenomas have generally been considered benign, and it is well known that their biological behavior cannot be predicted by histology. Hormonal production does

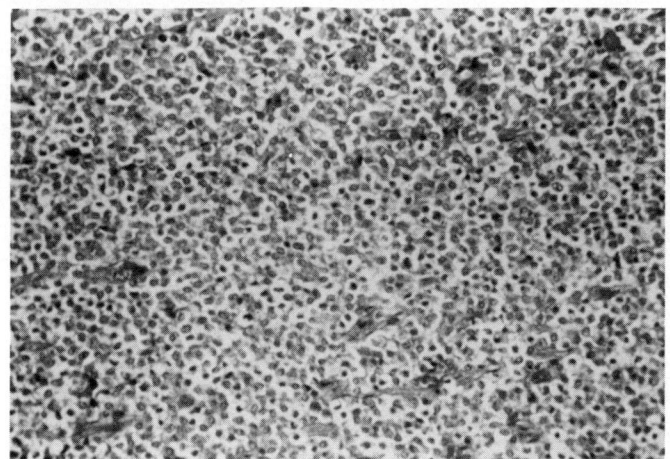

Figure 12–10 A photomicrograph of a prolactinoma showing monotonous-appearing cells. Note very few vascular channels.

not imply that a tumor is noninvasive.[32] Overall rate of gross invasion is thought to be about 35 percent.

Pituitary adenomas can metastasize throughout the subarachnoid spaces, as well as throughout the body.[33] Growth rates may be predicted by determining monoclonal antibody immunoreactivity[34,35]

The current classification of pituitary adenomas is based on the work of Horvath and Kovacs, which identifies (1) the specific hormones produced, (2) those tumors which produce multiple hormones, and (3) those which produce no identifiable hormones.[36] (See Table 12-4.) The classification requires a combination of electron microscopic and immunochemical investigations. (See Fig. 12-11.)

☐ TREATMENT OF PITUITARY ADENOMAS

Selection of the appropriate therapy for any specific lesion of the pituitary or in the area of the pituitary depends on the

Table 12–4
CLASSIFICATION OF PITUITARY ADENOMAS*

I. Growth hormone cell adenoma
    Sparsely granulated
    Densely granulated
II. Prolactin cell adenoma
    Sparsely granulated
    Densely granulated
III. Mixed prolactin cell
    Any combination of I and II
IV. ACTH-MSH cell adenomas
    Sparsely granulated
    Densely granulated
V. Undifferentiated cell adenomas
    Oncocytomas

*From Horvath and Kovacs.[36]

lesion. Controversy exists as to optimal treatment for some lesions. Options include conservative treatment by serial observation, medical therapy, surgical resection, and radiation therapy.

CONSERVATIVE THERAPY

An autopsy series of 100 consecutive examinations has reported and 8[4] percent incidence of pituitary microadenomas.[37] Serial observations of selected cases of microadenomas has indicated that some lesions may not expand at a significant rate. If they are *not* producing hormones which are detrimental to the patient's health or producing undesirable symptoms, serial observation may be the appropriate course. In addition, there are lesions contained within the sella, i.e., small craniopharyngiomas, resection of which is likely to produce severe endocrinological deficits. Such lesions may be followed on an annual or semiannual basis with repeated CT scans or MRI imaging. Periodic investigation of visual fields and hormonal assays should be obtained wherever appropriate.

MEDICAL THERAPY

Medical therapy is effective for the treatment of patients with prolactinomas. Bromocriptine will reduce the size of the neoplasms and reduce the level of prolactinemia.[38,39,40] However, the drug is not tumoricidal, and the mass of the tumor as well as hormonal production may return as soon as medication is discontinued. There is evidence that suggests long-term administration of bromacriptine reduces the chances for a surgical cure, perhaps because of the development of fibrosis in the adenoma.[41,42]

Bromocriptine may reduce the size of some adenomas that produce growth hormone. It may be that these adenomas produce prolactin as well. The dose of medication required to reduce the size of a growth hormone–producing tumor is greater than that required for prolactinomas.

A number of medications has been used for the treatment of Cushing's disease—with varying results. These include: mitotane, metyrapone, and aminoglutethimide.[1] Generally, they have proved to be adjunctive to surgical therapy rather than the basis for primary treatment. Serotonin antagonists, including cyproheptadine and metergoline, may prove to be the most efficacious in the long run. They also show promise in the treatment of Nelson's syndrome.

SURGICAL THERAPY

Indications for surgery on lesions of the pituitary or its surrounding structures include the *mass effect,* which may result in neurological impairment, rhinorrhea, or excesses in production of hormones. Impairment of visual fields, hypothalamic function, frontal lobe function, or the presence of

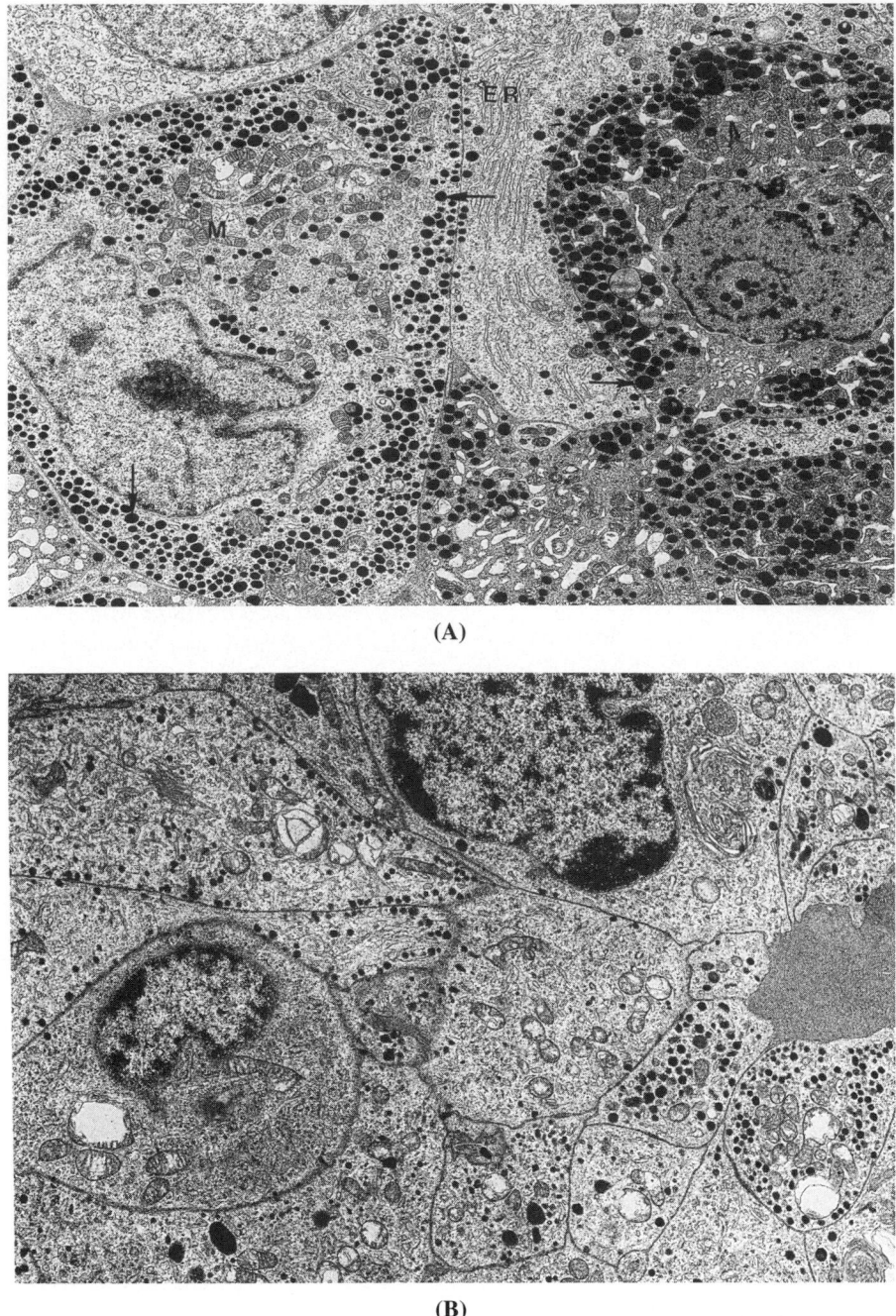

(A)

(B)

Figure 12–11 Electron microscopy of pituitary adenomas. Although application of immunoperoxidase markers has been of great help in functional histologic classification of pituitary adenomas, electron microscopy is still helpful in pathologic workup of these tumors, especially the functional tumors without stainable granules. Some of the electron microscopic features that determine the type of adenoma are secretory granules (arrows); their shape, size, surrounding membrane, abundance or sparseness, and extrusion between the adjacent cell membranes; quality of endoplasmic reticulum (ER); frequency of mitochondria (M); cytokeratin microfilaments; and other features. The photomicrograph *(A)* is from a "densely granulated growth hormone cell adenoma." ×7800.

A null cell adenoma (×10,000) is shown in *B*. Notice sparse small secretory granules. The mitochondria and RER are moderately developed and Golgi complexes are rare. This tumor showed focal rare eosinophilic granules in light microscopy (related to the mitochondria). The patient did not have appreciable elevation of serum levels of pituitary hormones.

hydrocephalus or seizures may lead to an ultimate diagnosis of a mass lesion in the area of the pituitary, and it will require surgical treatment. Before surgery, an evaluation should be directed toward identifying the origin and localizing the exact site of the lesion. Investigations usually include imaging by dynamic, high-definition CT scans and MRI, often with enhancement.

Excesses of prolactin, growth hormone, and ACTH may represent indications for ablation of lesions of the pituitary. Although prolactin-secreting tumors are the most common, excessive quantities of prolactin can often be controlled with bromocriptine. Medical therapy may be elected unless the adenoma is causing significant mass effects which are thought to be beyond the control of bromocriptine; or when the patient will not, or cannot, take bromocriptine; or unless pregnancy is desired without the limited risk of apoplexy.

Excessive growth hormone has been recommended as a clear indication for excising a pituitary adenoma, even when the mass is not important. Degenerative lesions of the cardiovascular system and degenerative arthritis are consequences of uncontrolled tumors producing growth hormone.

Cushing's disease represents a third endocrinologic indication for ablation of a recognizable adenoma. Adenomas of the pituitary producing ACTH rarely produce mass effects before there is demonstrable endocrinological evidence of such lesion. Microadenomas are sometimes too small to be seen in imaging studies. They may be best outlined by dynamic CT scans, but it is also good to bear in mind that cases of false-positive identification have been reported.

Lateralization of the source of elevated quantities of ACTH from the pituitary can be determined from blood samples aspirated simultaneously from the petrosal sinuses.[43]

Nelson's syndrome is progressive pigmentation of the skin in a patient who has undergone adrenalectomy in the presence of a pituitary adenoma secreting ACTH. This occurs in about 10 to 15 percent of patients and is associated with an aggressive tumor. The adenomas respond to surgical therapy, and the syndrome is considered definitive indication for resection of the pituitary tumor.[44]

PREPARATION FOR SURGERY IN THE REGION OF THE PITUITARY

Surgery in the region of the pituitary carries the risk of loss of adrenal function. Loading patients with adrenocortical steroids is indicated even when it is anticipated that resection will be limited to a microadenoma. Cortisone acetate, 100 mg, is administered 12 hours prior to surgery with another 100 mg just prior to surgery. Systemic antibiotics are used prophylactically; however, some surgeons prefer to use topical antibiotics on nasal mucosa. Prophylactic antibiotics may be administered during and after surgery. Steroids are tapered over a period of 3 to 7 days.

TRANSSPHENOIDAL RESECTION

Transsphenoidal resection of the pituitary is accomplished with the patient supine and the base of the nose turned to the side most convenient for the surgeon. The tip of the nose remains vertical.

While many surgeons utilize a sublabial approach, the authors use a purely septal approach—making an additional small incision in the ala of the nose if it is necessary to enlarge the nostril enough for the speculum. (See Fig. 12-12A and B.) After preparing the nose and oropharynx with an antiseptic solution, and packing the nose with a 4 solution of cocaine for 5 minutes, the nasal septum is infiltrated with 0.5 xylocaine-containing adrenaline, 1:2000.

After making a vertical incision in the septal mucosa, the mucosa is dissected free from the nasal cartilage and bony septum as high as the sphenoid sinus. (See Fig. 12-12C.) Segments of the septum are removed for implantation in the sella or sphenoid sinus at the time of closure. The mucosa is dissected from the anterior wall of the sphenoid sinus, which is penetrated on either side at the ostia. Mucosa is removed from the sinus and a Hubbard or Hardy retractor inserted.

The septum of the sphenoid sinus is removed and the floor of the sella inspected for penetrations. Any penetrating adenoma is removed. If the floor of the sella is intact, it is penetrated with a chisel, and the wall is removed laterally to the area of the cavernous sinus. (See Fig. 12-12D.) An X-shaped incision is made in the dura.

At this stage, the microscope is brought into the field. For macroscopic tumors, the sella is usually emptied and additional suprasellar extensions are brought down by insufflating the subarachnoid space with air or saline. For microadenomas, it is frequently necessary to make vertical incisions in the pituitary to search for an adenoma which is usually soft, reddish gray tissue without organization. This is curetted and sent for pathological examination.

The base of the tumor may be swabbed with absolute alcohol when the arachnoid remains intact. The sella is packed with fascia, and/or fat held in place by a fragment of the nasal septum. (See Fig. 12-12E.) The nasal mucosa falls into place when the retractor is removed and is sutured with through-and-through sutures of absorbable material, as is the incision in the nasal septum or sublabial mucosa. The nose is packed with gauze impregnated with petrolatum.

TRANSCRANIAL PROCEDURES

There are, basically, three transcranial approaches applicable to tumors in the region of the pituitary: *subfrontal, pterional,* and *subtemporal.*

Subfrontal For intrasellar masses with suprasellar extensions, the subfrontal approach is used most commonly, its primary purpose being to decompress the optic nerves.

Only by the subfrontal approach can one visualize *both* optic nerves and the carotid arteries, features which are very

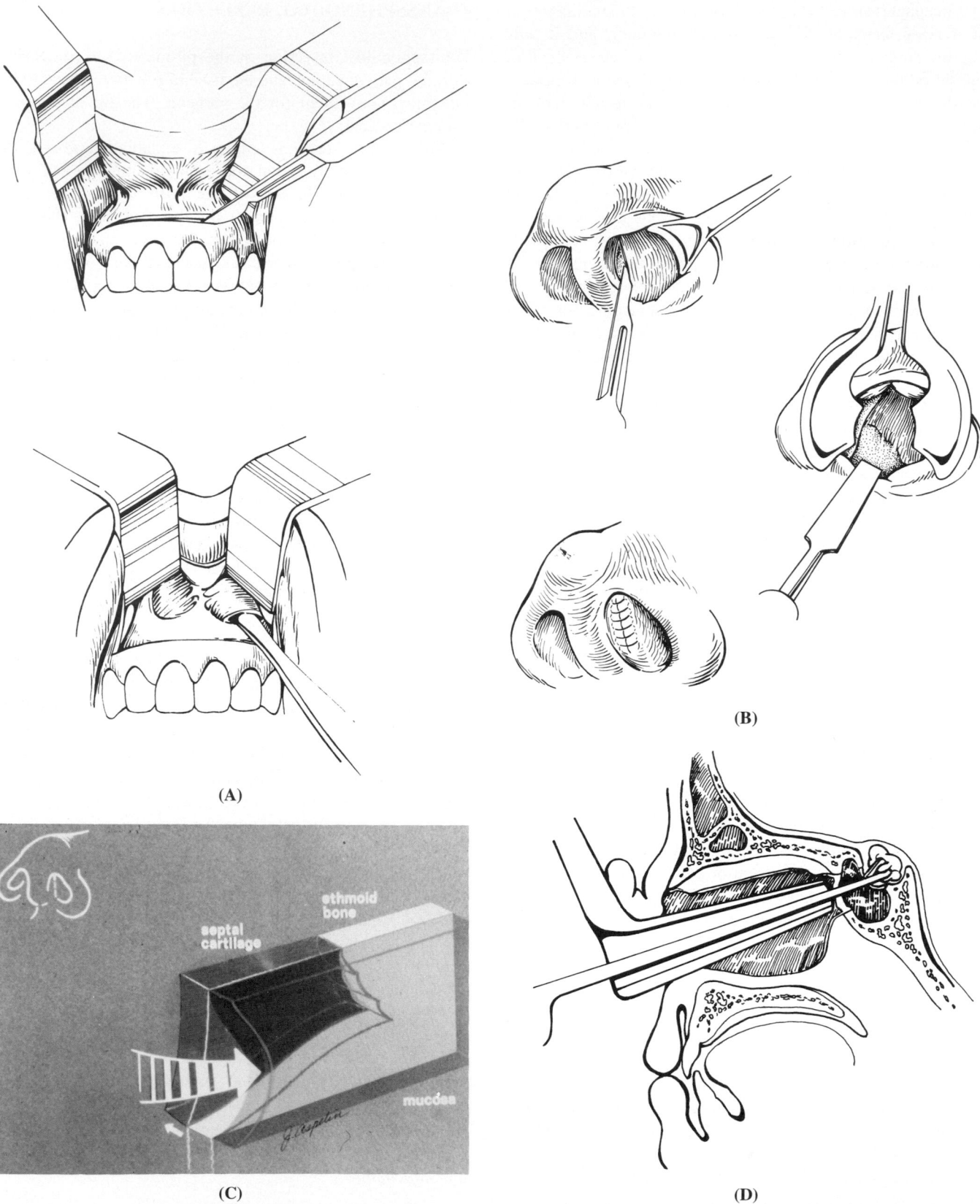

(A)

(B)

(C)

(D)

Figure 12–12 Schematic illustrations of tissue sphenoidal resection of pituitary. A sublabial approach to the nasal septum is illustrated in *A*. A submucosal approach to the nasal septum is illustrated in *B*. The submucosal dissection along the nasal septum is illustrated in *C*. Intrasellar removal of pituitary is illustrated in *D*. Opening the dura and the intrasella removal of pituitary tissue followed by replacement with fascia and fat that must be held in place by a segment of cartilage, bone, or plastic material are shown in *E*.

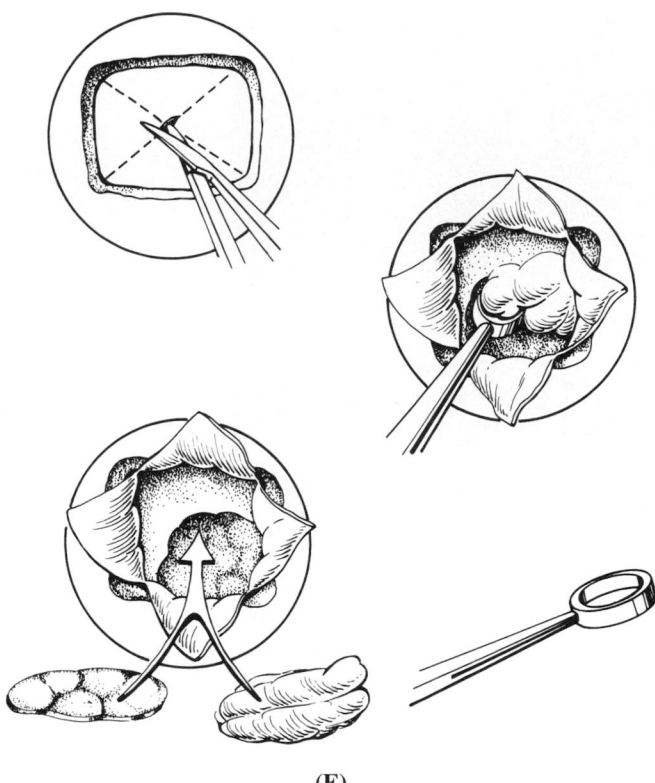

(E)

Figure 12–12 Continued.

important if the primary objective for the procedure is to preserve loss of vision from a lesion compressing the chiasm from below. The view of the mass of tumor may be severely limited if the chiasm is prefixed. This can be rectified by resecting the tuberculum sella and opening into the sphenoid sinus. Visualization of fragments of the mass which may have extended vertically or laterally into the cerebrum may be difficult by *any* approach.

The procedure is accomplished through a coronal incision, turning a frontal bone flap that may cross the midline. It is imperative to open the flap to the floor of the frontal fossa, even if this requires entering the frontal sinuses. When they are entered, they should be exenterated and packed. The frontal lobe is carefully retracted, exposing the optic nerves and the ipsilateral carotid artery. The tumor is usually visualized between the optic nerves or between the right optic nerve and the carotid artery. Curettage can decompress the optic nerves and resect much, if not all, of the mass.

Pterional and Subtemporal Pterional or subtemporal approaches may be necessary for neoplasms located in the parasellar areas, specifically for meningiomas of the medial sphenoid wing, chordomas, and other lesions involving the medial sphenoid wing, cavernous sinus, or dorsum sella. A supraorbital-pterional approach by which the zygomatic arch is displaced and an orbitocranial bone flap is raised has been recommended.[45,46] This gives excellent exposure to parasellar tumors in the region.

A midline, transcallosal approach may be substituted for treatment of lesions with extensions high in the third ventricle, usually craniopharyngiomas.

POSTOPERATIVE CARE

Postoperative care of patients having undergone surgery, who have compromised function of the adenohypophysis and/or posterior pituitary, requires prophylaxis against adrenal insufficiency. Monitoring, support for, and replacement of excessive urinary output and for insufficiency of antidiuretic hormone in the immediate postoperative period is necessary. Urinary output must be appropriately replaced during the first week after surgery. (See under postoperative care of patients with craniopharyngiomas.) Monitoring to determine deficiencies of anterior pituitary hormones in the early and late postoperative stages is also necessary. Steroids, in the form of hydrocortisone or synthetic steroids are administered throughout surgery and in tapering doses in the postoperative period. Prophylactic antibiotics are administered by many surgeons.

RADIATION THERAPY

Radiation therapy, initially popular as an adjunct to surgical treatment of pituitary lesions, has been used less frequently in recent years, but its popularity may be renewed with the availability of focused beams, i.e., proton beam, linear accelerator (LINAC), or "Gamma knife." The greatest limitations of radiotherapy are late complications, which may not be known for years, and problems related to panhypopituitarism. Focal irradiation is certainly appropriate in patients who have failed surgical therapy or who are poor candidates for surgical therapy.

COMBINATION THERAPIES

A combination of surgery and radiation therapy seems appropriate for many tumors of the pituitary in which mass is the presenting complaint. Medical therapy may be adjunctive to surgery in patients with Cushing's disease who have not obtained complete remission from the surgical therapy.

Many have advised the use of bromocriptine, at least temporarily, prior to resection of prolactinomas. This therapy will significantly reduce the size of many prolactin-secreting adenomas, but there is reason to question whether its administration reduces the chances of a curative resection. A trial of medical therapy may be indicated for adenomas producing both prolactin and growth hormones.

Craniopharyngiomas

Craniopharyngiomas are neoplasms which occur in the region of the sella turcica, thought to arise from Rathke's

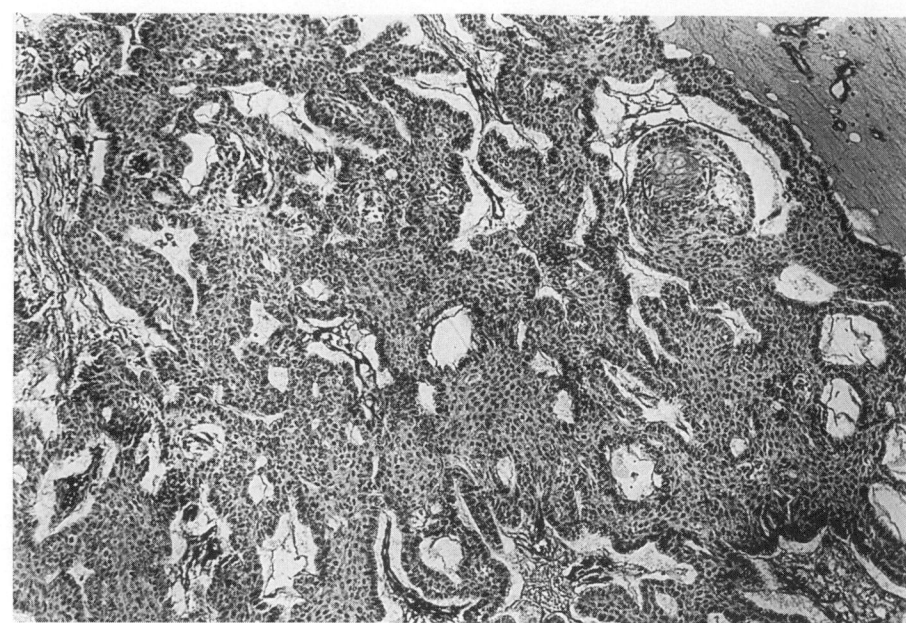

Figure 12–13 Photomicrograph of craniopharyngioma. Notice the basal cell layer (the single rows of darker cuboidal cells), which has given rise to the larger squamous cell layer forming the bulk of the cellular parts. Focally, the cells have further matured to an occasional "keratin pearl," one of which is seen in the right upper part. Microcystic cavities are scattered, and a macrocyst is seen in the right upper corner, with the "motor oil" content. H&E × 63.

pouch. While Rathke's pouch has long been considered the most likely source of craniopharyngiomas, metaplasia of adenomatous cells in the pituitary is also considered a possible source.[47] The predominant elements are nests of squamous epithelium, often standing alone but also often lining cysts which usually contain fluid that has the appearance of motor oil. The fluid contains cholesterol crystals, but there may be a high concentration of calcium.

Basal cells in the nests of epithelium are columnar or cuboidal, on which are two or three layers of polygonal or round cells. The flattened squamous cells lie next to the cyst or in the center of the nests. Collagen surrounds squamous cell nests. (See Fig. 12-13.)

☐ CLINICAL PRESENTATION

Craniopharyngiomas may become apparent in later life, but about half present before the age of twenty.[48–51]

Symptoms vary. In children, headaches are most likely to be the initial complaint; these are present in about half of diagnosed cases. Impairment of vision is common as well, often with temporal field defects apparent at the time of diagnosis. Hormonal deficiencies are not unusual.

Deficiencies in gonadal hormones are found in about 80 percent of adults, causing irregularities in cyclic sexual functions in women and loss of libido, often with sterility, in many patients.

Retarded and diminished growth is common in adolescents, and deficiencies in corticosteroids and thyroid function may result in lethargy, cold intolerance, and inability to

respond to stress. At least one mortality has been reported as a result of inability of a patient with a craniopharyngioma to respond to a metyrapone test.

Headaches are often the result of *hydrocephalus*. Craniopharyngiomas originate in the sella, in the suprasellar subarachnoid space, or in the third ventricle, and then may occlude the foramina of Monro. Shunting may be required, and it may be necessary to implant shunts bilaterally if both foramina are occluded.

Another cause for headaches is rupture of a cyst with escape of the contents into the cerebrospinal fluid. A chemical meningitis may result. Eighty percent of craniopharyngiomas in children and about 40 percent in adults are calcified to such an extent that they are demonstrated on plain radiographs.[52,53,54] Calcification is even more likely to be seen on CT and is almost routine on microscopy.

Collagenous elements are frequently adherent to adjacent structures in the parasellar area—especially blood vessels—and these are often difficult to separate. Craniopharyngiomas stimulate a significant glial response in areas where they come in contact with nervous elements. Fingers of epithelium often extend into the glial structures of the surrounding brain tissue, limiting the ability to effect a cure by surgery.[55] The surrounding glial reaction may provide an area wherein the surgeon is able to separate the neoplasm from the neural elements.

There is considerable variation in the growth rate of craniopharyngiomas.[56] While they are generally considered benign lesions, the growth potential in children usually far exceeds that in adults. An indication of the rate of growth is often estimated by reviewing the history of a patient. A patient who gives a long history of symptoms which are associated with the tumor is likely to survive a partial resection for a much longer period than a patient whose history is very short at a time when a large lesion is diagnosed.

☐ DIAGNOSTIC IMAGING

Plain radiographs frequently show evidence of distortion of the sella. When tumors are located within the sella, it is usually enlarged. When tumors are located in the suprasellar region, they may "sharpen" the clinoids. Calcification is apparent in about half the lesions and evidence of increased intracranial pressure is apparent when there is hydrocephalus. This may include thinning of the inner table of the skull and "splitting" of the sutures if they are not tightly fused.

CT scans, which are now becoming the primary imaging investigation, reveal suprasellar masses of soft tissue which frequently house islets of calcium and cysts that usually demonstrate decreased attenuation.[57]

However, on occasion, the cysts may contain major quantities of calcium and demonstrate increased attenuation. Soft-tissue elements may be enhanced. MRI discretely outlines the mass and reveals relationships to displaced neural elements, blood vessels, and dura.[58] Islets of calcification may not be as apparent as on CT scans. Cysts produce a high signal on T1- and T2-weighted images. Soft tissue is usually enhanced with gadolinium.

☐ TREATMENT OF CRANIOPHARYNGIOMAS

SURGICAL THERAPY

The primary treatment of craniopharyngiomas is generally surgical. For the more common lesions which originate in the subarachnoid space above the sella, a subfrontal approach is used. A coronal incision is made to open the scalp, and a frontal bone flap is raised.[57] Care should be taken to be sure that the flap extends to the floor of the frontal fossa. The frontal lobe is retracted, and the tumor exposed between the optic nerves beneath the optic chiasm or between an optic nerve and the adjacent carotid artery.

Cysts should be tapped and the tumor gradually mobilized. It is usually necessary to separate it from the carotid arteries by sharp dissection. The tumor will separate from the nervous tissue fairly readily, but there may be considerable difficulty exposing all of a lesion which extends high into the third ventricle. Steady traction must be applied. The tissue can be lost behind the chiasm if the tumor is released. Tissue behind the chiasm can be mobilized by dissecting through the lamina terminalis.

Care should be taken to identify and preserve the pituitary stalk whenever possible.[59] The stalk is identified behind the chiasm, but is often significantly displaced by the tumor. The incidence of diabetes insipidus can be reduced by preservation of the stalk. Even when the stalk cannot be preserved, the severity of diabetes insipidus may be minimized by limiting the damage to the stalk and preservation of even a remnant of it will provide a matrix for new portal veins to grow.[55]

A pterional approach may be required for lesions which extend onto the dorsum sella or into a temporal fossa. A transsphenoidal approach is very satisfactory for lesions contained within the sella.[59] For those lesions extending high in the third ventricle, a midline, transcallosal approach, passing into the third ventricle through a foramen of Monro or between the internal cerebral veins provides good access to the vertex of the tumor.[60] Dissection in the region of the hypothalamus is far removed from the operator, however. No matter which route is used, a microscope is helpful in determining lines of dissection and peripheral structures.

Experience has indicated that the best opportunity to obtain a complete removal of a craniopharyngioma is at the time of the original resection.[61,62,63] Removal of the entire tumor is desirable. A number of reports have urged radical resection of such lesions, and there is little doubt that the more tumor removed the longer the survival. However, craniopharyngiomas are located in a very restricted area, one in which injury to the surrounding elements produces serious consequences. Injury to the carotid arteries may be impossible to repair and injury to the hypothalamus may result in irreversible somnolence. Injury to the optic nerves results in producing the very neurological deficit that one is trying to prevent.

Resection of all of a craniopharyngioma at the time of a second exposure or following irradiation is quite difficult and complete resections at the time of a second exposure are not common.

RADIATION THERAPY

Craniopharyngiomas appear benign. Generally they behave as benign lesions and the efficacy of radiation therapy has been questioned. However, there are reports of long remissions of craniopharyngiomas following radiation therapy.[64,65,66] The consensus among most neurosurgeons is that one should remove as much of a craniopharyngioma as one can without significantly increasing the chances for neurological deficits, and use irradiation on those lesions where all of the tumor cannot be safely resected.

POSTOPERATIVE CARE

Diabetes insipidus should be anticipated routinely after resection of a craniopharyngioma. Hourly urinary output should be measured, and the urine fluid volume replaced. It may be necessary to replace fluids intravenously initially, but oral administration is desirable when the patient is alert.

Intravenous fluids are usually administered as glucose and water, but sugar is spilled in the urine when the glucose in intravenous infusions exceeds 15 g per hour.

It may be necessary to administer pitressin when more fluids are required, but pitressin administration should be kept at a minimum during the first week, when there may be considerable variation in the amount of pitressin that the patient releases. Long-acting pitressin (pitressin in oil) should be avoided during the first week after surgery. Usually two to three units of aqueous pitressin or minimal quantities of desmopressin, which may be administered intranasally, intramuscularly, or even intravenously, will reduce the requirements of water.

After initial care, desmopressin or vasopressin may be administered intranasally. In patients who have more limited needs for replacement of posterior pituitary hormones, chlorpropamide, hydrochlorthizide, or the two drugs in combination may be used to control diabetes insipidus. Chlorfibrate may be used in the place of chlorpropramide. It should be remembered that chlorpropramide produces hypoglyce-mia, and it may be necessary to supplement sugar intake when it is used.

Large doses of steroids should be administered in the early postoperative period. About 100 mg of hydrocortisone may be given at the end of the operation. This is repeated 4 to 6 hours later. A similar dose is given the next morning. Dexamethasone, 4.0 mg may be substituted. These doses are usually tapered over the period of about a week, to a maintenance dose with instructions that they be increased in the event of stress. Generally, a maintenance dose of cortisone acetate is about 25 to 37½ mg per day. Dexamethasone 0.5 mg per day may be substituted.

Testing for thyroid function may demonstrate deficiencies prior to surgery. If so, therapy should be instituted, desirably prior to surgery, but if a delay in surgery long enough to obtain normal metabolism is impossible, it should be instituted as soon as possible after surgery. If thyroid function is not known prior to surgery or if it is found to be normal, tests should be repeated after about a month to indicate whether administration of thyroxin is needed.

REFERENCES

1. Tindall GT, Barrow DL: Tumors of the sellar and sellar areas in adults, in Youmans JR (ed): *Neurological Surgery,* 3d ed. Philadelphia, Saunders, 1990, chap 119, pp 3447–3498.
2. Peyster RG, Hoover ED, Viscarello RR, Moshang T, Haskin ME: CT appearance of the adolescent and preadolescent pituitary gland. *AJNR* 4:411–414, 1983.
3. Bergland RM, Page RB: Pituitary-brain vascular relations: A new paradigm. *Science* 204:18–24, 1979.
4. Wilson CB: A decade of pituitary microsurgery: The Herbert Olivecrona Lecture. *J Neurosurg* 61:814–833, 1984.
5. Bernstein M, Hegele RA, Gentili F, et al: Pituitary apoplexy associated with a triple bolus test (case report). *J Neurosurg* 61:586–590, 1984.
6. Cusimano MD, Kovacs K, Bilbao JM, et al: Suprasellar craniopharyngioma associated with hyperprolactinemia, pituitary lactotroph hyperplasia, and microprolactinoma. *J Neurosurg* 69:620–623, 1988.
7. Lundberg PO, Osterman PO, and Wide L: Serum prolactin in patients with hypothalamus and pituitary disorders. *J Neurosurg* 55:194–199, 1981.
8. Balagura S, Frantz AG, Housepain EM, Carmel PW: The specificity of serum prolactin as a diagnostic indicator of pituitary adenoma. *J Neurosurg* 51:42–46, 1979.
9. Abboud CF, Laws ER Jr: Clinical endocrinological approach to hypothalamic-pituitary disease (review article). *J Neurosurg* 51:271–291, 1979.
10. Epstein N, Whelan M, Benjamin V: Acromegaly and spinal stenosis. *J Neurosurg* 56:145–147, 1982.
11. Wright AD, Hill DM, Lowry C, Fraser TR: Mortality in acromegaly. *QJ Med* 39:1–16, 1970.
12. Clemmons DR, Van Wyk JJ, Ridgeway EC, et al: Evaluation of acromegaly for radioimmunoassay of somatomedin-C. *N Engl J Med* 301:1138–1142, 1979.
13. Losa M, Oeckler R, Schopohl J, et al: Evaluation of selective transsphenoidal adenomectomy by endocrinological testing and somatomedin-C measurement in acromegaly. *J Neurosurg* 70:561–567, 1989.
14. Boggan JE, Tyrrell JB, and Wilson CB: Transsphenoidal microsurgical management of Cushing's disease: Report of 100 cases. *J Neurosurg* 59:195–200, 1983.
15. Martin JB: Management of hypersecretory pituitary adenomas. *Clin Neurosurg* 27:99–123, 1980.
16. King LW, Post KD, Yust I, Reichlin S: Suppression of cortisol secretion by low-dose dexamethasone testing in Cushing's disease (case report). *J Neurosurg* 58:129–132, 1983.
17. Liddle GW: Tests of pituitary-adrenal suppressibility in the diagnosis of Cushing's syndrome. *J Clin Endocrinol Metab* 20:1539–1560, 1960.
18. Liddle GW, Estep HL, Kendall JW Jr, et al: Clinical application of a new test of pituitary reserve. *J Clin Endocrinol Metab* 19:875–894, 1959.
19. Benoit R, Pearson-Murphy BE, Robert F, et al: Hyperthyroidism due to pituitary TSH secreting tumor with amenorrhea-galactorrhea. *Clin Endocrinol* 12:11–19, 1980.
20. Tolis G, Bird C, Bertrand G, et al: Pituitary hyperthyroidism: Case report and review of the literature. *Am J Med* 64:177–181, 1978.
21. Cunningham GR, Huckins C: An FSH and prolactin-secreting pituitary tumor. Pituitary dynamics and testicular histology. *J Clin Endocrinol Metab* 44:248–253, 1977.
22. Friend JN, Judge DM, Sherman BM, Santen RJ: FSH-secreting pituitary adenomas: Stimulation and suppression studies in two patients. *J Clin Endocrinol Metab* 43:650–657, 1976.
23. Peterson RE, Kourides IA, Horwith M, Vaughn ED Jr, et al: Luteinizing hormone and alpha subunit–secreting pituitary

tumor: Positive feedback of estrogen. *J Clin Endocrinol Metab* 52:692–698, 1981.

24. Demura R, Kubo O, Demura H, Shizume K: FSH and LH secreting pituitary adenoma. *J Clin Endocrinol Metab* 45:653–657, 1977.

25. Snyder PJ, Sterling FH: Hypersecretion of LH and FSH by a pituitary adenoma. *J Clin Endocrinol Metab* 42:544–550, 1976.

26. Klibanski A, Ridgway EC, Zervas NT: Pure alpha subunit-secreting pituitary tumors. *J Neurosurg* 59:585–589, 1983.

27. Black PMcL, Hsu DW, Klibanski A, Kilman B, et al: Hormone production in clinically nonfunctioning pituitary adenomas. *J Neurosurg* 66:244–250, 1987.

28. Miura M, Matsukado Y, Kodama T, Mihara Y: Clinical and histopathological characteristics of gonadotropin-producing pituitary adenomas. *J Neurosurg* 62:376–382, 1985.

29. Kaufman B, Arafah B, Selman WR: Advances in neuroradiologic imaging of the pituitary gland: Changing concepts. *J Lab Clin Med* 109:308–319, 1987.

30. Hasegawa T, Ito H, Shoin K, et al: Diagnosis of an "isodense" pituitary microadenoma by dynamic CT scanning. *J Neurosurg* 60:424–427, 1984.

31. Davis PC, Hoffman JC Jr, Spencer T, et al: MR imaging of pituitary adenomas: CT clinical and surgical correlation. *AJR* 148:797–802, 1987.

32. Scheithauer BW, Kovacs KT, Laws ER Jr, Randall RV: Pathology of invasive pituitary tumors with special reference of functional classification (review article). *J Neurosurg* 65:733–744, 1986.

33. Hashimoto N, Handa H, Nishi S: Intracranial and intraspinal dissemination from a growth hormone-secreting pituitary tumor (case report). *J Neurosurg* 64:140–144, 1986.

34. Landolt AM, Shibata T, Kleihues P: Growth rate of human pituitary adenomas. *J Neurosurg* 67:803–806, 1987.

35. Nagaskima T, Murovic JA, Hoshino T, et al: The proliferative potential of human pituitary tumors *in situ*. *J Neurosurg* 641:588–593, 1986.

36. Horvath E, Kovacs K. Ultrastructural classification of pituitary adenomas. *Can J Neurol Sci* 9–21, 1976.

37. Parent AD, Bebin J, Smith RR: Incidental pituitary adenomas. *J Neurosurg* 54:228–231, 1981.

38. Barrow DL, Tindall GT, Kovacs K, et al: Clinical and pathological effects of bromocriptine on prolactin-secreting and other pituitary tumors. *J Neurosurg* 60:1–7, 1984.

39. Hubbard JL, Scheithauer BW, Abboud CF, Laws ER Jr: Prolactin-secreting adenomas: The preoperative response to bromocriptine treatment and surgical outcome. *J Neurosurg* 67:816–821, 1987.

40. Fahlusch R, Buchfelder M, Schrell U: Short-term preoperative treatment of macroprolactinomas by dopamine agonists. *J Neurosurg* 67:807–815, 1987.

41. Landolt AM, Keller PJ, Froesch ER, Mueller J: Bromocriptine: Does it jeopardise the result of later surgery for prolactinomas? *Lancet* 2:657–658, 1982.

42. Landolt AM, Osterwalder V: Perivascular fibrosis in prolactinomas: Is it increased by bromocriptine? *J Clin Endocrinol Metab* 58:1179–1183, 1984.

43. Zovickian J, Oldfield EH, Doppman JL, et al: Usefulness of inferior petrosal sinus venous endocrine markers in Cushing's disease. *J Neurosurg* 68:205–210, 1988.

44. Wislawski J, Kasperlik-Zaluska AA, Jeske W, et al: Results of neurosurgical treatment by a transsphenoidal approach in 10 patients with Nelson's syndrome. *J Neurosurg* 62:68–71, 1985.

45. Al-Mefty O: Supraorbital-pterional approach to skull base lesions. *Neurosurgery* 21:474–477, 1987.

46. Al-Mefty O: Clinoidal Meningiomas. *J Neurosurg* 73:840–849, 1990.

47. Carmichael HT: Squamous epithelial rests in the hypophysis cerebri. *Arch Neurol Psychiatry* 26:966–975, 1931.

48. Tabaddor K, Shulman K, Dal Canto MC: Neonatal craniopharyngioma. *Amer J Dis Child* 128:381–383, 1974.

49. Arseni C, Martesis M: Craniopharyngioma. *Neurochir* (Stuttgart) 1:25–32, 1972.

50. Banna M: Craniopharyngioma in adults. *Surg Neurol* 1:202–204, 1973.

51. Garcia-Uria J: Surgical experience with craniopharyngioma in adults. *Surg Neurol* 9:11–14, 1978.

52. Banna M, Hoare RD, Stanley P, Till K: Craniopharyngioma in children. *J Pediatr* 83:781–785, 1973.

53. Michelsen WJ, Mount LA, Renaudin J: Craniopharyngioma: A thirty-nine year survey. *Acta Neurol Lat Amer* 18:100–106, 1972.

54. Sung DI, Chang CH, Harisiadis L, Carmel PW: Treatment results of craniopharyngiomas. *Cancer* 47:847–852, 1981.

55. Sweet WH: Recurrent craniopharyngiomas: Therapeutic alternatives. *Clin Neurosurg* 27:206–229, 1980.

56. Bartlett JR: Craniopharyngiomas: An analysis of some aspects of symptomatology, radiology and histology. *Brain* 94:725–732, 1971.

57. Carmel PW: Brain tumors of disordered embryogenesis, in Youmans JR (ed): *Neurological Surgery,* 3d ed. Philadelphia, Saunders, chap 111, 1990, pp 3223–3249.

58. Pusey E, Kortman KE, Flannigan BD, et al: MR of craniopharyngiomas: Tumor delineation and characterization. *AJNR* 8:439–444, 1987.

59. Carmel PW: Craniopharyngiomas, in Wilkins RH, Rengachary SS (eds): *Neurosurgery*. New York, McGraw-Hill, chap 106, 1985, pp 905–914.

60. Long DM, Chou SN: Transcallosal removal of craniopharyngiomas within the third ventricle. *J Neurosurg* 39:563–567, 1973.

61. Matson DD, Crigler JF: Management of craniopharyngioma in childhood. *J Neurosurg* 30:377–390, 1969.

62. Amacher AL: Craniopharyngioma: The controversy regarding radiotherapy. *Child's Brain* 6:57–64, 1980.

63. Hoffman JH, Hendrick EB, Humphreys RB, et al: Management of craniopharyngioma in children. *J Neurosurg* 47:218–227, 1977.

64. Kramer S, McKissock W, Concannon JP: Craniopharyngiomas: Treatment by combined surgery and radiation therapy. *J Neurosurg* 18:217–226, 1961.

65. Kramer S, Southard M, Mansfield CM: Radiotherapy in the management of craniopharyngiomas: Further experiences and late results. *AJR* 103:44–52, 1968.

66. Richmond IL, Wara WM, Wilson CB: Role of radiation therapy in management of craniopharyngiomas in children. *Neurosurgery* 6:513–517, 1980.

☐ STUDY QUESTIONS

I. A 9-year-old child was falling behind his classmates in size since he had started to school at about 5 years of age. He began complaining of difficulty seeing. When examined, he had severe field cuts in the lateral quadrants of both eyes and there was decreased acuity in the left eye. The patient had pale optic disks bilaterally. Plain skull x-rays showed suprasellar calcification which was stippled in the center, but there was a curvalinear line of calcification over the top which was some 4 cm above the sella. The sella was flattened.

1. What would be the most likely diagnosis? **2.** How should the lesion be treated? **3.** What should have been the cause of the field defects? **4.** What was the most likely status of the pituitary hormones when the patient was first seen? After surgery at which a grossly total removal was obtained? **5.** Would any residual tumor be amenable to irradiation therapy?

II. A 40-year-old female cotton mill worker began to notice that she was having to buy shoes every six months because her feet were getting bigger. She could no longer wear her wedding ring because her fingers were growing. She was also losing some vision and she had noticed that her nose was becoming larger and that the pores on her face were getting larger. Her voice was becoming deeper and on a recent examination for insurance, she had been told that she had diabetes. A growth hormone level was reported at 67.

1. What is the most likely diagnosis? **2.** What might plain skull x-rays show? **3.** Assuming a pituitary tumor was found and resected, what might be expected to happen to the enlarged nose, hands, and feet? **4.** What would be the indication for surgery on the tumor, assuming there were no visual changes? **5.** What laboratory tests would give the best indication of a cure of her lesion?

III. A 27-year-old female was on chlorpromazine for anxiety. She developed galactorrhea. Menstrual periods had become scanty and irregular. Physical and neurological examinations were normal. An MRI revealed a large subarachnoid space extending into the sella turcica but there was a small area of increased signal in the substance of the anterior pituitary lobe in the floor of the sella. A prolactin level was measured at 80 ng/ml.

1. What was the most likely cause of the galactorrhea and altered menstrual periods? **2.** What therapy should be administered? **3.** How should this patient be followed? **4.** Should surgical therapy be considered? Why or why not? **5.** Assuming the chlorpromazine was discontinued, the menses remained irregular, and a repeat galactorrhea was reported as 60 ng/ml, what other therapy might be considered?

IV. A 47-year-old male engineer had to stop driving because of his failing vision. On examination, he had bitemporal hemianopsia and a visual acuity of 20/60 bilaterally. His acuity was not correctable. A CT revealed an intrasellar mass extending 2 cm above the sella. An MRI revealed the carotid arteries deviated laterally on each side. A prolactin level was reported as 1200 ng/ml.

1. What is the most likely diagnosis? **2.** How should this be treated? **3.** Assuming bromocryptine was given and the tumor reduced in size by a few millimeters but there was no significant change in the visual fields, what steps should be considered? **4.** What are the advantages of a transsphenoidal over a transcranial approach to this lesion? What are the advantages of a craniotomy over transsphenoidal approach? **5.** What are the dangers of a transsphenoidal approach?

V. A 36-year-old female developed amenorrhea and galactorrhea along with some headache. Investigations revealed a small mass directly over a normally sized sella. The prolactin level was 85 ng/ml.

1. What diagnoses should be considered? **2.** Why is the prolactin elevated? **3.** What other pituitary hormones might be affected? Would they most likely be elevated or depressed? **4.** What treatment(s) might be considered? **5.** Assuming a transcranial resection of the suprasellar mass was performed, would this likely alter the prolactin? The antidiuretic hormone? How?

CHAPTER

13

Tumors of the Spinal Canal

Martin Greenberg
Dennis E. McDonnell
Herman F. Flanigin

Mass lesions that affect the function of the spinal cord are divided into: (1) *intramedullary,* those that originate within the spinal cord; (2) *intradural-extramedullary,* which is self-explanatory; and (3) *extradural,* those that arise outside the dura, most of which involve the vertebral column. Symptoms usually begin with local pain, which may be exacerbated at night and accompanied by a significant radicular component.[4–7,10,11,13] Paresis may become prominent. The rate of progression of the paresis varies greatly, depending on the degree of compromise of blood supply to the spinal cord, but paralysis below the level of involvement is associated with a grave prognosis—even with adequate decompression.

Virtually all neoplastic lesions located in or behind the spinal cord can be approached by unroofing the spinal canal (laminectomy), as can most neoplastic lesions located lateral to the spinal cord and most cystic lesions wherever they are located in the spinal canal.[1–13] Many lesions originating in the vertebral column are located anterior to the spinal cord and are best approached anteriorly or anterolaterally, depending on the vertical level of the lesion. For instance, lesions at the cervicomedullary junction may be attacked through a transoral or transcervical retroparapharyngeal approach,[14–16] while those lower in the neck are approached through an anterolateral cervical approach.[1–3,8,10,11] Lesions located in the thoracic and abdominal regions may be approached through a thoracotomy and retroperitoneal approach, although the costotransversectomy approach has also been popularized.[1,8,10,11] Generally, at least a part of, if not an entire, vertebral body must be removed to approach the spinal canal and, if so, it must be replaced with a graft or prosthesis. Malignant sacral tumors may require simultaneous anterior and posterior approaches in order to effect a cure.[10,11]

Risks to neurological function during surgery may be reduced by intraoperative monitoring, which at present is most commonly using somatosensory evoked potentials. Monitoring motor potentials may be more rewarding and is being developed with the use of magnetic field stimulators.

☐ CLINICAL PRESENTATION[1–16]

Most spinal tumors present with the onset of localized pain, often with a radicular component. Pain is often present at rest and severe at night, unrelieved by narcotics or analgesics. It may not be brought on by exertion and may also be exacerbated by vigorous exercise. Patients with intramedullary tumors may complain of burning dysesthesias in the hands or legs, often for months to years.[4,5,12,13] Metastases must be considered in patients with a history of malignancy. Patients with metastatic disease may have focal regions of tenderness with muscle cramps. Palpation often reproduces pain. Focal kyphoscoliosis or lordosis may be secondary to instability caused by a tumor infiltrating a vertebral body(ies). Patients may have a previous or current history of incidental trauma with a pathological compression fracture(s), associated with occult spinal tumor(s).

Along with pain, metastatic tumors present a variable course, with an abrupt onset below the lesion, of a demonstrable level of sensation to pinprick corresponding to the spinal segment involved and variable urinary retention with hyperreflexia and clonus corresponding to an upper motor neuronal deficit.[4,5,8] Metastatic tumors can present insidiously. When located posterior to the spinal cord, they cause proprioceptive deficits with early myelopathic signs.

Intramedullary tumors classically present with a dissociative sensory loss because of damage to crossing central commisural fibers of the spinothalamic tracts, sometimes secondary to a syrinx.[4,5] There is a marked disturbance of pain and temperature sensation typically at the level of the lesion but preservation of touch and position sense. There may be a history of accidental burns or a shoulder-cape distribution of loss to pinprick sensation.

Intradural-extramedullary tumors classically present with predominant motor and radicular symptoms. A neuroma or neurofibroma arising from a sensory nerve root sheath typically causes ipsilateral pain and weakness in the distribution of a root, as well as early spastic hemiparesis with hyperreflexia below the level of the lesion. As the neuroma expands, a Brown-Séquard syndrome may become evident. Meningiomas arising near the nerve root sheath from the dura-arachnoid present in a lateral or ventrolateral anatomic position with a combination of long-standing neurological signs and symptoms, particularly motor deficits.[9]

Both intramedullary and intradural-extramedullary tumors can present initially with signs and symptoms of increased intracranial pressure (ICP), particularly hydrocephalus, headaches, nausea and vomiting, papilledema, visual loss, obtundation, and gait apraxia.[65] Neurinomas and ependymomas secrete large amounts of proteins into the cerebral spinal fluid (CSF), which block or impede the flow in the spinal subarachnoid compartments. This block of CSF absorption results in increased ICP. Gardner hypothesized that such blockage accounts for hydrocephalus occulta, often seen as the presenting sign of primary intraspinal neoplasms.[65]

☐ DIAGNOSTIC STUDIES[1-16]

RADIOGRAPHY

Preliminary diagnostic examinations should include frontal (AP) and lateral x-rays, as well as oblique or swimmer's views to visualize the cervicothoracic region.[13] Absence, asymmetry, or overt destruction of a pedicle is suggestive of metastatic cancer. Extensive metastatic disease may present as a large paraspinal mass of soft tissue seen on plain radiographs. Malignant lesions have a predilection for vertebral bodies with consequent pathological compression fractures seen clearly on the lateral x-rays. Plain radiographs are positive in 80 to 90 percent of patients with spinal tumors, both extrinsic and intrinsic.[2,13]

Osteolytic lesions are most common with metastatic cancer, especially when the primary lesion is in the breast, lung, kidney, or colon.[4,5,10,11] Prostatic cancer produces an "ivory" vertebra or osteoblastic lesion with a sclerotic bone edge.

Primary bone tumors can be diagnosed by plain radiography.[2,6,7,10,11] Hemangiomas produce coarse vertical striations or trabeculae ("corduroy cloth" impression) while aneurysmal bone cysts and giant cell tumors produce multiloculated, lytic lesions. Osteoid osteomas and osteoblastomas are typically sclerotic. Osteosarcomas, chondrosarcomas, and multiple myelomas which are malignant (primary neoplasms) present with extensive bone destruction and paraspinal soft tissue masses. Chordomas produce gross destruction of the bone elements and amorphous, peripheral calcification, as well as a large soft tissue mass with epidural extension.

Intramedullary tumors, like ependymomas and astrocytomas, can attain considerable size and cause widening of the interpedicular distance, with enlargement of the canal on AP films or even kyphoscoliosis or lordosis in the lateral views.[4,5] Intradural-extramedullary neurofibromas can cause marked widening of the neural foramina and scalloping of the vertebral bodies. Dumbbell thoracic neurofibromas can be seen as masses on chest x-rays. Rarely, meningiomas are sufficiently calcified to be seen on plain radiographs, due to psammoma bodies commonly seen in intracranial tumors.[9] Bony hyperostoses are rare with spinal meningiomas.[9]

MAGNETIC RESONANCE IMAGING (MRI)[17]

Magnetic resonance imaging (MRI) has nearly supplanted computerized tomography (CT) in the diagnostic evaluation of spinal tumors.[17] MRI images the spine in three dimensions, (axial, sagittal, and coronal) and highlights the soft tissue and intraspinal changes.[17] It can be diagnostic for intrinsic cord lesions when gadolinium (Gd-DTPA) is administered.[17] Vascular tumors can be visualized as lesions with varying signals on MRI. Magnetic resonance angiography (MRA) further enhances the diagnostic capabilities of this imaging modality.

Metastatic cancer to vertebrae is visualized by MRI. As bone marrow is replaced by tumor, the tumor appears hypointense on the T1 image, hyperintense on the T2 image, and enhanced with gadolinium (Gd-DTPA).[17] MRI reveals soft tissue changes and epidural compression by lymphoma, multiple myeloma, and chordoma.

Intramedullary tumors are best imaged with MRI as the solid and cystic components of an astrocytoma or ependymoma can be defined on the T1, T2, and gadolinium-enhanced images.[17] Hemangioblastomas can be diagnosed by MRI since they demonstrate a vascular nodule and the tumor is associated with a syrinx or cystic mass. There are associated surface vessels, including arteries and veins leading to the nodule.

Intradural tumors are outlined by MRI.[17] Neurinomas and neurofibromas are hyperintense on T1 and T2 images, are enhanced with gadolinium, and often can be visualized arising from nerve sheaths in the neural foramina. Lipomas have a hyperintense signal on the T1 image. Meningiomas enhance with gadolinium, allowing definition of their ventral or ventrolateral orientation to the adjacent, compressed spinal cord.

A deficiency in MRI technology is that high sensitivity relies on direct imaging of the protons in body water, which is generally lacking in bone. Hence, tumors of bone and structural abnormalities are not imaged well by the MRI. There continues to be need for CT alone or in conjunction with myelography for diagnostic capabilities.

COMPUTERIZED TOMOGRAPHY (CT)

Although MRI has supplanted computerized tomography (CT) as the primary imaging technique for spinal tumors, there is still a key role for CT alone or in conjunction with myelography.[7,13] CT delineates involvement of pedicles, laminae, spinous processes, and vertebral bodies by primary bone tumors, i.e., multiple myeloma, chondrosarcoma, osteosarcoma, and chordoma.[7,13] It may demonstrate tumors or calcifications not seen by plain x-rays. Osteomas, osteoblastomas, giant cell tumors, meningiomas, and aneurysmal bone cysts or bone tumors are best visualized by thin-section CT.

MYELOGRAPHY[10,11,13]

Myelography followed by CT remains a useful imaging modality for spinal tumors. CT helps to differentiate intramedullary, intradural-extramedullary, and extradural lesions. Further, CT-myelography accurately delineates the ventral vs. dorsal or lateral spinal cord compression by outlining the contrast media in CSF or subarachnoid spaces. In clinical situations where the MRI indicates multiple levels of metastatic cancer, CT-myelography is helpful in determining the level producing deficits, especially if the neurological examination does not correlate closely with the MRI.

ANGIOGRAPHY

Spinal angiography can be helpful in localizing the artery of Adamkiewicz, typically on the left side between T8 and L3.[13] However, this procedure is not routinely necessary for preoperative evaluation. Vascular tumors such as metastatic renal cell carcinomas, hemangiomas, and aneurysmal bone cysts can be delineated by angiography, and preoperative embolization is helpful in reducing blood loss during surgery. Hemangioblastomas can be accurately diagnosed by spinal angiography. Arteriovenous (AV) shunting and highly vascular tumor nodules with large, draining veins are characteristically visualized.[17] Embolization may be helpful in the management of large or multiple hemangioblastomas.

At the cervicomedullary junction, vertebral angiography is warranted for meningiomas or neurofibromas that may encase a major vessel, signaling caution during tumor removal. It is important to know whether a dominant vertebral artery can be sacrificed. Extrinsic tumors like lymphomas, chordomas, and renal cell carcinomas which can present as extensive soft tissue masses palpable in the neck may have multiple tumor vessels arising from the muscular branches of the vertebral artery. Preoperative embolization may be useful.

BONE SCANS

Radioisotope bone scans are useful in locating sites of metastases.[7,10,11,13] Multiple metastases may affect the indications for, or type of, neurosurgical procedure. However, the isotope scan is nonspecific, and other radiological modalities are frequently required.

In primary benign bone tumors—e.g., osteoid osteomas and osteoblastomas—the bone scan is helpful in diagnosis, since it shows increased uptake in areas of active bone growth. With an aneurysmal bone cyst or hemangioma, there may be minimal, if any, uptake in the bone. In malignant bone tumors, particularly multiple myelomas, there may be decreased uptake or "cold" spots on radionuclide bone scanning, reducing the value of this modality in identifying sites of involvement in the spinal axis. A skeletal survey with plain x-rays is more helpful in myeloma for detecting occult lesions.

☐ LABORATORY INVESTIGATIONS

Several hematological investigations may be pertinent with suspected spinal tumors. Patients with metastatic lesions of the vertebrae may present with anemia, leukopenia, or thrombocytopenia due to involvement of the bone marrow.

Widespread bony metastases may lead to hypercalcemia and elevated serum alkaline phosphatase. Multiple myeloma can be diagnosed by the presence of the Bence Jones monoclonal antibody protein by urine or serum protein electrophoresis, a screening test that may be positive even with solitary plasmacytomas. Tumor markers can be diagnostic: prostatic specific antigen (PSA) with prostate cancer, CA 125 with ovarian cancer, carcinoembryonic antigen (CEA) with colon cancer, and vanillylmandelic acid (VMA) with neuroblastoma.[13] Elevated levels of alpha fetoprotein (a-FP) and beta human chorionic gonadotrophin (b-HCG) are diagnostic for tumors of germ cell origin, including seminomas, germinomas, embryonal carcinomas, endodermal sinus tumors, and mixed teratomas.[49]

Microscopic examination of the centrifuged sediment from CSF can be diagnostic for extramedullary tumors, especially lymphoma, leukemia (ALL), and in cases of "drop-metastases," including pinealoblastomas, medulloblastomas, ependymomas, germinomas, and other germ cell tumors.

The CSF should be routinely obtained at myelography and examined for protein, glucose, cell count, and cytology. The protein value is elevated with blocks of the subarachnoid space and is usually elevated in association with neurinomas and neurofibromas because of secretion of protein by the tumor. The elevated protein can distinguish neurinomas from meningiomas. CSF pleocytosis is a harbinger of leptomeningeal infiltration with metastatic or primary neoplasms.

☐ ADJUNCTIVE OPERATIVE MANAGEMENT[1–16]

STEROID ADMINISTRATION[18,19]

Glucocorticoids should be given to patients at least 24 h prior to surgery and should be continued postoperatively with tapering dosages beginning 3 to 5 days after surgery to decrease overall spinal cord edema.[18,19] Steroid tapering can be adjusted as the patient's neurobiological function is monitored. Ordinarily dexamethasone is administered at 4 mg q 6 h, but this dosage can be increased to 10 mg q 4 h. Protection of the gastrointestinal (GI) tract may be accomplished with ranitidine HCL [Zantac (H₂ blocker)] or an antacid. For patients with metastatic cancer to the spine and sudden, dramatic paraparesis or quadriparesis, an initial dose of 100 mg dexamethasone IV can be given, followed by 20 mg q 4 h. Glucocorticoids appear to have a beneficial effect on spinal cord edema from tumor cells, although it is unclear whether the mechanism of action is inhibition of cell growth or actual cytolysis.[18,19] Interestingly, there is evidence that glucocorticoids may have a direct oncolytic effect on lymphomas and leukemias through cell lysis.[19] Regardless of the mechanism, the administration of glucocorticoids to patients with spinal tumors appears to have a beneficial effect on neurological function.[18,19]

INTRAOPERATIVE (FROZEN) PATHOLOGY

Tumor specimens are usually examined microscopically during surgery. In patients with metastatic tumors with an unknown primary, the intraoperative frozen tissue will often be diagnostic. The biology of the metastatic tumor provides the opportunity to develop a rational management scheme. It may direct the type of surgery required. For example, in patients with metastatic lung cancer, it is important to know whether the tumor is undifferentiated carcinoma or oat-cell carcinoma as opposed to large cell or squamous cell carcinoma, since undifferentiated and oat cell tumors are associated with a very poor prognosis. Certain metastatic spinal neoplasms are quite radiosensitive, particularly lymphomas and seminomas, and postoperative irradiation will suppress or possibly eradicate residual tumor. Craniospinal irradiation is effective for intradural, radiosensitive tumors like medulloblastomas, germinomas, and pinealoblastomas, which may present as "drop-metastases."

Frozen tissue pathology is helpful during surgery for intramedullary tumors, particularly when differentiating astrocytomas from ependymomas. The neurosurgeon may be hesitant to attempt complete removal of an astrocytoma due to indistinct tumor margins, whereas ependymomas more readily peel away from normal spinal cord.

INTRAOPERATIVE SONOGRAPHY

The recent application of real-time ultrasonography to surgical explorations allows localization of spinal tumors by imaging the structural details.[13] The ultrasonic probe is applied to the epidural or intradural spaces. Then the full extent of an epidural mass, including ventral and ventrolateral extensions, is determined. In intramedullary tumors, the depth and extent of the tumor is ascertained, and any asso-

ciated syringes identified. Adequate decompression of a syrinx and division of septations can be followed by resolution or disappearance of an echogenic signal. After microsurgical resection, the spinal cord is examined by ultrasound for residual tumor, or the placement of a shunt is verified. Spinal cord pulsations demonstrating adequate decompression are monitored.[13]

☐ INTRINSIC TUMORS[4,5,8,11,12]

A recent retrospective review of primary intraspinal neoplasms in a defined population base imparts reasonably unbiased data and sheds light on the overall tumor biology.[20] Meningioma is the most-common spinal tumor (46.7 percent), followed by ependymoma (18.6 percent), neurinoma (10.8 percent), astrocytoma (6.0 percent), mixed glioma (5.3 percent), and glioblastoma (1.4 percent).[20] Oligodendroglioma was 0.7 percent and other miscellaneous tumors 6.3 percent.

The gender distribution of meningiomas was 6:1 female/male, and ependymomas were 2:1 male/female. Remaining types of spinal tumor were almost evenly distributed among males and females. The incidence of intraspinal tumor is 0.3 to 0.5 per 100,000 population per year, thus it is rare.[20] By comparison, this is the same percentage as that seen for male breast cancer in Norway.[20] In males, there is a peak of intraspinal tumors in the 15- to 29-year-old age range, whereas in females a similar peak is seen in the 60- to 74-year-old age group. Intraspinal meningiomas are associated with a very high 5-year survival rate of 99.5 percent, whereas the intracranial survival rate for meningiomas is significantly less, at 84 percent.[20] Similarly, the 5-year survival rate for intraspinal ependymomas is 88.9 percent, compared to 24.4 percent for the intracranial tumors.[20] Interestingly, there is an equivalent 5-year survival rate of 48 percent vs. 44.9 percent for intraspinal and intracranial astrocytomas. However, the intracranial mixed glioma has a survival rate of 28.1 percent, compared to 50.7 percent in the intraspinal mixed gliomas. In general, the prognosis is better in patients with primary intraspinal glial tumors as compared with intracranial tumors.[20]

☐ INTRAMEDULLARY TUMORS

EPENDYMOMAS[21–29]

Ependymoma is the most common intramedullary tumor of the spinal cord (Fig. 13-1, Plate 1). It is commonly found in cervical or cervicothoracic regions, but it is frequently found with a special predilection for the conus medullaris or filum terminale (56 percent).[21,23] Fusiform tumors extend from the medulla oblongata to the conus medullaris. Often the mean

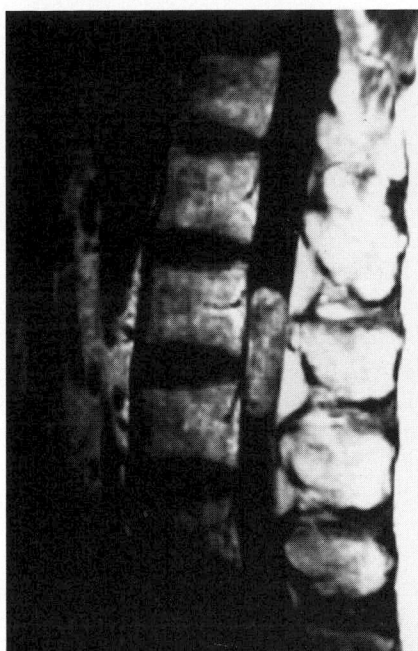

Figure 13–1A Myxopapillary ependymoma. A T2-weighted MRI in the sagittal plane with Gd-DTPA contrast shows a globular, inhomogeneous mass that enhances very intensely. It is adjacent to and spans the L2 and L3 vertebral bodies.

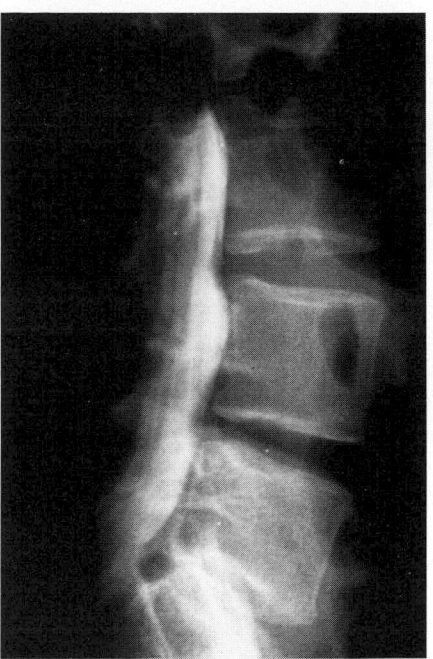

Figure 13–1B Myelographic image in the lateral view shows a spinal block at L2–L3 with a "capping" defect, or meniscus, due to an intradural-extramedullary mass. By comparison, an intramedullary ependymoma produces a fusiform enlargement of the entire spinal cord.

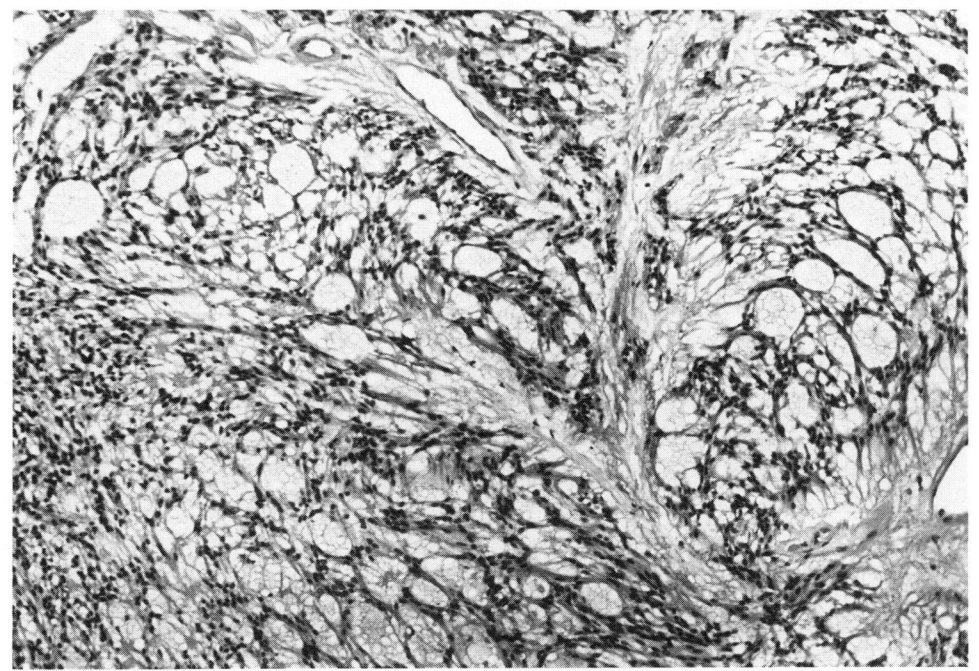

Figure 13–1C Microscopic features characteristic of the myxopapillary ependymoma usually found in the area of the filum terminale. Notice presence of streaming vessels with arrangements of tumor cells around them. The cystoplastic round vacuoles are filled with mucinous contents.

length of solid tumor is three to five spinal segments. Pain, sensory disturbance, and weakness are common symptoms, often preceding the diagnosis by 2 to 3 years. The age of presentation is typically 30 to 40 years old. The cauda equina ependymoma is particularly common in males. The tumor histology is 40 percent cellular, 2 percent epithelial, 21 percent myxopapillary, and 37 percent mixed.[4] A rare histologically malignant type of ependymoma is termed *ependymoblastoma.*

The cauda equina ependymoma is characterized by perineal pain; bowel, bladder, and sexual dysfunction; and paraparesis. Rarely, there is an associated symptom complex of acute subarachnoid hemorrhage with sciatica, termed *Fincher's syndrome,* which may be precipitated by pregnancy or trauma. Ependymomas arise from ependymal cell nests within the ventriculus terminalis and filum terminale. Very rarely, the myxopapillary ependymomas originate in ectopic sites outside the spinal canal, particularly in the sacrum and presacral tissues. They can even present as widespread metastases in the lymph nodes, lung, liver, and bone.

Syringomyelia and cystic fluid-filled cavitations are frequently found with intramedullary tumors.[24,26] The cystic fluid is yellow and proteinaceous when compared to the clear, colorless CSF obtained from syringomyelia cavities associated with the Arnold-Chiari malformation. There may be objective signs and symptoms of syringomyelia due to central canal destruction: amyotrophy in the upper extremities, "main-en-griffe," with concurrent hyporeflexia, and dissociated sensory loss in the face, neck ("Balaclava helmet"), shoulders, and arms, extending in a capelike distribution due to interruption of the crossing spinothalamic tracts. There may be scars from painless accidental burns, and Horner's syndrome from interruption of the central, anteromediolateral sympathetic fiber column at T1.

In the lower extremities, there is rigidity, hyperreflexia, clonus, and occasionally spasticity. In cervicomedullary tumors, there may be downbeat and vertical nystagmus; dizziness; vertigo; cough-syncope; occipital headaches; nuchal rigidity; hoarseness, dysphagia, and other bulbar signs; ataxia and dysmetria from cerebellar dysfunction; and spastic tetraparesis from bilateral involvement of the corticospinal tracts.

The neurosurgical rationale for treating intramedullary tumors was summarized by Elsberg's treatise in 1925.[25] Operative techniques including bipolar coagulation and use of the operating microscope were advanced by Greenwood, Kurze, and Malis in the period 1950–1970.[24,26,27]

Several recent series on the operative removal of the intramedullary and cauda equina ependymomas report complete removal in the majority of cases.[21,23,26,28,29] The intramedullary variant is a discrete tumor with a cleavage plane. It is well demarcated, allowing total removal, and there is a high incidence of cure evidenced by no recurrence of low-grade ependymomas 5 to 10 years postoperatively.[21,22,28,29]

However, the quality of the recovery depends on the degree of preoperative neurological impairment since patients who are paraplegic preoperatively usually do not regain motor function postoperatively. Further, dorsal column deficits due to midline myelotomy and dysesthetic pain syndromes are common complications. Overall, the sensorimotor deficit stabilizes after tumor removal without significant deterioration in the majority of cases.[21,22]

The role of radiation therapy in the treatment of ependymomas is relegated to infiltrative lesions or the malignant variant, ependymoblastoma, as radiation myelopathy is a serious complication. Reoperation is indicated for recurrent ependymomas; however, it may be complicated by a CSF fistula from an incompetent dural closure, with complicating meningitis and arachnoiditis.

A recent series of ependymomas of the cauda equina mirrors results similar to those seen in the intramedullary variant. Total tumor removal is the rule.[23] However, bowel and bladder dysfunction, present preoperatively, did not recover. Early surgery results in an excellent outcome in those patients presenting with pain only, as compared to pain with deficits and disturbance of sphincters. The role of chemotherapy in radioresistant tumors and the management of incompletely resected tumors are variable. There is no effective therapeutic regimen for infiltrating ependymomas or ependymoblastomas.

ASTROCYTOMA[30–33]

The *astrocytoma* is the second most common primary intramedullary tumor, followed by malignant astrocytoma and glioblastoma multiforme (Fig. 13-2, Plates 2 and 3).[20] It presents throughout the cord or as a fusiform tumor at the cervicomedullary junction in children.[33] Similar to the ependymoma, the astrocytoma occurs most commonly in the cervical and cervicothoracic regions and less commonly in the thoracolumbar region. The neurological signs and symptoms mirror those in the ependymomas, including corticospinal and spinothalamic tract involvement, paresis, and dysesthetic pain.

Also, cysts associated with tumors or large syringes are quite common, and they define the upper and lower extents of the tumor. They are readily identified by MRI. Cysts contain xanthochromic fluid, which is rich in protein, and they have a gliotic wall that is demarcated from normal spinal cord tissue. Classically, Schlesinger[4,5,8] advocated percutaneous drainage of these tumor cysts to alleviate neurological signs and symptoms, and this was performed both diagnostically and therapeutically at the time of myelotomy. However, the biology of the astrocytoma lends itself more readily to an open definitive resection.

Most spinal astrocytomas are low-grade. The mean duration of symptoms can go to up to 10 years, whereas less-common gliomas have a more-rapid course of 6 to 12 mo.[30] Benign astrocytomas are fibrillary or pilocytic and may contain Rosenthal fibers and microcysts. Gliomas show evidence of hypercellularity, vascular proliferation, necrosis, and hyperchromatic nuclei as seen in intracranial tumors.

Older series of surgically removed astrocytomas have stressed that radical, complete excision is rarely possible because of an absence of cleavage planes.[27,30] Few patients improved neurologically after subtotal excision or biopsy, and the lesions resumed their clinical course in 50 percent of cases after a period of as much as 5 years postoperatively. Recent reports, however, have indicated complete tumor removal in most instances, with improvement or stabilization of motor deficits in 70 to 80 percent of the patients.[28,29,33] The more extensive removal of intramedullary tumors has been attributed to advances in the microneurosurgical techniques.[28,29] Unfortunately, radical resection of intramedullary gliomas has but a transient effect on the natural history of the disease process.[29]

In striking contrast to ependymomas, recurrence is common despite near-complete tumor removal of astrocytomas, and a 50 percent recurrence rate is seen at 5 years.[29] This is accompanied by an increased mortality by 5 years postoper-

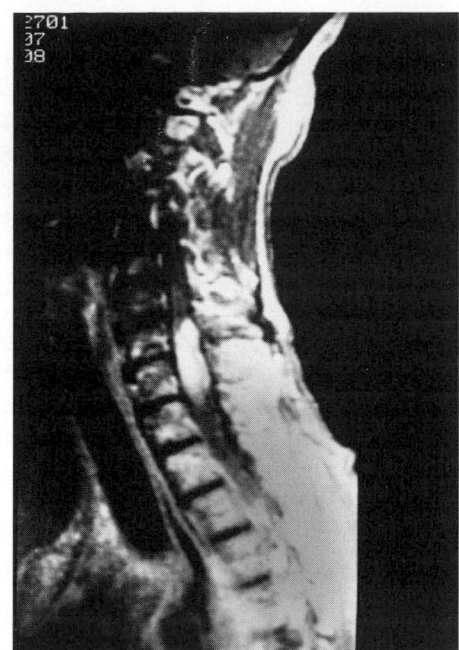 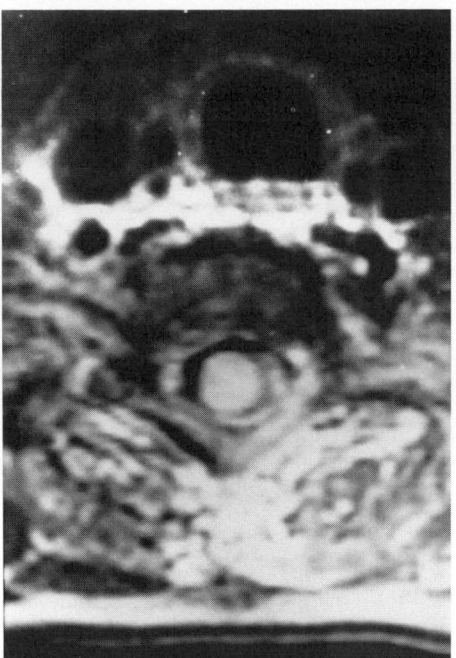 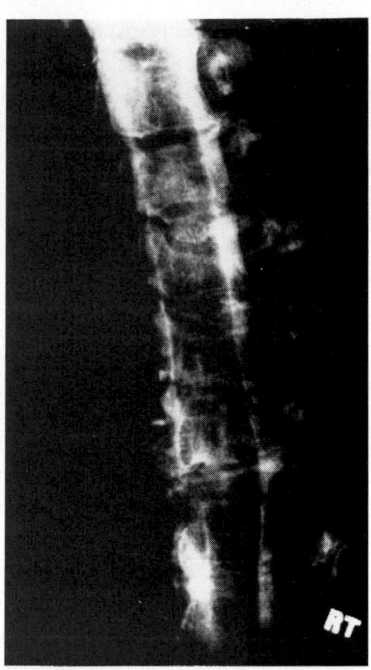

Figure 13–2A Astrocytoma. T2-weighted MRI in the sagittal plane with Gd-DTPA administration reveals an intrinsic, homogeneously enhancing tumor involving the entire spinal cord spanning the C6 and C7 vertebral levels.

Figure 13–2B Same case as 13–2A. T2-weighted MRI in the axial plane with Gd-DTPA administration reveals an intrinsic, enhancing tumor involving the entire spinal cord.

Figure 13–2C Myelographic image in the AP view showing a large intramedullary tumor that expands and nearly obliterates the spinal subarachnoid space.

atively. Several authors have stated that the outcome after treatment for astrocytomas is much poorer than that seen in the ependymomas, since ependymomas may be completely removed.[26,29] Patients with malignant tumors succumb within 5 to 6 months of onset.

In pediatric patients, intramedullary astrocytomas appear to be amenable to complete surgical excision, especially tumors localized at the cervicomedullary junction.[33] It appears that these tumors displace rather than invade normal neural tissue, and they may be clinically similar to cystic cerebellar astrocytomas, also seen in the pediatric population.[29,33]

The role of radiation therapy for treatment of astrocytomas is still controversial. To date, there has been a natural bias to treat those patients whose tumors have been subtotally resected or who have had recurrences.[29,31,32] So far there is no clear benefit to adjuvant radiation therapy, although the long natural history of astrocytomas and the rarity of such tumors make it difficult to answer this question definitively. Postoperative radiation therapy should be indicated in the glioma patient as a palliative treatment regimen.[29] Unfortunately, there is no specific chemotherapy for intramedullary astrocytomas or mixed gliomas.

HEMANGIOBLASTOMA[34,35]

Hemangioblastomas are rare, vascular, intramedullary benign tumors with a peak incidence in the fourth decade of life, an equal male-to-female ratio, and a preferential loca-

tion in the cervical and cervicomedullary regions.[4,5,34,35] Histologically, the stromal cell may be endothelial in origin with positive staining for factor VIII, thus accounting for the vascular mural nodules.

Hemangioblastoma has a high association with syringomyelia and tumor-associated cysts and a less common association (22 percent) with Lindau's disease or cystic cerebellar hemangioblastomas.[4,5,34,35] Von Hippel-Lindau's disease can include both retinal angiomas and cerebellar-spinal hemangioblastomas, indicating a wide genetic overlap for this clinical entity originally described as an autosomal dominant trait.

Sixty to seventy percent of hemangioblastomas are intramedullary and located preferentially on the dorsal surface of the spinal cord, whereas 20 to 30 percent are intradural, extramedullary, and present near the nerve root sheath, typically in the thoracic area.[4,5,34,35] These tumors are readily diagnosed by MRI and spinal angiography and have intensely shiny mural nodules that are highly vascular with rapid AV shunting.[17] The clinical presentation is like that of other intramedullary tumors, although subarachnoid hemorrhage with or without focal neurological deficits is a classic presentation and should be thought of in a young patient with new-onset of suboccipital headaches and nuchal rigidity.

Microneurosurgical techniques facilitate the complete excision of spinal hemangioblastomas, as seen in a series of twelve patients by Yasargil.[34] The CUSA, LASER, Malis CMC-III Bipolar, cautery, and cardiopulmonary bypass under hypothermia[35] are useful adjuncts in tumor removal.

Paradoxically, Stein[26] found a uniform enlargement of the spinal cord adjacent but caudal to the hemangioblastoma in his two cases, which resolved within several months after complete tumor removal. Edema of the spinal cord is postulated to be secondary to vascular shunting by the tumor.[26] Overall, surgical principles are similar to those used in treating arteriovenous malformations (AVMs). The arterial supply is secured first, and draining veins are preserved until the end of the resection for a total tumor removal.[26]

OLIGODENDROGLIOMA[36,37]

Oligodendrogliomas are very rare intramedullary tumors that are often calcified and can be intermixed with glial and cystic elements.[12] Occasionally, an intracranial oligodendroglioma is implicated as the origin of an intraspinal tumor by a "drop metastasis" throughout the spinal subarachnoid space.[37] Because of its rarity, the overall natural history of the intramedullary oligodendroglioma is poorly understood.[36,37]

LIPOMA, DERMOID, EPIDERMOID, TERATOMA[38–45]

These rare tumors are congenital lesions which typically present in the midline of the spinal cord in children, adolescents, and young adults, but they are also seen in the mature adult population. (These tumors are reported in Chap. 9, but a brief discussion is indicated here.)

In adults, the *lipoma* is most common in the cervical and thoracic regions, whereas in children the lumbosacral area is usually affected.[38,39,41] There is a high association with overlying cutaneous abnormalities, including nevi, dimples, skin hyperpigmentation, hypertrichosis, capillary angiomas, midline hairy patches, and subcutaneous lipomas—all indicative of an occult intraspinal tumor. There is a high incidence of underlying dysraphia. MRI is diagnostic for lipoma, with a very hyperintense signal on T1 imaging and a hypointense signal on T2 consistent with adipose tissue. Surgical excision is rarely complete, however, as the lipoma is often embedded within the pial substance of the spinal cord, making complete removal difficult.[38–41]

In children, the lumbosacral lipoma associated with spina bifida occulta is usually attached to the caudally displaced conus medullaris and adherent to the cauda equina rootlets.[41] There is no distinct cleavage plane between lipoma and spinal cord, prohibiting complete tumor removal.[41]

The *dermoid* is frequently associated with a fistulous sinus tract and occult spinal dysrhaphism, often with overlying skin hyperpigmentation or hypertrichosis.[42,43] The lesion contains skin with dermal appendages. It is most common in the lumbar and lumbosacral regions, and it can present with clinical evidence of meningitis due to rupture of the dermoid cyst into the subarachnoid space, with resultant chemical arachnoiditis. In contrast, the dermoid tumor presents classi-

cally as a midline cerebellar tumor in children, with a clinical history of repeated episodes of bacterial, or occasionally aseptic, meningitis. Total excision is often precluded by a diaphanous tumor capsule adherent to the spinal cord and with abundant through and through grumous hairs.[26,43]

Epidermoids are also associated with spina bifida occulta, but they predominate in the thoracolumbar region.[42] Epidermoid tumors contain four layers of normal skin. The epidermoid can be caused iatrogenically from repeated lumbar punctures or may be a remnant from a meningomyelocele repair. It has been produced experimentally in a rat model.[44] The *teratoma* is a rare congenital tumor with a predilection for the conus medullaris.[45] It contains skin and dermal appendages with abundant hair and cartilage, representing mesoderm and endodermal appendages. There is a tendency for malignant degeneration with occasional systemic metastases. This is a feature of teratomas in the sacrococcygeal region.

CANCER METASTASES[46–48]

These are rare intramedullary tumors with rapid clinical onset of signs and symptoms, typically in the cervical and thoracic spinal regions, usually presenting with progressive myelopathy of short temporal duration.[46] Lung cancer, followed by breast cancer and melanoma, are the most-common primary tumors, and spinal metastases may be the presenting feature of the occult cancer.[47,48] Most patients with intramedullary tumors have a previously diagnosed and widely metastatic malignancy at the time of presentation.[47,48] MRI will reveal an enhancing intramedullary metastatic nodule with surrounding edema not unlike that seen in astrocytoma or ependymoma. The intramedullary tumor can be completely resected through a definitive cleavage plane by microneurosurgical techniques, and surgery is recommended in patients with discrete solitary metastases and limited cancer.[46] Unfortunately, the long-term prognosis and outcome is still poor in patients who have metastatic cancer to the spine, despite surgery, palliative radiotherapy, and corticosteroid treatment.[47–49]

SPINAL METASTASES FROM INTRACRANIAL TUMORS

Several primary intracranial tumors have high rates of metastasis throughout the spinal subarachnoid space, producing drop metastases which present clinically with paraparesis or quadriparesis. Tumors in the pineal region—including pinealoblastoma, pinealocytoma, germinoma, and the malignant germ cell tumor (embryonal carcinoma, yolk sac tumor or endodermal sinus tumor, and choriocarcinoma)—can seed the entire neuraxis, prompting surveillance by panspinal MRI or myelography, CSF cytologic examination, and craniospinal irradiation with chemotherapy for chemosensitive tumors.[49] Medulloblastomas with spinal metastases can diffusely coat and expand the spinal cord, producing a desmoplastic reaction, or they present as multiple discrete tumor nodules on the nerve roots or on the surface of the cord.[17] Ependymomas of the fourth ventricle can spread through the subarachnoid spaces of the adjacent upper cervical cord, lending a "plastic" appearance by direct examination. Rarely, drop-metastases from an occult intracranial tumor can be the initial clinical presentation of the disease. It may be necessary to obtain an MRI of the brain in addition to an MRI of the spine.

PARAGANGLIOMA[7,50]

Paragangliomas are rare tumors of the cauda equina derived from the sympathetic ganglia and adrenal medulla, related phylogenetically to pheochromocytomas and carotid body tumors.[7,50] The tumors are intradural, intraarachnoid, hypervascular, and inherently benign, with "Zellballen" clusters histologically.[7,50] The incidence of paragangliomas is highest in the fifth decade of life, and there is a 2:1 male preference. A recent screening test includes radioactive metaiodo-benzyl-guanidine (MIBG) to image occult paragangliomas, carotid body tumors, and pheochromocytomas.[7]

ARACHNOID, EPENDYMAL, EPITHELIAL, ENTEROGENOUS, AND BRANCHIOGENIC CYSTS OF THE LEPTOMENINGES[51–55]

These rare congenital, developmental lesions are found predominantly in the cervical and thoracic regions, and they present as intramedullary or extramedullary intradural mass lesions. The most prominent symptom is pain with variable radiculopathies. Progressive myelopathy can result in a typically protracted clinical course over years.[51–55] These cysts usually present clinically by the fourth or fifth decade of life and show no gender predilection. MRI is diagnostic for the cystic mass, but histological examination is required to establish a definitive diagnosis. By myelography, cysts may or may not communicate with the CSF subarachnoid space, but the fluid will appear clear to colorless, similar to normal CSF.

The *arachnoid cyst* is the most-common intraspinal cyst. It has a single-layered arachnoid cell lining, without epithelium or cilia. It has a peak incidence in the fifth decade of life. It is typically located dorsal to the thoracic spinal cord but is less commonly ventral.[51,55] The *ependymal cyst* has a ciliated, cuboidal, or columnar epithelial lining and is common in children in the ventral, cervical spinal cord.[52] The *enterogenous cyst,* derived from the neurenteric canal or primitive endoderm, is common in the ventral cervicothoracic and thoracic canal, and it may be associated with duplication of the GI tract and dysraphic bony abnormalities of the vertebral body(ies). This cyst is lined by cilated, secretory columnar epithelium and can produce mucin, which is

diagnostic. Surprisingly, the neurenteric cyst has a predilection for the ventral cervicomedullary junction. The *branchiogenic cyst* has an associated respiratory epithelial lining and congenital vertebral anomalies in the thoracic spine as well.

Definitive treatment of intraspinal cysts includes microsurgical excision and/or fenestration of the intramedullary or extramedullary cyst, and occasional cystosubarachnoid, cystopleural, or cystoperitoneal shunting to divert the cystic fluid.[51,55] Recurrence is rare after definitive surgical treatment, and pain relief is common.[51,55]

☐ EXTRAMEDULLARY TUMORS[56–60]

MENINGIOMAS

Meningiomas are the most-common intradural spinal tumors, with 60 to 70 percent occurring most frequently at thoracic levels and 10 to 20 percent at cervical levels.[4,5,9,56] Lumbosacral and craniovertebral meningiomas are rare. Meningiomas have a 5:1 female-to-male predilection, and they are diagnosed at a mean age of 50 to 60 years.[4,5,9,56] They are typically intradural, extramedullary.[4,5,9,56,60] Over half are located laterally, the remainder being divided between dorsal and ventral segments of the canal (Fig. 13-3, Plate 4). Between 5 and 10 percent of spinal meningiomas have extradural components. Multiple meningiomas are associated with neurofibromatosis. Rarely, spinal meningiomatosis occurs in association with intracranial meningiomas.

Meningiomas arise from the arachnoid, near a nerve root sheath, and they are slow-growing, with a 1- to 2-year history of symptoms. The histology is typically of the syncytial or transitional type with whorls.[4,5] Angioblastic or hemangiopericytic types are rare. Calcification, *en plaque* growth, and hyperostosis are also rare.[9]

Long-tract signs, including paraparesis and quadriparesis, are common presentations, and because of the laterally positioned meningioma, a Brown-Séquard syndrome with a distinct sensory level to pinprick is frequent. Radicular pain is common and is often girdlelike in distribution near the involved root(s). Radicular pain is most prominent at night and may be exacerbated by Valsalva maneuvers. Foramen magnum meningiomas are uniquely associated with cold dysesthesias and clumsiness of the hands, as well as marked wasting of the intrinsic muscles. Suboccipital pain and nuchal rigidity are referable to involvement of the second cervical nerve root (C2), and eleventh nerve compression may cause weakness of the trapezius and sternocleidomastoid muscles.[9,58,59]

Surgically, meningiomas should be debulked anteriorly and laterally away from the compressed, displaced spinal cord. Sectioning of the dentate ligament ensures access to the tumor.[9] Meningiomas are frequently found attached to an insertion of the dentate ligament. Dorsal or sensory nerve

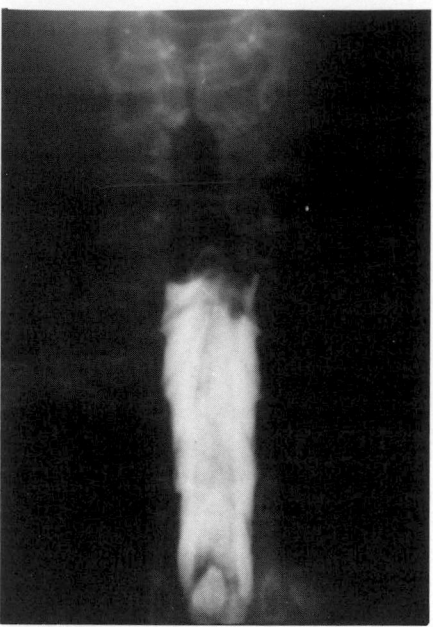

Figure 13–3A Meningioma. AP myelographic image reveals a complete block at C7 with classic "capping" or meniscus defect with the cord displaced to the left.

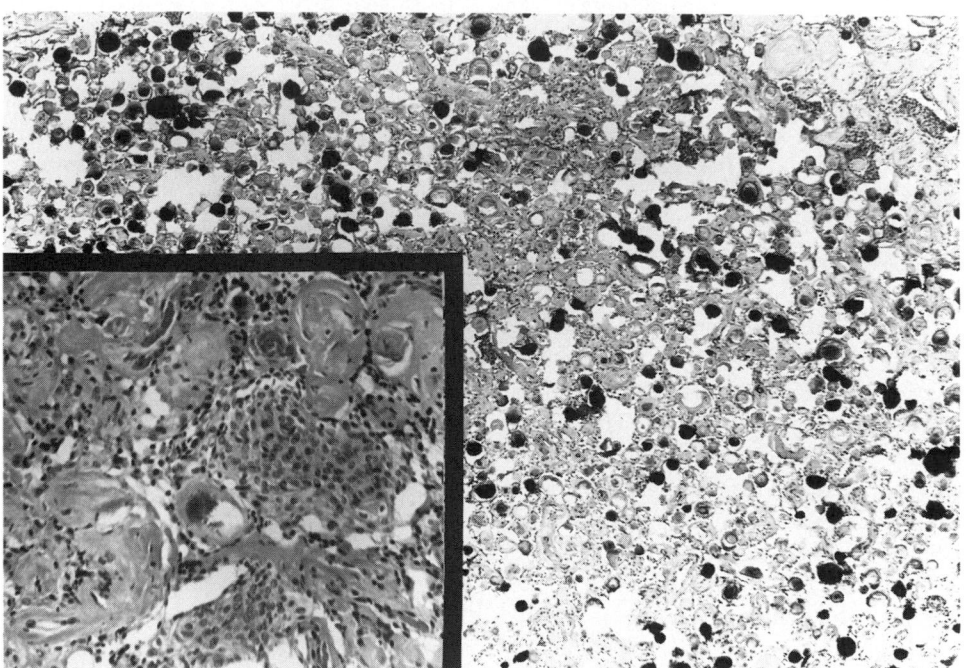

Figure 13–3B Spinal meningioma showing overwhelming abundance of psammomatous bodies forming the architecture of the tumor. Some are hyalinized (lighter spherules), and some are calcified (darker spherules). The inset represents rare areas of meningothelial tumor cells, revealing the true nature of the tumor as a meningioma.

roots can be sectioned, and traction sutures can be placed laterally in the dura mater for greater access to the tumor. Microsurgical excision of meningiomas is successful in 90 to 95 percent of patients.[56,57] A recurrence rate of only 6 percent after a period of 4 to 17 years has been reported.[56] The need for resection of the dural base is not clear, but the dura should be resected if it is easily accessible. When it is not feasible to resect the dura, the dura should be cauterized and scraped with microdissectors to reduce the risk of recurrence. Over 80 percent of patients treated for spinal meningiomas regain neurological normality, and only 5 percent have increased neurological deficits.[56,57] Even paraplegic patients may recover sufficiently to ambulate without assistance after surgery. Infrequent complications include CSF leak, meningitis, and arachnoiditis.

Ventrally placed meningiomas can be approached and

excised anteriorly or anterolaterally. This approach is particularly helpful for tumors in the region of the neck and at the cervicomedullary junction.[14–16,60] Crockard[14] has advocated a transoral approach to intradural tumors ventral to the cervicomedullary junction, particularly meningiomas and neurofibromas, whereas Stevenson[15] and, later, McDonnell[16] have favored a transcervical approach. Both techniques give similar results and represent methods for reaching formerly inaccessible lesions.

NEURINOMA, NEUROFIBROMA[61–65]

Neurinomas (*schwannomas*) and *neurofibromas* are the second most common intradural-extramedullary tumors. They occur most frequently at the thoracic level, followed by the cervical level, less commonly in the lumbosacral region, and rarely at the cervicomedullary junctions. About 70 to 80 percent are intradural extramedullary.[4,5,61] Ten to 20 percent are solely extradural.[4,5,61] Also, 10 to 20 percent are classically dumbbell, or hourglass, tumors.[4,5,61] Over 1 percent are wholly intramedullary. The male-to-female ratio is equal. The average duration of symptoms is almost 2 years before diagnosis (Fig. 13-4, Plates 5 and 6).

The sensory nerve root is the usual site of origin of the neurinoma or neurofibroma, but the ventral or motor root can be involved by local compression. A large cervical neurinoma or neurofibroma may be palpated in the neck by physical examination. Radicular pain and, occasionally, dysesthesias are reported in over 80 percent of patients. Motor and bladder dysfunction and sensory levels to pinprick are seen in less than 50 percent of patients. Rarely, neurofibromas present clinically with subarachnoid hemorrhage, causing sudden pain, fever, and meningismus.

Plain x-rays of the spine are abnormal in nearly half of patients, in marked contrast to meningiomas where changes are seen in only 15 to 20 percent of patients.[4,5,9] Common abnormalities include erosion and scalloping of pedicles and vertebral bodies (Fig. 13-5, Plates 7 and 8). Enlarged foramina may accompany dumbbell masses and, rarely, dural ectasia is seen by myelography in patients with von Recklinghausen's disease, with or without neurofibromas. In the case of a dumbbell neurofibroma, with intra- and extradural components, the extradural component may be large and readily visible as a soft tissue mass on chest or abdominal x-rays.

CSF may have markedly elevated levels of proteins, sometimes greater than 400 mg/100 ml, whereas meningiomas are associated with protein levels of 100 mg/100 ml. Nerve sheath tumors are markedly hyperintense on T2-weighted images compared to neural tissue. Tumor extension through an enlarged neural foramen is a characteristic feature.

Pathologically, schwannomas are typically limited to one nerve fascicle or bundle. The perineurium remains intact. Grossly, neurinomas may be cystic with nerve fibers absent, but Schwann cells grow out by tissue cultures. In contrast,

neurofibromas have extensive amounts of collagen or fibrous tissue with axons dispersed throughout the tumor, making tumor excision impossible without sacrificing nerve(s). Grossly, neurofibromas are firm and lobulated rather than cystic. They have an estimated 13 to 15 percent incidence of malignant degeneration to sarcoma. Like neurinomas, neurofibromas grow as Schwann cells in tissue cultures, identifying a common cellular type.

Gardner has postulated that intraspinal tumors can cause hydrocephalus and CNS symptoms by obstructing the spinal

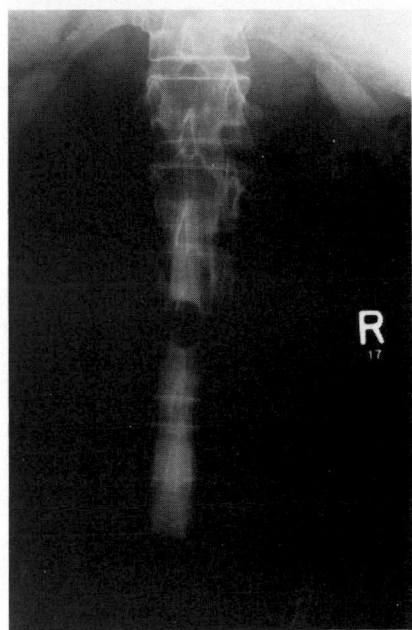

Figure 13–4A Schwannoma. AP myelographic image reveals an intradural tumor at L3 between the cauda equina roots and below the conus medullaris.

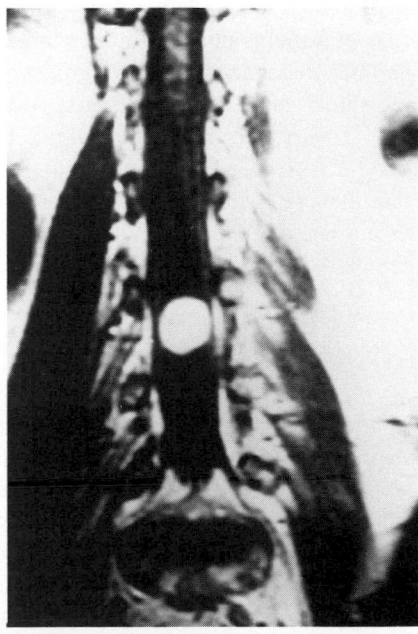

Figure 13–4B Same case as 13–4A. Coronal MRI with Gd-DTPA showing intradural tumor at L3 between the cauda equina roots.

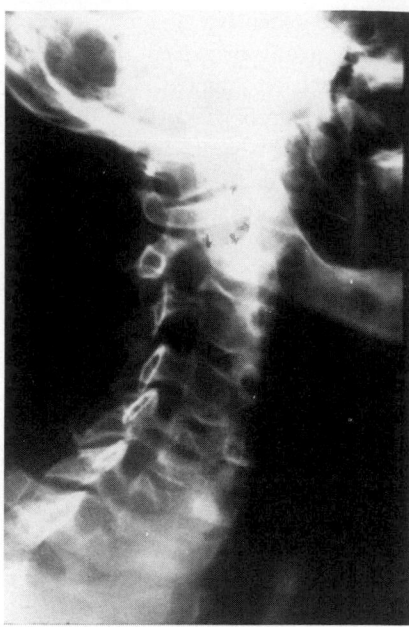

Figure 13–5 Neurofibroma. Right oblique x-ray showing extensive C1 to C2 bone erosion and foraminal enlargement with scalloping and a "silhouette" from a tumor mass.

subarachnoid space with large amounts of secreted protein.[65] This putative mechanism of altering the CSF dynamics postoperatively may cause the development of subdural hematomas.

Results following excision of neurinomas or neurofibromas are rewarding. In Levy's series of 66 neurofibromas, 80 percent had resolution of pain while 60 percent had full neurological recovery postoperatively and returned to work.[61] Only 5% experienced worsening of neurological deficits after surgery. No tumors recurred during follow-up of 1 to 7 years. In Kim's series,[62] in 86 cases where the nerve root was resected to achieve complete tumor removal, only 23 percent of patients developed detectable sensory or motor deficits, and these deficits were minimal. They concluded that the spinal nerve roots giving rise to the schwannoma, typically sensory, are frequently nonfunctional at the time of surgery. Risks of incurring disabling neurological deficits are minimal. The studies indicate that radical resection of a neurinoma or neurofibroma is indicated for an excellent outcome.

SARCOIDOSIS[66,67]

Sarcoidosis is a rare manifestation of systemic disease, characterized by a noncaseating, granulomatous infiltration. Involvement of the spinal cord including meninges is about 1 percent clinically and can present as three entities: multiple intramedullary lesions with focal arachnoiditis; large intradural-extramedullary tumors with marked mass effects and focal neurologic deficits or myelopathy; or as an extradural mass from sarcoid infiltration of the spinal cord and dura (Fig. 13-6, Plate 9).

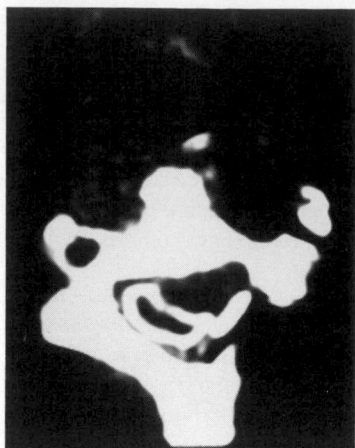

Figure 13–6 Sarcoidosis. Myelographic CT axial image reveals an intradural-extramedullar mass compressing and displacing the cord to the right. There is also infiltration of the vertebral body and dura.

The typical presentation is progressive, painless paraparesis. The thoracic spine is the most common site of involvement. Surgical treatment is laminectomy, biopsy and, if indicated, decompression of the granuloma coupled with the administration of corticosteroids, known to be an effective medical treatment in this disease. Serum and CSF levels of angiotensin converting enzyme (ACE) can be followed to assess the progression of the disease.[66,67] The natural history of spinal sarcoidosis is remission and relapse, and corticosteroids are the cornerstone of continuing medical treatment.

☐ EPIDURAL TUMORS

CANCER METASTASES[68–72]

About 5 percent of cancer patients develop clinical signs of compression of the spinal cord or a nerve root due to metastases.[2,4,5,7,10,11,13,68–72] In nearly 10 percent of patients presenting for the first time with spinal metastases, the primary site is unknown and a surgical resection is undertaken to establish a tissue diagnosis.[2,4,5,7,10,11,13,68–72]

The majority of spinal tumors, i.e., greater than 80 percent, are cancer metastases most commonly from lung, breast, kidney, prostate, colon, thyroid, melanoma, lymphomas, or sarcoma.[2,4,5,7,10,11,13,68–72] Postmortem studies of cancer victims show that 50 to 70 percent have clear-cut evidence of vertebral metastases. A smaller percentage have dural encroachment and spinal cord compression.

The vertebral body is often involved first in metastasis. Posterior elements are affected only one-fifth to one-seventh as often as vertebral bodies.[4,5,7,10,11,13,68–72] Many metastases are believed to be spread through Batson's venous plexus. Even more than vertebral bodies, pedicles appear to be infiltrated first as they are composed of cortical bone only,

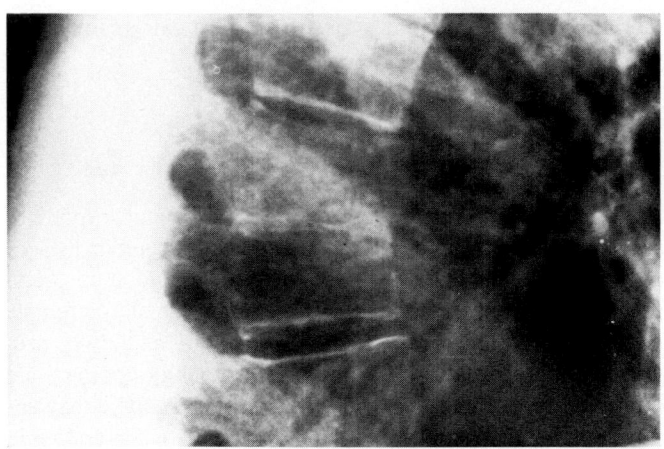

Figure 13–7 Metastatic hypernephroma. Lateral thoracic x-ray shows a 25 percent compression fracture of the T8 vertebral body.

and metastatic disease is manifested by pedicle erosion or enlargement on AP x-ray films of the spine. Nearly 50 percent of the vertebral bodies, which are primarily cancellous bone, are infiltrated by metastases by the time abnormalities are seen on plain x-rays of the spine,[4,5,7,10,11,13,68–72] i.e., collapse, of a vertebral body or a compression fracture (Fig. 13-7). Usually, lung, breast, and colon metastases affect the thoracic spine, whereas prostate, testicular, and ovarian or uterine carcinoma affect the lumbosacral spine. Metastasis to the cervical spine is slightly less common.

Spinal cord compression is most likely to occur at the thoracic level; here the diameter of the canal is, at most, 1 cm, making little room for tumor mass.[11] The lumbosacral canal typically spans 1.5 to 3.0 cm, allowing room for metastatic deposits that cause subtle lumbosacral radiculopathy or symptoms of cauda equina compression.[10,11] Myelopathic changes are acutely apparent in metastases at thoracic levels. The cervical cord averages 1.5 to 2.0 cm in diameter.[2,3] It is also the site of progressive myelopathic changes due to metastatic disease.

Symptoms of metastatic disease may begin with sharp, unremitting pain, localized and occasionally radicular, exacerbated by deep direct palpation. The localized site of pain will be associated with focal abnormalities on x-ray in 60 percent of patients, including pedicular erosion and a "winking owl" sign on AP films, collapse of vertebral bodies, wedge compression fracture and subluxation, kyphoscoliosis and/or a paraspinal soft tissue shadow.[4,5,10,11,13] Devastating myelopathy is seen in over 50 percent of patients, and bowel/bladder dysfunction occurs in 25 percent.[4,5,10,11,13,68–72] The level of motor loss is a more-dependable diagnostic indicator than the sensory level. Subtle neurological findings include hyperreflexia, Hoffman, or Babinski signs, and proprioceptive or dorsal column deficits provide additional diagnostic indications.

MRI imaging with Gd-DTPA enhancement reveals more than 95 percent of all spinal metastases, and it is the diagnostic test of choice after plain x-rays of the spine. MRI delineates the extent of spinal cord compression, detects any multilevel involvement, differentiates tumor and infection if

the clinical history is unclear, and identifies contiguous organ or tissue involvement, including lung or uterine cancer. If the MRI does not coincide with the clinical history and examination, a myelogram followed by CT, above and below a presumed level of spinal block, is the gold standard of radiographic examinations (Fig. 13-8).

The surgical indications are manifold and should consist of a thorough analysis and evaluation of the cancer biology, including prognosis, life expectancy, and extent of disease as assessed in concert with the oncologist and radiation therapist. Spinal instability or compression fractures with compression of the neural elements should prompt urgent decompression and stabilization in a combined or staged procedure.

The presence of a radiosensitive metastatic tumor—e.g., lymphoma, leukemia, seminoma, plasmacytoma, myeloma, or neuroblastoma, which has progressed rapidly with marked neurological deterioration despite emergency radiation therapy—should prompt early surgical intervention. The immediate salutary effect of radiation therapy may be seen in 24 to 48 h, at best. However, many metastatic tumors are

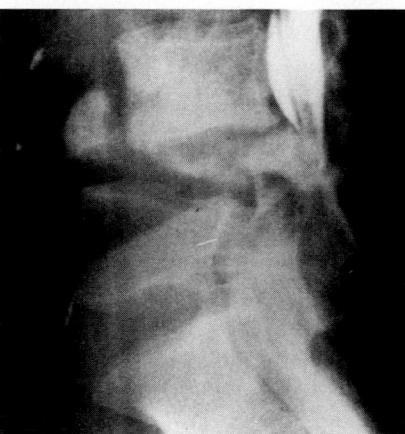

Figure 13–8A Metastatic seminoma. Lateral lumbosacral myelogram showing a complete extradural block at L4 with the classic "paintbrush" tapering of the contrast seen in extradural lesions.

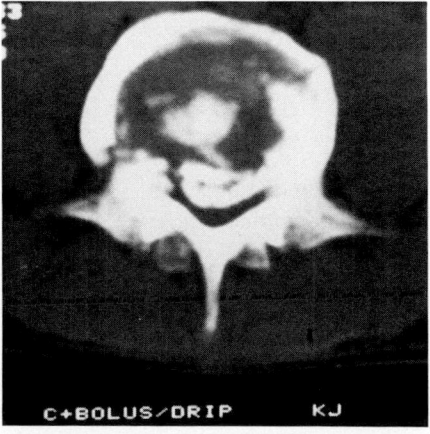

Figure 13–8B Axial CT image through pathological fracture at L4. There is bone, disk, and tumor extruded within the canal producing a complete block.

radioresistant, unfortunately. Commonly the neurosurgeon will be consulted and presented with a case of a patient with known metastatic disease who has deteriorated neurologically despite emergent radiation therapy as a palliative measure. It is less common for a metastatic tumor to present with an unknown or occult primary, and surgery is indicated for decompression and definitive diagnosis.

Postoperative radiation therapy and the administration of corticosteroids may be palliative, adjunctive treatments for metastatic tumors. The neurosurgeon's zeal to provide decompression should be tempered in any patient who has a life expectancy limited to a few months because of widespread metastases.

In older surgical series of metastatic cancer to the spine, laminectomy was the procedure of choice. But there was little difference in outcome between decompressive laminectomy and conservative radiation therapy, and the surgical approach was decried, particularly by Posner.[72] However, more recent advanced surgical techniques to the vertebral body—including the transthoracic, transpedicular, retroperitoneal, and lateral, extracavitary approaches to anterior spinal metastatic disease—have revealed excellent results and overall outcomes.[68–71]

Sundaresan treated 54 patients with documented spinal metastases in a prospective study,[68] using anterior resection of the vertebral body in 45 patients and laminectomy in 7 patients, and all patients became ambulatory after surgery, with the majority of patients surviving after 2 years and remaining ambulatory. This is significant since 24 patients were nonambulatory before surgical treatment. Primary tumors were soft tissue sarcoma, kidney, breast, and lung. Unfortunately, there was a 25 percent recurrence rate at the site of surgery, precluding a long-term cure. Nevertheless, pain and motor deficits were markedly improved, and Siegal,[70] Overby,[69] and Harrington[71] reported excellent surgical results in extensive series.

It might be concluded that *de novo* surgery should be considered for selected patients with cancer metastases to the spine, while external beam radiation therapy is reserved as the second phase of treatment after extensive surgical resection of the tumor.

LIPOMATOSIS[73,74]

Epidural lipomatosis is a rare disease, characterized by excessive fatty accumulation with spinal cord compression.[73,74] The symptoms and signs are those of acute pain and progressive myelopathy. Lipomatosis is typically seen in the thoracic spine and described in patients with a history of chronic exogenous steroid usage, for various clinical disorders, particularly Cushing's syndrome, morbid obesity, and hypothyroidism.[7,73,74] MRI is diagnostic with a very high intensity signal on T2-weighted images in the posterior, epidural space, consistent with fat accumulation. Treatment is wide decompressive laminectomy and debulking of the adipose tissue, with or without significant weight loss in the morbidly obese patient.[7,73,74] The surgical results are good.[73,74]

ANGIOLIPOMA, ANGIOMYOLIPOMA[75]

Angiolipoma is a rare tumor composed of mature lipocytes and angiomatous proliferation, with or without other mesenchymal elements (e.g., muscles, cartilage), and it is found predominantly in the thoracic spine with no male or female predilection.[75] The neurological presentation is slowly progressive paraparesis.[75] Commonly, the angiolipomas are multiple, cystic, and encapsulated; less commonly, they infiltrate the entire vertebral body and epidural space and recur after excision.[75] Since infiltrating angiolipomas do not undergo malignant transformation, there is no role for postoperative radiation therapy (Fig. 13-9, Plate 10).

Anterior vertebrectomy or posterior laminectomy is necessary to obtain total excision.[75] Differential diagnosis includes vertebral hemangioma, since the angiolipoma also presents as a coarse trabecular pattern on plain x-ray and CT scan. However, MRI reveals a high-signal intensity in the vertebral body, consistent with fatty infiltration from the angiolipoma.[75]

☐ MALIGNANT OSSEOUS TUMORS

CHORDOMA[76–78]

Chordomas are rare malignant tumors arising from primitive notochord with a predilection for the clivus, specifically the spheno-occipital synchondrosis and sacrococcygeum, and, less commonly, the cervical spine.[2–5,7,10,11,76–78] Chordoma is slightly more common in males, from 1.5:1 to 2:1, with a peak incidence at about 50 to 60 years of age. The tumor is locally invasive and slow-growing. Local pain is seen in over 70 percent of patients.[2–5,7,10,11,76–78]

Cervical chordomas present classically as a palpable prevertebral or retropharyngeal soft tissue mass with dysphagia and neck pain, whereas sacrococcygeal chordomas present as a presacral or pelvic mass with lower back and rectal pain and dysfunction that involves the bowel and bladder. Constipation is common. Clivus chordomas present with localized pain, headache, dysfunction of multiple lower cranial nerves, and a foramen magnum syndrome with gait ataxia.

The classic radiological features are expansile, destructive tumors with significant osteolytic destruction of bone, coupled with focal calcification. The presence of a large soft tissue mass is diagnostic, and chordomas can extend locally to the epidural space, but they rarely extend intradurally to cause compression of the spinal cord. MRI reveals a high-signal, soft tissue extradural mass, whereas CT and plain films of the spine highlight the extensive osteolytic effects and scattered focal calcification.[17] All chordomas demon-

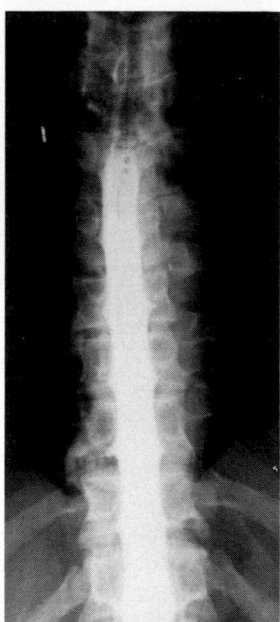

Figure 13–9A Angiolipoma. Thoracic myelogram shows a complete extradural block at T5 with the classic tapering or "paintbrush" and highlights the right T5 pedicle erosion.

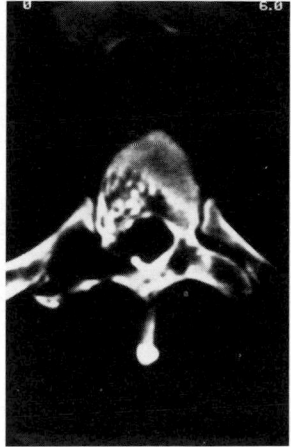

Figure 13–9B Axial CT image cut through the block at T5 shows no contrast visible secondary to marked bone destruction of the vertebral body, pedicles, and lamina on the right with cord compression.

strate high-signal images on T2-weighted MRIs (Fig. 13-10, Plate 11).

Pathologically, chordomas form soft tissue masses with pseudocapsules. They are composed of two cell types: (1) compact stellate cells and (2) physaliphorous cells, which are jellylike, vacuolated, with characteristic "signet-ring" nuclei displaced eccentrically. Tumors of the physaliphorous type have a tendency toward recurrence. They infiltrate locally and have distant metastases, with a poor prognosis despite palliative radiation therapy, investigational chemotherapy, and even experimental interstitial brachytherapy.

The surgical management of chordomas is still difficult as there is an 80 to 90 percent recurrence rate despite grossly complete tumor removal.[76–78] Unfortunately, com-

plete tumor excision is often impossible, and debulking procedures with spinal stabilization are necessary. Chordomas are radioresistant, although there are still preliminary attempts with interstitial brachytherapy using radioactive iodine seeds to halt tumor growth.[77] Overall, there is a 15 percent 10-year survival despite radiation therapy,[76–78] and, unfortunately, chemotherapy is not promising to date. There is a significant tendency to metastatic spread.

MULTIPLE MYELOMA, PLASMACYTOMA

Multiple myeloma is the most common primary malignant bone tumor of the spine, with a peak incidence in the sixth to eighth decade.[2–5,7,10,11] There is a slight predominance in males. The vertebral bodies are replaced by malignant plasma cells, a B-cell lymphoproliferative disorder, resulting in local pain and systemic symptoms including weight loss, anorexia, and malaise. There is resultant anemia, hypercalcemia, and an elevated sedimentation rate (ESR).

Multiple myeloma can be detected by urine or serum protein electrophoresis as a monoclonal gamma-spike pattern, the Bence Jones protein. Plain x-rays of the spine and CT reveal multiple round, "punched-out" or "moth-eaten" appearances secondary to widespread osteolysis, with patho-

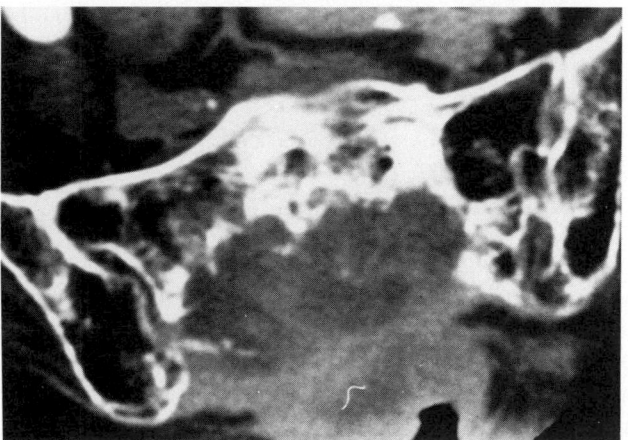

Figure 13–10A Chordoma. Axial bone window CT image of the sacrum shows the large mass with extensive bone destruction and focal sites of calcification characteristic of chordoma.

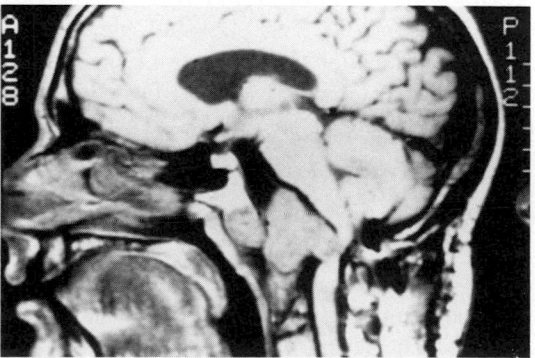

Figure 13–10B MRI in the sagittal plane showing a large chordoma indenting the pons and cervicomedullary junction.

logical fractures and dislocation. MRI reveals decreased signal intensity in multiple vertebral bodies secondary to myeloma infiltration, although these features are also commonly seen in cancer metastases. The bone scan is often negative in contradistinction to scans of patients with metastases, which show multiple "hot" spots.

The primary treatment of multiple myeloma is medical, specifically, multiregimen chemotherapy and radiation therapy to the affected spine. Pain can be alleviated dramatically by local radiotherapy and corticosteroids. If patients develop spinal cord compression, surgery is indicated by an anterior or a posterior approach, with spinal reconstruction. Despite adjunctive treatment, the prognosis for survival in patients with disseminated multiple myeloma is only about 30 percent at 5 years after diagnosis.[2–5,7,10,11]

Less commonly, a single vertebral body is infiltrated by malignant plasma cells, a *plasmacytoma*.[79] Radiologically, the plasmacytoma presents as a single lytic lesion. In these cases the disease is self-limited and has a better prognosis, but 10 to 20 percent of patients progress to multiple myeloma, with systemic effects and multilevel spinal involvement. The treatment is vertebrectomy, spinal reconstruction, and local radiation therapy, with careful follow-up for signs of multilevel malignancy while maintaining routine spine x-rays, MRI, CT, and laboratory studies.[79] With aggressive treatment, the plasmacytoma has a 5-year survival of greater than 60 percent, since tumors are radiosensitive and unlikely to dedifferentiate to myeloma.[79]

OSTEOSARCOMA (OSTEOGENIC SARCOMA)[7,10,11,80]

Osteogenic sarcoma is a rare, bone-forming tumor, which can arise *de novo* in 50 percent of cases, or secondarily, as metastases from a limb extremity.[7,10,11,80] It occurs at a site of earlier irradiation but is commonly associated with Paget's disease. The median age of presentation is 40 years, with a slight male preponderance and an equal distribution among spinal segments. Intractable pain is a uniformly ominous symptom, and neurological deficits are seen in 70 percent of patients.[7,10,11,80] Osteosarcoma usually involves the vertebral body primarily, with areas of additional lysis and dense sclerosis with calcification seen radiographically by plain x-rays and CT scan. Despite aggressive surgical debulking, focal radiation therapy, and multiregimen chemotherapy, the overall prognosis is poor. Less than 10 percent of patients survive at 5 years.[7,10,11,80]

CHONDROSARCOMA[7,10,11,81,82]

Chondrosarcomas are rare malignant tumors that form cartilage. They are commonly found in long bones, pelvis, and skull base with 6 percent distributed throughout the spinal column.[7,10,11,81,82] Chondrosarcomas typically involve vertebral bodies, and the age distribution is 40 to 60 years. Pain is

a frequent and constant finding, as in the case of osteosarcoma. Radiographically, there are characteristic "fluffy" globular areas of sclerotic tumor, combined with lucent areas secondary to bone lysis; angiography reveals a very vascular tumor. As with osteosarcoma, despite surgery and *en bloc* radical excision, radiation therapy, and chemotherapy, local recurrence and metastases are common, leading to a dismal overall prognosis.

☐ BENIGN BONE TUMORS[7,10,11,83]

OSTEOCHONDROMA

Osteochondromas are common benign single or multiple bone tumors.[7,10,11,83] Osteochondromas rarely occur in the spine, but when they do occur they present as mass lesions that cause spinal cord compression or radiculopathy. They occur typically in males under 30 years of age and are found predominantly in the spinous processes and, particularly, the posterior neural arches. Pain is not a predominant feature, but slowly progressive myelopathy has been described repeatedly. Tumors have a characteristic appearance radiographically, showing a round bony exostosis with a radiolucent, cartilagenous cap. They are found predominantly in the cervical spine and less commonly in the thoracic spine. Surgical decompression by laminectomy is curative, with recovery of neurological function and rare recurrences. Malignant degeneration occurs in at least 10 percent of patients with the genetically inherited Ollier's disease or Maffucci's syndrome, multiple chondromatosis, or exostoses, with a distinct tendency toward the chondrosarcoma and, very rarely, the osteosarcoma.[7,10,11,83]

OSTEOBLASTOMA, OSTEOID OSTEOMA[7,10,11,84–86]

Osteoblastomas are common benign tumors seen in males, with a peak incidence below 30 years of age.[7,10,11,84–86] They have a predilection for the posterior spinal elements, specifically spinous and transverse processes and lamina. Osteoblastoma is commonly accompanied by scoliosis or spinal stiffness, and it has an equal distribution throughout the spinal column. Classically, symptoms described are dull aching pains, neither nocturnal nor relieved by aspirin.

By plain x-rays and CT, the tumors have a central, radiolucent, or lytic, area surrounded by a sclerotic rim, and its size is usually greater than 1.5 cm in diameter. Although most frequently in the femur and tibia, 35 percent of osteoblastomas occur in the spine.[7,10,11,84–86] MRIs of osteoblastomas show enhancement with Gd-DTPA on T1 images and present a high signal on T2 images. The technetium bone scan has intense, or "hot," uptake with radioisotopes.

Osteoblastoma is locally aggressive and can attain considerable size, causing spinal cord compression associated with

THE COLOR PLATES

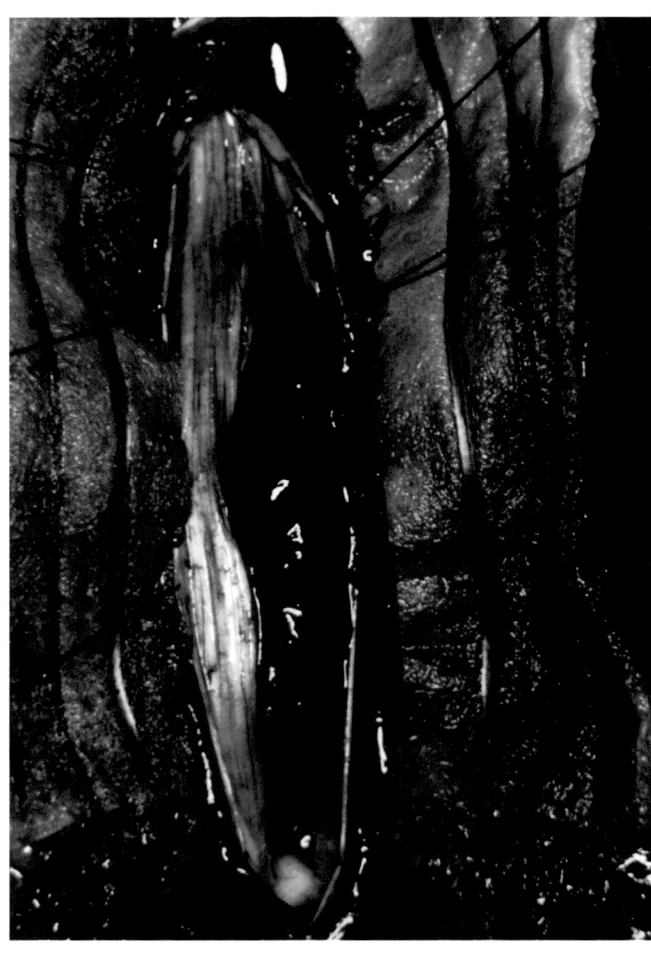

1. Intraoperative photograph of a hemorrhagic myxopapillary ependymoma arising along the filum terminale and displacing the cauda equina roots.

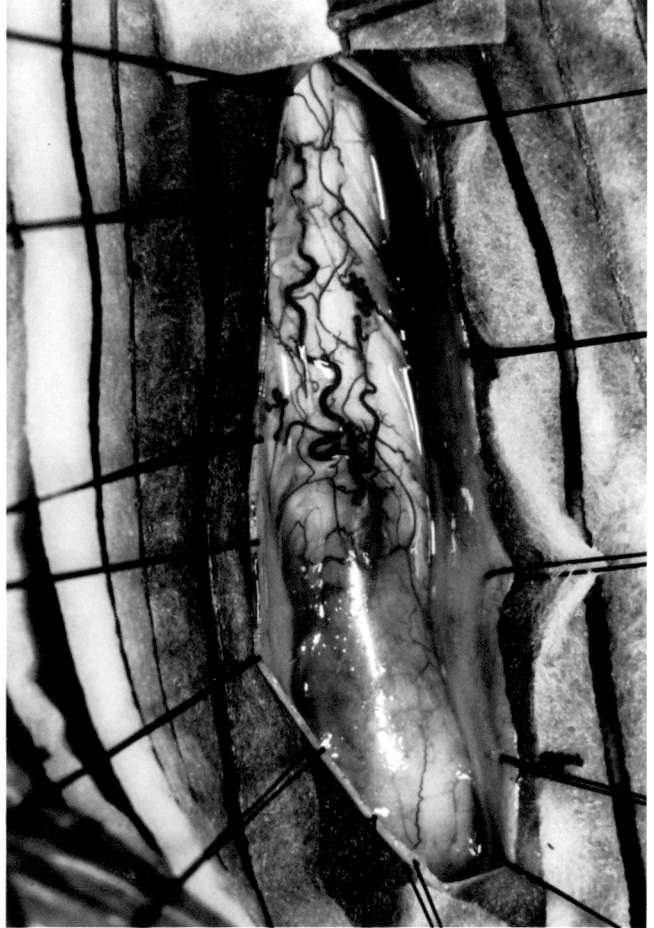

2. Intraoperative photograph demonstrating a fusiform intramedullary tumor with prominent tumor vessels at the caudal end of the pial surface.

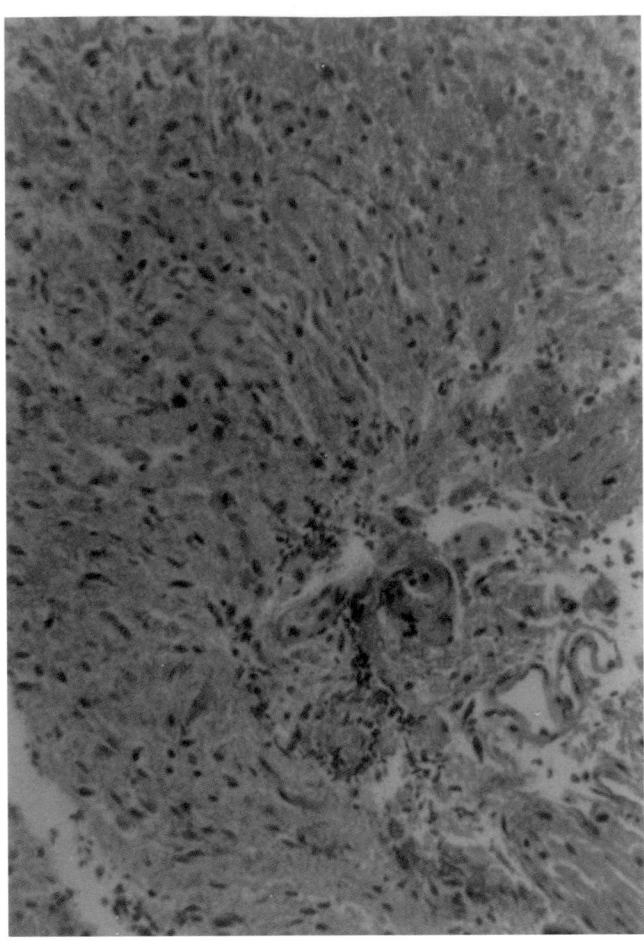

3. Microscopic features of a low-grade pilocytic astrocytoma.

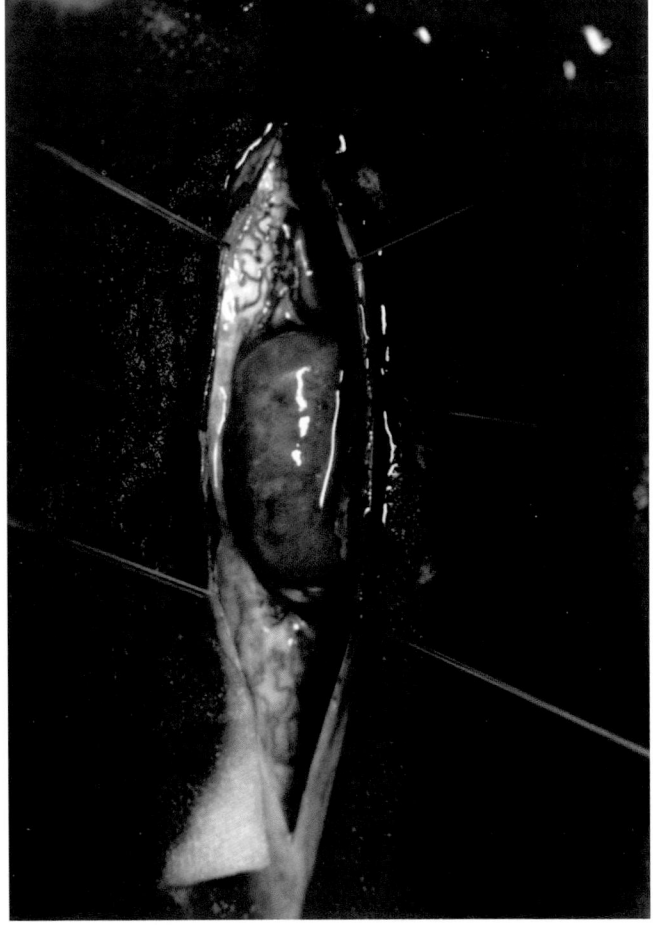

4. Intraoperative photograph showing a large dorsal meningioma compressing the midthoracic spinal cord.

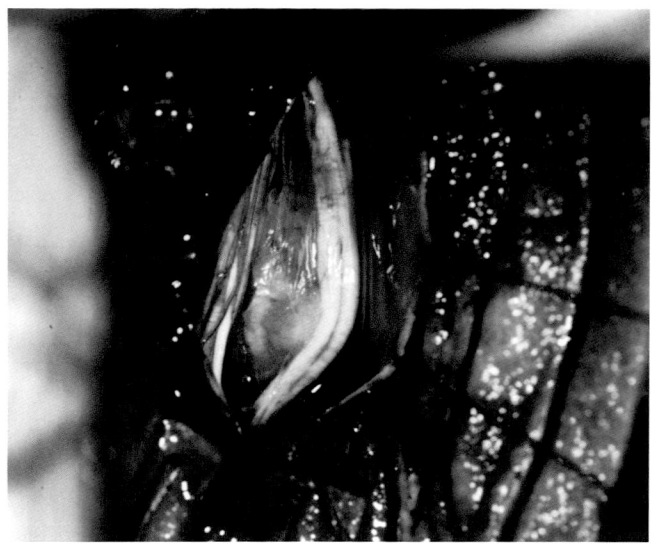

5. Intraoperative photograph of cauda equina schwannoma.

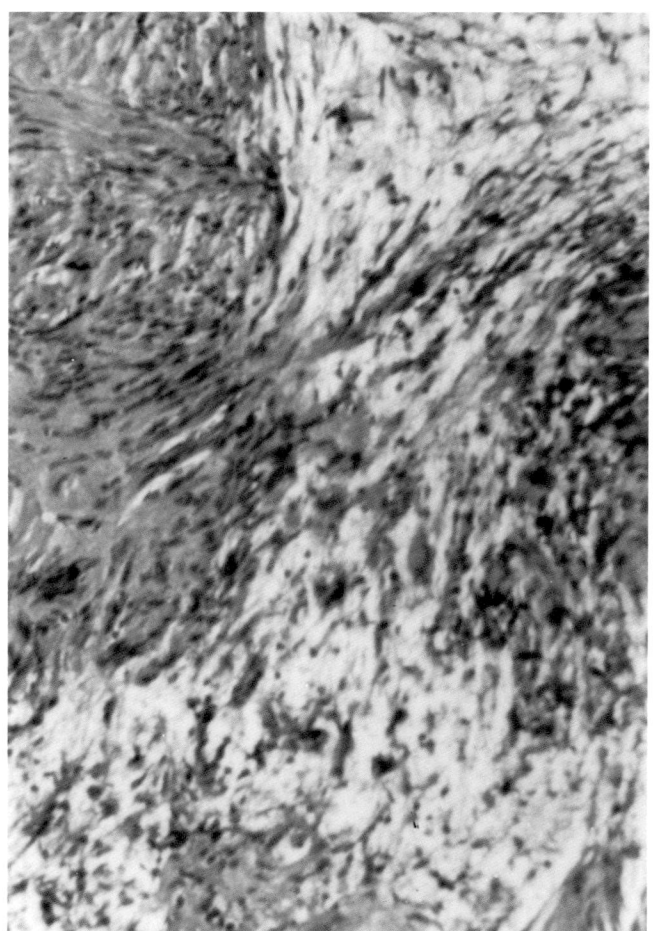

6. Photomicrograph of schwannoma showing classic palisading with Antoni A and B patterns.

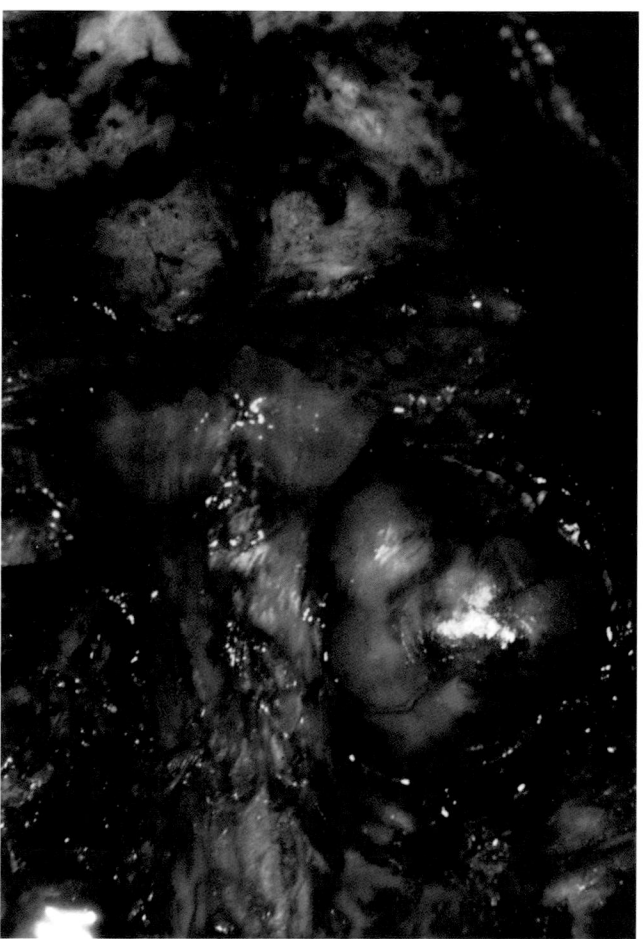

7. Intraoperative photograph following suboccipital craniectomy and C1-3 laminectomy showing an extradural portion of a large extradural/intradural "dumbbell" neurofibroma of C2.

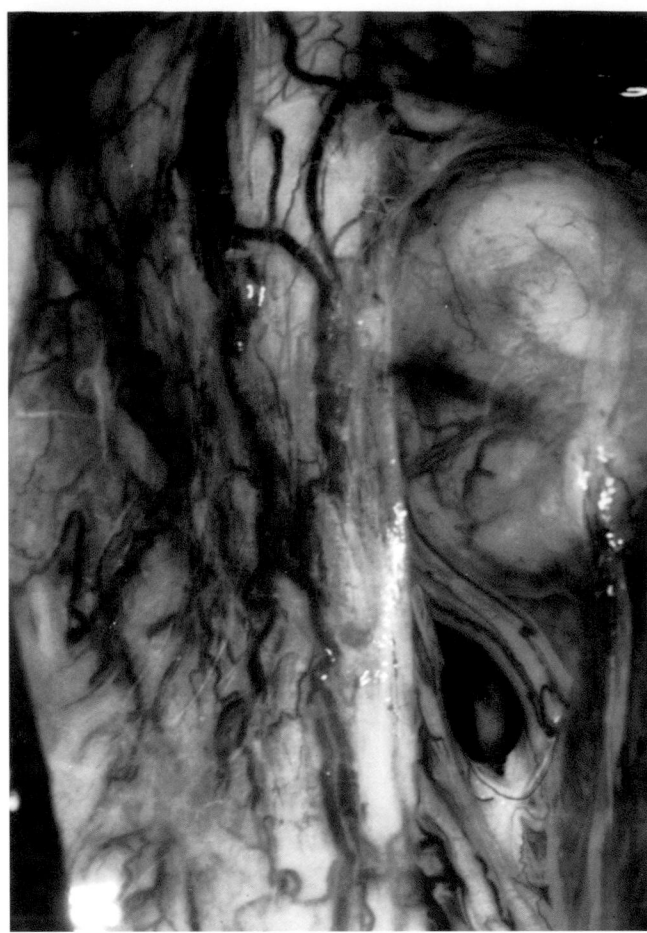

8. Same case as Plate 7. Intradural portion of "dumbbell" neurofibroma with intradural compression of the upper cervical spinal cord.

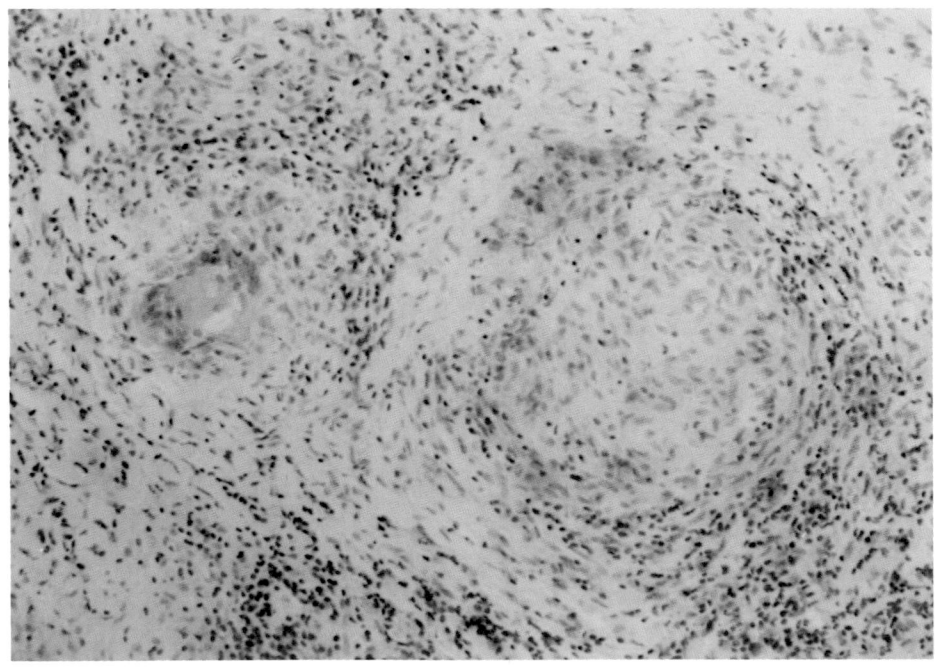

9. Photomicrograph shows noncaseating granulomas with Langhans cells, diagnostic of sarcoid, or Boeck's disease.

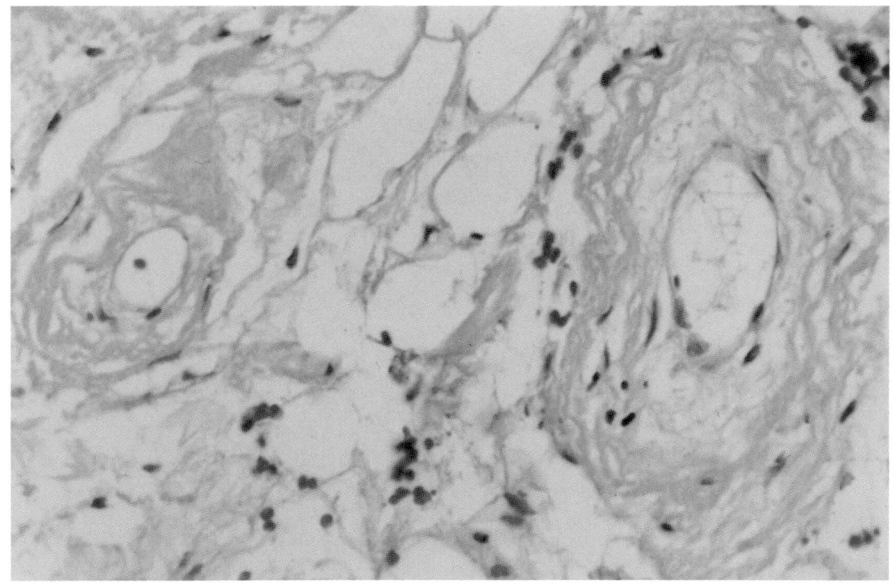

10. Photomicrograph shows classic histological findings of mature vascular and fatty channels or "sinusoids" of angiolipoma (H&E stain).

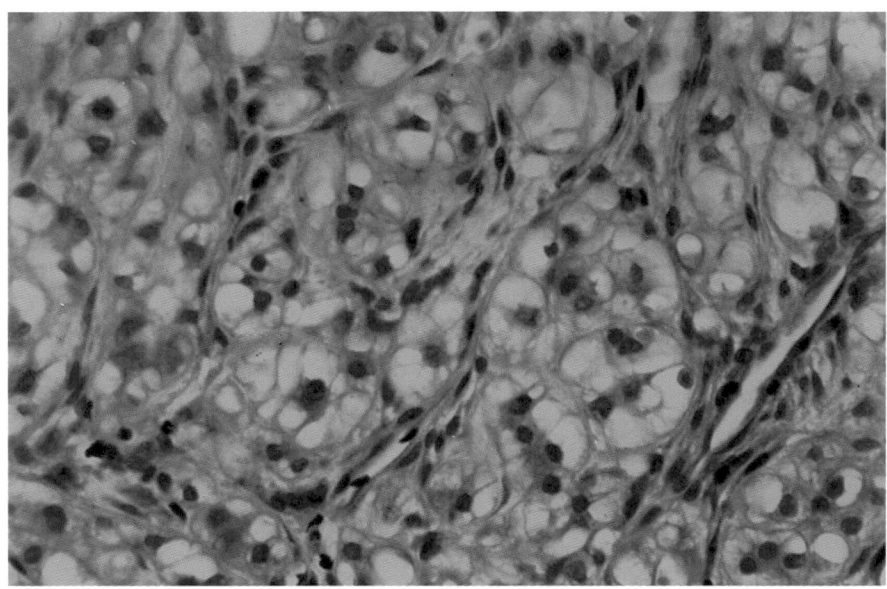

11. Photomicrograph of a chordoma reveals the classic physaliphorous or "bubble bearing" cells with characteristic "signet ring" eccentric nuclei.

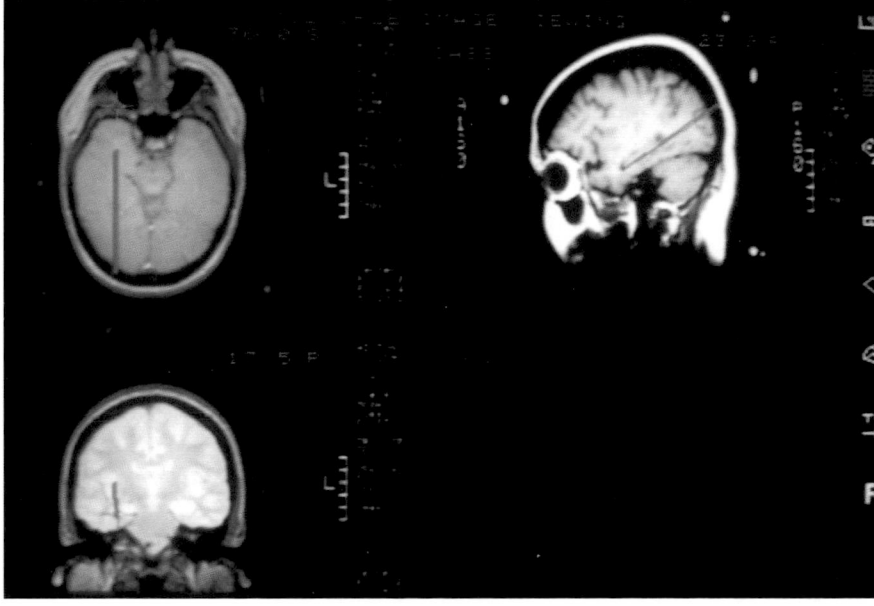

12. Multiplanar graphic rendering of an MRI-guided stereotactic right temporal lobe procedure.

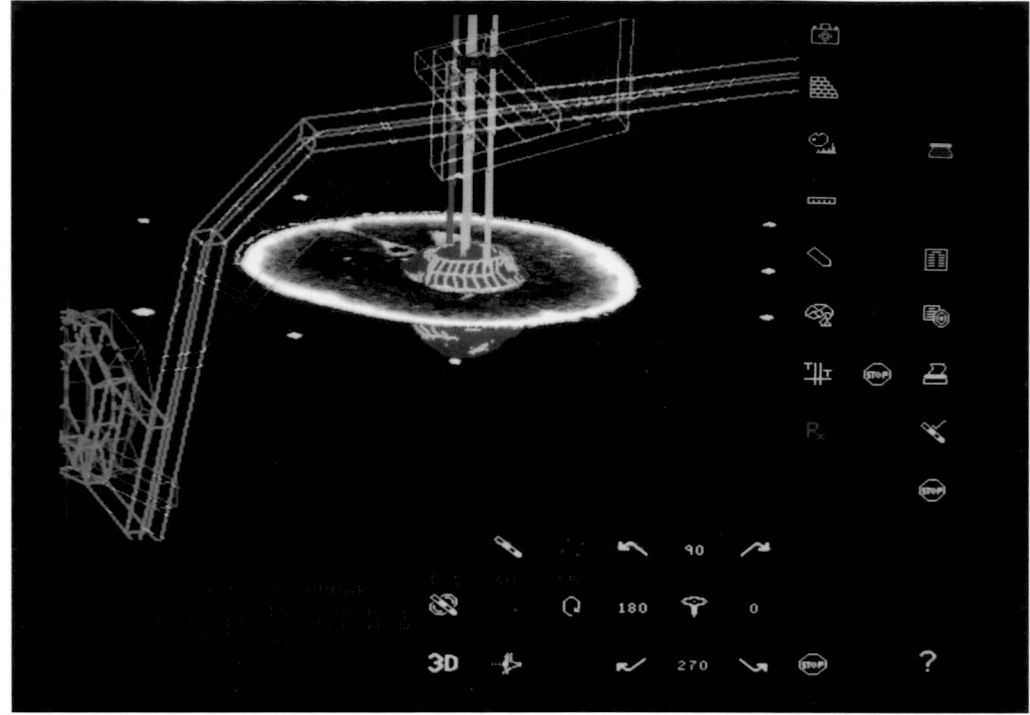

13. Computer graphic display of interstitial brachytherapy implant. The afterloading catheters are pink and green. The tumor mass is wire frame rendered in light blue. The 100 percent isodose zones are solid red. The CRW stereotactic frame is seen as a wire-frame rendering in multiple colors. *(Courtesy of MIDCO, Inc.)*

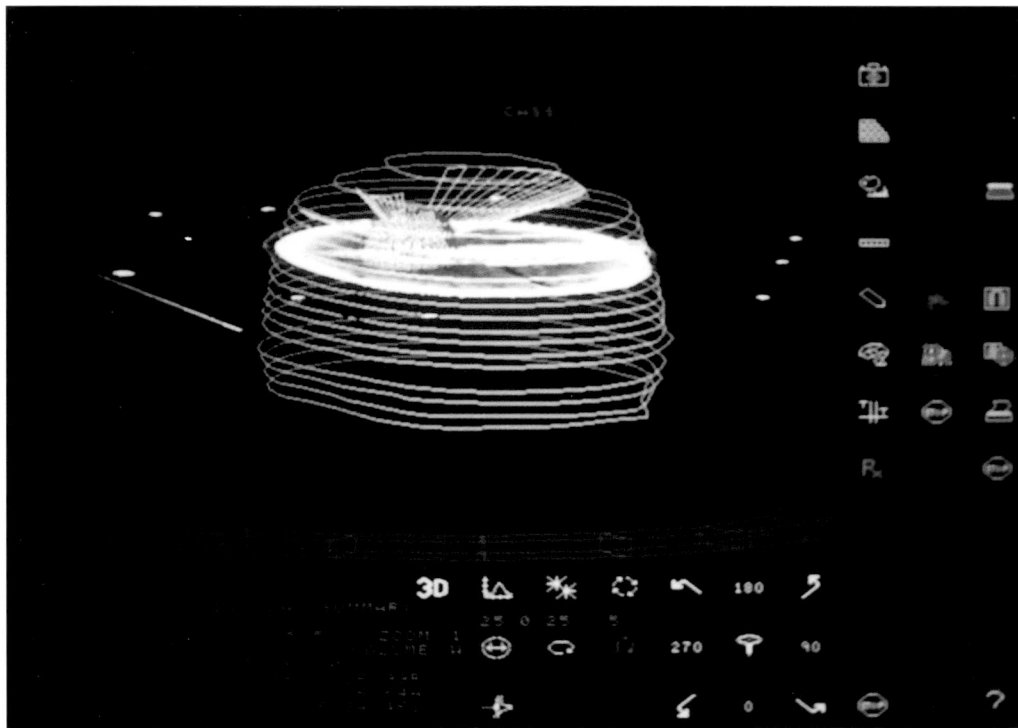

14. Computer graphic simulation of a radiosurgery treatment plan. Skull contour for each CT slice is outlined in yellow. The five radiosurgery treatment arcs are in taupe. Tumor mass is light blue. The 80 percent isodose is in solid red. The image can be rotated 360° and viewed from various perspectives. In this way, adequacy of coverage of the lesion within a given isodose zone can be determined, as can overlap of the isodose zone onto critical local structures, for example, the internal capsule, optic chiasm, etc. *(Courtesy of MIDCO, Inc.)*

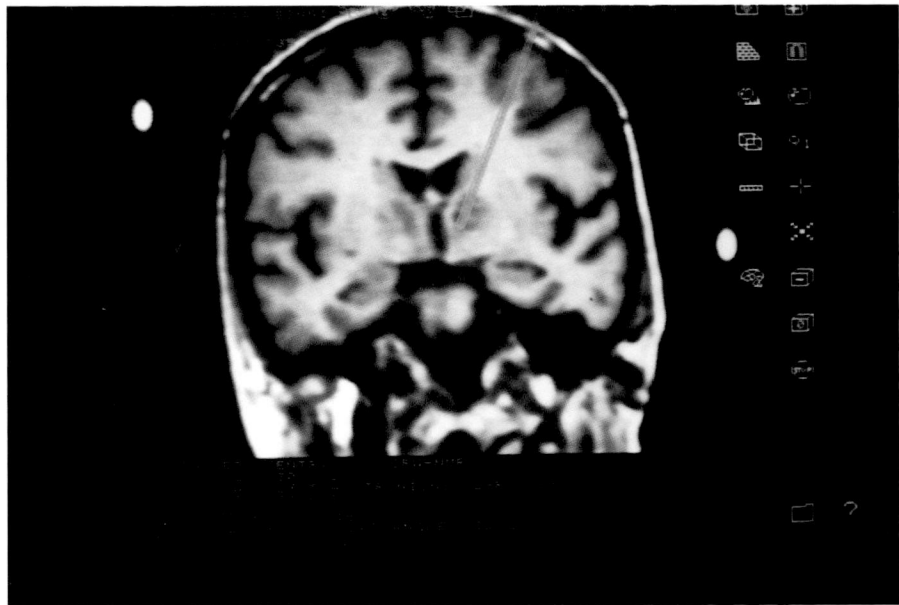

15. Immediate postoperative coronal MRI scan of an MRI-guided, computer-assisted stereotactic frontothalamic tractotomy. The lesions are in the proximal inferior anterior limb of the internal capsule. The probe trajectory for the left-sided lesion is seen.

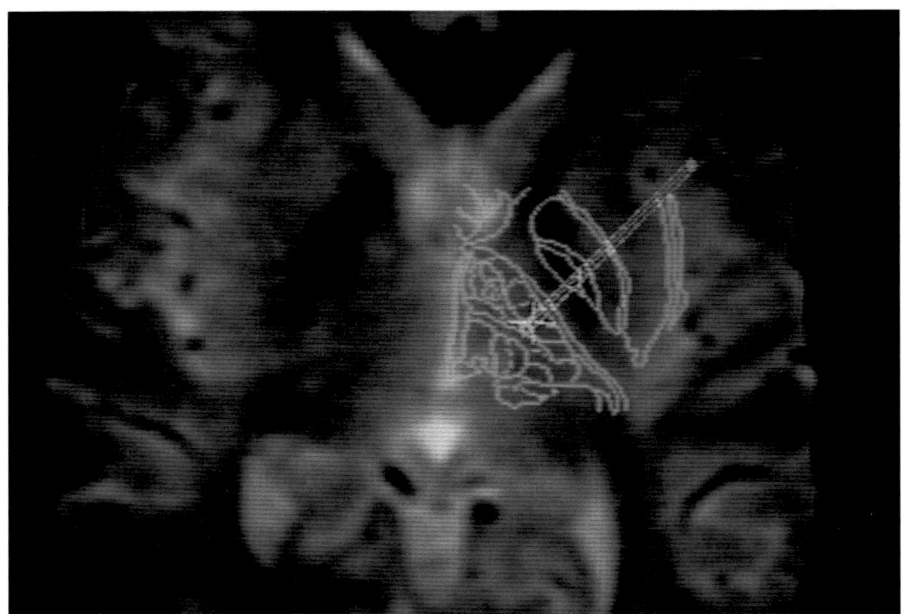

16. Axial MRI slice in the plane of the anterior and posterior commissures. A digitized horizontal atlas map has been scaled and onlayed over the right thalamus. The cursor is located at the junction of the middle and posterior thirds of the VL nucleus. The lateral angle of the trajectory is indicated.

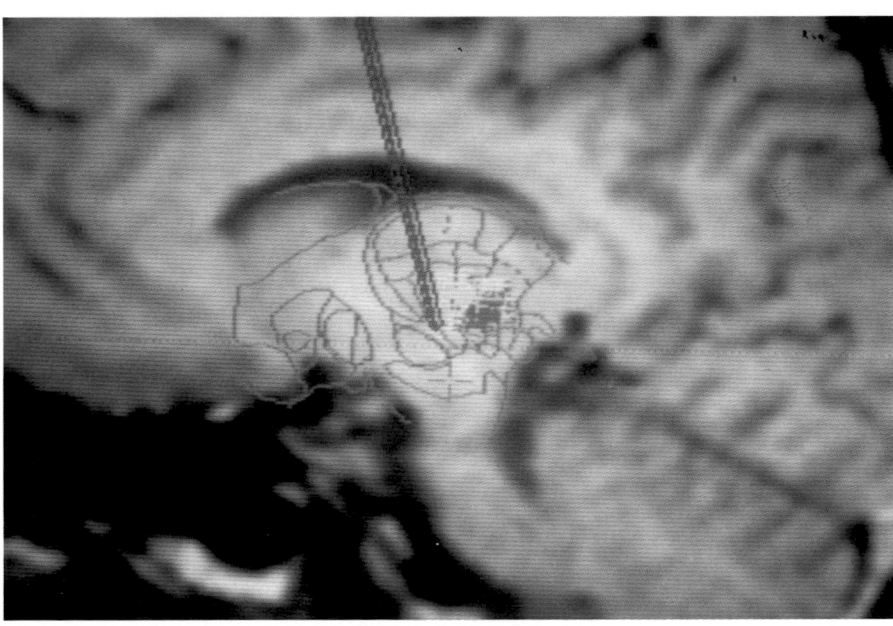

17. Same case as in Plate 16. Sagittal slice approximately 13 mm to the right of midline. The probe tip is positioned at the same target as in Plate 16. The AP angle of trajectory is indicated. The yellow letters represent sites in other cases where stimulation produced contralateral facial paresthesias, and the green letters indicate sites where stimulation produced contralateral finger paresthesias. The thalamic target for tremor alleviation should be just anterior to such sites. Location of the cursor beyond the probe tip indicates that the target, which was first defined on the axial view in Plate 16, was not precisely in this scan plane.

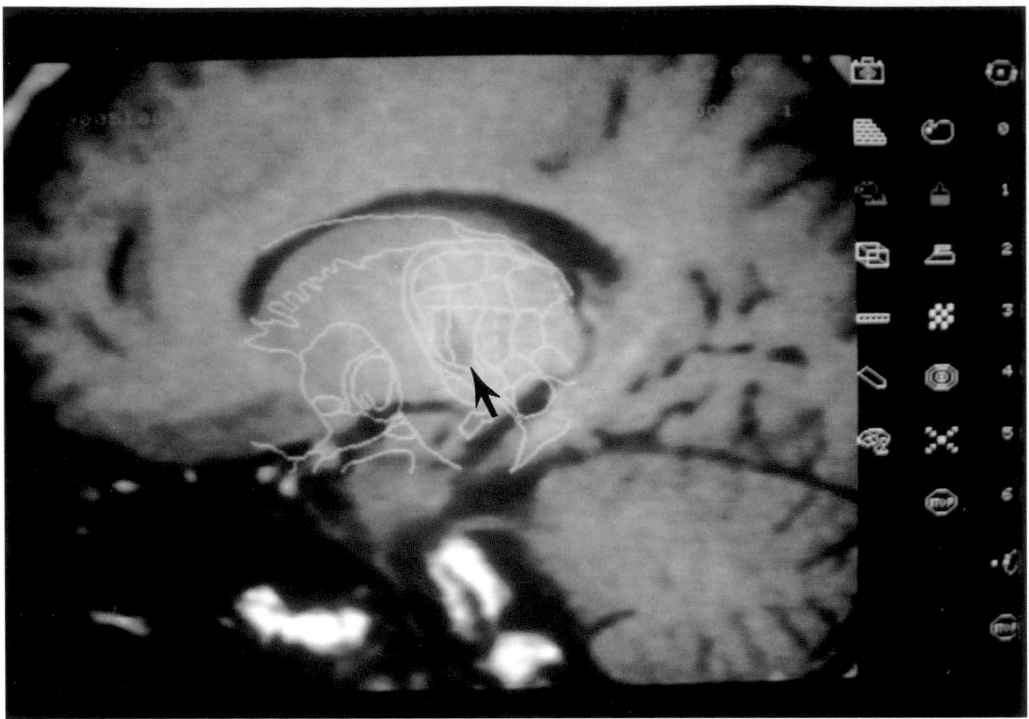

18. Postoperative sagittal MRI scan of the same case as in Plate 16. The thalamotomy lesion (arrow) involves the posterior two-thirds of the VL nucleus.

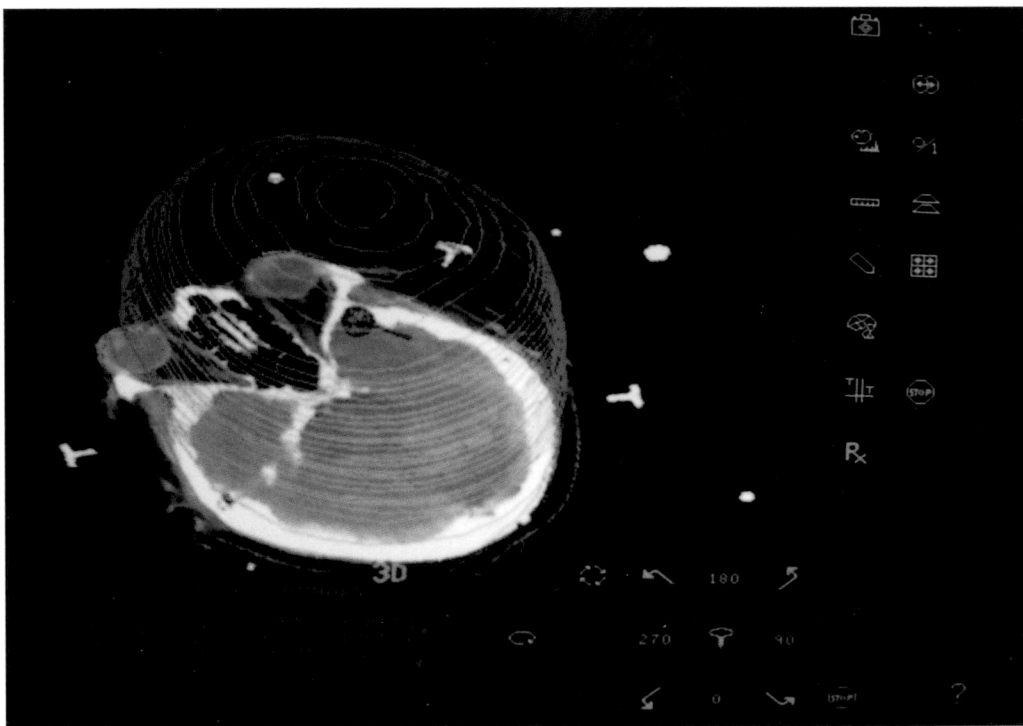

19. An interictal epileptiform magnetic dipole (maroon) has been recorded from the right temporal lobe. The blue arrow indicates the direction of the dipole. The location of the dipole in stereotactic space was derived using nasion and the two tragi to divide the reference plane. The position of the 37-channel magnetoencephalograph is shown in red as a wire-frame rendering to the upper right of the patient's head. The recording was performed in a magnetically shielded room. *(Courtesy of MIDCO, Inc.)*

local scoliosis. Treatment consists of *en bloc* resection and spine stabilization, and recurrence is common because of aggressive tumor infiltration and inability to achieve complete removal surgically. Both anterior and posterior procedures may be required for total tumor removal; curettage and bone grafting are very successful.[7,10,11,84–86] Local irradiation is ineffective and may cause malignant transformation to sarcoma.

Osteoid osteoma is histologically identical to osteoblastoma, yet it is characterized classically by nocturnal pain well-alleviated by aspirin and arbitrarily defined in size as less than 1.5 cm in diameter. Although frequently located in the femur and tibia, approximately 10 percent of osteoid osteomas are located in the spine.[7,10,11,84–86] The technetium bone scan is very sensitive, as the central lucent nidus is "cold" and the sclerotic rim "hot," allowing confirmation of complete removal of th nidus intraoperatively by testing the surrounding bone with the radioactive counter for any residual "hot" spots. MRIs seem to enhance vividly the nidus with Gd-DTPA contrast agent.

Osteoid osteoma is seen in even younger patients, particularly males, with an average age of 19 years, and it has a preference for the lumbar spine, followed by the cervical spine. As with osteoblastoma, the osteoid osteoma involves preferentially the posterior spinal elements, i.e., lamina and pedicles. Painful scoliosis is a common symptom (>60 percent) in adolescents with osteoid osteoma.[7,10,11,84–86]

Surgical excision of osteoid osteomas is often complete and curative without recurrence due to its small size; scoliosis will resolve spontaneously with time. However, long-standing lesions may require spinal instrumentation to correct the scoliosis. Pain resolution is a gratifying end-result.[7,10,11,84,86]

GIANT CELL TUMORS OR OSTEOCLASTOMAS[7,10,11,87,88]

These are rare benign bone tumors composed of multinucleated giant cells with a fibrous stroma consisting of mononuclear cells.[7,10,11,87,88] They are most common in long bones, epiphyses, and metaphyses, occurring in young adults and adolescents, with a female preponderance, and they are found less commonly, but preferentially, in the thoracic spine with a predilection for the vertebral body. Giant cell tumors grow rather large and are highly vascular. They cause localized or radicular pain with slowly progressive spinal cord compression. Radiographically, these tumors are large, osteolytic masses termed *soap bubbles,* with evidence of destruction on plain x-rays or CT. MRI delineates the extensive vertebral bone and soft tissue components of the tumor, with a low signal intensity by T2 image due to marrow replacement.

Surgery is aimed at radical en bloc excision or curettage with reconstruction of the involved vertebra and tumor mass, but the rate of local recurrence is very high, nearly 50 percent,[87,88] and giant cell tumors can metastasize at a rate of

15 percent.[87,88] Postoperative radiotherapy is routinely indicated to halt metastases.

ANEURYSMAL BONE CYSTS[7,10,11,89,90]

These are benign lesions of bone. Approximately 10 to 20 percent of aneurysmal bone cysts occur in the spine, most commonly in the lumbar region.[7,10,11,89,90] The cyst presents in the 10- to 30-year-age range, and there is a slight preference for females, with predilection for the posterior neural arches and pedicles. Less commonly, these cysts involve several vertebral bodies. Painful scoliosis in the back is commonly seen, and tumors enlarge as soft tissue masses into the spinal canal, causing neurological deficits in 60 percent of cases.[7,10,11,89,90]

Histologically, aneurysmal bone cysts contain cystic, fluid-filled spaces with fibrous septae. Radiographically, there is a honeycomb trabeculated pattern with an eggshell-thin cortical margin by plain x-ray and CT. Angiography reveals multiple vascular "lakes." MRI confirms the expansile soft tissue mass with internal septations and lakes containing fluid levels.

Complete surgical excision should be attempted, but a recurrence rate of 15 to 25 percent is reported despite extensive curettage and reconstruction.[7,10,11,89,90] Low-dose radiation therapy (20 to 30 cGy) prevents recurrence and should be considered in cases where complete excision is not possible.[7,10,11,89,90]

HEMANGIOMAS[7,10,11,91,92]

Hemangiomas are the most common benign bone tumor with asymptomatic lesions in autopsy series, ranging from 9 to 13 percent.[7,10,11,91,92] Hemangiomas are vascular tumors arising from newly formed blood vessels of diverse sizes. In about 33 percent of cases, multiple vertebra are involved, and the thoracic and thoracolumbar regions are most often affected.[7,10,11,91,92] Hemangiomas are frequently incidental findings on x-ray, and the majority of patients are asymptomatic. There is a slight female preponderance of 1.5:1, and the age at presentation is typically 30 to 50 years.[7,10,11,91,92]

Hemangiomas become symptomatic, with progressive vertebral body collapse, fracture, and, rarely, epidural hemorrhage. They cause focal pain and tenderness with muscle spasms, with or without neurological deterioration, and myelopathy is commonly seen.

Plain radiographs or CT scans show coarse vertical striations, or trabeculae. Dilated vascular spaces are easily seen by CT, and they give a characteristic spotted appearance. Typically, hemangiomas are confined to the vertebral bodies but can extend into the neural arches.

MRI is very sensitive and shows bright high-intensity signals on both T1- and T2-weighted images. MRI readily shows the paravertebral and epidural extension of the tumor, and it outlines spinal cord compression. Hemangiomas have vascular lacunae on angiography and multiple tumor vessels, which are readily amenable to embolization.[91,92]

Most hemangiomas can be treated symptomatically with low-dose radiation therapy and external bracing, alleviating local pain and tenderness. Vertebrectomy and stabilization of the spine are considered in cases of spinal cord compression from an enlarging hemangioma, but intraoperative hemorrhage is a concern, and preoperative embolization of tumor feeders is recommended. Asymptomatic hemangiomas are left untreated, but they are followed since there is a low incidence of new-onset signs or symptoms in these patients. Early surgical intervention in a neurologically compromised patient leads to a good outcome postoperatively and a successful result, with rare recurrence.[7,10,11,91,92]

EOSINOPHILIC GRANULOMAS[7,10,11,93]

Eosinophilic granulomas are the most common benign bone tumors of children, particularly males, with a peak incidence at 5 to 10 years of age.[7,10,11,93] The bone is infiltrated and destroyed by histocytes and eosinophils. The lesion can be representative of one end of a diagnostic spectrum of systemic diseases, including Letterer-Siwe and Hand-Schiller-Christian disease, the last being a malignant reticuloendotheliosis akin to cancer. Solitary eosinophilic granulomas are described commonly in the skull as "punched-out" lesions, but vertebral involvement occurs in 10 to 15 percent of cases.[7,10,11,93]

Eosinophilic granuloma occurs frequently in the thoracic spine, with acute onset of chest or back pain, focal sprain, torticollis, kyphoscoliosis, and, rarely, neurological compromise. The classic radiographic appearance is the *"vertebra plana,"* or vertebral body, which is symmetrically flattened and thinned compared with the adjacent vertebrae.[7,10,11,93]

Treatment includes a diagnostic needle biopsy and curettage. Patients with a solitary eosinophilic granuloma are immobilized in a spinal orthosis and given low-dose radiation therapy, 5 to 10 cGy. Systemic eosinophilic granulomas are treated with multiregimen chemotherapy.[7,10,11,93] Rarely, eosinophilic granulomas cause myelopathy or radiculopathy, necessitating spinal decompression and/or stabilization.[93]

REFERENCES

1. Seeger W: *Microsurgery of the Spinal Cord and Surrounding Structures.* New York, Springer-Verlag, 1982.
2. Bailey RW, Sherk HH: *The Cervical Spine.* The Cervical Spine Research Society, Philadelphia, Lippincott, 1983.
3. Dunsker SB: *Cervical Spondylosis.* New York, Raven, 1981.
4. Youmans JR: *Neurological Surgery,* vols 1 to 6. Philadelphia, Saunders, 1982.
5. Wilkins RH, Rengachary SS: *Neurosurgery,* vols 1 to 3. New York, McGraw-Hill, 1985.
6. Wilkins RH, Rengachary SS: *Neurosurgery,* Update I. New York, McGraw-Hill, 1991.
7. Wilkins RH, Rengachary SS: *Neurosurgery,* Update II. New York, McGraw-Hill, 1991.
8. Schmidek HH, Sweet WH: *Operative Neurosurgical Techniques,* vols 1 and 2. New York, Grune and Stratton, 1982.
9. Al-Mefty O: *Meningiomas.* New York, Raven, 1991.
10. Rothman RH, Simeone FA: *The Spine.* Philadelphia, Saunders, 1982.
11. Frymoyer JW: *The Adult Spine.* New York, Raven, 1991.
12. Rand RW, Rand CW: *Intraspinal Tumors of Childhood,* Springfield, Charles C. Thomas, 1960.
13. Congress of Neurological Surgeons: *Clin Neurosurg Proc,* vols 30, 37, and 38. Baltimore, Williams & Wilkins, 1983, 1991, 1992.
14. Crockard HA, Sen CN: The transoral approach for the management of intradural lesions at the craniovertebral junction: Review of 7 cases. *Neurosurgery* 28:88–97, 1991.
15. Stevenson GC, Stoney RJ, Perkins RK, Adams JE: A transcervical transclival approach to the ventral surface of the brain stem for removal of a clivus chordoma. *J Neurosurg* 24:544–551, 1966.
16. McDonnell DE: Anterolateral cervical approach to the craniovertebral junction, in Rengachary SS, Wilkins RH (eds): *Neurosurgical Operative Atlas,* vol 1, no 3. Baltimore, Williams & Wilkins, pp 147–164, 1991.
17. Kucharczyk W: MRI: *Central Nervous System,* Philadelphia, Lippincott, 1990.
18. Gutin P: Corticosteroid therapy in patients with cerebral tumors: Benefits, mechanisms, problems, practicalities. *Seminars in Oncology* 2:49–56, 1975.
19. Thompson EB, Srivistava D, Johnson BH: Interaction of the phenylpyrazolo steroid cortivazol with glucocorticoid receptors in steroid-sensitive and steroid-resistant human leukemia cells. *Cancer Res* 49:2253–2258, 1989.
20. Helseth A, Mork S: Primary intraspinal neoplasms in Norway. *J Neurosurg* 71:842–845, 1989.
21. McCormick PC, Torres R, Post KD, Stein BM: Intramedullary ependymoma of the spinal cord. *J Neurosurg* 72:523–532, 1990.
22. Fischer G, Mansuy L: Total removal of intramedullary ependymoma: Follow-up study of 16 cases. *Surg Neurol* 14:243–249, 1980.
23. Schweitzer JS, Batzdorf U: Ependymoma of the cauda equina region: Diagnosis, treatment, and outcome in 15 patients. *Neurosurgery* 30:202–207, 1992.
24. Greenwood J Jr: Total removal of intramedullary tumors. *J Neurosurg* 11:616–621, 1954.
25. Elsberg CA: *Tumors of the Spinal Cord.* New York, Paul B. Hoeber, 1925.
26. Stein BM: Surgery of intramedullary spinal cord tumors. *Clin Neurosurg* 26:529–542, 1979.

27. Malis LI: Intramedullary spinal cord tumors. *Clin Neurosurg* 25:512–539, 1978.
28. Cooper PR, Epstein F: Radical resection of intramedullary spinal cord tumors in adults. *J Neurosurg* 63:492–499, 1985.
29. Cooper PR: Outcome after operative treatment of intramedullary spinal cord tumors in adults: Intermediate and long-term results in 51 patients. *Neurosurgery* 25:855–859, 1989.
30. Guidetti B, Mercuri S, Vagnozzi R: Long-term results of the surgical treatment of 129 intramedullary spinal gliomas. *J Neurosurg* 54:323–330, 1981.
31. Sandler HM, Papadopoulos JM, Thornton AF, Ross DA: Spinal cord astrocytomas: Results of therapy. *Neurosurgery* 30:490–493, 1992.
32. Rossitch E, Jr, Zeidman SM, Burger PC, et al: Clinical and pathological analysis of spinal cord astrocytomas in children. *Neurosurgery* 27:193–196, 1990.
33. Epstein F, Wisoff J: Intraaxial tumors of the cervicomedullary junction. *J Neurosurg* 67:483–487, 1987.
34. Yasargil MG, Antic J, Laciga R, et al: The microsurgical removal of intramedullary spinal hemangioblastomas: Report of twelve cases and a review of the literature. *Surg Neurol* 6:141–148, 1976.
35. Silverberg GD, Reitz BA, Ream AK: Hypothermia and cardiac arrest in the treatment of giant aneurysms of the cerebral circulation and hemangioblastoma of the medulla. *J Neurosurg* 55:337–346, 1981.
36. Sloof JL, Kernohan JW, McCarty CS: *Primary Intramedullary Tumors of the Spinal Cord and Filum Terminale.* Philadelphia, Saunders, 1964.
37. Velthovan VV, Culliauw L, Caemaert J: Intramedullary spread of a cerebral oligodendroglioma. *Surg Neurol* 30:476–481, 1988.
38. Ehni G, Love JG: Intraspinal lipomas: Report of cases, review of the literature, and clinical and pathologic study. *Arch Neurol Psychiatr* 53:1–28, 1945.
39. Rogers HM, Long DM, Chou SN: Lipoma of the spinal cord and cauda equina. *J Neurosurg* 34:349–354, 1971.
40. Heary RF, Bhandari Y: Intradural cervical lipoma in a neurologically intact patient: Case report. *Neurosurgery* 29:468–471, 1991.
41. McLone DG, Naidich TP: Laser resection of fifty spinal lipomas. *Neurosurgery* 18:611–615, 1986.
42. Manoin J, Uihlen A, Kernohan JW: Intraspinal epidermoids. *J Neurosurg* 19:754–765, 1962.
43. Guidetti B, Gagliardi FM: Epidermoid and dermoid cysts. Clinical evaluation and late surgical results. *J Neurosurg* 47:12–18, 1977.
44. Van Gilder JC, Schwartz HG: Growth of dermoids from skin implants to the nervous system and surrounding spaces of the newborn rat. *J Neurosurg* 26:14–20, 1967.
45. Garrison JE, Kasdon DL: Intramedullary spinal teratoma: Case report and review of the literature. *Neurosurgery* 7:509–512, 1980.
46. Findlay JM, Bernstein M, Vanderlinden RG, Resch L: Microsurgical resection of solitary intramedullary spinal cord metastases. *Neurosurgery* 21:911–915, 1987.
47. Edelson RN, Deck MDF, Posner JB: Intramedullary spinal cord metastases: Clinical and radiographic findings in nine cases. *Neurology* 22:1222–1231, 1972.
48. Grem JL, Burgess J, Trump DL: Clinical features and natural history of intramedullary spinal cord metastases. *Cancer* 56:2305–2314, 1985.
49. Bruce JN, Stein BM: Pineal tumors. *Neurosurg Clin North Am* 1:123–138, 1990.
50. Llena JF, Wisoff HS, Hirano A: Gangliocytic paraganglioma in cauda equina region with biochemical and neuropathological studies. *J Neurosurg* 56:280–282, 1982.
51. Osenbach RK, Godersky JC, Traynelis VC, Schelper RD: Intradural extramedullary cysts of the spinal canal: Clinical presentation, radiographic diagnosis, and surgical management. *Neurosurgery* 30:35–42, 1992.
52. Rousseau M, Lesoini F, Combelles G, et al: An intradmedullary ependymal cyst in a 71-year-old woman *Neurosurgery* 13:52–54, 1983.
53. Miyagi K, Mukawa J, Mekaru I, et al: Enterogenous cyst in the cervical spinal canal. Case report. *J Neurosurg* 68:292–296, 1988.
54. Findler G, Hadani M, Tadmor R, et al: Spinal intradural ependymal cyst: A case report and review of the literature. *Neurosurgery* 17:484–486, 1985.
55. Andrews BT, Weinstein PR, Rosenblum ML, Barbaro NM: Intradural arachnoid cysts of the spinal canal associated with intramedullary cysts. *J Neurosurg* 68:544–549, 1988.
56. Solero CL, Fornari M, Giombini S, et al: Spinal meningiomas: Review of 174 operated cases. *Neurosurgery* 25:153–160, 1989.
57. Levy WJ, Jr, Bay J, Dohn D: Spinal cord meningioma. *J Neurosurg* 57:804–812, 1982.
58. Stein BM, Leeds NE, Taveras JM, Pool JL: Meningiomas of the foramen magnum. *J Neurosurg* 20:740–751, 1963.
59. Meyer FB, Ebersold MJ, Reese DF: Benign tumors of the foramen magnum. *J Neurosurg* 61:136–142, 1984.
60. Giroux JC, Nohra C: Anterior approach for removal of a cervical intradural tumor: Case report and technical note. *Neurosurgery* 2:128–130, 1978.
61. Levy WJ, Latchaw J, Hahn JF, et al: Spinal neurofibromas: A report of 66 cases and a comparison with meningiomas. *Neurosurgery* 18:331–334, 1986.
62. Kim P, Ebersold MJ, Onofrio BM, Quest LM: Surgery of spinal nerve schwannoma. *J Neurosurg* 71:810–814, 1989.
63. Bruni P, Esposito S, Oddi G, et al: Subarachnoid hemorrhage from multiple neurofibroma of the cauda equina: Case report. *Neurosurgery* 28:910–913, 1991.
64. Cantore G, Ciappetta P, Delfini R, et al: Intramedullary spinal neurinoma. *J Neurosurg* 57:143–147, 1982.
65. Gardner WJ, Spitler DK, Whitten C: Increased intracranial pressure caused by increased protein content into the cerebrospinal fluid. An explanation of papilledema in certain cases of small intracranial and intraspinal tumors, and in the Guillain-Barré syndrome. *N Engl J Med* 250:932–936, 1954.
66. Day AL, Sypert GW: Spinal cord sarcoidosis. *Ann Neurol* 1:79–85, 1977.
67. Hitchon PW, Haque AU, Olson JJ, et al: Sarcoidosis presenting as an intradmedullary spinal cord mass. *Neurosurgery* 15:86–90, 1984.
68. Sundaresan N, Digiacinto GV, Hughes JEO, et al: Treatment of neoplastic spinal cord compression: Results of a prospective study. *Neurosurgery* 29:645–650, 1991.
69. Overby MC, Rothman AS: Anterolateral decompression for metastatic epidural spinal cord tumors: Results of a modified costotransversectomy approach. *J Neurosurg* 62:344–348, 1985.
70. Siegal T, Siegal T: Current consideration in the management of neoplastic spinal cord compression. *Spine* 14:223–229, 1989.
71. Harrington KD: Current concepts review metastatic disease of the spine. *J Bone Joint Surg* (Am) 68:1110–1115, 1986.
72. Gilbert RW, Kim JH, Posner JB: Epidural spinal cord compression from metastatic tumor. Diagnosis and treatment. *Ann Neurol* 3:40–51, 1978.
73. Haddad SF, Hitchon PW, Godersky JC: Idiopathic and glucocortcoid induced spinal epidural lipomatosis. *J Neurosurg* 74:38–42, 1991.
74. Kaplan JG, Barasch E, Hirschfeld A, et al: Spinal epidural lipomatosis: A serious complication of iatrogenic Cushing's syndrome. *Neurology* 39:1031–1034, 1989.

75. Kuroda S, Abe H, Akino M, et al: Infiltrating spinal angiolipoma causing myelopathy: Case report. *Neurosurgery* 27:315–318, 1990.

76. Sundaresan N, Galicich JH, Chu FCH, Huvos AG: Spinal chordomas. *J Neurosurg* 50:312–319, 1979.

77. Gutin PH, Leibel SA, Hosobuchi Y, et al: Brachytherapy of recurrent tumors of the skull base and spine with Iodine-125 sources. *Neurosurgery* 20:938–945, 1987.

78. O'Neill P, Bell BA, Miller JD, et al: Fifty years of experience with chordoma in southeast Scotland. *Neurosurgery* 16:166–170, 1985.

79. Loftus CM, Michelsen CB, Rapoport F, Antunes JL: Management of plasmacytoma of the spine. *Neurosurgery* 13:30–36, 1983.

80. Sundaresan N, Rosen G, Huvos AG, Krol G: Combined treatment of osteosarcoma of the spine. *Neurosurgery* 23:714–719, 1988.

81. Camins MB, Duncan AW, Smith J, Marcovic RC: Chondrosarcoma of the spine. *Spine* 3:202–209, 1978.

82. Hirsch LF, Thanki A, Spector HB: Primary spinal chordosarcoma with eighteen-year followup: Case report and literature review. *Neurosurgery* 14:747–749, 1984.

83. Palmer FJ, Blum PW: Osteochondroma with spinal cord compression: A report of three cases. *J Neurosurg* 52:842–845, 1980.

84. Janin Y, Epstein JA, Carras R: Osteoid osteomas and osteoblastomas of the spine. *Neurosurgery* 8:31–38, 1981.

85. Shikata J, Yamamuro T, Iida H, Kotoura Y: Benign osteoblastoma of the cervical vertebra. *Surg Neurol* 27:381–385, 1987.

86. Bucci MN, Feldenzer JA, Phillips WA, et al: Atlantoaxial rotational limitations secondary to osteoid osteoma of the axis. *J Neurosurg* 70:129–131, 1989.

87. Dilorenzo N, Spallone A, Nolletti A, Nardi P: Giant cell tumors of the spine. A clinical study of six cases, with emphasis on the radiological features, treatment and follow-up. *Neurosurgery* 6:29–34, 1980.

88. Dahlin DC: Giant cell tumor of the vertebra above the sacrum: A review of 31 cases. *Cancer* 39:1350–1356, 1977.

89. Ohry A, Lipschitz M, Shemesh Y, et al: Disappearance of quadriparesis due to a huge cervicothoracic aneurysmal bone cyst. *Surg Neurol* 29:307–310, 1988.

90. Podos PN Jr, White RJ: Aneurysmal bone cyst of the cervical spine: A twelve-year followup after surgical treatment. *Surg Neurol* 14:259–262, 1980.

91. Feuerman T, Dwan PS, Young RF: Vertebrectomy for treatment of vertebral hemangioma without preoperative embolization: Case report. *J Neurosurg* 65:404–406, 1986.

92. Healy M, Herz DA, Pearl L: Spinal hemangioma. *Neurosurgery* 13:689–691, 1983.

93. Acciarri N, Paganini M, Fonda C, et al: Langerhans' cell histiocytosis of the spine causing cord compression: Case report. *Neurosurgery* 31:965–968, 1992.

☐ STUDY QUESTIONS

I. A 38-year-old female is referred because of localized interscapular pain with radiation in a band around to the right breast. This is worse at night. There is a strip of hyperesthesia along the distribution of the right fifth intercostal nerve. There are hyperactive reflexes in the right lower extremity and decreased sensation to pin prick on the left. X-rays show a enlarged neural foramen at T4–L5 on the right.

1. What is the most likely diagnosis? **2.** What imaging structures might be considered to outline the lesion? **3.** What image might be produced by myelography? **4.** How might the lesion be approached? **5.** Would the lesion most likely be dorsal or ventral to the dentate ligament? Why?

II. A 60-year-old male has a long history of upper lumbar back pain and progressive weakness of his lower extremities. X-rays and CT scan reveal a sharp kyphosis centered at T10. Disk spaces are preserved. There is compression of the tenth thoracic vertebra. There are multiple lesions throughout the chest. An endotracheal biopsy shows evidence of squamous cell carcinoma.

1. What is the most likely cause of the paraparesis? **2.** How might the spinal cord be decompressed? **3.** What is the objective of corpectomy? **4.** How can the spine be

stabilized surgically? **5.** What part might irradiation therapy play in the treatment of this patient?

III. A 52-year-old female is seen because of progressive weakness and ataxia in all four extremities, but most severe **2.** What is the microscopic appearance? **3.** How might this appearance differ if the lesions involved the upper spinal in the upper extremities. She has difficulty eating, and there is paresis and severe atrophy of the right side of the tongue. MRI shows a mass lesion on the anterior lip of the foramen magnum.

1. What is the most likely diagnosis? **2.** From what approach might the lesion be attacked surgically, anteriorly or posteriorly? **3.** What are the variations to the anterior approach that might be used? **4.** What adjunctive therapy might be necessary? **5.** What form of radiation therapy might be effective?

IV. A 43-year-old male is experiencing weakness of his hands and lower extremities. He has decreased motor function and pinprick in the hands but fast reflexes in lower extremities. He is spastic in the lower extremities and has intrinsic muscle wasting of the hands. An MRI shows intrinsic mass effect in the lower cervical area. The spinal cord is enhanced only moderately. There is no cystic component.

1. What is the differential diagnosis? **2.** How might this patient obtain definitive diagnosis? **3.** What surgical therapy might be considered? **4.** How could radiation play a part in the treatment of this lesion? **5.** How might his course change if syringomyelia became a problem?

V. A 30-year-old male complains of severe lumbar back pain radiating into both buttocks. Sphincter control has been lost. MRI reveals an intraspinal mass fanning out into the paraspinal area. Microscopically, the lesion is myxomatous. It has infiltrated the cauda equina.

1. What intrinsic spinal tumor fits this description? **2.** What is the microscopic appearance? **3.** How might this appearance differ if the lesions involved the upper spinal cord? **4.** What forms of therapy might be considered? **5.** What is the prognosis?

CHAPTER 14

DIAGNOSIS AND TREATMENT OF STROKES
Ischemic Lesions and Intraparenchymal Hemorrhages of the Brain

Dennis E. McDonnell
Marshall B. Allen, Jr.

Cerebrovascular disease is the third leading cause of death among adults in the United States, ranking behind cancer and heart disease.[1] Although on the decline, it is the most important cause of chronic disability.[2,3] Ischemic cerebrovascular disease accounts for about 75 percent of the cases while lesions resulting from hemorrhage into the brain or subarachnoid space account for about 16 percent.[4,5] The role of surgery in the prevention of stroke and the treatment of various clinical afflictions is becoming clearly defined. In this chapter, we will discuss ischemic lesions and spontaneous intraparenchymal hemorrhages of the brain. Cerebrovascular diseases have been classified and detailed both clinically and pathologically.[6]

☐ MECHANISMS OF CEREBRAL ISCHEMIA

Cerebral infarction occurs when blood flow drops below critical levels in regions of brain irrigated by specific vessels that are occluded or when there is a global reduction of bulk flow resulting from systemic hypoperfusion. This critical level is approximately 18 ml/100 g per minute compared to a normal average resting flow rate of 60 ml/100 g per minute.[7] Emboli originating from intraluminal lesions of the extracranial carotid artery account for two-thirds of infarcts in the middle cerebral artery distribution (Fig. 14-1).[8] Surgery may be utilized to excise or repair constriction, remove lesions that might be a source of emboli, bypass occlusions, or augment collateral flow.[9–12] Surgical attempts to reopen complete occlusions often fail clinically.[13] Bypass revascularizations, once popular, are presently much more restricted.[14,15] Decompressive resections of intracranial hematoma or edematous or infarcted brain may be life-saving, by relieving mass effect and preventing tentorial herniation.

LOCALIZATION

Cerebral infarction occurs in the distribution of tissue supplied by one of the four major arteries that supply the brain,

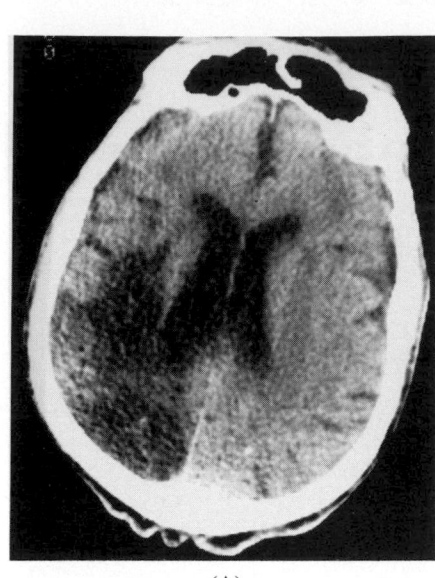

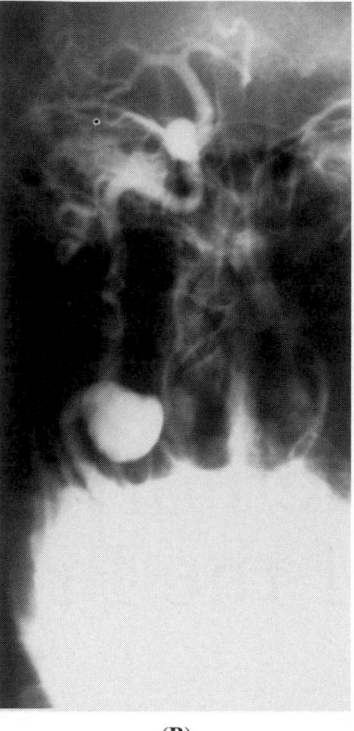

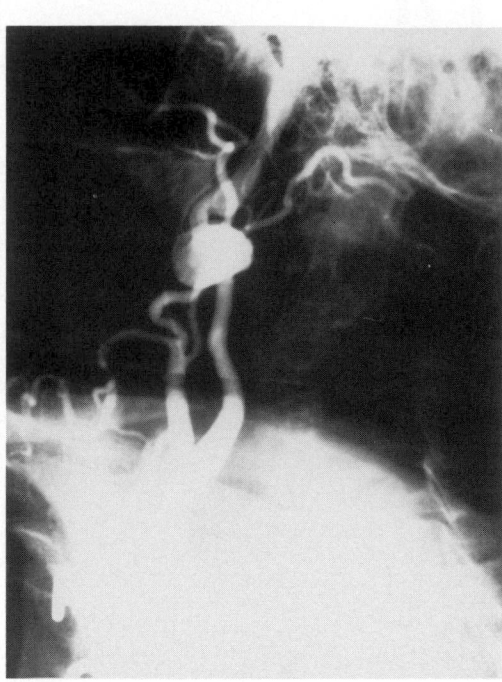

| (A) | (B) | (C) |

Figure 14–1 Infarction of the right temporal and occipital lobes due to emboli from an aneurysm of the right extracranial internal carotid artery. *(A)* CT scan shows decreased attenuation due to encephalomalacia of infarct; *(B)* right carotid angiogram frontal projection; and *(C)* lateral projection shows the aneurysm and mural thrombus, source of emboli, within it.

a major arterial branch such as the middle cerebral artery or posterior inferior cerebellar artery, or a cortical or penetrating branch. Infarction may occur in zones of limited perfusion within the watershed distribution between areas supplied by two cerebral arteries—for example, parenchyma at the peripheral zone of supply by the middle cerebral artery (Fig. 14-2). Infarction in the primary distribution of a major vessel is most likely the result of occlusion of that vessel. Most occlusions of major vessels supplying the brain result from emboli, but other causes include propagation of an intraluminal clot, dissection of the wall of a vessel, thrombosis within a vessel containing a plaque, or progressive narrowing of the vessel.

The occurrence, size, and distribution of the infarction may be assured or even expanded by the development and propagation of an antegrade intraluminal thrombus which progresses to compromise collateral conduits. On the other hand, an efficient collateral circulation may limit the size and distribution of an infarct. Thus occlusion of a carotid or a vertebral artery may be of no clinical consequence in the presence of a competent circle of Willis or other collaterals. In many instances, occlusion of a proximal segment of the middle cerebral artery proves to be inconsequential in the presence of adequate collateral circulation from the anterior and posterior cerebral arteries.

Most strokes that occur in the distribution of the middle cerebral artery are not due to a local lesion in the middle cerebral artery but arise from propagation of a thrombus or an embolus released from a proximal extracranial artery or endocardium.[13] In some cases of occlusion of the circle of Willis, the entire cerebrum may be irrigated by collaterals, often supplied from the vertebral arteries. When the collateral circulation is less efficient, clinical consequences of vascular obstructions may be severe. When acute occlusion of the carotid artery produces a stroke, only 2 to 12 percent of patients will recover, 40 to 69 percent will be disabled with severe neurological deficits, and 16 to 55 percent will die.[13]

Penetrating arteries are generally "end" arteries with no collateral circulation, and occlusion is likely to result in "lacunar" infarcts, i.e., *small infarcts deep within the white matter.*[16,17]

Infarction in a watershed area is usually the result of reduced bulk flow from a devastating cardiovascular event such as cardiac arrest, hypovolemic shock, occlusion of an extracranial internal carotid artery, or widespread disturbances in the microvascular circulation.[3]

PATHOGENESIS

Emboli may originate from the endocardium within the heart, from plaques on the endothelial walls of proximal arteries, from fresh thrombi originating in acutely occluded major proximal arteries, or from systemic sources passing through defects in the heart (paradoxical emboli) such as

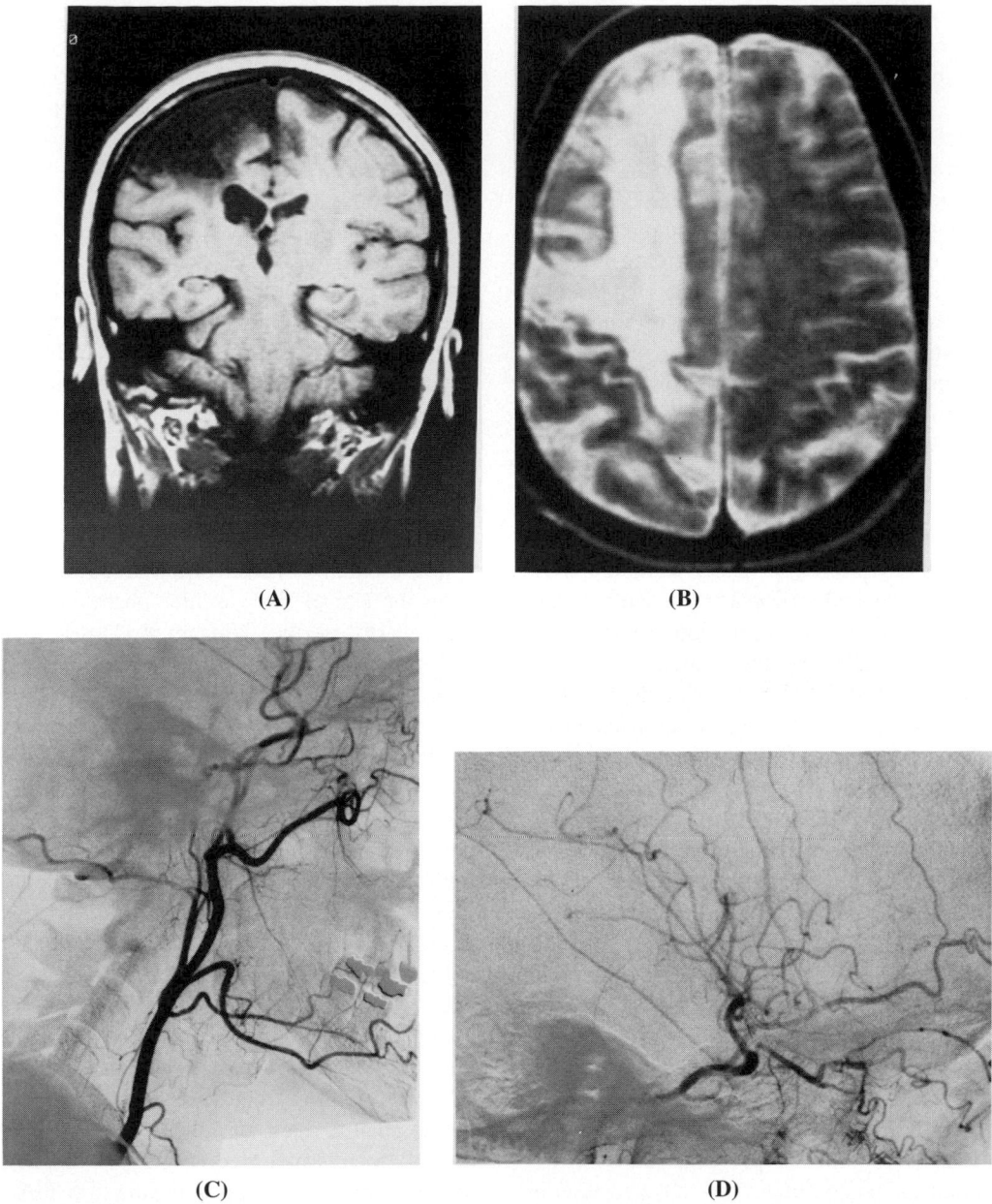

(A)   **(B)**

(C)   **(D)**

Figure 14–2   Infarction within the right cerebral hemisphere in a 36-year-old female who suffered an acute left hemiparesis due to sudden occlusion of the right internal carotid artery while using cocaine 10 years previously. *(A)* MRI T1-weighted image coronal view and *(B)* MRI T2-weighted image axial view show location and extent of the infarct. The right carotid angiogram lateral view shows *(C)* no filling of the extracranial internal carotid artery and prominent meningeal collaterals from ascending pharyngeal and internal maxillary branches of the external carotid artery reconstituting the petrous and cavernous segments of the internal carotid artery, *(D)* additional collateral flow from the ophthalmic artery augmenting intracranial internal carotid flow with reconstitution of the middle cerebral artery.

occur in the course of pulmonary embolization. Emboli may be bland or septic. Bland emboli may be platelet aggregates, clots, or acellular debris having developed in proximal segments of the vascular tree, as in the case of thrombi occurring within the heart following myocardial infarction or in blood vessels that have been partially occluded, or they may be the result of atheromatous calcification or ulcerated plaques in proximal vessels. Periarterial inflammatory reaction to an atheroma is often intense enough to produce dense adherence between the carotid artery and the adjacent tissues.[12] Other sources of emboli are vegetations or calcific deposits on the mitral valves. Emboli may also be iatrogenic, due to thrombi forming on intravascular catheters used for infusions and shunts or from thrombi released during the course of intracardiac or intravascular injections, monitoring, or surgery.

Emboli pass distally, usually lodging at bifurcations. There they may occlude the vessel temporarily and then resolve. They may break up into smaller fragments and pass more distally. After a vessel is occluded, an infarction may result and yet the embolus resolve, leaving a patent vessel supplying an area of infarction. Arteritis with a resulting aneurysm or brain abscess is often the end result of a septic embolus.

Occlusion of penetrating vessels is usually the result of thickening of the walls by hyalin degeneration, most commonly the result of long-standing hypertension.[3,16,17]

The brain is somewhat resistant to ischemia and can recover if blood flow is reestablished before irreversible neuronal damage occurs.[18] A focal volume of infarcted cerebral tissue is surrounded by an ischemic region that is nonfunctional but still viable and potentially recoverable, the penumbra.[19] Complex interactions occur at the cellular level under conditions of acute ischemia. Over time, they lead to irreversible damage of cells. Neuronal membrane depolarization occurs with loss of detectable electrical activity within 20 sec. Several minutes after this, major ionic shifts occur with influx of sodium into the cells and efflux of potassium into the extracellular space. Calcium is released from mitochondria and endoplastic reticulum, further impairing cellular energy transformation. Extracellular edema and astrocytic swelling results, which further impedes oxygen transfer. Additionally there is depletion of energy stores with loss of phosphocreatine and adenosine triphosphate (ATP), leading to build up of anaerobic metabolites and lactic acid. These changes evolve over several hours and can potentially be reversed if oxygenated blood flow is reestablished. However, ischemia tends to potentiate more ischemia because of edema, reduced cellular oxygen delivery, and increased metabolic demand of the ischemic tissue.[20,21]

The main cause of neuronal dysfunction and cell death in ischemia is failure of ATP synthesis with loss of cellular ion homeostasis and acid-base balance. Ion fluxes with buildup of intracellular Ca^{2+}, Na^+, and H^+ are associated with a leaking cell membrane so that ATP is wasted and dissipated further by futile cycling of ions. Acidosis is caused by increased glycolysis over oxidative phosphorylation where pyruvate is converted to lactate rather than CO_2 and H_2O by the normal oxidative reactions in the mitrochondria. This is followed by lipolysis, proteolysis, and inhibition of protein synthesis. Cell death rapidly follows.[20–22]

The metabolites of arachidonic acid (AA) also have a direct effect on cell membrane integrity, platelet aggregation, and microvascular patency in cerebral ischemia. These include prostaglandins (PGs), thromboxane (TXA), and leukotrienes (LTs), which are compounds derived from 20-carbon polyunsaturated fatty acids collectively known as *eicosanoids*.[23] Prostaglandins and thromboxane have opposing actions on platelets and vessel walls. Leukotrienes are chemotactic agents that increase cell permeability. PGs and LTs interact to cause edema. Several reactions catalyze the conversion of AA to PGs, TXA, and LTs. Free oxygen radicals are also generated by these reactions, which have direct deleterious effects on cell membrane integrity. PG conversions can be inhibited by aspirin and other nonsteroidal anti-inflammatory drugs. Thromboxane is a major AA meta-

bolite in platelets and named for its platelet aggregating effects; it is also a potent vasoconstrictor. PGs tend to inhibit platelet aggregation and are vasodilators. Leukotrienes are released in immune reactions and anaphylaxis. They react slowly, stimulate smooth muscle contraction, and increase vascular permeability. LTs stimulate TXA synthesis, and PGs tend to inhibit synthesis of LTs.[23]

In cerebral ischemia, cell breakdown leads to release of fatty acids, including AA. These are converted to eicosanoids. A predominance of TXA synthesis contributes to platelet microthrombi and impaired cerebral microcirculatory perfusion as well as aggravate ischemia.[23] Intervention to impede or reverse these reactions offers modes of therapy.

CLINICAL FEATURES

Clinical features of ischemic cerebrovascular disease depend upon the site of the vascular obstruction, its duration, and the severity of the damage produced. The term *transient ischemic attack (TIA)* has been applied to episodes of neurological deficits of vascular origin, lasting for less than 24 h. When the duration of such episodes exceeds 24 h but lasts for less than 3 weeks, the name *reversible ischemic neurological deficit (RIND)* is applied. The name *stroke in evolution*, or *progressing stroke,* is applied to a neurological deficit thought to be of ischemic origin which progresses for 6 h or more. The differential etiology of such clinical experiences must include infarction, hemorrhage, and neoplasm. The name *completed stroke* is applied when the neurological deficit has been stable for 72 h or longer.

The incidence of cerebral infarction is greatly increased in patients with TIAs although *TIAs precede infarction in less than 10 percent of cases.*[24] They are likely to be indicative of carotid lesions when the neurological symptoms are limited to an arm, a leg, or aphasia rather than when a combination of these is involved (Fig. 14-3).[25] The risk of stroke is highest during the month after the first TIA.[22] Headache is a common premonitory symptom of cerebral ischemia and is prominent in 25 percent of patients with TIAs.[26] When symptoms and deficits build over several hours, this implies an acute unstable cerebral ischemic event that is termed *crescendo TIA*; this is an uncommon event and may be reversed with urgent medical or surgical treatment. Unfortunately, there is a tendency for patients suffering stroke to delay seeking medical care. The majority of patients with infarcts (64 percent) and subarachnoid hemorrhage (54 percent) do not present within 24 h of stroke onset.[27] This delay may preclude the benefits of some treatments for acute stroke.

Ischemic lesions in the distribution of one of the internal carotid arteries result in hemiparesis—most marked in the upper extremity—and hemianopsia. Aphasia with its associated features of acalculia and right-left disorientation is associated with lesions in the dominant hemisphere while dyspraxia, loss of initiative, and parietal lobe signs are

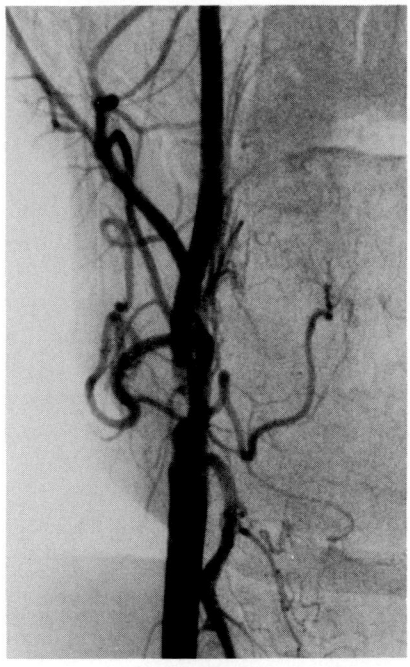

(A)

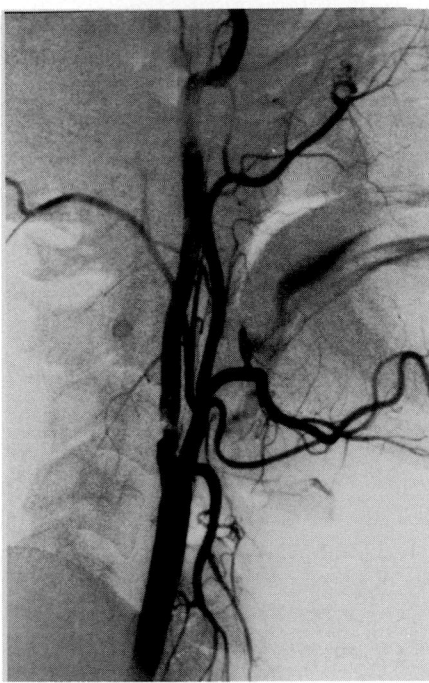

(B)

Figure 14–3 Atherosclerotic plaque with intraluminal thrombus in the proximal internal carotid artery is seen on *(A)* frontal and *(B)* lateral views of a right carotid angiogram, as a source of emboli causing multiple focal TIAs.

prominent when lesions affect the nondominant hemisphere. Consciousness is impaired in 25 percent of patients with acute infarction in the distribution of the carotid arteries.[3] Involvement of the middle cerebral artery at the level of the trifurcation causes a faciobrachial motor and sensory disturbance with dysphasia or dyspraxia, depending on the side.

Isolated monocular transient visual loss, *amaurosis fugax (AF)*, is the ocular equivalent of a TIA. The majority (79 percent) of patients with AF have plaques in the ipsilateral carotid artery, although only 16 percent of these are severe enough to impede flow.[28] Even though the prognosis in this group is much better, they should be evaluated by carotid ultrasonography.

Occlusions of the anterior cerebral artery result in motor and sensory disturbances of the lower extremities on the contralateral side. There may be behavioral changes as well. Bilateral anterior cerebral artery occlusion results in akinetic mutism with infarction of the septal nuclei, medial head of caudate nuclei, anterior cingulate gyri, and corpus callosum.[29]

Epilepsy complicates cerebral infarction in 3 percent of cases in the early period after infarction.[30] Seizures may be a late consequence of infarction, commencing as late as 5 years after the infarct. An incidence of 9.5 percent has been reported.[31]

Hemorrhage may complicate acute infarction when the involved tissue is exposed to normal perfusion pressures.[32] This is rare in the natural state but is a potential complication that has limited the use of fibrinolytic therapy and revascularization procedures.

Massive cerebral infarction frequently results in death, usually as a result of hemispheric edema and tentorial herniation if death occurs within the first week.[33] Massive edema may result in compartmental shifts or further decrease in cerebral perfusion. Death after a week is likely to result from a complication such as pneumonia, renal infection, or septicemia.

RISK FACTORS

Habits, lifestyles, and diseases that potentiate cerebrovascular disease are sought in the clinical history. Behavioral factors include smoking cigarettes, drinking alcohol, and abusing drugs (particularly cocaine).[34,35] Constitutional factors include age, sex, race, familial factors, abnormal serum lipids, diabetes mellitis, hypertension, sickle cell disease, elevated fibrinogen, polycythemia, migraine, hypothyroidism, and cardiac disease (congenital, atherosclerotic, or dysrhythmic).[4,24]

EVALUATION

Indications for evaluating patients with respect to stroke prevention and treatment include episodes of temporary deficit (TIAs or RINDs) and bruits in the neck of those over 40 years of age. Similarly, patients who have recently experienced clinically evident ischemic episodes should be evaluated as they often have risk factors for vasculopathy and hypercoagulability, which potentiate strokes.

Workup includes computed tomography (CT) with and without contrast enhancement, magnetic resonance imaging

(MRI) with and without gadolinium, electroencephalography (EEG), direct Doppler or B-scan ultrasound examinations of the neck, angiography, cardiac investigation, and hematological studies.

The evaluation of patients who have recently experienced strokes has been greatly simplified by the advent of CT.[36] CT identifies the site and size of areas of infarction so that it readily differentiates lacunar infarcts from those produced by cortical vessels. It differentiates those that are in the primary distribution of a major feeding vessel from those that are located in watershed areas. CT with contrast enhancement shows areas of compromise of the blood brain barrier (BBB). CT also demonstrates the site and degree of edema and compartmental shift, which may be a major factor in determining the need for surgery (Fig. 14-4). In the posterior fossa, cerebellar infarction with swelling or hemorrhage and presence of acute hydrocephalus are readily detected by CT; this is very important in determining the need for surgical intervention. Occasionally, CT may demonstrate an unexpected mass lesion such as a neoplasm or intracranial hematoma.

MRI is very sensitive to the presence of edema and may demonstrate evidence of infarction even before CT.[37] There is less often need for contrast media with MRI than there is with CT. MRI may indicate whether blood is flowing in large vessels supplying the brain by the "flow void" image. The primary disadvantages of MRI relate to the length of time required for scanning, its cost, and its interference with cardiac pacemakers.

EEG is normal in only 25 percent of patients having recently experienced a stroke.[3] A slow-wave focus is the most common abnormality and may last for several weeks after a stroke, even in a patient who has not experienced seizures. A seizure focus is more likely to be present when seizures occur late or are remote to the ictus. Seizures may be helpful in differentiating lacunar from striatocapsular lesions.[38]

Although ophthalmodynamometry and orbital Doppler investigations can demonstrate the laterality of severe stenosis or occlusion of the carotid artery, duplex Doppler and color Doppler ultrasonic examinations of the cervical carotid artery have proved to be accurate, noninvasive indicators of the local site of pathology in these vessels.[3,39] Accuracy depends on the skill of the technician and diagnostician. The Doppler indicates the speed of blood flow and evidence of turbulence, from which the presence and amount of stenosis within the carotid artery can be determined. Noninvasive procedures are preferred for screening and initial evaluation. Duplex Doppler ultrasonographic examination of the cervical carotid artery is accurate and specific for detecting lesions that obstruct flow.[28,40] Transcranial Doppler (TCD) has been shown to be as accurate in evaluating obstructive lesions in the intracranial arteries. The most important clinical application is detection of moderate to severe stenosis in asymptomatic but high-risk patients, such as those with sickle cell disease.[41]

Angiography remains the most definitive indicator of arterial lesions of the neck that might be the cause of ischemic cerebral disease. However, angiography in the patient who has recently experienced an acute cerebrovascular ischemic event is associated with increased morbidity and is not advocated as a routine study. It is clearly indicated in the presence of: (1) a stenotic lesion in the cervical carotid artery imaged by ultrasound, (2) cerebral infarction following trauma, (3) symptoms of cerebral ischemia suggesting intimal dissection, (4) symptoms occurring in a youth, and (5) symptoms of stroke that progress atypically. Angiography is not necessary for lacunar strokes or when a cardiac source for emboli has been demonstrated, and it may also be contraindicated by age, debility, or associated diseases. Venous digital subtraction angiography may be used as the first angiographic study since it avoids manipulating the vessel housing an obstructive lesion.[42] However, image resolution is poor using this modality, making it difficult to assess vascular pathology accurately. It also requires larger amounts of contrast, with resultant adverse effects in patients who have impaired renal function. Arterial contrast injections usually provide clearer images of arterial lesions required when surgery is anticipated.[42,43] Generally it is desirable to limit the amount of contrast material used for angiography so that intraarterial injections are preferable to venous digital subtraction angiography.

Routine cardiac evaluation for a patient who has recently had a stroke includes a 12-channel electrocardiogram and chest x-ray. Abnormalities will be seen in about 50 to 60 percent of patients who have had a recent cerebral infarction.[3] An indicator of a cardiac origin for a recent cerebrovascular embolus is the presence of atrial fibrillation or evidence of a recent myocardial infarction.[44] Evidence of an old, large anterior and apical myocardial infarction may indicate an adynamic wall from which mural thrombi might develop. Most patients also undergo a treadmill stress test or a thallium isotope test with dipyridamole cardiac imaging to define concomitant coronary arterial atherosclerosis.

Other investigations that may provide indication of a cardiac origin of stroke include echocardiogram and prolonged ECG cardiac monitoring. Echocardiograms can be used to evaluate the heart valves, motility in cardiomegaly, and evidence of myxoma.[45] Extended ECG monitoring using a Holter-type cardiac monitor can detect intermittent arrhythmias such as episodes of prolonged asystole or transient tachycardia that affect cardiac output, resulting in impaired cerebrovascular perfusion.

Common hematological disorders associated with cerebral infarction are: abnormalities in clot lysis, presence of lupus anticoagulants, abnormal platelet function, hyperviscosity, and hemoglobin abnormalities. Specific cellular aberrations linked to stroke include sickle cell disease, erythrocytosis, thrombocytosis, and high white cell counts (leukemia). The presence of most of these is determined by routine blood counts and a coagulation profile. An occult hematological disorder should be considered when a stroke occurs in a very young individual, when infarction occurs in more than one arterial territory, and when a cause for arterial occlusive disease or embolic source cannot be determined.[3]

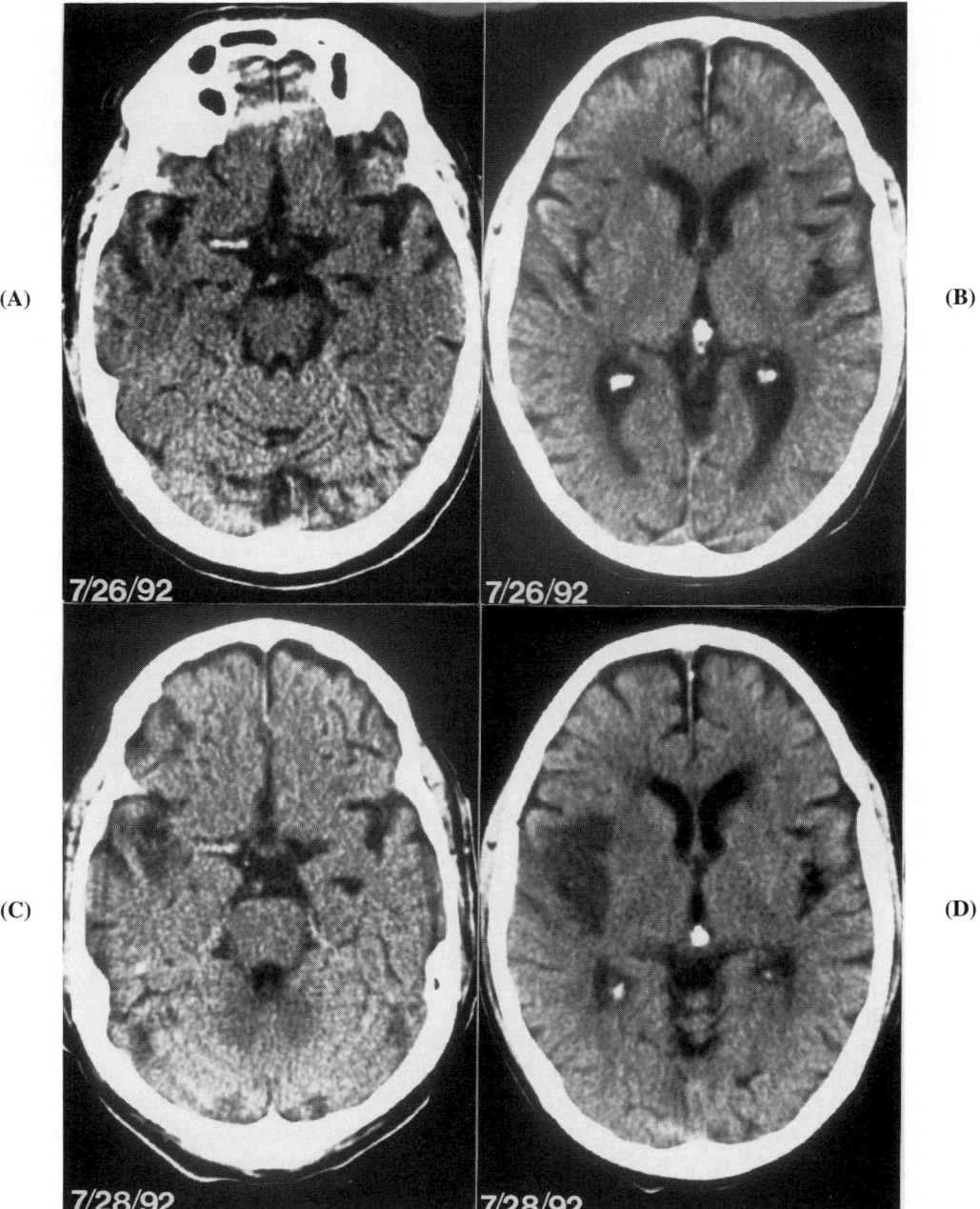

Figure 14–4 Developing infarction with positive "cord sign" in a 58-year-old male presenting with acute onset of left hemiplegia as seen on noncontrasted CT; *(A)* and *(B)* on 7/26/92 show thrombosis of the M-1 segment of the middle cerebral artery along with diffuse atrophy. Repeat study 48 h later on 7/28/92 at comparable levels *(C)* and *(D)* respectively shows decreased attenuation in the right temporal and frontal lobes as well as the striatum. The smaller frontal horn of the right lateral ventricle in the later CT suggests associative edema.

Lupus anticoagulants are frequently associated with a hypercoagulable state.[46] They are a group of antibodies found in only 5 to 10 percent of patients with lupus erythematosus and commonly occur in patients with autoimmune disorders and malignant neoplasms. These antibodies are seen in patients receiving drugs such as phenothiazine, penicillin derivatives, hydralazine, phenytoin, procainamide, and isoniazid. These antibodies are immunoglobulins with antibody specificity to phospholipids found in several spontaneous and drug-induced autoimmune states. They may be associated with thrombosis of deep veins, recurrent intravascular thrombosis, and myocardial and/or cerebral infarction. These antibodies may cause prolongation of the partial thromboplastin time, false-positive serological tests, and mild thrombocytopenia. Such reactions result from specific phospholipids that are activity-directed.

Other common systemic disorders that are complicated by an increased incidence of stroke include diabetes mellitus, essential hypertension, peripheral vascular arteriosclerosis, and the group of hyperlipidoses. Uncommon conditions such as fibromuscular dysplasia, inflammatory arteritis, Takayasu's syndrome, and moyamoya disease will occasionally present.

☐ SOME SPECIFIC SYNDROMES ASSOCIATED WITH CEREBROVASCULAR INSUFFICIENCY

MOYAMOYA DISEASE

Moyamoya disease is a progressive cerebrovascular occlusive disease involving the siphon and proximal intracranial portion of the carotid arteries (Fig. 14-5). There is a bimodal age incidence in children and adolescents and again in adults peaking in the fourth decade. It was first described in Asians by Takeuchi in 1957.[50] Occlusion of vessels supplying the circle of Willis results in the development of a variety of transdural, leptomeningeal anastomotic vessels, as well as dilated perforating vessels that supply the basal ganglia. The angiographic appearance of these vessels inspired the name of the disease, *moyamoya*—Japanese for mist, fog, or puffs of smoke. There also may be a history of inflammation in the head or neck.[47]

Patients experience repeated attacks of motor weakness, speech disturbance, alteration in mental status, and organic mental syndromes. These may be in the form of TIAs but more commonly are completed strokes. Intermittent ocular symptoms of amaurosis, impaired acuity, scotomata, diplopia, and hemianopsia can accompany the symptoms of cerebral ischemia; however, intraocular findings are rare.[48] Older patients may present with intracranial hemorrhage. Aneurysms occur frequently and can be a source of hemorrhage.[49,50] The more common source of bleeding is from collateral vessels that develop near the ventricular walls.[47]

Surgical treatment is directed to augmenting collateral blood flow by intracranial-extracranial bypass. Dural synangiosis is technically simple and is reported to be an effective procedure but not without complications.[51,52] Nevertheless, moyamoya is a progressive disease, and repeated TIAs and seizures may eventually result in permanent severe deficits unless there is surgical intervention.[53]

FIBROMUSCULAR DYSPLASIA

Fibromuscular dysplasia is a nonatherosclerotic and noninflammatory stenotic arterial disease commonly affecting the renal and internal carotid arteries. It occurs most frequently in young women, and the trait appears to be inherited. Patients are often asymptomatic but may have hypertension, stroke, or other evidences of vascular insufficiency, depending on the severity of stenosis and the arteries affected. It involves different parts of the arterial wall, the intima, media, or adventitia. Medial fibromuscular dysplasia is the most-frequent form, representing 70 to 90 percent of cases.

The angiographic appearance of fibromuscular dysplasia, characteristically, is corrugated or beaded. The internal carotid artery is usually involved at the level of C2, where the artery can be mechanically irritated by repeated stretching with extension or rotation of the neck. Intimal fibroplasia has a similar angiographic appearance to the medial type, but it may present as a long tubular narrowing of the artery, particularly in young patients.[54]

Fibrous dysplasia may remain stable, but the form seen in renal arteries has been shown to progress in 35 percent of patients. It may also be aggravated by smoking. Ergotamines have produced similar arterial changes. Although oral contraceptives may induce some increased stenosis, pregnancy does not worsen it. Renal artery aneurysms may occur alone or in combination with stenosis and hypertension. Angiotensin-converting enzyme inhibitors are reportedly effective in managing associated hypertension.[54] In the cerebrovascular form, patients complain of headache, vertigo, tinnitus, or fatigue. More serious TIAs, stroke, and subarachnoid hemorrhage occur in about 30 percent of patients, and spontaneous dissections can occur.[55,56] The long-term prognosis for these patients is good, as they tend not to progress over the years.[54] This benign course should be remembered when managing these patients.

VERTEBROVASCULAR INSUFFICIENCY

Stenosis in the vertebrobasilar system most commonly arises at the vertebral artery origin. Thrombosis can occur at the site of stenosis and extend distally or act as a source of emboli. Since signs of ischemia present distal to the site of occlusion, the site of the vascular lesion cannot be localized. Also, an intact contralateral vertebral artery does not necessarily protect against a brainstem or cerebellar stroke.[57]

Vertebral arteries may be compromised within the serial

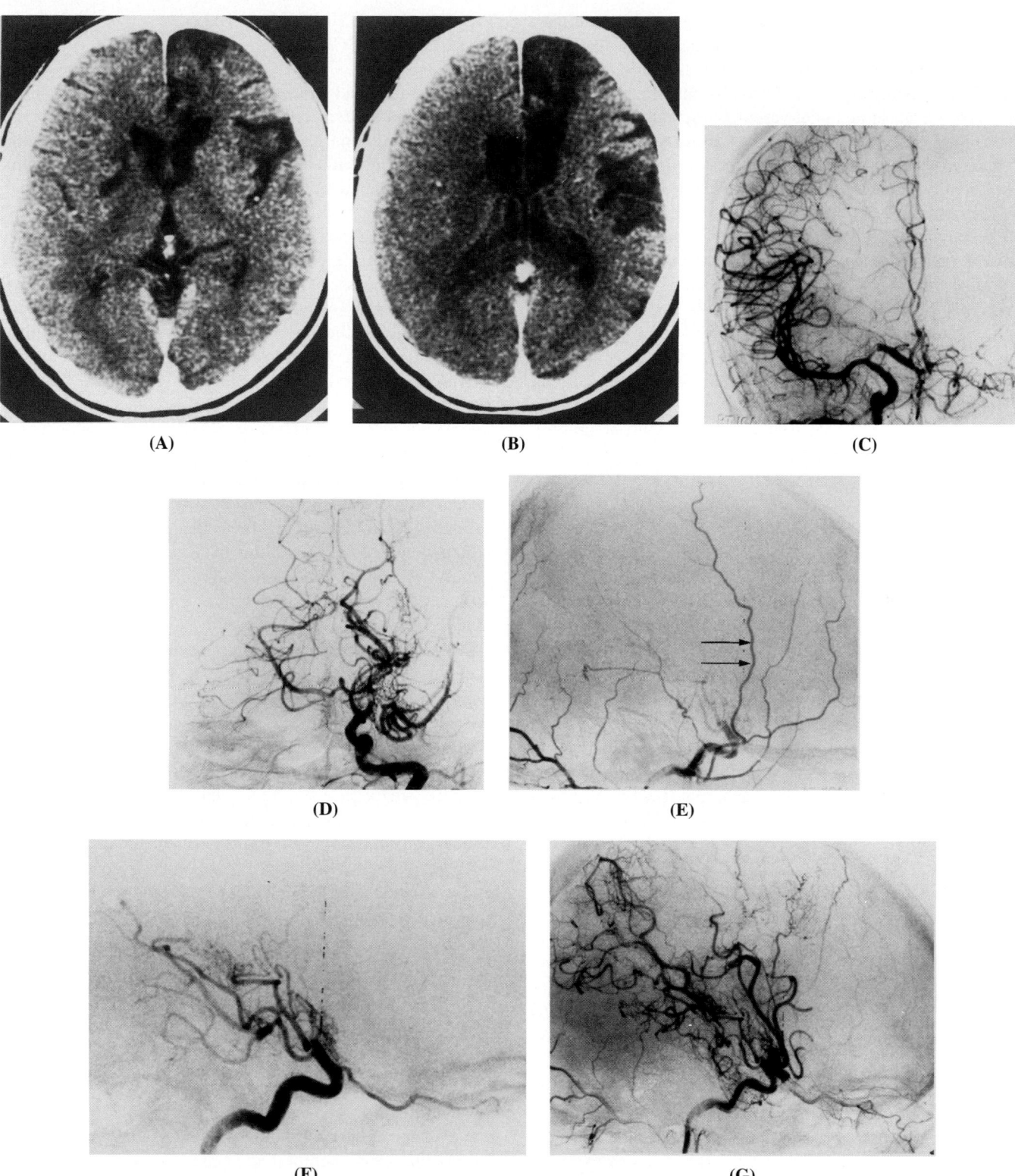

(A)　　　　　　　　(B)　　　　　　　　(C)

(D)　　　　　　　　(E)

(F)　　　　　　　　(G)

Figure 14–5　A 19-year-old female who had transient episodes of confusion, aphasia, and sialorrhea along with progressive intellectual decline; her left supraclinoid internal carotid artery was found to be occluded. *(A)* CT shows a right striatal lacunar infarct along with left frontal and sylvian infarcts. *(B)* CT shows extension of the left frontal lobe infarcts; *(C)* anterior-posterior (AP) view right carotid angiogram shows tight stenosis of proximal A-1 segment that may explain the lacunar infarct in the striatum; *(D)* AP view of the left vertebral artery reconstitutes the left middle cerebral artery via the posterior communicating artery and other collaterals; *(E)* lateral view left carotid angiogram shows retrograde filling of the occluded internal carotid artery and prominent meningeal vessels. The large superficial temporal artery (arrows) was subsequently used for a dural synangiosis procedure as an additional source to augment collateral flow. *(F)* Left internal carotid is occluded; "whispery" collaterals are typical for moyamoya disease. *(G)* Lateral view left carotid angiogram shows reconstituted middle cerebral artery with leptomeningeal, dural, and ophthalmic artery collaterals. The patient recovered speech and intellectual function after additional augmentation of collateral flow with a scalp to dura arterial synangiosis procedure.

foramina transversae through which they course rostrally. This may be the result of traumatic dislocation of the cervical spine or encroachment on the vessels by flaring vertebral osteophytes. Generally, vertebrobasilar insufficiency results more often from intracranial vasculopathy as opposed to the extracranial vascular disease of the carotid system. Stenosis of the vertebral or basilar arteries results in hemodynamic insufficiency rather than emboli, and there is less collateral flow beyond the vertebral arteries than in the carotid system.

The etiology can be confirmed by angiography. Symptoms of vertebrobasilar insufficiency are often characterized by transient "dizziness" and/or a loss of consciousness. There may be transient visual loss or dizziness when extending the neck or turning the head. Clinical examination alone fails to localize the vascular pathology. Symptoms of vertebrobasilar insufficiency have multiple causes; stenotic and occlusive lesions have been found at every level of the vertebrobasilar system. To study it adequately, at present, requires four-vessel angiography.

SUBCLAVIAN STEAL

The transience and variability of vertebrobasilar insufficiency is seen in the manifestation of flow changes with subclavian steal syndrome. Here the subclavian or innominate artery is occluded proximal to the origin of the vertebral artery, and the distal subclavian artery is supplied by retrograde flow from the vertebral artery that fills from the contralateral vertebral artery. Vertigo occurs in over one-half of the patients, while about one-third have binocular visual disturbances, paresis of a limb, and/or paresthesias. Ataxia, diplopia, syncope, and monocular visual changes are frequent complaints.[58]

BASILAR ARTERY OCCLUSION

Basilar artery occlusion was described in 1946.[59] Many patients have chronic hypertension. The prognosis is usually grave, and anticoagulant treatment is probably ineffective.[60] Circulatory characteristics of the penetrating branches of the basilar artery are the critical factors determining the severity of the symptoms and outcome of this disease. These are 100 μm or less and arise at right angles from the basilar artery; they are also vulnerable to a reduction in flow, as well as to atherosclerosis at their origin from the basilar artery. Although they are considered end arteries, there are collateral channels between adjacent territories.[61]

Patients usually have a prodrome of vertigo, headache, nausea, hemiparesis, diplopia, dysarthria, and other symptoms in various combinations that clear before the definitive clinical onset, which is often sudden. Patients often deteriorate to a "locked-in" syndrome or to coma, indicating an advanced form of the disease. Noninvasive evoked potentials and transcranial Doppler can assist in early recognition of this disease.

TRAUMATIC EXTRACRANIAL VASCULAR OCCLUSION

Trauma to the head and neck can result in significant injury to the carotid and/or vertebral arteries along their extracranial course. Such injuries may result from blunt or penetrating injuries. The morbidity of neurological deficits from trauma lesions is high, about 52 percent, and mortality is 40 percent.[62]

The carotid artery is most commonly involved proximal to the base of the skull at C2. With proximity to the transverse process of C2, the internal carotid artery is stretched over it by any injury involving hyperextension and rotation of the head and neck. This may result in intimal disruption with platelet aggregation and occlusion or embolization or the development of an intimal flap with dissection and occlusion, rupture and hemorrhage, or development of a pseudoaneurysm with embolism.[63,64] The carotid artery can also be injured by a direct blow or blunt intraoral trauma, or it can be affected in conjunction with a basilar skull fracture. The vertebral arteries in their course through the paravertebral foramina are also subject to stretch or contusion, resulting in dissection, pseudoaneurysm, or occlusion. This may lead to focal ischemic lesions of the cervical spinal cord, brainstem, cerebellum, and/or occipital lobes.

Diagnosing traumatic vascular occlusions before symptoms of cerebral ischemia occur is difficult because the diagnosis is made by angiography, which is rarely performed in head and neck trauma, having been replaced by CT and MRI. One should remain suspicious of such injuries in appropriate cases. Auscultation is a poor screening tool. The presence of Horner's syndrome and focal deficits are prominent clues to diagnosing carotid injury. The initial CT scan is frequently normal. Any trauma patient having focal neurological deficits that cannot be explained from the imaging studies should undergo early cerebral angiography to diagnose carotid artery dissection.[65,66]

☐ TREATMENT OF CEREBRAL ISCHEMIA

Treatment of transient neurological deficits is directed toward providing dependably adequate blood supply to the brain. In most cases, this involves eradicating or bypassing lesions that cause cerebral ischemia. The heart is the most frequent source of cerebral emboli, so an embolic stroke should be considered an indication of heart disease. Cardiac or vascular sources of bland emboli may be treated by antiplatelet factors or anticoagulants. Intensive antibiotic therapy is required for septic cardiovascular disease. Surgical correction of intracardiac masses or valvular lesions may be required. Endarterectomy may be indicated for stenotic lesions or eroded plaques in major arteries supplying the brain.[9–12] Treatment of cerebral ischemia must be categorized into prophylaxis against potential infarction and treatment of the completed infarction.

Symptoms that point to the need for prophylaxis usually relate to episodes of temporary neurological deficits such as TIAs or RINDs. The occurrence of these symptoms is indication enough for determining the cause. Demonstration of a source of emboli should lead to treatment of that source. A cardiac cause of emboli may require anticoagulation, correction of arrhythmias, or repair of valves. Extracranial carotid stenosis becomes hemodynamically significant when the constriction is 80 percent or greater, and it may require surgical reconstruction to remove impedance of flow.

Ulcerated plaques in the cervical carotid artery are a common source of cerebral embolism and may be treated medically by anticoagulant and antiplatelet agents or by surgical endarterectomy. Septic embolism from subacute bacterial endocarditis, pulmonary or other systemic infection, or other sources of septicemia usually requires aggressive parenteral antibiotic therapy for specific organisms.

MEDICAL TREATMENT

A significant advancement in understanding cerebrovascular disease is the recognition and management of risk factors such as hypertension, diabetes, and hyperlipidemia; as well as control of smoking, drug abuse, and obesity. Once the cerebrovascular event occurs, methods of management are determined by the presence and amount of cerebral tissue damage incurred, with the object of limiting or preventing infarction. Directions of treatment are toward the heart, blood, arterial wall, and brain tissue. Treatment of lesions that may be producing symptoms of cerebral ischemia is usually accomplished by the person or team most experienced with the treatment of the particular lesion.

Cardiac sources include arrhythmias, myocardial infarction with global flow deficiency due to low cardiac output, or mural thrombi which produce emboli, valvular obstruction due to stenosis, or endocardiac vegetations, which may produce emboli. Each must be managed individually. Anticoagulation may protect against emboli from a prosthesis of the aortic valve, mitral stenosis, and certain instances of atrial fibrillation.[70] Anticoagulants should be avoided in the face of septic emboli because of the increased risk of hemorrhage. Patients who are subjects of septic emboli are best managed by sensitivity-specific antibiotics.

Blood-clotting characteristics may be the cause of cerebral ischemia, and treatment by anticoagulation is applied cautiously because of the risk of complications from bleeding and intracerebral hemorrhage. Therapeutic anticoagulation requires (1) an accurate diagnosis, (2) physician understanding of anticoagulants, (3) accurate laboratory clotting tests, and (4) no contraindication to treatment.[66,67] Intravenous heparin by continuous infusion is the generally accepted treatment for acute TIAs, major arterial thrombosis without infarction, and emboli of cardiac origin.[71] The activated partial prothrombin time is maintained at two times the control values. However, both retrospective and prospective studies have failed to demonstrate a difference between patients treated with and without heparin.[68,69]

Anticoagulants may be prescribed in specific circumstances to prevent further embolization or propagation of thrombi.[70] Recombinant genetic technology has allowed tissue plasminogen activator (TPA) to be available for clinical use. TPA induces the conversion of plasminogen to active plasmin, the main fibrinolytic enzyme. The TPA binds to the surface of fibrin and enhances the affinity and action of plasminogen, which accelerates the thrombolytic process. Clinical experience in the treatment of cerebrovascular thrombi has been limited, but TPA remains an attractive thrombolytic agent.[71,72] It has a half-life of about 4 min. It is nonimmunogenic and has no hemodynamic effects.

Oral anticoagulants, warfarin compounds, and, specifically sodium warfarin (Coumadin), are used for chronic anticoagulation and are effective in eliminating TIAs.[70] The feared complication of this therapy is intracerebral hemorrhage, which occurs in 4 percent of cases.[24]

Antiplatelet agents have special application in prophylaxis against stroke. Aspirin is the current standard medical treatment for patients who are prone to strokes. Aspirin irreversibly inhibits platelet function by blocking cyclooxygenase and the conversion of AA to prostaglandin endoperoxides and, ultimately, TXA. Taking 325 mg every other day reduces the risk for myocardial infarction, nonfatal stroke, and cardiovascular death by 18 percent, although hemorrhagic strokes may be increased.[73] Dipyridamole, a phosphodiesterase inhibitor, when combined with aspirin was found to reduce stroke risk by 30 percent.[74] Ticlopidine is a new powerful platelet suppressor that inhibits the adenosine diphosphate pathway of the platelet membrane. The dose is 250 mg twice a day, and the effect lasts the lifetime of the platelet. It has been shown to reduce the risk of cerebral ischemia by 21 to 46 percent, but it can cause diarrhea, skin rash, and neutropenia.[75] Platelet suppression is effective in reducing the incidence of stroke.

Systemic supportive measures are directed toward increasing collateral flow by increasing blood pressure and cardiac output. This includes parenteral fluids, lactated Ringer's solution, and plasmanate colloid to increase circulating blood volume. The risk of aggravating cerebral edema and hemorrhage requires close monitoring and balance of fluids and electrolytes. Hyperglycemia is to be avoided because it increases lactic acid concentrations in the regions of cerebral ischemia, aggravating edema and tissue infarction.[22,74] Hemodilution and reduction of hematocrit have been advocated to reduce viscosity and improve rheologic qualities of blood for better capillary flow.[76,80] These measures do not increase oxygen metabolism or change clinical status.[74] Laboratory studies suggest that normovolemic hemodilution avoids the edema associated with hypervolemic hemodilution and reduces the size of infarction.[77] This treatment is precluded by signs, symptoms, or CT evidence of increased intracranial pressure.[80]

There is a general consensus that corticosteroids are of no

benefit in attenuating either the cytotoxic or vasogenic edema of cerebral ischemia.[74]

MANAGEMENT OF STROKE PATIENTS

Generally, management of stroke patients is directed toward minimizing neurological deficits, treating complications, and managing concomitant medical problems. Supplemental O_2 and maintaining the PO_2 at or above 100 torr assures adequate oxygenation. Optimizing circulating blood volume with parenteral fluids (lactated Ringer's Solution) and oncotic agents (6% hetastarch) along with exogenous pressor amines (dopamine) will assist in maintaining adequate cardiac output. This, in turn, is directed toward maintaining cerebral perfusion pressure and cerebral blood flow even in the otherwise normotensive stroke patient. Anticoagulation is rarely indicated for patients who have recently sustained cerebral infarction. Patients having cerebral ischemia without infarction due to intraarterial constriction or emboli may benefit from continuous intravenous heparin while awaiting endarterectomy, and long-term oral anticoagulation may be indicated for chronic cardiac conditions such as atrial fibrillation, as well as for patients with prosthetic heart valves, mitral valvular disease, or atrial fibrillation with mitral valve prolapse. Long-term anticoagulation is rarely recommended for intracranial vascular occlusive disease.

Activated tissue thromboplastin and urokinase are agents under investigation for lysis of acute thrombotic vascular occlusions. They show promise in reestablishing flow in acutely occluded cerebral arteries, and they may reduce or prevent infarction. Hemorrhage into the infarction is the major concern and limiting factor; however, preliminary results with this mode of therapy are encouraging.

Surgical therapy is usually reserved for endarterectomy, arterial ligation or reimplantation, and treatment of complications such as severe intracerebral edema or hemorrhage when there is a danger of herniation and brainstem compression. Expeditious evacuation of a hematoma may be life-saving. Basilar artery occlusion is now potentially treatable with local intraarterial fibrinolytic thrombolysis.[78] Patients who have been in coma for more than 6 h are no longer candidates for this treatment.

The vertebral artery is compromised by local compression or distortion in the neck. This can occur with cervical spine dislocation, spondylotic spurs, or chiropractic manipulation. Treatment is usually directed toward reestablishing cervical alignment or surgically opening the foramina transversae. When vertebrobasilar insufficiency is caused by atheromatous stenosis at the origin of the vertebral arteries, it produces symptoms similar to those of intermittent postural hypotension. This can be treated surgically by bypassing the stenotic lesion with a carotid-vertebral anastomosis.

Treatment of traumatic vascular occlusions is individualized. Most patients can be managed nonoperatively. Usually, heparinization for 3 weeks followed by oral anti-coagulation for 6 months prevents progression. Carotid ligation will prevent embolization from intimal flaps, but ligation will not be tolerated unless cross-filling is adequate.[79] Rarely carotid bypass will prevent disabling stroke.[80] Follow-up angiography frequently demonstrates progressive pseudoaneurysm formation and delayed changes on the contralateral side.[64]

Penetrating injuries of the neck may be associated with severe blood loss. Patients with knife, gunshot, or other penetrating injuries to the cervical vessels are hemodynamically unstable and demand aggressive blood volume replacement with emergency operative exploration. If the injuries are in the midcervical region, they should be surgically explored. If they are above the mandible or below the level of the cricoid tracheal cartilage and the patients are hemodynamically stable, angiography is performed before any surgical procedure in order to plan management.[81]

CAROTID ENDARTERECTOMY

Endarterectomies remove arteriosclerotic plaques commonly developing at the bifurcation of the common carotid artery (see Fig. 14-3). The American Symptomatic Endarterectomy Trial (NASCET) and the European Carotid Surgery Trial (ECST) have concluded that carotid endarterectomy reduces risk of stroke in patients with tight stenosis of the extracranial carotid artery who are symptomatic with symptoms of cerebral ischemia due to the focal stenotic lesion.[81,82] There is still a question regarding patients with tight lesions who are asymptomatic, and study of this situation is ongoing.[83] Long-term follow-up of endarterectomy has shown 10 percent restenosis compared to 26 percent progression of stenotic lesions on the opposite side. The cumulative stroke or ischemic episode probability was 4 percent at 1 month and 8 percent at 5 years, or less than 1 percent after the first month.[84]

Technique of Endarterectomy. The carotid artery is isolated initially by dissection of the distal 3 to 5 cm of the common carotid artery for proximal control. The bifurcation of the common carotid and the proximal 2 to 3 cm of the external and internal carotid arteries are then dissected. The patient is anticoagulated with heparin, 100 U/kg body weight. The common carotid artery is then clamped, followed sequentially by clamping the external and internal carotid arteries. Some surgeons routinely insert a shunt immediately upon opening the artery. Others insert the shunt only in the event that there is evidence of inadequate blood supply to the brain when the vessel is occluded. This may be indicated by altered consciousness when the patient is operated on under local anesthesia, diminished "back-flow" when the distal carotid artery is opened, or, most commonly, focal or hemispheric decline in cortical electrical activity with continuous intraoperative EEG monitoring.

The atherosclerotic plaque is excised by sharp and blunt dissection. Most important to the success of carotid endarterectomy is the fixation of the distal intimal flap to the vessel wall with tacking sutures, preventing elevation of an intimal flap that can be a source of emboli or luminal occlusion. Heparin may be reversed at the termination of the procedure with protamine sulfate; however, it is preferable to allow the anticoagulant effect of heparin to resolve spontaneously, thus impeding immediate postoperative thrombus formation. A review of many series indicates that the fewest complications in carotid endarterectomy occur when operations are performed by the most experienced surgeons. Dissections of intimal flaps along the intraluminal course of the carotid may require permanent ligation to avoid distal embolism. Excision of the involved segment and interposition of a graft to maintain intraluminal flow is an alternative measure when the patient cannot tolerate carotid occlusion.

Patients presenting with symptomatic carotid stenosis often have accompanying occlusive disease of the coronary arteries. Therefore they undergo cardiac evaluation to include a stress test. Some may present with severe coronary occlusive disease requiring a coronary artery bypass graft (CABG). Such patients may have carotid Doppler studies to evaluate risk of stroke occurring during the CABG. Simultaneous carotid endarterectomy with CABG has been performed to avoid a perceived risk of stroke. A retrospective study concludes that carotid stenosis does not increase the risk of stroke during CABG.[85]

CEREBRAL ARTERY BYPASS

Cerebral revascularization procedures were introduced in 1967 to reestablish perfusion of regions of the brain with diminished flow due to proximal arterial obstruction when the obstruction was not directly accessible. Superficial temporal to middle cerebral artery anastomosis (STA-MCA) became a popular bypass procedure. However, in 1985, an international cooperative study concluded that strokes were not prevented by STA-MCA bypass surgery.[14] This led to a virtual shutdown of bypass surgery, but considerable controversy regarding the study's design, method, performance, and conclusions has followed. The study failed to separate any subgroup of patients with symptoms of cerebral ischemia due to demonstrable perfusion deficits but having viable residual tissue in the region of ischemia. Positron emission tomography (PET) offers the capability of determining the presence of ischemic nonfunctional but viable cerebral tissue. The response of such tissues to revascularization is under study. Another question is whether the standard STA-MCA will deliver enough bulk flow to correct a clinically significant perfusion deficit. A conventional STA-MCA bypass delivers initial flows of 25 to 50 ml/min compared to potentially 100 ml/min or more by a larger vein graft bypass.[86] Thus, the study may not have separated the population that might have been benefited by a STA-MCA bypass.

There is risk of acute and delayed cerebral ischemia with carotid ligation: 49 percent after internal carotid and 28 percent after common carotid ligation.[87] Bypass may prevent ischemic stroke in the cerebral distribution of a major artery, giving origin to an unclippable giant aneurysm that requires ligation of the parent artery and distal runoff (trapping the aneurysm).[88,89] It remains the best treatment for moyamoya disease, particularly in adults, along with other measures previously discussed here.[53,90]

A bypass may have a role in limiting the extent of acute stroke. Use of the procedure is limited by the possibility of aggravating edema or the chance of precipitating hemorrhage by increasing flow to infarcted brain tissue that is no longer protected by an intact blood-brain barrier. This results in a "luxury perfusion syndrome."[91] The low flow rates of STA-MCA may be an advantage in this case and offer enough flow to preserve the penumbra.[92] Vertebrobasilar insufficiency with the limited available collateral flow may be best ameliorated by a bypass when medical treatment fails.[93–95] However a bypass using the proximal superior cerebellar artery as the recipient should be considered with caution because of the technical difficulties involved and the risk of complications.[96]

Finally, there may be a small select group of patients with multiple carotid and vertebral occlusions sustained by isolated collateral flow and suffering recurrent TIAs while on medical treatment who would benefit from a bypass.[97] Regional cerebral blood flow has been demonstrated to be improved along with the clinical course in this patient population.[98]

Limitations of STA-MCA bypass are due to inadequate donor arteries and insufficient flow through the small diameter of the anastomosis. Placement of the anastomosis within the sylvian fissure along the proximal middle cerebral artery close to the trifurcation allows for a larger anastomosis and greater flow rates.[99] Alternatively, saphenous vein interposition grafts have been advocated as a solution to these limitations. This eliminates uncertainties by having a donor vessel of a size large enough to bring ample bulk flows to the cerebral tissues immediately after construction of the bypass.[100,101] The drawbacks are that interposition vein grafts are technically demanding and subject to occlusion because of a size discrepancy between vein and recipient artery, as well as kinking or compression along the course of the graft and endothelial reaction within the vein graft.[102] Technical advances to limit these impediments include care in dissecting the vein and limiting distension pressure within the graft while it is harvested.[103,104] These measures are effective in augmenting flow to the brain.

The conclusion of the cerebral artery bypass study is that it has only limited application, although it may have dramatic effects in selected circumstances. Meanwhile, a specific surgical procedure that resulted in 95 percent patency rate after anastomosis has generally been retired for lack of purpose except for selected, relatively rare, indications.

☐ CAROTID OCCLUSION STUDIES

Carotid ligation is a classic operation, but indications for it have changed. Classically, it was used most often to treat otherwise nonoperable aneurysms of the carotid artery. About 30 percent of the population will not tolerate carotid ligation without a stroke because of incompetent collateral flow through the circle of Willis.[105] Clamps such as the Crutchfield and Selverstone were designed to be gradually closed over several days. These theoretically allow collateral flow to develop so that closure of the carotid can be tolerated. Carotid occlusion is performed less often for treatment of aneurysms now because microsurgical techniques and multiple designs and forms of clips allow for direct aneurysm obliteration and parent artery reconstruction. With the advancement of "skull base" surgical techniques and radical resections of tumors located along the intracranial course of the internal carotid artery, the carotid artery may require occlusion for cure or hemostasis. If there is a potential need to occlude the carotid artery, it is first necessary to predetermine the patient's tolerance to carotid occlusion in order to plan for bypass or other procedures.

TEMPORARY BALLOON OCCLUSION

After cerebral angiography, a nondetachable balloon is positioned in the internal carotid artery under local anesthesia. The patient is anticoagulated with heparin, 100 U/kg of body weight. Adequacy of anticoagulation is verified by obtaining serial activated clotting times, which should be twice the control time. The balloon is expanded and occlusion of flow verified angiographically. The patient is examined neurologically throughout the procedure. Additionally, the scalp EEG is monitored and any slowing or change in symmetry of activity is critically observed. A transcranial Doppler is used to observe changes in direction and velocity of flows through the major cerebral arteries. Regional cerebral blood flow studies are performed as additional verification of adequacy of collateral flow. Inhalation xenon gives quantitative volumetric flow rates. Recently, single-photon emission computed tomography (SPECT) using the isotope, ^{99m}Tc-hexamethylpropyleneamine oxime (^{99m}Tc-HMPAO) has given quick and accurate semiquantitative cerebral perfusion rates during balloon occlusion of the carotid artery.[107,108] There has been a 3.7 percent overall complication rate due to this procedure. Asymptomatic carotid dissection was discovered in 2 percent. The rate of permanent neurologic deficit was 0.33 percent. Approximately 9 percent of patients fail the clinical portion of the occlusion test, and they inevitably would have experienced a stroke if the carotid artery had been permanently occluded.[106]

An algorithm is presented that is a synopsis for a clinical approach to evaluation and management of cerebrovascular ischemia (Fig. 14-6).

☐ VENOUS SINUS THROMBOSIS

GENERAL CONSIDERATIONS

Cerebral venous drainage is characterized by ample collaterals so that disorders of cerebral function are uncommon. If superior sagittal sinus occlusion occurs gradually as by neoplastic invasion, many alternate collateral drainage routes including the scalp veins are recruited, thus avoiding cerebral edema and symptoms of elevated intracranial pressure.[109]

Acute thrombosis of the cerebral venous outflow is an uncommon but difficult problem to manage, particularly when complicated by venous infarction, which may be disabling or even life-threatening. Infections and septic phlebitis such as cavernous sinus thrombosis (cavernous sinus syndrome) and lateral sinus thrombosis (otic hydrocephalus)[110] are causes of venous obstruction that can be dramatic. These conditions are uncommon with modern antibiotic treatment of intracranial infection. Other etiologies include hypercoagulable states associated with oral contraceptives, pregnancy, and protein S deficiency.[111] Surgical occlusion by jugular vein resection, depression of a skull fracture so that it protrudes into and occludes a major dural sinus, or surgical transection of a dominant cortical or deep draining vein are other mechanisms resulting in venous congestion and major neurological morbidity. Venous infarction has a greater tendency for hemorrhage than ischemic infarction of arterial occlusion.[112] Surgical management of traumatic injury or neoplastic evolvement is a major challenge requiring considerable skill to avoid an impairment or even fatal outcome. Cortical veins may be incorporated in the dura, forming dural lakes or sinuses before entering the superior sagittal sinus. Cortical veins can be anastomosed or connected by tubes, but veins 2 to 3 mm in diameter should be carefully dissected or avoided.[113]

SYMPTOMS

Headache is a prominent initial symptom of occlusion of a venous sinus. This progresses and seizures supervene. Focal deficits follow, depending on the location. Signs of cavernous sinus occlusion are fever, proptosis, and variable ophthalmoplegia. Papilledema and altered sensorium may be noted as the condition advances.

DIAGNOSIS

Multiple findings of edema and hemorrhage on the unenhanced and contrast-enhanced CT give strong indications to dural sinus thrombosis. The "empty delta" sign on enhanced CT, indicating venous engorgement around a thrombosed superior sagittal sinus, is the most specific finding on CT

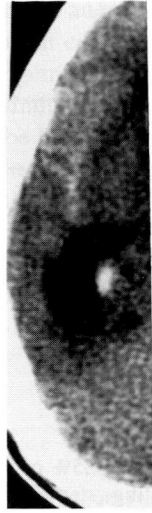

Figure 14–7
hypertension su...
plane CT (A) s...
horns of the lat...

hemisensory ...
cuts suggests ...

DIAGNOSTI...

Diagnostic ev...
around CT sca...
ence of mass e...
will also indic...
cause of hemo...
gression or re...
trast may reve...
other abnorma...
pertension is o...
including plat...
thromboplastin...
mechanism. Pa...
agement probl...
gists and repla...

MRI is less h...
globin, which i...
nent imaged, h...

TREATMEN...
INTRACRAN...

General. T...
rhage deep with...
uation of large...
deeply stuporou...
orrhages may n...
gressive deteric...
caused by fur...

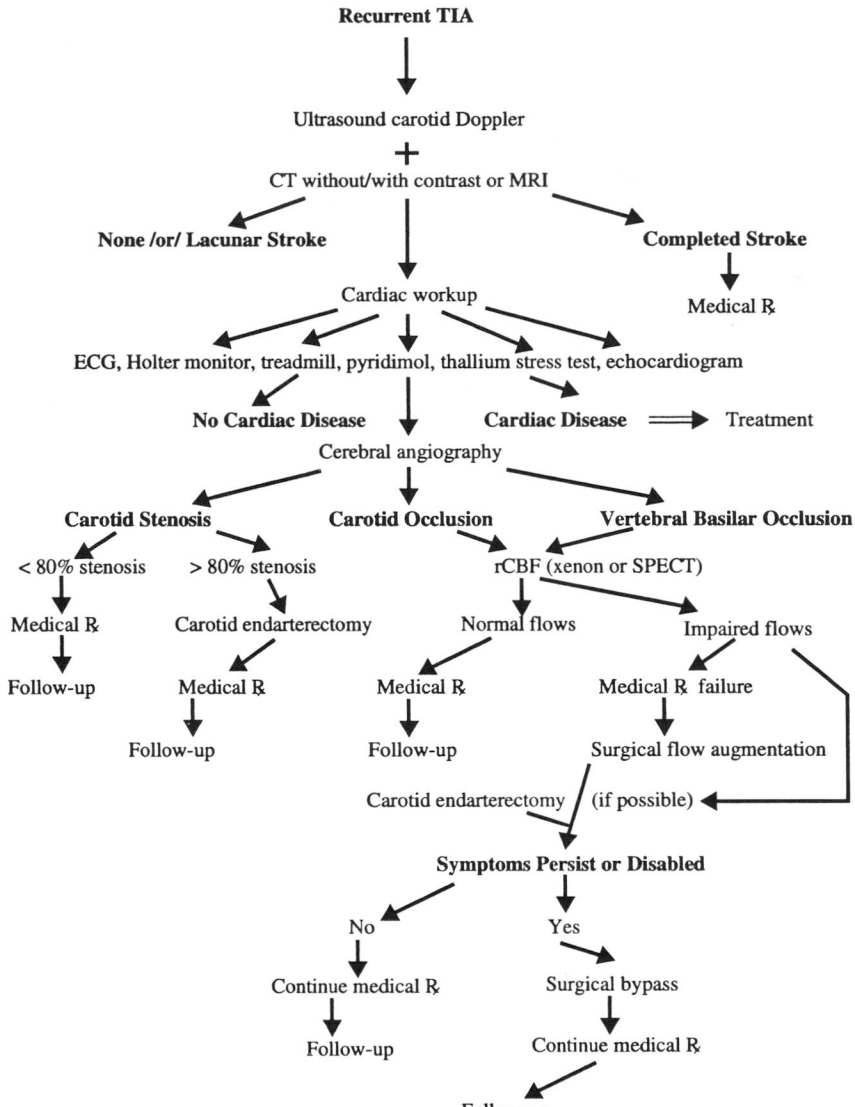

Figure 14–6 This algorithm outlines a clinical approach for the evaluation and management of cerebrovascular ischemic and occlusive disease.

and carries an ominous prognosis.[114] Cerebral angiography, apart from surgery or autopsy, has been the definitive diagnostic procedure for this condition. Digital subtraction arterial angiography is a refinement that nicely demonstrates the venous system.[115] However, MRI angiography using phase-sensitive gradient-echo imaging is an accurate noninvasive method that can measure flow velocities within the dural sinuses, and it may replace contrast injection angiography as the preferred method for evaluating the cerebral venous system.[116]

TREATMENT

General supportive care with parenteral fluids, intensive care monitoring, and systemic anticoagulation with hep-

arin and warfarin are the usual measures of management for patients with acute venous sinus thrombosis. The dilemma is whether anticoagulation will aggravate the hemorrhagic infarction that characteristically accompanies acute sinus occlusion. Aggressive direct intervention by surgical clot removal has met with only limited success. More success in reestablishing venous sinus patency has been reported using direct sinus perfusion of thrombolytic enzymes, i.e., urokinase or streptokinase.[117-120] Activated tissue plasminogen may have some advantage in local treatment of sinus thrombosis, but a definitive conclusion awaits further trials. Many patients recover with supportive measures. It is the patient who continues to decline in spite of these measures and faces a grim prognosis that may be salvaged by local enzymatic manipulation of the sinus.

□ SPO
HEM
STR

INCIDEN

The incide
the brain
strokes fro
cocaine ab
the accura
diagnosis
mate of h
cent.[121]

ETIOLO

Causes of
tion defec
venous thi
frequent c
hypertensi

DISTRIB

The vesse
mal hemo
proximal r
nicating a
(Fig. 14-7
monly inv
intraparen
location o
posterior
Intraparen
in the por
junction o
tions, ven
Midbrain
in other p
tentorial h

Table 1
lar ischem
lesions, a
from Capl

The site
shown in

Degene
ous materi
basal nucl
aging. The
thickening
Thinned re
chard, whi

breakdown of the BBB seen consistently in SAH.[32] Changes in reactivity of the cerebral arteries can be closely correlated with the presence of blood in the subarachnoid space.[33] There is extensive disturbance of permeability in the walls of the major cerebral arteries within the basal cisterns. The most important mechanism for breakdown of the BBB is opening of endothelial tight junctions. SAH appears to activate endothelial pinocytosis, which contributes to the breakdown of the barrier of the arterial wall to blood. The breakdown of the barrier of the major cerebral arteries allows plasma factors to penetrate the arterial walls to produce the thickening that follows the SAH in these arteries.[32] The vessels may be sensitized to the effects of the catecholamines and prostaglandins that concentrate in the CSF following SAH. The contrast enhancement seen on CT patterns associated with delayed vasospasm, which can last for several days, may be explained by these changes in the arterial walls.[34,35] Delayed alterations of vasoreactivity affect autoregulation, particularly when vasospasm in major central arteries is compensated by vasodilatation in the distal vessels. Cerebral perfusion pressures fall to tolerably reduced arterial pressure.[33]

Acutely, there is an alteration of the arterial barrier to blood immediately after SAH, induced by the sudden elevation of ICP, transient systemic hypertension, and blood collecting around the arterial wall.[35] Acute arterial hypertension causes increased permeability of the cerebral capillaries.[36] Such changes occur in the major cerebral arteries as well. Permeation of serum products into the subendothelial layers of the vessel wall occur through the endothelial cells directly rather than through the endothelial cell junctions, as is seen in the delayed phases of alteration of the BBB by SAH.[35] This results in the transient dysautoregulation acutely and may potentiate the vasospasm that occurs later.

Loss of autoregulation and vasoreactivity to CO_2 is called *vasoparalysis.* This occurs in association with SAH. The severity of vasoparalysis is related to the severity of the SAH and the patient's clinical grade.[37] Autoregulation can be restored with hyperventilation and resultant hypocapnia in most cases.[38] The exact mechanism for this is not known, but it is postulated to be related to perivascular acidosis. Vasoparalysis in patients with minimal deficits may lead to delayed ischemic neurologic deficits, even when the aneurysm is clipped before the onset of vasospasm. Lost CO_2 reactivity can be detected intraoperatively using thermal conduction probes.[37]

CARDIAC CHANGES

The heart is affected by central autonomic provocations from the hypothalamus caused by acute SAH, and it may require specific medical attention. Cardiac changes are implicated in sudden unexpected death precipitated by SAH.[39] Electrocardiographic (ECG) changes occur in 50 to 70 percent of patients experiencing SAH.[40] Catecholamines are the predominant mediator of these cardiac events, causing an in-

crease in sympathetic tone. The ECG abnormalities seen more commonly with SAH are: (1) large broad T waves, (2) prolonged QT intervals, (3) pathological Q waves, (4) prominent U waves, (5) various conduction arrhythmias, and even changes compatible with myocardial infarction.[41–44] The ECG changes mimicking myocardial infarction that occur with akinesis of a cardiac wall have been termed *stunned myocardium,* and they may be caused by coronary vasospasm.[44,45] MB isoenzymes may be elevated but not to levels of transmural infarction. There is profound ischemia without death of the cells, causing the involved myocardium to become electrically inert.

Myocardial lesions are seen at autopsy. These consist of subendocardial hemorrhages and other structural changes including subendocardial myocytolytic, myofibrillar, and fuchsinophilic degeneration.[40,44] Endogenous outflow of norepinephrine from SAH is the probable cause of myocardial damage from strain due to systemic hypertension or by direct myocardial toxicity.[40]

NATURAL HISTORY

Aneurysms have been found in up to 8 percent of persons who have died from other causes. Such lesions may be found in 4 to 6 percent of the general population.[46] This figure probably includes many small aneurysms found in older patients with hypertension. Small aneurysms have a low incidence of rupture. Most aneurysms (95 percent) are asymptomatic until they rupture. The clinical behavior and predictability between ruptured and unruptured aneurysms are quite different.[47–49] There are three types of unruptured aneurysms: (1) *incidental,* asymptomatic, and imaged by radiologic procedures for unrelated conditions; (2) *multiple* (most asymptomatic), discovered concurrently in patients who have experienced SAH from rupture of another aneurysm; and (3) *symptomatic, unruptured,* diagnosed for clinical signs or symptoms other than SAH (mass effect, cranial nerve compression, embolism). There are no prospective randomized studies on the behavior of incidental aneurysms, and conclusions are inferred from autopsy studies and clinical behavior of ruptured aneurysms.[2,50] The chances of rupture of an aneurysm less than 5 mm in diameter have been estimated to be less than 2 percent per year, but the figure for those between 6 and 10 mm is higher.[51] Spontaneous thrombosis of ruptured cerebral artery aneurysms can occur without intervention, but this is rare—too infrequent to be anticipated with any confidence.[52]

INCIDENTAL ANEURYSMS

About 5 percent of the population harbors at least one aneurysm, so that about 12 million persons in the United States are at risk of SAH from a ruptured aneurysm. The annual incidence of SAH is 10 per 100,000, so that the annual rate of rupture is about 1 percent. Approximately 20 percent of patients with SAH have multiple aneurysms. These rupture at a rate of 1.5 to 3 percent per year.[48,51] The most predictive factor is aneurysm size. The critical size for rupture is from 4 to 7 mm in diameter. Several factors in addition to the size of the aneurysm play a roll in determining the likelihood of an aneurysm to rupture, including the age of the patient, the location of the aneurysm, the presence of hypertension, previous rupture, and the shape of the lesion. Aneurysms in patients less than 50 years of age most often have ruptured by the time they are first recognized. Aneurysms with secondary lobules are twice as likely to bleed as smooth aneurysms. Chances for repeat hemorrhage from an aneurysm which has previously bled are 3 to 5 percent per year, almost 10 times the chances for hemorrhage from a small aneurysm that has never bled. Generally, operative treatment is recommended for incidental aneurysms 5 mm or more in diameter.[50]

☐ CLINICAL COURSE

GENERAL CONSIDERATIONS

Over 75 percent of symptomatic aneurysms that have not bled are larger than 10 mm in diameter. Headache is a common symptom. Localization of the headache is of little value, although periorbital pain is common. Aneurysms of the internal carotid artery are most likely to present localizing signs which, in addition to headache, may include evidences of oculomotor involvement (Fig. 15-1). Lesions on the internal carotid artery at the posterior communicating artery junction are most likely to produce oculomotor paresis, although diplopia may be produced by lesions at the anterior choroidal or at the bifurcation of the carotid. Aneurysms at the origin of the ophthalmic artery are likely to produce headache and orbital pain as well as impairment of vision due to involvement of the optic nerve.

Hemorrhage from aneurysms along the internal carotid artery may extend into adjacent brain, producing contralateral hemiparesis. Hemorrhage from anterior communicating arteries may cause spasm of the anterior cerebral arteries, producing weakness of the lower extremities, or extension of the hemorrhage into the cerebral hemisphere may result in hemiparesis on the side contralateral to the one into which the hemorrhage has extended. The side of intracerebral hemorrhage depends on the direction in which the aneurysm is pointing (Fig. 15-2). Disruption of frontal lobe connections to the thalamus can result in changes in mental status or cause cognitive and memory deficits that may persist. Hemorrhage from an aneurysm of the middle cerebral artery may extend into the adjacent hemisphere, producing signs of pressure and hemiparesis.

Clinical suspicion of intracranial aneurysms is aroused by the symptoms caused by the three events that occur: (1) *aneurysmal enlargement:* localized headache, cranial

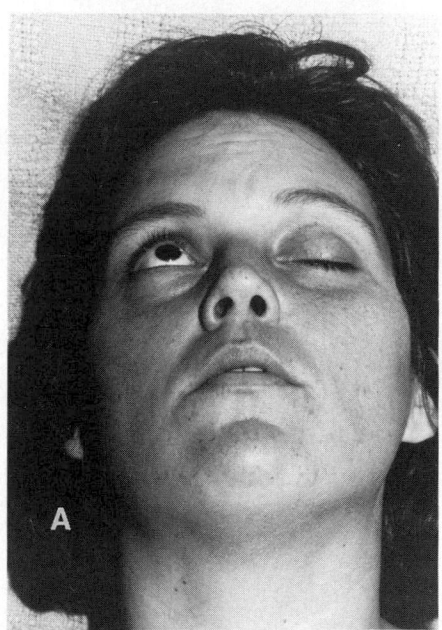

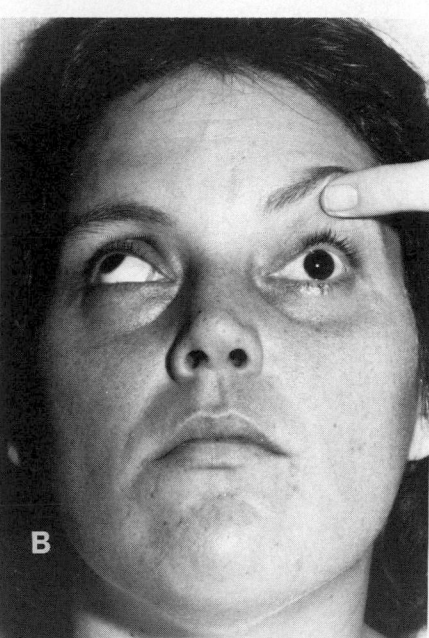

Figure 15-1 A 32-year-old woman 5 days after acute headache, vomiting, and stiff neck. Her left eye closed 24 h after onset of symptoms (*A*). Left oculomotor nerve palsy is evident with paralysis of upward gaze, the pupil was 5 mm and not reactive to light (*B*). Her neurological examination was otherwise normal. Cerebral angiography verified an aneurysm arising from the left internal carotid artery at the origin of the posterior communicating artery.

nerve palsy, and visual defects; (2) *warning leak:* sudden severe headache, nausea, back pain; and (3) *ischemia:* transient cerebral ischemic attack and focal neurological findings.[53,54] Certainly, symptoms of photophobia and signs of meningeal irritation and stiff neck are important clues to the diagnosis of SAH, but they may not appear until 4 to 8 h

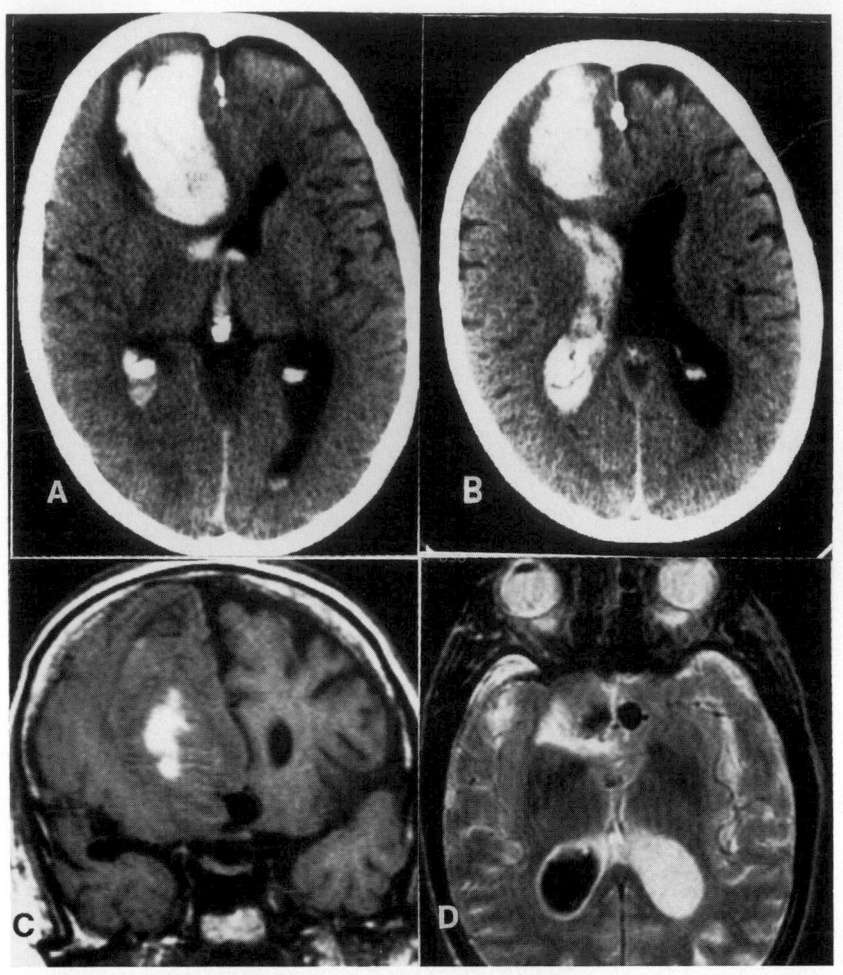

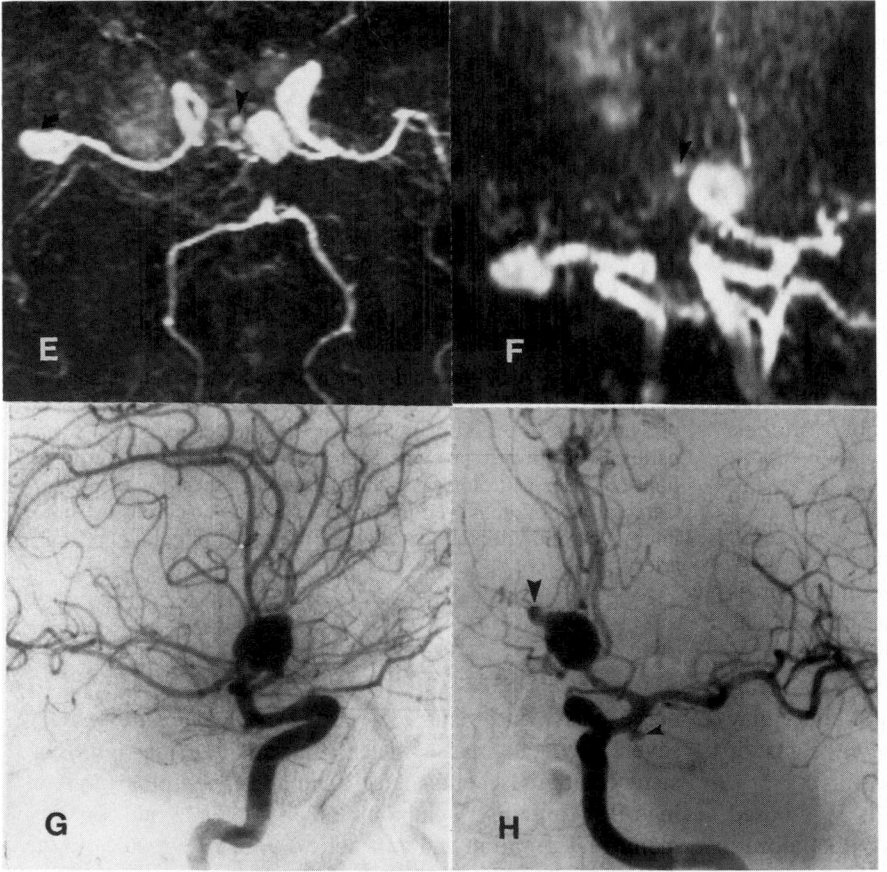

Figure 15-2 A 48-year-old man with massive hemorrhage from a large anterior communicating aneurysm; he was clinically grade 3. CT shows a large hematoma in the right frontal lobe with fresh blood in the third ventricle (*A*). Higher cut CT shows subependymal extension of hemorrhage along the right lateral ventricle (*B*). MRI coronal cut shows flow void in the aneurysm at the base of the interhemispheric fissure and mass effect with shift of the right frontal lobe (*C*). T2 MRI horizontal cut shows aneurysm and hematoma in the right lateral ventricle (*D*). MR angiogram axial view shows aneurysm and expanded rupture point (*arrowhead*) and incidental right middle cerebral aneurysm (*curved arrow*) (*E*). Same study coronal view (*F*). Left carotid angiogram lateral view shows anterior communicating artery aneurysm, filling exclusively from the left internal carotid artery (*G*). Left carotid angiogram coronal view shows aneurysm and rupture point (*large arrowhead*) and another small incidental anterior choroidal artery aneurysm (*small arrowhead*) (*H*). Compare with *F* for resolution and detail of similar view.

after hemorrhage. The initial presentation can be missed. Signs and symptoms of these events are misinterpreted as tension headache, migraine, or "the flu."[54,55]

CLINICAL PICTURE OF SUBARACHNOID HEMORRHAGE

The classical clinical picture of a person having an SAH is the sudden onset of a severe headache that is incomparable to any previously experienced, followed by nausea and vomiting. Loss of consciousness for a variable period of time may occur, but consciousness may not be affected. If coma occurs, it usually develops soon after aneurysm rupture.[56] The acute form of headache is often described as "getting hit in the head by a hammer." The headache may occur while straining at stool, during coitus, or during some other form of physical stress. The headache may awaken the patient from sleep as well, so that physical stress is not necessary to precipitate a hemorrhage. The headache is often generalized but may be localized behind an eye, usually associated with rupture of an aneurysm on an ipsilateral carotid artery, or the headache may be bifrontal, often associated with hemorrhage from an aneurysm of the anterior communicating or an anterior cerebral artery. Pain from hemorrhage of an aneurysm in the posterior fossa may be referred to the back of the neck, but none of these sites of referred pain is dependable for the localization of the site of hemorrhage. The headache is often unremitting, lasting for several days to a week or more. Nausea may last for a few hours.

WARNING LEAK

A careful history taken at the time of SAH may reveal the occurrence of an earlier episode, a headache occurring 10 days to 2 weeks prior to the SAH. Sentinel headaches are premonitory signs of an impending catastrophic SAH. These warning symptoms are more common in women and can occur in 60 to 70 percent of cases.[54] They may be due to stretching the fibers within the aneurysmal wall or limited bleeding from the aneurysm.[57,58] Sentinel headaches are recognized as unusual in the patient's experience, and they are warning of an impending major hemorrhage when recognized for what they are. The median time between a minor leak and major rupture is 14 days, and the interval ranges from 1 day to 4 months.[59] These early presentations are frequently atypical so that the diagnosis is often missed and the gravity of the ultimate outcome is not appreciated[55,60] (Table 15-1).

PHYSICAL FINDINGS

When hemorrhages remain subarachnoid, there may be no localizing signs. The most common localizing sign is that of a third nerve palsy, usually involving the pupillary constric-tory fibers most prominently. This is most often caused by direct compression from an aneurysm at the junction of the internal carotid and posterior communicating arteries, but the third nerve can also be compressed by aneurysms of the cavernous and supracavernous carotid artery. Other localizing signs are likely to result from intracerebral extension of hemorrhage from an anterior communicating artery aneurysm into the frontal lobe or from a hemorrhage from an aneurysm of the middle cerebral artery within the sylvian fissure. Intracerebral extensions of SAH can also result from vascular malformations or from aneurysms of inflammatory origin.

Meningismus is a common feature of SAH in alert patients. In addition to stiff neck, the stretch signs of Brudzinski and Kernig may appear a few hours after hemorrhage. There may be mild elevation of temperature along with photophobia. Increased intracranial pressure can cause traction along the course of a sixth cranial nerve with loss of abduction of an eye—a sign that bears little relationship to the site of the aneurysm.

Ophthalmological findings are reported in over one-third of patients with ruptured intracranial aneurysms. These can include abnormalities of visual fields, blurred vision, hemorrhage along the sheath of the optic nerve, and intraocular hemorrhage. Terson's syndrome or extension of subhyaloid hemorrhage into the vitreous is associated with loss of visual acuity.[61,62] Hemorrhage into the vitreous usually clears spontaneously.

DIAGNOSTIC EVALUATION

Evaluation of a patient suspected of having an SAH includes CT followed by angiography. MRI may add significant information but currently is not considered a routine part of the evaluation. CT, performed soon after an SAH, can reveal blood in the subarachnoid space, often locally concentrated at the site of the bleed (Fig. 15-3). The CT also detects hematomas, brain shifts, and early hydrocephalus following aneurysm rupture. When intravenous contrast media is injected just prior to the CT, the aneurysm may be identified (Fig. 15-4). Thus when there are multiple aneurysms, CT may be of great help in identifying the one which has hemorrhaged. CT will also demonstrate a hematoma within the parenchyma, and when performed with contrast material, it can image a vascular malformation.[63] Usually the CT is performed first without contrast material. This is followed by a tomogram made after the injection of contrast material, which will outline vascular defects when compared to the image made without contrast.

Limited hemorrhages and hemorrhages that have occurred 2 to 3 days or more prior to CT may not be apparent. Lumbar puncture may be helpful by demonstrating blood cells in the CSF in the early period after hemorrhage, and xanthochromia may still be present after the hemoglobin has broken down.[64]

The amount of blood imaged in the subarachnoid space by

Table 15-1
HEMORRHAGIC VASCULAR LESIONS

	Subarachnoid	Intracerebral
Risk factors	Often none, hypertension, bleeding disorders, drugs, trauma, cigarette smoking, alcohol abuse, anticoagulants	Hypertension, bleeding disorders, drugs, trauma
Onset	Sudden, often during exertion, "worst headache of my life"	Gradually progressive during minutes or hours, occasional onset with exertion or stress
Anatomic characteristics	Subarachnoid (no major focal neurologic signs), occasionally meningocerebral, photophobia, nuchal rigidity	Deep brain structures, basal ganglia, cerebral white matter, thalamus, pons, cerebellum
Accompanying signs	Headache, vomiting, transient interruption in activity or loss of consciousness	When large, headache, vomiting decreased level of consciousness, seizures
Imaging: CT or MRI	Location: In subarachnoid space CT: hyperdensity (white) MRI: on T1-weighted images lesion is black; on T2-weighted images, lesion is white	Location: Within brain, often spreading to surfaces and/or ventricles CT: focal hyperdensity (white) MRI: acute hematomas are black on T1-weighted images; chronic hematomas are white on T1- and T2-weighted images

the initial CT has predictive value with respect to the development of vasospasm, infarction, and functional outcome (Table 15-2).[65] Most grading systems are subjective but can be modified for interobserver agreement and accuracy.[66]

Group 3 shows almost 100 percent incidence of severe vasospasm.

MRI can detect acute blood in CSF and may be more sensitive than CT in all phases of SAH. It can detect early hydrocephalus as well as small infarcts.[66,67] The greatest disadvantage to MRI is the long time required for imaging, which results in movement artifacts in the acutely ill patient.

Angiography outlines specific lesions that produce SAH. While an aneurysm may be identified on a CT and MRI, the size, configuration, relationship to its parent vessels, and the presence or absence of a neck are best demonstrated by angiography (see Fig. 15-2). Angiography may be digitalized, but the best images are obtained from subtraction of films made by direct exposure. In alert patients, these are usually performed as soon after hemorrhage as is practical. The complication rate from angiography is less when performed within 3 days of the ictus.[68]

Angiography will demonstrate an etiology for the SAH in

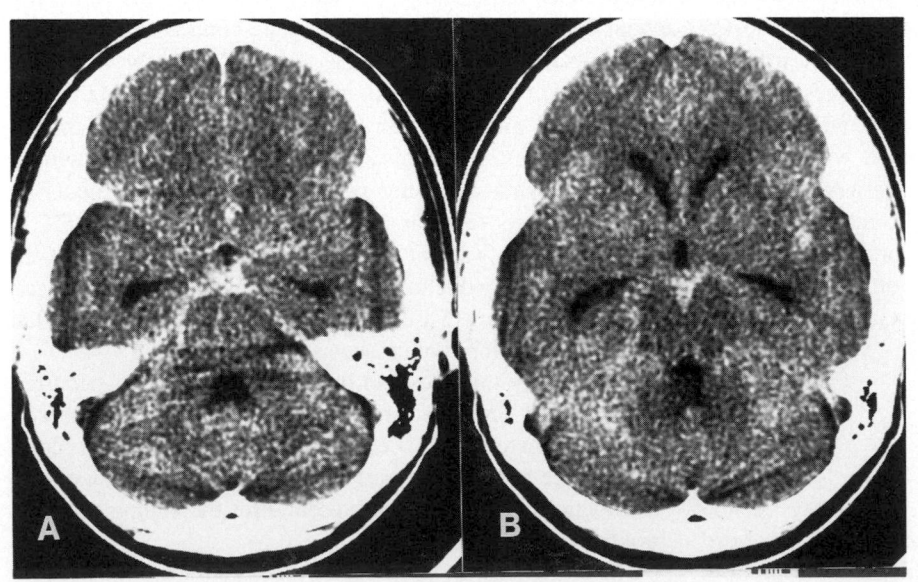

Figure 15-3 A 30-year-old woman with history of hypertension had an acute severe headache, nausea, and vomiting; there was no loss of consciousness or neurological deficit. CT at pons, without contrast enhancement, shows fresh blood in the prepontine cistern with apparently more volume of blood in the right parapontine cistern (*A*). Same study at mesencephalic level shows blood in the interpeduncular fossa and right ambient cistern (*B*). Angiography confirmed a 7 × 6 × 6 mm aneurysm on the left internal carotid–ophthalmic artery junction. These demonstrate appearance of SAH on CT and lack of correlation of blood and site of hemorrhage as demonstrated on CT.

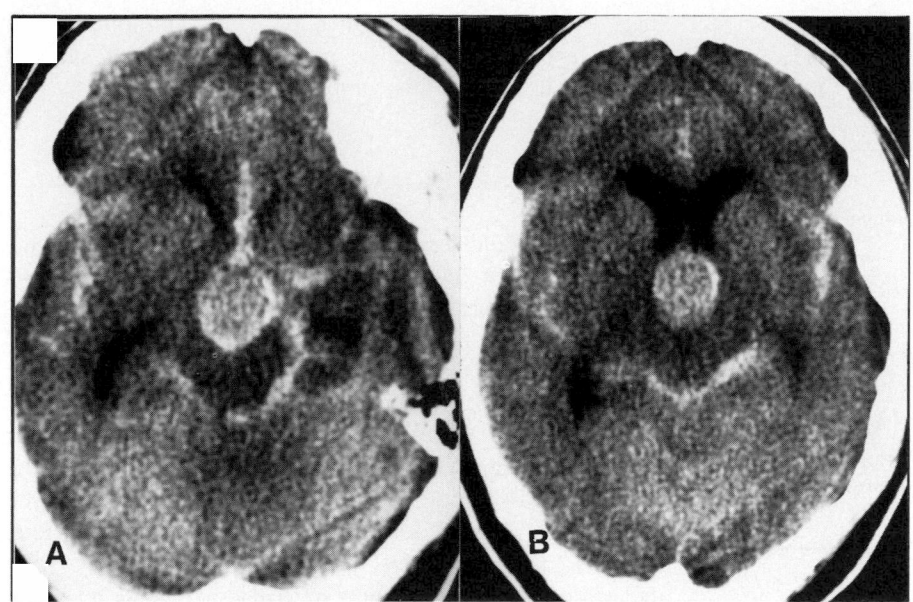

Figure 15-4 A 32-year-old obese woman with acute onset of severe headache followed shortly by loss of responsiveness. Upon arrival she was grade 4. Unenhanced CT shows fresh blood in the cisterns (*A*). Shows a large aneurysm of the basilar artery bifurcation, with atheroma plaque in the wall (*B*). The patient failed to recover and expired within 24 h on supportive nonoperative care.

about 80 percent of patients. Current methods of selective retrograde arterial catheterization, subtraction fluoroscopy, digitized images, magnification, and nonionic contrast media have greatly improved the safety and diagnostic accuracy of cerebral angiography.[69] Since SAH may result from malformations in the spinal canal, consideration should be given to myelography in the event that no intracranial lesion is found.

The cause of SAH may not be found on the initial arteriogram. Rarely a delayed angiogram after spasm has subsided may demonstrate an aneurysm.[70] In about 20 percent of patients presenting with SAH, no vascular lesion is found despite repeated angiography and myelography. Such patients are usually treated as though they have not had SAH. The rate of rebleeding in such patients is relatively low.[71]

Some patients with SAH develop hydrocephalus.[72] A subgroup of these have acute hemorrhagic necrosis of a pituitary adenoma. The sella should be studied with high-resolution thin-cut CT and pituitary hormonal studies to detect evidence of pituitary apoplexy presenting as SAH that might have otherwise been missed.[73]

CLINICAL GRADING

The ultimate clinical outcome for intracranial aneurysms is closely related to the neurological status of the patient prior to treatment. Grading systems have been developed to determine the feasibility of surgical treatment on an intracranial aneurysm at any given time. The first of these was developed by Botterell and his colleagues in 1956.[74] This was then modified by Hunt and Hess in 1968 (Table 15-3).[75] Hunt's system has proved to be most popular through the years although there are other modifications.[75,76] A review of the application of grading systems has demonstrated considerable variation, most being in the assignment of grade III in the Hunt and Hess scale.

A further revision and clarification of the classification was provided by Nibbelink et al. in 1977, and acceptance of this classification might reduce the confusion (Table 15-4).[3]

The advantage of these scales is that they indicate the presence of deficits which may compromise the immediate outcome of surgery and give some indication of the long-term neurological status of survivors. Some deficits are transient and some are permanent. Transient deficits may be

Table 15-2
Blood Predictive Value on CT

Group 1	No subarachnoid blood
Group 2	Diffuse subarachnoid blood with no clots
Group 3	Clotted or thick-layered blood
Group 4	Diffuse SAH with cerebral or ventricular blood[65]

Table 15-3
CLASSIFICATION OF STATUS FOLLOWING SUBARACHNOID HEMORRHAGE ACCORDING TO HUNT AND HESS[75]

Grade 1	Asymptomatic or minimal headache and slight nuchal rigidity
Grade 2	Moderate to severe headache, nuchal rigidity, no neurological deficit other than cranial nerve palsy
Grade 3	Drowsiness, confusion, or mild focal deficit
Grade 4	Stupor, moderate to severe hemiparesis, possible early decerebrate rigidity, and vegetative disturbances
Grade 5	Deep coma, decerebrate rigidity, moribund appearance

Table 15-4
DEFINITION OF NEUROLOGICAL CONDITION ACCORDING TO NIBBELINK[3]

Grade 1	Symptom-free
Grade 2	Minor symptoms (headache, meningeal irritation, diplopia)
Grade 3	Major neurological deficit but fully responsive
Grade 4	Impaired state of alertness but capable of protective or other adaptive responses to noxious stimuli
Grade 5	Poorly responsive but stable vital signs
Grade 6	No response to address or shaking, nonadaptive response to noxious stimuli, and progressive instability of vital signs.

due to vasospasm or intracranial hypertension, both of which are associated with a poor outcome. While intracranial hypertension and vasospasm frequently occur simultaneously, their treatment may require different approaches. If the intracranial hypertension is due to hydrocephalus, it may require shunting. The level of consciousness is a good indication of the success of treatment of both these entities, so that as the patient's state of consciousness improves, he or she may become a better candidate for surgery.

☐ COMPLICATIONS OF SUBARACHNOID HEMORRHAGE

RECURRENT HEMORRHAGE

The most dreaded complication of aneurysmal SAH is rebleeding because of the devastating morbidity and mortality. Recurrent hemorrhage is suspected when there is a sudden deterioration in the patient's neurological condition. This is verified by noting an increase in fresh hemorrhage on CT or increased blood content in the CSF on lumbar puncture. The mortality from recurrent hemorrhage may be as high as 80 percent.[77,78] Peak interval for recurrence is reportedly within the first 24 h with the rate at 4.1 percent.[79] Reportedly, the cumulative rebleeding rate at 14 days can be 20 percent. The rate in patients treated with antifibrinolytics is reduced by 50 percent.[78,79] The cooperative study suggested a peak incidence for recurrent hemorrhage at the end of the first week.[4] A later peak of 2 percent on the ninth day has been noted.[77,78] Patients with good clinical grades tend to have fewer repeat hemorrhages whereas those with poorer grades are at greater risk.[78] These statistics have important bearing on treatment strategy, particularly in the timing of surgical therapy. Repeat hemorrhage within the first hours after the initial hemorrhage implies that surgical therapy should be accomplished as an emergency, which is often logistically difficult.[79] Clinical evidence indicates that recurrent hemor-

rhage is a catastrophic complication with high mortality and overall poor prognosis. The primary objective of surgical therapy is to combat this complication.

CEREBRAL ARTERIAL VASOSPASM

Vasospasm would seem to have a protective effect on recurrent hemorrhage, but it appears to worsen the prognosis because of cerebral ischemia and infarction. Vasospasm is the most common cause of postoperative morbidity and mortality in patients with ruptured intracranial aneurysms. Vasospasm is defined variously as: (1) narrowing of one or more of the major cerebral arteries in the basal cisterns due to muscular contractions or morphological changes in the arterial wall in response to injury of the vessel, (2) delayed onset of neurological deficit after SAH because of ischemia, or (3) a combination of these.[80] The cause is not fully understood and most attempts to treat it have failed, at least clinically. Large amounts of blood clot within the cisterns, and contrast enhancement of the cisterns evidenced by CT are predictors of vasospasm.[34,66] Transcranial Doppler determination of increasing flow velocities in the major cerebral arteries is indicative of vasospasm. Antifibrinolytic agents, epsilon-aminocaproic acid, and tranexamic acid tend to aggravate vasospasm.[81–83]

The cerebral blood vessels have no vasovasorum but have an adventitial rete vasorum in continuity with the CSF and are permeable to large proteins.[84] The vessels are nourished by this adventitial system, perhaps in preference to the endovascular route. The adventitial stomas of this rete vasorum appear to be mechanically blocked by blood clots and debris from SAH. In spite of this, the arterial walls become permeable through the various layers to the endothelial layer when in contact with blood from SAH.[85] This suggests that disruption of the arterial wall barrier to blood allows access of spasmogenic factors from SAH into the arterial muscular layer.

The severity of cerebral vasospasm depends on the volume of blood released into the subarachnoid space and the time the blood is released. The arteries are sensitized by SAH so that spasm is enhanced by recurrent hemorrhage even of small volumes.[86] Spasm begins on the third day and becomes maximal around the seventh day. It tends to resolve around the fourteenth day but may persist several weeks. Spasm is resistant to any pharmacological maneuvers to reverse it. Arterial narrowing is primarily due to contraction within the media that produces longitudinal convolutions of the intima. There are degenerative changes in all layers of the arterial wall that may indicate temporary resistance to reversal.[87] The intimal thickening and medial rigidity and damage may be the result of intense prolonged smooth muscle contraction of the arterial media.[88]

Cerebral vasospasm results from release of spasmogenic compounds from subarachnoid clot. Oxyhemoglobin (OxyHb) is an important mediator when it is released from red blood cells (RBC). The other products of hemolysis, methemoglobin (MetHb) and bilirubin, are not vasoreactive. Thus when OxyHb is oxidized to MetHb, it is no longer spasmogenic. There may be cycling of MetHb back to OxyHb through the action of other RBC products such as MetHb reductase that converts the ferric iron of MetHb to ferrous iron of OxyHb.[89] Vasospasm is probably produced by prolonged release of OxyHb from hemolysis of RBCs of the SAH along with other factors such as superoxide free radicals, eicosanoids, perivascular denervation, release of endothelin, and perhaps other factors from RBCs, endothelium, and platelets.[89–93]

Reversal of vasospasm by medications has failed. Measures to prevent vasospasm before it develops show more promise. The calcium channel blocker specific for cerebral vasculature, nimodipine, has been partially effective when administered systemically but not when applied intrathecally.[94] Direct clearing of blood from the subarachnoid space using plasminogen fibrinolytics has shown dramatic effects, experimentally.[95] Direct application of papaverine intraoperatively may be of benefit as well.

The current treatment for chronic vasospasm appears to be reduction of the viscosity of blood and increasing the systemic blood pressure, both maneuvers contraindicated in patients harboring intracranial aneurysms that have recently hemorrhaged. Since these maneuvers can only be applied after aneurysms have been obliterated, the need for treatment of vasospasm has led to a more aggressive approach to the treatment of intracranial aneurysms. Another maneuver that has recently been recommended is the use of angioplasty.[96]

Measurement of cerebral flow velocities by transcranial Doppler offers an invaluable noninvasive method for monitoring vasospasm and determining when it is present before it is evident clinically so that measures which minimize cerebral ischemia can be initiated.[97,98]

INTRAVENTRICULAR HEMORRHAGE

Extension of intracranial hemorrhage from a ruptured aneurysm into the ventricular system can occur from lesions on the internal carotid, anterior cerebral, and vertebrobasilar arteries (see Fig. 15-2). This phenomenon is commonly associated with intracerebral, subarachnoid, and/or subdural hematomas (over 50 percent). Patients with such lesions are usually grade III or worse and the outcome is poor, with 75 percent being disabled or dead.[99]

The ventriculocranial ratio (VCR) is a helpful guide in gauging associated hydrocephalus. The VCR, as determined by CT, measures the frontal horns between the caudate nuclei and the brain width at the inner table.[100,101] The size of the intraventricular clot is of no prognostic significance, but patients whose ventricles are filled with blood tend to do poorly.[99,101] The VCR is a sensitive indicator of outcome. There are no survivors with a ratio greater than 0.25.[99] External ventricular drainage (EVD) should be considered as the initial management, and the ventricular dilatation may require conversion of the EVD to a permanent shunt for management of persistent hydrocephalus.

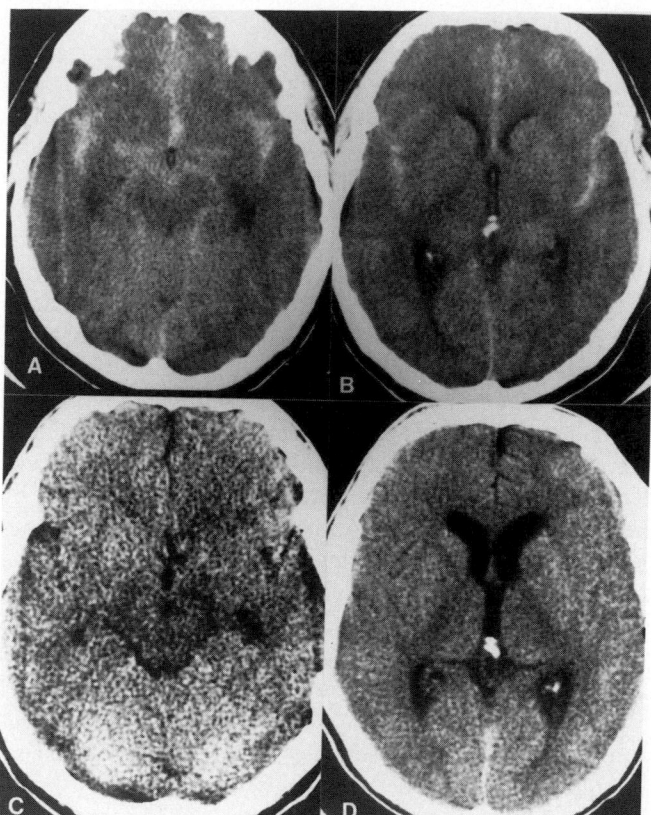

Figure 15-5 A 52-year-old man with acute SAH and clinical grade 3 from rupture of an anterior communicating artery aneurysm. Noncontrast CT on admission, Sept. 2, shows fresh blood filling the basal cisterns (*A*). The same study at the level of the third ventricle shows fresh blood in the sylvian fissures (*B*). Noncontrast CT on Sept. 25 at comparable sections shows ventricular enlargement (*C*). The patient's clinical grade deteriorated to grade 4. A study of Sept. 25 shows diffuse dilatation of the ventricles (*D*). This temporary hydrocephalus cleared spontaneously without shunt. The patient's clinical status cleared slowly as the ventricular size slowly resolved toward normal.

HYDROCEPHALUS

Dilatation of the ventricles within hours to a few days after SAH is common and responsible for unexpected decline in mental status or occurrence of seizures, agitation, and pyramidal signs that may be reversed by drainage of CSF.[102,103] Acute hydrocephalus following SAH is probably due to blood collecting within the basal cisterns or the exit foramina of the fourth ventricle and mechanically obstructing outflow of CSF. There is a direct relationship between the amount of blood in the CSF and the development of hydrocephalus.[104] Hydrocephalus is a common complication of SAH and closely linked to vasospasm since both sequelae are caused by blood in the basal cisterns and CSF pathways.[105] Some have noted hydrocephalus occurring when blood was intraventricular.[106] Obstruction of the CSF pathways is one of the factors leading to neurological decline in the early period after hemorrhage.[104] It is diagnosed by CT. The earliest and most consistent CT finding is ballooning of the frontal horns of the lateral ventricles followed by generalized ventricular enlargement[107] (Fig. 15-5). These changes may be subtle, and they are often overlooked. Recognizing symptomatic hydrocephalus is important, because the neurological decline can be arrested or even reversed by controlling ICP with early EVD placement.[103,104,106] A ventricular drainage tube allows for intermittent drainage of CSF to control ICP as well as a means of monitoring ICP. Observation of the amplitude of pulsation of the ventricular fluids infers intracranial compliance. One can calculate the pressure-volume index. The pressure-volume index is determined by challenging the CSF compartment with a volume change and recording the amplitude and time course of ICP change. It is a measure of cerebral elastance and intracranial compliance.[108,109] Most patients can be effectively treated by temporary external drainage and will not require a permanent shunt. This has generally not been complicated by precipitating recurrent hemorrhage.[107] However, a recent report has directly linked a relationship of ventricular drainage to aneurysmal rebleed.[110] The risk of recurrent hemorrhage in patients undergoing ventricular drainage is suspected to result from a rise in transmural pressure gradient and increased stress on the fibrin patch at the sealed rupture site.

Chronic hydrocephalus following SAH is usually communicating because of obstruction of the arachnoid villi. There is evidence that blood accumulates in these structures shortly after the SAH and that the blood is subsequently replaced by fibrosis. Clinical evidences include ataxia, urinary incontinence, and intellectual deterioration.

Ventriculostomy should be considered for acute hydrocephalus, and shunting may be necessary to treat chronic hydrocephalus. In the presence of an unclipped aneurysm, the use of ventriculostomy must be considered cautiously by balancing the risk of recurrent hemorrhage with the clinical improvement expected by reducing ICP by ventricular drainage. Since the etiologies of acute and chronic hydrocephalus following SAH are probably different, the occurrence of acute hydrocephalus does not necessarily imply that the hydrocephalus will be permanent, and thus a permanent shunt may not be required. Commercial EVD systems allow for precise control of the fluid pressure, which may reduce the risk of recurrent hemorrhage by maintaining intraventricular pressures between 15 and 20 torr.

☐ MEDICAL THERAPY OF SUBARACHNOID HEMORRHAGE

The objective of treatment is to prevent recurrent hemorrhage and combat the effects of SAH as well as to preserve neurological function by maintaining adequate cerebral blood flow. Therapeutic measures vary according to clinical grade.

INITIAL MANAGEMENT

Patients with SAH of all grades are maintained at rest in a quiet room, preferably in an intensive care environment

Table 15-5
LINES OF ACCESS
(POOR GRADE PATIENTS)

1. Indwelling Foley catheter for hourly urine output
2. Intraarterial catheter (radial artery) for continuous blood pressure monitoring and blood analysis sampling
3. Peripheral venous catheter for fluid infusion
4. Nasogastric tube to vent gastric secretion
5. Nasojejunal tube for intestinal alimentation
6. Central venous catheter for central venous pressure (CVP) monitor is placed in good grade patients
7. Swan-Ganz catheter in pulmonary artery for monitoring pulmonary wedge pressures (PWP) and verifying cardiac output or cardiac index (CI) in poor grade patients
8. Nasotracheal intubation and ventilator assistance for pulmonary support
9. Intracranial pressure monitor: subdural bolt or preferably an intraventricular catheter for more direct ICP control; due to risk of rebleed keep ICP above 15 torr, if aneurysm is unprotected

where physiological parameters of heart rate, electrocardiogram, blood pressure, respiratory rate, and intracranial pressure are readily monitored. Frequent observation of cognitive responsiveness by skilled nursing staff is required for all patients with SAH.

The position is that of comfort, usually with the head up at 30°. Visitors are limited to immediate family. Blood pressure and cardiac output are regulated to maintain normal cerebral perfusion pressure (CPP). Antihypertensive medications may be needed if CPP exceeds 80 torr. Headache and neck stiffness can be relieved with codeine (30 to 60 mg) or a nonsteroidal anti-inflammatory drug (NSAID) such as ketorolac tromethamine (30–60 mg), either of which can be given orally or by intramuscular injection. Morphine SO_4 (2 mg) or meperidine (25–50 mg) by intravenous injection every 2 h is an effective alternative and can be reversed by naloxone HCL if depression of sensorium warrants. Lines of access are listed in Table 15-5. Laboratory investigations are listed in Table 15-6.

PULMONARY MANAGEMENT

Supplemental oxygen by mask or nasal prong is given to the somnolent patient. The airway must be maintained for the comatose patient, usually by tracheal intubation. For long-term airway control tracheostomy may be required. Humidified air and intermittent positive pressure treatments may be helpful. Frequent blood gas analysis assists in detecting atelectasis, pneumonia, pulmonary embolism, and acidosis or alkalosis.

GASTROINTESTINAL MANAGEMENT

Patients in neurological grades 1 or 2 can take clear liquids orally. Phenothiazines such as promethazine HCl, 25 to 50 mg,

Table 15-6
LABORATORY STUDIES TO BE OBTAINED

1. Hemoglobin, hematocrit, white blood count, and differential
2. Sedimentation rate
3. Partial thromboplastin time and prothrombin time
4. Blood urea nitrogen (BUN) and creatinine
5. Fasting blood sugar
6. Serum sodium, potassium, carbon dioxide, chloride, magnesium
7. Cholesterol, glycerides, uric acid
8. Stools for occult blood
9. Urinalysis for sugar, protein, specific gravity, and microscopic exam for cells and casts
10. CT of head and chest x-ray on admission
11. Electrocardiogram (12-lead) with rhythm strip if indicated
12. Total cerebral angiography with magnification and subtraction techniques within 24 h of admission

are effective in relieving nausea. Intravenous fluids may be necessary if nausea is persistent to maintain fluid balance and optimal cardiac output. Fluid and general nutritional intake can be facilitated with continuous infusion through a nasogastrojejunal feeding tube in patients who are stuporous. Feeding tubes specifically designed for jejunal placement can be positioned within a few hours so that alimentary nutrition can be readily established to combat the catabolic state that potentiates complications of infection and nutritional depletion that otherwise occur in the poorly responsive patient. Exertions such as straining at stool should be avoided with stool softeners such as docusate sodium 200 mg and laxatives such as Milk of Magnesia (30 ml) and bisacodyl (10 mg). A bedside commode requires less straining than a bed pan and is preferred for patients who are able to get out of bed.

CARDIOVASCULAR MANAGEMENT

A fluid intake of at least 1500 to 2500 cc per day is necessary to maintain hydration, circulating blood volume, and improved rheological qualities of blood for capillary flow unless there is evidence of inappropriate antidiuretic hormone secretion. The use of antihypertensive medications in patients who have sustained SAH requires analytical considerations. While reduction of intravascular pressure reduces the stress placed on an aneurysm, maintenance of cerebral perfusion is critical. In an alert patient, the state of consciousness may be used as a guide to the level of cerebral perfusion. Hypotensive medications may be administered up to a level that the patient begins to experience drowsiness. Short-term reduction of hypertension can be achieved with a calcium channel blocker such as nifedipine, 10 to 20 mg, sublingually. Intravenous medications, such as nitroglycerine or sodium nitroprusside, by continuously titrated infusion are usually reserved for patients whose blood pressures cannot be controlled by more moderate means.

PROPHYLAXIS AGAINST RECURRENT HEMORRHAGE

Inhibition of clot lysis with agents that interfere with activation of plasminogen has been advocated for the prevention of recurrent hemorrhage. Epsilon-aminocaproic acid (EACA), 1.5 g hourly, or tranexamic acid (tranaminoethylcyclohexane carboxylic acid, AMCA), 6 g daily, have been shown effective in reducing the incidence of aneurysmal rebleed.[111,112] However, these agents are not effective in preventing hemorrhage in the first 3 days after SAH, which is the period of highest recurrence rate.[113,114] There is reduced clearance of blood from the CSF and increased incidence of cerebral ischemia due to enhanced intravascular sludging and fibrin emboli, causing microthrombosis with use of these agents.[115,116] Antifibrinolytics have *little* role in the management of aneurysmal SAH.[117,118] The most effective means of preventing hemorrhage from aneurysms is early surgical occlusion of the aneurysm.[114]

PROPHYLAXIS AGAINST VASOSPASM

Calcium Channel Blockers Cells communicate with their environment through receptors or channels on the cell membrane. Ion channels control intracellular ion concentrations.[119] Calcium ions (Ca^{2+}) are required for smooth muscle contraction. Agents blocking Ca^{2+} cause relaxation of smooth muscle of the vascular wall resulting in vasodilatation. Calcium channel blockers have been shown to produce vasodilatation of cerebral arteries. Nimodipine (60 mg every 4 h) is known to have specific action on cerebral vasculature.[120,121] It has been advocated for prophylaxis against delayed cerebral ischemia from vasospasm.[120] Nimodipine has reduced mortality without increasing cerebral perfusion pressure (CBF), suggesting a protective effect apart from vasodilatation.[122] It has a significant effect in reducing delayed ischemia in patients undergoing early surgical clipping.[123] There is no uniform agreement on the effectiveness of nimodipine.[124] Treatment is effective only when initiated early after SAH. It has no effect on reversing chronic vasospasm once that has started. Treatment is continued with therapeutic drug levels maintained through the period of highest risk, the first 21 days. Patients on beta blockers should be treated with caution, using nimodipine so as to avoid facilitated cardiac conduction blockade and aggravation of cardiac arrhythmias.[124,125]

SURGICAL REMOVAL OF SUBARACHNOID CLOTS

Early operation (within 48 h of SAH) with evacuation of cisternal blood clots surrounding major arteries has been advocated to reduce or prevent vasospasm.[126] Technically, it is difficult to mechanically remove clots extensively from the subarachnoid spaces. The bifrontal interhemispheric approach offers better access to clot removal than does the pterional approach. It has been concluded that clot removal may ameliorate vasospasm, although the overall effect does not seem significant.[127]

ACTIVATED TISSUE PLASMINOGEN SUBARACHNOID THROMBOLYSIS

Experimental use of intracisternal recombinant tissue plasminogen activator (rt-PA) has resulted in dramatic clearing of blood from the subarachnoid space and significant amelioration of vasospasm.[128,129] Limited clinical experience suggests that rt-PA can be safely instilled into the cisterns, and it can effectively clear blood from the CSF and thereby prevent vasospasm.[130] This seems promising, but further clinical investigation is required before intracisternal rt-PA can be established as being effective in the prevention of stroke due to the vasospasm of SAH.

PROPHYLAXIS AGAINST SEIZURES

A loading dose of phenytoin sodium, 1 g or 15 mg/kg by slow intravenous infusion followed by 300 mg daily maintenance, is usually adequate for prevention of seizures. The infusion rate should not exceed 50 mg/min to avoid cardiac arrhythmia. Regular blood levels are monitored and the dosage altered to maintain a therapeutic range of 10 to 20 μg/ml. If there is adverse reaction to phenytoin, carbamazepine or phenobarbital can be substituted.

PROPHYLAXIS AGAINST THROMBOEMBOLISM

Thigh-length elastic stockings supplemented with sequential pneumatic hose are indicated in poor-grade patients. We are reluctant to use subcutaneous heparin or any drug that may potentiate hemorrhage in patients with SAH.

PROPHYLAXIS AGAINST SKIN BREAKDOWN

An "egg crate" sponge or an air mattress helps to redistribute concentration of pressure and focal myodermal ischemia that leads to decubitus ulcers. In some cases the rotokinetic bed facilitates skin care as well as mobilization of pulmonary secretions.

BLOOD, FLUIDS, AND ELECTROLYTES

There is controversy over the effectiveness of hypervolemic versus normovolemic hemodilution to balance oxygen carrying capacity and reduce rheologic shear forces, improving capillary flow.[131,132] It is clear that negative fluid balance must be avoided. Hypovolemia and fluid restriction are associated with cerebral ischemia and infarction in patients with SAH and are particularly hazardous when vasospasm is present.[133,134] Hypovolemia (reduced red cell mass and plasma volume) in SAH is common and insidious. It has many causes: dehydration, catabolism, reduced erythropoiesis, iatrogenic blood loss, supine diuresis, natriuresis, and neuroendocrine disturbances.[133,135,136] Higher-grade patients with CT findings compatible with high ICP (midline shift or hydrocephalus) are hypovolemic. The hypovolemia is induced by increased sympathetic activity leading to a reduced vascular capacitance.[136] Such hypovolemia is more common in women and is often not evident in results of routine clinical blood studies. Hyponatremia occurring with SAH is more likely due to natriuresis or "cerebral salt wasting" than abnormal antidiuretic hormone function.[137] Vigorous, active fluid maintenance including correction of sodium loss that occurs from central autonomic responses to SAH is the primary focus of fluid balance therapy.[133,138] All patients with ruptured aneurysms should be given adequate fluid loads to prevent hypovolemia.

Requirements must be individualized. Crystalloid, generally lactated Ringer's solution, or 5% dextrose in normal saline along with 5% human plasma protein fraction at a 3:1 ratio is given in volumes of 150 to 200 cc/h. Colloid in the form of plasma, albumin, or hetastarch along with blood transfusion is an important supplement, expanding plasma volume and keeping fluids within the intravascular compartment.[139] Dextran is not used as an oncotic agent because of induced coagulopathy noted with this agent.[140] Volumes of infused fluids are adjusted to hourly urine outputs, serum electrolytes at 6 hourly intervals, central venous or pulmonary wedge pressures (PWPs), and daily weights. Bolus volumes of 250 to 500 ml are given if neurologic decline is noted under conditions of normal or low PWPs.[141] The normal PWP range is 10 to 12 torr and gives a reasonable approximation of intravascular volume.

Reduction of hematocrit to 33 to 35 percent can improve rheologic characteristics of cerebral capillary flow and may be helpful. Reduction of hematocrit must not be at the expense of circulating blood volume.[132] Red cell mass is replaced with a packed RBC transfusion if the hematocrit falls to or below 28 percent.

The use of hypervolemia and suppression of diuresis with vasopressin, 5 units by intramuscular injection, along with induced hypertension and vagal blockade has been advocated, particularly in the face of established vasospasm.[140,142] This has an inherent risk of recurrent hemorrhage if the aneurysm is not clipped and there are significant cardiopulmonary complications of hemothorax, pulmonary edema, and myocardial infarction. Nevertheless, such measures can overcome cerebrovascular resistance of vasospasm to elevate CPP and reverse regional ischemia in order to prevent cerebral infarction. Usually replenishing circulating blood volume to normal parameters as reflected by PWP is sufficient to improve CPP. Occasionally dopamine HCl titrated by continuous infusion is needed to maintain adequate CPP above 50 torr.

☐ SURGICAL MANAGEMENT OF INTRACRANIAL ANEURYSM

CAROTID ARTERY OCCLUSION

Ligation of a carotid artery for treatment of an intracranial aneurysm was applied by Horsley over a hundred years ago.[143] The rationale for the procedure is reduction of intravascular pressure on the aneurysm. Occlusion of the common carotid artery (CCA) may result in reversal of flow in the internal carotid artery.[144]

Occlusion of the CCA is an effective treatment for unclippable aneurysms of the internal carotid artery such as giants or those located in the cavernous sinus.[145] Follow-up studies have demonstrated that some aneurysms reduce in size or even disappear from angiographic studies after such therapy.[146] Ligation of the internal carotid artery (ICA) accomplishes the above objectives more efficiently than ligation of the CCA. However, it also carries a risk of cerebral ischemia and absence of recurrent hemorrhage is not assured.[146,147] The use of adjustable clamps for gradual occlusion of the carotid artery has been an accepted technique, the assumption being that slow occlusion allows more time for collateral circulation to increase. Two such systems are in common use.[146] To apply the clamps, the carotid artery is exposed. A clamp is applied about 2 cm below the bifurcation of the CCA. After applying the screwdriver, the clamp is closed, under local anesthesia. The closure is reversed by three to four turns of the screwdriver and the system left in place. The clamp is ultimately closed by gradual turns of the screwdriver over three or four days. This system continues to be used for selected patients with aneurysms of the internal carotid artery.[148]

TRIAL INTERNAL CAROTID OCCLUSION STUDY

Formal tests of carotid occlusion while the patient is alert under local anesthesia, using temporary retrograde femoral ICA balloon occlusion, are performed when CCA ligation is planned. With this test, the patient's clinical response is supplemented by monitoring with EEG, transcranial Doppler ultrasound, and isotope regional cerebral blood flow measurements (either SPECT or inhalation xenon). Occlusion is tolerated by 70 percent of the population with the help of collateral flow. With evidence that the patient tolerates occlusion of the CCA, the artery can be ligated and even transected without the incremental clamping. If the patient fails to tolerate the test by exhibiting a transient focal deficit, an extracranial-intracranial bypass procedure is performed to augment collateral flow so that carotid occlusion can be tolerated.[149]

With the advent of microsurgical techniques by which normal anatomy may be restored with minimal neurological deficits, carotid ligation has been virtually abandoned except for lesions inside the cavernous sinus, broad-based or giant aneurysms on the internal carotid artery, or, rarely, aneurysms beneath the anterior clinoid.[145]

ANEURYSMAL CLIPPING

Surgical clipping or wrapping a cerebral artery aneurysm is the most effective means of preventing rupture and SAH. Timing of surgery has changed from delaying 2 weeks to proceeding within 72 h. This has been prompted by the discovery that aneurysms tend to have recurrent hemorrhage early within the first few days rather than later. If the patient is diagnosed within the first 24 to 48 h and graded 2 or less or has a mass hematoma, urgent surgery is performed.[150–154] For higher grades in the Hunt-Hess classification, surgery is delayed until the patient improves. Grade 3 patients will frequently be operated on early. Some authors advocate that higher-grade patients be operated on early, suggesting that overall outcome for this group might be improved by such measures.[155]

Surgery is usually accomplished under general anesthesia with the patient lying supine on the operating table, the head turned away from the operator. The anesthesiologist must have good access to the airway, urinary catheter, and CSF drainage if that has been instituted. The patient should be comfortable on the table with the head slightly elevated, and there must be no obstruction to venous flow. Mild hypothermia may be used to reduce the chances of neurological deficits if temporary occlusion of intracranial vessels is required. Steroids may be administered prior to surgery, and a hyperosmolar solution or a diuretic is administered about time the incision is begun.

Some aneurysms do not have necks. On occasion, it is possible to clip the fundus of such a lesion. At other times it may be necessary to wrap the aneurysm and parent artery with muslin gauze. Plastic coating has been recommended by some surgeons, but none of the plastics has been approved for routine application. All appear to have some toxic effects on tissue.

Alternative forms of management have included implantation of sclerosing materials and, more recently, navigation of wire coils or balloons into the aneurysms, thereby obliterating them.[156] Advances in interventional radiology are bringing promise and success in managing nonoperative lesions using intravascular manipulations.

Once the lesion has been adequately treated, postoperative care is directed toward minimizing complications such as hematomas, cerebral vasospasm, pneumonia, and thrombophlebitis. Progressive ambulation and respiratory assistance play a role in minimizing the chances of pulmonary complications. Treatment of vasospasm is best accomplished by reducing the viscosity of the blood, by increased fluid intake or by use of plasma expanders and by maintaining a normal to slightly elevated blood pressure, while continuing adequate cerebral perfusion. Use of thromboembolic stockings or intermittent pneumatic sleeve compression of the calves may reduce the incidence for pulmonary embolism.

MICROSCOPE

Stereoscopic magnification and coaxial lighting during surgery provided by a surgical microscope reduce the mortality and morbidity previously attendant in surgery for cerebral aneurysms. The precision of experienced surgical hand movements and control are limited by the surgeon's vision. The microscope essentially brings the eye closer to the surgical field.[157]

A counterbalanced support stand that is maneuverable in an infinite number of spacial planes and can be locked by electromagnetic switches is preferred. Binocular eye pieces are 12.5× and the objective lens with a focal length of 300 mm allows good magnification at a reasonable working distance. Individual preferences may include other choices.

ANEURYSM CLIPS

Temporary Clips Development of the clips with a low closing force for temporary arterial occlusion allows deflation of the aneurysm and diminished flow limited only to the region of supply from the occluded parent artery.[158] Collateral flow is potentially available to irrigate the area of brain supplied by the occluded vessel. This is preferable to systemic hypotension that provides reduced flow to the entire CNS. Normotension or induced hypertension can be maintained while the temporary clip is in place to maximize flow to the cerebral tissue supplied by the occluded artery. Temporary occlusion of a major cerebral artery risks immediate ischemia and infarction due to reduced flow. This is time-related; occlusion exceeding 20 min has been found to result in infarction.[159] Repeated clip application is more frequently associated with a permanent deficit.[160] Temporary clips also risk segmental vascular injury because of pressure disruption of the arterial wall, particularly the intima. This could lead to platelet and fibrin emboli or delayed vascular occlusion and stroke. Generally, temporary occlusion using the clips with minimum pressure is well tolerated. Temporary clips are applied whenever feasible to soften the aneurysm during dissection of the neck. Aspiration and collapse of the aneurysm sac is another maneuver that can facilitate manipulation of the aneurysm under the influence of a temporarily occluded parent artery.[161]

Permanent Clips Permanent clips of nonmartensitic steel alloy have high closing pressures that are measured.[162] Clips of martensitic alloys are ferromagnetic and can fracture from corrosion; use of these should be avoided.[163] Aneurysm clips are manufactured in multiple sizes from "mini" to large with multiple shapes and configurations. Fenestrated clips allow for encircling an artery, another clip, or the aneurysm.[164] The Sundt "graft clip" can be used to close a rent in a cerebral artery while maintaining flow. Clip appliers are designed for specific clips by the manufacturer allowing not only application of the clip but also removal. The jaws of the applier are of the same metal as the clip, so as to avoid transfer of a different metal type to the clip.[165] It

is preferable that the surgeon have a multiple array of clips available, so that the exigencies of each patient can be individually met. There are "booster" clips that clamp the tips and add force to the closing of the original clip (Fig. 15-6). This may be necessary when clips are applied over an atheroma in the aneurysm wall.[166] Most current clips are nonferromagnetic and MRI compatible, but this should be individually checked.[163,167–169]

PTERIONAL CRANIOTOMY (PREFERRED APPROACH FOR TREATMENT OF ANEURYSMS)

All aneurysms of the circle of Willis and upper basilar artery can be approached through a "frontolateral, sphenoidal craniotomy" or the pterional approach promoted by Yasargil.[157,170,171] Its advantages are: (1) maximal surface exposure, (2) expendable wide bone removal from the cranial base, (3) wide arachnoid and basal cistern dissection, and (4) minimal brain retraction. The patient lies supine, with the head elevated, turned 45° away, extended 15°, and secured in a three-pin head rest. The incision is behind and parallel to the hairline, extending from midline to the zygoma just anterior to the tragus so as to avoid the ascending frontotemporal branch of the facial nerve and the superficial temporal artery. The scalp flap is reflected with periosteum, which is separated from the superior temporal line, forward and retracted with sutures tensed by rubber bands. The temporal fascia which is separated into an outer layer attached to the lateral zygoma surface of the temporal bone and a deeper layer attached to the medial zygomatic border is opened and split close to the frontozygomatic process. The outer fascial layer is reflected forward toward the orbit and forms a sleeve to protect the nerve to the frontalis muscle.[172] The inner fascial layer is reflected along with the bulk of the temporalis muscle inferior-posteriorly toward the ear and is retracted with sutures tensed with rubber bands. An alternative is to reflect the temporalis muscle forward.[173] This exposes the bony surface of the lateral orbital ridge and temporal fossa.

The first and most important burr hole is drilled just behind the zygomatic process of the frontal bone so that cosmesis is protected by preserving the orbital and superior temporal bony ridges. This exposes the dura along the floor of the anterior fossa. Three to four additional burr holes are drilled along the circumference of the exposure frontally and temporally to raise a free bone flap and expose the anterior and middle fossae separated by the lesser wing of the sphenoid bone as it merges laterally with the greater wing at the pterion. The lesser wing of the sphenoid is removed with rongeurs after careful epidural dissection, until the dural reflection of the superior orbital fissure is exposed. The middle meningeal artery is coagulated with a bipolar cautery and transected. Bone removal of the lateral sphenoid wing and orbital plate gives access to the sylvian fissure and basal cisterns with minimal retraction of the frontal lobe and temporal pole. The dura is opened in a "semilunar" fashion to span the sylvian region from frontal to temporal base and

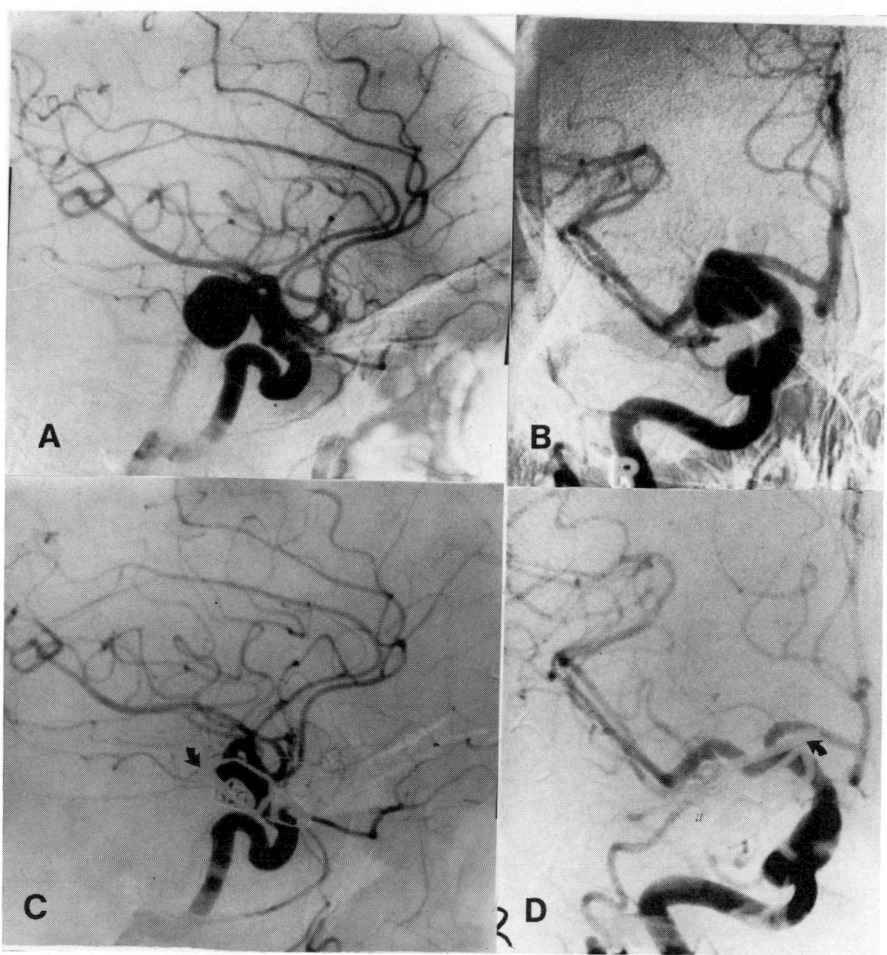

Figure 15-6 A 69-year-old man with progressively severe headache. Essential hypertension had been medically controlled for many years. Neurologically, the patient was intact. An MR scan of the head revealed a large flow void, which prompted a cerebral angiogram. A right carotid angiogram (lateral view) shows a giant aneurysm projecting posteriorly from the internal carotid artery bifurcation (*A*). Right carotid angiogram, anterior-posterior view (AP), shows the aneurysm to involve the proximal M1 segment also (*B*). (The aneurysm was surgically clipped via a pterional approach. Temporary clips on ICA, A1, and M1 trapped and collapsed the aneurysm so that a 15-mm McFadden clip could be positioned on the aneurysm neck. An atheroma in the wall prevented closure of the clip jaws. Closure of the clip was achieved with a Sundt booster clip positioned on the jawtips of the McFadden clip). Postoperative angiogram (lateral view) shows no filling of the aneurysm and booster clip on jaws of McFadden clip (*arrow*) (*C*). The same study (AP view) shows reconstitution of ICA bifurcation and booster clip on tips of the McFadden clip (*arrow*) (*D*).

sutured to the exposed temporalis muscle. Retraction is accomplished with a self-retaining cable system that is attached to the pin head holder. Retractor blades are bent and cables adjusted to lay flat so as to project a low and unencumbered surface profile. The microscope enclosed in a sterile cover is brought into the field.

The frontal lobe is gently lifted from the orbital plate until the optic nerve is seen. The ipsilateral optic nerve identifies the chiasmatic cistern medially and carotid cistern laterally. The arachnoid enclosing these cisterns is opened by sharp dissection to release CSF and ease retraction. Fine-tip adjustable suction is used to evacuate CSF and gently displace fine vessels and arachnoidal trabeculae. The cistern furthest from the aneurysm is dissected first to gain exposure and avoid disturbing the aneurysm prematurely. Sharp dissection with knife or scissors is safer and less traumatic than bluntly tearing the arachnoidal attachments. Lifting the arachnoid with a micro-hook and cutting with a no. 11 pointed knife blade works well. The internal carotid artery (ICA) is isolated at the dural base just lateral to the optic nerve so that it can be controlled with a temporary clip, if necessary. Control of the ICA should be the first strategic maneuver. This may require dissecting dura of the anterior clinoid process and gradually drilling the clinoid away to expose the rostral fibrous ring of the carotid. Sometimes this dura must be

opened to gain access to the anterior superior compartment of the cavernous sinus (CVS). The membrane of Liliequist (arachnoid sheet from mammillary bodies to posterior clinoids) is opened sharply to release CSF and gain access to the interpeduncular and prepontine cisterns en route to the basilar artery.

When dissecting the carotid cistern, the small arteriolar feeders supplying the optic nerve and chiasm should be preserved. The ophthalmic artery arises from the anterior carotid wall and is ventral to the optic nerve and often not in view. The posterior communicating artery (PCA) is seen coursing posterolaterally from the lateral carotid wall close to the tentorial edge. The oculomotor cranial nerve (CN III) is seen lateral to PCA as it enters the superior lateral wall of the CVS. Multiple arterial perforating branches course rostrally from the PCA. It is not necessary to disturb these unless approaching the basilar artery. Aneurysms arising at the ICA-PCA junction are most common (60 percent).[174] They may locally compromise the third nerve. The aneurysms usually project posterolaterally. The neck is dissected circumferentially and must be separated from the take off of the PCA and the anterior choroidal artery. When a microdissecting instrument can be passed between the aneurysmal neck and adjacent branches, the neck can be clipped without disturbing the fundus or dome. The anterior choroidal artery

(AChA) arises from the ICA just rostral to the PCA. It is protected as dissection of the ICA is continued rostrally. Retractor blades are readjusted to distract the opened cisterns and expose the rostral ICA at its bifurcation. The arachnoidal shelf at the medial sylvian fissure is opened sharply, facilitating a view of the proximal anterior cerebral (A1) and proximal middle cerebral arteries (M1).

Dividing the arachnoid overlying the A1 and M1 arteries opens the sylvian fissure. Multiple perforating branches supplying the basal ganglia and internal capsule arise along the posterior-superior walls of A1 and M1. They must be preserved by sharp dissection.

Aneurysms arising from the ICA at the takeoff of the AChA or bifurcation are visualized. Sharp or semisharp clearing of arachnoid and adventitial adhesions defines the aneurysmal neck. Retractors are adjusted to retract the lateral frontal lobe. The olfactory tract is preserved. The temporal pole may require retraction also. The sylvian veins can be freed and retracted. If these veins are not freed, traction may tear them as they enter their dural sinus at the sphenoid wing. The ICA bifurcation should be viewed. Carotid bifurcation aneurysms must be freed from perforating arterioles before they can be clipped. The dome projects into the anterior perforated substance and, thus, may be adherent to the perforators supplying this region. They can be freed at the level of the neck without disturbing the fundus of the aneurysmal sac. The neck can be gently cauterized so that it will accept a clip without kinking the origin of A1 and M1 (Fig. 15-6).

Dissection is continued laterally from the ICA bifurcation along M1 toward the limbus of the sylvian fissure. Progressive dissection laterally leads to the main branching of the M1 segment to the frontal and temporal lobes from M2, the site of origin of most middle cerebral aneurysms. Middle cerebral aneurysms may be large and complex. The necks of these aneurysms may be broad and incorporate takeoffs of the main branches. Atheromatous plaques within the aneurysm wall may prevent effective closure or cause slippage of the clip jaws. The clip must be effectively closed without embarrassing flow in the M2 arteries.

From the ICA bifurcation medially, dissection is carried along A1 to the anterior communicating artery (ACA) and the junction of A1 and A2. Anatomic variations of the A1 and the ACA are common, including hypoplasia of A1 and duplications of ACA. The optic chiasm and lamina terminalis of the third ventricle are met along the way. As the ACA is approached, the recurrent artery of Heubner is visualized. The contralateral A1 is seen coursing over the contralateral optic nerve and chiasm. With both A2 arteries dissected, flow to aneurysms of the ACA can be controlled. Multiple small perforators are seen from the distal A1s and ACA. They are preserved while isolating the A1, ACA, and A2 segments. This is accomplished *before* attempting to dissect an ACA aneurysm. Aneurysms arising from the ACA arise on the side of the dominant A1 and project toward the contralateral side. The neck must be separated from the adjacent vessels. Temporary clips on both A1s will facilitate

dissection and soften the aneurysm for safer application of the clip. The anatomy of the aneurysm neck must be determined, and both A2s must be freed before attempting to clip the aneurysm. The fundus is freed so that the entire aneurysm can be folded to inspect the back wall.

INTRAOPERATIVE CONTROL OF BRAIN BULK

Brain bulk is initially reduced with an intravenous infusion of mannitol, 0.5 to 1.5 g/kg and furosemide (10 to 30 mg). Hyperventilation to a PCO_2 of 28 torr is also helpful, but PCO_2's below 28 torr are avoided to maintain adequate cerebral blood flow.

Central venous pressure is maintained at about 3 cmH_2O. If these measures are not successful in providing adequate intracranial space, intravenous sodium pentothal with doses that induce burst suppression on the electroencephalographic monitor (EEG) should provide further space. Once the basal cisterns are reached, CSF can be released to complete the process of decompression so that exposure of the internal carotid can be achieved and the treatment of aneurysms accomplished. Lumbar CSF drainage is rarely required to achieve adequate surgical conditions—even with surgery during the first 3 days after hemorrhage.

LESION EXPOSURE

Sharp, wide dissection of the natural anatomical planes of the sulci, fissures, and cisterns allows retraction of overlying brain to expose the aneurysm. Anatomical landmarks such as dural reflections, major arachnoidal planes, cranial nerves, and arterial trunks provide appropriate orientation. Limited resection of brain tissue may produce less injury to normal overlying brain tissue than retraction for treatment of aneurysms in selected locations.[175]

MIDDLE CEREBRAL BIFURCATION

For aneurysms of the middle cerebral artery bifurcation, an alternative to proximal exposure of the ICA and M1, described earlier, is direct exposure of the sylvian fissure. Resection of the superior temporal gyrus gives access to the trunks of M2 and subsequently M1 without disturbing the aneurysmal sac. An aneurysm must be dissected so that it can be rotated to visualize the complex arrangement of branches adjacent to the aneurysm, which is common in this location. This approach is not applicable for aneurysms where the M1 is short or aneurysms are located in the proximal sylvian fissure.[176]

ANTERIOR COMMUNICATING ARTERY

The pterional approach allows adequate exposure of aneurysms of the ACA in most instances. Resection of the gyrus

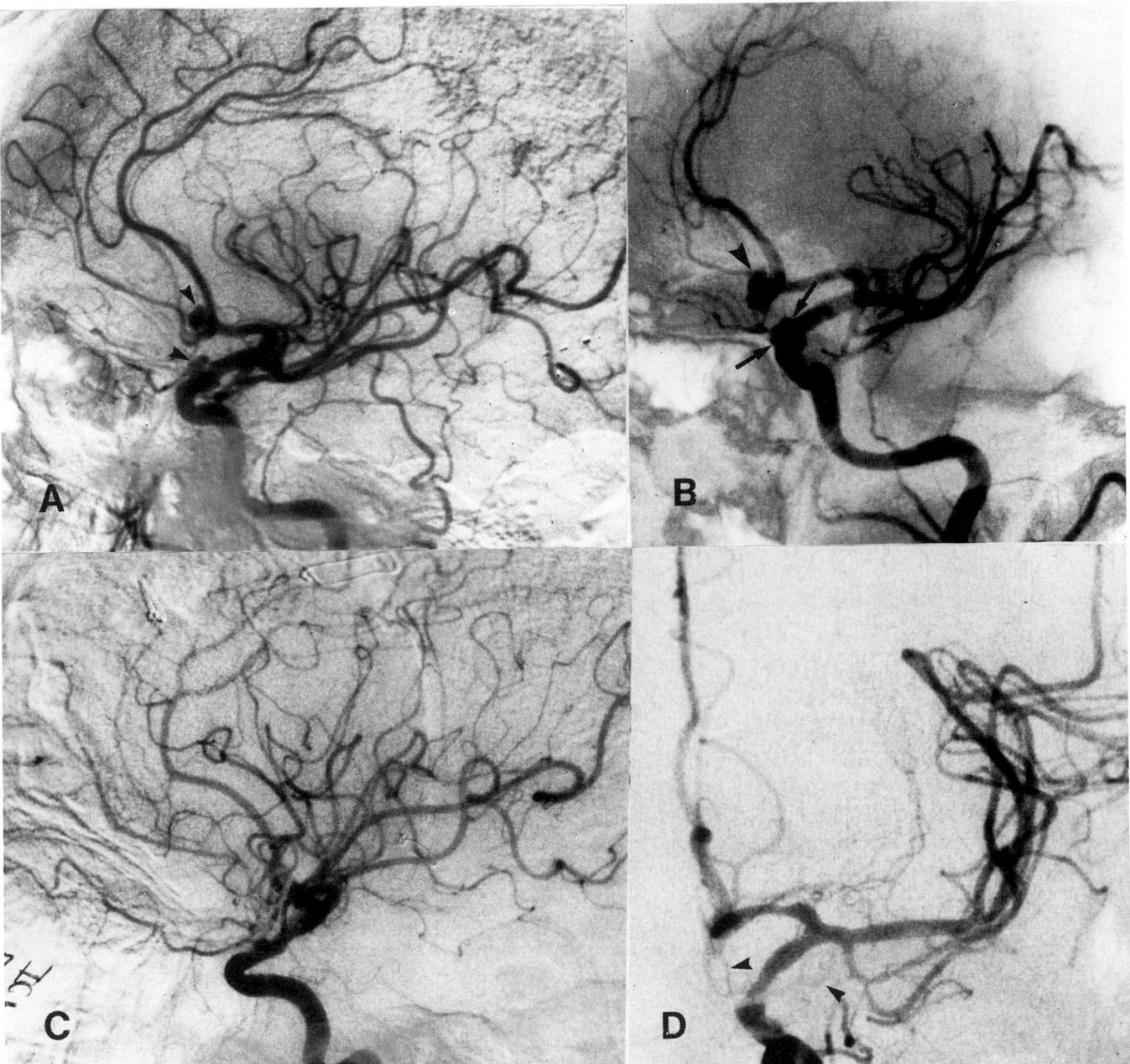

Figure 15-7 The patient described in Fig. 15–5 was studied 48 h after occurrence of SAH. Left carotid angiogram, lateral view, shows aneurysms of the anterior communicating artery and ICA-OpthA junction (*arrowheads*) with no spasm (*A*). Same study (oblique view) shows variation of aneurysm appearance and broad base of the ICA-OpthA aneurysm (*between arrows*) (*B*). The larger anterior communicating artery aneurysm (*arrowhead*) was the origin of the SAH. Postoperative left carotid angiogram (lateral view) shows no filling of clipped aneurysms (*C*). Same study (AP view) shows clips (*arrowheads*) and spasm in ICA and A1 (*D*). Spasm is more when compared with the preoperative study (*B*) of similar projection.

rectus, which lies just medial to the olfactory tract, provides ready access into the interhemispheric fissure and both A2 segments. This may provide an advantage when the aneurysm projects anteriorly and inferiorly.[157,177] There are no neurological deficits associated with this maneuver. Anatomic variations include hypoplasia of A1, duplication of ACA, and multiple A2s (including the median artery of the corpus callosum)[178] (Fig. 15-7). The bifrontal interhemispheric approach also offers good exposure to this region and is advantageous in sorting out anomalous A2s.[179]

PERICALLOSAL ARTERY

About 5 percent of aneurysms are on the pericallosal or distal anterior cerebral artery (DACA) and are associated with anomalous A2s, multiple aneurysms (50 percent), and AVMs.[180] They are most common at the genu of the corpus callosum. These aneurysms are treacherous, deceptive, and require a carefully planned approach, which varies in angle of access according to the position of the aneurysm along the course of the distal anterior cerebral artery.[181] The frontal interhemispheric route must be low enough to expose the parent A2 *proximal* to the aneurysm.[182,183] The coronal interhemispheric transcallosal approach is preferred if the lesion is above the genu of the corpus callosum.[184] Lesions inferior to the genu can be accessed through the corpus callosum so that A2 proximal to the aneurysm is controlled.[185]

BASILAR ARTERY BIFURCATION

Two approaches to the basilar artery bifurcation are the subtemporal transtentoral and the transylvian approach.[186–189] The transylvian is the authors' preference as it avoids the third nerve and views both superior cerebellar arteries (SCA) and proximal posterior cerebral arteries (P1 and P2) as well as the junction of the aneurysm neck with both P2s. It requires wide dissection of the sylvian fissure and basal cisterns as well as retraction on the ICA or M1, which is the major disadvantage of this route.

For high or giant basilar bifurcation lesions, removal of the zygoma and orbital plate may afford better exposure of this region with less frontal lobe retraction.[190]

BASILAR ARTERY TRUNK

The combined subtemporal retrolabyrinthine transtentorial route allows access of the basilar trunk from the anterior inferior cerebellar artery (AICA) in the cerebellopontine angle (CPA) to the superior cerebellar artery (SCA) and the prepontine cistern.[191] This also offers access to aneurysms of the P2, P3, and P4 segments of the posterior cerebral artery in the ambient cistern and beyond.

VERTEBRAL ARTERY BRANCHES AND BIFURCATION

The far lateral transcondylar approach to the medullary cistern and caudal CPA provides access to aneurysms of the vertebral artery with minimal retraction of the cerebellum.[192–196]

INTRAOPERATIVE COMPLICATIONS

Intraoperative rupture of the aneurysm before clipping can be a source of increased morbidity. It is usually due to technical matters. Insight into the mechanisms may help in avoiding them.[197,198] When unexpected rupture occurs, direct exposure of the bleeding site with suction and use of focal tamponade with microfibrillar collagen, bipolar coagulation of the site, or temporary clips to trap the aneurysm is safer and more effective than hurried packing with multiple large cottonoids, since bleeding may continue unnoticed under the packs, resulting in acute progressive intracerebral hemor-

rhage and aggravation of injury. Larger tears tend to occur with blunt dissection using microdissectors, hooks, and forceps.[198] The urge to place a clip in haste before the bleeding aneurysm is completely dissected should be resisted since this may extend the tear and convert a salvageable to an unsalvageable complication.

MANEUVERS THAT FACILITATE SAFE ANEURYSMAL CLIPPING: AVOIDING PITFALLS

1. Mount EEG needle scalp electrodes—provides opportunity to monitor cortical activity.
2. Select and load temporary clips at start—prepares for the unexpected.
3. Dissect wide arachnoidal planes and cisterns—reduces tension of retraction.
4. Identify and define anatomy of adjacent arteries—allows control of lesion.
5. Use sharp dissection of neck of the aneurysm—reduces tension pull that may tear neck wall.
6. Preserve adjacent perforators—avoids unexpected deficit.
7. Use temporary clips on parent artery—a soft aneurysm allows neck manipulation.
8. Complete circumferential neck dissection—enables full neck visualization.
9. Aspirate a bulky aneurysm after trapping—facilitates clipping.[161]
10. Use light bipolar coagulation of neck—develops clip seat without kinking.
11. Visualize a trial of multiple clip configurations—ensures "best fit."
12. Wiggle clip jaws like a dissector upon application—prevents tears. (*Not* a substitute for adequate dissection *prior* to clip application.)
13. Inspect tips after clip is in place—ensures against incomplete clipping.
14. Remove and reapply clip if in doubt—guarantees optimal clip placement.
15. Use booster clip or double clip—eliminates delayed clip slip or migration.

These measures are not universal and each circumstance must be individualized, but they will serve as a guide and be helpful in the majority of circumstances.

MANEUVERS FOR CEREBRAL PROTECTION

Since cerebrovascular surgery often requires temporary reduction or suspension of cerebral blood flow, either regionally or globally, steps to protect the ischemic tissues from infarction are often critical for preventing permanent deficits. The basic rational for such steps is reducing or eliminating the metabolic demand of the tissues, decreasing the cerebral metabolic rate ($CMRO_2$), and inhibiting or reversing the ischemic progression to infarction. This can be accomplished pharmacologically with anesthetic agents or physically with induced hypothermia, but there are striking differences in the effect on adenosine triphosphate (ATP) depletion between the two modalities.[199]

Continuous EEG monitoring with these steps helps to guide dosage and gauge level of cerebral activity; it infers the degree of cerebral metabolic demand. Metabolic requirements beyond isoelectric cortical activity are those needed for maintaining neuronal integrity itself. Pharmacological agents do not protect the brain in conditions of total ischemia such as cardiac arrest.[200] It should be understood that no measure presently available for protecting cerebral tissues from infarction under conditions of temporary ischemia is consistently effective or without limitation and risk.

Osmotic Agents Hyperosmolar agents increase cerebral blood flow in both normal and ischemic cerebral tissue.[201] They not only reduce edema but also improve rheological characteristics of blood.[202] Mannitol (20 percent) by intravenous infusion in a dose of 1 g/kg of body weight given 5 min prior to temporary clipping of parent artery serves to protect the ischemic cerebral tissues from infarction for 30 min.[203,204]

Anesthetic Agents *Isoflurane* Isoflurane, an inhalation anesthetic agent reduces electrocortical activity to burst suppression with increasing systemic concentration, progressing to a flat (isoelectric) EEG.[205] Additional anesthetic concentrations beyond these levels do not lower $CMRO_2$ further. Isoflurane does not protect primates from infarcts to the extent that barbiturates do under the same experimental conditions.[202] This implies that there are additional factors beyond pharmacological metabolic suppression that protect cerebral tissues from ischemia. Clinical experience suggests that isoflurane is effective in protecting against infarction during conditions of temporary ischemia.[206] The advantage of isoflurane over barbiturates is its short duration of effect so that patients can be neurologically assessed before leaving the operating room. It is the preferred anesthetic agent for aneurysm surgery.[199]

Barbiturates Barbiturates produce a dose-related reduction of $CMRO_2$ while preserving the cerebral energy state under conditions of focal incomplete ischemia. Anesthetic doses of thiopental lower the $CMRO_2$ by 52 percent and CBF by 48 percent.[207] Incremental doses of thiopental produce EEG burst suppression and, ultimately, an isoelectric state.[199,208] The $CMRO_2$ is not reduced further beyond EEG burst suppression. Therefore, EEG burst suppression is the dosage end point. It is maintained by titration of a continuous intravenous infusion.

Barbiturates have better protective effects against cerebral ischemia than other anesthetic agents.[202] They redistribute blood flow to ischemic regions, a "reversed steal" phenomenon.[209] They scavenge free radicals and inhibit peroxidation of fatty acids.[210,211] Thiopental is the agent of choice in

protecting against effects of focal temporary ischemia because it rapidly produces maximal metabolic suppression without totally disrupting cardiovascular hemodynamics. The initial "sleep dose" is 3 to 5 mg/kg followed by subsequent maintenance with 1 to 2 mg/kg. A bolus dose of 6 to 8 mg/kg can produce hypotension to a mean of 30 to 40 torr in case of acute aneurysmal rupture.[208] Thiopental affords cerebral protection from the focal ischemia of temporary arterial clipping for intraoperative vascular control.[209,210] Such therapy should be restricted to conditions where flow is restored in a reasonable period of time.[212]

Hypothermia with Cardiopulmonary Bypass Profound hypothermia with circulatory arrest has recently gained resurgence and become more commonly used as an adjunct to facilitate surgical management of complex or giant intracranial aneurysms that would otherwise be considered inoperable.[213-216] It offers vascular control and protection of the perfusion bed of the aneurysm and its parent artery. The aneurysm can be opened and debulked in a bloodless field. The clipping can be accomplished with precision.

At times, an exsanguinated collapsed aneurysm under circulatory arrest can be a disadvantage. Small perforating branches become transparent and blend imperceptively with the aneurysm wall so that the origin of the perforator near the neck cannot be visualized. Safe dissection may be difficult if not impossible. In this circumstance, low perfusion rather than total circulatory arrest may be preferable.

Advances in technique, equipment, knowledge, and experience have improved safety and tolerance to the patient so that profound hypothermia is an established and available service in many major centers. Heparin anticoagulation is monitored by repeated measurements of activated clotting time. Coagulopathy can be controlled by reinfusion of autologous whole blood procured before the bypass and, possibly, elective autologous donation drawn in advance to scheduling the procedure. This preserves platelets and clotting factors, which supplements the usual control and reversal of heparinization. The addition of fresh frozen plasma, concentrated clotting factors from cryoprecipitated plasma extracts, and pooled platelet transfusion ensures adequate clotting factors to eliminate the coagulopathy associated with *rewarming coagulopathy*. This has been a major encumbrance of hypothermia in the past.[217,218]

Bypass can be achieved by open thoracotomy and cannulation of the right atrium and ascending aorta or by cannulation of the femoral artery and vein in the groin.[214-216] There may be potential drawbacks with femoral cannulation due to small vessels and lower flow volumes, which are avoided by thoracotomy.[213,216] This is usually not a problem, but the chest is always prepared in the surgical field so that direct cardiac and aortic cannulation can be achieved if the need arises.

The times of estimated safe circulatory arrest as measured by potassium (K) concentrations in CSF, which rises during experimental circulatory arrest, are: (1) $37°C = 3.5$ min,

(2) 19°C = 31 min, and (3) 13°C = 65 min.[219] Core temperatures of 17° to 18°C are used clinically, and the time limit for arrest at these levels is less than 60 min. Therefore, as much dissection as possible is completed before arrest is instituted. Steps are planned in coordination with the anesthesia and cardiothoracic teams before commencing. It is preferable for the attending physicians of the respective teams to remain constant in these procedures in order to ensure that there is a mutual understanding and that routines are familiar to all personnel.

☐ SPECIAL CONSIDERATIONS

GIANT ANEURYSMS

Cerebral artery aneurysms larger than 2.5 cm (1 in) in diameter are classified as giant aneurysms. They comprise about 5 percent of cerebral aneurysms; they are more common in women.[220] They may arise by enlargement of saccular aneurysms or expand from atherosclerotic weakening of the arterial wall as the fusiform type. As the lesions enlarge, they broaden the parent artery, and branches are splayed along the base and walls of the aneurysms. Atherosclerotic and calcified plaques may form in the wall, and a mural thrombus may be deposited within the fundus in irregular layers. Aneurysms will expand and compress brain tissue locally as a tumor. Florid edema of surrounding white matter aggravates the mass effect of the aneurysm, even to the point of increasing the intracranial pressure. Contrary to some impressions these lesions tend to bleed at the same rate as smaller lesions. Massive mural thrombus in a giant fundus does not protect it from bleeding.[221] The CT scan provides images for the diagnosis. Giant aneurysms bleed, grow to compress vital structures, and cause pain as well as develop thrombi that can embolize and cause focal deficits. The aneurysms should be obliterated if possible. The clinical evaluation includes CT and MRI, followed by complete cerebral angiography. The angiogram should include cross compression and temporary balloon occlusion of the involved carotid artery to determine adequacy of collateral flow. Both direct and indirect methods of treatment are used to manage these lesions.

The Hunterian principle (*ligation of the parent artery*) is often an effective indirect maneuver. Internal carotid artery ligation is recommended over ligation of the CCA because giant aneurysms of the carotid system can continue to enlarge over the years after CCA ligation. Tourniquet occlusion using 3-O plastic suture cinched around the artery can be applied for graded occlusion of the parent artery as recommended by Drake as an alternative for managing giant aneurysms. The ends of the suture are threaded through a P.E. 190 polyethylene tubing cut to appropriate length and brought through a stab wound in the scalp. Protocol for clinical and physiological monitoring is required during closure of the tourniquet to assess accurately the patient's tolerance. Ischemic signs usually are reversed with release of the tourniquet.[221]

Extracranial-intracranial (EC-IC) bypass may be required to supplement collateral flow when the parent artery is occluded or the aneurysm is trapped.[222] A small-volume scalp artery or large-volume vein graft may be considered, depending on individual circumstances of aneurysm location and sources of collateral flow.[223] EC-IC bypass may fail to prevent infarction in acute occlusion of the middle cerebral artery because of the low flow rate of the bypass in the acute phase (20 to 60 ml/min).[224]

Direct measures are the same as for smaller lesions and include clipping, trapping, wrapping, or intraluminal clotting.[220,221,225,226] These measures do not reduce the mass effect or local tissue compression produced by the aneurysm. Aneurysmorrhaphy involves temporary trapping and opening the aneurysm with removal of thrombus and plaque, followed by clipping of the neck or suture closure to reconstruct the parent artery and remove the aneurysmal mass.[227] The neck of the aneurysm is a major determinant of whether a lesion can be clipped. Often, the neck is small and thin-walled so that it can be ligated or clipped. Selection of a clip allows for individual creative application of multiple configurations so that the neck of the aneurysm is selectively secured while preserving the parent artery and adjacent perforating vessels. Most complications occurring in the management of giant aneurysms are due to ischemia from occlusion of the parent artery, damage to adjacent perforating vessels, and/or inadequacy of collateral flow.[225]

CAVERNOUS CAROTID ANEURYSMS

Aneurysms of the cavernous sinus are extradural and become symptomatic when they expand to compress the cranial nerves in the wall of the cavernous sinus. Retroorbital pain may precede cranial nerve dysfunction. The sixth nerve is often initially involved; this is followed by impairment of the third nerve and the ophthalmic division of the fifth nerve. Rarely, cavernous sinuses may hemorrhage, causing epistaxis or otorrhagia. The aneurysm may be a source of embolism or spontaneous carotid cavernous fistula generally. Lesions in this area do not hemorrhage but may be a source of intractable pain. Usually, if aneurysms in this location are to be treated, the carotid artery is investigated for tolerance to temporary occlusion in preparation for permanent carotid occlusion. However, direct surgical approach to the cavernous sinus with dissection and clipping of the aneurysm and preservation or reconstruction of the carotid artery is the preferred treatment in selected cases.[228]

PARACLINOID-SUPRACLINOID CAROTID (CAROTID-OPHTHALMIC) ANEURYSMS

This is the most-common site for a giant aneurysm of the carotid artery. Such aneurysms present with compression of the optic pathways and visual loss. This is reportedly the location of only 5 percent of aneurysms. Multiple aneurysms tend to occur more commonly here with mirror locations on the opposite side. It may be difficult to determine the exact angiographic origin of the larger lesions. Surgical exposure is equally difficult, often requiring resection of the anterior clinoid and enlarging the optic canal to expose the optic nerve, along with dissection of the carotid fibrous rings so as to enter into the superior cavernous sinus. This combined extra and intradural exposure offers proximal control of the ICA and full access to the base and neck of the aneurysm.[229]

CAROTID BIFURCATION

Aneurysms at the carotid bifurcation comprise 5 percent of aneurysms, many of which progress to giants. Rarely, lesions in this location enlarge to produce hydrocephalus, which is another complication of giant aneurysms.[230] Surgical management of these lesions is particularly hazardous because perforating branches to the striatum and thalamus as well as vessels originating on the A1 and M1 trunks must be preserved. The Drake tourniquet and EC-IC bypass are adjunctive procedures for treatment of lesions at the ICA bifurcation.

BASILAR ARTERY

Lesions of the basilar bifurcation usually project upward to compress the midbrain or pons. They can impair memory, induce personality changes, or cause dementia, ataxia, pseudobulbar palsy, and hydrocephalus (Fig. 15-8). The neck may be atheromatous and incorporate the origin of P1. Digital carotid occlusion during vertebral angiography to demonstrate retrograde filling of the posterior communicating arteries is helpful in assessing collateral circulation.[221,231] Management of these lesions incurs a high morbidity and mortality even with current technical advances. Profound hypothermia with cardiac bypass is adjunctive for controlling flow during manipulation of large aneurysms in this location. EC-IC bypass can be established with the proximal posterior cerebral artery prior to ligation of the basilar artery by tourniquet.[231]

VERTEBRAL BASILAR SYSTEM

Like lesions at the basilar bifurcation, giant aneurysms in this location are hazardous because of the proximity to the medulla and pons and to vascular branches supplying these vital structures. A staged combination of vertebral artery occlusion and direct aneurysmal clipping can control these lesions. Proximal vertebral artery ligation is often well-tolerated because of collateral flow to the brainstem and cerebellum from the posterior communicating arteries and the contralateral vertebral artery. Intraaneurysmal thrombectomy is necessary to decompress the brainstem.[232,233] Staging these

procedures in multiple steps may yield better and often dramatic neurological recovery. The far lateral suboccipital approach will give access to lesions of the vertebral artery.[193,195,196,233,234] The subtemporal retrolabyrinthine transtentorial approach is more suitable for aneurysms of the basilar arterial trunk and junction of the anterior inferior cerebellar artery.[191]

ATHEROSCLEROTIC FUSIFORM ANEURYSMS

Atherosclerotic fusiform aneurysms and generalized ectasia of the major cerebral arteries often present a dilemma for the patient and physician. They reflect a systemic vasculopathy. The diseased arterial wall involves the origin of its branches. There is no neck, occlusion of which can isolate the lesion from the parent artery. Aneurysmal formation is relentlessly progressive. Treatment is control of a systemic disease such as diabetes mellitis and hyperlipidemia. Surgical maneuvers are limited to trapping and bypass. This is an option if the lesion is in a more-peripheral artery such as the MCA.[221,235] Lesions of the basilar and internal carotid arteries are less amenable to such management.

SERPENTINE ANEURYSMS AND MIDDLE CEREBRAL ARTERY ANEURYSMS

Serpentine aneurysms are giant partially thrombosed aneurysms that have recanalized with tortuous channels. They can occur in arteries other than the middle cerebral artery.[236] When left to their natural course, these lesions act as masses and may hemorrhage. They can lead to death of the patient.[237] Most giant aneurysms of the MCA have slowed circulation which has induced development of ample collateral flow through leptomeningeal channels that can protect against infarction, even when aneurysms are trapped, particularly when the aneurysm is excised and the mass effect is removed.[237]

Giant aneurysms of the middle cerebral artery can reach enormous size, which is compounded by surrounding edema and mass effect.[238,239] They commonly present with headache, seizures, hemiparesis, and dysphasia. They may also bleed. Edema and mass effects must be addressed when managing these lesions. In situ sources of collateral, such as a branch of the MCA, can be anastomosed side-to-side to reestablish distal flow.[239,240] Excision of the aneurysm followed by end-to-end or branch reconstruction of the parent artery is an ideal goal that can be achieved at times, particularly in MCA lesions.[222,241]

☐ TRAUMATIC ANEURYSMS

Saccular aneurysms resulting from cerebral arterial trauma are uncommon but can occur from blunt, penetrating, or

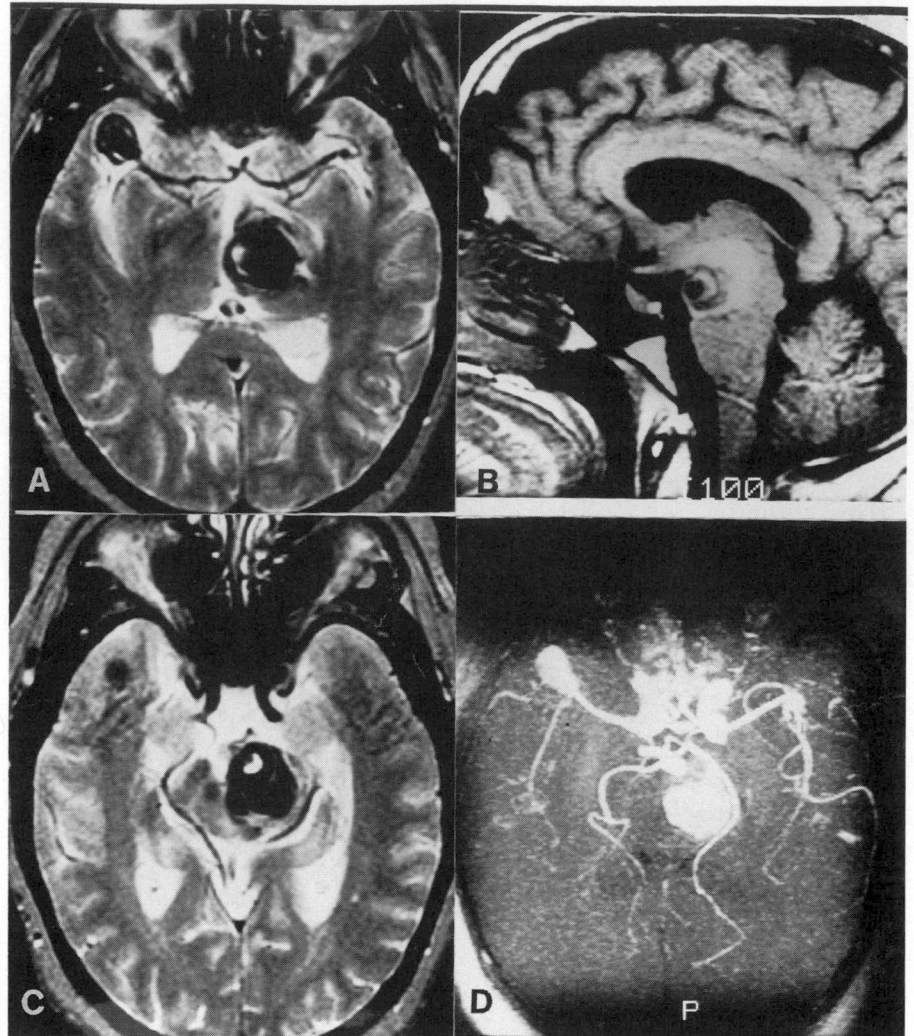

Figure 15-8 A 54-year-old woman who was a chronic smoker with hypertension and hyperlipidemia had recurrent headaches, intermittent unsteadiness, and loss of recent memory. She had two automobile accidents, which prompted a CT scan and then an MR scan. Her gait was spastic and unsteady; dysmetria was present on the left. An MR scan (axial view) shows a large aneurysm of the right M1-M2 junction and a giant aneurysm of the basilar artery embedded in the diencephalon (*A*). Both aneurysms contained a laminated mural thrombus. An MR scan, (sagittal cut) shows giant basilar artery aneurysm with signal void of active flow, lamination of mural thrombus, and aneurysmal mass expanding into the mesencephalon and rostral pons (*B*). An MR scan (axial view) through the mesencephalon shows chronic compression and almost total replacement of the left mesencephalon by the giant aneurysm (*C*). An MR angiogram of similar view and section level as *C* is given for comparison (*D*). Note discrepancy of sizes due to mural thrombus seen on MR and active flow as seen on an MR angiogram. A right carotid angiogram (lateral view) shows a large middle cerebral artery aneurysm (*E*). A composite of both carotid angiograms (AP view) shows bilateral "mirror" middle cerebral aneurysms (*F*). A vertebrobasilar angiogram (lateral view) shows a basilar artery bifurcation aneurysm and "flow jet" from the parent artery trunk into the sac (*G*). A vertebrobasilar angiogram (AP view) shows a projection of the aneurysm to the left and suggests that the neck wall is relatively thin without thrombus—and thus capable of accepting a clip (*H*).

surgical trauma.[242–245] There are different types: (1) *true form*: aneurysm wall comprises an intact adventitia; (2) *false form*: lacerated arterial wall occluded by hematoma within which the aneurysm forms, the aneurysm wall having no normal arterial structure; (3) *dissecting aneurysm*: another form, which is caused by formation of a false lumen between the intima and internal elastica.

Most traumatic aneurysms are associated with skull frac-

ture. There is frequently an associated severe brain injury. Typically, the patient has an injury, producing coma that resolves to a subsequent lucid interval after a few hours to days (average, 14 days). This is followed by neurological decline in the form of seizures, third nerve palsy, impaired mental status, paralysis, or decerebrate posturing as the aneurysm enlarges to compress local structures or hemorrhages.[246] Discovery of traumatic aneurysms is usually de-

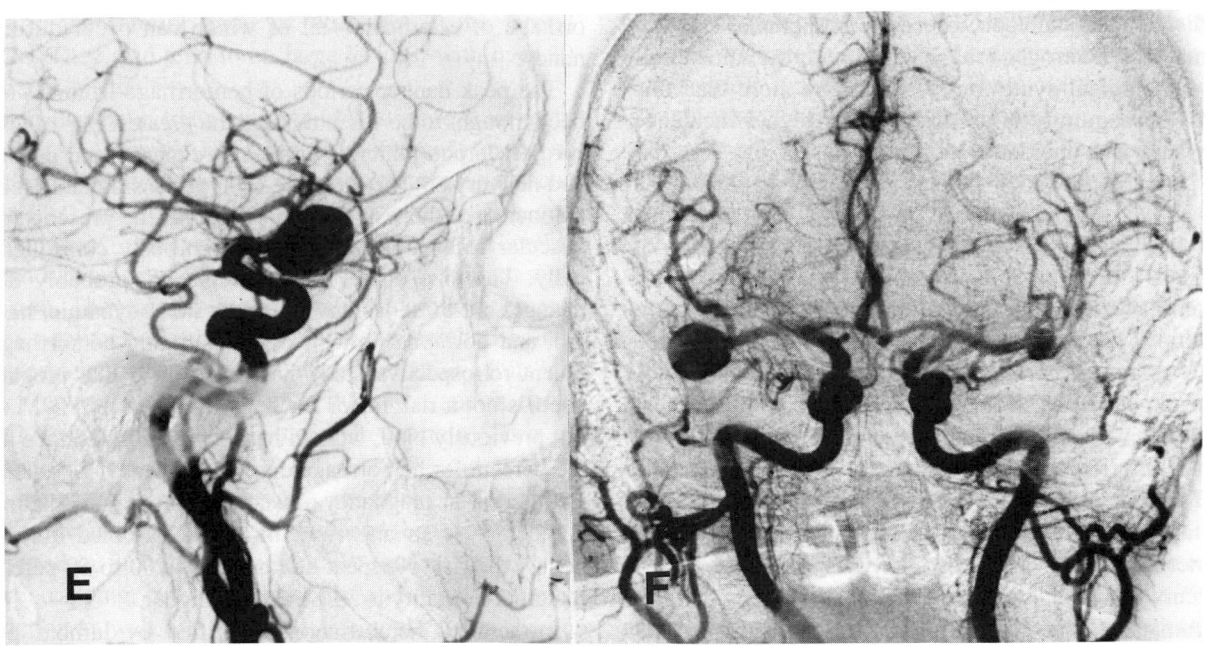

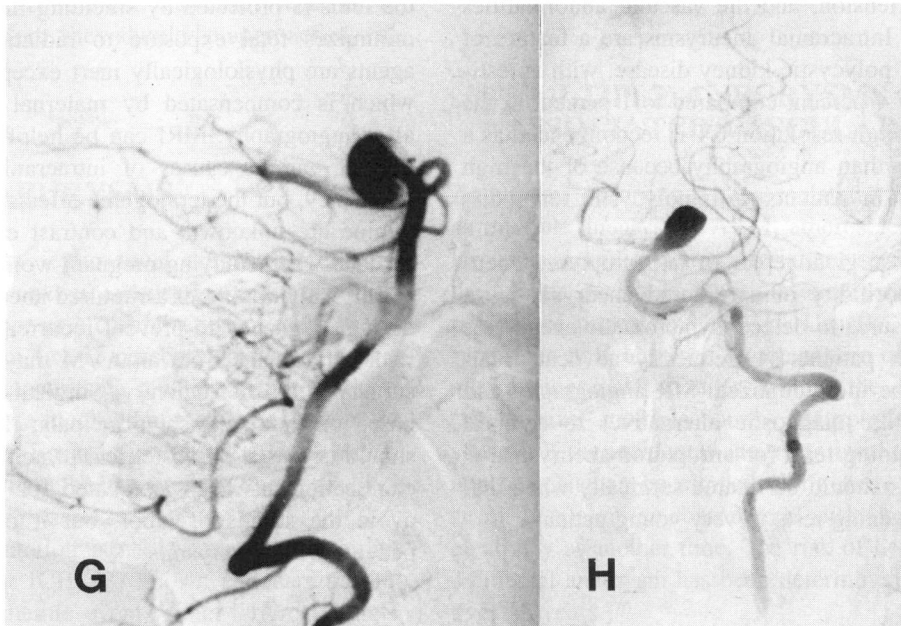

Figure 15-8 *Continued*

layed and often missed—particularly in this era of CT and MRI when angiography is rarely employed in evaluating head trauma—until an unexpected neurological event occurs. For this reason, these are treacherous lesions with high mortality (50 percent). In penetrating injuries, fragments penetrating the temporal, temporoparietal, or pterional areas have a significant chance of causing arterial injury.[243] Intracerebral hematoma may harbor and simultaneously obscure a traumatic aneurysm. Angiography is the diagnostic procedure of choice and should be performed if there is suspicion of a traumatic aneurysm.

Traumatic aneurysms also occur in children and are relatively more common in children than adults. Penetrating injuries such as gunshot wounds are found in teenage boys. Blunt trauma with basilar skull fractures more commonly cause aneurysms of the carotid artery along the petrous, cavernous, or clinoid portions, depending on the course of the fracture. Peripheral aneurysms occur along the course of the distal anterior cerebral artery, which can be traumatized at the falcine edge.[247] Patients suffering stab wounds to the head should undergo routine angiography because of the increased risk of a life-threatening traumatic aneurysm.

☐ FAMILIAL ANEURYSMS

Aneurysms are known to occur in families and are associated with different inherited conditions such as polycystic

intracranial aneurysms. When the aneurysm is on the internal carotid system, the stenosis may have a "protective effect" on the aneurysm. Endarterectomy can risk increasing exposure of the aneurysm to increased hemodynamic stress and potentiate rupture.[274] Elective clipping of the aneurysm followed by endarterectomy as a subsequent staged procedure should be considered in selected patients having this combination of lesions.

☐ OUTCOME AND SUMMARY

The diagnosis and treatment of SAH and intracranial aneurysms have made great strides during the past 20 to 30 years. Much is now known about the natural history of patients having recently experienced SAH, about the problems associated with, and the treatment of, chronic vasospasm, and about the natural history of incidental aneurysms as well as aneurysms having previously bled. There are very few aneurysms that cannot be approached and treated surgically. Most can be clipped, but alternative modes of treatment include isolation of the lesion, supplementing residual blood

flow by anastomosis of distal vessels, and obliterating the fundus of the aneurysms using coils, balloons, or various mechanisms of lesion thrombosis.

Mortality rates associated with the treatment of aneurysms are now acceptably low, rarely reaching as high as 3 to 5 percent for most aneurysms. This compares favorably with the complication rate of hemorrhage of a previously ruptured aneurysm and even lower than that of rupture from an incidental aneurysm.

Timing of treatment for an aneurysm remains controversial. Development of current techniques for treatment of vasospasm has prompted earlier treatment of vasospasm. Most patients can withstand surgical obliteration of the aneurysm, following which systemic blood pressure may be maintained at normal or even slightly hypertensive levels, while hemodilution and volume expansion are being instituted. This provides optimal cerebral perfusion during the critical period of vasospasm. Ancillary support mechanisms, such as bypass procedures, may be used in conjunction with plastic procedures on intracranial vessels in order to obliterate these treacherous lesions. The future of patients harboring intracranial aneurysms is much brighter than in past years.

REFERENCES

1. Weibers DO, Torner JC, Meissner I: Impact of unruptured intracranial aneurysms on public health in the United States. *Stroke* 23:1416–1419, 1992.
2. McCormick WF, Acosta-Rua GJ: The size of intracranial saccular aneurysms: An autopsy study. *J Neurosurg* 33:422–427, 1970.
3. Nibbelink DW, Torner JC, Henderson WG: Intracranial aneurysms and subarachnoid hemorrhage—Report on a randomized treatment study. IV-A. Regulated bed rest. *Stroke* 8:202–218, 1977.
4. Locksley HB: Report on the Cooperative Study of Intracranial Aneurysms and Subarachnoid Hemorrhage: Section V, Part II. Natural history of subarachnoid hemorrhage, intracranial aneurysms, and arteriovenous malformation. Based on 6368 cases in the Cooperative Study. *J Neurosurg* 25:321–368, 1966.
5. Heros RC, Kistler JP, Intracranial aneurysm—An update. *Stroke* 14:628–631, 1983.
6. Longstreth WT Jr, Nelson LM, Koepsell TD, Van Belle G: Cigarette smoking, alcohol use, and subarachnoid hemorrhage. *Stroke* 23:1242–1249, 1992.
7. Stehbens WE: Review article: Etiology of intracranial berry aneurysms. *J Neurosurg* 70:823–831, 1989.
8. Ostergaard JR: Review article: Risk factors in intracranial saccular aneurysms. Aspects on the formation and rupture of aneurysms, and development of vasospasm. *Acta Neurol Scand* 80:81–98, 1989.
9. Glynn LE: Medial defects in the circle of Willis and their relation to aneurysm formation. *J Pathol Bacteriol* 51:213–221, 1940.
10. Sahs AL: Observations in the pathology of saccular aneurysms. *J Neurosurg* 24:792–806, 1966.
11. Ferguson GG: Physical factors in the initiation, growth, and rupture of human intracranial saccular aneurysms. *J Neurosurg* 37:666–677, 1972.
12. Kamiya K, Kuyama H, Symon L: An experimental study of the acute stage of subarachnoid hemorrhage. *J Neurosurg* 59:917–924, 1983.
13. McCormick PW, McCormick J, Zimmerman R, et al: The pathophysiology of acute subarachnoid hemorrhage. *BNI Quarterly* 7(3):18–26, 1991.
14. Trojanowski T: Early effects of experimental arterial subarachnoid haemorrhage on the cerebral circulation: I. Experimental subarachnoid haemorrhage in cat and its pathophysiological effects. Methods of regional cerebral blood flow measurement and evaluation of microcirculation. *Acta Neurochir* 72:79–94, 1984.
15. Steiner L, Lofgren J, Zwetnow NN: Characteristics and limits of tolerance in repeated subarachnoid hemorrhage in dogs. *Acta Neurol Scand* 52:241–267, 1975.
16. Suzuki J, Ohara H: Clinicopathological study of cerebral aneurysms: Origin, rupture, repair, and growth. *J Neurosurg* 48:505–514, 1978.
17. Forbus WD: On the origin of miliary aneurysms of the superficial cerebral arteries. *Bull Johns Hopkins Hosp* 47:239–284, 1930.

18. Ferguson GC: Physical factors in the initiation, growth, and rupture of human intracranial saccular aneurysms. *J Neurosurg* 37:666–677, 1972.

19. Sekhar LN, Heros RC: Origin, growth, and rupture of saccular aneurysms: A review. *Neurosurgery* 8:248–260, 1981.

20. Sekhar LN, Sclabassi RJ, Sun M, et al: Intra-aneurysmal pressure measurements in experimental saccular aneurysms in dogs. *Stroke* 19:352–356, 1988.

21. Yamaki T, Yoshino E, Higuchi T: Rapidly growing aneurysm. *Surg Neurol* 26:301–305, 1986.

22. Austin GM, Schievink W, Williams R: Controlled pressure-volume factors in the enlargement of intracranial aneurysms. *Neurosurgery* 24:722–730, 1989.

23. McMenemey WH: The significance of subarachnoid bleeding. *Proc Roy Soc Med* 47:701–704, 1954.

24. DuPont JR, Van Wart CA, Kraintz L: The clearance of major components of whole blood from cerebralspinal fluid following simulated subarachnoid hemorrhage. *J Neuropath Exp Neurol* 20:450–455, 1961.

25. Tourtellotte WW, Somers JF, Parker JA, et al: A study of traumatic lumbar puncture. *Neurology* (Minneapolis) 8:129–134, 1958.

26. Tourtellotte WW, Metz LN, Bryan ER, DeJong RN: Spontaneous subarachnoid hemorrhage. Factors affecting the rate of clearing of the cerebrospinal fluid. *Neurology* 14:301–306, 1964.

27. Paoletti P, Gaetani P, Grignani G, et al: CSF leukotriene C_4 following subarachnoid hemorrhage. *J Neurosurg* 69:488–493, 1988.

28. Mabe H, Suzuki S, Mase M, et al: Serum neuron-specific enolase levels after subarachnoid hemorrhage. *Surg Neurol* 36:170–174, 1991.

29. Scarna H, Delafosse B, Steinburg R, et al: Neuron-specific enolase as a marker of neuronal lesions during various comas in man. *Neurochem Int* 4:405–411, 1982.

30. Persson L, Hardemark H-G, Gustafsson J, et al: S-100 protein and neuron-specific enolase in cerebrospinal fluid and serum: markers of cell damage in human central nervous system. *Stroke* 18:911–918, 1987.

31. Dilraj A, Botha JH, Rambiritch V, et al: Levels of catecholamine in plasma and cerebralspinal fluid in aneurysmal subarachnoid hemorrhage. *Neurosurgery* 31:42–51, 1992.

32. Sasaki T, Kassel NF, Yamashita M, et al: Barrier disruption in the major cerebral arteries following experimental subarachnoid hemorrhage. *J Neurosurg* 63:433–440, 1985.

33. Boisvert DP, Overton TR, Weir B, Grace MG: Cerebral arterial responses to induced hypertension following subarachnoid hemorrhage in the monkey. *J Neurosurg* 49:75–83, 1978.

34. Fox JL, Ko JP: Cerebral vasospasm: A clinical observation. *Surg Neurol* 10:269–275, 1978.

35. Sasaki T, Kassell NF, Zuccarello M, et al: Barrier disruption in the major cerebral arteries during the acute stage after experimental subarachnoid hemorrhage. *Neurosurgery* 19:177–184, 1986.

36. Nagy Z, Mathison G, Huttner I: Blood-brain barrier opening to horseradish peroxidase in acute arterial hypertension. *Acta Neuropathol* 48:45–53, 1979.

37. Dernbach PD, Little JR, Jones SC, Ebrahim ZY: Altered cerebral autoregulation and CO_2 reactivity after aneurysmal subarachnoid hemorrhage. *Neurosurgery* 22:822–826, 1988.

38. Paulson OB, Olesen J, Christensen MS: Restoration of autoregulation of cerebral blood flow by hypocapnia. *Neurology* 22:286–293, 1972.

39. Estanol BV, Marin OSM: Cardiac arrhythmias and sudden death in subarachnoid hemorrhage. *Stroke* 6:382–385, 1975.

40. Marion DW, Segal R, Thompson ME: Subarachnoid hemorrhage and the heart. *Neurosurgery* 18:101–106, 1986.

41. Burch GE, Meyers R, Abildskov JA: A new electrocardiographic pattern observed in cerebrovascular accidents. *Circulation* 9:719–723, 1954.

42. Weintraub BM, McHenry LC Jr: Cardiac abnormalities in subarachnoid hemorrhage: A résumé. *Stroke* 5:384–392, 1974.

43. Keren A, Tzivoni D, Gavish D, et al: Etiology, warning signs and therapy of torsade de pointes: A study of 10 patients. *Circulation* 64:1167–1174, 1981.

44. Yuki K, Kodama Y, Onda J, et al: Coronary vasospasm following subarachnoid hemorrhage as a cause of stunned myocardium. *J Neurosurg* 75:308–311, 1991.

45. Braunwald E, Kloner RA: The stunned myocardium: prolonged, postischemic ventricular dysfunction. *Circulation* 66:1146–1149, 1982.

46. McCormick WF, Rosenfield DB: Massive brain hemorrhage. A review of 144 cases and an examination of their causes. *Stroke* 4:946–954, 1973.

47. Graf CJ: Prognosis for patients with nonsurgically-treated aneurysms: Analysis of the Cooperative Study of Intracranial Aneurysms and Subarachnoid Hemorrhage. *J Neurosurg* 35:438–443, 1971.

48. Winn HR, Richardson AE, Jane JA: The long-term prognosis in untreated cerebral aneurysms: I. The incidence of late hemorrhage in cerebral aneurysms. A 10-year evaluation of 364 patients. *Ann Neurol* 1:358–370, 1977.

49. Winn HR, Richardson AE, O'Brien W, Jane JA: The long-term prognosis in untreated cerebral aneurysms: II. Late morbidity and mortality. *Ann Neurol* 4:418–426, 1978.

50. Kassell NF, Torner JC: Size of intracranial aneurysms. *Neurosurgery* 12:291–297, 1983.

51. Wiebers DO, Whisnant JP, Sundt TM Jr, O'Fallon WM: The significance of unruptured intracranial saccular aneurysms. *J Neurosurg* 66:23–29, 1987.

52. Edner G, Forster DMC, Steiner L, Bergvall U: Spontaneous healing of intracranial aneurysms after subarachnoid hemorrhage: Case report. *J Neurosurg* 48:450–454, 1978.

53. Ojemann RG, Heros RC, Crowell RM: Intracranial aneurysms and subarachnoid hemorrhage: Incidence, pathology, clinical features, and perioperative management, in Ojemann RG, Heros RC, Crowell RM (eds): *Surgical Management of Cerebral Vascular Disease,* 2d ed. Baltimore, Williams & Wilkins, 1988, pp 147–177.

54. Waga S, Ohtsubo K, Handa H: Warning signs in intracranial aneurysms. *Surg Neurol* 3:15–20, 1975.

55. Adams HP, Jr, Jergenson DD, Kassell NF, Sahs AL: Pitfalls in recognition of subarachnoid hemorrhage. *JAMA* 244:794–796, 1980.

56. Toole JF: Subarachnoid hemorrhage, in Toole JF (ed): *Cerebrovascular Disorders,* 3d ed. New York, Raven Press, chap 24, pp 347–360, 1984.

57. Okawara SH: Warning signs prior to rupture of an intracranial aneurysm. *J Neurosurg* 38:575–580, 1973.

58. Ball MJ: Pathogenesis of the "sentinel headache" preceding berry aneurysm rupture. *Can Med Assoc J* 112:78–79, 1975.

59. Juvela S: Minor leak before rupture of an intracranial aneurysm and subarachnoid hemorrhage of unknown etiology. *Neurosurgery* 30:7–11, 1992.

60. Leblanc R: The minor leak preceding subarachnoid hemorrhage. *J Neurosurg* 66:35–39, 1987.

61. Khan SG, Frenkel M: Intravitreal hemorrhage associated with rapid increase in intracranial pressure (Terson's syndrome): *Am J Ophthalmol* 80:37–43, 1975.

62. Garfinkle AM, Danys IR, Nicolle DA, et al: Terson's syndrome: A reversible cause of blindness following subarachnoid hemorrhage. *J Neurosurg* 76:766–771, 1992.

63. Rusyniak WG, Peterson PC, Okawara SH, et al: Acute subdural hematoma after aneurysmal rupture. Evacuation with

aneurysmal clipping after emergent infusion computed tomography: Case report. *Neurosurgery* 31:129–132, 1992.

64. Hillman J: Should computed tomography scanning replace lumbar puncture in the diagnostic process in suspected subarachnoid hemorrhage? *Surg Neurol* 26:547–550, 1986.

65. Fisher CM, Kistler JP, Davis JM: Relation of cerebral vasospasm to subarachnoid hemorrhage visualized by computerized tomographic scanning. *Neurosurgery* 6:1–9, 1980.

66. Hijdra A, Brouwers PJ, Vermeulin M, Van Gijn J: Grading the amount of blood on computed tomograms after subarachnoid hemorrhage. *Stroke* 21:1156–1161, 1990.

67. Matsumura K, Matsuda M, Handa J, Todo G: Magnetic resonance imaging with aneurysmal subarachnoid hemorrhage: Comparison with computed tomography scan. *Surg Neurol* 34:71–78, 1990.

68. Perret G, Nishioka H: Report on the Cooperative Study of Intracranial Aneurysms And Subarachnoid Hemorrhage: Cerebral angiography. An analysis of the diagnostic value and complications of carotid and vertebral angiography in 5,484 patients. *J Neurosurg* 25:98–115, 1966.

69. Hesselink JR: Radiology: I. Investigation of intracranial aneurysms, in Fox JL (ed): *Intracranial Aneurysms,* New York, Springer-Verlag, chap 17, pp 497–548, 1983.

70. Iwanaga H, Wakai S, Ochiai C, et al: Ruptured cerebral aneurysms missed by initial angiographic study. *Neurosurgery* 27:45–51, 1990.

71. Brismar J, Sundbarg G: Subarachnoid hemorrhage of unknown origin: Prognosis and prognostic factors. *J Neurosurg* 63:349–354, 1985.

72. Juul R, Frediksen TA, Ringkjob R: Prognosis in subarachnoid hemorrhage of unknown etiology. *J Neurosurg* 64:359–362, 1986.

73. Bjerre P, Videbaek H, Lindholm J: Subarachnoid hemorrhage with normal cerebral angiography: A prospective study on sellar abnormalities and pituitary function. *Neurosurgery* 19:1012–1015, 1986.

74. Botterell EH, Lougheed WM, Scott JW, Vandewater SL: Hypothermia, and interruption of carotid, or carotid and vertebral circulation, in the surgical management of intracranial aneurysms. *J Neurosurg* 13:1–42, 1956.

75. Hunt WE, Hess RM: Surgical risk as related to time of intervention in the repair of intracranial aneurysms. *J Neurosurg* 28:14–20, 1968.

76. Sano K, Tamura A: A proposal for grading of subarachnoid hemorrhage due to aneurysm rupture, in Auer LM (ed): *Timing of Aneurysm Surgery,* New York, Walter de Gruyter, pp 3–7, 1985.

77. Juvela S: Rebleeding from ruptured intracranial aneurysms. *Surg Neurol* 32:323–326, 1989.

78. Rosenorn J, Eskensen V, Schmidt K, Ronde F: The risk of rebleeding from ruptured intracranial aneurysms. *J Neurosurg* 67:329–332, 1987.

79. Kassell NF, Torner JC: Aneurysmal rebleeding: A preliminary report from the Cooperative Aneurysm Study. *Neurosurgery* 13:479–481, 1983.

80. Wilkins RH: Attempts at prevention or treatment of intracranial arterial spasm: An update: Review article. *Neurosurgery* 18:808–825, 1986.

81. Fodstad H, Forssell A, Liliequist B, Schannong M: Antifibrinolysis with tranexamic acid in aneurysmal subarachnoid hemorrhage: A consecutive controlled clinical trial. *Neurosurgery* 8:158–165, 1981.

82. Kassell NF, Torner JC, Adams HP, Jr: Antifibrinolytic therapy in the acute period following subarachnoid hemorrhage: Preliminary observations from the Cooperative Aneurysm Study. *J Neurosurg* 61:225–230, 1984.

83. Vermeulen M, Lindsay KW, Murray GD, et al: Antifibrino-lytic treatment in subarachnoid hemorrhage. *N Engl J Med* 311:432–437, 1984.

84. Zervas NT, Liszczak TM, Mayberg MR, Black PMcL: Cerebrospinal fluid may nourish cerebral vessels through pathways in the adventitia that may be analogous to systemic vasa vasorum. *J Neurosurg* 56:475–481, 1982.

85. Ohata T, Satoh G, Kuroiwa T: The permeability change of major cerebral arteries in experimental vasospasm. *Neurosurgery* 30:331–336, 1992.

86. Zabramski JM, Spetzler RF, Bontelle C: Chronic cerebral vasospasm: Effect of volume and timing of hemorrhage in a canine model. *Neurosurgery* 18:1–6, 1986.

87. Findlay JM, Weir BKA, Kanamaru K, Espinosa F: Arterial wall changes in cerebral vasospasm. *Neurosurgery* 25:736–746, 1989.

88. MacDonald RL, Weir BKA, Young JD, Grace MGA: Cytoskeletal and extracellular matrix proteins in cerebral arteries following subarachnoid hemorrhage in monkeys. *J Neurosurg* 76:81–90, 1992.

89. MacDonald RL, Weir BK, Runzer TD, Grace MG, et al: Etiology of cerebral vasospasm in primates. *J Neurosurg* 75:415–424, 1991.

90. Harada T, Suzuki Y, Satoh S, et al: Blood component induction of cerebral vasospasm. *Neurosurgery* 27:252–256, 1990.

91. Juvela S: Cerebral infarction and release of platelet thromboxane after subarachnoid hemorrhage. *Neurosurgery* 27:929–935, 1990.

92. Yamaura I, Tani E, Maeda Y, et al: Endothelin-1 of canine basilar artery in vasospasm. *J Neurosurg* 76:99–105, 1992.

93. Suzuki R, Masaoka H, Hirata Y, et al: The role of endothelin-1 in the origin of cerebral vasospasm in patients with aneurysmal subarachnoid hemorrhage. *J Neurosurg* 77:96–100, 1992.

94. Lewis PJ, Weir BKA, Nosko MG, et al: Intrathecal nimodipine therapy in a primate model of chronic cerebral vasospasm. *Neurosurgery* 22:492–500, 1988.

95. Findlay JM, Weir BKA, Kassell NF, et al: Intracisternal recombinant tissue plasminogen activator after aneurysmal subarachnoid hemorrhage. *J Neurosurg* 75:181–188, 1991.

96. Barnwell SL, Higashida RT, Halbach VV, et al: Transluminal angioplasty of intracerebral vessels for cerebral arterial spasm: Reversal of neurological deficits after delayed treatment. *Neurosurgery* 25:424–429, 1989.

97. Sekhar LN, Wechsler LR, Yonas H, Luyckx K, Obrist W: Value of transcranial Doppler examination in the diagnosis of cerebral vasospasm after subarachnoid hemorrhage. *Neurosurgery* 22:813–821, 1988.

98. Becker G, Greiner K, Kaune B, et al: Diagnosis and monitoring of subarachnoid hemorrhage by transcranial color-coded real-time sonography. *Neurosurgery* 28:814–820, 1991.

99. Mohr G, Ferguson G, Kahn M, et al: Intraventricular hemorrhage from ruptured aneurysm: Retrospective analysis of 91 cases. *J Neurosurg* 58:482–487, 1983.

100. Hahn FJY, Rim K: Frontal ventricular dimensions on normal computed tomography. *Am J Radiol* 126:593–596, 1976.

101. Vassilouthis J, Richardson AE: Ventricular dilatation and communicating hydrocephalus following spontaneous subarachnoid hemorrhage. *J Neurosurg* 51:341–351, 1979.

102. Raimondi AJ, Torres H: Acute hydrocephalus as a complication of subarachnoid hemorrhage. *Surg Neurol* 1:23–26, 1973.

103. VanGijn J, Hijdra A, Wijdicks EFM, et al: Acute hydrocephalus after aneurysmal subarachnoid hemorrhage. *J Neurosurg* 63:355–362, 1985.

104. Kusske JA, Turner PT, Ojemann GA, Harris AB: Ventriculostomy for the treatment of acute hydrocephalus following subarachnoid hemorrhage. *J Neurosurg* 38:591–595, 1973.

105. Black PMCL: Hydrocephalus and vasospasm after subarachnoid hemorrhage. *Neurosurgery* 18:12–16, 1986.

106. Auer LM, Mokry M: Disturbed cerebral spinal fluid circulation after subarachnoid hemorrhage and acute aneurysm surgery. *Neurosurgery* 26:804–809, 1990.

107. Milhorat TH: Acute hydrocephalus after aneurysmal subarachnoid hemorrhage. *Neurosurgery* 20:15–20, 1987.

108. Kosteljanetz M: Pressure-volume conditions in patients with subarachnoid and/or intraventricular hemorrhage. *J Neurosurg* 63:398–403, 1985.

109. Marmarou A, Shulman K, Rosende M: A nonlinear analysis of the cerebralspinal fluid system and intracranial pressure dynamics. *J Neurosurg* 48:332–344, 1978.

110. Pare' L, Delfino R, Leblanc R: The relationship of ventricular drainage to aneurysmal rebleed. *J Neurosurg* 76:422–427, 1992.

111. Mullan S, Dawley J: Antifibrinolytic therapy for intracranial aneurysms. *J Neurosurg* 28:21–23, 1968.

112. Garijo JAA, Vilches JJ, Aznar JA: Preoperative treatment of ruptured intracranial aneurysms with tranexamic acid and monitoring of fibrinolytic activity. *J Neurosurg* 52:453–455, 1980.

113. Kassell NF, Torner JC, Adams HP, Jr: Antifibrinolytic therapy in the acute period following aneurysmal subarachnoid hemorrhage: Preliminary observations from the Cooperative Aneurysm Study. *J Neurosurg* 61:225–230, 1984.

114. Ausman JI, Diaz FG, Malik GM, et al: Current management of cerebral aneurysms: Is it based on facts or myths? *Surg Neurol* 24:625–635, 1985.

115. Vermeulin M, Lindsay KW, Murrasy GD, et al: Antifibrinolytic treatment in subarachnoid hemorrhage. *N Engl J Med* 311:432–437, 1984.

116. Kassell NF, Torner JC: Aneurysmal rebleeding: A preliminary report from the Cooperative Aneurysm Study. *Neurosurgery* 13:479–481, 1983.

117. Weir B: Antifibrinolytics in subarachnoid hemorrhage: Do they have a role? No. *Arch Neurol* 44:116–118, 1987.

118. Ausman JI, Diaz FG, Malik GM, et al: Management of cerebral aneurysms: Further facts and additional myths. *Surg Neurol* 32:21–35, 1989.

119. Lewis DL, Lechleiter JD, Kim D, et al: Intracellular regulation of ion channels in cell membranes: Subject review. *Mayo Clin Proc* 65:1127–1143, 1990.

120. Allen GS, Ahn MS, Preziosi TJ, et al: Cerebral arterial spasm—a controlled trial of nimodipine in patients with subarachnoid hemorrhage. *N Engl J Med* 308:619–624, 1983.

121. Meyer FB, Anderson RE, Yakish TL, Sundt TM, Jr: Effect of nimodipine on intracellular brain Ph, cortical blood flow, and EEG in experimental focal cerebral ischemia. *J Neurosurg* 64:617–626, 1986.

122. Mee E, Dorrance D, Lowe D, Neil-Dwyer G: Controlled study of nimodipine in aneurysm patients treated early after subarachnoid hemorrhage. *Neurosurgery* 22:484–491, 1988.

123. Ohman J, Heiskanen O: Effect of nimodipine on the outcome of patients after subarachnoid hemorrhage and surgery. *J Neurosurg* 69:683–686, 1988.

124. Pellettieri L, Bolander H, Carlsson H, Sjolander U: Nimodipine treatment of selected good-risk patients with subarachnoid hemorrhage: No significant difference between present and historical results. *Surg Neurol* 30:180–186, 1988.

125. Abramowicz M (ed): Felodipine—another calcium-channel blocker for hypertension. *Medical Letter* 33(859)115, 1991.

126. Mizukami M, Kawase T, Usami T, Tazawa T: Prevention of vasospasm by early operation with removal of subarachnoid blood. *Neurosurgery* 10:301–307, 1982.

127. Inagawa T, Yamamoto M, Kamiya K: Effect of clot removal on cerebral vasospasm. *J Neurosurg* 72:224–230, 1990.

128. Findlay JM, Weir BKA, Steinke D, et al: Effect of intrathecal thrombolytic therapy on subarachnoid clot and chronic vasospasm in a primate model of SAH. *J Neurosurg* 69:723–735, 1988.

129. Findlay JM, Weir BKA, Kanamaru K, et al: The effect of timing of intrathecal fibrinolytic therapy on cerebral vasospasm in a primate model of subarachnoid hemorrhage. *Neurosurgery* 26:201–206, 1990.

130. Zabramski JM, Spetzler RF, Lee KS, et al: Phase I trial of tissue plasminogen activator for the prevention of vasospasm in patients with aneurysmal subarachnoid hemorrhage. *J Neurosurg* 75:189–196, 1991.

131. Yamakami I, Isobe K, Yamaura A: Effects of intravascular volume expansion on cerebral blood flow in patients with ruptured cerebral aneurysms. *Neurosurgery* 21:303–309, 1987.

132. Wood JH, Simeone FA, Kron RE, Litt M: Rheological aspects of experimental hypervolemic hemodilution with low molecular weight dextran: Relationships of cortical blood flow, cardiac output, and intracranial pressure to fresh blood viscosity and plasma volume. *Neurosurgery* 11:739–753, 1982.

133. Solomon RA, Post KD, McMurty JG, III: Depression of circulating blood volume in patients after subarachnoid hemorrhage: Implications for the management of symptomatic vasospasm. *Neurosurgery* 15:354–361, 1984.

134. Wijdicks EFM, Vermeulen M, Hijdra A, van Gijn J: Hyponatremia and cerebral infarction in patients with ruptured intracranial aneurysms: Is fluid restriction harmful? *Ann Neurol* 17:137–140, 1985.

135. Maroon JC, Nelson PB: Hypovolemia in patients with subarachnoid hemorrhage: Therapeutic implications. *Neurosurgery* 4:223–226, 1979.

136. Nelson RJ, Roberts J, Rubin C, et al: Association of hypovolemia after subarachnoid hemorrhage with computed tomographic scan evidence of raised intracranial pressure. *Neurosurgery* 29:178–182, 1991.

137. Nelson PB, Seif SM, Maroon JC, Robinson AG: Hyponatremia in intracranial disease. Perhaps not the syndrome of inappropriate secretion of antidiuretic hormone (ISADH). *J Neurosurg* 55:938–941, 1981.

138. Wijdicks EF, Vermeulon M, ten Haaf JA, et al: Volume depletion and natriuresis in patients with a ruptured aneurysm. *Ann Neurol* 18:211–216, 1985.

139. Kudos T, Suzukai S, Iwabuchi T: Importance of monitoring the circulating blood volume in patients with cerebral vasospasm after subarachnoid hemorrhage. *Neurosurgery* 9:514–520, 1981.

140. Kassell NF, Peerless SJ, Durward QJ, et al: Treatment of ischemic deficits from vasospasm with intravascular volume expansion and induced arterial hypertension. *Neurosurgery* 11:337–343, 1982.

141. Finn SS, Stephensen SA, Miller CA, et al: Observations on the perioperative management of aneurysmal subarachnoid hemorrhage. *J Neurosurg* 65:45–62, 1986.

142. Kosnik EJ, Hunt WE: Postoperative hypertension in the management of patients with intracranial aneurysms. *J Neurosurg* 45:148–152, 1976.

143. Horsley V: Aneurysms of the larger cerebral artery. *Brain* 30:285–386, 1907.

144. Bakay LJ, Sweet WH: Intra-arterial pressure in the neck and brain. Late changes after carotid closure, acute measurements after vertebral closure. *J Neurosurg* 10:353–359, 1953.

145. Swearingen B, Heros RC: Common carotid occlusion for unclippable carotid aneurysms: An old but still effective operation. *Neurosurgery* 21:288–295, 1987.

146. Odom GL, Tindall GT: Carotid ligation in the treatment of certain intracranial aneurysms. *Clin N Surg* 15:101–116, 1968.

147. Jha AN, Butler P, Lye RH, Fawcitt RA: Carotid ligation: What happens in the long term? *J Neurol Neurosurg Psychiatr* 49:839–898, 1986.

148. Perret GE, Nibbelink DW: Randomized treatment study. Carotid ligation, in Sahs AL, et al (eds): *Aneurysmal Subarachnoid Hemorrhage: Report of the Cooperative Study*, Baltimore, Urban & Schwartzenberg, chap 8, pp 121–143, 1981.

149. Miller JD, Jawad K, Jennet B: Safety of carotid ligation and its role in the management of intracranial aneurysms. *J Neurol Neurosurg Psych* 40:64–72, 1977.

150. Wheelock B, Weir B, Watts R, et al: Timing of surgery for intracerebral hematomas due to aneurysm rupture. *J Neurosurg* 58:476–481, 1983.

151. Milhorat TH, Krautheim M: Results of early and delayed operations for ruptured intracranial aneurysms in two series of 100 consecutive patients. *Surg Neurol* 26:123–128, 1986.

152. Disney L, Weir B, Petruk K: Effect of management mortality of a deliberate policy of early operation on supratentorial aneurysms. *Neurosurgery* 20:695–701, 1987.

153. Ohman J, Heiskanen O: Timing of operation for ruptured supratentorial aneurysms: A prospective randomized study. *J Neurosurg* 70:55–60, 1989.

154. Solomon RA, Onesti ST, Klebanoff L: Relationship between the timing of aneurysm surgery and the development of delayed cerebral ischemia. *J Neurosurg* 75:56–61, 1991.

155. Railes JE, Spetzler RF, Hadley MN, Baldwin HZ: Management morbidity and mortality of poor-grade aneurysm patients. *J Neurosurg* 72:559–566, 1990.

156. Alksny JF, Smith RW: Iron-acrylic compound for stereotaxic aneurysm thrombosis. *J Neurosurg* 47:137–141, 1977.

157. Yasargil MG, Fox JL: The microsurgical approach to intracranial aneurysms. *Surg Neurol* 3:7–14, 1975.

158. Jabre A, Symon L: Temporary vascular occlusion during aneurysm surgery. *Surg Neurol* 27:47–63, 1987.

159. Ogawa A, Sato H, Sakurai Y, Yoshimoto T: Limitation of temporary vascular occlusion during aneurysm surgery: Study by intraoperative monitoring of cortical blood flow. *Surg Neurol* 36:453–457, 1991.

160. Sakaki T, Tsunoda S, Morimoto T, et al: Effects of repeated temporary clipping of the middle cerebral artery on pial arterial diameter, regional cerebral blood flow, and brain structure in cats. *Neurosurgery* 27:914–920, 1990.

161. Flamm ES: Suction decompression of aneurysms. *J Neurosurg* 54:275–276, 1981.

162. Atkinson JLD, Anderson RE, Piepgras DG: A comparative study in opening and closing pressures of cerebral aneurysm clips. *Neurosurgery* 26:80–85, 1990.

163. Dujovny K, Kossovsky N, Kossowsky R, et al: Aneurysm clip motion during magnetic resonance imaging: In vivo experimental study with metallurgical factor analysis. *Neurosurgery* 17:543–548, 1985.

164. Sugita K, Kobayashi S, Inoue T, Banno T: New angled fenestrated clips for fusiform vertebral aneurysms. *J Neurosurg* 54:346–350, 1981.

165. Kossowsky R, Dujovny M, Kossovsky N: Metallurgical evaluation of the compatibility of surgical clips with their appliers. *Acta Neurochir* 59:95–109, 1981.

166. Sundt TM, Jr, Piepgras DG, Marsh WR: Booster clips for giant and thick-based aneurysms. *J Neurosurg* 60:751–762, 1984.

167. Holtas S, Olsson M, Romner B, Larsson: Comparison of MRI and CT in patients with intracranial aneurysm metal clips. *AJNR* 9:891–897, 1988.

168. Shellock FG: MR imaging of metallic implants and materials: A compilation of the literature. *Am J Radiol* 151:811–814, 1988.

169. Romner B, Olsson M, Ljunggren B, et al: Magnetic resonance imaging and aneurysm clips. Magnetic properties and image artifacts. *J Neurosurg* 70:426–431, 1989.

170. Peerless SJ: The surgical approach to middle cerebral and posterior communicating aneurysms. *Clin Neurosurg* 21:151–165, 1974.

171. Fox JL: Microsurgical exposure of intracranial aneurysms. *J Microsurg* 1:2–31, 1979.

172. Yasargil MG, Reichman MV, Kubik S: Preservation of the frontotemporal branch of the facial nerve using the interfascial temporalis flap for the pterional craniotomy: Technical article. *J Neurosurg* 67:463–466, 1987.

173. Chehrazi BB: A temporal transsylvian approach to anterior circulation aneurysms. *Neurosurgery* 30:957–961, 1992.

174. Hacker RJ, Krall JM, Fox JL: Data. I, in Fox JL (ed): *Intracranial Aneurysms*, vol 1, New York, Springer-Verlag, chap 3, 1983, pp 19–62.

175. Heros RC: Technical note: Brain resection for exposure of deep extra-cerebral and paraventricular lesions. *Surg Neurol* 34:188–195, 1990.

176. Heros RC, Ojeman RG, Crowell RM: Superior temporal gyrus approach to middle cerebral artery aneurysms: Technique and results. *Neurosurgery* 10:308–313, 1982.

177. VanderArk GD, Kempe LG, Smith DR: Anterior communicating aneurysms: The gyrus rectus approach. *Clin Neurosurg* 21:120–133, 1974.

178. Ogawa A, Suzuki M, Sakurai Y, Yoshimoto T: Vascular anomalies associated with aneurysms of the anterior communicating artery: Microsurgical observations. *J Neurosurg* 72:706–709, 1990.

179. Suziki J, Mizoi K, Yoshimoto T: Bifrontal interhemispheric approach to aneurysms of the anterior communicating artery. *J Neurosurg* 64:183–190, 1986.

180. Wisoff JH, Flamm ES: Aneurysms of the distal anterior cerebral artery and associated vascular anomalies. *Neurosurgery* 20:735–741, 1987.

181. Ohno K, Monma S, Suzuki R, et al: Saccular aneurysms of the distal anterior cerebral artery. *Neurosurgery* 27:907–913, 1990.

182. Yasargil MG, Carter LP: Saccular aneurysms of the distal anterior cerebral artery. *J Neurosurg* 39:218–223, 1974.

183. Yoshimoto T, Uchida K, Suzuki J: Surgical treatment of distal anterior cerebral artery aneurysms. *J Neurosurg* 50:40–44, 1979.

184. Ellenbogen RG, Scott RM: Transfalcine approach to a callosomarginal artery aneurysm. *Neurosurgery* 29:140–143, 1991.

185. Dickey PS, Bloomgarden GM, Arkins TJ, Spencer DD: Partial callosal resection for pericallosal aneurysms. *Neurosurgery* 30:136–137, 1992.

186. Drake CG: The treatment of aneurysms of the posterior circulation. *Clin Neurosurg* 26:96–144, 1979.

187. Yasargil MG, Antic J, Laciga R, et al: Microsurgical pterional approach to aneurysms of the basilar bifurcation. *Surg Neurol* 6:83–96, 1976.

188. Kobayashi S, Sugita K, Nakagawa F: An approach to a basilar aneurysm above the bifurcation of the internal carotid artery: Case report. *J Neurosurg* 59:1082–1084, 1983.

189. Sugita K, Kobayashi S, Shintani A, Mutsuga N: Microneurosurgery for aneurysms of the basilar artery. *J Neurosurg* 51:615–620, 1979.

190. Fujitsu K, Kuwabara T: Zygomatic approach for lesions in the interpeduncular cistern. *J Neurosurg* 62:340–343, 1985.

191. Samii M, Ammirati M: The combined supra-infratentorial pre-sigmoid sinus avenue to the petro-clival region. Surgical technique and clinical applications. *Acta Neurochirurg* 95:6–12, 1988.

192. Heros RC: Lateral suboccipital approach for vertebral and vertebrobasilar artery lesions. *J Neurosurg* 64:559–562, 1986.

193. George B, Dematons C, Cophignon J: Lateral approach to the anterior portion of the foramen magnum: Application to surgical removal of 14 benign tumors: technical note. *Surg Neurol* 29:484–490, 1988.

194. Sen CN, Sekhar LN: An extreme lateral approach to intradural lesions of the cervical spine and foramen magnum. *Neurosurgery* 27:197–204, 1990.

195. Spetzler RF, Grahm TW: The far-lateral approach to the inferior clivus and the upper cervical region: Technical note: *BNI Quarterly* 6:25–38, 1990.

196. Bertalanffy H, Seeger W: The dorsolateral, suboccipital, transcondylar approach to the lower clivus, and anterior portion of the craniocervical junction. *Neurosurgery* 29:815–821, 1991.

197. Yasu N, Suzuki A, Ohta H, et al: Pitfalls in aneurysm surgery—management of aneurysm rupture, in Auer LM (ed): *Timing of Aneurysm Surgery,* Berlin/New York, Walter de Gruyter, 1985, pp 349–355.

198. Batjer H, Samson D: Intraoperative aneurysmal rupture: Incidence, outcome, and suggestions for surgical management. *Neurosurgery* 18:701–707, 1986.

199. Michenfelder JD: Cerebral preservation for intraoperative focal ischemia. *Clin Neurosurg* 32:105–113, 1985.

200. Michenfelder JD, Milde JH: Failure of prolonged hypocapnia, hypothermia, or hypertension to favorably alter acute stroke in primates. *Stroke* 8:87–91, 1977.

201. Little JR: Modification of acute focal ischemia by treatment with mannitol. *Stroke* 9:4–9, 1978.

202. Nehls DG, Todd MM, Spetzler RF, et al: A comparison of the protective effects of isoflurane and barbiturates in a primate model of temporary cerebral ischemia. *Anesthesiology* 66:453–464, 1987.

203. Suzuki J: New brain protective agents and clinical use, in Suzuki J (ed): *Advances in Surgery for Cerebral Stroke.* Tokyo: Springer, 1988.

204. Ausman JI, Diaz FG, Malik GM, et al: Management of cerebral aneurysms: Further facts and additional myths. *Surg Neurol* 32:21–35, 1989.

205. Newberg LA, Milde JH, Michenfelder JD: The cerebral metabolic effects of isoflurane at and above concentrations that suppress the electroencephalogram. *Anesthesiology* 59:23–28, 1983.

206. Meyer FB, Muzzi DA: Cerebral protection during aneurysm surgery with isoflurane anesthesia: Technical note: *J Neurosurg* 76:541–543, 1992.

207. Pierce EC, Jr, Lambertsen CJ, Deutsch S, et al: Cerebral circulation and metabolism during thiopental anesthesia and hyperventilation in man. *J Clin Invest* 41:1664–1671, 1962.

208. Michenfelder JD, Milde JH: Influence of anesthetics on metabolic, functional, and pathological responses to regional cerebral ischemia. *Stroke* 6:405–410, 1975.

209. Branston NM, Hope DT, Symon L: Barbiturates in focal ischemia of primate cortex: Effects on blood flow distribution, evoked potential and extracellular potassium. *Stroke* 10:647–653, 1979.

210. Majewska MD, Strosznajder J, Lazarewicz J: Effect of ischemic anoxia and barbiturate anesthesia on free radical oxidation of mitochondrial phospholipids. *Brain Res* 158:423–434, 1978.

211. Selman WR, Spetzler RF: Therapeutics for focal cerebral ischemia. *Neurosurgery* 6:446–452, 1980.

212. Spetzler RF, Selman WR, Roski RA, Bonstelle C: Cerebral revascularization during barbiturate coma in primates and humans. *Surg Neurol* 17:111–115, 1982.

213. Silverberg GD, Reitz BA, Ream AK: Hypothermia and cardiac arrest in the treatment of giant aneurysms of the cerebral circulation and hemangioblastoma of the medulla. *J Neurosurg* 55:337–346, 1981.

214. Spetzler RF, Hadley MN, Rigamonti D, et al: Aneurysms of the basilar artery treated with circulatory arrest, hypothermia, and barbiturate cerebral protection. *J Neurosurg* 68:868–879, 1988.

215. Michenfelder JD, Kirklin JW, Uihlein A, et al: Clinical experience with a closed-chest method of producing hypothermia and total circulatory arrest in neurosurgery. *Ann Surg* 159:125–131, 1964.

216. Chyatte D, Elefteriades J, Kim B: Profound hypothermia and circulatory arrest for aneurysm surgery: Case report. *J Neurosurg* 70:489–491, 1989.

217. Drake CG, Barr HWK, Coles JC, Gergely NF: The use of extracorporeal circulation and profound hypothermia in the treatment of ruptured intracranial aneurysm. *J Neurosurg* 21:575–581, 1964.

218. Kirklin JF, Chenoweth DE, Naftel DC, et al: Effects of protamine administration after cardiopulmonary bypass on compliment, blood elements, and the hemodynamic state. *Ann Thorac Surg* 41:193–199, 1986.

219. Bering EA, Jr: Effects of profound hypothermia and circulatory arrest on cerebral oxygen metabolism and cerebralspinal fluid electrolyte composition in dogs. *J Neurosurg* 39:199–205, 1974.

220. Hosobuchi Y: Direct surgical treatment of giant intracranial aneurysms. *J Neurosurg* 51:743–756, 1979.

221. Drake CG. Giant intracranial aneurysms: Experience with surgical treatment in 174 patients. *Clin Neurosurg* 26:12–95, 1979.

222. Ausman JI, Diaz FG, Sadasivan B, et al: Giant intracranial aneurysm surgery: The role of microvascular reconstruction. *Surg Neurol* 34:8–15, 1990.

223. Gelber BR, Sundt TM Jr: Treatment of intracavernous and giant carotid aneurysms by combined internal carotid ligation and extra- to intracranial bypass. *J Neurosurg* 52:1–10, 1980.

224. Samson DS, Neuwalt EA, Beyer CW, Ditmore QM: Failure of extracranial-intracranial arterial bypass in acute middle cerebral artery occlusion: Case report. *Neurosurgery* 6:185–188, 1980.

225. Sundt TM, Jr, Piepgras DG: Surgical approach to giant intracranial aneurysms: Operative experience with 80 cases. *J Neurosurg* 51:731–742, 1979.

226. Ojemann RG, Heros RC, Crowell RM: Giant aneurysms, in Ojemann RG, Heros RC, Crowell RM (eds): *Surgical Management of Cerebral Vascular Disease,* 2d ed. Baltimore, Williams & Wilkins, 1988, chap 20, pp 297–336.

227. Hylton PD, Reichman OH: Endaneurysmal microendarterectomy in the treatment of giant cerebral aneurysms: Technical note. *Neurosurgery* 23:674–679, 1988.

228. Dolenc V: Direct microsurgical repair of intracavernous vascular lesions. *J Neurosurg* 58:824–831, 1983.

229. Dolenc V: A combined epi- and subdural direct approach to carotid-ophthalmic artery aneurysms. *J Neurosurg* 62:667–672, 1985.

230. Morota N, Ohtsuka A, Kameyama S, et al: Obstructive hydrocephalus due to a giant aneurysm of the internal carotid bifurcation. *Surg Neurol* 29:227–231, 1988.

231. Hopkins LN, Budny JL, Castellani D: Extracranial-intracranial arterial bypass and basilar artery ligation in the treatment of giant basilar artery aneurysms. *Neurosurg* 13:189–194, 1983.

232. Beck DW, Boarini DJ, Kassell NF: Surgical treatment of giant aneurysm of the vertebral-basilar junction. *Surg Neurol* 12:283–285, 1979.

233. Sugita K, Kobayashi S, Takemae T, et al: *J Neurosurg* 68:960–966, 1988.

234. Heros RC: Lateral suboccipital approach for vertebral and vertebrobasilar artery lesions. *J Neurosurg* 64:559–562, 1986.

235. Tognetti F, Andreoli A, Testa C: Giant fusiform aneurysm of

the middle cerebral artery treated with extracranial-intracranial arterial bypass and Drake tourniquet. *Surg Neurol* 22:33–35, 1984.

236. Belec L, Cesaro P, Brugieres P, Gray F: Tumor-simulating giant serpentine aneurysm of the posterior cerebral artery. *Surg Neurol* 29:210–215, 1988.

237. Kunabe T, Kaneko U, Ishibashi T, et al: Two cases of giant serpentine aneurysm. *Neurosurgery* 26:1027–1033, 1990.

238. Heros RC, Kolluri S: Giant intracranial aneurysms presenting with massive cerebral edema. *Neurosurgery* 15:572–577, 1984.

239. Fuji K, Fukui M, Matsubara T, et al: Microsurgical procedures for management of giant middle cerebral aneurysm causing increased intracranial pressure. *Surg Neurol* 32:366–371, 1989.

240. Bederson JB, Spetzler RF: Anastomosis of the anterior temporal artery to a secondary trunk of the middle cerebral artery for treatment of a giant M_1 segment aneurysm. *J Neurosurg* 76:863–866, 1992.

241. Bojanowski WM, Spetzler RF, Carter LP: Reconstruction of the MCA bifurcation after excision of a giant aneurysm. *J Neurosurg* 68:974–977, 1988.

242. Teal JS, Bergeron RT, Rumbaugh CL, Segall HD: Aneurysms of the petrous or cavernous portions of the internal carotid artery associated with nonpenetrating head trauma. *J Neurosurg* 38:568–574, 1973.

243. Aarabi B: Traumatic aneurysms of the brain due to high-velocity missle head wounds. *Neurosurgery* 22:1056–1063, 1988.

244. Haddad FS, Haddad GF, Taha J: Traumatic intracranial aneurysms caused by missiles: Their presentation and management. *Neurosurgery* 28:1–7, 1991.

245. Cosgrove GR, Villemure JG, Melancon D: Traumatic intracranial aneurysm due to arterial injury at surgery. *J Neurosurg* 58:291–294, 1983.

246. Parkinson D, West M: Traumatic intracranial aneurysms. *J Neurosurg* 52:11–20, 1980.

247. Buckingham MJ, Crone KR, Ball WS, et al: Traumatic intracranial aneurysms in childhood: Two cases and a review of the literature. *Neurosurgery* 22:398–408, 1988.

248. Bannerman RM, Ingall GB, Graf CJ: The familial occurrence of intracranial aneurysms. *Neurology* 20:283–292, 1970.

249. Hashimoto I: Familial intracranial aneurysms and cerebral vascular anomalies. *J Neurosurg* 46:419–427, 1977.

250. Norrgard O, Angquist KA, Fodstad H, et al: Intracranial aneurysms and heredity. *Neurosurgery* 20:236–239, 1987.

251. Rubinsk MK, Cohen NH: Ehlers-Danlos syndrome associated with multiple intracranial aneurysms. *Neurology* 14:125–132, 1964.

252. Muhonen MG, Godersky JC, VanGilder JC: Cerebral aneurysms associated with neurofibromatosis. *Surg Neurol* 36:470–475, 1991.

253. Chapman AB, Rubinstein D, Hughes R, et al: Intracranial aneurysms in autosomal dominant polycystic kidney disease. *N Eng J Med* 327:916–920, 1992.

254. Schievink WI, Limberg M, Dreissen JJR, et al: Screening for unruptured familial intracranial aneurysms: Subarachnoid hemorrhage 2 years after angiography negative for aneurysms. *Neurosurgery* 29:434–438, 1991.

255. Dias MS, Sekhar LN: Intracranial hemorrhage from aneurysms and arteriovenous malformations during pregnancy and the puerperium. *Neurosurgery* 27:855–866, 1990.

256. Robinson JL, Hall CS, Sedzimir CB: Arteriovenous malformations, aneurysms, and pregnancy. *J Neurosurg* 41:63–70, 1974.

257. Uchide K, Terada S, Akasofu K, Higashi S: Cerebral arteriovenous malformations in a pregnancy with twins: Case report. *Neurosurgery* 31:780–782, 1992.

258. Horton JC, Chambers WA, Lyons SL, et al: Pregnancy and the risk of hemorrhage from cerebral arteriovenous malformations. *Neurosurgery* 27:867–872, 1990.

259. Ostergaard JR, Volby B: Intracranial arterial aneurysms in children and adolescents. *J Neurosurg* 58:832–837, 1983.

260. Lipper S, Morgan D, Krigman MR, Staab EV: Congenital saccular aneurysm in a 19-day-old neonate: Case report and review of the literature. *Surg Neurol* 10:161–165, 1978.

261. Cedzich C, Schramm J, Rockelein G: Multiple middle cerebral artery aneurysms in an infant: Case report. *J Neurosurg* 72:806–809, 1990.

262. Meyer FB, Sundt TM, Jr, Fode NC, et al: Cerebral aneurysms in childhood and adolescence. *J Neurosurg* 70:420–425, 1989.

263. Lansen TA, Kasoff SS, Arguelles JH: Giant pediatric aneurysm treated with ligation of the middle cerebral artery with the Drake tourniquet and extracranial-intracranial bypass. *Neurosurgery* 25:81–85, 1989.

264. Bohmfalk GL, Story JL, Wissinger JP, Brown WE, Jr: Bacterial intracranial aneurysm. *J Neurosurg* 48:369–382, 1978.

265. Molinari GF, Smith L, Goldstein MN, et al: Pathogenesis of cerebral myocotic aneurysms. *Neurology* 23:325–332, 1972.

266. Piotrowski WP, Pilz P, Chuang I-H: Subarachnoid hemorrhage caused by a fungal aneurysm of the vertebral artery as a complication of intracranial aneurysm clipping: Case report. *J Neurosurg* 73:962–964, 1990.

267. Mielke B, Weir B, Oldring D, von Westarp C: Fungal aneurysm: Case report and review of the literature. *Neurosurgery* 9:578–582, 1981.

268. Bingham WF: Treatment of mycotic intracranial aneurysms. *J Neurosurg* 46:428–437, 1977.

269. Day AL: Extracranial-intracranial bypass grafting in the surgical treatment of bacterial aneurysms: Report of two cases. *Neurosurgery* 9:583–588, 1981.

270. Heiskanen O: Risk of bleeding from unruptured aneurysm in cases with multiple intracranial aneurysms. *J Neurosurg* 55:524–526, 1981.

271. Batjer H, Suss RA, Samson D: Intracranial arteriovenous malformations associated with aneurysms. *Neurosurgery* 18:29–35, 1986.

272. Brown RD, Jr, Wiebers DO, Forbes GS: Unruptured intracranial aneurysms and arteriovenous malformations: Frequency of intracranial hemorrhage and relationship of lesions. *J Neurosurg* 73:859–863, 1990.

273. Cuna E, Sa MJ, Stein BM, Solomon RA, McCormick PC: The treatment of associated aneurysms and arteriovenous malformations. *J Neurosurg* 77:853–859, 1992.

274. Denton IC, Jr, Gutmann L: Surgical treatment of symptomatic carotid stenosis and asymptomatic ipsilateral intracranial aneurysm: Case report. *J Neurosurg* 38:662–665, 1973.

☐ STUDY QUESTIONS

I. A 28-year-old female screams out with a headache while in the bathroom. When the door is opened, she is found lying on the floor, responding only to painful stimuli. She is taken to the emergency room. While on the way she awakens and complains of a severe headache. She is nauseated and vomits twice. On examination she is still drowsy and has a stiff neck but is otherwise neurologically normal.

1. What is the most likely cause of the headache? **2.** What diagnoses should be considered? **3.** What ways might one consider finding proof of an intracranial hemorrhage? **4.** What is the most likely explanation for the loss of consciousness? **5.** Once a subarachnoid hemorrhage is proved, what can be done to determine the cause?

II. A 10-year-old female is taken to the emergency room because of severe headache of sudden onset, nausea, and vomiting. She has nuchael rigidity, and she is agitated but otherwise normal. A noncontrasted CT reveals SAH.

1. What diagnoses should be entertained? **2.** What might be accomplished with the CT to determine the specific cause of the hemorrhage? **3.** What features of the noncontrasted CT might indicate the specific lesion? **4.** Assuming there is indication of hemorrhage from an aneurysm and no evidence of a vascular malformation, what other diagnoses should be considered? **5.** How should an aneurysm be treated?

III. A 30-year-old male experiences a severe SAH and remains drowsy for a couple of days at a small local hospital, after which he is transferred to a neurosurgical unit where, on angiography, he is found to have an anterior communicating artery aneurysm with severe vasospasm. At the termination of the angiogram he becomes more stuporous. This occurs 3 days after the initial ictus.

1. What is the most likely cause of the increasing stupor? **2.** What other possibilities might be considered? **3.** Assuming vasospasm is the proven cause of the stupor, what courses might be considered? **4.** How would the surgical risk be affected by the vasospasm? **5.** Assuming the aneurysm was clipped before the onset of vasospasm, how might the vasospasm be treated?

IV. A 36-year-old male has an acute onset of severe headache from which he recovers within 3 days. In the meantime, a CT reveals a small amount of SAH in the basal cisterns. A contrasted CT scan fails to demonstrate a lesion. A four-vessel angiogram likewise fails to demonstrate a lesion.

1. What further procedures might be considered? **2.** Assuming a repeat angiogram 2 weeks later along with a myelogram are normal, how should the patient be treated? **3.** Why should one consider doing a myelogram? **4.** Why might a late angiogram show an aneurysm not shown on the original study? **5.** What other causes of SAH might be considered?

V. A 48-year-old female is admitted with stupor coming on 3 days after a severe headache. A CT reveals blood between the hemispheres along both sylvian fissures and throughout the ventricular system.

1. Where is the most likely site of an aneurysm? **2.** How might the blood have found its way into the ventricular system? **3.** When would be the optimum time for clipping such an aneurysm? **4.** What would be an alternate means of treating such an aneurysm assuming there was no neck? **5.** When are the optimum times for clipping aneurysms, assuming they are seen at the time of the initial ictus?

CHAPTER
16

Diagnosis and Treatment of Arteriovenous Malformations of the Brain and Spinal Cord

Dennis E. McDonnell
Marshall B. Allen, Jr.

Vascular malformations are the second most common cause for spontaneous subarachnoid hemorrhage.[1] They are the most common cause of subarachnoid hemorrhage in children. In addition, intracranial malformations are associated with seizures in a high percentage of cases, and both intracranial and intraspinal malformations are responsible for serious neurological deficits which may be the result of the "steal" phenomenon, pressure by the mass of the malformation or increased venous pressure resulting in decreased perfusion of the neural tissues. Death may result from intracranial hemorrhage, or even cardiac failure, due to shunting of blood in infants and, occasionally, older persons.

☐ INTRACRANIAL VASCULAR MALFORMATIONS

Arteriovenous malformations (AVMs) are congenital vascular hamartomas forming direct connections between cerebral arterial and venous channels, bypassing the normal capillaries. They arise early (3-week gestation) with the development of primitive vessels. Arrest in development results in direct arterial to venous communications without intervening capillary beds.[2]

McCormick has classified vascular malformations of the brain into four categories: AVMs, cavernous malformations,

venous malformations, and telangiectasias.[3,4] A recent review of cases has led to the recommendation that cavernous malformations and capillary telangiectasias represent the extremes of one group.[5] There are also dural arteriovenous shunts and carotid-cavernous fistulae that occur spontaneously or result from trauma.

Clinically, AVMs are the most frequently recognized vascular malformation, and are composed of a central angiomatous nidus supplied by varying numbers of feeding arteries and draining veins. Inside the malformation are often cavernous channels that cannot be classified as arteries or veins (Fig. 16-1). Evidence of hemorrhage with macrophages and neuronal loss, as well as ischemia, may be present in the adjacent parenchyma.[6] Many vessels have thick hyalinized walls and they may spontaneously thrombose. The presence of elastica in the walls of vessels is variable (Fig. 16-2).

The vessels are focused on a nidus, which may be restricted to cortical areas, or more commonly they form a "pyramid" in the white matter with the apex directed toward the lateral ventricle. The nidus consists of numerous thin-walled, tortuous channels with poorly developed elastica and muscularis (Fig. 16-2). When the lesion projects into the ventricle, the protruding ventricular vessels are covered only by thin ependyma. This may explain the tendency for intraventricular hemorrhage.

Cerebral malformations are most commonly fed by

311

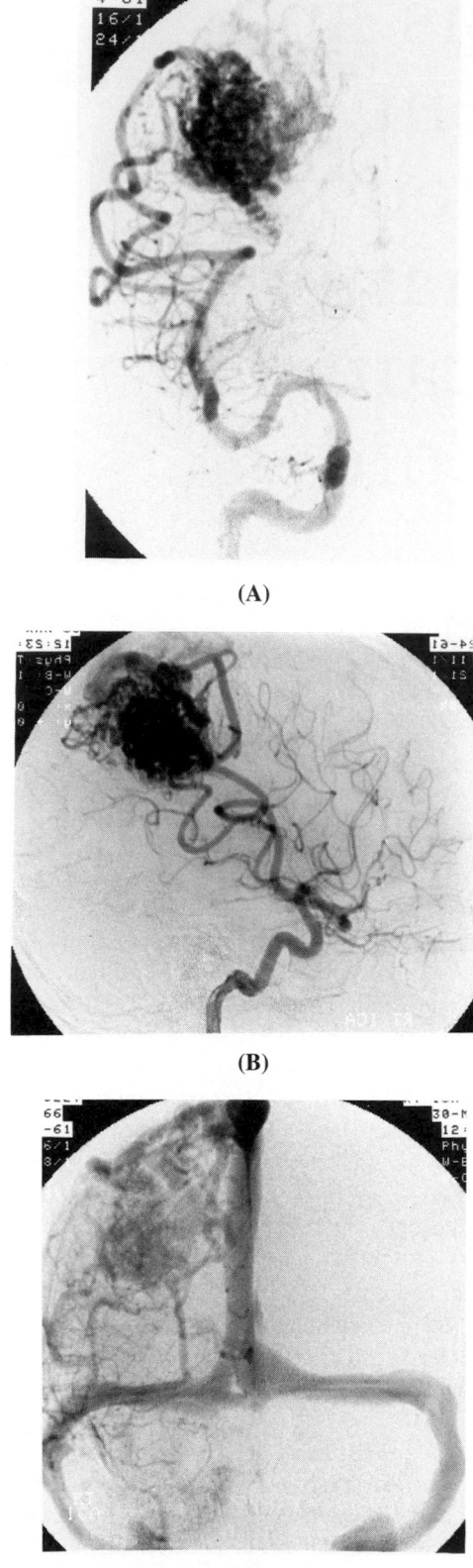

(A)

(B)

(C)

Figure 16–1 Digital right parietal arteriogram showing an arteriovenous malformation in a 32-year-old female with intractable headaches. There was no history of hemorrhage. The frontal *(A)* and lateral *(B)* views of the arterial phase of the right carotid arteriogram outline, feeding branches of the middle cerebral artery. The right anterior cerebral artery is not visualized. The frontal *(C)* venous phase of the angiogram demonstrates drainage into the superior and transverse sinuses.

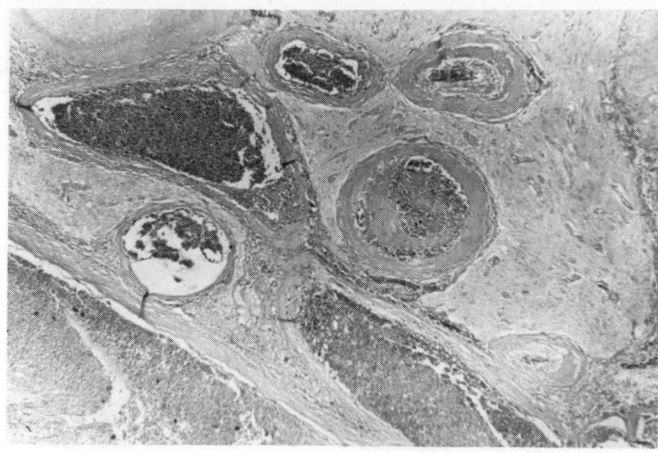

Figure 16–2 Microscopic view of an arteriovenous malformation of the cerebrum. There is an admixture of thick-walled arteries and veins and arterialized veins making up this vascular malformation, which is the most common. The entrapped brain matter among the vessels is typical of these AVMs.

branches of the middle cerebral artery, followed in order by the anterior and posterior cerebral arteries. Arterial feeders may run a serpentine course through sulci before entering the nidus of the malformation. In most cases, neural tissue within the confines of the malformation is gliotic and nonfunctional. AVMs may be diffuse, with normal-appearing parenchyma between the vascular channels.[7] These lesions follow the spectrum of cerebral AVMs and are more difficult to remove totally because they tend to be large and complex. They present in the older pediatric group, with a mean age of 18.5 years, and they represent a high risk. AVMs of the anterior and posterior cerebral arteries may drain directly into the vein of Galen, causing it to dilate in an aneurysmal fashion.

The incidence of AVMs in the general population is not clear. McCormick reported an incidence of about 1/2 percent in a consecutive autopsy series of nearly 6000.[4] Symptomatic vascular malfunctions are about one tenth as common as aneurysms, with only 2000 new cases diagnosed in the United States each year.[8]

Multiple AVMs have been reported rarely; their discovery may require very careful scrutiny of the complete cerebral angiogram. Surgical removal of one lesion may be followed by hemorrhage from another previously unruptured AVM.[9]

CLINICAL PRESENTATION

Hemorrhage and seizures are the most-common clinical presentations of AVMs. These clinical presentations occur with about equal frequency, although the mean age for seizures is slightly younger than that of hemorrhage. Seizures usually have a focal component.

Hemorrhages are generally intraparenchymal but may extend into the subarachnoid space. Initial hemorrhages are usually less devastating than hemorrhage from aneurysms. The mortality from hemorrhage is much lower than for aneurysm, and early-repeat hemorrhage is also less frequent in AVMs.[10] AVMs are the most-common cause of spontaneous subarachnoid hemorrhage in children.

Recurrences are infrequent, usually months to years apart, but, frequently, there is progressive deterioration. Recurrent hemorrhages reportedly occur, about 2 to 3 percent per year. Progressive neurological deterioration may occur even in the absence of hemorrhage and is thought to result from relative ischemia in regions around the lesion owing to steal of blood flow. Some surgeons believe that asymptomatic hemorrhages occur more frequently. These may be reasons for aggressive therapy.

Headaches, typical of migraine but lateralized to the side of the lesion, frequently accompany vascular malformations. Rarely, AVMs reportedly present with intermittent headache, obscuration of vision, and papilledema (symptoms and signs of intracranial hypertension). These changes occur without hemorrhage or hydrocephalus and are compatible with pseudotumor cerebri. This has been attributed to highly elevated dural sinus pressure, transmitted to the draining cortical veins. Elevated dural sinus pressure can interfere with CSF absorption through arachnoid villi. Increased blood volume and hormonal factors related to estrogens may be involved in this process. The pseudotumor phenomenon resolves after AVM removal.[11]

NATURAL HISTORY

There is limited information on the natural history of untreated patients with AVMs. This, along with the variability of features and behavior of such lesions, makes it difficult to assess their natural history. Troupp has reported that of 134 patients with an average follow up of 12 years, only one-fourth were normal; one-fourth were disabled, and close to one-third were deceased.[12] Svien's series of 95 patients showed that 50 percent had hemorrhaged, and 25 percent had either died or were disabled, but 68 percent lived "normal lives."[13] Ondra reviewed Troupp's series after 24 years of follow up and determined that the overall mortality from hemorrhage was 23 percent, the annual rate of major repeat hemorrhage was 4 percent, and the combined major morbidity and mortality was 2.7 percent per year.[14]

The mortality rate from the first hemorrhage of an AVM is 10 percent, for the second hemorrhage it is 13 percent, and for subsequent hemorrhages, the mortality ranges from 20 to 40 percent.[15,16] A recent series showed overall good outcome in 74 percent of patients. Children under the age of 15 years had a better prognosis.[17] Characteristics that potentiate hemorrhage are small size, location, and high hemodynamic resistance.[18] Another series of 168 patients with unruptured AVMs ultimately showed a hemorrhage rate of 18 percent, occurring at 2.2 percent per year. Death from rupture was 29 percent, and 23 percent of survivors were impaired.[15] With these figures, practice in recent years has been to treat the majority of such lesions surgically, where feasible, often in conjunction with embolization. Elective surgical resection is

justified in many patients before hemorrhage from the AVM occurs, particularly in young patients where the AVM has a favorable location, size, and venous drainage. Models have been described to assist in risk assessment and decision making for elective surgical removal of unruptured cerebral AVMs.[19,20]

A rare and poorly understood aspect of natural history for intracranial AVMs is the potential for spontaneous regression. Three females with medium- to large-size lesions, each supplied by a single feeding artery and drained principally through a single vein, thrombosed spontaneously.[21] Usually, when regression occurs, there are associated factors such as hemorrhage, surgery, radiation treatment, or a thrombotic event heralded by new neurological deficits. The most-common factor associated with this phenomenon is hemorrhage within the lesion. Some had an associated aneurysm, suggesting vascular flow strain, but this may be incidental and unrelated to resolution of the AVM.[22] A series of patients with AVMs followed angiographically over many years was found to have 20 percent that enlarged, 20 percent that decreased in size, 20 percent that totally resolved, and 40 percent that remained unchanged; the time span ranged from 5 to 28 years (median, 15 years).[23] There was a 35 percent recurrence of hemorrhage in this series. Enlargement tended to occur in younger patients, and regression tended to occur in the older patients. Another prominent feature of regression was the presence of a single major feeding vessel. The smaller lesions were the ones that tended to regress. On the other hand, a very large lesion resolved after massive hemorrhage.[24] Some of the mechanisms that have been postulated in the involutional process of AVMs have been hemorrhage and clot compression, vasospasm, thromboembolism from aneurysms, hypercoagulability, and progressive vascular fibrosis. It must be emphasized that spontaneous resolution of an AVM is rare. Over the course of time an AVM tends to bleed, cause focal cerebral ischemia, and produce neurological impairment.

DIAGNOSTIC TECHNIQUES

The computerized tomographic scan (CT) may be the first study that demonstrates an AVM. When there is hemorrhage, the location of a lobar hematoma or intraventricular hematoma may be the first clue of rupture.[25] In the absence of hemorrhage, AVMs are suggested by contrast-enhanced CT that demonstrates the lesion without mass effect. CT scans are performed initially without and then with contrast media, and the two studies are compared for retention of contrast within the lesion.

Usually the AVM is not detected on the noncontrasted CT. A noncontrasted CT scan demonstrates evidence of cerebral atrophy, subarachnoid blood, and intracerebral hemorrhage. A repeat scan after the injection of intravenous contrast media demonstrates the extent of the lesion and outlines vessels that might be difficult to differentiate from

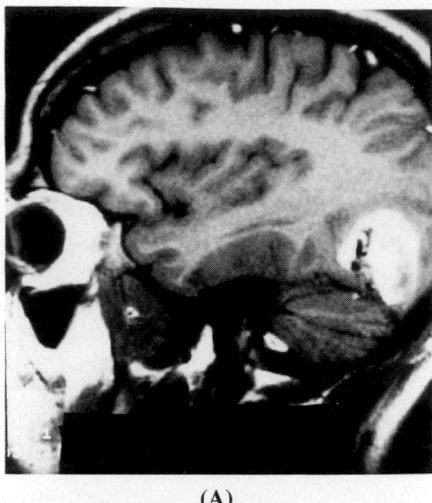

(A)

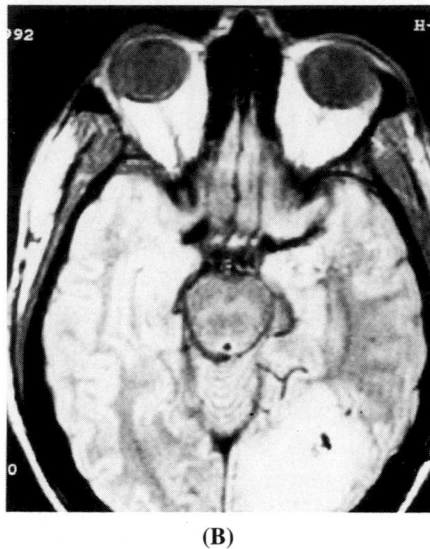

(B)

Figure 16–3 Arteriovenous malformation of the left posterior temporo-occipital area fed by a branch of the posterior cerebral artery. The malformation is seen in the sagittal *(A)* and axial *(B)* views of the MRI. Images are T1 weighted. Recent hemorrhage and the flow void of patent abnormal blood vessels are evident.

hematoma unless one is able to compare the contrasted scan with one made before contrast was injected.

Magnetic resonance imaging (MRI) is a valuable supplement to CT and angiography. It demonstrates the nidus of the lesion and its relationship to arterial, venous, parenchymal, and cerebral topographical structures. The nidus has a "honeycomb" appearance, and its relationship to feeding arteries and draining veins is imaged by MRI. Even small AVMs are detected by MRI (Fig. 16-3). The morphology and volumetric extent of the AVM, along with tortuous tubular arteries and serpiginous veins, are readily detected by MRI.[26] In the presence of hemosiderin, the signal also may give evidence of previous hemorrhage. MRI angiography further defines these lesions and some of their flow characteristics.

Angiography is the diagnostic procedure that provides the most-precise information required for determining whether

surgery is reasonable and the appropriate techniques to be employed. The nidus of the malformation, the origins and courses of the arterial feeders, and the size and locations of the draining veins must be identified. Location of individual feeding vessels is possible by detailed angiography. A balloon catheter can be used to block noncontributing vessels. It is during the course of detailed angiography that embolization of feeding vessels may be accomplished. Feeding vessels may be occluded by embolization, thereby reducing the shunt flow (Fig. 16-4). Multiple substances have been used. Polyvinyl alcohol or gelfoam particles in a slurry may be directed into the nidus with the use of balloon catheters. Generally, embolization is considered a technique for reducing the blood flow for an AVM as an adjunct to surgical excision, the maximal effects occurring over several days.[27,28]

Transcranial Doppler ultrasound permits noninvasive documentation of blood flow velocities through the major cerebral arteries. Normally, there is essentially no variation in time–mean value and pulsatility of the velocity spectrum

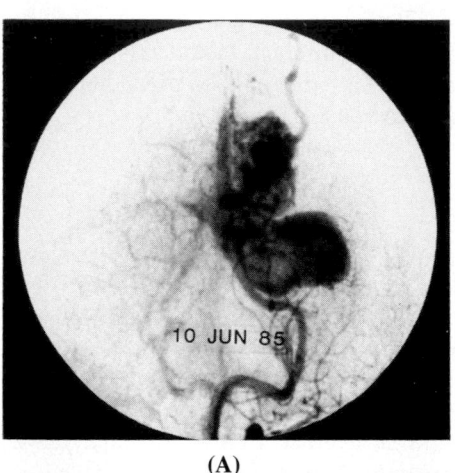

(A)

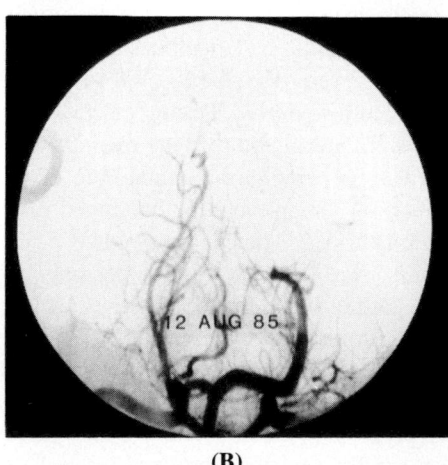

(B)

Figure 16–4 Digital angiogram of a "high-flow" AVM of the medial left parietal lobe fed by the posterior cerebral artery embolized preoperatively with bucrylate. A frontal view before *(A)* and after *(B)* embolization is shown. This malformation had bled before embolization and the patient had a right homonymous hemianopsia. The AVM was almost obliterated by the embolization.

that are measured in different basal cerebral arteries in the same patient. Usually, identical hemodynamic conditions occur in different regions of the normal brain as a reflection of cerebrovascular autoregulation. In response to reduced inflow pressures, cerebral autoregulation maintains blood flow by lowering cerebrovascular resistance. Usually, there is a wide range of flow velocities in the basal arteries.[29] In AVMs, the resistance of flow is low compared to cerebrovascular resistance under normal conditions. Therefore, there is increased bulk flow through arteries feeding an AVM. Reactivity of cerebral and AVM feeding arteries can be tested by comparing velocity flow changes with changes induced by PCO_2 within the vessels as a means of identifying feeding arteries to an AVM, which are relatively nonreactive. Flow velocities can be related to flow volumes. Also chronically low perfusion pressure in areas of normal brain is evidence of steal and predicts postoperative brain swelling.[30] Assessment of flow characteristics of an AVM by transcranial Doppler gives preoperative hemodynamic insights into individual AVMs that may aid in safer removal of such lesions. Real-time evaluations by Doppler are helpful in identifying surface-feeding arteries and veins intraoperatively.[31]

GRADING SYSTEMS

It is important to advise patients of the risk-benefit ratio when advocating treatment of an AVM, whether it be embolization, surgical excision, radiosurgery, or no treatment. Grading systems have been devised to standardize parameters of arterial supply, size, location, and venous drainage so that morbidity and mortality can be statistically estimated for the individual patient.[32,33] The system assessing size, location, and venous drainage proposed by Spetzler and Martin is presently the most popular. It comprises six grades, and each grade incorporates the three parameters of size, location, and venous drainage.[33] The size of the AVM is measured as the largest diameter of the nidus indicated by the angiogram. The location is factored according to adjacent cerebral function and "eloquence." Location is a factor when the AVM is in sensorimotor, language, or visual cortex; the diencephalon; the internal capsule; the brainstem; or deep cerebellum. Venous drainage is factored when the deep galenic venous system is part of the AVM drainage (see Table 16-1). Surgical morbidity is a significant factor in grades III and higher. Surgical mortality is a factor in grade V lesions, and grade VI lesions are considered inoperable. Preoperative embolization and staged surgical excision reduce the risks of surgical excision; in effect, they may reduce the grade.[34,35]

SPECIFIC LOCATIONS

Eloquent cortical areas such as sensorimotor cortex in the posterior frontal region, speech areas of the frontal and

Table 16–1
DETERMINING FACTORS FOR GRADING ARTERIOVENOUS MALFORMATIONS*

Factor	Point Weight
AVM Size	
Small <3 cm	1
Medium 3–6 cm	2
Large >6 cm	3
Functional Eloquence of Location	
Noneloquent	0
Eloquent	1
Venous Drainage Complex	
Surface cortical only	0
Deep or galenic component	1

*Total grade score = sum of 3 factors: 1 through 5.

temporal lobes, and visual cortex of the calcarine occipital lobe present additional challenge and risk when involved by AVMs. Other areas of concern require special consideration as well. Such regions as the striatum, thalamus, brainstem, and cerebellum present exceptions to grading systems and will be discussed separately. These locations inherently present greater risk of morbidity and may be more amenable to radiosurgery than formal surgical resection. Nevertheless, lesions in these locations are amenable to surgical removal under restricted circumstances, and they will be individually discussed.

Striatum and Thalamus AVMs in the striatum comprise 8 to 18 percent of all AVMs, and surgical excisions are reported (Fig. 16-5).[36,37] The morbidity involved with surgical excision is formidable: hemiplegia, aphasia, hemianopsia, memory impairment, and hydrocephalus. However, these deficits are part of the natural course of lesions that hemorrhage into the basal ganglia and internal capsule. Intraventricular hemorrhage is also common with such lesions. Usually, the arterial supply is through lenticulostriate branches from the proximal middle cerebral artery, the anterior choroidal artery, cortical branches from middle cerebral and anterior cerebral arteries, the recurrent artery of Heubner, and the posterior choroidal artery. They usually drain through the thalamostriate vein and basal vein of Rosenthal into the galenic system. The surgical approach involves opening of the sylvian fissure and microsurgical isolation of the perforating vessels that feed the malformation.[38] The lateral ventricle is opened and the lesion excised including the choroid plexus, which carries the deep arterial supply to the nidus. A mortality of 6 percent and increased deficits were described in a series of 16 cases.[39] Profound neurological deficits can resolve if the surrounding parenchyma is preserved, owing to the rich collateral supply that naturally accompanies AVMs.[40] One should embark on surgical excision of lesions in this region with extreme caution because of the formidable risk. Microsurgical technique is mandatory. AVMs can be approached from a variety of directions: transfrontal-transventricular, transcallosal-

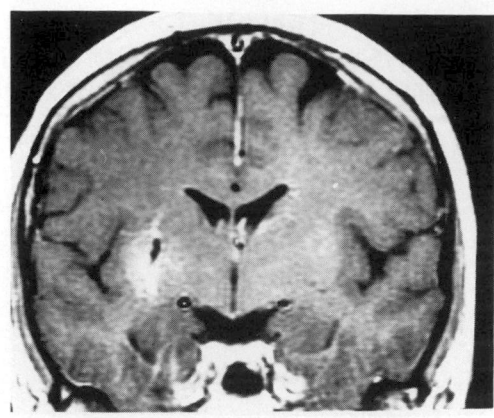

Figure 16–5 Arteriovenous malformation involving the right corpus striatum in a 37-year-old male seen on MRI projections in the coronal view. The image is T1 weighted. A flow void is seen in the view. Hemorrhage has occurred. This patient was asymptomatic.

transventricular, and transsylvian-transinsular.[37] Thalamic AVMs are accessed through interhemispheric approaches—transcallosal or transsplenial, depending on location.[41,42]

Brainstem Cryptic and angiographically demonstrable AVMs occur in the brainstem and are a source of brainstem and cerebellopontine hemorrhage with acute and often catastrophic presentation.[43,44] As with hemorrhage from AVMs in other locations, the hemorrhage is often self-limited so that the patient recovers from the insult and is subject to recurrence. Primary pontine hemorrhage most commonly occurs with hypertension, but an AVM must be excluded. MRI is the most helpful diagnostic procedure, as the malformation can be imaged and separated from the hematoma by presence of flow void. Angiography may not demonstrate these lesions.[45] Now that the location and adjacent anatomy of these brainstem AVMs are being imaged by MRI and digital angiography, successful microsurgical resection is being reported with greater frequency. These lesions are also amenable to radiosurgery. A gliotic interface at the periphery of the nidus allows for a plane of dissection to be developed, offering surgical extirpation with minimal deficits, even in this delicate location.[45–47] Lesions in the brainstem are best dealt with through the combined subtemporal-suboccipital-retrolabyrinthine-transtentorial approach.[48]

Vein of Galen Aneurysms of the vein of Galen are usually associated with AVMs of the pericallosal arteries and may involve the corpus callosum, with arterial feeders from the ambient and quadrigeminal segments of the posterior cerebral and superior cerebellar arteries, and from thalamic perforating branches of the basilar-posterior communicating arterial system.[49] These lesions are rare. Symptoms and signs involve the cardiovascular and central nervous systems. There are four clinical categories based on time of onset.[50] Group I presents in the neonatal period with a cranial bruit and cardiac failure; cyanosis and cardiac failure occur at or shortly after birth. The mortality rate is high in

this group. Group II has a cranial bruit and mild cardiac failure in the neonatal period, and cardiac enlargement occurs 1 to 6 months later. Group III presents with cardiomegaly at 1 to 12 months with a variable or intermittent cranial bruit. Group IV presents after some years with headache and syncope on exercise. There may be subarachnoid hemorrhage. Treatment of these lesions is directed to removing the shunt and eliminating the threat of high-output cardiac failure. Megalocephaly (head enlargement) is due to obstructive hydrocephalus, which is present in over 80 percent of patients with this condition.[51] Operative mortality in the neonatal group is high, and preoperative correction of cardiac failure is critical.[52] For AVMs, excision is the treatment of choice. With aneurysms of the vein of Galen, basically there is a fistulous tract from the arterial side to the venous side. Occlusion of the fistula is all that is required to cure the lesion, and surgery has been recommended.[53,54] Percutaneous transtroclear embolization of the galenic aneurysm from the venous side using wire coils (Gianturco coils) via a tethering plunger system that allows precise positioning of the coils is an effective alternative to open surgical occlusion of the fistula.[55] Complete anatomical occlusion may not always be achieved, but cardiac failure can be reversed by reducing the shunt, and approaches from the arterial or venous side are individualized. Long-term good results can be achieved in over 60 percent of patients, using combinations of endovascular and surgical techniques.[56]

Posterior Fossa Infratentorial AVMs are uncommon, 5 to 7 percent in most series, so that less is known about the behavior of lesions in this location. They are likely to involve critical areas. The large arteries that feed the AVMs have branches that supply the normal cerebellum and brainstem. Branches can be surgically occluded only if they clearly enter the nidus. Occlusion of an artery proximal to a normal branch could lead to a devastating infarct in the brainstem or cerebellum.[57] Hemorrhage is the most-common presentation of these lesions. Generally they are best handled surgically, although AVMs in the posterior fossa are listed in the nonoperated group in many series. The combined operative morbidity and mortality is 20 percent or more.[58,59] AVMs in the posterior fossa tend to rebleed frequently, although lesions presenting with ischemic steal symptoms may have less tendency to bleed.[58] It is generally recommended that AVMs of the cerebellum be surgically removed because the natural course of such lesions is treacherous. The approach is tailored to the specific location, and a transtentorial route may be preferable for lesions around the tectum and superior cerebellum.[60]

TREATMENT

The indications for treatment of an AVM are (1) to eliminate life-threatening hemorrhage, (2) to prevent progressive neurological and cognitive deficits, (3) to control or prevent seizures, (4) to prevent enlargement of the shunt that produces hemodynamic effects and cardiovascular strain, and (5) to eliminate the mental anguish of living with the knowledge of incurring an unpredictable cerebral hemorrhage and the attendant effects on patient and family.[61] To prevent the effects of natural outcome, an AVM must be totally eliminated with less morbidity than would occur without treatment. Residual AVM, persisting after completion of treatment, is subject to hemorrhage.

Treatment of an AVM of the brain may require radiosurgical techniques, embolization, or resection, or it may incorporate a combination of these techniques. Selection of appropriate therapy considers age of the patient, history of hemorrhage, and size and location of the lesion. Since there is a tendency for deficits associated with vascular malformations to progress and since malformations recognized in younger individuals are more likely to hemorrhage than those found in older individuals, more aggressive treatment is recommended for younger patients. Resection of a small polar AVM is associated with a much lower complication risk than resection of an AVM from a more-eloquent site, and thus surgical removal is more likely to be considered for a polar lesion. Vascular malformations that have previously bled are more likely to rebleed than are malformations that have not previously bled. Finally, resection of malformations deep within the cerebrum such as the basal ganglia, the thalamus, or brainstem may be hazardous and should be undertaken by surgeons experienced in treatment of AVMs.

Embolization is accomplished during the course of angiography. Embolization is rarely the definitive procedure but is often a prelude to definitive surgery. Several materials can be used to embolize malformations, including silastic beads, Gelfoam, polymers that harden upon exposure to electrolytes, and wire coils. Embolization reduces flow through the malformation, thereby reducing the hazards associated with definitive surgery. Unless the entire malformation is eradicated, new feeding vessels and gliotic scar will make future surgical procedures more difficult. Generally, definitive surgery is performed within a week of embolization. New neurological deficits may complicate patients undergoing embolization of AVMs. Fortunately, most of these deficits are temporary. Permanent deficits of major consequence occur in about 2 to 3 percent of cases.[27,28]

SURGICAL TECHNIQUE

Definitive treatment for AVMs is excision without injury to adjacent brain tissue. For lesions on the surface of the brain, the ideal procedure is to divide the arterial supply, excise the nidus, and isolate and excise the draining veins, taking precautions to maintain the microvascular circulation of the remaining brain. Techniques using the surgical microscope assist with these objectives. There are *circumferential, terminal,* and *penetrating* types of feeding arteries, which are 0.5 to 2 mm in diameter. These are distinguished from the *shunting arterioles,* which are transitional, and penetrating arterioles that have multiple branches to vessels of 50 to 200 μm and connect directly to the venules of the nidus. Feeding arteries may supply branches to the adjacent cerebral parenchyma. They must be preserved. The terminal feeding artery is often dilated and courses without branches to the parenchyma for some distance before connecting through shunting arterioles with the venous loops of the nidus.[62,63]

Insight into the individual anatomy and flow characteristics is critical for the safe surgical removal of an AVM. Two strategies of approach are advocated: (1) the tractional *en bloc* method is directed to peripheral isolation of the feeding arteries with marginal resection of the nidus; (2) central retrograde isolation of the major draining vein is used as a guide to nidus to collapse of the lesion from within.[64,65] Electrocortical stimulation and surface electroencephalographic recording techniques under local anesthesia are useful in delineating specific cortical function and seizure focus localization, respectively.[66] This allows for removal of lesions with preservation of function. It also allows for more effective seizure control. Such techniques are not without risk, including precipitation of a seizure during the procedure.[65]

Approaching the lesion from the venous side has the merit of collapsing the lesion from within. Cortical veins drain arterialized blood radially from the lesion. The major draining vein is often in the center and is initially identified and localized. This is matched with the angiogram. The central draining vein is followed into the nidus and carefully preserved. The venous drainage may be through single or multiple cerebral or dural veins.[67] This is opposed to the technique of isolating feeding arteries, which are subcortical. Brain tissue must be removed to expose them. Shunting venules and arterioles are cauterized and cut along the central vein. A cleavage plane is developed around the nidus, which is incrementally isolated. The larger lesions are separated into zones or compartments and can be isolated and collapsed as separate units. The draining vein can be a guide to these compartments. The venules are thin-walled and tear easily. They are occluded by multiple bipolar coagulations under saline irrigation along with topical hemostatic-cottonoid pledget tamponade.[63] Extreme caution is needed because premature occlusion of venous drainage from an incompletely resected nidus results in severe and possibly uncontrolled hemorrhage.

Controlled hypotension during the course of surgery and maintenance of a mean arterial pressure in the range of 40 to 60 mmHg reduces blood loss significantly while maintaining metabolic stability. Embolization of feeding vessels prior to definitive surgery may also reduce the blood loss and may significantly shorten the procedure since less time may be required to locate feeding vessels.[65]

The same objectives and techniques are applied to large AVMs and lesions in more eloquent areas of the brain. Fortunately, the glial elements surrounding these lesions are usually nonfunctional and can be removed without producing additional deficits. Removal of the vascular malformation may be followed by progressive neurological improvement, apparently a result of better tissue perfusion.

Consideration should be given for selective definitive embolization or radiosurgery to treat AVMs involving the thalamus or brainstem, but surgical extirpation is also possible in selected cases, using microsurgical techniques and cerebral protection.[35,68]

STAGED PROCEDURES

Large AVMs present a formidable risk and challenge. They may be successfully removed by staging therapy. Such lesions are associated with flow steal from adjacent tissues, and many have supply from dural branches of the external carotid system. They are typically greater than 6 cm in diameter and located in highly functional areas, with deep venous drainage (Spetzler Grade 5). Obliteration of the major feeding arteries is achieved with selective embolization, using slurry that can be directed by a catheter guided selectively into the interstices of the nidus. This maneuver does not eliminate flow in the lesion, and surgical excision is necessary to completely eliminate the AVM. Surgical removal can be staged as well. Fibrotic adhesions can be minimized by leaving the dura intact over a major portion of an AVM, presenting on the cortical surface and occluding penetrating feeding arteries from the periphery. Reduction of flow into the AVM causes reduction in venous pressure and an increase in local cerebral perfusion pressure. Neural deficits can resolve with improved regional cerebral capillary blood flow.[34,69] Gradual reduction of the shunt by staging the treatment can reduce risk of *normal perfusion pressure breakthrough* or *postocclusion hyperemia*.[70] Objections to staged AVM removal have been raised. They include risk of interval hemorrhage, rapid recruitment of collateral vessels, and converting feeders to less-accessible deep vessels and stretching thin-walled vessels, thus increasing the difficulty of resection.[71] Staging procedures should be reserved for large high-flow lesions.

SURGICAL COMPLICATIONS AND PERFUSION BREAKTHROUGH

Complications of the treatment of arteriovenous malformations of the brain focus on edema and hemorrhage in the early postoperative period. A comparison of several reported series implies an operative morbidity of 20 percent and mortality of 3.6 percent.[72] Possible causes include parenchymal ischemia from retraction, venous infarction due to occlusion of draining veins, residual AVM that bleeds, and increased flow through adjacent cerebral vessels with relative loss of autoregulation, resulting in parenchymal hyperperfusion. Decreased perfusion of the neural elements in the region of an arteriovenous malformation has already been mentioned.[34,69,73] Hypoperfusion is a result of the shunting of arterial blood through the malformation. In many cases this shunting results in loss of autoregulation. Interruption of the feeders to the vascular malformation results in immedi-

ate return of normal perfusion pressure to the surrounding brain tissue. Since the vessels penetrating the brain in the area are not prepared for the rise in perfusion pressure, serum may leak out of the vessels, producing edema. Frequently, hemorrhages will occur, often large. They present by sudden spontaneous, profuse swelling and generalized hemorrhage from the bed of the AVM. Swelling occurs later during the surgical resection, unrelated to technical error. There may be concealed intraventricular hemorrhages.[74] Staging resections of vascular malformations has been recommended as a means of avoiding this complication. This is one reason for the recommendation that embolization be performed a few days before the resection of a vascular malformation. Unfortunately, postoperative edema and hemorrhage still plague the resection of vascular malformations, the assumption being that it requires weeks to months for the brain to adapt to the alterations in blood flow in many cases.

VENOUS COMPLICATIONS

Venous outflow pattern is a significant factor in the occurrence of hemorrhage from an AVM. Analysis of venous anatomical risk factors shows that a single draining vein, stenosis or occlusion of a draining vein, and drainage through the deep venous system are associated with increased resistance to flow and increased venous pressure. Increased pressure transmitted though the shunt leads to hemorrhage.[75] Cerebral veins are in jeopardy during surgical resection. Venous occlusion is a cause for postoperative hemorrhage but is differentiated from other causes by diffuse, massive multifocal hemorrhage through cortex and white matter, which occurs a few days after surgical resection.[76] Caution and extreme care must be afforded the venous drainage of not only the AVM but also adjacent regional cerebral parenchyma.

ASSOCIATED ANEURYSMS

Another complication of the resection of AVMs is rupture of aneurysms. Saccular aneurysms are associated with AVMs in about 10 percent of cases. Four types of aneurysms are described with AVM: type I—proximally located on an ipsilateral major artery; type IA—proximally located on a contralateral major artery; type II—distally located on a superficially feeding artery; type III—proximally or distally located on a deep-feeding artery; and type IV—located on an artery unrelated to the AVM.[77]

Type I is the most common. Multiple aneurysms occur in about 30 percent of patients with AVMs with aneurysms. When hemorrhage occurs, it is due to the aneurysm about half of the time. There is an increase in the resistance of the vessels that have fed an AVM after the AVM is removed. If saccular aneurysms are not recognized and treated before or at the time the vascular malformation is treated, they may hemorrhage in the postoperative period. Generally, it is best to treat the lesion that has bled first. If it is safe to extirpate the other lesion in the same operation, it is done. If there is doubt about which lesion bled, usually the aneurysm is treated first because of the increased morbidity associated with aneurysms. Hemorrhage occurs in about 20 percent of cases. CTs showing intraparenchymal clot usually indicate hemorrhage from AVM whereas subarachnoid hemorrhage usually implies rupture of the aneurysm. Mortality rates of 2 to 10 percent are reported for the larger series of AVMs and aneurysms with about 10 percent morbidity.

HEMODYNAMICS OF AVMS

Flow shunted through an AVM is extremely pressure-dependent (no autoregulation) and follows the conditions described by the Hagen-Poiseuille equation where flow (Q) is directly related to the pressure difference (ΔP) and the fourth power of the radius (r) and is inversely related to the length of the tube (L) and viscosity (n):

$$Q = \frac{\Delta P + \sim r^4}{8 \cdot L \cdot n}$$

Intraoperative Doppler studies have determined that these parameters and bulk flow rates vary according to size and anatomy, varying from 150 to 900 ml/min (average, 490 ml/min).[78] AVM feeders have low intravascular pressure, high flow velocity, low peripheral stream resistance, and very poor vasomotor reactivity. Pressure within the feeding arteries rises by about 60 percent to normal values as the AVM is resected.[77,79] Normal CO_2 reactivity is established in adjacent cerebral vessels immediately after AVM removal, which is a factor against the perfusion breakthrough theory.[78] In vitro studies have demonstrated reactivity in AVM feeders to direct stimulation by vasoconstrictors such as serotonin and that there is a wide variability of responses in feeding arteries, with no histologic correlation to such reactivity. The complication rate is higher in cases where the feeding arteries are least reactive.[80]

RADIATION THERAPY

Another form of therapy recommended for arteriovenous malformations is the use of stereotaxic radiosurgery. This utilizes a high concentration of radiation focused upon the nidus of the malformation. Techniques include the "gamma knife," the linear accelerator, and the proton beam.[81–84] Results using these techniques appear to be relatively similar. Treated malformations are occluded in about 80 percent of cases after 2 years. Several months are required for the shunts to be occluded, and a small incidence of hemorrhage occurs in the interval, or "incubation period," which lasts 2 years. There are relative limitations to the size of lesions amenable to radiosurgery. Ideally, lesions are less than 3 cm in diameter. Conventional radiation has been used to treat

larger AVMs, and this modality is estimated to effectively obliterate the lesion in only 20 percent of cases with an annual hemorrhage rate of 3 percent, equal to the natural history of an AVM.[85]

SEIZURE CONTROL

The incidence of AVMs presenting as epilepsy without hemorrhage is 17 to 40 percent. Secondary epileptogenesis and kindling can persist after removal of the AVM in about one third of patients.[86] A remote independent epileptogenic focus persists, the amygdala being the most sensitive site for this. It has been postulated that seizures with AVMs are due to (1) ischemia of adjacent cerebral cortex because of flow shunting, (2) gliosis that may result from subclinical hemorrhage and hemosiderin deposits, and (3) secondary seizure foci, particularly in the temporal lobe. These sites can be determined by depth electrode recordings. There is a low incidence of new seizure disorders following surgical excision. The prospect for seizure control after AVM removal is good, and this result can be expected more frequently with the smaller lesions. Seizures may persist after removal of larger lesions. There is also a good capacity to recover from preoperative neurological deficits.[87] Early surgery for AVMs in young patients presenting with seizures may prevent secondary epileptogenesis for better long-term control of seizures.[88] Patients are maintained on anticonvulsant medications after treatment of the AVM is accomplished.

RISKS WITH PREGNANCY

Pregnancy apparently does not increase the risk of hemorrhage in women having an AVM that has not previously hemorrhaged. Such women have a 3.5 percent risk of hemorrhage. The risk increases to almost 6 percent if the AVM has previously hemorrhaged.[89] When hemorrhage occurs during pregnancy, it usually occurs in younger women (18 to 25 years of age), during the sixteenth to twenty-fourth week, shortly before labor, during delivery, or in the early puerperium. Also once hemorrhage occurs during the pregnancy there is approximately a 25 percent chance of recurrent hemorrhage.[90] Intracranial hemorrhage during pregnancy is due to AVM in 20 to 48 percent of cases. The overall maternal mortality rate for angiomatous hemorrhage is 28 percent.[91] Surgical management of intracranial hemorrhage during pregnancy should be based on neurosurgical principles. If the AVM hemorrhage causes a massive shift and progressive neurological deterioration, angiography and surgical excision of the hematoma and AVM is considered. The AVM should be proved resectable before embarking on such a course. The majority of such hemorrhages can be managed nonoperatively until delivery. The method of delivery should be determined by obstetrical principles. A cerebral AVM does not preclude normal vaginal delivery.[90]

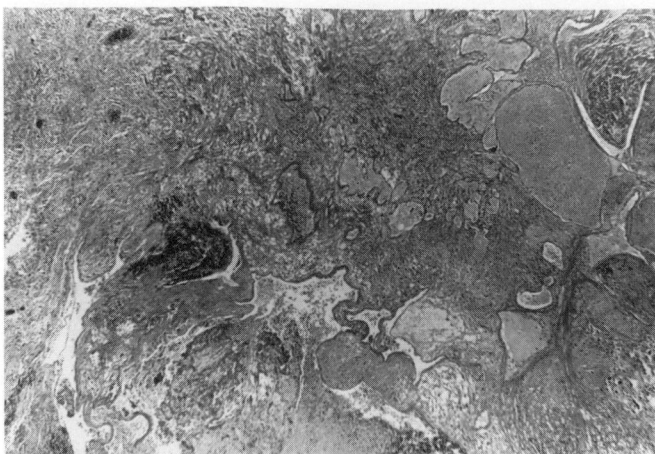

Figure 16–6 Microscopic view of a cavernous hemangioma. This vascular malformation is formed of large, thin-walled dilated venous channels and dilated capillary-like structures. Adjacent scarred brain tissue and evidence of old hemorrhage are seen in this surgical specimen.

☐ CAVERNOUS ANGIOMAS

Cavernous malformations, until recently, have been considered relatively rare, comprising 5 to 13 percent of vascular malformations. They occur at any location within the central nervous system. They are being detected with greater frequency with current imaging technology, and there is a an increased incidence and multiplicity among Mexican-American families.[92] Familial intracranial cavernous angiomas may be accompanied by similar lesions in the spinal cord.[93] They present with seizures, hemorrhage, and mass lesions in about equal frequency.[94] They are made up of dilated sinusoidal vascular spaces varying in size from a millimeter to many centimeters. Vascular walls are often hyalinized and contain calcium. Hemosiderin staining due to multiple small subclinical hemorrhages is common (Fig. 16-6). They contain varying amounts of clotted and unclotted blood. These features lead to characteristic pictures on CT or MRI. The MRI is most-sensitive in detecting these lesions, particularly on the T2-weighted images.[95] Arterial feeders are small and rarely visible on angiography. Cavernous malformations are well-circumscribed, expand slowly, and may be multiple.

Cavernous angiomas are hamartomatous collections of vascular spaces lined by thin walls devoid of smooth muscle.[96,97] They are usually located within the parenchyma of the brain but rarely may be located within the dura.[98] Those lesions located within the substance of the brain rarely have glial elements between the vascular channels, but lobules of the cavernous elements may invade adjacent brain. Surrounding brain tissue is often gliotic, stained with hemosiderin, and may contain feeding arteries and draining veins that accommodate the slow blood flow.

Cavernous angiomas were formerly diagnosed only at autopsy or surgery since they do not present a typical appearance on angiography or CT. They often went undiagnosed, but the use of MRI has substantially increased the frequency of their discovery. The characteristic appearance

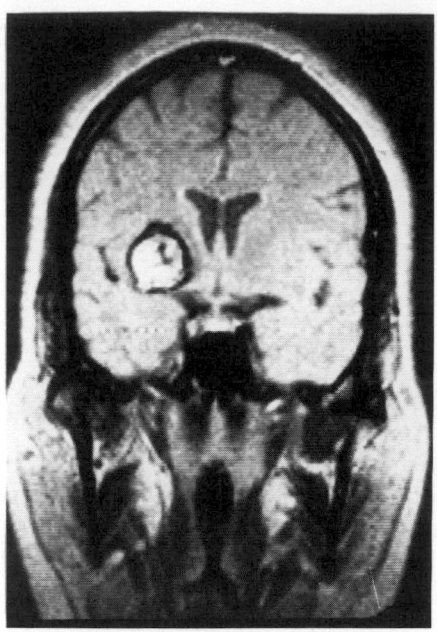

Figure 16–7 Cavernous hemangioma of the right basal ganglia in a 35-year-old black female who had hypertension and sickle cell trait. The patient had a history of right frontal headaches. A coronal image of the T1-weighted MRI shows the typical "cavernous" center with included vessels. The nidus is surrounded by hemosiderin, suggesting previous hemorrhage(s). A CT scan (not included) shows stippled calcification. An angiogram was normal.

on MRI includes a reticulated core of mixed-signal intensity, which is surrounded by a rim of decreased-signal intensity, largely hemosiderin (Fig. 16-7).[95,99] Small lesions may be recognized as black dots.

Seizures are the most frequently occurring symptoms for supratentorial cavernous angiomas. Asymptomatic angiomas have a 40 percent chance of eventually causing symptoms.[97] Lesions within the brainstem present with focal neurological deficits with progressive morbidity from recurrent hemorrhage (Fig. 16-8).[99] Headaches are prominent wherever the angiomas are located. Cavernous angiomas are distributed roughly by volume of the cerebral tissue, 80 to 90 percent above and 10 to 20 percent below the tentorium. Lesions above the tentorium are more frequently associated with seizures while infratentorial lesions are more likely to be associated with focal neurological deficits.[99,100] Patients occasionally present with acute exacerbations due to overt hemorrhage, which is more likely to occur in women, especially early in pregnancy.[97]

Hemorrhage from cavernous angiomas occurs at a rate of about 0.1 to 1.0 percent per year.[94] There appears to be little relationship between the size of the lesion and the rate of hemorrhage, and there is no identifiable relationship between the age of the patient and the occurrence of hemorrhage. Cavernous angiomas have been demonstrated to enlarge over a period of months to years because of capsule formation and recurrent hemorrhage.[101] Hemorrhages may be severe enough to result in mortality or long-term disability and may represent an indication for excision. Uncontrolled sei-

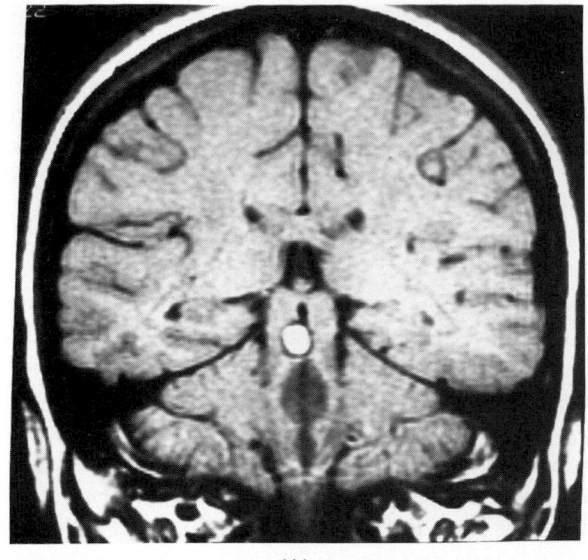

(A)

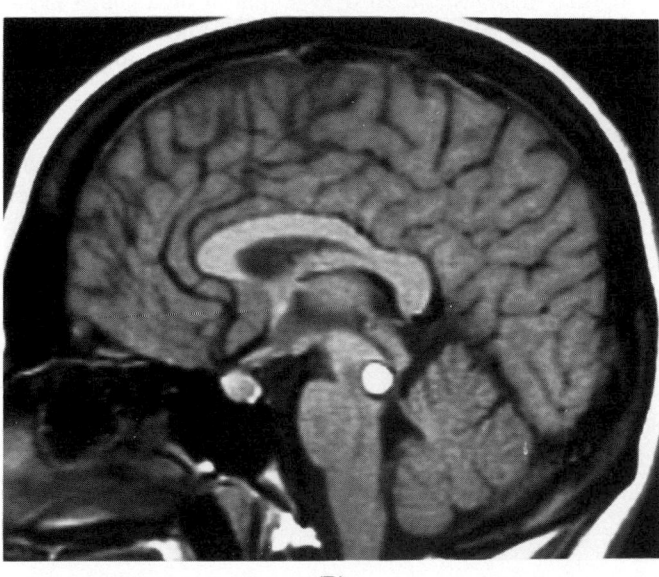

(B)

Figure 16–8 Cavernous hemangioma of tectum, slightly to the right of midline in a 19-year-old female who complained of intermittent headaches. She had internuclear ophthalmoplegia. Hemorrhages were accompanied with exacerbations of the headaches. Coronal *(A)* and sagittal *(B)* views of the MRI in the T1-weighted sequence show evidence of recent and old hemorrhage. Note the circular area of hemorrhage.

zures are the most-common indication for surgical therapy of angiomas above the tentorium.

Treatment of cavernous angiomas is controversial. Surgical excision is the treatment of choice when seizures are intractable or hemorrhages are recurrent. Neurological deficits may be reversed by the surgical evacuation or removal of a lesion that can be approached safely. Intraoperative cortical electroencephalographic recording is helpful during excision of cavernous angiomas that are the site of a seizure focus. Lesions located superficially within the brainstem that have hemorrhaged are probably best treated by microsurgical excision as this is curative.[99]

Radiosurgery has been rarely used for the treatment of cavernous angiomas since the surgical indications are usually seizures or mass effect, which may be the result of recurrent hemorrhage. These lesions are somewhat resistant to radiosurgery.[102]

Dural cavernous malformations may take on the appearance of mass lesions on CT and may have significant vascularity, leading to profuse bleeding when excision is attempted. Preoperative radiation may reduce the size and vascularity of such lesions so that they can be surgically removed more safely.[103]

☐ CAPILLARY TELANGIECTASIAS

Telangiectasias are small collections of capillaries containing no smooth muscle or elastic tissue, separated by glial background, usually located in the basis pontis or roof of the fourth ventricle. They usually accompany the Sturge-Weber syndrome or Rendu-Osler disease and rarely cause subarachnoid hemorrhage. They are rarely seen on CT.

Capillary telangiectasias are described as "typically small solitary malformations, usually encountered incidentally at necropsy."[3]

They have been recognized most commonly in the posterior fossa on various parts of the brainstem, but they occur on the cortex as well. These malformations are only rarely associated with large hemorrhages but may be found by microscopic examination of the cavity of some intracerebral hematomas.[16]

Telangiectasias are composed of blood vessels, walls of which vary from saccular dilatations of capillaries to ectatic, dilated groups of capillaries that may resemble cavernous spaces.[43,104] They are not seen on angiograms, a feature that these lesions share with cavernous angiomas and cryptic AVMs. The only feature that differentiates capillary telangiectasias from cavernous angiomas is the presence of brain parenchyma between the vascular channels of capillary telangiectasias.[5] Some cavernous angiomas have been identified with parenchyma between the vessels. A recent review presents convincing evidence that capillary telangiectasias and cavernous angiomas represent two pathological extremes of the same entity. Patients with multiple lesions have cavernous malformations, capillary telangiectasias, and transitional forms. The difference between these entities appears to be arbitrary. Telangiectasias rarely come to surgical attention.[4,5]

☐ CRYPTIC VASCULAR MALFORMATIONS

Cryptic AVMs are small fistulas that are clinically silent and occur with equal frequency in both supratentorial and infratentorial components of the brain.[43] They can bleed spontaneously. They may be found unexpectedly in the wall of an intracerebral hematoma evacuated surgically, even when associated with an aneurysm.[105,106] AVMs are not seen on angiography because of their small size, thrombosis, or pressure from a hematoma. CT and MRI have improved the detection of these lesions. The CT shows moderately hyperdense lesions that enhance unevenly with contrast. MRI shows one or more bright areas interspersed with foci of low or no signal located in the center or at the periphery of the main defect on both T1- and T2-weighted images.[107] There are other types of vascular lesions which are not seen angiographically that can present with hemorrhage.[108] Surgical removal is indicated if they are accessible so as to prevent recurrent hemorrhage.

When compared with AVMs seen angiographically, cryptic AVMs tend to occur more frequently in males and in slightly younger age groups. They are associated with less severe but more frequently recurrent hemorrhage because of delayed diagnosis. The cryptic lesions are therefore associated with higher nonoperative morbidity. Seizures occur in both types of AVMs with an equal incidence of 27 percent.[109] Small spontaneous hemorrhages and uneven bright lesions on MRI can also be due to neoplasms, which are best handled by surgical removal.

VENOUS ANGIOMAS

Venous malformations have no arterial elements. There may be a single draining vein originating deep within the white matter. Although anomalous, they may take the place of normal venous drainage; this fact is critical when surgical excision is considered. They occur in the posterior fossa and above the tentorium. They rarely hemorrhage and are usually asymptomatic. With contrast-enhanced CT, these lesions appear as a linear enhancement. The vein may be large and serpentine and may displace adjacent structures. A slow flow signal is apparent on MRI.

Cerebral venous malformations are composed of anomalous medullary veins arranged radially and converging on a centrally located large venous trunk that usually empties into a venous complex located on the surface of the brain.[110] Some venous angiomas drain centrally into enlarged periventricular veins. Glial tissue is usually located among the medullary veins. The angiographic picture is that of a "caput medusa," resembling the head of the mythical gorgon Medusa. Histologically, the veins contain limited numbers of muscular fibers but no elastic fibers, and arterial elements are not in increased numbers.[111]

These lesions have been considered incidental findings at autopsy, usually without significance clinically, but numerous recent reports have indicated that massive hemorrhage may result from them.[112,113]

Venous angiomas are seen angiographically in the late arterial or early capillary phase in many cases, but they may be seen in the venous phases of an angiogram.[114]

The clinical presentations of venous angiomas depend in large part on their location. Seizures are frequent with those located within the frontal lobes, and the seizures may be followed by postictal paresis. A significant number of venous angiomas are located within the posterior fossa, in the brainstem or cerebellum, where they may produce ataxia, diplopia, or even paresis. Although hemorrhage has been considered unusual in the past, there are many reports of such occurrences.[115]

Diagnosis of venous angiomas is definitively made by angiography. CT can frequently suggest the diagnosis as a linear, spotty, or nodular enhancement. The vessels may be delineated with contrast medium. Various stages of hemorrhage may be apparent. CT is considered by some to be the best imaging modality.[116]

MRI may be even more definitive. The venous malformation is sited as a tubular area of decreased signal in the white matter of the brain (Fig. 16-9).[117] MRI on T2-weighted imaging may demonstrate an oval region of high signal intensity extending toward the centrum semiovale.[118]

Treatment of cerebral venous angiomas is still controversial. When they were considered asymptomatic or of no clinical consequence, treatment was thought not to be indicated, but with growing numbers of hemorrhages being reported, more surgeons are being aggressive with the excision of such lesions. Associated seizures are difficult to control at times. Surgical resection is considered particularly if there has been recurrent hemorrhage. Venous angiomas are more likely to be coincidentally associated with other conditions that are the true cause of symptoms. This should be thoroughly evaluated before surgical excision is performed. The fact that these anomalus veins may serve as the definitive venous drainage for functional cerebral parenchyma should be considered.[110]

CAROTID-CAVERNOUS AND DURAL ARTERIOVENOUS FISTULAE

Carotid-cavernous fistulae are most commonly the result of severe head trauma resulting in basilar fractures, but many are spontaneous.[119,120] Etiologies differ according to the type of onset. Those occurring spontaneously are frequently caused by ruptured cavernous internal carotid aneurysms or adjacent dural fistulae with tributaries feeding the cavernous sinus.[42,121,122] Other dural arteriovenous fistulae may be located adjacent to and drain into the sagittal, transverse, or inferior sagittal sinus or into adjacent cortical veins.

Posttraumatic carotid-cavernous fistulae present with a bruit, usually loudest in the adjacent ear, and edema of the ipsilateral conjunctiva and periorbital soft tissues, along with congested conjunctival vessels of one or both eyes. An affected eye may be proptotic. Visual impairment in the affected eye may progress over a period of days or weeks. Cerebral venous infarction may occur as a result of increased

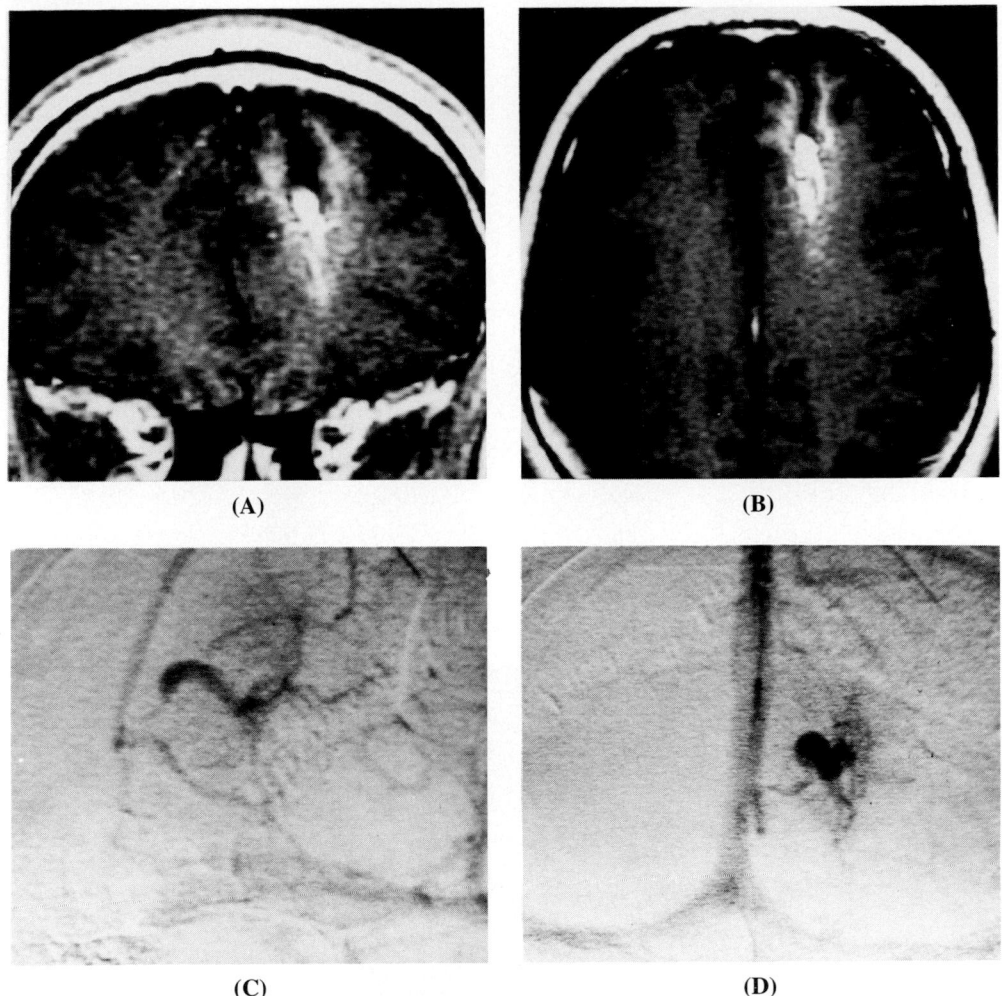

(A)

(B)

(C)

(D)

Figure 16–9 Left frontal venous angioma in a 36-year-old male. Frontal *(A)* and coronal *(B)* views in the T1-weighted sequence of the MRI and lateral *(C)* and frontal *(D)* views of the digital angiogram are shown. The patient had recent onset of frontal headache.

venous pressure and resultant ischemia from decreased perfusion pressure.

Posttraumatic arteriovenous shunting from the carotid artery into the cavernous sinus may be through a tear in the carotid arterial wall or through a tear of a branch from the carotid artery within the cavernous sinus.[123,124] Some dural arteriovenous fistulae may begin as a traumatic tear in a branch of the middle meningeal, intraorbital or even occipital, artery.[125–127] Drainage into a venous sinus may develop later.

Spontaneous carotid-cavernous fistulae present clinical pictures similar to posttraumatic lesions but may be divided into direct and dural fistulae.[128] Direct fistulae are usually the result of communications with high levels of flow between the internal carotid artery and the cavernous sinus, often the result of rupture of an intracavernous aneurysm. Dural cavernous-carotid-cavernous fistulae are low-flow communications between branches of the internal or external carotid arteries and the cavernous sinus. Alternately, drainage may occur into a cortical vein. Drainage into a vein may develop as a result of a previous thrombosis of the cavernous

sinus. Some carotid-cavernous fistulae are due to abnormal collagen within the leaves of the dura.

An atypical spontaneous carotid-cavernous fistula occurs in elderly women with no history of trauma, the *red-eyed shunt syndrome*. This is a variant of a dural fistula. Usually there is no bruit and only mild proptosis. There is a prominent episcleral and conjunctival vascular congestion, causing the red eye. The only major complication is open-angle glaucoma, which should be considered in these patients. The majority of these lesions resolve spontaneously.[129]

Precise delineation of the site of the carotid-cavernous sinus fistula is accomplished with angiography using high-speed digital subtraction imaging in multiple views. Both internal and external carotid arterial injections are required for spontaneous fistulae.[130,131]

The treatment of carotid-cavernous fistulae has gone through many stages of evolution. Initial efforts involved the simple ligation of the internal carotid artery, followed by occlusion of the supracavernous segment of the carotid artery in order to prevent the fistula from stealing blood from

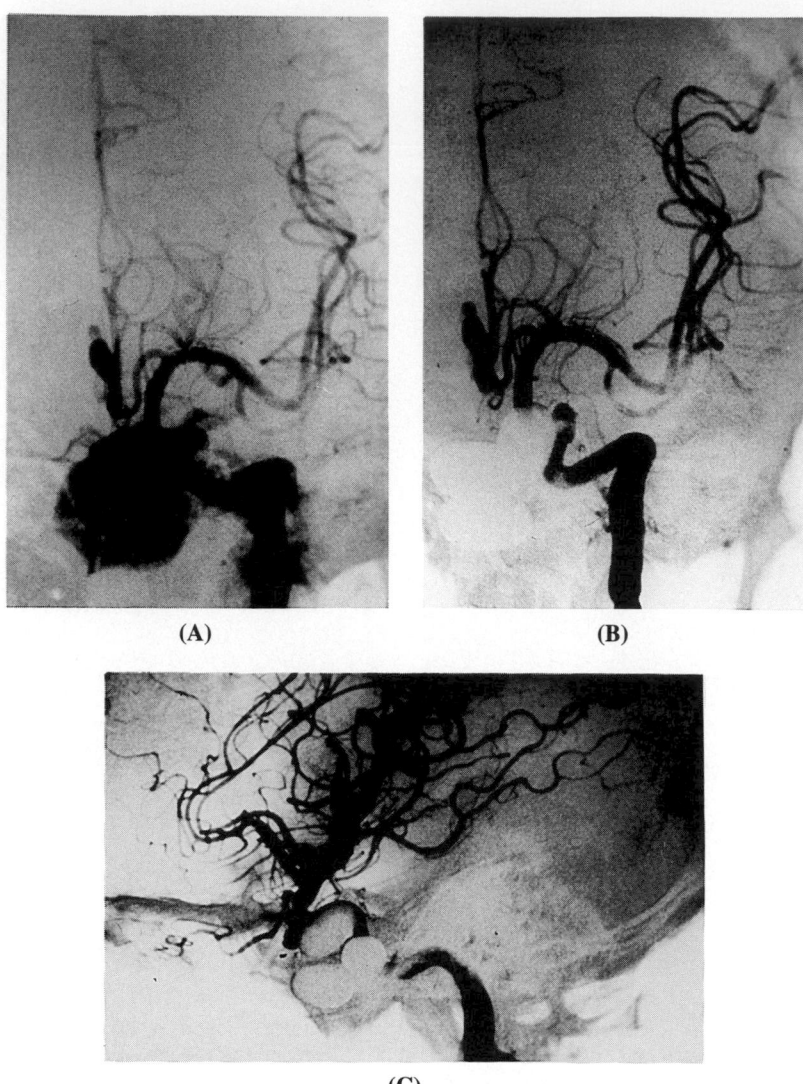

Figure 16–10   Traumatic carotid-cavernous fistula in an adult male. The frontal *(A)* projection of the diagnostic arteriogram is shown. Frontal *(B)* and lateral *(C)* projections of the angiogram after occlusion of the fistula with balloons are seen. Note that three balloons were required to occlude the fistula while leaving the carotid artery patent.

the cerebral vasculature. Subsequently, Hamby clipped the supracavernous carotid artery intracranially, proximal to the posterior communicating artery, after which a fragment of muscle was embolized into the fistula from the cervical internal carotid artery. Both the fistula and the internal carotid artery are occluded by these methods.[120]

Subsequently, Serbinenko and then Debrun introduced interventional radiologic techniques whereby detachable balloons are introduced through retrograde femoral or direct carotid catheters.[132,133] The balloon is maneuvered into the fistulous tract or into the cavernous sinus, after which it is detached. In most cases, patency of the carotid artery can be preserved (Fig. 16-10). An alternate technique introduces balloons into the cavernous sinus through the venous route.[134,135] Techniques by which direct attacks are made on the cavernous sinus have also been introduced by Parkinson.[123,124] Knowledge of the cavernous

sinus anatomy is essential for these procedures.[136–138] Parkinson used hypothermia and cardiac bypass during such procedures, but others have performed the transcavernous interruption of these fistulae without interrupting blood flow.[139] Presently, the balloon technique for treatment of posttraumatic carotidcavernous fistulae is preferred in most centers.

A significant number of low-flow fistulae will occlude spontaneously. Therefore, if a fistula is found to be fed through the external carotid artery, it may be desirable to observe the patient for a period before attempting to occlude the fistula. The primary danger is loss of vision. If there is evidence of loss of visual acuity, consideration should be given to occluding the dural tract. Frequently, it is impossible to maneuver an endovascular catheter into a dural fistula, in which case the external carotid feeders may be occluded, which facilitates a direct attack on the dural fistula.[140]

☐ VASCULAR MALFORMATIONS WITHIN THE SPINAL CANAL

Spinal vascular malformations are currently classified according to location and anatomy as dural fistulae and intradural vascular malformations.[141–143] Intradural malformations are subdivided into cavernous angiomas and "juvenile" malformations, the later name carried over from previous classifications. Previous classifications have typed vascular malformations according to their pathological appearance.[144] Selective angiography has lead to specificity of type.[145,146] Type 1 was described as a single vessel attached to the dorsum of the spinal cord, usually originating in the lower thoracic area and extending cephalad for varying distances. Type 1 spinal vascular malformations were recognized as the most common. Type 2 was called "glomus" or "nidus" and was described as a tightly collected group of blood vessels lying on the surface of the spinal cord or extending into the spinal cord for varying depths and fed by small branches of the medullary vasculature. Some such lesions are wholly contained within the spinal cord. Type 3, the "juvenile," or "diffuse," type, was described as a diffuse collection of arteries and veins, usually almost completely replacing a segment of the spinal cord. Juvenile was the name applied because lesions were usually recognized in children or young adults. With careful observations and analysis of diagnostic procedures, type 1 malformations have proved to be dural fistulae, type 2 lesions have, at least in many instances, proved to be cavernous angiomas, and type 3 lesions closely resemble classical intracranial AVMs.

Diagnosis of vascular malformations of the spinal canal has been difficult by classical techniques and many, most prominently, type 2, or glomus, lesions were missed.[147] Frequently, the only identifying feature on myelography is widening of the spinal cord, and this may not be apparent in some cases. Angiography of glomus lesions may not have identifying features in the case of cavernous hemangiomatous lesions.[148] The development of MRI has simplified the diagnosis of isolated lesions of the spinal canal and has lead to more-frequent diagnosis of isolated lesions that lie within the spinal cord.

Epidural vascular malformations most commonly originate in the vertebrae, and many may be recognized by the radiographic appearance of the vertebrae. They usually produce neurological changes by mass effects. Those will not be further considered here.

Dural fistulae are collections of arteries and veins located on the surface or between the leaves of the dura, which cuff a nerve root.[149,150] The fistulae may extend into adjacent areas of dura. Usually, there is a single arterial feeder connecting with venous components that pass through a neural foramen; but sometimes multiple feeders are present. These continue intradurally to rest on the dorsal surface of the spinal cord. They continue cephalad along the spinal canal for varying distances, usually as a single arterialized serpentine vein. This dorsal vein has intimate connections with the coronal venous plexus, which drains blood from the spinal cord. While valves are normally present in the spinal medullary veins, these valves become incompetent under a number of conditions. The arterialized veins transmit abnormally elevated pressure back into the coronal veins, thus reducing the perfusion pressure within the spinal cord and ultimately producing ischemia and myelopathy.[151,152] This phenomenon can occur with intracranial fistulae that drain into spinal medullary veins.[153]

Spinal dural fistulae usually occur at lower thoracic and lumbar levels. They are more common in men than women and present in middle age. Clinical symptoms are usually those of progressive sensory and motor deficits below the level of the lesion, although radicular symptoms related to the nerve root compromised by the fistula have been reported.[154] Spinal dural fistulae are reported to be the most-common type of vascular malformation affecting the spinal cord. Diagnosis is usually initiated by myelography, which demonstrates the single serpentine vein lying on the dorsum of the spinal cord. Confirmation is obtained by selective angiography through intercostal and lumbar vessels. Blood flow within this draining vein is routinely quite slow, and there is some obstruction in its communications with the extrathecal venous complexes. Vessels supplying the dural fistulae are usually separate from the radicular vessels supplying the spinal cord. MRI reveals a high signal intensity in the T2-weighted image at levels where venous delay is encountered.[155] However, myelography may be more sensitive in detecting these lesions, showing a typical serpentine filling defect in the contrast column.

Treatment of spinal dural fistulae involves interruption of the fistulous connection between the feeding arteries and the arterialized vein. Several methods have been reported, including embolization of feeding vessels, surgically interrupting the arterialized veins within or near the sleeve of the nerve root, excision of the arterial-venous connections, or coagulating the vessels about the nerve root.[156] Questions have been raised about the permanency of embolization.[157] In the past, practice has been to remove the serpentine vein from the dorsum of the spinal cord, but it is now recognized that this vessel will thrombose if all or even most of the radicular fistulous connections have been interrupted.

Intradural cavernous malformations are small collections of poorly formed vessels lying on the surface of, or within, the spinal cord. Many of those located on the surface of the spinal cord extend for various depths into the cord. Although most cavernous angiomas, or "cavernomas," are located on or within the spinal cord, they have been reported to occur within the substance of the dura, and one lesion has been reported on a segment of the cauda equina.[158] These lesions resemble cavernous angiomas anywhere else in the nervous system, that is, a collection of blood vessels with thin, poorly developed walls. Those cavernous angiomas lying within the medullary substance are surrounded by a layer of glial tissue that usually contains hemosiderin. There are often cystic pockets of old blood nearby, signifying previous hemorrhage. Small arterial feeders and draining veins

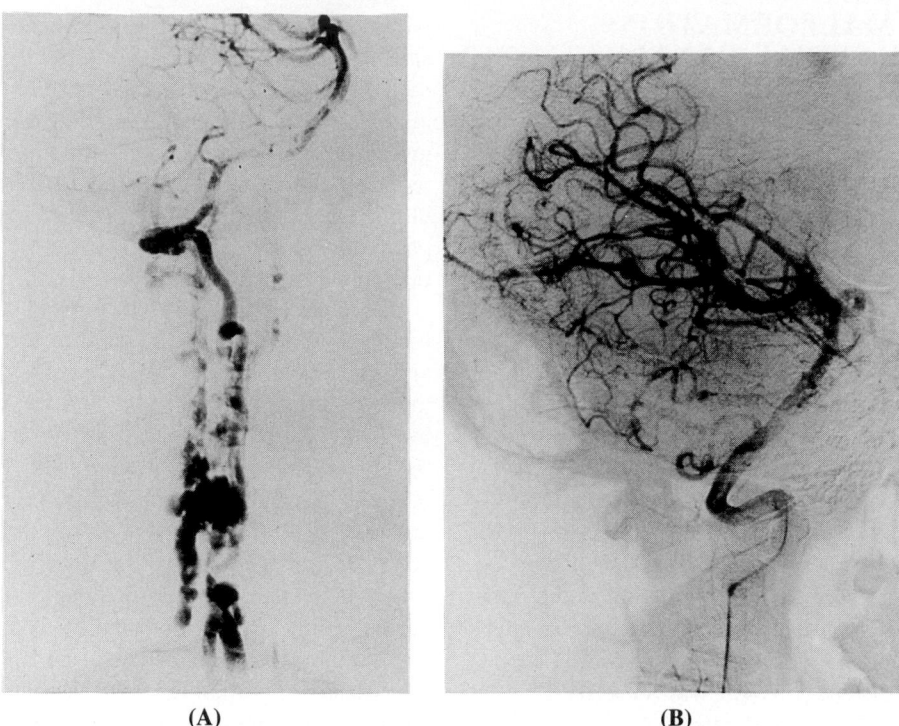

(A)   **(B)**

Figure 16–11   Juvenile vascular malformation of the spinal cord in a 19-year-old female fed by branches of the right vertebral artery. Complaints were severe headaches, nausea, and vomiting. The patient had meningismus. A lateral *(A)* view of a right vertebral arteriogram shows the nidus in the upper spinal canal. The malformation was treated by embolization of the branches of the right vertebral artery. An angiogram 2 years later *(B)* showed no residual malformation.

traverse the surrounding glial tissue. However, blood flow in these vessels is quite slow, reducing the incidence of complications during surgical resection.[159]

Cavernous angiomas of the spinal cord usually present clinically as gradual motor and sensory deterioration, often with exacerbations. Pain may be prevalent with exacerbations. Most exacerbations are assumed to be due to hemorrhage. Slowly progressive deterioration may be due to the mass effect of the lesion, but more rapid deterioration between exacerbations may be due to secondary effects of hemorrhage.

Microsurgical excision may be curative without increasing the neurological deficits. Intramedullary lesions are approached through a myelotomy, usually in the midline unless the lesion is located to one side, in which case the myelotomy may be performed through a dorsal root entry zone.[159] Dissection should remain very close to the nidus. Since blood vessels supplying angiomas are small and flow is slow, bleeding at the time of surgery is rarely a problem.

Juvenile or *diffuse malformations* of the spinal cord closely resemble AVMs within the cranium (Fig. 16-11). They are likely to become clinically apparent in children or young adults. Since these lesions are commonly found in the neck and upper thoracic area, it is common for the neurological deficits to involve the upper extremities.

Juvenile malformations are composed of collections of feeding arteries and draining veins, and the lesions may nearly replace segments of the spinal cord.[64] Contrary to cavernous angiomas, there may be glial tissue interspersed between the angiomatous vessels. These lesions are fed by arteries with high flow rate and, similarly, the flow within the veins is rapid. Aneurysms are common to both the arteries and veins. Most juvenile malformations present by acute exacerbations, suggesting hemorrhage, although progressive neurological deterioration occurs as well since the lesions are so diffuse. Diagnostic features of juvenile malformations include widening of the interpeduncular distance on plain radiographs. There may be obstruction to flow of contrast media on myelography. Large vessels may be apparent. Selective angiography, initiated through the vertebral arteries and aorta, usually provides the definitive diagnosis and identifies the feeding vessels.[159-161] So much of the cord is involved by these lesions, it is rare that they can be removed with any degree of confidence. Embolization has been successful in reducing blood flow through such lesions and, interestingly enough, in reducing the size of aneurysms.[162,163]

REFERENCES

1. Stein BM, Solomon RA: Arteriovenous malformations of the brain, in Youmans JR (ed): *Neurological Surgery,* 3d ed. Philadelphia, Saunders, 1990, pp 1831–1863.
2. McLone DG, Naidich TP: Embryology of the cerebral vascular system, in Edwards MSB, Hoffman HJ (eds): *Cerebral Vascular Disease in Children and Adolescents.* Baltimore, Williams & Wilkins, 1989, pp 1–16.
3. McCormick WF: The pathology of vascular ("Arteriovenous") malformations. *J Neurosurg* 24:807–816, 1966.
4. McCormick WF: Pathology of vascular malformations of the brain, in Wilson LB, Stein BM (eds): *Intracranial Arteriovenous Malformations.* Baltimore, Williams & Wilkins, 1984, pp 44–63.
5. Rigamonti D, Johnson PC, Spetzler RF, et al: Cavernous malformations and capillary telangiectasia: A spectrum within a single pathological entity. *Neurosurgery* 28:60–64, 1991.
6. Fink GR: Effects of cerebral angiomas on perifocal and remote tissue: A multivariate positron tomography study. *Stoke* 23:1099–1105, 1992.
7. Chin LS, Raffel C, Gomez IG, et al: Diffuse arteriovenous malformations: A clinical, radiological, and pathological description. *Neurosurgery* 31:863–869, 1992.
8. Stein BM, Wolpert SM: Arteriovenous malformations of the brain: I. Current concepts and treatment. *Arch Neurol* 37:1–5, 1980.
9. Nakayama Y, Tanaka A, Yoshinaga S, et al: Multiple intracerebral arteriovenous malformations: Report of two cases. *Neurosurgery* 25:281–286.
10. Graf CJ, Perret GE, Torner JC: Bleeding from cerebral arteriovenous malformations as part of their natural history. *J Neurosurg* 58:331–337, 1983.
11. Barrow DL: Unruptured cerebral arteriovenous malformations presenting with intracranial hypertension. *Neurosurgery* 23:484–490, 1988.
12. Troupp H, Marttila I, Halonen V: Arteriovenous malformations of the brain. Prognosis without operation. *Acta Neurochir* 22:125–128, 1970.
13. Svien HJ, McRae JA: Arteriovenous anomalies of the brain. Fate of patients not having definitive surgery. *J Neurosurg* 23:23–28, 1965.
14. Ondra SL, Troupp H, George ED, Schwab K: The natural history of symptomatic arteriovenous malformations of the brain: A 24-year follow-up assessment. *J Neurosurg* 73:387–391, 1990.
15. Faults D, Kelly DL, Jr: Natural history of arteriovenous malformations of the brain: A clinical study. *Neurosurgery* 15:658–662, 1984.
16. Wilkins RH: Natural history of intracranial vascular malformations: A review. *Neurosurgery* 16:421–430, 1985.
17. Itoyama Y, Uemura S, Ushio Y, et al: Natural course of unoperated intracranial arteriovenous malformations: Study of 50 cases. *J Neurosurg* 71:805–809, 1989.
18. Brown RD, Weibers DO, Forbes G, et al: The natural history of unruptured intracranial arteriovenous malformations. *J Neurosurg* 68:352–357, 1988.
19. Fisher WS III: Decision analysis: A tool of the future: An application to unruptured arteriovenous malformations. *Neurosurgery* 24:129–134, 1989.
20. Auger RG, Weibers DO: Management of unruptured intracranial arteriovenous malformations: A decision analysis. *Neurosurgery* 30:561–569, 1992.
21. Omojola MF, Fox AJ, Vinuela FV, Drake CG: Spontaneous regression of intracranial arteriovenous malformations. Report of three cases. *J Neurosurg* 57:818–822, 1982.
22. Nehls DG, Pittman HW: Spontaneous regression of arteriovenous malformations. *Neurosurgery* 11:776–780, 1982.
23. Minakawa T, Tanaka R, Koike T, et al: Angiographic follow-up study of cerebral arteriovenous malformations with reference to their enlargement and regression. *Neurosurgery* 24:68–74, 1989.
24. Ezura M, Kagawa S: Spontaneous disappearance of a hugh cerebral arteriovenous malformation: Case report. *Neurosurgery* 30:595–599, 1992.
25. Leblanc R, Ethier R, Little JR: Computerized tomography findings in arteriovenous malformations of the brain. *J Neurosurg* 51:765–772, 1979.
26. Leblanc R, Levesque M, Comair Y, Ethier R: Magnetic resonance imaging of cerebral arteriovenous malformations. *Neurosurgery* 21:15–20, 1987.
27. Purdy PD, Batjer HH, Risser RC, Samson D: Arteriovenous malformations of the brain: Choosing embolic materials to enhance safety and ease of excision. *J Neurosurg* 77:217–222, 1992.
28. Jafar JJ, Davis AJ, Berenstein A, et al: The effect of embolization with N-butyl cyanoacrylate prior to surgical resection of cerebral arteriovenous malformations. *J Neurosurg* 78:60–69, 1993.
29. Lindegaard KF, Bakke S, Grolimund P, et al: Assessment of intracranial hemodynamics in carotid disease by transcranial Doppler ultrasound. *J Neurosurg* 63:890–898, 1985.
30. Lindegaard KF, Gromlimund P, Aaslid R, Nornes H: Evaluation of cerebral AVM's using transcranial Doppler ultrasound. *J Neurosurg* 65:335–344, 1986.
31. Hitchon PW, Kassell NF, Carlstrom TA, McDonnell DE: The Doppler ultrasonic flowmeter as an adjunct to operative management of cerebral arteriovenous malformations. *Surg Neurol* 11:345–347, 1979.
32. Luessenhop AJ, Gennarelli TA: Anatomical grading of supratentorial arteriovenous malformations for determining operability. *Neurosurgery* 1:30–35, 1977.
33. Spetzler RF, Martin NA: A proposed grading system for arteriovenous malformations. *J Neurosurg* 65:476–483, 1986.
34. Spetzler RF, Martin NA, Carter LP, et al: Surgical management of large AVM's by stages embolization and operative excision. *J Neurosurg* 67:17–28, 1987.
35. U SH, Kerber CW, Todd MM: Multimodality treatment of deep periventricular cerebral arteriovenous malformations. *Surg Neurol* 38:192–203, 1992.
36. Andreussi L, Cama A, Grossi G, et al: Microsurgical excision of a strio-insular arteriovenous malformation. *Surg Neurol* 12:499–502, 1979.
37. Malik GM, Umansky F, Patel S, Ausman JI: Microsurgical removal of arteriovenous malformations of the basal ganglia. *Neurosurgery* 23:209–217, 1988.
38. Sugita K, Takemae T, Kobayashi S: Sylvian fissure arteriovenous malformations. *Neurosurgery* 21:7–14, 1987.
39. Shi YQ, Chen XC: Surgical treatment of arteriovenous malformations of the striatothalamocapsular region. *J Neurosurg* 66:352–356, 1987.
40. Sang H, Rosenberg J: Complete recovery from hemiplegia following excision of a giant basal ganglia arteriovenous malformation. *Surg Neurol* 15:328–330, 1981.
41. Solomon RA, Stein BM: Interhemispheric approach for the

surgical removal of thalamocaudate arteriovenous malformations. *J Neurosurg* 66:345–351, 1987.

42. Lee JP: Surgical treatment of thalamic arteriovenous malformations. *Neurosurgery* 32:498–504, 1993.

43. McCormick WF, Nofziger JD: Cryptic vascular malformations of the central nervous system. *J Neurosurg* 24:865–875, 1966.

44. Russell B, Rengachery SS, McGregor DM: Primary pontine hematoma presenting as a cerebellopontine angle mass. *Neurosurgery* 19:129–133, 1986.

45. Kashiwagi S, van Loveren HR, Tew JM Jr, et al: Diagnosis and treatment of vascular brain-stem malformations. *J Neurosurg* 72:27–34, 1990.

46. Chyatte D: Vascular malformations of the brain stem. *J Neurosurg* 70:847–852, 1989.

47. Heffez DS, Zinreich SJ, Long DM: Surgical resection of intrinsic brain stem lesions: *Neurosurgery* 27:789–798, 1990.

48. Samii M: The combined supra-infratentorial presigmoid avenue to the petro-clival region. Surgical technique and clinical applications. *Acta Neurochirurg* 95:6–12, 1988.

49. Asargil MG, Antic J, Laciga R, et al: Arteriovenous malformations of the vein of Galen: Microsurgical treatment. *Surg Neurol* 6:195–200, 1976.

50. Amacher AL, Shillito J Jr: The syndromes and surgical treatment of aneurysms of the great vein of Galen. *J Neurosurg* 39:89–98, 1973.

51. Massey CE, Carson LV, Beveridge WD, et al: Aneurysms of the great vein of Galen: Report of two cases and review of the literature, in Smith RR, Haerer A, Russell WF (eds): *Vascular Malformations.* New York, Raven, pp 163–179, 1982.

52. Menezes AH, Graf CJ, Jacoby CG, Cornell SH: Management of vein of Galen aneurysms. Report of two cases. *N Neurosurg* 55:457–462, 1981.

53. Hoffman HJ, Chuang S, Hendrick EB, Humphreys RP: Aneurysms of the vein of Galen. Experience at the hospital for Sick Children, Toronto. *J Neurosurg* 57:316–322, 1982.

54. Hernesniemi J: Arteriovenous malformations of the vein of Galen: Report of three Microsurgically treated cases. *Surg Neurol* 36:465–469, 1991.

55. Mickle JP, Quisling RG: The transtorcular embolization of vein of Galen aneurysms. *J Neurosurg* 64:731–735, 1986.

56. Lylyk P, Vinuela F, Dion JE, et al: Therapeutic alternatives for vein of Galen vascular malformations. *J Neurosurg* 78:438–445, 1993.

57. Drake CG, Friedman AH, Peerless SJ: Posterior fossa arteriovenous malformations. *N Neurosurg* 64:1–10, 1986.

58. McCormick WF, Hardiman JM, Boulter TR: Vascular malformations ("angiomas") of the brain, with special reference to those occurring in the posterior fossa. *J Neurosurg* 28:241–251, 1968.

59. Batjer H, Samson D: Arteriovenous malformations of the posterior fossa. Clinical presentation, diagnostic evaluation, and surgical treatment. *J Neurosurg* 64:849–856, 1986.

60. Salcman M, Nudelman RW, Bellis EH: Arteriovenous malformations of the superior cerebellar artery: Excision via an occipital transtentorial approach. *Neurosurgery* 177:749–756, 1985.

61. Troupp H: Arteriovenous malformations of the brain: What are the indications for operation? in Morley TP (ed): *Current Controversies in Neurosurgery.* Philadelphia, Saunders, pp 210–216, 1976.

62. Parkinson D: Cerebral arteriovenous aneurysms: Surgical management. *Can J Surg* 1:313–325, 1958.

63. Yamada S: Arteriovenous malformations in the functional area: Surgical treatment and regional cerebral blood flow. *Neurol Res* 4:283–322, 1982.

64. Pool JL: Excision of cerebral arteriovenous malformations. *J Neurosurg* 29:312–321, 1968.

65. Yamada S. Brauer FS, Knierim DS: Direct approach to arteriovenous malformations in functional areas of the cerebral hemisphere. *J Neurosurg* 72:418–425, 1990.

66. Burchel KJ, Clarke H, Ojeman GA, et al: Use of stimulation mapping and corticography in the excision of arteriovenous malformations in sensorimotor and language-related neocortex. *Neurosurgery* 24:322–327, 1989.

67. Hubschmann OR, Krieger AJ: The perivenous technique of resection of arteriovenous malformations from vital areas of the brain. *Surg Neurol* 27:323–330, 1987.

68. Masayuki E, Takahashi A, Yoshimoto T: Successful treatment of an arteriovenous malformation by chemical embolization with estrogen followed by conventional radiotherapy. *Neurosurgery* 31:1105–1107, 1992.

69. Andrews BT, Wilson CB: Staged treatment of arteriovenous malformations of the brain. *Neurosurgery* 21:314–323, 1987.

70. Mullan S, Brown FD, Patronas NJ: Hyperemic and ischemic problems of surgical treatment of arteriovenous malformations. *J Neurosurg* 51:757–764, 1979.

71. Morgan MK, Sundt TM Jr: The case against staged operative resection of cerebral arteriovenous malformations. *Neurosurgery* 25:429–436, 1989.

72. Morgan MK, Johnston IH, Hallinan JM, Weber NC: Complications of surgery for arteriovenous malformations of the brain. *J Neurosurg* 78:176–182, 1993.

73. Spetzler RF, Wilson CB, Weinstein P, et al: Normal perfusion pressure breakthrough theory. *Clin Neurosurg* 25:651–672, 1977.

74. Batjer HH, Devous MD Sr, Seibert GB, et al: Intracranial arteriovenous malformation: Relationship between clinical factors and surgical complications. *Neurosurgery* 24:75–79, 1989.

75. Miyasaka Y, Yada K, Ohwada T, et al: An analysis of the venous drainage system as a factor in hemorrhage from arteriovenous malformations. *J Neurosurg* 76:239–243, 1992.

76. Miyasaka Y, Yada K, Ohwada T, et al: Hemorrhagic venous infarction after excision of an arteriovenous malformation: Case report. *Neurosurgery* 29:265–268, 1991.

77. Cunha E, Sa MJ, Stein BM, et al: The treatment of associated intracranial aneurysms and arteriovenous malformations. *J Neurosurg* 77:853–859, 1992.

78. Nornes H, Grip A: Hemodynamic aspects of cerebral arteriovenous malformations. *J Neurosurg* 53:456–464, 1980.

79. Hassler W, Steinmetez H: Cerebral hemodynamics in angioma patients: An intraoperative study. *J Neurosurg* 67:822–831, 1987.

80. Muraszko K, Wang HH, Pelton G, Stein BM: A study of the reactivity of feeding vessels to arteriovenous malformations: Correlation with clinical outcome. *Neurosurgery* 26:190–200, 1990.

81. Steiner L, Lindqvist C, Adler JR, et al: Clinical outcome of radiosurgery for cerebral arteriovenous malformations. *J Neurosurg* 77:1–8, 1992.

82. Friedman WA, Bova FJ: Linear accelerator radiosurgery for arteriovenous malformations. *J Neurosurg* 77:832–841, 1992.

83. Kjellberg RN, Hanamura T, Davis KR, et al: Bragg-Peak proton-beam therapy for arteriovenous malformations of the brain. *N Engl J Med* 309:269–274, 1983.

84. Hosobuchi Y, Fabricant J, Lyman J: Stereotactic heavy-particle irradiation of intracranial arteriovenous malformations. *Appl Neurophysiol* 50:248–252, 1987.

85. Redekop GJ, Elisevich KV, Gaspar LE, et al: Conventional radiation therapy of intracranial arteriovenous malformations: long-term results. *J Neurosurg* 78:413–422, 1993.

86. Yeh H, Privitera MD: Secondary epileptogensis in cerebral

arteriovenous malformations. *Arch Neurol* 48:1122–1124, 1991.

87. Piepgras DG, Sundt TM Jr, Ragoowansi AT, Stevens L: Seizure outcome in patients with surgically treated cerebral arteriovenous malformations. *J Neurosurg* 78:5–11, 1993.

88. Yeh H, Tew JM Jr, Gartner M: Seizure control after surgery on cerebral arteriovenous malformations. *J Neurosurg* 78:12–18, 1993.

89. Horton JC, Chambers WA, Lyons SL, et al: Pregnancy and the risk of hemorrhage from cerebral arteriovenous malformations. *Neurosurgery* 27:867–872, 1990.

90. Robinson JL, Hall CS, Sedzimir CB: Arteriovenous malformations, aneurysms, and pregnancy. *J Neurosurg* 41:63–70, 1974.

91. Dias MS, Sekhar LN: Intracranial hemorrhage from aneurysms and arteriovenous malformations during pregnancy and the puerperium. *Neurosurgery* 27:855–866, 1990.

92. Rigamonti D, Hadley MN, Drayer BP, et al: Cerebral cavernous malformations: Incidence and familial occurrence. *N Engl J Med* 319:343–347, 1988.

93. Lee KS, Spetzler RF: Spinal cord cavernous malformation in a patient with familial intracranial cavernous malformations. *Neurosurgery* 26:877–880, 1990.

94. Simard JM, Bengochea FG, Ballinger WE Jr, et al: Cavernous angioma: A review of 126 collected and 12 new clinical cases. *Neurosurgery* 18:162–172, 1986.

95. Rigamonti D, Drayer B, Johnson PC, et al: The MRI appearance of cavernous malformations (angiomas). *J Neurosurg* 67:518–524, 1987.

96. Curling OD, Jr, Kelly DL, Jr, Elster AD, Craven TE: An analysis of the natural history of cavernous angiomas. *J Neurosurg* 75:702–708, 1991.

97. Robinson JR, Awad IA, Little JR: Natural history of the cavernous angioma. *J Neurosurg* 75:709–714, 1991.

98. Isla A, Roda JM, Alvarez F, et al: Intracranial cavernous angioma in the dura. *Neurosurgery* 25:657–659, 1989.

99. Zimmerman RS, Spetzler RF, Lee KS, et al: Cavernous malformations of the brain stem. *J Neurosurg* 75:32–39, 1991.

100. Rigamonti D, Drayer B, Johnson S, et al: Cavernous malformations, MRI, and epilepsy. *Neurology* 37:322, 1987.

101. Pozzati E, Giuliani G, Nuzzo G, Poppi M: The growth of cerebral cavernous angiomas. *Neurosurgery* 25:92–97, 1989.

102. Lindquist C, Guo WY, Karlsson B, Steiner L: Radiosurgery for venous angiomas. *J Neurosurg* 78:531–536, 1993.

103. Shibata S, Mori K: Effect of radiation therapy on extracerebral cavernous hemangioma in the middle fossa: Report of three cases. *J Neurosurg* 67:919–922, 1987.

104. Rigamonti D, Johnson PC, Spetzler RF, et al: Cavernous malformations and capillary telangiectasia: A spectrum within a single pathological entity. *Neurosurgery* 28:60–64, 1991.

105. Golden JB, Kramer RA: The angiographically occult cerebrovascular malformation. *J Neurosurg* 48:292–296, 1978.

106. Deruty R, Guyotat IP, Mottolese S, Soustiel JF: Ruptured occult arteriovenous malformation associated with unruptured intracranial aneurysm: Report of three cases. *Neurosurgery* 30:603–607, 1992.

107. Ogilvy CS, Heros RC, Ojemann RG, New PF: Angiographically occult arteriovenous malformations. *J Neurosurg* 69:350–355, 1988.

108. Lobato RD, Perez C, Rivas JJ, Cordobes F: Analysis of 21 cases and review of the literature. *J Neurosurg* 68:518–531, 1988.

109. Lobato RD, Rivas JJ, Gomez PA, et al: Comparison of the clinical presentation of symptomatic arteriovenous malformations (angiographically visualized) and occult vascular malformations. *Neurosurgery* 31:391–397, 1992.

110. Rigamonti D, Spetzler RF, Medina M, et al: Cerebral venous malformations. *J Neurosurg* 73:560–564, 1990.

111. Wendling LR, Moore JS Jr, Kieffer SA, et al: Intracerebral venous angioma. *Radiology* 119:141–147, 1976.

112. Sawar M, McCormick WF: Intracerebral venous angioma: Case report and review. *Arch Neurol* 35:323–325, 1978.

113. Malik GM, Morgan JK, Boulos RS, Ausman JI: Venous angiomas: An underestimated cause of intracranial hemorrhage. *Surg Neurol* 30:350–358, 1988.

114. Moritake K, Handa H, Mori K, et al: Venous angiomas of the brain. *Surg Neurol* 14:95–105, 1980.

115. Numaguchi Y, Kitamura K, Fuki M, et al: Intracranial venous angiomas. *Surg Neurol* 18:193–202, 1982.

116. Cammarata C, Han JS, Haaga R, et al: Cerebral angiomas imaged by MR: *Radiology* 155:639–643, 1985.

117. Rigamonti D, Spetzler RF, Drayer BP, et al: Appearance of venous malformations on magnetic resonance imaging. *J Neurosurg* 69:535–539, 1988.

118. Scott JA, Augustyn GT, Gilmor RL, et al: Magnetic resonance imaging of a venous angioma. *AJNR* 6:284–286, 1985.

119. Debrun GM, Vinuela F, Fox AJ, et al: Indications for treatment and classification of 132 carotid-cavernous fistulas. *Neurosurgery* 22:285–289, 1988.

120. Hamby WB: Carotid cavernous fistulae. Springfield, Il. Charles C Thomas, 1966.

121. Barrow DL, Spector RH, Braun IF, et al: Classification and treatment of spontaneous carotid-cavernous fistulas. *J Neurosurg* 62:248–256, 1985.

122. Barnwell SL, Halbach VV, Dowd CF, et al: A variant of arteriovenous fistulas within the wall of dural sinuses: Results of combined surgical and endovascular therapy. *J Neurosurg* 74:199–204, 1991.

123. Parkinson D: Carotid cavernous fistula: Direct repair with preservation of the carotid artery: Technical note. *J Neurosurg* 38:99–106, 1973.

124. Parkinson D: A surgical approach to the cavernous portion of the carotid artery: Anatomical studies and case report. *J Neurosurg* 23:474–483, 1965.

125. Hayes GJ: External carotid-cavernous sinus fistulas. *J Neurosurg* 20:692–700, 1963.

126. Mingrina S, Moro F: Fistula between the external carotid artery and cavernous sinus: Case report. *J Neurosurg* 27:157–160, 1967.

127. Mahalley MS Jr, Boone SC: External carotid-cavernous fistula treated by arterial embolization: Case report. *J Neurosurg* 40:110–114, 1974.

128. Schievink WI, Peipgras DG, Earnest F IV, Gordon H: Spontaneous carotid-cavernous fistulae in Ehlers-Danlos syndrome IV. *J Neurosurg* 74:991–998, 1991.

129. Phelps CD, Thompson HS, Ossoinig KC: The diagnosis and prognosis of atypical carotid-cavernous fistula (red-eyed shunt syndrome). *Am J Ophthalmol* 93:423–436, 1982.

130. Debrun G, Lacour P, Vinuela F, et al: Treatment of 54 traumatic carotid-cavernous fistulas. *J Neurosurg* 55:678–692, 1981.

131. Taniguchi RM, Goree JA, Odom GL: Spontaneous carotid-cavernous shunts presenting diagnostic problems. *J Neurosurg* 35:384–391, 1971.

132. Serbinenko FA: Balloon catheterization and occlusion of major cerebral vessels. *J Neurosurg* 41:125–145, 1974.

133. Debrun G, Lacour P, Caron JP, et al: Detachable balloon and calibrated-leak balloon techniques in the treatment of cerebral vascular lesions. *J Neurosurg* 49:635–649, 1978.

134. Shimizu T, Waga S, Kojima T, Tanaka K: Transvenous balloon occlusion of the cavernous sinus: An alternative therapeutic choice for recurrent traumatic carotid-cavernous fistulas. *Neurosurgery* 22:550–553, 1988.

135. Teng MMH, Guo WY, Huang CI, et al: Occlusion of arteriovenous malformations of the cavernous sinus via the superior ophthalmic vein. *AJNR* 9:539–546, 1988.

136. Rhoton AL Jr, Hardy DG, Chambers SM: Microsurgical anatomy and dissection of the sphenoid bone, cavernous sinus, and sellar region. *Surg Neurol* 12:63–104, 1979.

137. Umansky F, Nathan H: The lateral wall of the cavernous sinus: With special reference to the nerves related to it. *J Neurosurg* 56:228–234, 1982.

138. Sekhar LN, Burgess J, Akin O: Anatomical study of the cavernous sinus emphasizing operative approaches and related vascular and neural reconstruction. *Neurosurgery* 21:806–816, 1987.

139. Dolenc V: Direct microsurgical repair of intracavernous vascular lesions. *J Neurosurg* 58:824–831, 1983.

140. Albert P, Polaina M, Trujillo F, et al: Treatment of carotid-cavernous fistulas by embolization of the cavernous sinus through venous affluents or direct pressure. *Acta Neurochir* (suppl) 42:88–92, 1988.

141. Kendall BE, Logue V: Spinal epidural angiomatous malformations draining into intrathecal veins. *Neuroradiology* 13:181–189, 1977.

142. Logue, V: Angiomas of the spinal cord: Review of the pathogenesis, clinical features, and results of surgery. *J Neurology, Neurosurg, and Psychiatr* 42:1–11, 1979.

143. Rosenblum G, Oldfield EH, Doppman JL, DiChiro G: Spinal arteriovenous malformations: A comparison of dural arteriovenous fistulas and intradural AVMs in 81 patients. *J Neurosurg* 67:795–802, 1987.

144. Antoni N: Spinal vascular malformations (angiomas) and myelomalacia. *Neurology* 12:795–804, 1962.

145. Ommaya AK, DiChiro G, Doppman J: Ligation of arterial supply in the treatment of spinal cord arteriovenous malformations. *J Neurosurg* 30:679–692, 1969.

146. DiChiro G, Werner L: Angiography of the spinal cord: A review of contemporary techniques and applications. *J Neurosurg* 29:1–29, 1973.

147. McCormick PC, Michelsen WJ, Post KD, et al: Cavernous malformations of the spinal cord. *Neurosurgery* 23:459–463, 1988.

148. Cosgrove GR, Bertrand G, Fontaine S, et al: Cavernous angiomas of the spinal cord. *J Neurosurg* 68:31–36, 1988.

149. Cahan LD, Higashida RT, Halbach VV, Hieshima GB: Variants of radiculomeningeal vascular malformations of the spine. *J Neurosurg* 66:333–337, 1987.

150. Symon L, Kuyama H, Kendall G: Dural arteriovenous malformations of the spine. *J Neurosurg* 60:238–247, 1984.

151. Aminoff MJ, Barnard RO, Logue V: The pathophysiology of spinal vascular malformations. *J Neurol Sci* 23:255–263, 1974.

152. Choi IS: Commentary: Spinal dural arteriovenous fistula: The role of PVA embolization. *AJNR* 13:941–942, 1992.

153. Wrobel CJ, Oldfield EH, DiChiro G, et al: Myelopathy due to intracranial dural arteriovenous fistulas draining intrathecally into spinal medullary veins: Report of three cases. *J Neurosurg* 69:934–939, 1988.

154. Tanaka K, Waga S, Kojima T, et al: Spinal dural arteriovenous malformations: Report of an unusual case. *Neurosurgery* 24:915–918, 1989.

155. Isu T, Iwasaki Y, Akino M, et al: Magnetic resonance imaging in cases of spinal dural arteriovenous malformation. *Neurosurgery* 24:919–923, 1989.

156. Nichols DA, Ruenacht DA, Jack CR Jr, Forbes GS: Embolization of spinal dural arteriovenous fistula with polyvinyl alcohol particles: Experience in 14 patients. *AJNR* 13:933–940, 1992.

157. Hall WA, Oldfield EH, Doppman JL: Recanalization of spinal arteriovenous malformations following embolization. *J Neurosurg* 70:714–720, 1989.

158. Pagni CA, Canavero S, Forini M: Report of a cavernoma of the cauda equina and review of the literature. *Surg Neurol* 33:124–131, 1990.

159. Ogilvy CS, Louis DN, Ojemann RG: Intramedullary cavernous angiomas of the spinal cord: Clinical presentation, pathologic features, and surgical management. *Neurosurgery* 31:219–229, 1992.

160. Biondi A, Merland JJ, Hodes JE, et al: Aneurysms of the spinal arteries associated with intramedullary arteriovenous malformations: I. Angiographic and clinical aspects. *AJNR* 13:913–922, 1992.

161. Biondi A, Erland JJ, Hodes JE, et al: Aneurysms of the spinal arteries associated with intramedullary arteriovenous malformations: II. Results of AVM endovascular treatment and hemodynamic considerations. *AJR* 13:923–931, 1992.

162. Spetzler RF, Zabramski JM, Flom RA: Management of juvenile spinal AVM's by embolization and operative excision. *J Neurosurg* 70:628–632, 1989.

163. Touho H, Karasawa J, Shishido H, et al: Sucessful excision of a juvenile-type spinal arteriovenous malformation following intraoperative embolization: Case report. *J Neurosurg* 75:647–651, 1991.

☐ STUDY QUESTIONS

I. A 23-year-old female is seen in the hospital because of the sudden onset of lumbar back pain and weakness in her lower extremities. The patient has a past history of an episode of back pain for which she had a diskectomy at age 16 years. At that time there had been severe weakness of her left lower extremity. Weakness had been gradual over a period of 6 months. With the current episode, the patient had suddenly experienced the pain, followed by progressive weakness in both lower extremities, worse on the left. She is experiencing "numbness" in both lower extremities. Examination reveals decreased sensation to pinprick in both lower extremities, but more marked on the right.

1. What is the most likely diagnosis? **2.** What investigations might be considered? In what order? **3.** Assuming the finding of a dural fistula with a nidus at T10 on the left with a draining vein extending up to the cervical area, what therapy might be considered? **4.** What would be the anticipated result? **5.** What explanations might be made for the sudden onset of paresis?

II. A 23-year-old male suddenly experiences a series of five seizures, leading to a CT without contrast, which is normal. A repeat with contrast reveals an arteriovenous malformation in the right frontal area, measuring 2 cm in diameter. Review of the seizure history reveals that each ictus begins with a stiffening of the left arm, followed by loss of consciousness and a generalized convulsion. An EEG reveals an interictal seizure focus in the posterior right frontal area, near the AVM.

1. How should the lesions be treated? **2.** Would excision of the vascular lesion assure termination of seizures? **3.** How can the seizures be explained? **4.** Would the seizure focus be found directly beneath the AVM? Why or why not? **5.** What are the chances of hemorrhage from the AVM if the seizures are treated by medication alone?

III. A 19-year-old right-handed-male has the sudden onset of a mild headache, right hemiparesis, and impairment of sensation to pinprick on the right. A CT scan reveals an AVM measuring 1.5 cm in the left thalamus with a small hemorrhage in the area, distorting the thalamus but not altering the position of the ventricles or midline structures. The patient is alert but mildly dysphasic.

1. What are the chances of repeat hemorrhage if the lesion is left untreated? **2.** What are the treatment options? **3.** Assuming that "radiosurgery" is selected, how long will it take to obtain obliteration of the lesion? **4.** What are the chances of repeat hemorrhage in the meantime? **5.** What are the possible consequences of a direct surgical attack upon such a lesion?

IV. A newborn is found to have a bruit within the head at the time of his initial examination. Twelve hours later he is short of breath and is in congestive heart failure.

1. What is the most likely diagnosis? **2.** What is his prognosis? **3.** What treatments might be considered? **4.** What are the chances of success? **5.** Assuming the congestive failure did not occur until the patient was 1 year old, how might this affect the prognosis?

CHAPTER
17

Interventional Neuroradiology

José A. Bauzá

Interventional neuroradiology is a new discipline that is gaining acceptance in medicine as an alternate form of therapy for selected neurological lesions. It has been made possible because of the development of small catheters and guidewires that can be navigated into selected branches of the intracranial or extracranial vasculature.[1] Embolic materials have become available that allow vascular occlusion of very small vessels. Catheters and guidewires, as small as 2 and 3 French, allow selective catheterization of even the smallest arteries. This permits the angiographer to investigate lesions discretely. Embolic materials, now available, include solid agents (polyvinyl alcohol particles, Gelfoam powder, coils, or balloons) or liquid agents (cyanoacrylates or dehydrated ethanol). The choice of embolic material is dictated by the location of the lesion and the end point or goal of the procedure.

☐ INDICATION

Interventional neuroradiology may be indicated in the nonoperative treatment of some solid tumors of the central or peripheral nervous system. This includes meningiomas and the intraarterial chemotherapy of malignant brain tumors. Many vascular lesions, such as some arteriovenous malformations, dural arteriovenous fistulae, traumatic arteriovenous fistulae, vein of Galen malformations, intracranial aneurysms, and spinal vascular malformations are ideally suited for interventional neuroradiology.[4] Thrombolysis of intracranial vascular disease is a new form of therapy that is gaining favor for use of interventional radiology in the treatment of cerebrovascular disease. Likewise percutaneous transluminal angioplasty of major branches of the carotid and vertebrobasilar systems is indicated in selected cases of blood vessel spasm or occlusive vascular disease.

☐ SOLID LESIONS

MENINGIOMAS

These vascular lesions arise from the meningothelial cells located throughout the meninges, most commonly adjacent to the arachnoid villae and the dura which surrounds the exit of the cranial nerves.[2] They receive their blood supply from dural vessels but may parasitize pial vessels to supply their surface.[3] The definitive treatment of a meningioma is surgical resection. Selective embolization of supplying branches can result in devascularization of the lesion, causing tumor necrosis and a decrease in size. Preoperative embolization will shorten the operative time and reduce the surgical blood loss.[4]

Preoperative embolization consists of selectively catheterizing and performing angiograms of all arterial feeders to the meningioma. Embolization is usually performed using polyvinyl alcohol microparticles (PVA) 150 to 300 μm (Fig. 17-1). Smaller particles (Gelfoam powder) or liquid agents may provide a deeper penetration into the tumor but carry increased risk of undesirable side effects. The cranial nerves are also supplied by branches of the external carotid artery. Preservation of the petrosal branch that supplies the facial nerve is paramount.[3,5]

PARAGANGLIOMAS

Paragangliomas, also known as glomus tumors or chemodectomas, arise from nonchromaffin paraganglioma cells located at the carotid artery bifurcation, middle ear, or the ganglion nodosum of the vagus nerve. Less-common locations include the larynx, orbit, nose, or aortic arch.[6] The majority of these lesions are nonsecretory, but in 5 percent of cases where the lesion secretes catecholamine, manipula-

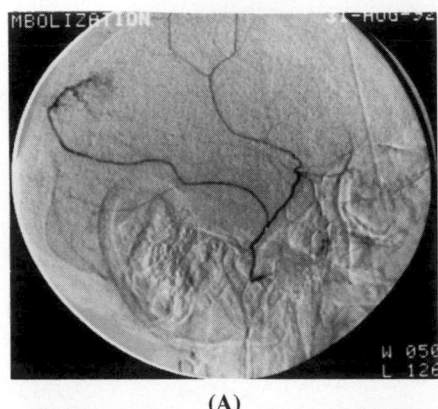

(A)

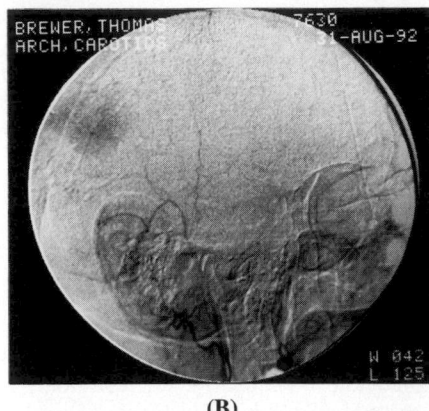

(B)

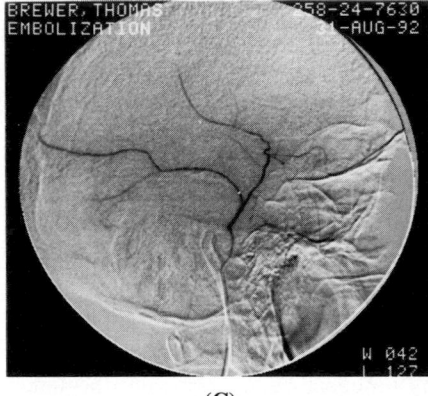

(C)

Figure 17–1 Meningioma. **A.** Selective middle meningeal artery injection shows early tumoral blush from posterior branch. **B.** Capillary phase shows tumoral blush. **C.** Microparticles show absence of tumoral blush.

tion can precipitate a hypertensive crisis.[5,7] Rarely surgical removal or embolization of these lesions can produce severe hypotension. Because of these two worrisome features of paragangliomas, suspected secretors should be evaluated for urinary vanillylmandelic acid (VMA) or 5-hydroxyindole-acetic acid (5-HIAA), and patients should be treated with alpha blockers and volume expanders prior to any surgical procedure.

Tumors involving the carotid body and vagus nerve ganglion are usually supplied by the external carotid artery, while those located in the jugulotympanic region receive their blood

supply primarily from the ascending pharyngeal branch of the external carotid artery, occasionally parasitizing blood from the vertebrobasilar system. Selective catheterization of the internal and external carotid arteries should be accomplished in the vascular territory of the lesion. Embolization can be performed immediately after the diagnostic angiogram. Microparticles or liquid agents can be utilized.[7,8]

INTRAARTERIAL CHEMOTHERAPY OF BRAIN TUMORS

The systematic administration of chemotherapeutic agents is frequently part of the overall surgical treatment of primary malignant brain tumors. Because of the toxic side effects of chemotherapeutic agents, the intraarterial approach has often been recommended.[8] Interventional neuroradiologists are often called upon to catheterize selectively arteries supplying a malignant brain tumor so that chemotherapeutic agents may be infused intraarterially.[9] This can be done by one of two approaches. In the first, the catheter is placed in the internal carotid artery with its tip in the cervical segment of the vessel. Injections in this location can produce optic complications including pain, increased intraocular tension, and visual loss.[10] The second approach is to place the intraarterial catheter beyond the origin of the ophthalmic artery. While this protects the ophthalmic artery and the eyes, it increases the neurotoxic effects of the chemotherapeutic agents.[8] The neurotoxic effects include progressive dysfunction in the ipsilateral hemisphere.[11,12] The neurotoxic effects are dose-related and are dependent on the interval between procedures and the cumulative dose. Nitrosoureas appear to have the least-adverse side effects.[12]

☐ VASCULAR LESIONS

ARTERIOVENOUS MALFORMATIONS (AVMs)

Central nervous system arteriovenous malformations (AVMs) may be fed entirely from branches of the internal carotid artery (purely pial malformations) or fed entirely by branches of the external carotid artery system (purely dural malformations). In many instances, the blood supply to the AVM comes from branches of both the internal and external carotid systems (mixed pial-dural malformations).[13]

Definitive treatment of AVMs may require surgery alone, surgery after endovascular occlusion, radiosurgery and surgery, or radiosurgery and endovascular occlusion. Interventional neuroradiology for AVMs involves supraselective catheterization and arteriography of each suspected feeding vessel. If branches to normal brain arise from the blood vessel feeding the malformation, that blood vessel cannot be embolized. In those instances where vital portions of the brain are thought to be irrigated by the same vessels supplying the malformation, sodium amytal may be injected and the patient evaluated for

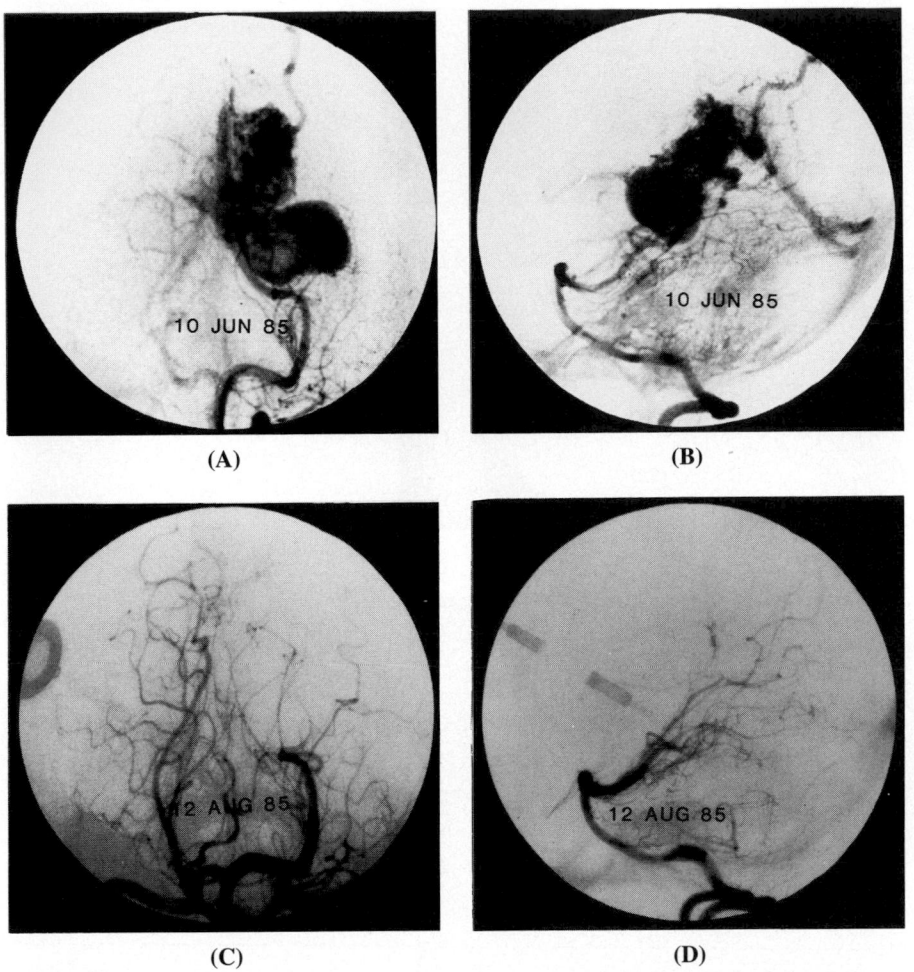

(A)   (B)

(C)   (D)

Figure 17–2 Arteriovenous malformation. *A, B.* AP and lateral projection reveal an AVM with its main supply from the left posterior cerebral artery with early venous drainage. *C, D.* Arteriogram after embolization with cyanoacrylates shows obliteration of the AVM. *(Case courtesy of Paul Pevsner.)*

alterations in the electroencephalogram (EEG) and the neurological picture.[14] Embolization of those malformations will be performed only if no adverse effects are noted on the EEG or the neurological examination.

Acrylics are the most popular materials used in embolizing AVMs because of their ability to penetrate deeply into the nidus of the malformation and permanently occlude it. Other materials used include PVA, silk sutures, and balloons. The use of acrylics decreases the chances of embolizing the venous drainage of the malformation or allowing embolic particles to become pulmonary emboli.[15]

Small AVMs can be completely obliterated by embolization alone (Fig. 17-2). Larger lesions with multiple feeding vessels usually require surgical excision or radiosurgery.[15,16] In many of these cases, preoperative embolization reduces a portion of the blood flow to the malformation.

DURAL ARTERIAL FISTULAE

Dural arterial fistulae are abnormal connections between arteries and veins that occur within the dura, most often within the wall of a dural sinus. The arterial inflow is usually from meningeal vessels, although on occasion pial recruitment may occur.[17–19] Therapeutic methods for these lesions include vascular compression, transarterial embolization, transvenous embolization, or surgical excision. If the lesion involves the transverse or the sigmoid sinus, the initial treatment may consist of manual compression of the occipital artery behind the mastoid for up to 30 min.[18] The diminished inflow can induce thrombosis. This technique should not be performed on patients with cortical venous drainage, hemorrhage, or infection. In patients with cavernous sinus fistulae, manual compression of the carotid jugular vessels can be attempted. Again, patients with carotid artery atherosclerotic disease, underlying hypercoagulable states, high platelet counts, or patients receiving epsilon-aminocaproic acid (EACA) should not be treated in this manner.

If compression techniques fail, transarterial embolization of the feeders should be attempted. PVA particles should be used since liquid and polymerizing agents carry a great risk of producing cranial nerve paralysis or stroke.[17]

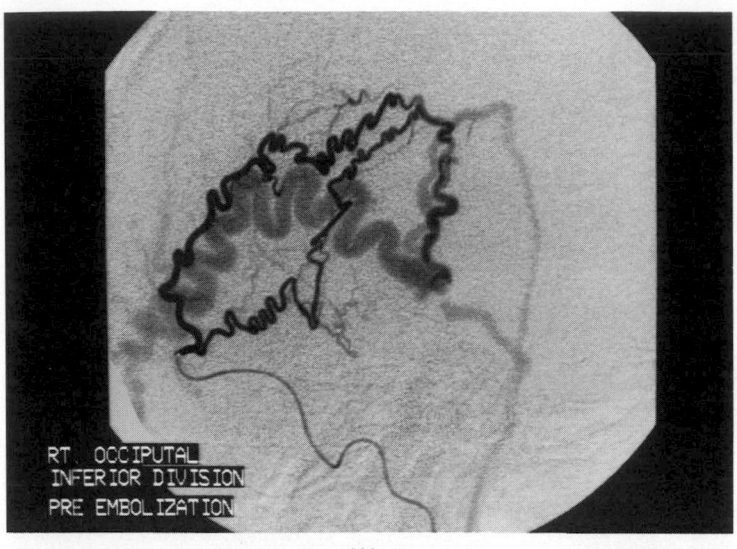

(A)

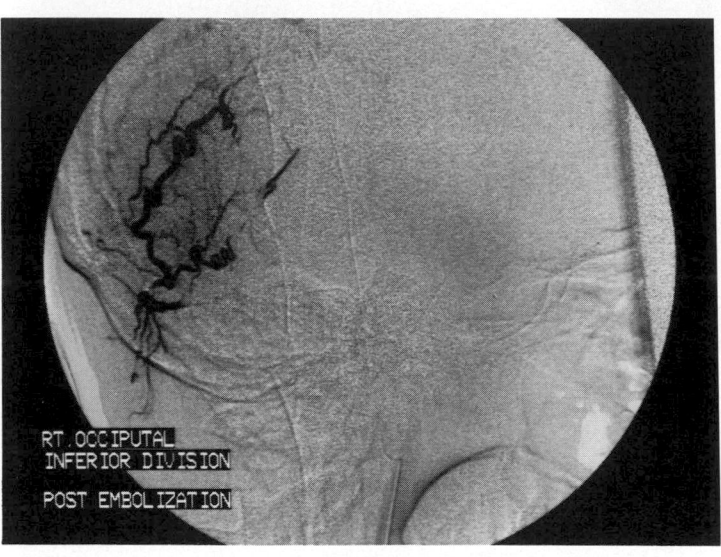

(B)

Figure 17–3 Traumatic arteriovenous (AV) fistula. **A.** Supraselective arteriogram of the occipital artery shows two prominent branches draining directly to a markedly dilated draining vein. **B.** Arteriogram after embolization with PVA microparticles and coils show nonfilling of the draining vein. (*Case courtesy of Victor Toro.*)

TRAUMATIC ARTERIOVENOUS FISTULAE

Traumatic arteriovenous fistulae represent abnormal communications between an artery and a vein secondary to traumatic laceration of the vessels (Fig. 17-3). Rarely they arise spontaneously from preexisting aneurysms or angiodysplasia.[20] The most-common example of these is the traumatic carotid-cavernous fistula. Treatment of carotid cavernous fistulae is through endovascular occlusion with detachable balloons. This is performed through a transfemoral approach with inflation of the balloon within the cavernous sinus itself (Fig. 17-4).[20,21] In selected cases, a transvenous approach can be performed through the inferior petrosal sinus with deposition of coils into the cavernous sinus.[22] Rarely, a retrograde ophthalmic vein catheterization is performed with the deposition of coils within the cavernous sinus.[23] Emergency treatment of carotid cavernous fistulae should be considered if the patient presents progressive visual loss, rapidly increased intraocular pressure, severe epistaxis, sphenoid sinus pseudoaneurysm, acute hemiplegia without intracerebral hematoma, or subarachnoid hemorrhage.

Fistulae involving the vertebral system often involve the vertebral artery and its epidural venous plexus or the internal carotid artery and the adjacent internal jugular vein. These may be treated with balloons, PVA, liquid agents, or coils.[24]

VEIN OF GALEN MALFORMATIONS

Yasargil divides vein of Galen aneurysms into four types: type I: fistulae located in the wall of a varix arising from feeders from the anterior and posterior choroidal and/or the pericallosal arteries; type II: fistulae with feeders from transmesencephalic and transdiencephalic arteries; type III: a combination of types I and II; type IV: diencephalic and mesencephalic arteriovenous malformations draining into an enlarged, but otherwise normal, vein of Galen.[25]

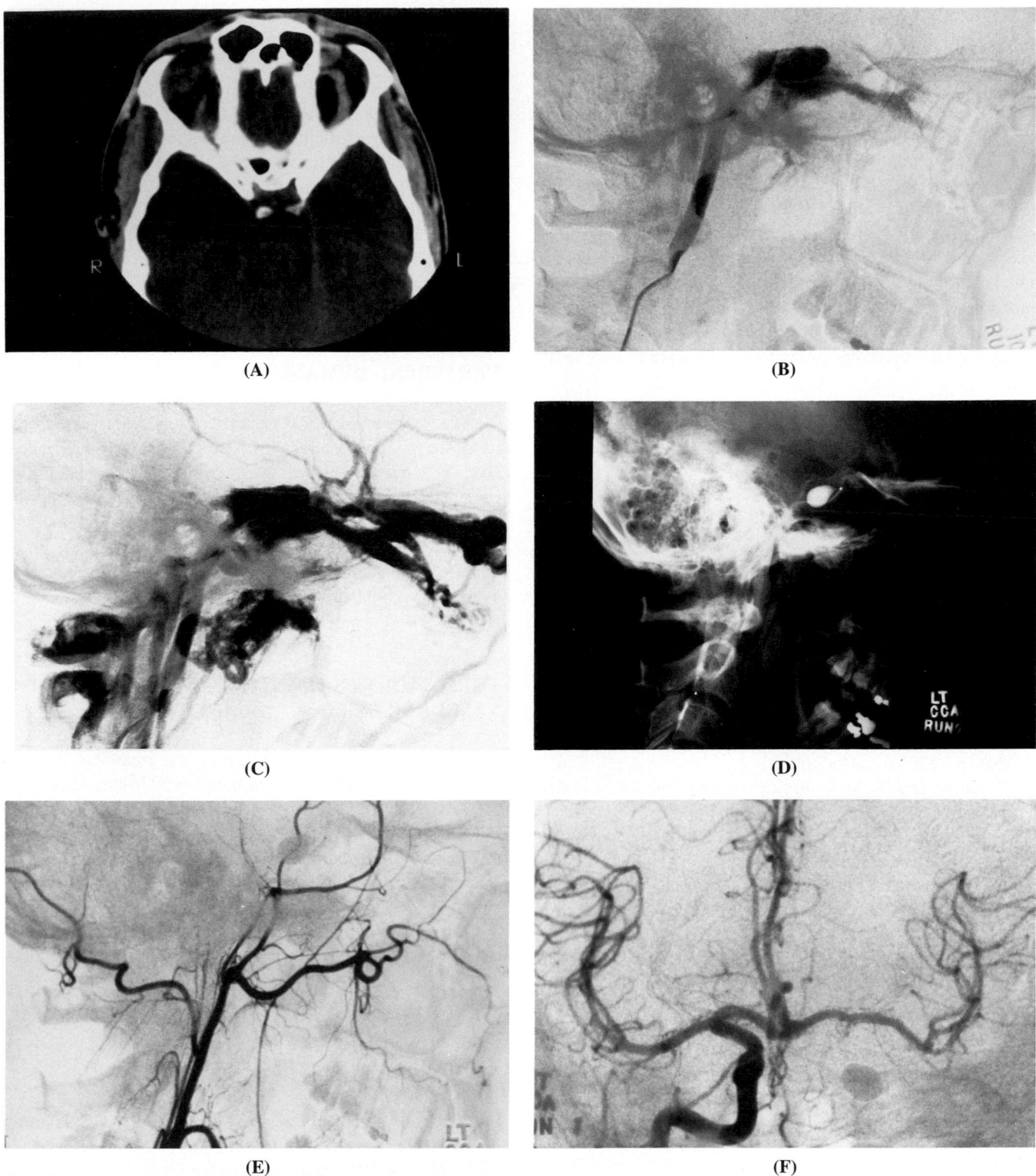

Figure 17–4 Carotids—cavernous fistula. *A.* Contrast-enhanced CT through orbit demonstrates an enlarged left superior ophthalmic vein (SOV). *B, C.* Lateral projection of left internal carotid artery with opacification cavernous sinus and SOV. *D.* Lateral skull film showing a balloon with radiopaque contrast material. *E.* Lateral projection of left common carotid shows occlusion of the internal carotid due to balloon placement. *F.* Right common carotid shows crossflow to the left internal carotid artery territory.

Vein of Galen malformations may be approached through transarterial or transvenous routes. They can be approached transvenously through a retrograde femoral vein catheterization or through a transtorcular approach following craniectomy. The approach will depend on the type of lesion, the patient's condition, and the experience of the interventional neuroradiologist.

Emergent embolization of vein of Galen malformations should be considered in newborns with refractile congestive heart failure, symptomatic hydrocephalus, or severe neurological symptoms.[26,27]

The type of embolic material will depend on the interventional neuroradiologist's experience. For those lesions requiring a transarterial approach, liquid glue or coils can be used. These should be placed as close to the fistula as possible. In the transvenous approach, coils are usually used.

ENDOVASCULAR TREATMENT OF INTRACRANIAL ANEURYSMS

The endovascular treatment of intracranial aneurysms was first described by Serbinenko in 1974.[28]

Indications for endovascular treatment include:[28,29]

1. Prior surgical exploration of an aneurysm with inability to clip the neck
2. Anatomic locations that are difficult to approach surgically
3. Fusiform aneurysms without a well-defined neck
4. Inability of the patient to tolerate general anesthesia
5. Patients with poor collateral circulation for whom bypass surgery is not possible
6. Aneurysms with high surgical risk because of their size or location

Currently, a retrograde transfemoral approach is used; the most widely used embolic agents are silicone balloons filled with liquid glue. One or several balloons may be needed for complete obliteration of the aneurysm lumen. Occasionally coils are used to supplement the balloons.[29–31]

Incomplete occlusion of the lumen of the aneurysm may allow regrowth of the aneurysm or shift of the balloon within the aneurysm lumen.[29] Other complications of balloon occlusion of aneurysms include premature detachment of the balloon, which may result in parent vessel occlusion or distal embolization; aneurysm rupture during balloon inflation; or delayed thromboembolic events in an incompletely treated aneurysm.

Gulielmi has developed a platinum coil system coupled with electrothrombosis, which induces clot formation within the coil after the application of an electric current.[32]

ENDOVASCULAR TREATMENT OF SPINAL VASCULAR MALFORMATION

Spinal cord AVMs are true vascular lesions of congenital origin.[33] The nidus may be purely intraparenchymal, on the surface of the spinal cord or perimedullary. The blood supply is usually from the anterior and posterior radiculomedullary arteries.

Embolization should be considered a first-line technique in the treatment of spinal arteriovenous malformations.[33–35] Currently, microparticles are the embolic agents of choice since they present little risk to the patient. Their drawback is a high frequency of arterial recanalization. Embolization with liquid acrylic may produce permanent occlusion but is more likely to cause acute ischemia. Spinal cord infarction can occur, particularly when the anterior spinal artery is involved in the malformation.

VERTEBRAL HEMANGIOMAS

These tumors involve a vertebral body and may extend into its posterior arch. They may be quiescent or quite aggressive. For the aggressive lesions, embolization should be considered prior to surgical intervention. This can be accomplished by percutaneously puncturing the vertebral body and injecting acrylic within it (vertebroplasty). Particulate embolization of the tumor can reduce or eliminate the compression of the spinal cord frequently seen with this lesion.

THROMBOLYSIS IN INTRACRANIAL OCCLUSIVE VASCULAR DISEASE

Fibrinolytic therapy has a place in the treatment of acute stroke due to a thrombus or embolus.[36,37] Urokinase or tissue plasminogen activator (tpa) has been used for this purpose but it is not indicated for many cerebral infarctions.

The thrombolytic agent is delivered by infusion through a microcatheter positioned as closely to the site of the occlusion as possible.

Complications of this form of therapy include intraparenchymal hemorrhage or propagation of a secondary thrombus.

PERCUTANEOUS TRANSLUMINAL ANGIOPLASTY (PTA)

Percutaneous transluminal angioplasty (PTA) is an established, efficacious method of treating arterial occlusive vascular disease.[38,40] Angioplasty of the carotid artery has been performed in patients who are poor surgical candidates or those in whom intensive anticoagulation therapy has failed to control neurological symptoms. Some patients with severe vasospasm secondary to subarachnoid hemorrhage have successfully undergone PTA.[39] Subclavian artery PTA has been performed on stenotic subclavian arteries as well as homolateral and contralateral vertebral arteries.[40]

Complications of PTA include transient ischemia during angioplasty or arterial spasm after angioplasty.

REFERENCES

1. Rufenacht DA, Latchaw RE: Principles and methodology of intracranial endovascular access. *Neuroimaging Clinics of North America* 2:251–267, 1992.

2. Hodges FJ, III: Meningioma, in Taveras JM, Ferrucci JT (eds): *Radiology, Diagnosis-Imaging-Intervention.* Philadelphia, Lippincott, 1986, vol 3, chap 4, pp 1–11.

3. Sheporaitis LA, Osborn AG, Smirniotopoulus JG, et al: Intracranial meningioma. *AJNR* 13:29–37, 1992.

4. Lasjaunias P, Berenstein A: *Surgical Neuroangiography.* New York, Springer-Verlag, 1987, vol 2, chap 2, pp 88–96.

5. Halbach VV, Hieshima GB, Higashida RT, David C: Endovascular therapy of head and neck tumors, in Vinuela F, Halbach VV, Dion JE (eds): *Interventional Neuroradiology: Endovascular Therapy of the Central Nervous System,* New York, Raven, 1992, chap 2, pp 17–28.

6. Duncan AW, Lack EE, Deck MF: Radiological evaluation of paragangliomas of the head and neck. *Radiology* 132:9–105, 1979.

7. Lasjaunias P, Berenstein A: *Surgical Neuroangiography.* New York, Springer-Verlag, 1987, vol 2, chap 4, pp 127–162.

8. Valvanir A: Preoperative embolization of the head and neck: Indications, patient selection, goals and precautions. *AJNR* 7:943–952, 1986.

9. Chiras J, Chedid G, De Busche-Depriester C: Intraarterial chemotherapy of brain tumors, in Fernando Vinuela, Halbach VV, Dion JE (eds): *Interventional Neuroradiology: Endovascular Therapy of the Central Nervous System.* New York, Raven, 1992, chap 14, pp 181–192.

10. Miller DF, Bay JW, Lederman RJ, et al: Ocular and orbital toxicity following intracarotid injection of BCNU and cisplatinum for malignant gliomas. *Ophthalmology* 92:402–400, 1985.

11. Shapiro WR: Reevaluating the efficacy of intraarterial BCNU. *J Neurosurg* 66:313–316, 1987.

12. Poisson M, Chiras J, Fauchon F, et al: Treatment of malignant recurrent glioma by intra-arterial infra ophthalmic infusion of HECNI [1-(2-chloroethyl)-1-nitroro-3-(2-hydroxyethyl)urea]. *J Neurooncol* 8:255–262, 1990.

13. Debrun GM: Arteriovenous malformation, in Taveras JM, Ferrucci JT (eds): *Radiology, Diagnosis-Imaging-Intervention.* Philadelphia, Lippincott, 1986, vol 3, chap 42, pp 1–11.

14. Rauch R, Vinuela F, Dion J, et al: Preembolization functional evaluation in brain arteriovenous malformations: The ability of superselective amytal test to predict neurologic dysfunction before embolization. *AJNR* 13:309–314, 1992.

15. Vinuela F: Functional evaluation and embolization of intracranial arteriovenous malformation, in Fernando Vinuela, Halbach VV, Dion JE (eds): *Interventional Neuroradiology: Endovascular Therapy of the Central Nervous System.* New York, Raven, 1992, chap 6, pp 77–86.

16. Dawson R, Tarr R, Hecht S, et al: Treatment of arteriovenous malformations of the brain with combined embolization and stereotactic radiosurgery: results after 1 and 2 years. *AJNR* 11:857–864, 1990.

17. Duckwiler G: Dural Arteriovenous Fistula. *Neuroimaging Clinics of North America* 2:291–307, 1992.

18. Halbach VV, Higashida RT, Hieshima GB, David C: Endovascular therapy of dural fistulas, in Vinuela F, Halbach VV, Dion JE (eds): *Interventional Neuroradiology: Endovascular Therapy of the Central Nervous System.* New York, Raven, 1992, chap 3, pp 29–50.

19. Pierot L, Chiras J, Meder JF, et al: Dural arteriovenous fistulas of the posterior fossa draining into subarachnoid veins. *AJNR,* 13:315–323, 1992.

20. Lasjaunias P, Berenstein A: *Surgical Neuroangiography.* New York, Springer-Verlag, 1987, vol 2, chap 6, pp 175–233.

21. Debrun G: Management of traumatic carotid-cavernous fistulas, in Vinuela F, Halbach VV, Dion JE (eds): *Interventional Neuroradiology: Endovascular Therapy of the Central Nervous System.* New York, Raven, 1992, chap 8, pp 107–112.

22. Halbach VV, Higashida RT, Barnwell ST, et al: Transarterial platinum coil embolization of carotid cavernous fistulas. *AJNR* 12:429–433, 1991.

23. Monsein L, Debrun G, Miller N, et al: Treatment of dural carotid-cavernous fistulas via the superior ophthalmic vein. *AJNR* 12:435–439, 1991.

24. Dion J: Acquired cervicocranial arteriovenous fistulas. *Neuroimaging Clinics of North America* 2:319–335, 1992.

25. Yasargil MG: *Microneurosurgery,* Thieme, Stuttgart, 1987, vol 3B, pp 18–19.

26. Lylyk P, March AD, Kohan GA, Vinuela F: Alternative therapeutic approaches in intravascular embolization of Veins of Galen vascular malformation, in Vinuela F, Halbach VV, Dion JE (eds): *Interventional Neuroradiology: Endovascular Therapy of the Central Nervous System.* New York, Raven, 1992, chap 10, pp 129–139.

27. Garcia-Monaco R, Lasjaunias P, Berenstein A: Therapeutic management of veins of the Galen aneurysmal malformation, in Vinuela F, Halbach VV, Dion JE (eds): *Interventional Neuroradiology: Endovascular Therapy of the Central Nervous System.* New York, Raven, 1992, chap 9, pp 113–127.

28. Serbinenko FA: Balloon catheterization and occlusion of major cerebral vessels. *J Neurosurg* 41:125–145, 1974.

29. Higashida RT, Halbach VV, Barnwell SL: Treatment of intracranial aneurysms with preservation of the parent vessel: Results of percutaneous balloon embolization in 84 patients. *AJNR* 11:633–640, 1990.

30. Nakahara I, Taki W, Nishi S, et al: Treatment of giant anterior communicating artery aneurysm via endovascular approach using detachable balloons and occlusive coils. *AJNR* 11:1195–1197, 1990.

31. Higashida RT, Halbach VV, Dowd C, et al: Endovascular detachable balloon embolization therapy of cavernous carotid artery aneurysms: Results in 87 cases. *J Neurosurg* 72:857–862, 1990.

32. Guglielmi G, Vinuela F, Dion J, Duckwiler G: Electrothrombosis of saccular aneurysms via endovascular approach: II. Preliminary clinical experience. *J Neurosurgery* 75:8–14, 1991.

33. Casasco AE, Houdart E, Gobin YP, et al: Embolization of spinal vascular malformations. *Neuroimaging Clinics of North America* 2:337–358, 1992.

34. Merland JJ, Reizine D, Laurerot A, et al: Embolization of spinal cord vascular lesions, in Vinuela F, Halbach VV, Dion JE (eds): *Interventional Neuroradiology: Endovascular Therapy of the Central Nervous System.* New York, Raven, 1992, chap 12, pp 153–165.

35. Biondi A, Merland JJ, Hodes JE, et al: Aneurysms of spinal arteries associated with intramedullary arteriovenous malformations: I. Angiographic and clinical aspects. *AJNR* 13:933–940, 1992.

36. Zeumer H, Freitag HJ, Knospe V: Intravascular thrombolysis in central nervous system cerebrovascular disease. *Neuroimaging Clinics of North America* 2:359–369, 1992.

37. Levy DE: Medical treatment of acute, ischemic stroke. *Neuroimaging Clinics of North America* 3:597–605, 1992.
38. Tsai FY, Higashida R, Meoli C: Percutaneous transluminal angioplasty of extracranial and intracranial arterial stenosis in head and neck. *Neuroimaging Clinics of North America* 2:371–384, 1992.
39. Pistoia F, Horton JA, Sekhar L, Horowitz M: Imaging of blood glow changes following angioplasty for treatment of vasospasm. *AJNR* 12:446–448, 1991.
40. Theron AJ: Angioplasty of brachiocephalic vessels, in Vinuela F, Halbach VV, Dion JE (eds): *Interventional Neuroradiology: Endovascular Therapy of the Central Nervous System.* New York, Raven, 1992, chap 13, pp 167–180.

☐ STUDY QUESTIONS

I. A 27-year-old female had the sudden onset of headache followed by a left hemiparesis and left-sided apraxia, which persisted. A CT scan reveals a vascular malformation in the left occipital lobe measuring 7 cm in greatest diameter. There is a small subcortical hematoma in the posterior parietal area. The malformation is fed by the right middle and posterior cerebral arteries.

1. How could the malformation be most clearly outlined? **2.** What alternate method might be used to outline the lesion? **3.** What method might be considered to reduce blood flow to the malformation? **4.** How would endovascular occlusion assist the surgeon? **5.** What is the alternate therapy?

II. A 38-year-old male is seen in the emergency room because of seizures involving the left face and arm. The seizures have been occurring for about 3 mo but were now followed by a left hemiparesis. A noncontrasting MRI shows an isodense mass in the right sylvian fissure, which is quite vascular. After injection of contrast, the tumor takes on a high signal. It includes not only the temporal fossa but also extends into the calvarian. Angiography reveals blood supply from the branches of the right middle cerebral artery and the temporal branch of the external carotid.

1. What is the most likely diagnosis? **2.** What is the definitive therapy? **3.** How can the feeding vessels be best identified? **4.** How can the feeding vessels be occluded? **5.** What substances might be used to occlude the feeding vessels?

III. A 22-year-old male sustains a closed head injury with loss of consciousness for about 30 min. When he recovers he notes a "buzzing" in the left ear, and there is swelling of the left eye, which persists. There is infection of the conjunctiva on the left.

1. What is the most likely diagnosis? **2.** How can the lesion be outlined? **3.** What forms of treatment have been used? **4.** What interventional consideration might be considered? **5.** Using current techniques, what are the chances for occluding the fistula leaving the carotid artery patent?

IV. A hydrocephalic male infant is found to have an aneurysmal mass above the quadrigeminal plate. The mass is fed by branches of the posterior choroidal artery and branches of the ipsilateral pericollosal artery.

1. What is the lesion? **2.** What is the most likely cause of the hydrocephalus? **3.** What forms of therapy might be considered (*a*) for the hydrocephalus and (*b*) for the malformation? **4.** Where are the most common complications of a vein of Galen aneurysm? **5.** How might these be prevented?

V. A 26-year-old female develops a left foot drop at the time of an acute episode of back pain. An MRI suggests a spinal AVM with a nidus located posteriorly behind the twelfth thoracic vertebra. The lesion is fed by a radicular branch located between T11 and T12 on the right.

1. What are the alternative forms of treatment? **2.** How might the lesion be embolized (technically)? **3.** What materials might be considered for embolization? **4.** When should this patient be treated? **5.** Where is the artery of Adamkiewicz most likely located?

CHAPTER 18

Cranial Trauma of Children and Adults

Marshall B. Allen, Jr.
Ann Marie Flannery

Head injury is a major cause of morbidity and mortality in the United States. According to the Center for Disease Control, there were about 17 deaths per 100,000 population, or about 40,000 deaths per year, from head injuries in the United States during the period 1979–1986.[1]

Head injury is the most common cause of death in children and young adults. Deaths from head injury were 3 times more common in males than in females, and there was a peak incidence in the 15- to 24-year-old age group. Over half resulted from automobile accidents, but 14 percent resulted from firearms. Fatal trauma may be isolated to the head or associated with additional injuries to viscera and/or extremities.

Specialized centers for treatment of patients with acute head injuries have been developed in the United States and abroad; however, the mortality rates for victims of head injury remains high. One report from San Diego suggests that the greatest influence on reduction of death rates there had resulted from an "improvement in the county's prehospital emergency ground and air evacuation services." A comparison of the survival rates of two institutions in The Netherlands reports higher survival in the more conservative institution.[2,3] At least some of the difference in survival rates in those two centers was probably related to severity of injuries. Still, overall mortality from severe head injury remains high.

Head injuries are categorized according to whether they are "open" or "closed," whether open wounds are a result of blunt trauma or penetrating missiles, and whether injuries are accompanied by discrete intracranial lesions, such as hematomas or contusions. Hematomas are categorized according to location—i.e., outside the dura, beneath the dura, or in the brain substance; whether they are above or below the tentorium; and the number and size of the collections.

Victims of head injury are categorized according to the severity of their neurological deficits, especially the level of consciousness.

In this chapter, various brain lesions and head injury states are defined, followed by a review of the evaluation, treatment, and disposition of the patient with head injury. Cerebral edema and the resultant increased intracranial pressure (ICP) represent such a unique position in head injury and monitoring of ICP is so important that the care of patients and the techniques of ICP monitoring, along with methods of treatment, must be reviewed before we discuss the evaluation and treatment of specific intracranial lesions.

☐ DEFINITIONS

OPEN HEAD INJURY

The term *open head injury* indicates there is communication between intracranial contents and the atmosphere. Open head injuries can result from penetrating missiles or blows to the head by sharp or blunt objects with consequent lacerations and/or severe abrasions to the scalp. (See Fig. 18-1.)

A CSF fistula may result from blunt injury that produces fractures at the base of the skull, involving the paranasal sinuses or mastoid air cells. While the scalp itself may not be violated, basilar skull fractures present problems similar to open injuries in which the scalp *and* skull are penetrated.

Open head injuries are sites of possible contamination of the intracranial spaces at the time of injury, or later. Surgical treatment involves debridement of the tract and closure of the wound, preferably with living tissue. In addition to

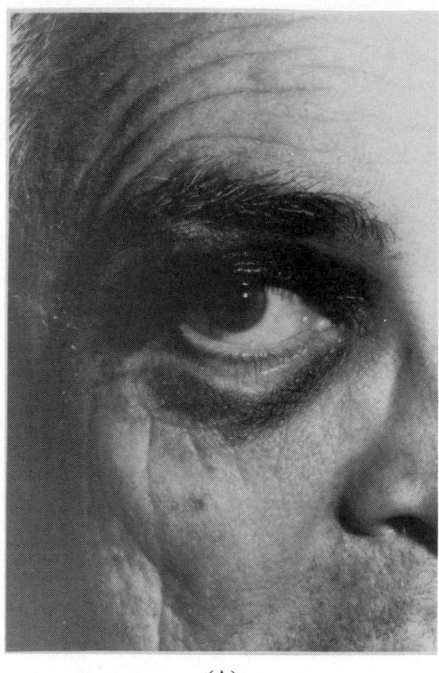

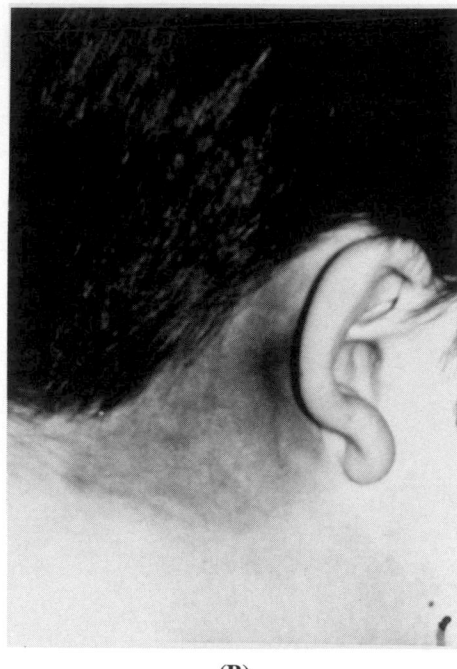

(A)   (B)

Figure 18–1 Photograph of periorbital (*A*) and retroauricular ecchymosis (*B*) in patients with basilar skull fractures.

infection, open injuries involve most of the problems that are associated with closed head injuries.

CLOSED HEAD INJURY

Closed head injuries result from blunt trauma. The scalp and/or skull remain intact so that there are no tracts connecting the intracranial contents and the atmosphere. There may be fractures of the skull, even with bone fragments depressed or driven into subarachnoid spaces or brain substance. Likewise, there may be defects in the scalp but not connected with kull fractures.

Concerns of closed head injuries relate to: the severity of injury to intracranial structures, the occurrence of intracranial hematomas, cerebral edema, and axonal or vascular disruption.

CEREBRAL CONCUSSION

Cerebral concussion is a term used to indicate temporary loss of consciousness due to injury to the head. Limitations on the period of impaired consciousness are implied but imprecise. Although definitions in the past indicated that there was no structural damage, there probably is, at least, damage to cellular membranes when there is loss of consciousness. The exact site(s) are debated, but neurophysiological knowledge and observations would suggest that changes occur in the reticular activating system (RAS), in the midbrain. Treatment is generally supportive and expectant.

CEREBRAL CONTUSION

Contusions of the brain are injuries to cerebral substance, usually accompanied by hemorrhage into the substance of the brain with adjacent edema. (See Fig. 18-2.) In a closed head injury, contusions are most frequent at the bases of the

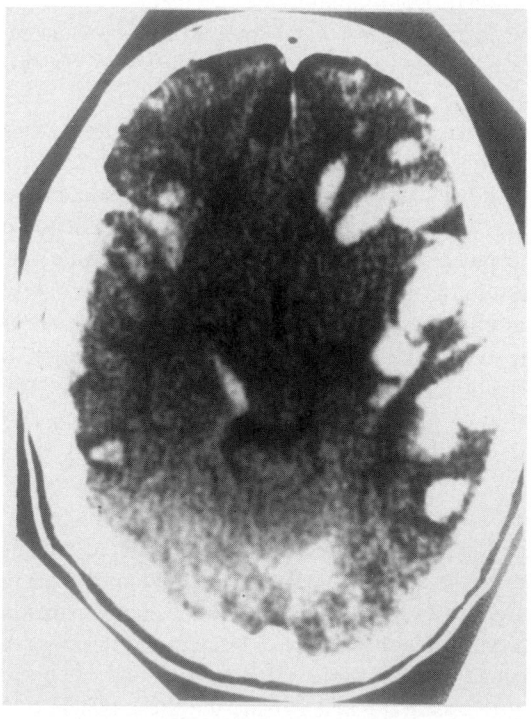

Figure 18–2 Computerized tomogram of brain following closed head injury showing multiple contusions.

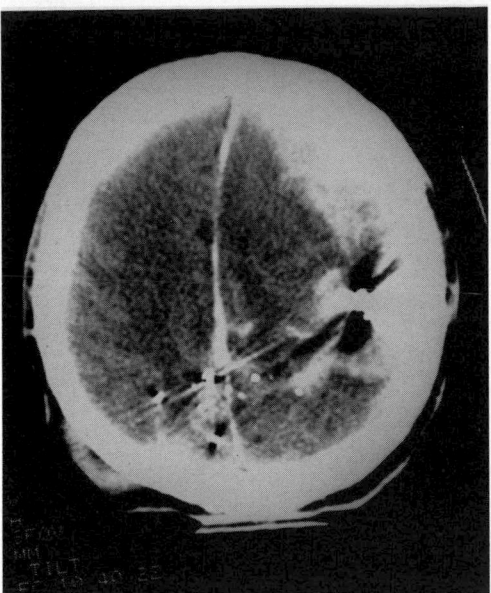

Figure 18–3 Computerized tomogram showing contusion along the course of a gunshot wound.

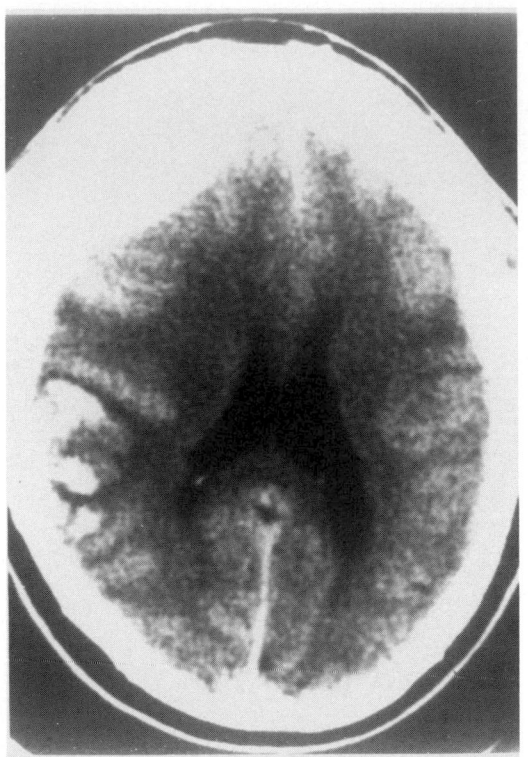

Figure 18–4 Computerized tomogram showing epidural hematoma in the right frontal area.

frontal and temporal lobes, as a result of surfaces of the brain being "slapped" against the base of the skull.

Contusions may occur elsewhere as well. Computerized tomograms demonstrate such lesions in the brain stem, along the falx and the tentorium, and beneath the surface of the brain. Contusions are common beneath a depressed skull fracture, and they routinely accompany missile injuries—the extent depending on the velocity of the missile, movement characteristics, temperature, and the number and size of in-driven bony fragments. (See Fig. 18-3.)

EPIDURAL HEMATOMA

Epidural hematoma, as the name signifies, is a collection of blood located immediately above the dura but beneath the inner table of the skull. (See Fig. 18-4.) In the acutely injured patient, epidural hematomas are usually the result of a tear in a meningeal artery, most commonly the middle meningeal, although they can result from tears in other vessels as well. Epidural hematomas occasionally develop hours or days after trauma—apparently the result of temporary intracranial hypotension.[4] They also result from fractures crossing the venous sinuses, from bleeding beneath a bone flap following craniotomy, or from bleeding at the periphery of a craniotomy where the dura has been separated from the inner table of the skull. If the hematoma is chronic, the collection may liquify, but this is rare.

SUBDURAL HEMATOMA

Subdural hematoma usually results from tears in veins bridging from the surface of the brain to the inner surface of the dura, where they connect with the sinuses. They are most common over the cerebral hemispheres but may be present in the middle or posterior fossae as well, often resulting composed of clotted blood. (See Fig. 18-5.) Subdural hematomas usually liquify within a week and can be treated as chronic lesions thereafter. (See Fig. 18-6.)

INTRACEREBRAL HEMATOMA

Intracerebral hematomas are collections of blood within cerebral tissue. Those which follow head injury are usually the result of a coalition of multiple petechial hemorrhages resulting from cerebral contusion. (See Fig. 18-7.) They are most common in the anterior temporal lobe and the base of the frontal lobe when they result from blunt trauma. When associated with a penetrating injury, intracerebral hematomas may occur wherever vessels are interrupted along the tract of the missile. They usually include a considerable amount of contused brain tissue mixed with the blood.

CEREBRAL EDEMA

Cerebral edema is a most serious consequence of head injury. Edema, may be localized, often in association with

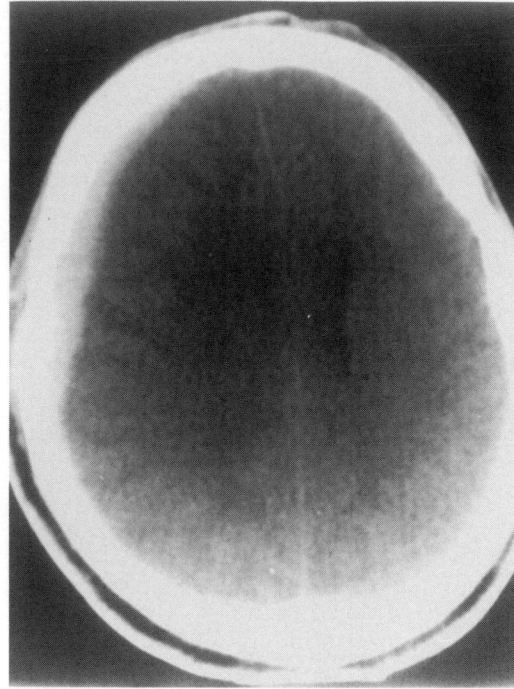

Figure 18–5 Computerized tomogram following acute subdural hematoma. Note increased attenuation of acute hemorrhage. Many hematomas in the subacute phase may be isodense and difficult to differentiate from brain substance.

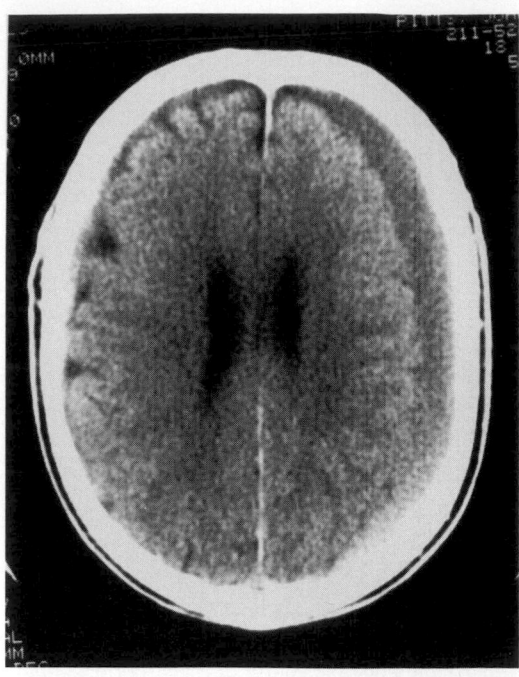

Figure 18–6 Computerized tomogram showing chronic subdural hematoma. Note that the attenuation is decreased and easily differentiated from the brain substance. Note increased attenuation in occipital area due to increased hemoglobin content.

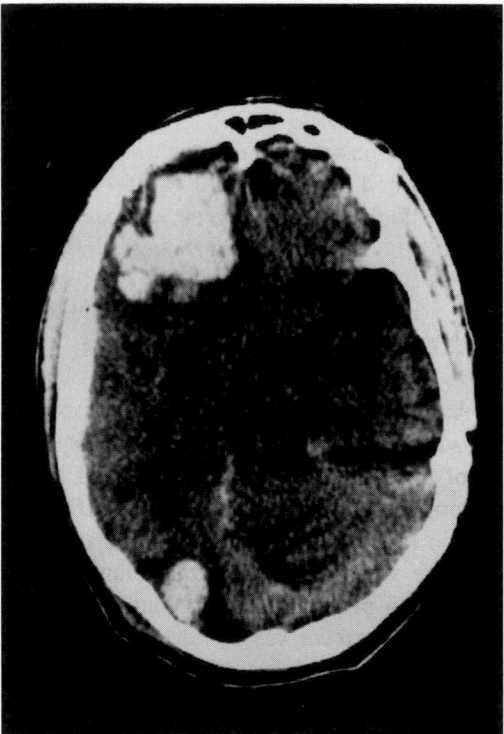

Figure 18–7 Computerized tomogram showing posttraumatic intracerebral hematoma. Note contusions at periphery and in occipital lobe.

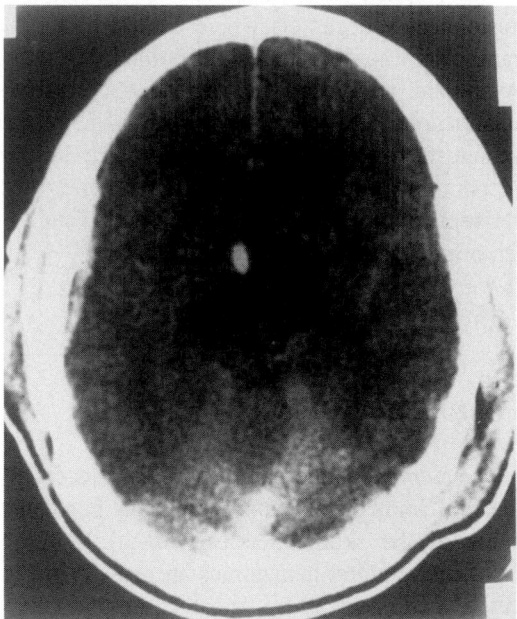

Figure 18–8 Computerized tomogram showing a small subdural hematoma and cerebral edema sufficient to obliterate the lateral ventricle and reduce the size of the cisterns in a patient following an acute head injury.

other lesions, such as hematomas or infarction; however, it may be diffuse. Evidences of edema are often apparent on computerized tomography (CT) by decreased attenuation and loss of basal cisterns.[6,7] (See Fig. 18-8.) Cerebral edema is responsible for increased intracranial pressure and resultant decreased cerebral perfusion.[8]

TREATMENT OF CEREBRAL EDEMA AND INTRACRANIAL PRESSURE MONITORING

Cerebral edema of "differing" types apparently responds differently to treatment. "Vasogenic edema," associated with brain tumors and even chronic subdural hematomas, responds to the administration of steroids, whereas the response of cerebral edema associated with trauma to medical therapy is less obvious.

Cerebral edema results in increased mass in a rigidly enclosed space. The result is increased intracranial pressure (ICP), which leads to decreased cerebral perfusion and further ischemia if the increased ICP persists, unless systemic blood pressure becomes elevated. Intracranial contents, in addition to brain tissue, include blood contained in the arteries, veins, and sinuses, and the cerebrospinal fluid (CSF).

When swelling of the brain occurs, the CSF and blood in the veins and venous sinuses become displaced. The ventricles and cisterns become smaller. When the venous sinuses collapse, resistance to blood flow out of the cranium increases, leading to retention of blood in the arteries and capillaries and further decompensation.[11] Once fluid spaces of the brain have been replaced, there is a rapid rise in intracranial pressure in response to any further increments in mass.[12]

Treatment possibilities are limited to: (1) removal of more CSF, (2) reducing the quantity of blood in the arteries, (3) reducing fluid in the brain substance, (4) providing more space for the brain tissue, or (5) reducing the amount of brain substance. There are severe limitations to each of these options. Even though much CSF is displaced as the brain swells, there is usually some fluid in the ventricles that can be removed by ventricular drainage.

The amount of blood contained in the arteries within the cranium is controlled by the size of the vessels, and this is controlled by the level of carbon dioxide Pa_{CO_2}. Vessels dilate as the level of CO_2 rises. The normal Pa_{CO_2} is in the low 30s. Reducing the Pa_{CO_2} to about 25 results in contraction of the arterioles and reduces the ICP.[13] Reduction below this level results in reduced cerebral blood flow, which may add to the ischemia.[14]

Mannitol, furosemide, and albumin have been used to reduce tissue edema.[15,16,17] Mannitol increases the osmolarity of the blood, which draws fluid from surrounding tissues, including the brain. This results in reducing brain volume, initially; however, these results may be temporary. Recurrence of swelling requires repeated administration.

For treatment of cerebral edema, an initial dose of 40 to 50 g is administered in the adult.[18] This is followed by about 20 g every 4 to 6 h if the intracranial hypertension recurs. Administration must be withheld if the serum osmolarity reaches 310 mOsm/liter. There is a similar response to infusion of urea or furosemide, although the mechanism of action of furosemide may be primarily hemoconcentration.[15] Rebound phenomenon is thought to be greater with urea than mannitol.

Following closed head injury, mass lesions (hematomas) should be removed early. An edematous or contused lobe can be removed, but the possibility of increasing neurological deficits limits the amount of brain substance that can be excised. Expansion of the intracranial spaces by craniectomy has been employed in the past with very limited success.

INTRACRANIAL PRESSURE MONITORING

The indication for intracranial pressure (ICP) monitoring is suspicion of elevated ICP in a patient who has, or is expected to have, an impaired state of consciousness. In severely traumatized patients, this includes all those with mass lesions demonstrated by CT; and in patients above the age of 40 years, those with systolic blood pressures less than 90 mmHg, as well as those who are posturing.

Narayan and Becker have recommended monitoring any patient who meets two or more of these criteria.[19] Monitoring may be discontinued in patients with normal CTs whose pressures have remained normal for 24 h.[20] ICP monitoring is mandatory in a patient who is being treated for increased ICP with paralysis and who is receiving controlled respiration or mannitol.

Three types of apparatus are available for monitoring ICP. The most accurate is a catheter inserted into a lateral ventricle and connected to an electronically controlled pressure transducer. (See Fig. 18-9.) The tubing usually has extensions coming off the sides by which CSF collected from the ventricular space can be evacuated and by which the catheter can be connected to a vertical column of fluid to check the accuracy of the electronic monitor.

The system has two limitations: (1) Insertion of the catheter into a lateral ventricle is difficult when the ventricles are reduced in size, as many are when there is elevated ICP. In addition, the ventricles are often displaced when there is a localized effect of cerebral edema or there is a mass lesion. Repeated attempts to insert the catheter can produce further injury to the brain. Intraventricular catheters are usually inserted on the nondominant side unless this is contraindicated. (2) *Infection* is the most common serious complication of monitoring intraventricular pressure by catheter.[21] The rate of ventriculitis rises with the length of time a catheter is in place. The incidence of infection may be reduced by tunneling the tube beneath the scalp for several centimeters and applying antiseptic ointments about the site of penetration. But even then, infection is still a frequent complication. Catheters should be changed about every 5

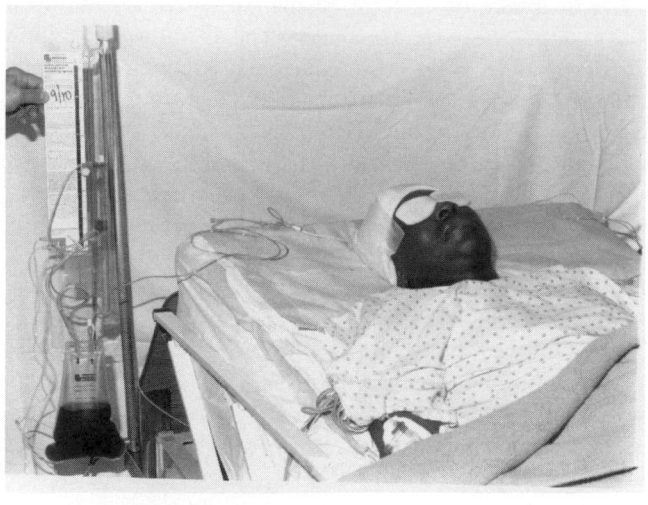

(A)

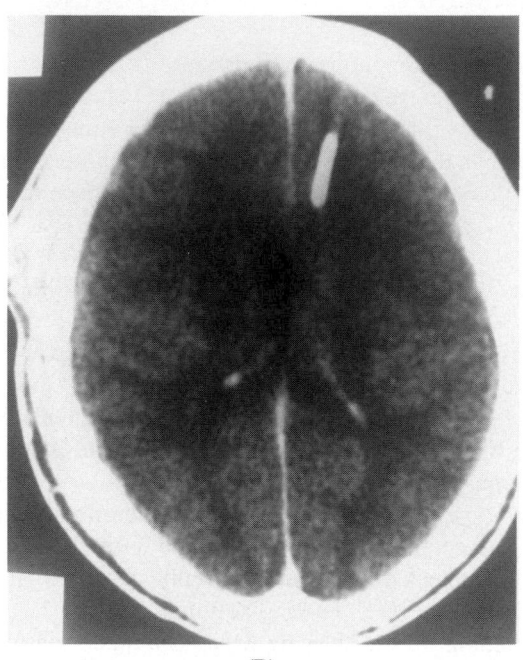

(B)

Figure 18–9 *A*. Photograph of a patient whose intracranial pressure is being monitored by a ventricular catheter and fluid column. Note that the base of the fluid column is at the head of the patient's head. The intracranial catheter is directed toward the lateral ventricle in *B*.

days to reduce the chances of infection when monitoring is required for longer periods.

Ventriculostomy permits continuous monitoring of the ICP and periodic evacuation of CSF. The pressure transducer and the head must remain at the same level. A pressure of less than 20 mm of mercury—even with a small hematoma seen on CT—rarely requires surgery, whereas hemorrhagic lesions seen in association with a monitored pressure above 30 mmHg require evacuation.[22]

Alternate mechanisms for measuring ICP are surface screws placed in subdural or subarachnoid spaces and spring-type monitors which are placed into the epidural space, usually through twist drill-burr holes.[23,24,25] Measurements made through screws are less accurate than measurements through ventricular catheters; they underestimate the pressure by more than 10 mmHg in from 25 to 40 percent of patients.[26] Obstructions at the end of the screw result from blockage of the opening by a fragment of dura or gyrus of the brain. Obstructions may be identified by alterations in the wave form. The normally pulsatile recording becomes flattened. Examination of the wound may reveal leaks around the screws. Screws are less likely to be associated with intracranial infection than are ventricular catheters, but they require penetrations of the dura and have the potential for carrying infection into the subarachnoid spaces. CSF cannot be evacuated through screws. The accuracy of epidural recording devices, like subarachnoid screws, is repeatedly questioned. They have the advantage of rarely being associated with serious intracranial infection. They provide no route for evacuating CSF.

Any intracranial mass lesion in a patient with ICP pressures above 30 mmHg should be removed. If the pressure remains elevated, the patient should have an endotracheal tube or tracheostomy and should be paralyzed if he or she is not able to cooperate with respiratory assistance. Respiratory assistance is provided with machine settings that will provide a P_{CO_2} of 25, and the P_aO_2 should be maintained between 80 and 100 mmHg. If the ICP remains significantly above 20 mm of mercury when the patient is at rest, the administration of mannitol intravenously should be initiated. For this purpose, 40 to 50 grams of mannitol may be given at the start, followed by 10 to 20 grams as needed, usually at about every 4 to 6 h. The serum osmolarity must be monitored. If the osmolarity of the blood exceeds 310 mOsm/liter, the mannitol must be discontinued.

Pentabarbital coma has been recommended as a treatment of cerebral ischemia in association with head injury. Barbiturates reduce the oxygen requirement of the brain. However, prolonged coma is associated with a high incidence of pneumonia and other medical problems. Recent reports have indicated that, while the use of barbiturates may have a beneficial effect in some cases of severe anoxia, barbiturate use in patients subjected to severe trauma is probably not warranted.[27,28]

Use of steroids to combat cerebral edema as a result of trauma has been recommended by many. Steroids are clearly effective in the treatment of edema in association with intracranial neoplasms, and steroids often reduce the neurological deficits associated with chronic subdural hematomas.[29,30] However, there has been no statistical evidence that steroids benefit patients with head injury, despite a number of studies.[31,32,33,34] Recent statistical evidence that steroids are advantageous in the treatment of acute spinal injury doubtlessly will reopen the question.[35,36]

Table 18-1
GLASGOW COMA SCALE

Eye Opening (E)
4 Opens eyes spontaneously
3 Opens eyes to voice
2 Opens eyes to pain
1 No eye opening

Best Motor Response (M)
6 Obeys commands
5 Localizes pain
4 Withdraws to pain
3 Abnormal flexor response
2 Abnormal extensor response
1 No movement

Best Verbal Response (V)
5 Appropriate and oriented
4 Confused conversation
3 Inappropriate words
2 Incomprehensible sounds
1 No sounds

☐ THE EVALUATION OF PATIENTS HAVING SUSTAINED AN INJURY TO THE HEAD

Assurance of adequate respiration and circulatory function must be the first consideration for any patient who has sustained a recent injury. *A patent airway is critical.* Aspiration of the oropharynx may be necessary. An endotracheal tube or tracheostomy may be required if the patient is stuporous.

Adequate circulation must be assured. This may require fluids, cardiac stimulants, control of bleeding, administration of blood, or even treatment of cardiac tamponade. Fluids infused under these circumstances should be crystalloid—that is, saline or Ringer's lactate solution—since cerebral edema is a major concern. This is the appropriate time to obtain samples of blood for cell counts, blood gas determinations, cross-match, blood chemistries, and determination of levels of intoxicants if this is appropriate and has not been accomplished earlier.

A rapid evaluation of the overall status of the patient is the next requirement. There *must* be rapid evaluation for the presence of other injuries that may include deformities or swelling of the extremities. There must also be examination of the chest and abdomen with appropriate efforts to find evidence of bleeding, perforations of the gut or its appendages such as the liver and other intra-abdominal organs, or injuries to the genitourinary system and/or spine. Plain radiographs of the chest, spine, and extremities may be indicated to complete some of these evaluations. This may be the appropriate time to obtain plain films of the skull as well.

The next evaluation is that of the nervous system, and the Glasgow coma scale has become the standard for evaluation in most trauma centers. (See Table 18-1.)[37] A rating is given for the capabilities of the patient for eye movement, motor function, and verbal response. There are a possible 15 points of the scale. The lower the score, the poorer the state of cerebral function, and follow-up studies have indicated that low scores are associated with a poor prognosis, although they may not predict intellectual capabilities.

Although there have been many criticisms of the Glasgow scale, it is one that is known to most personnel who care for patients with severe head injuries; consequently, it forms a standard for communication as well as care.[38,39,40]

Additional observations are required for unilateral pupillary dilatation and/or oculomotor palsy and lateralized paresis. *A dilated pupil in a stuporous patient who has recently experienced injury to the head is a surgical emergency,* heralding the possibility of an acute intracranial hemorrhage. Lateralized paresis emphasizes the urgency for consideration of surgical therapy.

COMPUTED TOMOGRAPHY

Computed tomography (CT) is almost routine for patients who have had a head injury severe enough to alter consciousness. The overall time required for the procedure can be reduced to 5 or 10 min and the time required for individual scans can be reduced to a few seconds so that interpretable scans can usually be obtained even in patients who are uncooperative. The procedures can be performed on patients requiring respiratory assistance or circulatory support.

Scans provide invaluable information for the differentiation of lesions causing stupor, and they often demonstrate unsuspected hematomas, providing information that reduces the risk of releasing patients with unsuspected intracranial hemorrhages. CT localizes intracranial hemorrhages, providing information for pinpointing the site of a craniotomy to evacuate the lesion. Intraventricular hemorrhage in a closed head injury suggests brain damage and carries a very poor prognosis.[41] Areas of decreased attenuation and decreased size or absence of cisterns are indications of cerebral edema and increased ICP. Scans also frequently demonstrate fractures which may not be apparent on plain radiographs. Displacement or distortion of ventricles may help to localize the site of mass lesions or edema which might not be apparent on the scan. CTs performed to evaluate patients with acute head injury do *not* require intravenous contrast material since the primary purpose is demonstration of fresh blood, distortion of ventricles, or fractures; however, contrast material may be required to outline subacute or chronic hematomas.

Retained metallic fragments of missiles distort CT scans, but the scans may reveal bone driven into the cranium, identify sites and sizes of hematomas, and demonstrate evidence of surrounding edema. (See Fig. 18-10.) Tracts through the ventricles, leaving a significant collection of intraventricular blood, are associated with a particularly poor

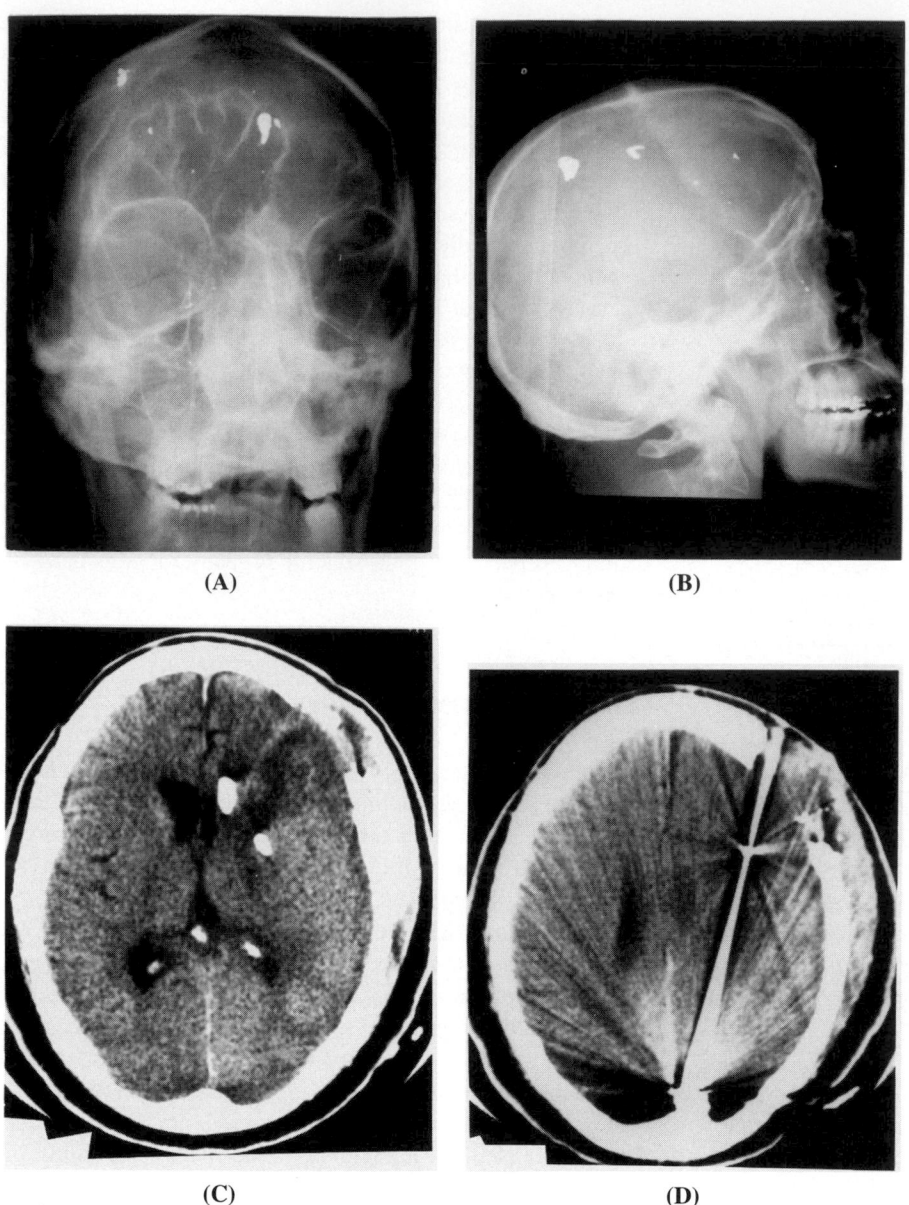

(A)

(B)

(C)

(D)

Figure 18–10 *A* and *B*. Plain radiographs of a patient having sustained a gunshot wound of the head. The missile fragments are seen behind the coronal suture in *B*. CT of another patient showing missile fragments are seen in *C* and *D*.

prognosis.[42] The CT also demonstrates evidence of damage to parts of the brain that may be far removed from the tract of the missile.[43]

Preliminary observations comparing the identification of lesions by CT, magnetic resonance imaging (MRI), and positron emission tomography (PET) indicate that the latter forms of imaging may provide additional information, but for practical reasons—particularly, rapid examination in an uncooperative patient—CT remains the examination of choice.[44]

The need for plain x-rays has been questioned.[45] But plain radiographs of the chest are required for patients being considered for surgery. Plain films of the neck are usually taken in patients who have impaired consciousness as a result of a head injury. The authors usually obtain plain radiographs of the head as well. While CTs often demonstrate fractures in such patients and outline depressions better than plain films, an overall picture of the location and extent of a fracture may be more apparent on plain films. The tract of a missile may be better projected on a plain radiograph than on CT, although the reverse may also be true. (See Fig. 18-11.)

PLANNING THERAPY

Examination of the patient, radiographs and CT scanning give a good indication of intracranial lesions from head injury that will require urgent therapy. Planning necessitates a knowledge of associated injuries and the general condition of the patient, including: cardiac function, status of the lungs, liver and renal function, and the presence of any major bleeding problems.

Blood for determining the status of pulmonary function and liver and renal function, as well as a sample for cross-

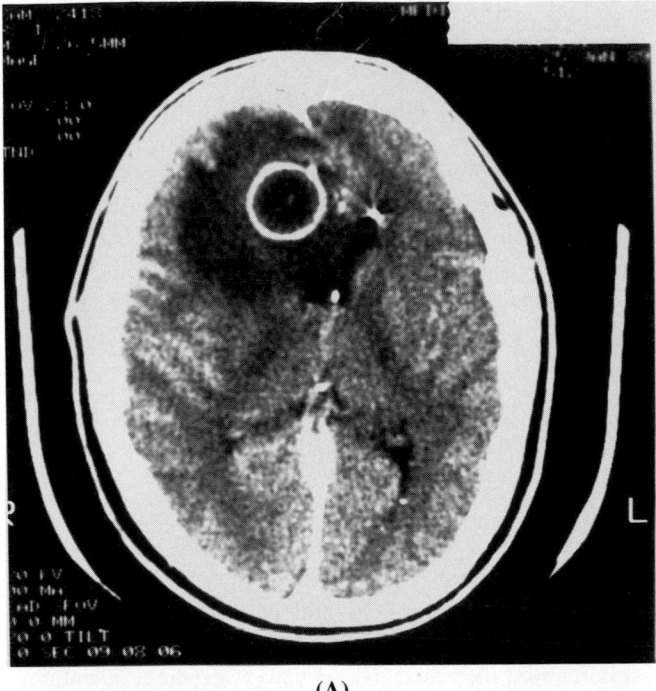

(A)

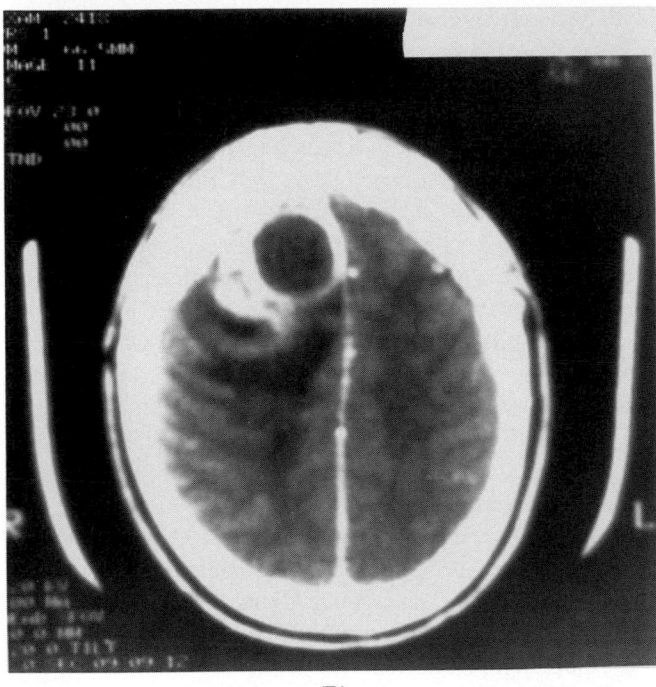

(B)

Figure 18–11 Computerized tomograms showing abscess within the tract of a gunshot wound developing several days after the injury.

match, is collected as the patient arrives in the emergency room, and the results of laboratory investigations are usually available by the time the radiographic investigations have been completed.

Cardiac monitoring occurs in the operating room. There may be inadequate time to do a detailed cardiac workup, but abnormalities in rhythm or evidence of congestive failure should be apparent in the routine evaluation. Likewise, evidence of irregularity in clotting mechanisms and major dis-

turbances in liver or renal function should be apparent from the initial profile of blood chemistries.

The presence of concomitant lesions will alter significantly the plan of therapy for intracranial lesions. Major sources of bleeding must be controlled. It may be necessary for one surgical team to remove an expanding intracranial hematoma while another team is repairing defects in major blood vessels in other parts of the body. Repair of lesions of internal organs may also be necessary, although it usually adds to confusion in the operating room for several teams to be working at the same time. In addition, there may be difficulty in getting the patient positioned optimally when more than one operative procedure is in progress.

Thus, priorities must be developed on the basis of acuteness of individual lesions. A plan of therapy of cranial lesions must be initiated. Scalp wounds must be closed. Nondisplaced fractures which are closed and do not communicate with sinuses or air cells and are not associated with underlying hematomas do *not* require therapy other than observation of the patient for concomitant lesions. Patients with nondisplaced fractures entering sinuses or mastoid air cells may be treated expectantly, investigating evidences of a CSF fistula. Fractures of the paranasal sinuses with displacement require early repair. Hematomas, large enough to produce mass effects and areas of contusion of significant size should be resected. Usually intracranial pressure monitoring is instituted at the close of the procedure.

Patients who are stuporous but have no major intracranial mass lesions several hours after having sustained a head injury, as well as those who have radiographic evidence of increased intracranial pressure such as small ventricles or small cisterns, are candidates for ICP monitoring. An intraventricular catheter or subdural screw (bolt) is implanted. Patients, then, will be treated as though they have cerebral edema if the ICP is elevated. Determination of ICP may be a major factor in deciding whether patients with small hematomas should undergo evacuation of their lesions.

☐ TREATMENT OF SPECIFIC LESIONS OF THE HEAD

CEPHALOHEMATOMA AND SUBGALEAL HEMATOMAS

When blood collects beneath the scalp in infants and children, accumulation occurs subperiosteally, or in the subgaleal loose areolar tissue. *Cephalohematomas* are subperiostal hematomas commonly found in newborns following birth trauma. Characteristically, this collection of fluid-blood is limited by the periostial insertion at suture lines.

Cephalohematomas commonly resolve without treatment; however, they occasionally calcify. Calcified cephalohematomas are cosmetic deformities, which are self-correcting. The calcified tissue is gradually absorbed by the expanding calvarium and appearance becomes normal before 1 year of age, usually.

Subgaleal hematomas are commonly seen following fractures, or even mild head injury. Parents note a soft fluctuant swelling which is not limited by periostial insertions. Even if the hematoma is large, the indicated therapy is observation. This is because needle or incisional drainage may result in infection in an otherwise benign and self-limiting condition.

PENETRATING WOUNDS

Penetrating wounds of the head are generally treated by culture, debridement, control of hemorrhage, and closure. Powder burns on the scalp of victims of gunshot wounds indicate that missiles were fired at close range. This may imply a large energy expenditure in the cranium, and the presence of powder burns may have legal significance.

Wounds of entrance and exit, if the latter is present, should be debrided. Debridement usually requires a craniectomy at the site of entrance, since there are frequently in-driven fragments of bone beneath the penetration of the skull. The scalp incision may incorporate the site of the penetration, but it is often better to locate it away from the penetration so that the least possible scarring will overlie the site of any future cranioplasty. Scarring may be of cosmetic concern in the area of the forehead.

Once the scalp and periosteum have been dissected free from the cranium, examination of the site of skull penetration will indicate whether the defect can be enlarged to debride the intracranial tract or whether it is necessary to drill a burr hole adjacent to the penetration.

The dura must be separated and the debridement accomplished. It may be necessary to enlarge the dural defect. Specimens for culture and sensitivity are taken. The tract of the missile will be inspected and all fragments of in-driven bone removed wherever possible.[46] Ultrasonic imaging is helpful in finding retained fragments or hematomas.[47]

The tract is then irrigated. Any continuing hemorrhage must be controlled. If the missile has passed out of the cranium, the site of exit should be debrided. In this case, the entire wound may need to be irrigated. If it is not practical to expose wounds of entrance and exits simultaneously, separate debridements will be necessary, but in any event it is important to be sure that thorough irrigation is accomplished.

Following this, irrigating fluids must be evacuated. The dura should be closed tightly, using a graft if necessary. The patient's fascia or periosteum may be used. If periosteum is used, it should be positioned so that the surface which has been against bone is directed away from the brain. Some surgeons prefer the use of preserved tissues or dural substitutes. After hemostasis, all layers of the wound are closed tightly. Drains are added when hemostasis is not absolute.

Penetrating wounds are considered contaminated, as are all open wounds. Antibiotics, prophylactic against gram-positive organisms, are started at the time anesthesia is ad-

ministered. Antibiotics with a broader spectrum of coverage might be considered if the missiles have passed through mucosal membranes or there is reason to suspect contamination from organisms other than those usually found on the skin.

The secondary removal of retained fragments is controversial, but it appears that the complication rate for repeat exploration may exceed the rate of complications of retained fragments.[48,49] The authors are currently not reexploring wounds unless there is evidence of an unusually large retained fragment or another specific reason.

FRACTURES OF THE SKULL DUE TO DIRECT TRAUMA

Nondisplaced fractures of the skull in adults, uncomplicated by hemorrhage, may be of limited consequence. The thin and vascular skull of infants and young children alters the management of skull fractures in this age group. Infants and children are at increased risk of venous epidural hematomas derived from fractures of any portion of the skull, unlike adults, who are more at risk when the skull fracture crosses a vascular groove. Infants less than 1 year of age, whose heads are large in proportion to the rest of the body, are at risk for anemia as a result of hemorrhage beneath the scalp associated with a skull fracture or scalp hematoma. The hematocrit should be checked every 12 to 24 h after injury to detect a decline.

Generally, the same principles and techniques apply to treating open fractures as apply to the treatment of penetrating wounds of the head. (See Fig. 18-12.) The name "open fracture" implies that there is a laceration of the scalp overlying the fractured cranium. The least scarring will result from simply extending the laceration for the scalp incision. An extension of the incision should not cross major vessels supplying the scalp when interruption of these vessels can be avoided.

Small compound linear, but nondisplaced, fractures of the skull represent a special group which are treated by opening the laceration in the emergency room. The fracture is cultured, curetted, and irrigated. The scalp is then closed, as it is for other compound fractures.

Complex frontal fractures that extend into the paranasal sinuses represent a special group. Although the scalp may not be penetrated, these are treated as "open fractures" because of their communication with the paranasal sinuses. Usually the back wall of the frontal sinus is fractured. For these wounds, an adequate scalp flap is opened.[51] A craniectomy or craniotomy is necessary.

After cultures are taken, the paranasal sinus(es) is exenterated and occluded with muscle, fat, or Gelfoam soaked in an antibiotic solution. The dura in this region is usually quite thin, but it can be grafted with periosteum or fascia. The graft may be performed on the outer surface of the dura, but it is frequently easier to perform it from the inner surface

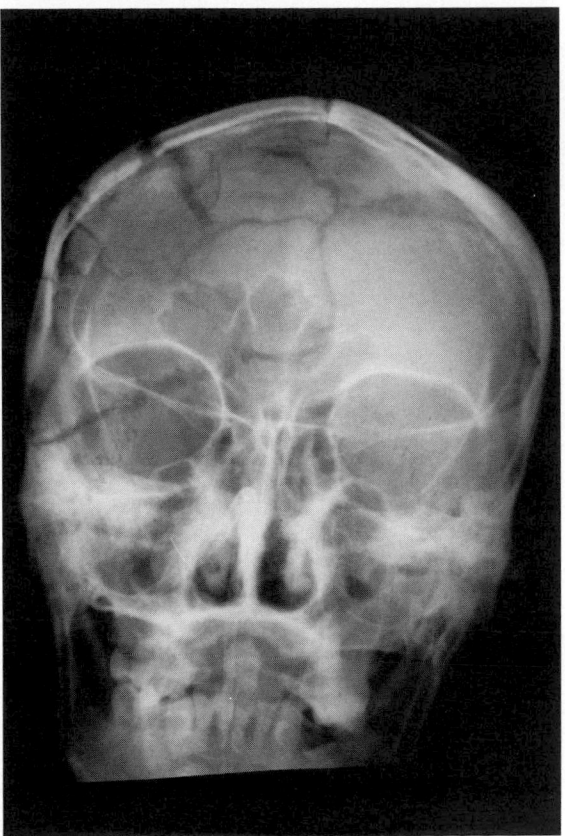

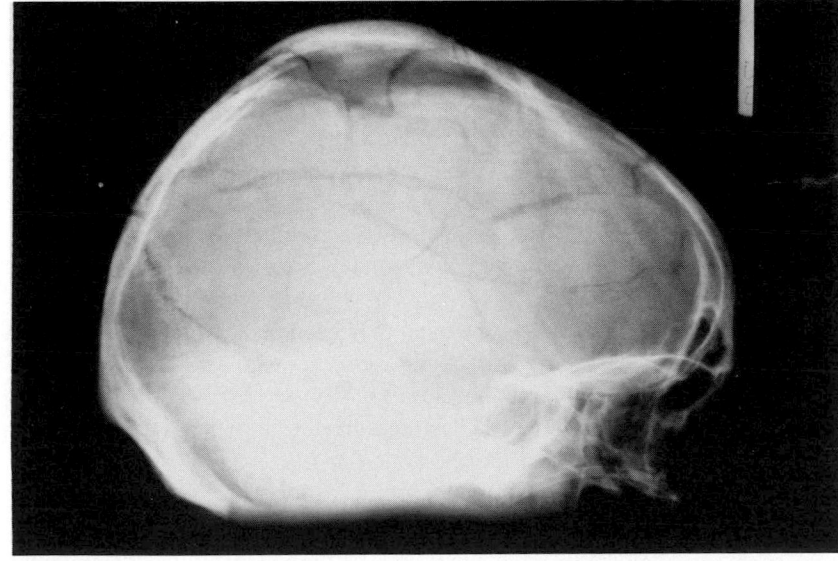

Figure 18–12 Computerized tomogram showing a comminuted skull fracture beneath a scalp laceration.

after the dura has been opened and the frontal lobe(s) retracted.

It may be necessary to ligate the anterior extent of the saggital sinus if it has been injured or if it requires division to expose both frontal fossae. If the cleaned bone fragments are large, they may be replaced. If the bone is severely contaminated or fragmented, fragments should be left out and a cranioplasty performed later. Cranioplasty using methyl methacrylate is usually performed 6 months after a craniotomy with no evidence of infection. About a year should pass after all infection has cleared, following a cran-

iotomy performed in the presence of infection or when infection complicates the debridement.

CLOSED HEAD INJURIES

Closed head injuries include several anatomical lesions, many of which alter consciousness and some of which may require surgical intervention. Alteration of consciousness implies inadequate functioning of the brainstem,[52] which could be the result of injury or ischemia, the latter being most likely due to increased pressure. Injury to the midbrain may result in concussion or contusion. Increased ICP following head injury and resulting from edema, contusions of the cerebral hemispheres, or hematomas can account for ischemia. Although serial physical examinations may suggest such lesions by change in mental or neurological status, the CT scan is quite specific and may demonstrate lesions before the patient's neurological status has changed.

EPIDURAL HEMATOMAS

The typical clinical picture of an *acute epidural hematoma* is that of an individual who has had a head injury—perhaps with loss of consciousness—and recovery, but who develops a headache with progressive hemiparesis contralateral to the side of the lesion and a dilated pupil ipsilateral to the lesion.[53] Unfortunately, this picture cannot be relied on since patients with more severe head injuries may not experience any "lucid interval" and other patients will experience a more subtle course.[54]

Usually the middle meningeal artery is the source of hemorrhage in an acute epidural hematoma. It lies in the outer layer of the dura and is usually partially embedded in a grove in the inner table of the skull. When the skull is fractured, it may lacerate the artery, resulting in hemorrhage into the potential space between the dura and the skull. The developing hematoma displaces the dura and consequently tears penetrating vessels, both arterioles and venules, which will add to the hematoma.

Epidural hematomas can grow rapidly. They typically lie low in the middle cranial fossa. Since the accumulation of blood is clotted in most cases, a craniectomy or craniotomy is required for evacuation. Rapid, safe exposure of the area is achieved through a vertical scalp incision about 1 cm anterior to the tragus, with its lower limit at the zygomatic arch. A craniectomy is accomplished by rongeuring around a burr hole placed in the squamosal part of the temporal bone. If a craniotomy flap is preferred, this vertical incision can be curved anterior to the region of the hairline and an osteoplastic flap turned inferiorly.

Once the hematoma has been evacuated, the bleeding points are controlled by coagulating the middle meningeal artery and any penetrating vessels which may be bleeding from the outer surface of the dura. It may be necessary to follow the artery to the foramen spinosum, where it can be controlled by plugging the foramen with cotton, bone wax, or a swab stick. Stay sutures are used to tack the dura to the surrounding bone edges or the overlying periosteum. A Jackson-Pratt drain may be left in place if the wound is not dry. The temporalis muscle and scalp are closed in layers. Epidural hematomas occasionally occur in the frontal fossa and even in the posterior fossa. The surgical treatment varies only in its location.[55]

SUBDURAL HEMATOMAS

Subacute or *chronic subdural hematomas* usually result from tearing of bridging veins. Acute subdural hematomas are frequently the result of hemorrhage from an artery on the surface of the cortex or from a penetrating wound.[5] Chronic subdural hematomas are often quite subtle in their clinical appearance and may not become apparent for days to weeks after a head injury.[56]

In many cases, a history of head injury may not be obtainable. Paresis is inconstant and may be ipsilateral to the lesion because of Kernohan's notch. *Kernohan's notch* is a defect in the cerebral peduncle, contralateral to a mass in or over a cerebral hemisphere.[57] The cerebral peduncle opposite to the site of the mass is forced against the tentorium contralateral to the side of the lesion, and the pressure causes paresis ipsilateral to the mass. A third-nerve palsy may be inconstant. Papilledema is common although not dependable.

Acute subdural hematomas, although less common than chronic, are usually diagnosed within 24 h of the injury, perhaps more frequently now than in the past because of computed tomography. They consist of fresh clotted blood which, if not evacuated, liquifies in 10 days. Chronic subdural hematomas may continue to collect fluid, further stretching bridging veins and resulting in a combination acute and chronic subdural lesion.

Treatment of subdural hematomas varies according to acuteness of the lesion. An acute subdural hematoma requires craniotomy to remove the hematoma and to control the bleeding points that may be bridging veins or cortical arteries if the lesion accompanies a severe contusion, laceration, or penetration of the brain. The craniotomy flap should encompass nearly the extent of the hematoma. If the hematoma extends near the temporal fossa, the bone flap may be hinged on the temporalis muscle, but usually the dura is turned toward the saggital sinus. The hematoma peels off the surface of the brain. Segments of hematoma, not directly exposed, can be irrigated. Bleeding points must be meticulously controlled. Once hemostasis has been accomplished, routine closure of the craniotomy is accomplished.

Acute cerebral edema may become apparent at the time of evacuation. This is an ominous sign. Subtotal temporal and/or frontal lobectomies may be carried out in order to develop space. The authors have usually sutured in a periosteal graft and left the bone flap out.

The treatment of chronic subdural hematomas is much easier. It requires two or three burr holes, preferably over the extents of the hematoma. The dura is coagulated beneath the burr hole, following which a cruciate incision is made. Further coagulation causes the edges to retract. The subdural space is irrigated. If the holes are placed too near the extremes of the hematoma, drainage may be blocked by the brain. It may be necessary to depress the surface of the brain with a spatula to obtain adequate drainage. The wound is irrigated until the saline returns clear. A Jackson-Pratt drain may be placed in the wound by attaching it to a Gigli saw guide passed between burr holes. The drain is left in place until the drainage has diminished in amount.

It may be difficult to determine whether subacute subdural hematomas will require craniotomy before exposure at the time of evacuation. A good indication may come from the CT scan, which will show a horizontal line of demarcation at the site of settled hemoglobin. If residual clots cannot be evacuated at the time of surgery, a craniotomy may be required.

Chronic subdural hematomas may resolve.[58] Patients whose primary complaints are headache, and even some with hemiparesis, may become asymptomatic when placed on high doses of steroids. Patients who are well-compensated may be treated with steroids until the hematomas resolve, but significant neurological deficits favor early surgical treatment. All patients treated with steroids are closely monitored for progression of symptoms.

CHRONIC SUBDURAL HEMATOMAS IN INFANTS AND CHILDREN

Most surgically correctable lesions caused by head trauma in the pediatric age group—such as an acute subdural or epidural hematoma—are treated as described for adults. Chronic subdural hematomas may occur in children as well as adults.

Pediatric subdural hematomas have three unique features: (1) Chronic subdural hematomas in infants who do not yet walk should raise concerns about child abuse. (2) A chronic subdural hematoma may cause symmetrical or asymmetrical cranial enlargement in children. (3) Chronic subdural hematomas may require prolonged drainage, usually via a subdural-peritoneal shunt.

Chronic subdural hematomas in children may present as an acute triad of findings which includes a full fontanel, seizures, and retinal hemorrhages. A CT scan will often reveal subdural hematomas of various ages, acute, subacute, and chronic. The infant, usually between 6 months and 1 year of age, is often lethargic. Child abuse should be considered, especially the "shaken baby" syndrome.[3]

Associated injuries will include fractures of the skull or ribs. The injury in "shaken baby" syndrome is thought to result from grasping the infant around the thorax, squeezing tightly, and shaking the head back and forth. Recent studies have shown that the simple act of shaking is probably insufficient to cause a subdural hematoma. These children probably sustain a deceleration injury when they are slammed onto a surface, even a padded surface.

Treatment, when chronic, is surgical drainage of the subdural fluid by burr holes. If acute blood is present, a craniotomy is performed. The prognosis for these infants is guarded, depending on the amount of cortical damage they have sustained from abuse and neglect.

Chronic subdural hematomas also occur in otherwise healthy infants who are noted to have an increasing head circumference. The anterior fontanel is often full, and the eyes tend to appear slightly protuberant. CT scanning reveals a subdural collection with the density of cerebrospinal fluid. With infusion of iodinated contrast, the surrounding membrane enhances. Although burr holes and drainage are occasionally effective treatment for these collections, treatment usually includes burr holes, with drainage of 4 to 7 days, or a subdural-peritoneal shunt for approximately 6 months. Often, children with chronic subdural fluid collections are developmentally normal or only slightly delayed prior to therapy. The outlook for recovery following surgery is good. The etiology of large chronic subdural collections in children is not infrequently linked to head trauma or abuse.

INTRACEREBRAL HEMATOMAS

Intracerebral hematomas as a result of head injury are usually due to shearing forces in the white matter adjacent to the cortex.[59] They are most likely to be located near the surfaces of the frontal or temporal lobes. They may be mixed with injured brain substance, and there is usually considerable edema surrounding the area. If left in place and the patient survives for months to years, the hematomas will resolve but may be replaced by gliosis. Seizures may follow within a few days or months.[60] However, in the acute phase, the size of the lesions may add to, if not be the primary cause of increased ICP, at least in the local area, leading to cerebral decompensation in the form of depressed consciousness or even herniation.

Localized intracerebral hemorrhages may continue to bleed, but usually expand in part because of localized edema. They frequently do not reach their maximum size for 2 to 3 days following head injury, so that sites of cerebral contusion should be observed by serial CT scans.[61]

The treatment of intracerebral hematomas is evacuation whenever they reach a size such that they are causing significant elevation of ICP or displacement of the brain. This is usually accomplished through a formal craniotomy over the site of the lesion and aspiration of the hematoma and surrounding traumatized brain.

Temporal lobe hematomas may be bilateral. Removal of both temporal lobes will produce the Kluver-Bucy syndrome, which includes visual agnosia, compulsive oral behavior in which the individual places inappropriate objects in his mouth, reaction to visual stimuli, a change from aggressive to passive behavior, and increased sexual activity.[62,63] In addition, injury or resection of more than 5 cm of the temporal lobe of the dominant hemisphere may result in dysphasia.[64] Consequently, bitemporal resections are avoided wherever possible, but if bilateral intracerebral hematomas are present, resection is limited to fresh blood on the dominant side, although the resection might be more generous on the nondominant side.

☐ PROGNOSIS OF PATIENTS WITH SEVERE HEAD INJURY

Despite well-organized aggressive therapy, Clifton et al.[65] reported a mortality rate of 52 percent of 167 patients seen with a Glasgow coma scale score of 8 or less due to head injury. However, when patients with gunshot wounds and those who met criteria for brain death were excluded, the mortality rate fell to 29 percent. He recalled that Becker et al.[66] had reported comparable results and contrasted this to the 50 percent rate reported from a large international series. A mortality rate of 28 percent reported by Marshall et al.[67] in patients, some of whom were treated with barbiturates, was also recalled. These figures have not significantly changed in the past 10 years. In summary, a mortality rate of between 25 and 30 percent can be anticipated from patients admitted with severe impairment of consciousness.

Several factors enter into the prediction of outcome. According to a later report from Richmond, when the age of the patient, the Glasgow coma scale score on admission, the pupillary response, the presence of mass lesions, extraocular motility, and posturing were all considered, the prognostic accuracy was about 82 percent.[68] Use of computed tomography alone was a poor prognosticator, but when added to the clinical information listed above it improved prognostic capability considerably. The capability was even further improved by data obtained from multimodel evoked potentials. As for prognostic features of the CT scan, van Dongen et al.[69] found that "the state of the basal cisterns . . . proved to be a very powerful prognosticator." A multicenter study, however, indicated that the worst outcomes came with acute subdural hematomas, while patients with coma of 6 to 24 h associated with diffuse injury had a good recovery.[70] Diffuse injury with coma lasting longer than 24 h carried a poor prognosis. Epidural hematomas evacuated early have a high incidence of excellent recovery.[71]

From this cursory review, it is apparent that patients with head injuries who are deeply stuporous must be evaluated and treated for localized lesions. Those who have diffuse swelling but who show improvement within 24 h do well. Those who have diffuse brain injury and prolonged coma have a very guarded prognosis.

SUPPORTIVE CARE

Any patient who is immobilized for a prolonged period requires support for respiration, nutrition, evacuation of bowels and bladder, and care of skin, joints, and veins.

SUPPORT FOR RESPIRATION

Support of pulmonary function is routinely required in patients with severe head injuries. Ischemia is a major cause of cerebral edema and patients with serious head injuries tolerate hypoxia poorly. Impairment of respiration is also common among patients with head injury.[72]

Neurogenic causes of pulmonary insufficiency appear to involve "diffuse pulmonary shunting," the basis of which is unclear.[73] Pulmonary edema frequently accompanies acutely increased ICP and may significantly contribute to impaired function.[74] Injury to the chest and lungs may contribute as well to impaired ventilation. Perfusion of gases through the alveoli can be impaired by contusion or pneumonia, whether due to aspiration, bacterial infection, or embolism.[75] These conditions, alone or collectively, result in development of the "adult respiratory distress syndrome," which is a consequence of pulmonary edema. Unless the edema can be resolved within a few days, the mortality rate approaches 100 percent.[76]

Treatment requires removal of the inciting factors and the use of positive end-expiratory pressure. Diuretics may be helpful.[75] Respiratory support requires use of supplemental oxygen to keep the P_{O_2} above 80 mmHg. Mechanical ventilation is usually accomplished at about 12 breaths per minute with a tidal volume in the range of 705 cm^3. When the intracranial pressure is elevated, the P_{CO_2} is usually maintained between 25 and 30 mmHg. PEEP up to 10 cm of water pressure may be used if the patient's head is elevated.[77] Elevation of the inspiratory pressure will elevate the intracranial pressure.

Discontinuation of respiratory assistance must be accomplished incrementally with frequent blood gases being used as a guide. Tracheostomy has been recommended when endotracheal intubation is expected to exceed a week, but a recent report has suggested that the complications of tracheostomy may exceed those of leaving an endotracheal tube in place for up to 3 weeks.[78] Frequent pulmonary toilet and cultures of aspirates are a part of the routine care of an endotracheal airway and are especially important in the event of unexplained fever or radiographic evidence of pneumonia.

NUTRITION

Average daily requirements for an adult are about 2500 calories, 3000 cm^3 of water, $4\frac{1}{2}$ g of salt, 40 mEq of potassium, and 70 g of protein. A minimum of 100 g of glucose is required to prevent ketosis.[79]

The usual response of the body to head injury is similar to that of injury to the body in general: increased loss of nitrogen, usually lasting for 8 to 10 days; increase in the level of blood sugar; retention of water, sodium, and chloride, usually lasting for 2 to 3 days; and decreased body weight.[80] An increase in the output of corticosteroids doubtlessly accounts for many of these changes, which are exacerbated by multiple trauma, severe brain injury, infection, fever, posturing, and seizures.[81]

The nitrogen loss may be related to decreased synthesis of protein as well as catabolism.[81] A negative nitrogen balance for a few days is not harmful, but prolonged nitrogen imbalance will seriously jeopardize recovery. The value of early enteral feedings is well-established, but in the event that these are prevented by regurgitation, abdominal injury, or distension, hyperalimentation may be necessary.[82,83] It should be remembered that hyperalimentation often potentiates hyperglycemia, which may be prominent in patients with severe head injuries. Generally, maintenance quantities of fluids, electrolytes, and vitamins should be included, but quantities of salt and potassium must be tailored according to serum levels. Excessive quantities of water or hypotonicity can add significantly to cerebral edema.

Tube feedings are usually administered in solutions containing about 1 calorie per milliliter. The presence of diarrhea may require that this concentration be reduced. Hydrolyzed proteins permit higher concentrations of enteral feedings.

SKIN CARE

Patients who are immobile must be turned side-to-side at least every 2 h. Decubitus ulcers have been reported when patients were left in one position for as much as 4 h. Maintenance of skin care may be assisted by the use of rocking beds or mattresses which alternate levels of pressure every few moments. Fluctuating air mattresses are usually more comfortable and less disturbing to patients, but rocking beds provide a stable surface for traction. The rocking beds have doors at the base which may be opened to allow for nursing care.

EVACUATION OF BOWELS AND BLADDER

An indwelling catheter is usually required initially in patients whose head injuries are severe enough to produce coma for more than a few moments. The catheter should be the smallest size consistent with adequate drainage of the bladder. It should be fixed to the skin of the abdomen or thigh so that it will not erode the urethra or produce ulcers in the trigone of the bladder.

In men, a transurethral catheter may be replaced by a condom-type catheter as soon as spontaneous voiding is acquired. It may be necessary to maintain a catheter in women until patients are able to have volitional control of bladder functions.

Bowel movements may be interrupted by devastating injuries. They are usually resumed by the second or third day, but periodic checks for impaction may be necessary unless evacuations occur every day or two days. Impactions require digital removal. Suppositories or laxatives may be necessary. Enemas are difficult in uncooperative patients.

PREVENTION OF THROMBOPHLEBITIS

Thrombophlebitis and subsequent pulmonary embolism are the most feared complications of immobilization. Prevention of thrombophlebitis is clearly indicated whenever possible. Two techniques are commonly utilized in patients recently subjected to trauma; (1) prophylactic use of heparin, usually administered in doses of 5000 units every 8 h, or (2) use of external pneumatic compression of the lower extremities.[84,85] Although therapeutic heparinization is not generally used in patients who have recently been subjected to intracranial procedures (within 3 days), use of "low dose" heparin in many services is accepted.[86,87] Hemorrhagic complications appear to be minimal. Many physicians feel more comfortable with external pneumatic compression that not only mechanically "milks" the veins in the legs but also contributes to the production of fibrinolysis.[88,89,90] Complications are rare but must be recognized and treated appropriately.

PHYSICAL THERAPY

The goals of physical therapy in patients who have been subjected to head injury are: (1) to prevent loss of motion and flexibility of joints, (2) to prevent deformity, (3) to increase strength, and (4) to maximize function. To accomplish these objectives there must be early intervention and mobilization wherever possible. Physical therapists establish a treatment program that is appropriate for the individual case based on the individual's cognitive and functional capabilities. Treatment patterns are adapted to the level of cognitive functioning, graded according to the scale devised at the Division of Neurological Sciences of the Rancho Los Amigos Hospital.[91,92]

Participation of the physical therapist must begin early to maintain flexibility of joints and maintain muscle length. Passive range-of-motion exercises may be used initially, but active motion is instituted when the patient can cooperate. Serial casting and splinting may be required.

The upright position is assumed as soon as the medical condition permits. This facilitates head control, control of the trunk, a sitting posture and maintenance of balance, midline orientation, weight bearing and transference.[93,94] Functional activities out of the bed are begun as quickly as possible.

Evaluation and identification of problems by the physiotherapist continue through the phases of rehabilitation. The treatment plan must be continuously revised according to the patient's stage of recovery. Therapists emphasize patient and family education and try to involve the family in the rehabilitation from the start of the treatment program through discharge planning. Additional comments relating to speech therapy, occupational therapy, and vocational rehabilitation are presented in Chap. 27.

☐ LATE COMPLICATIONS OF HEAD INJURY

Late complications of head injury include hydrocephalus, dementia, and seizures, as well as specific neurological deficits that will not be reviewed here.

HYDROCEPHALUS

Head injury is the most common cause of subarachnoid hemorrhage. Blood in the subarachnoid pathways occludes the pathways to the arachnoid villi. Ventricular dilitation and intracranial hypertension are common during the first month after subarachnoid hemorrhage.[95]

Ventricular dilitation after head injury producing hydrocephalus is differentiated from atrophy radiographically by the presence of decreased attenuation around the ventricles and the small sulcal markings over the surface of the brain on CT scans.[96] If the failure of CSF absorption is marked, shunting may be required.

In more chronic hydrocephalus, the triad of ataxia, incontinence, and dementia, usually without headache, occurs.[97] The only dependable radiographic signs are ventricular dilitation with evidence of transependymal absorption and decrease to absence of sulci.[96] Treatment requires shunting. In the authors' experience, lumbar subarachnoid-peritoneal shunts are quite satisfactory provided the subarachnoid pathways are open. If there is a question of patency of the subarachnoid pathways, a ventriculoperitoneal shunt is implanted. Techniques used for ventriculoperitoneal shunting are no different from those used for shunting hydrocephalus from other causes. (See Chap. 8.)

DEMENTIA AND DISCRETE NEUROLOGICAL DEFICITS

Head injuries may result in irreparable damage to specific parts of the central nervous system, sometimes leading to dementia but often leaving discrete injuries which must be differentiated. Chronic hydrocephalus has been mentioned. Dysphasia, deafness, anosmia, blindness, hemiparesis, movement disorders, and behavioral disorders have resulted from head injuries.

Treatment of these disabilities, sometimes by surgery, and sometimes by training or adaptive tools, such as hearing aids, can result in improved quality of life for many victims of head injury and enable them to be productive despite severe injuries. Function of the cerebral hemispheres of such patients may be impaired; however, all disabilities must be differentiated by careful physical, and often psychological, evaluation. (See Chap. 4.)

EPILEPSY

Epileptic seizures occur in the early period after injury in about 5 percent of patients having experienced head injury.[98] Seizures occurring during the first week after head injury have been classified separately from those occurring more than 3 months later.[99] There is evidence that seizures occurring in the early post-injury period signal an increased likelihood that they are more likely to occur later. However, temporal lobe seizures that are common in late epilepsy are

Table 18-2
GUIDELINES FOR DECLARATION OF BRAIN DEATH

A. An individual with irreversible cessation of circulatory and respiratory function is dead.
   1. Cessation is recognized by an appropriate clinical examination.
   2. Irreversibility is recognized by a persistent cessation of functions during an appropriate period of observation and/or results of therapy.
B. An individual with irreversible cessation of all functions of the entire brain, including the brain stem, is dead.
   1. Cessation is recognized when evaluation discloses findings of a and b:
      a. Cerebral functions are absent.
      b. Brain stem functions are absent.
   2. Irreversibility is recognized when evaluation discloses findings of a, b, and c:
      a. The cause of coma is established and is sufficient to account for the loss of brain functions.
      b. The possibility of recovery of any brain functions is excluded.
      c. The cessation of all brain functions persists for an appropriate period of observation and/or trial of therapy.

Complicating Conditions
   A. Drug and metabolic intoxication
   B. Hypothermia
   C. Children
   D. Shock

Source: Guidelines of the Medical Consultants on the Diagnosis of Death to the President's Commission for the Study of Ethical Problems in Medicine and Biomedical and Behavioral Research.[102]

rare in the early post-injury phase. Definitive risk factors are associated with the development of late epilepsy. These include intracranial hematomas and penetrating wounds, as well as infections, which frequently complicate head injuries.

The consequences of seizures should not be underestimated. Seizures are indications of increased neuronal function, albeit abnormal. They are associated with increased metabolism and may contribute to ischemia. Seizures *must* be treated aggressively. Valium and Dilantin are the drugs used most commonly in seizures occurring in the early post-injury phase. More specific anticonvulsants are administered in patients who develop seizures late after head injury. (See Chap. 22.)

☐ BRAIN DEATH

Unfortunately, despite well-organized, efficient, and aggressive therapy, the mortality rate among patients with severe head injuries remains high. Declaration of brain death should be considered whenever it is apparent that a victim of a head injury cannot survive. Thus, the basic procedure may be instituted in the emergency room or at any one of a number of steps along the evaluation and therapy of patients with severe head injury. The object is to specifically identify patients who have experienced brain death. The need for this declaration is emphasized by the need for tissues for transplantation, but also by the need to preserve resources that might be expended without hope for recovery.

Declaration of brain death in the United States is made upon the demonstration that there is irreversible loss of cortical and brain stem activity.[100,101] Guidelines for such a declaration were published in the report of the Medical Consultants on the Diagnosis of Death to the President's Commission for the Study of Ethical Problems in Medicine and Biochemical and Behavioral Research.[102] They are shown in Table 18-2.

Absence of cerebral function is indicated by absence of spontaneous—or any other—movement except spinal reflexes. Brain stem reflexes include pupillary, corneal, oculocephalic, oculovestibular, oropharyngeal, cough, and respiratory reflexes. The oculovestibular reflex is tested by irrigating external ear canals which are devoid of debris with 30 ml of ice water. The patient's head should be elevated 30 degrees and irrigations should be accomplished with a syringe and cannula. The respiratory reflex is evaluated by the apnea test. O_2 is administered via an endotracheal tube at 100 percent for 10 min. P_{CO_2} is maintained at 40 mmHg or above.[103] Repetition of the test at least once in 6 h is required; 12 h is recommended.

Absence of electrical activity of the cortex may be demonstrated by EEG. Absence of blood flow can be demonstrated by angiography or ultrasound.

Drug intoxication is ruled out by history and laboratory analysis for barbiturates and antidepressants. Respiratory effort may be abolished by neuromuscular blocking agents. Elevated levels of ammonia and lowered levels of phosphates should be ruled out by laboratory examinations. The body temperature should measure at least 35°C or 95°F. Hypothermia may be reversed by a heating blanket. Blood pressure should be at least 95 mmHg systolic.

Clinical examinations are accepted in most cases. Some institutions require examinations by two staff members who are neurologists or neurosurgeons. Confirmation of the clinical evaluation may be accomplished by EEG using a minimum of eight electrodes and reference electrodes with interelectrode distances of at least 10 cm. Resistance of 100 to 10,000 ohms is necessary. The gain is increased from 7 microvolts to 2 microvolts per mm.

Declaration of brain death has been accepted in the United States. It is necessary for harvesting organs for transplantation or for withdrawal of support mechanisms.

REFERENCES

1. Sosin DM, Sacks JJ, Smith SM: Head injury—Associated deaths in the United States from 1979 to 1986. *JAMA* 262:2251–2255, 1989.
2. Klauber MR, Marshall LF, Toole BM, et al: Cause of decline in head-injury mortality rate in San Diego County, California. *J Neurosurg* 62:528–531, 1985.
3. Gelpke GJ, Braakman R, Habbema DF, Hilden J: Comparison of outcome in two series of patients with severe head injuries. *J Neurosurg* 59:745–750, 1983.
4. Borovich B, Braun J, Guilburd JN, et al: Delayed onset of traumatic extradural hematoma. *J Neurosurg* 63:30–34, 1985.
5. Shenkin HA: Acute subdural hematoma: Review of 39 consecutive cases with high incidence of cortical artery rupture. *J Neurosurg* 57:254–257, 1982.
6. Yoshino E, Yamaki T, Higuchi T, et al: Acute brain edema in fatal head injury: Analysis by dynamic CT scanning. *J Neurosurg* 63:830–839, 1985.
7. Toutant SM, Klauber MR, Marshall LF, et al: Absent or compressed basal cisterns on first CT scan: Ominous predictors of outcome in severe head injury. *J Neurosurg* 61:691–694, 1984.
8. Obrist WD, Lanffitt TW, Jaggi JL, et al: Cerebral blood flow metabolism in comatose patients with acute head injury: Relationship to intracranial hypertension. *J Neurosurg* 61:241–253, 1984.
9. Clasen RA, Penn RD: Traumatic brain swelling and edema, in Cooper PR (ed): *Head Injury,* 2d ed. Baltimore, Williams & Wilkins, 1987, pp 285–313.
10. Hubschmann OR, Nathanson DC: The role of calcium and cellular membrane dysfunction in experimental trauma and subarachnoid hemorrhage. *J Neurosurg* 62:698–703, 1985.
11. Martins AN, Kobrine AI, Larsen DF: Pressure in the sagittal sinus during intracranial hypertension in man. *J Neurosurg* 40:603–608, 1974.
12. Lofgren J, Zwetnow NN: Influence of a supratentorial expanding mass on the intracranial pressure-volume relationships. *Acta Neurol Scand* 49:599–612, 1973.
13. Raichle ME, Posner JR, Plum F: Cerebral blood flow during and after hyperventilation. *Arch Neurol* 23:394–403, 1970.
14. Muizelaar JP, Obirst WP: Cerebral blood flow and brain metabolism with brain injury, in Becker DP, Povlishock JT (eds): *Central Nervous System Trauma Status Report.* Bethesda, National Institutes of Communicative Disorders and Stroke, 1985, pp 123–138.
15. Albright AL, Latchaw RE, Robinson AG: Intracranial and systemic effects of osmotic and oncotic therapy in experimental cerebral edema. *J Neurosurg* 60:481–489, 1984.
16. Muizelaar JP, Lutz HA III, Becker DP: Effect of mannitol on ICP and CBF and correlation with pressure autoregulation in

severely head-injured patients. *J Neurosurg* 61:700–706, 1984.

17. Nath F, Galbraith S: The effect of mannitol on cerebral white matter water content. *J Neurosurg* 65:41–43, 1986.

18. Smith HP, Kelly DL, Jr, McWhorter JM, et al: Comparison of mannitol regimens in patients with severe head injury undergoing intracranial monitoring. *J Neurosurg* 65:820–824, 1986.

19. Narayan RK, Kishore PRS, Becker DP, et al: Intracranial pressure: To monitor or not to monitor? A review of our experience with severe head injury. *J Neurosurg* 56:650–659, 1982.

20. Narayan RK, Becker DP: Selection of patients for ICP monitoring. *J Neurosurg* 62:624–625, 1985.

21. Mayhall CG, Archer NH, Lamb VA, et al: Ventriculostomy-related infections: A prospective epidemiologic study. *N Engl J Med* 310:553–559, 1984.

22. Galbraith S, Teasdale G: Predicting the need for operation in the patient with an occult traumatic intracranial hematoma. *J Neurosurg* 55:75–81, 1981.

23. Vries JK, Becker DP, Young HF: A subarachnoid screw for monitoring intracranial pressure (technical note). *J Neurosurg* 39:416–419, 1973.

24. Swann KW, Cosman ER: Modification of the Richmond subarachnoid screw for monitoring intracranial pressure (technical note). *J Neurosurg* 60:1102–1103, 1984.

25. Dearden NM, McDowall DG, Gibson RM: Assessment of Leeds device for monitoring intracranial pressure. *J Neurosurg* 60:123–129, 1984.

26. Mendelow AD, Rowan JO, Murray L, Kerr AE: A clinical comparison of subdural screw pressure measurements with ventricular pressure. *J Neurosurg* 58:45–50, 1983.

27. Ward JD, Becker DP, Miller JD, et al: Failure of prophylactic barbiturate coma in the treatment of severe head injury. *J Neurosurg* 62:383–388, 1985.

28. Abramson NS, Safar P, Detre KM, et al: Randomized clinical study of thiopental loading in comatose survivors of cardiac arrest. *N Engl J Med* 314:397–403, 1986.

29. Beks JWF, Doorenbos H, Walstra GJM: Clinical experiences with steroids in neurosurgical patients, in Reulen HJ, Schurmann K (eds): *Steroids and Brain Edema.* New York, Springer-Verlag, 1972, pp 233–238.

30. Braughler JM, Hall ED: Current application of "high-dose" steroid therapy of CNS injury: A pharmacological perspective. *J Neurosurg* 62:806–810, 1985.

31. Gudeman SK, Miller JD, Becker DP: Failure of high-dose steroid therapy to influence intracranial pressure in patients with severe head injury. *J Neurosurg* 51:301–306, 1979.

32. Braakman R, Schouten HJA, Dishoeck MB, Minderhoud JM: Megadose steroids in severe head injury. Results of a prospective double-blind clinical trial. *J Neurosurg* 58:326–330, 1983.

33. Jennett B, Teasdale G, Fry J, et al: Treatment for severe head injury. *J Neurol Neurosurg Psychiatry* 43:289–295, 1980.

34. Dearden NM, Gibson JS, McDowall DG, et al: Effect of high-dose dexamethasone on outcome from severe head injury. *J Neurosurg* 64:81–88, 1986.

35. Hall EB, Braughler JM: Glucocorticoid mechanisms in acute spinal cord injury: A review and therapeutic rationale. *Surg Neurol* 18:320–327, 1982.

36. Bracken MB, Shepard MJ, Collins WF, et al: A randomized, controlled trial of methylprednisolone or naloxone in the treatment of spinal-cord injury: Results of the second national acute spinal cord injury study. *N Engl J Med* 322:1405–1411, 1990.

37. Teasdale G, Jennett B: Assessment of coma and impaired consciousness. A practice scale. *Lancet* 2:81–84, 1974.

38. Stanczak DE, White JG, Gouview WD, et al: Assessment of level of consciousness following severe neurological insult: A comparison of the psychometric qualities of the Glasgow coma scale and the comprehensive level of consciousness scale. *J Neurosurg* 60:955–960, 1984.

39. Levati A, Farina ML, Vecchi G, et al: Prognosis of head injuries. *J Neurosurg* 57:779–783, 1982.

40. Young B, Rapp RP, Norton JA, et al: Early prediction of outcome in head-injured patients. *J Neurosurg* 54:300–303, 1981.

41. Cordobes F, De La Fuente M, Lobato RD, et al: Intraventricular hemorrhage in severe head injury. *J Neurosurg* 58:217–222, 1983.

42. Grahm TW, Williams FC, Harrington T, Spetzler RF: Civilian gunshot wounds to the head: A prospective study. *Neurosurg* 27:696–700, 1990.

43. Carey ME, Tutton RH, Strub RL, et al: The correlation between surgical and CT estimates of brain damage following missile wounds. *J Neurosurg* 60:947–954, 1984.

44. Langfitt TW, Obrist WD, Alavi A, et al: Computerized tomography, magnetic resonance imaging, and positron emission tomography in the study of brain trauma: Preliminary observations. *J Neurosurg* 64:760–767, 1986.

45. Cooper RR, Ho V: Role of emergency skull x-ray films in the evaluation of the head-injured patient: A retrospective study. *Neurosurgery* 13:136–140, 1983.

46. Schwartz HG, Roulhac GE: Craniocerebral war wounds. Observations on delayed treatment. *Ann Surg* 121:129–151, 1945.

47. Enzmann DR, Britt RH, Lyons B, et al: Experimental study of high-resolution ultrasound imaging of hemorrhage, bone fragments, and foreign bodies in head trauma. *J Neurosurg* 54:304–309, 1981.

48. Meirowsky AM: Secondary removal of retained bone fragments in missile wounds of the brain. *J Neurosurg* 57:617–621, 1982.

49. Pitlyk PJ: Removal of retained bone fragments. *J Neurosurg* 54:624, 1983.

50. Jennett B, Miller JD. Infection after depressed fracture of skull: Implications for management of nonmissile injuries. *J Neurosurg* 36:333–339, 1972.

51. Arendall REH, Meirowsky AM: Air sinus wounds: An analysis of 163 consecutive cases incurred in the Korean War, 1950–1952. *Neurosurg* 13:377–380, 1983.

52. Jane JA, Steward O, Gennarelli T: Axonal degeneration induced by experimental noninvasive minor head injury. *J Neurosurg* 62:96–100, 1985.

53. Gallagher JP, Browder EJ: Extradural hematomas. Experiences with 167 patients. *J Neurosurg* 29:1–12, 1968.

54. Hirsh, LF: Chronic epidural hematomas. *Neurosurgery* 6:508–512, 1980.

55. Garza-Mercado R: Extradural hematoma of the posterior cranial fossa: Report of seven cases with survival. *J Neurosurg* 59:664–672, 1983.

56. Shields CB, Stites TB, Garretson HD: Isodense subdural hematoma presenting with paraparesis. *J Neurosurg* 52:712–714, 1980.

57. Kernohan JW, Woltman HE: Incisura of the crus due to contralateral brain tumor. *Arch Neurol Psychiat* 21:274–287, 1929.

58. Bender MB, Christoff N: Nonsurgical treatment of subdural hematomas. *Arch Neurol* 31:73–79, 1974.

59. Gadi GF, Becker DP, Miller JD, Dwan PS: Pathology and pathophysiology of head injury, in Youmans JR (ed): *Neurological Surgery,* 3d ed. Philadelphia, Saunders, 1990, chap 66, pp 1965–2016.

60. Jennett B, Miller JD, Braakman R: Epilepsy after nonmissile depressed skull fracture. *J Neurosurg* 41:208–217, 1974.

61. Zimmerman RA, Bilaniuk LT: Computer tomography of trau-

matic intracerebral hemorrhagic lesions: The change in density and mass effect with time. *Neuroradiol* 16:320–321, 1978.

62. Talbert OR: General methods of clinical examination, in Youmans JR (ed): *Neurological Surgery,* 3d ed. 1990, Philadelphia, Saunders, chap 1, pp 3–36.

63. Terzian H, Ore GD: Syndrome of Kluver and Bucy reproduced in man by bilateral removal of the temporal lobes. *Neurol* 5:373–380, 1955.

64. Rasmussen T, Milner B: Clinical and surgical studies of the cerebral speech areas in man, in Zulch KJ, Creutzfeldt O, Galbraith GC (eds): *Cerebral Localization.* New York, Springer-Verlag, 1975, pp 238–257.

65. Clifton GL, Grossman RG, Makela ME, et al: Neurological course and correlated computerized tomography findings after severe closed head injury. *J Neurosurg* 52:611–624, 1980.

66. Becker DP, Miller JD, Ward PD, et al: The outcome from severe head injury with early diagnosis and intensive management. *J Neurosurg* 47:491–502, 1977.

67. Marshall LF, Smith RW, Shapiro HM: The outcome with aggressive treatment in severe head injuries. Part I: The significance of intracranial pressure monitoring. *J Neurosurg* 50:20–25, 1979.

68. Narayan RK, Greenberg RP, Miller JD, et al: Improved confidence of outcome prediction in severe head injury. A comparative analysis of the clinical examination, multimodality evoked potentials, CT scanning, and intracranial pressure. *J Neurosurg* 54:751–762, 1981.

69. van Dongen KJ, Braakman R, Gelpke GJ: The prognostic value of computerized tomography in comatose head-injured patients. *J Neurosurg* 59:951–957, 1983.

70. Gennarelli TA, Spielman GM, Langfitt TW, et al: Influence of the type of intracranial lesion on outcome from severe head injury: A multicenter study using a new classification system. *J Neurosurg* 56:26–32, 1982.

71. Lobato RD, Cordobes F, Rivas JJ, et al: Outcome from severe head injury related to the type of intracranial lesion: A computerized tomography study. *J Neurosurg* 59:762–774, 1983.

72. Becker DP, Gader GF, Young HF, Feuerman TF: Diagnosis and treatment of head injury in adults, in Youmans JR (ed): *Neurological Surgery,* 3d ed. Philadelphia, Saunders, 1990, pp 2017–2148.

73. Frost EAM, Arancibia CV, Shulman K: Pulmonary shunt as a prognostic indicator in head injury. *J Neurosurg* 50:768–772, 1979.

74. Ducker TB: Increased intracranial pressure and pulmonary edemas. Part I: Clinical study of 11 patients. *J Neurosurg* 28:112–117, 1968.

75. Geisler FH, Salcman M: Respiratory system: Physiology, pathophysiology, and management, in Wirth FP, Ratcheson RA (eds): *Neurological Critical Care,* Baltimore, Williams & Wilkins, chap 1, pp 1–50, 1987.

76. National Heart, Lung, and Blood Institute: Extracorporal support for respiratory insufficiency: A collaborative study. Bethesda, MD, National Institutes of Health, 1979, p 10.

77. Cooper KR, Boswell PA, Choi S: Safe use of PEEP in patients with severe head injury. *J Neurosurg* 63:552–555, 1985.

78. Berlauk JF: Prolonged endotracheal intubation versus tracheostomy. *Crit Care Med* 14:742–745, 1986.

79. McCredie JA: Fluid, electrolyte and acid-base balance, in McCredie JA: *Basic Surgery.* New York, MacMillan, 1977, pp 92–102.

80. Rowlands BJ, Litofsky NS, Kaufman HA: Metabolic physiology, pathophysiology and management, in Wirth FP, Ratcheson RA (eds): *Neurosurgical Critical Care.* Baltimore, Williams & Wilkins, 1987, pp 81–1081.

81. Gadisseux P, Ward, JP, Young HF, Becker DP: Nutrition and the neurosurgical patient: Review article. *J Neurosurg* 60:219–232, 1984.

82. Clifton GL, Roberston CS, Contant CF: Enteral hyperalimentation in head injury. *J Neurosurg* 62:186–193, 1985.

83. Rapp RP, Young B, Twyman D, et al: The favorable effect of early parenteral feeding on survival in head-injured patients. *J Neurosurg* 58:906–912, 1983.

84. Black PMcL, Crowell RM, Abbott WM: External pneumatic calf compression reduces deep venous thrombosis in patients with ruptured intracranial aneurysms. *Neurosurg* 8:25–28, 1986.

85. Zelikovski A, Zucker G, Eliashiv A, et al: A new sequential device for the prevention of deep vein thrombosis. *J Neurosurg* 54:652–654, 1981.

86. Kakkar VV, Corrigan TP, Fossard DP: Prevention of fatal postoperative pulmonary embolism by low doses of heparin. *Lancet* 2:45–51, 1975.

87. Clarke-Pearson DL, DeLong E, Synan IS, et al: A controlled trail of two low-dose heparin regimens for the prevention of postoperative deep vein thrombosis. *Obstet Gynecol* 75:684–689, 1990.

88. Knight MTN, Dawson R: Effect of intermittent compression of the arms on deep venous thrombosis in the legs. *Lancet* 2:1265, 1976.

89. Nicolaides AN, Miles C, Hoak M, et al: Intermittent sequential pneumatic compression of the legs and thromboembolism deterrent stockings in the prevention of postoperative deep venous thrombosis. *Surgery* 94:21–25, 1983.

90. Salzman EW, McManama GP, Shapiro AH, et al: Effect of optimization of hemodynamics on fibrinolytic activity and antithrombotic efficacy of external pneumatic calf compression. *Ann Surg* 206:636–641, 1987.

91. Hagen C, Nalkmus D, Durham P: Levels of Cognitive Functioning. Communication Disorders Service, Rancho Los Amigos Hospital, 1972.

92. Malkmus D, Stenderup K: Communication Disorders Service, Rancho Los Amigos Hospital, 1974.

93. Management of clinical problems, in Umphred D (ed): *Neurological Rehabilitation,* Mosby, chap 10, 1985.

94. Texas Head Injury Foundation: Comprehensive rehabilitation of the head injured person: A family education manual.

95. Black PMcL: Hydrocephalus and vasospasm after subarachnoid hemorrhage from ruptured intracranial aneurysms. *Neurosurg* 18:12–16, 1986.

96. Kishore PRS, Lipper MH, Miller JD, et al: Postraumatic hydrocephalus in patients with severe head injury. *Neuroradiology* 16:261–265, 1978.

97. Ojemann RC: Normal pressure hydrocephalus. *Clin Neurosurg* 18:337–370, 1971.

98. Bricola A: Electroencephalography in neurotraumatology. *Clin Electroenceph* 7:184–197, 1976.

99. Jennett B, Miller JD, Braakman R: Epilepsy after non-missile-depressed skull fracture. *J Neurosurg* 41:208–216, 1974.

100. Black PMcL: Brain death, in Youmans JR (ed): *Neurological Surgery* 3d ed. Philadelphia, Saunders, chap 20, pp 602–619.

101. Black, PMcL: Brain death (part I). *New Eng J Med* 299:338–344, 1978.

102. President's Commission: Guidelines for the determination of death. Report of the medical consultants on the diagnosis of death to the president's commission on the study of ethical problems in medicine and biomedical and behavioral research. *JAMA* 246:2184–2186, 1981.

103. Ropper AH, Kennedy SK, Russell L: Apnea testing in the diagnosis of brain death: Clinical and physiological observations. *J Neurosurg* 55:942–946, 1981.

☐ STUDY QUESTIONS

I. A 16-year-old male is involved in an automobile accident and sustains blunt trauma to the head. When seen in the emergency room, his pupils are 2 mm and slightly reactive. He is breathing. He has posturing on the right and minimal flexor response to painful stimulation on the left. He does not vocalize to any stimulus. A CT reveals diffuse cerebral edema on the left.

1. What is his Glasgow coma score? **2.** What might be told the relatives regarding the patient's chances for recovery at this time? **3.** What types of therapy might be considered for the head injury? **4.** Assuming a ventricular catheter is inserted into the right lateral ventricle and the ventricular pressure measures 25 mmHg, what courses should be considered in what sequence? **5.** Should this patient have sequential CT scans? Why or why not?

II. A 40-year-old female becomes depressed and shoots herself in the head. The missile is of a small calibre and lodges in the right hemisphere near the vertex. The patient has a left hemiparesis. A CT reveals the missile and several depressed bone fragments in the right temporal area and a moderate-sized (8 mm thick) acute subdural hematoma.

1. What procedures should be carried out in the emergency room? **2.** Should this patient's head be debrided? **3.** What consideration should be given to the subdural hematoma? **4.** What are the chances of seizures as a complication? **5.** What should be accomplished at the site of the missile entrance at the time of debridement?

III. A 20-year-old female sustains a blunt head injury, is stuporous for a few minutes but recovers, then begins to notice drainage of clear fluid from her left nostril.

1. What is the most likely cause? **2.** How can one identify the source of the fluid? **3.** What are the dangers of such a fluid leak? **4.** Should consideration of repair be given? If so, when? **5.** If the fluid leak had begun spontaneously without the history of head injury, would the considerations for its treatment be different? If so, why?

IV. A 60-year-old laborer has a minor head injury and continues to work, but he notes a progressive headache over a period of 3 weeks before he becomes stuporous and is taken to the emergency room. By the time he arrives, he is found to have a right hemiparesis and a dilated pupil on the right. A CT scan shows a subdural hematoma.

1. On which side is the hematoma most likely located? **2.** How can it be evacuated? **3.** What is the explanation for the pupillary dilatation and the hemiparesis being on the same side? **4.** What is the most likely source of the hematoma? **5.** Can an acute hemorrhage have complicated the chronic hematoma without additional trauma in the presence of normal clotting factors? Why?

V. A depressed fracture occurs over the saggital sinus.

1. What are the options for therapy? **2.** Is there a difference in the neurological deficits which might occur after ligation of the sagittal sinus at different points? **3.** How can hemorrhage from the saggital sinus on the operating table be controlled? **4.** What are the dangers of elevating the head to control the hemorrhage? **5.** Is the presence of a simple fracture across the sinus an indication for exposing the sinus?

Trauma to the Spine and Spinal Cord

Marshall B. Allen, Jr.
J. Allan Goodrich

☐ ANATOMY AND CLASSIFICATION OF INJURIES

Twenty-four *vertebrae* are incorporated into the spinal column between the base of the skull and the sacrum. Vertebral bodies are composed of cancellous bone surrounded by a more rigid cortex. Completing the canal behind the vertebral bodies are the pedicles and laminae, from which project the spinous processes, a pair of transverse processes, and pairs of superior and inferior articular facets. (See Fig. 19-1*A* and *B*.)

Intimately attached on the anterior and posterior surfaces of the vertebral bodies are the respective longitudinal ligaments, which also blend into the intervertebral disks and connect the spinal column to the base of the skull and the sacrum. There is a progressive increase in size of the vertebrae from the base of the skull to the sacrum.

The *facets* and the *ligamentous attachments* connecting the posterior elements play a most important role in maintaining the alignment of the vertebral column. At the cervical and thoracic levels, the facets are arranged like shingles, so that inferior facets of a more cephalic vertebra lie superior and dorsal to the superiorly projecting facets of the more caudal vertebra, separated only by cartilaginous plates. They are joined by their *joint capsules*. In the lumbar area the facets are larger. Their orientation is rotated so that the major portion of the superior facets lies more lateral to the inferior facets, but medial projections of the superior facets are directed toward the spinal canal ventral to the inferior facets. About 80 percent of the vertical strength of the spinal column is assumed by the vertebral bodies and the intervertebral disks, with the remainder being provided by the facets.[1]

The support of the posterior longitudinal ligament is augmented by the ligamentum flavum, which connects the laminae, the interspinous and supraspinous ligaments, and the capsules of the facets. The attached paraspinal muscles—the psoas, longus coli, and scalene muscles—participate in the orientation of the spinal column.

While the spinal cord extends throughout the spinal canal at the time of embryological development, its growth rate is exceeded by the vertebral column, so that it comes to lie at the lower level of the first lumbar vertebra by the time skeletal growth is complete. In the distal spinal canal, the *cauda equina* connects the spinal cord to respective nerve roots. While both the spinal cord and the cauda equina are soft tissues and subject to significant injury by trauma, the spinal cord is much more vulnerable than is the cauda equina, and it does not exhibit the regenerative properties of peripheral nerves.

Protection of the neural elements is a most important role of the spinal column. This role is thwarted by compromise of the neural canal by penetration, malalignment, angulation or stenosis, or by intrusion into the canal of bony parts or soft tissues.

VASCULAR SUPPLY TO THE SPINAL CORD

Arterial Supply The primary arterial blood supply to the spinal cord comes from the *anterior spinal artery,* which originates as paired branches of the vertebral arteries that join just below the *basilar artery.* The anterior spinal artery and its branches provide blood supply to the anterior two-thirds of the spinal cord, including the grey matter and the long tracts, with the exception of the posterior columns.

The posterior columns are supplied by the paired *posterior spinal arteries,* which originate as branches of the posterior-inferior cerebellar arteries. The posterior spinal arteries have fewer tributaries and a less extensive area to supply with blood than does the anterior spinal artery.

Both the anterior and posterior spinal arteries are supplied by radicular branches of the vertebral and intercostal arteries, which are irregular in number and size. (See Fig. 19-2.) The largest and most prominent of these is the *magnus ramus radicularis anterior,* or *artery of Adamkiewicz,* which arises usually on the left between the ninth thoracic and first lumbar levels. There is usually a feeding radicular branch high in the thoracic area and another in the lumbar area entering the spinal canal in association with the cauda equina.

Venous Drainage *Venous drainage* of the spinal cord is more haphazard and highly variable. *Batson's plexus* is a large complex venous channel extending from the base of

Table 19-1
CLASSIFICATION OF FRACTURES OF THE THORACOLUMBAR SPINE

Compressive Flexion
Compression through anterior elements.

Patterns of failure
1. Wedge fracture anteriorly.
2. Anterior wedge fracture plus tension disruption of posterior elements.
3. Anterior wedge fracture plus middle element failure. Neural canal compromised by bony elements. Neurological deficits may progress.

Instrumentation. Harrington system or segmental instrumentation if there is failure of the anterior and posterior elements but the middle elements are intact. Failure of the middle elements (bone in the spinal canal) may require Harrington distraction.

Distractive Flexion
Failure of all three elements.

Examples
1. Chance fracture
2. Pure distraction

Neurological injuries proportional to amount of translation.

Instrumentation. Compression system (Harrington or Knodt). May use segmental instrumentation over L-rods if neurological recovery unlikely.

Lateral Flexion
Compressive force caused by lateral bending in compression.

Patterns of failure
1. Anterior and middle elements, unilaterally (usually stable)
2. All three elements fail.

Neurological deficits likely to progress.

Instrumentation. Segmental instrumentation or Harrington distraction. Distraction preferred if there is middle column failure.

Translation
Results from displacement of vertebral body, anteriorly, posteriorly, or laterally.
All connecting processes and ligaments likely disrupted if displacement exceeds 25%.
Neurological deficits are usual.

Instrumentation. Segmental.

Torsional Flexion
Torsion with compression of anterior elements and tension and torsion of posterior elements.
Involvement of middle elements inconstant.
Neurological deficits likely. May progress.

Instrumentation. Harrington or segmental.

Vertical Compression
Shortened vertebral body.

Patterns of protrusion into canal.
1. Wall may bulge into canal.
2. Wall may enfold with apex at superior or inferior segment of vertebral body.

Instrumentation. Harrington distraction or anterior decompression.

Table 19-1
(*continued*)

Distractive Extension
Tension disruption of anterior elements and compression failure of posterior elements.
Rare except in cervical area. Displacements may reduce sponstaneously.

Source: Ferguson and Allen.[7]

McAfee and his colleagues used CT to determine three modes of "middle column failure," including axial compression, axial distraction, and translation.[6] They concluded that CT provided a very accurate means of demonstrating disruption of the posterior elements in unstable and burst injuries.

Sagittal reconstructions are useful in identifying failure of the facet joints in distraction injuries. CT also provides great assistance in the identification of structural injuries of the spine. MRI has proved efficacious in demonstrating hemorrhage and damage to soft tissues, as well as bony alignment—although bony imaging is superior when CT is used.

In a recent review of spinal injuries, substituting the term "elements" for "columns" as defined by Denis, Ferguson and Allen devised a comprehensive classification with the proposed therapies outlined in Table 19-1.[7] (See Figs. 19-4 through 19-10.)

Luque rods, in conjunction with sublaminar wires, were the most commonly used form of segmental fixation when this classification was published. Recently, several forms of anterior fixation, involving some form of plating, have become popular. Use of pedicle screws, with plates or rods, is often favored for segmental fixation from a posterior approach.

The basic anatomy of the vertebrae and their ligamentous attachments *below* the third cervical vertebra exhibits similar features throughout, although the environment of the spine and its vulnerability to injury vary according to the level. The presence of the vertebral arteries in the neck, the size of the vertebrae, and the response of cervical fracture-dislocations to skeletal traction, as well as the ease of access to anterior portions of the vertebral column by surgery, dictate variations in the management of injuries. However, an understanding of the basic mechanisms of injury and the importance of residual structures, particularly the middle column, to stability of the vertebral system, applies throughout. This is important to the surgeon who is planning to apply manipulative therapy—whether by skeletal traction, instrumentation, or surgical decompression of the spinal canal. In applying instrumentation, it is important to remember that failure of any one of the vertebral columns may involve a compression effect (failure of vertical strength) or failure of the ligamentous strength (failure of the capability to oppose distraction).

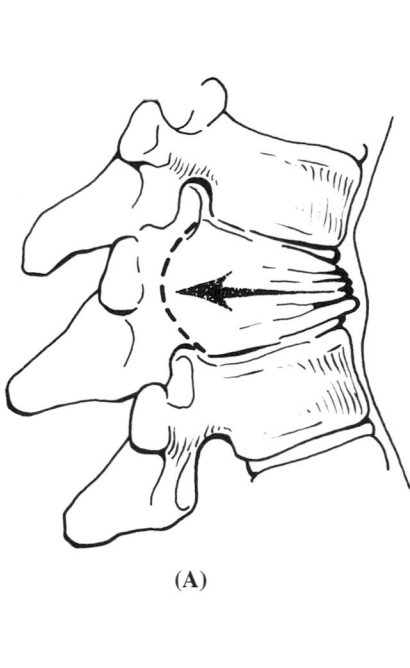

(A)

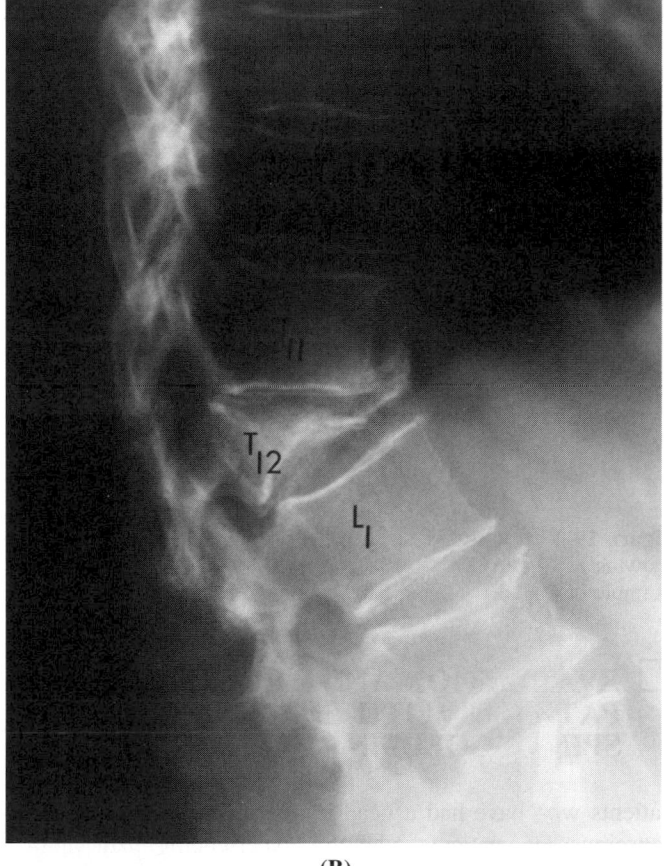

(B)

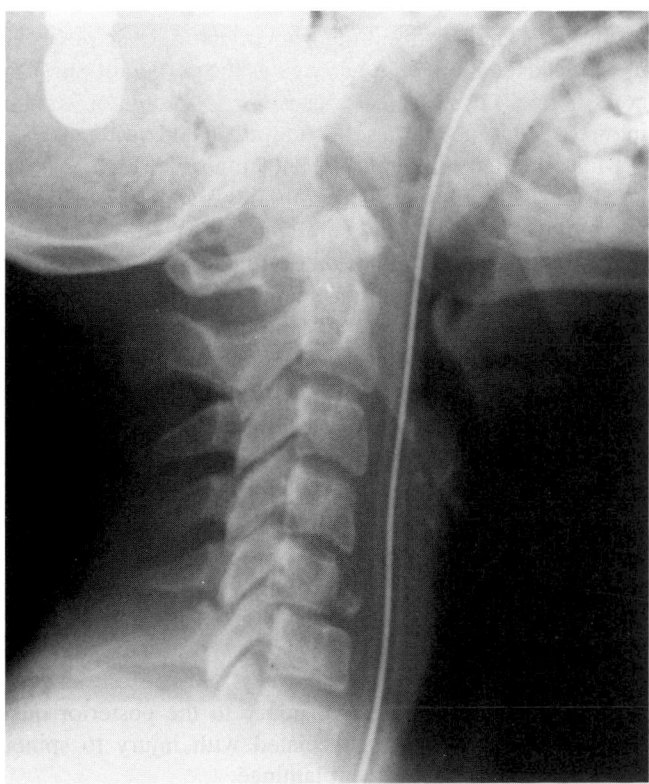

(C)

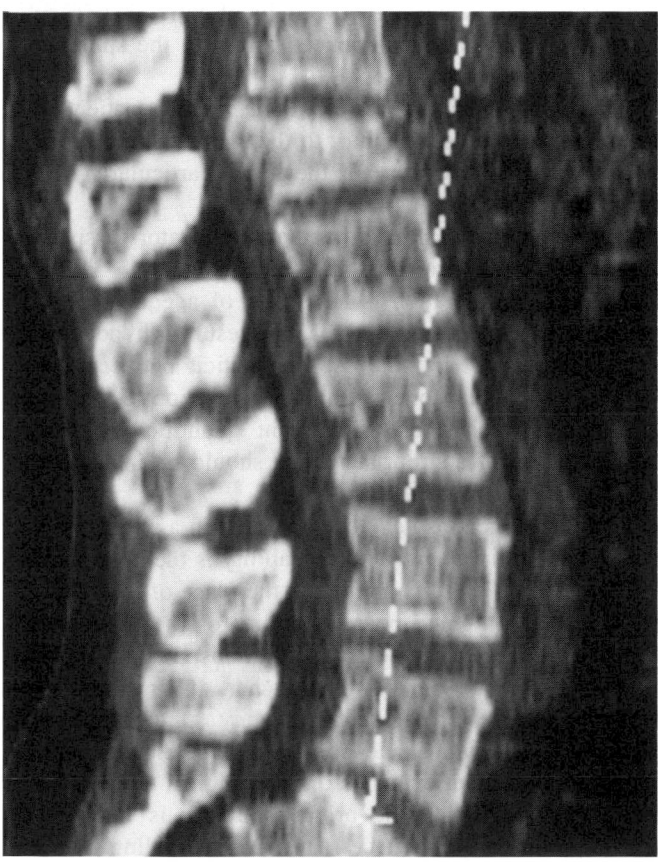

(D)

Figure 19–4 Compression flexion injury of spinal column in an illustrative sketch *(A)*, in a lateral radiograph, showing collapse of the twelfth thoracic vertebra in an elderly osteoporotic patient *(B)*, compression fracture of the fifth cervical vertebra with slight separation of the spinous processes between C5 and C6 *(C)*, and a reconstructed sagittal CT scan, showing compression of the anterior element and failure of the middle element with displacement of a fragment of the superior posterior lip of the vertebral body into the spinal canal *(D)*.

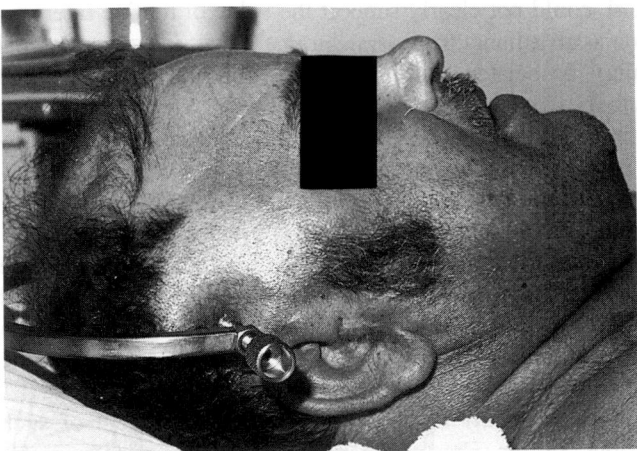

Figure 19–12 Photograph of a patient, showing the Gardner-Wells tongs for distraction and/or stabilization of an injury to the cervical vertebrae.

skull and the third cervical vertebra result in special considerations that set them aside from lesions in lower parts of the spinal column. They will therefore be discussed as separate lesions. Treatment of most malalignments of the cervical spine requires cervical traction, and treatment of many lesions requires fixation, which is frequently accomplished by a halo apparatus. The application and use of equipment required for these forms of therapy will be described first.

CERVICAL TRACTION

Cervical traction is administered with a fabricated halter which applies traction beneath the chin and behind the occiput, or by an apparatus applied to the cranium. Halter traction can be used for temporary stabilization of neck injuries, but it should be replaced by skeletal traction as early as possible, and weights should not exceed 10 lb for more than 2 h.

Gardner-Wells tongs are most commonly used to apply *skeletal traction.* The area chosen for application is prepared with an antiseptic and infiltrated with a local anesthetic. (See Fig. 19-12.)

Spring-loaded pins are driven into the skull below its broadest width above the pinnae of the ears, usually at a point above a line extending from the mastoid process through the external auditory meatus.[12]

A more anterior placement will provide traction with the neck in extension, which is often desirable when treating dislocations of the odontoid. A more posterior placement will provide traction with the neck in flexion which may be desirable when trying to "unlock" facets. Otherwise, traction is usually applied in a straight line.

A general rule for application of weights is to apply initially 5 lb per vertebra between the base of the skull and the site of injury. However, amounts of traction must be closely monitored by neurological observation and by fre-

quent radiographs or fluoroscopy. It may be necessary to administer a mild sedative such as diazepam, and/or an analgesic when attempting to unlock facets.

Traction for patients without neurological deficit is usually applied in a hospital bed, with the head of the bed elevated enough to counter the weight of the traction. For patients with paresis, paraplegia, or quadriplegia, traction is usually accomplished in a rotating bed to minimize the risks of decubiti. Prophylaxis against venous thromboses is provided patients with paralysis of the lower extremities by intermittent venous compression or low-dose heparin.

For patients who have sustained severe injuries to the skull, traction may be applied to the posterior zygomas using sterilized fish hooks which are attached to a crossbar over the head.

APPLICATION OF A HALO JACKET SYSTEM

There are several commercially available halo-vest systems.[13,14] All systems consist of a halo ring and pins, a plastic vest, and uprights which connect the two. The uprights may be adjusted for the proper alignment of the halo.

Rings may be applied to the cranium when an unstable fracture of the neck is diagnosed and used for traction, or they may be applied after a period of initial traction with Gardner-Wells tongs. (See Fig. 19-13.) Four sites for pin placement are shaved, sterilely prepared, and infiltrated with local anesthetic. Sites are located about 1 cm above the lateral segments of the eyebrows—and in the posterior parietal skull in such a position that the ring will be about 1 cm above the pinnae of the ears.

The ring is usually applied with the patient lying supine on a thin narrow board that holds the head. Rings should be of such a size that there will be about $1\frac{1}{4}$ cm between the ring and the scalp.

Sterilized pins are passed through threaded sites in the halo ring and applied to the skull through the anesthetized scalp with a torque screwdriver. They are tightened to about 8 to 10 lb and then locked in place with hexagonal nuts.

After the vest is applied, connecting bars are employed in such a manner as to hold the head in a neutral position. Pins should be tightened a second time in 24 to 48 h. Radiographs are obtained following the application of the halo apparatus. Local pin care with hydrogen peroxide 3 times daily will minimize problems with infections of the pin sites.

☐ TREATMENT OF SPECIFIC INJURIES

JEFFERSON FRACTURE

A *Jefferson fracture* is a fracture through the ring of the atlas.[15] Since the atlas is ring-shaped, there are usually

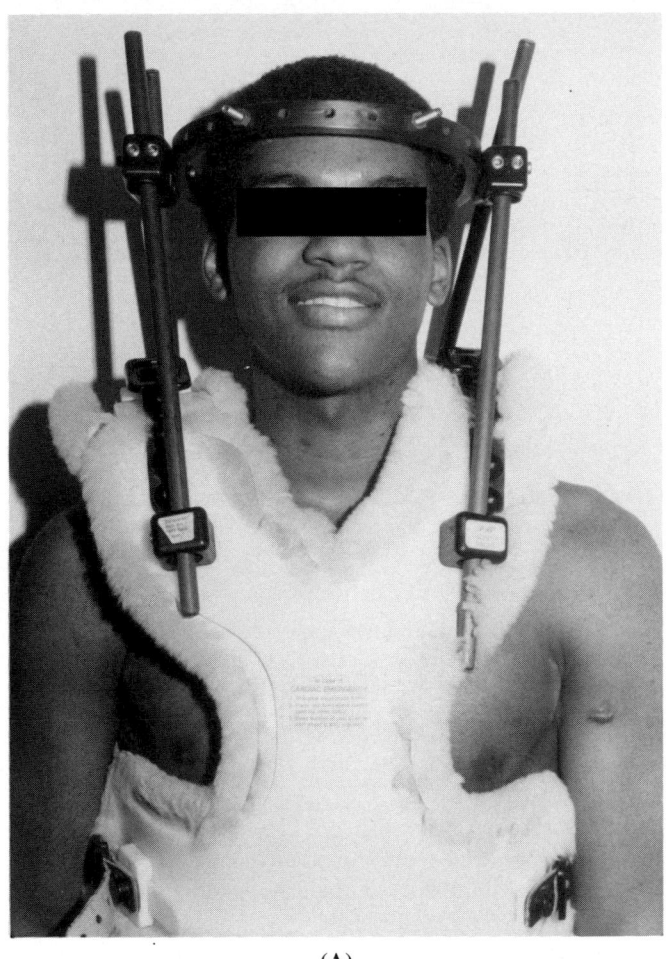

(A)

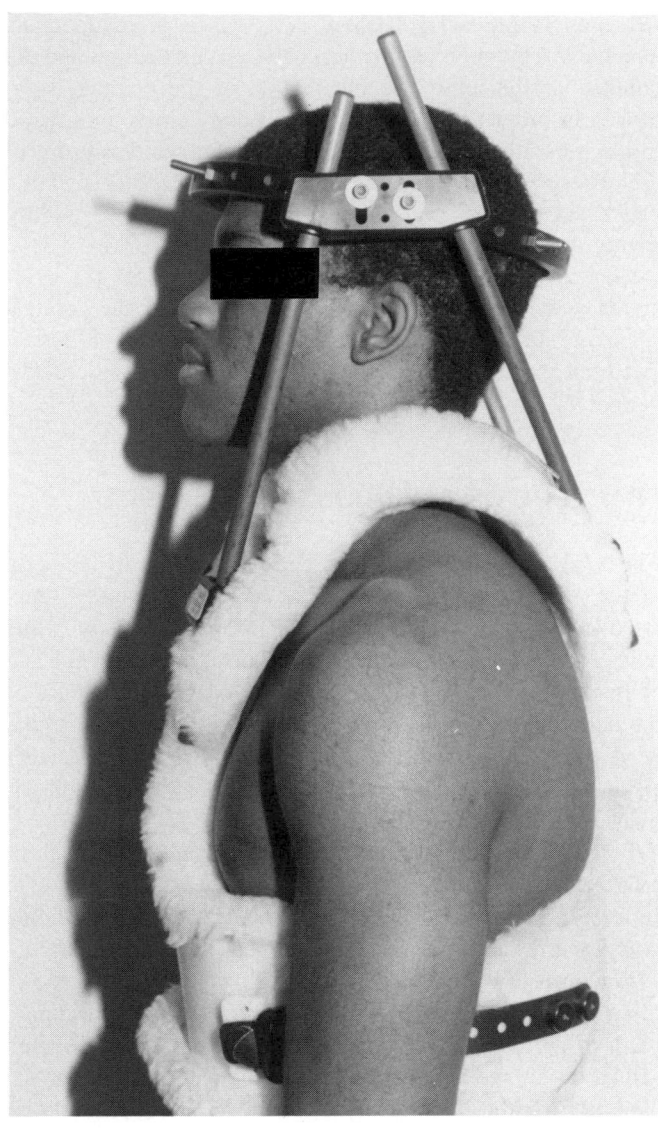

(B)

Figure 19–13 Photographs of a patient in a halo apparatus for stabilization of cervical fractures.

fractures at two sites, one anterior and one behind the lateral masses. (See Fig. 19-14.) This fracture usually occurs as a result of a blow to the vertex of the head.

The lateral masses of the atlas are wedge-shaped, with the apex of the wedge being directed toward the neural canal. A

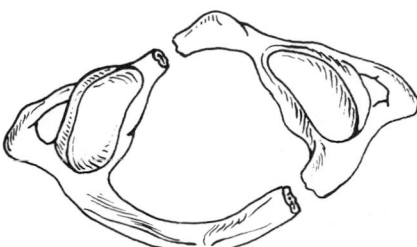

Figure 19–14 Schematic illustration of a Jefferson fracture. Note that there are fractures in both the anterior and posterior segments of the ring. Injury to the ligamentous elements in such a fracture is variable.

blow to the vertex causes these masses to be forced apart. If the load is so great that connecting bony elements fail, the masses separate and fractures in the ring occur. If lateral masses appear separated more than 6.9 mm on a frontal projection radiograph, there is likely to be injury to the transverse ligaments as well.[16] A recent study by Heller et al. considers the effects of radiographic magnification and suggests that the number may be close to 8 mm.[16a]

Confirmation of ligamentous injury is obtained by radiographic demonstration of abnormal motion between the odontoid and the atlas. (Note measurements in section on dislocation of the odontoid in text following.)

Symptoms of fracture of the atlas are usually limited to localized pain. Neurological deficits are rarely significant in patients with injuries of this type.

If there is no evidence of ligamentous injury, mild skeletal traction may be applied initially, but a halo brace is used for long-term stabilization.[17]

Fusion is necessary if there is evidence of ligamentous damage.[18] This requires fixation between the occiput and the laminae of the axis. The outer table of the occiput is removed in order to obtain fusion, and bony struts are affixed to the remaining occipital bone and decorticated laminae of C2. These bony struts are supported by wires or metallic plates. External fixation with a halo brace assures stability during the healing process.

Careful inspection of images should be made for associated defects since fractures in other parts of the cervical spine are found in 50 percent of patients with Jefferson fractures, particularly fractures involving the second cervical vertebrae.

FRACTURE OF THE ODONTOID PROCESS

The *odontoid process* develops embryologically as the body of the atlas. During development, the body becomes separated from the ring of the atlas and fuses to the body of the axis. There is usually some cartilaginous material at the site of fusion until maturity is reached. Separation at the base of the odontoid may occur with a relatively slight injury to the head during childhood. The resulting bony segment is called an *os odontoidium*. Stabilization of the dens in proper alignment is necessary, usually by a halo brace.[19]

Fractures of the odontoid in adults are usually the result of relatively severe trauma, frequently to the occiput. As with Jefferson fractures, patients seen initially with odontoid process fracture rarely have significant neurological deficits.

Fractures of the odontoid are typed according to the site of the fracture. (See Fig. 19-15.) Fractures through the upper mass of the dens are classified as type I and are considered stable, but a recent report indicates that such lesions may be associated with atlanto-occipital instability and will require fusion.[20]

Type II fractures are through the base of the dens. They may render the dens ischemic and are associated with a high incidence of nonunion.[21] Fusion between the laminae of C1 and C2, often incorporating C3, is indicated. (See Fig. 19-16.)

Stabilization may be accomplished by wire loops between the lamina of C1 and the spinous process of C2, or with Halifax clamps.[21,22]

Fusion requires decorticating the respective laminae and overlaying the remaining bony elements with chips of cancellous and cortical bone. Added strength may be acquired by placing fragments of bone between the decorticated segments of laminae and spinous processes of the two vertebrae.

An alternative form of fixation which is reported to have a high degree of success is the application of methylmethacrylate into the area after the bony cortex has been denuded.[23] The authors have had no personal experience with this technique.

Another alternative procedure for the treatment of type II fractures of the odontoid is application of screws through the bony axis into the odontoid process.[24] This is accomplished through an anteriolateral approach. Wire pins are inserted

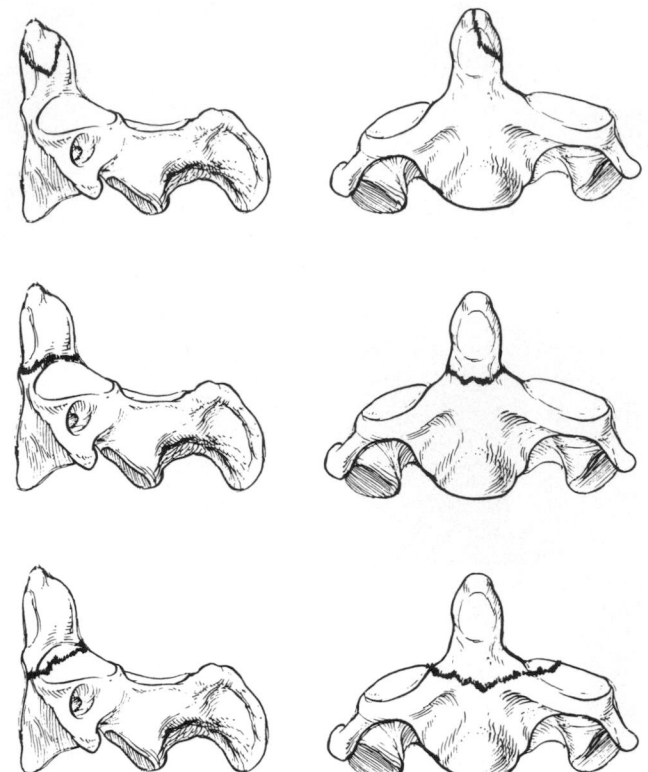

Figure 19–15 Schematic illustrations of the three types of fractures of the odontoid. Type I (upper) involves the apex of the odontoid. This is rare but may be associated with significant ligamentous injury. Type II (middle), across the neck, is often associated with ischemic necrosis of the odontoid process. Type III extends into the body of the axis.

under fluoroscopy. (See Fig. 19-17.) These are replaced by screws. Fusion rates are reportedly high. The procedure should be accomplished during the first 6 weeks after a fracture; its success is diminished in cases of nonunion.

Type III fractures of the odontoid extend into the body of the axis. Such lesions usually heal when stabilized, so appropriate treatment is traction until alignment is obtained and the patient is physiologically stable. A halo apparatus is then applied. (See Fig. 19-18.) A 15 percent incidence of malunion or nonunion may also occur with this type of fracture.

DISLOCATION OF THE ODONTOID

The dens may become dislocated as a result of congenital abnormalities; trauma to the cruciate ligament; an inflammatory process, either rheumatoid arthritis or a retropharyngeal infection; or in association with Downs syndrome.[25,26,27]

The distance between the dens and the anterior rim of the atlas may be as much as 4.5 mm in a child but should not exceed 2.5 mm in the adult.[28] Displacements greater than 5.0 mm are associated with tears in the alar ligaments as well. Left untreated, displacements of the odontoid may progress so that the dens compresses the medulla, often in or above the foramen magnum.[29]

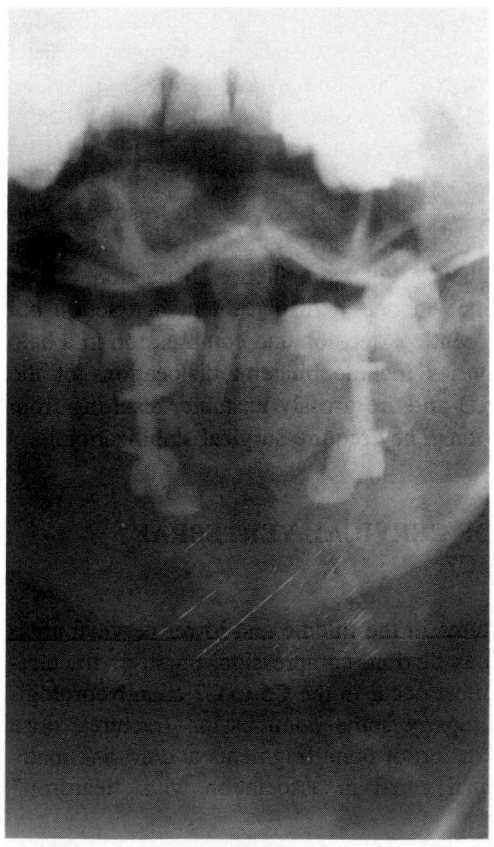

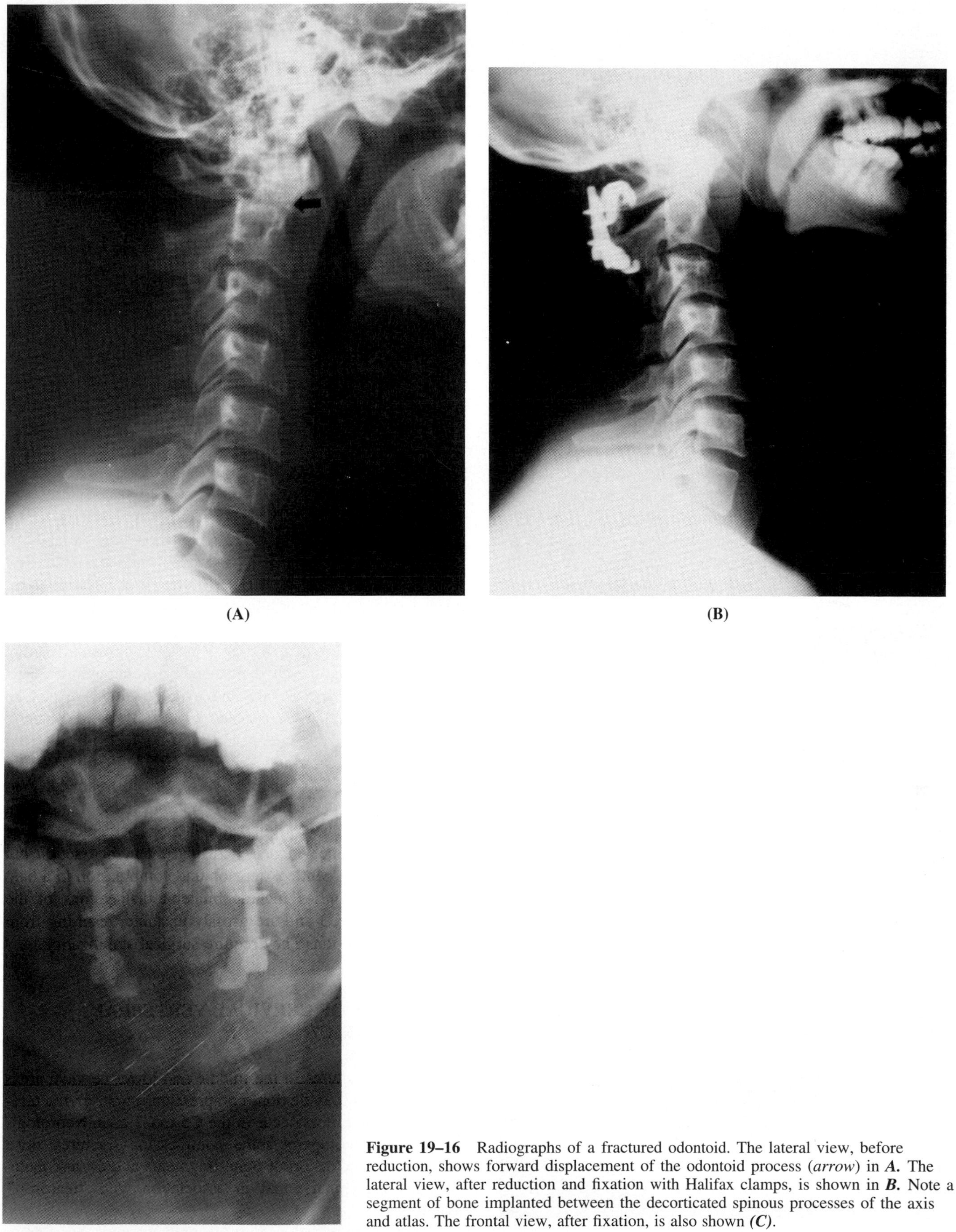

(A)

(B)

(C)

Figure 19–16 Radiographs of a fractured odontoid. The lateral view, before reduction, shows forward displacement of the odontoid process (*arrow*) in *A.* The lateral view, after reduction and fixation with Halifax clamps, is shown in *B.* Note a segment of bone implanted between the decorticated spinous processes of the axis and atlas. The frontal view, after fixation, is also shown *(C).*

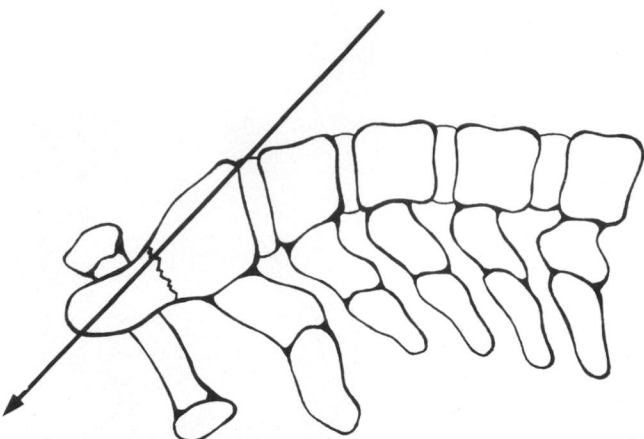

Figure 19–17 A schematic illustration of fixation of the odontoid process with one or two screws. This form of fixation is reportedly quite effective early but frequently met with failure when delayed.

The ideal treatment is to reduce displacement of the odontoid process and perform a posterior fusion as described for a fractured odontoid.[27] This may be accomplished by traction, with the neck in extension. On occasion, reduction is impossible and the odontoid must be removed by drilling through a transoral or anterolateral approach.[30,31,32,33,34]

Fusion must be accomplished when the odontoid is removed. This is done posteriorly with wiring or metallic plates and bony struts, as described in the previous section,

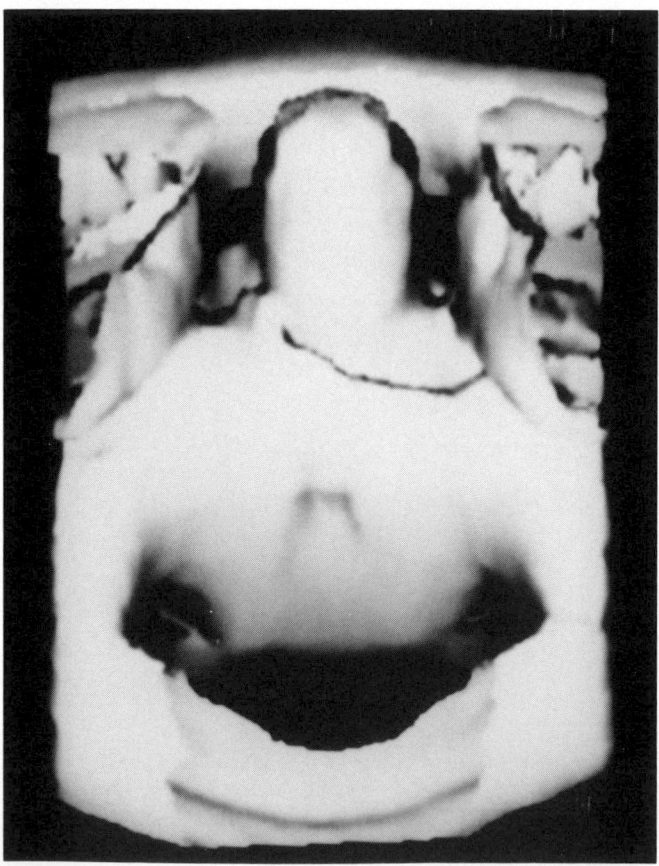

Figure 19–18 A 3-dimensional recontruction of a type III fracture of the odontoid.

or by placing bony chips between the denuded articular surfaces between C1 and C2. The laminae and spine of C3 are incorporated if the fusion is accomplished from behind. Patient immobilization is required, often in a halo for 3 to 4 months. In severe cases, an anterior strut graft may be necessary. (See Fig. 19-19*A* through *E*.)

HANGMAN'S FRACTURE

A hangman's fracture is a fracture through the pedicles of the second cervical vertebra that may be accompanied by anterior translocation of the body of C2 on C3.[35] The fracture results from hyperextension of the neck. Its name is derived historically from injuries sustained during the course of judicial hangings, when the noose was secured beneath the chin.

Most hangman's fractures today result from sudden deceleration of an automobile, causing the driver's chin to catch on the steering wheel or a passenger's chin to catch on the dashboard. Since there is fracture *and* separation between the body of C2 and posterior elements, compression of neural elements is unlikely and neurological deficits are rarely significant.

Separation of bony fragments may be quite variable. A recent report by Levine and Edwards has added a great deal to the understanding of these fractures, and it summarizes their classification according to stability.[36] (See Fig. 19-20*A* and *B*.)

There are three types. A type 1 stable hangman's fracture is one with insignificant displacement or angulation. This results from hyperextension and axial loading and can be adequately treated by a cervical collar. A type 2 fracture shows significant angulation and translation. It results from initial hyperextension and axial loading injury followed by hyperflexion. These patients respond well to treatment with a halo. Type 2A fractures have no translation but severe angulation, and they result from flexion-distraction. These fractures experience increased displacement in traction but are reduced with gentle extension and compression in a halo vest. Type 3 injuries include bilateral dislocations of the facets of C2 or C3 and are grossly unstable, resulting from flexion-compression. They require surgical stabilization.

FRACTURES OF CERVICAL VERTEBRAE C3 THROUGH C7

Most major fractures in the middle and lower cervical areas can be classified as flexion, compression, burst, or fracture-dislocation, and most occur in the C5 to C7 area. Neurological deficits accompany some compression fractures since there may be extrusion of bone fragments and/or disk material into the spinal canal in association with "teardrop" fractures.

Severe neurological deficits accompany most burst fractures and a high percentage of fracture-dislocations. Major

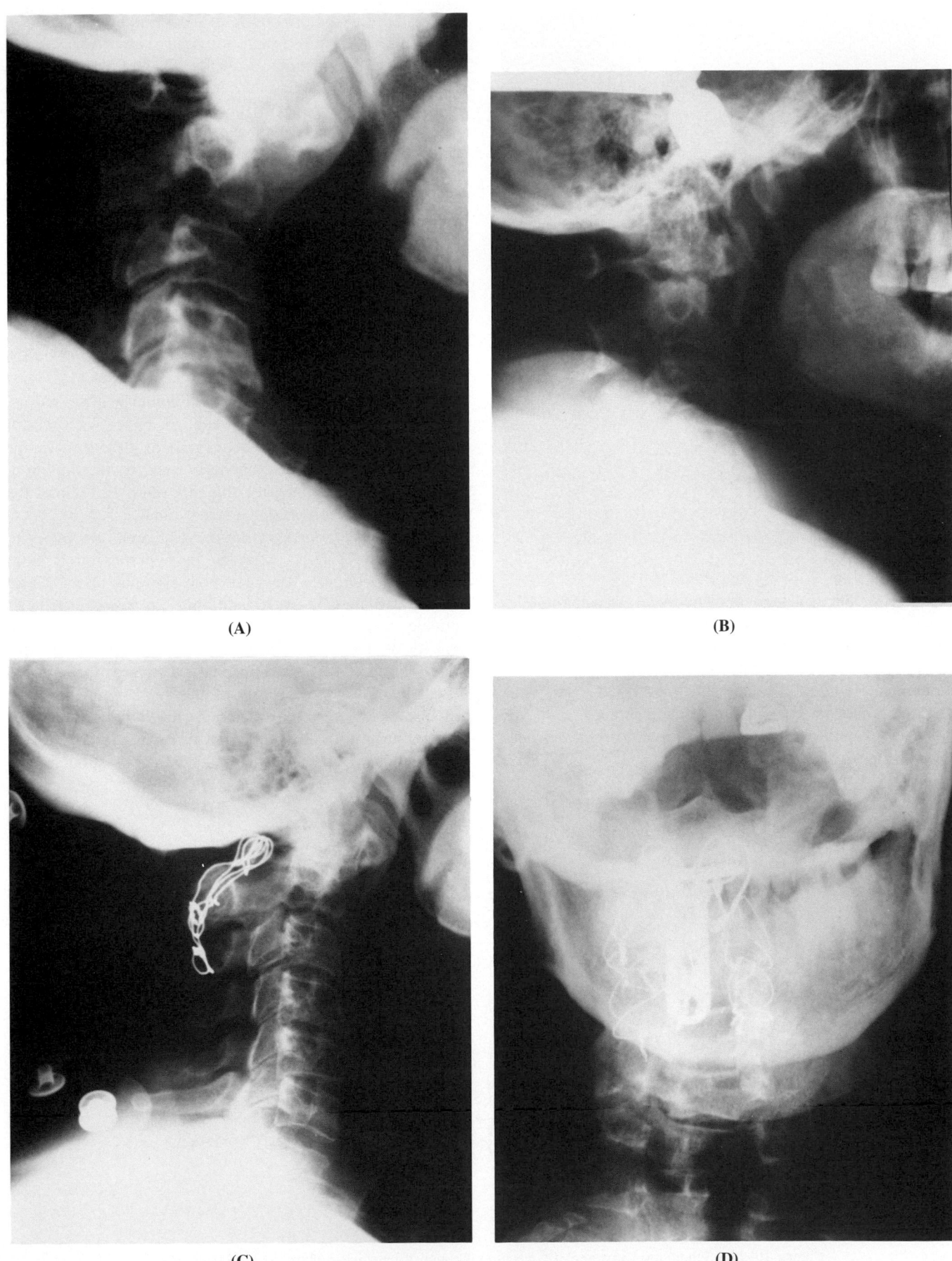

(A)

(B)

(C)

(D)

Figure 19–19 A dislocated odontoid in a patient with rheumatoid arthritis seen in the lateral view before reduction *(A)* and after reduction *(B)*, after wiring failed to maintain reduction *(C)* and after fixation with a posteriorly placed plate held in place with sublaminar and occipital wires *(D, E)*.

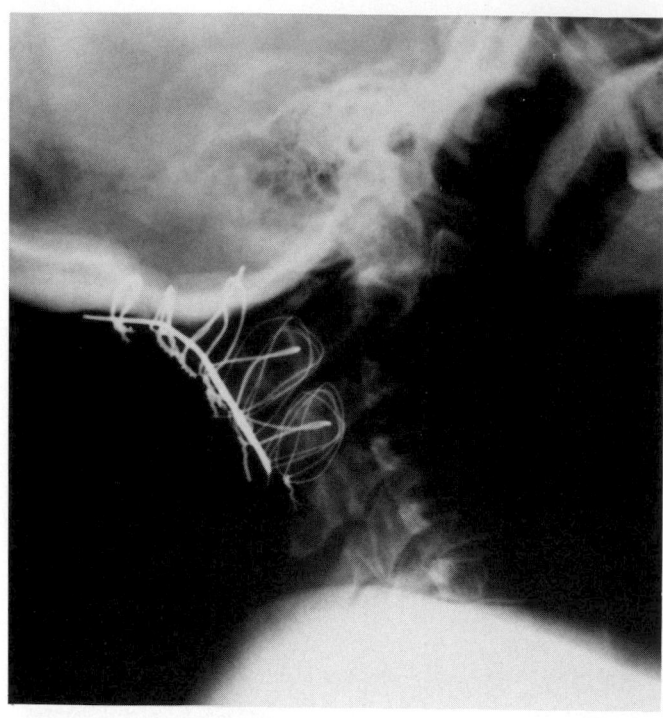

(E)

Figure 19–19 Continued

neurological deficits also accompany hyperextension injuries in the neck when the canal is narrow—despite no radiographic evidence of structural damage. The injury is to the central portion of the spinal cord and motor and sensory involvement being most prominent in the distal parts of the upper extremities.[9] Imaging of the spinal cord with MR demonstrates evidence of edema with inconsistent evidence of contusion.[37]

Sensitivity to the possibility of flexion injuries must arise when there is localized pain and tenderness. (See Fig. 19-21A and B.) Radiographic evidence of abnormal separation of spinous processes may appear on plain films, but is more evident on films made in the lateral projection, with the patient holding his or her neck in flexion for comparison with another lateral projection that is made while the patient holds the neck in extension. The importance of diagnosis here is in its value as a predictor of subsequent dislocation.

Compression fractures are usually stable, but impingement of fragments of bone or disk on the spinal canal may indicate the need for resection of the vertebral body and/or disk material—usually by an anterior approach. A bone graft, which is obtained from iliac crest or fibula, or from an allograft, may be implanted. The strength and stability of the graft is supplemented by use of a metallic plate.[38,39,40,41] (See Fig. 19-22A through C.)

Severe neurological deficits are common with burst fractures. Skeletal traction may be applied, but replacement of the vertebral body with a bone graft as described in the paragraph above provides long-term stability. In addition to providing structural integrity, this procedure also allows the opportunity to decompress the spinal canal.

Fracture-dislocations, in the cervical area, are likely to be the result of hyperextension or hyperflexion with or without rotation.[42,43] They are most common at the C5 to C6 and C6 to C7 levels, and they are associated with variable degrees of neurological deficit, depending on the severity of damage to underlying neural elements. In this injury, facets of the more cephalic vertebra become displaced anterior to the facets of the caudal vertebra. The articular facets are often fractured, and there may be associated injury to the intervertebral disk.

Reduction is accomplished by cervical traction, which

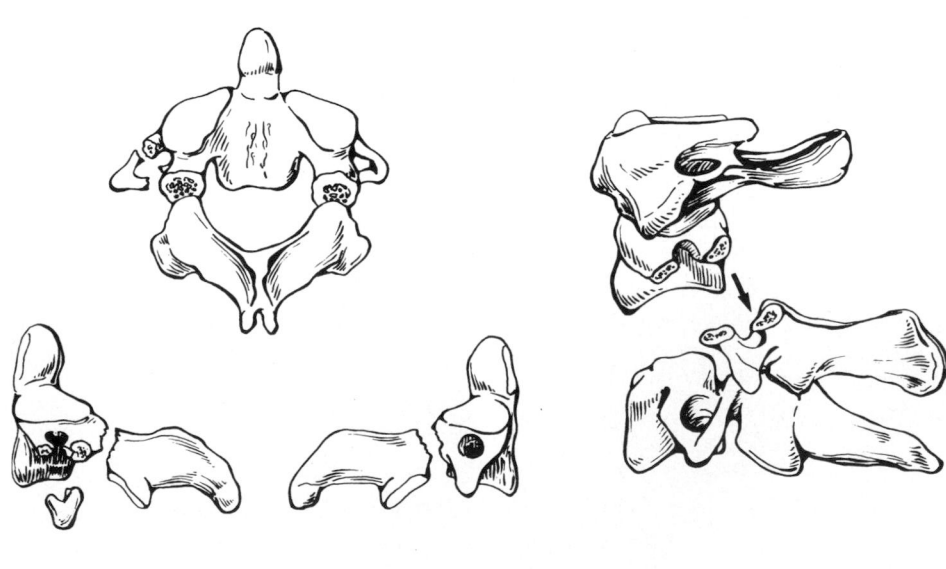

(A)   **(B)**

Figure 19–20 Schematic illustration of fractures through the pedicles of the axis (Hangman's fracture) *(A)*, showing potential dislocation *(B)*.

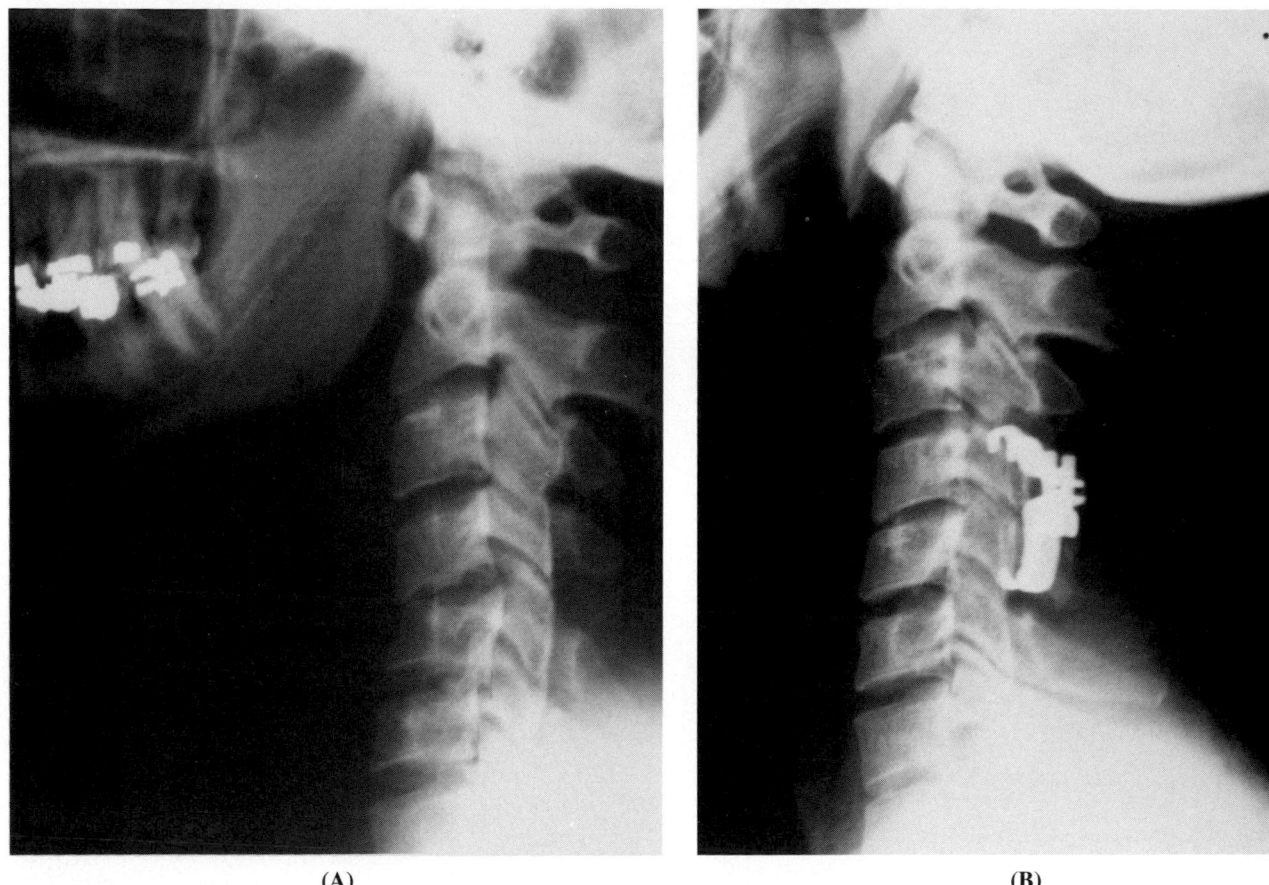

(A)   **(B)**

Figure 19–21 Compression flexion injury with ligaments torn between the spinous processes of C4 and C5 *(A)* fixed with Halifax clamps and fusion *(B)*.

should be carefully monitored.[44,45] If reduction has not been achieved with traction of 40 to 60 lb, open reduction is to be considered. Open reduction is accomplished, usually through a posterior approach, by manipulating the facets. Stabilization is achieved by (1) wiring a superior lamina to a subjacent spinous process, (2) wiring adjacent spinous processes together using Wisconsin wires, or (3) with Halifax clamps.[46]

Fusion is accomplished by the implantation of fragments of cancellous and cortical bone over decorticated laminae and between the laminae and spinous processes. This may be supplemented by placing fragments of bone in the facet joints after removing the cartilaginous plates.

Occasionally, the ligaments are so severely torn that posterior clamping or wiring will not maintain stability. This fixation may be supplemented by plating anteriorly. (See Fig. 19-23A and B.) An alternative mechanism is to fix the reduced fracture over rib struts with sublaminal wires, a procedure the authors' colleagues have named after Dr. Herbert Locksley.

Another alternate method of fixation is accomplished with methylacrylate, a technique often used to treat fractures resulting from metastatic disease.[47]

When there is evidence of injury to the intervertebral disk, a diskectomy by the anterior approach should be considered first. It may be possible to disengage facets from an anterior approach, followed by interbody fusion.[48] This is supplemented by posterior stabilization when there is evidence of incompetence of the posterior ligaments. Failure to recognize herniation of a cervical disk prior to reduction of subluxed facets can result in increased neurological deficits.

CENTRAL CORD SYNDROME WITH HYPEREXTENSION INJURIES

A central cord syndrome incorporates the neurological findings associated with injury to the central portion of the spinal cord, usually in the cervical area. Sensations of pain and temperature as well as motor function in the distal parts of the upper extremities are lost. There may be variable loss of function of the lower extremities. Bowel and bladder control may be lost.

This injury is usually the result of hyperextension of the neck in the presence of a narrow spinal canal. Radiographs demonstrate narrowing of the spinal canal, often the result of severe spondylosis. Initial treatment is conservative, with significant degrees of recovery being the rule, although often there are residual neurological deficits that may be disabling. Since the spinal canal is narrow in its anterior-posterior diameter, laminectomy may serve as prophylaxis. If performed, it is accomplished as an elective procedure.

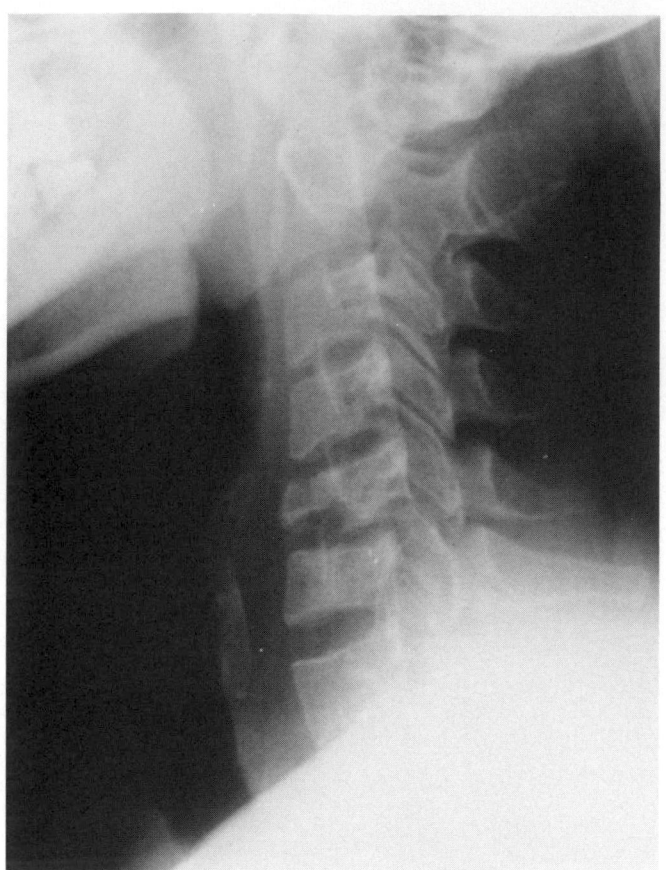

(A)

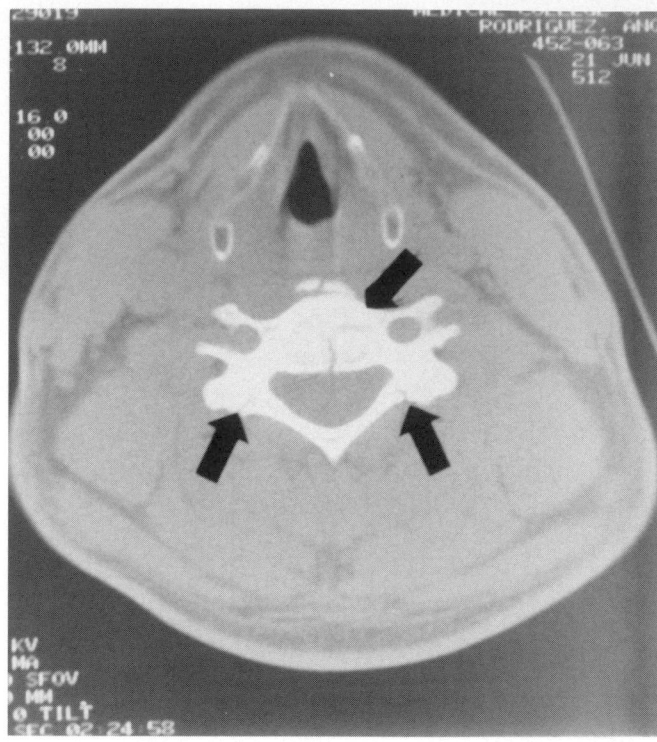

(B)

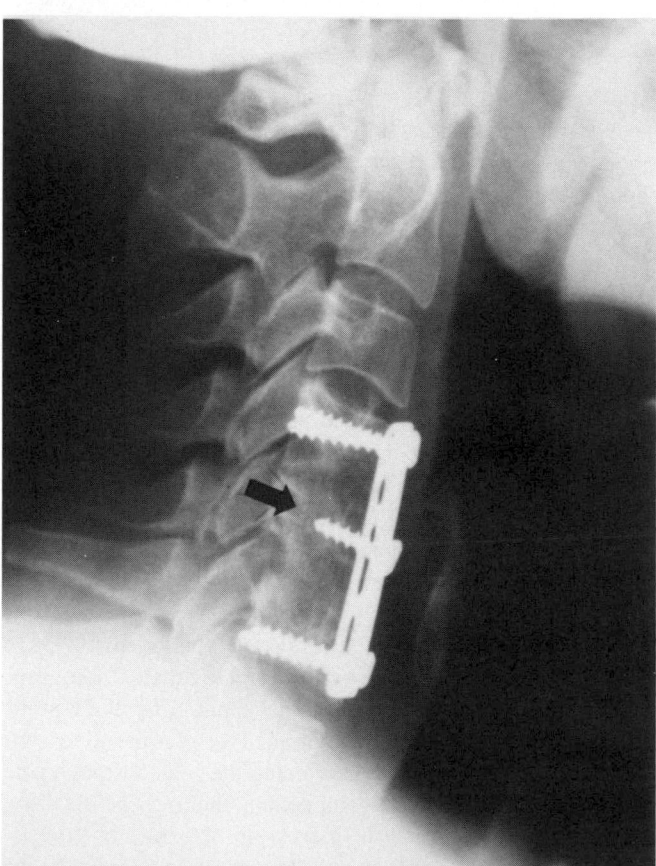

(C)

Figure 19–22 Flexion compression fracture of C5 seen in the lateral radiograph *(A)* and on axial CT *(B)* fixed by corpectomy and fusion maintained with a Caspar plate *(C)*.

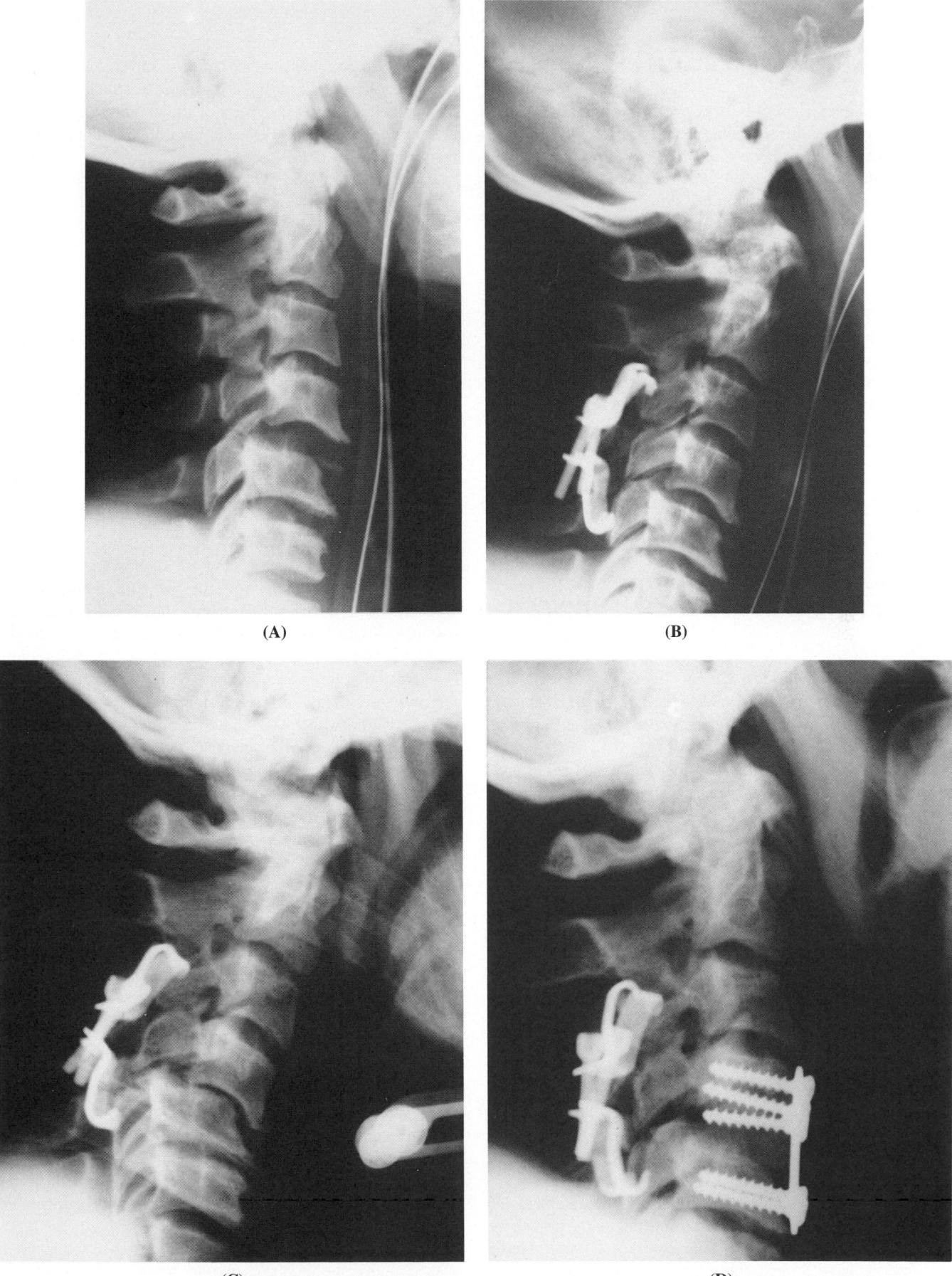

(A)

(B)

(C)

(D)

Figure 19–23 Severe ligamentous injury between C4 and C5 after reduction in *A*. Note the separation between the vertebrae. The dislocation was fixed with Halifax clamps *(B)*, which slipped because of the severe ligamentous damage *(C)*. Final fixation was obtained by an anterior fusion held in place with a Caspar plate *(D)*.

AVULSION OF THE BRACHIAL PLEXUS

The brachial plexus may be torn from the spinal cord, an injury that must be differentiated from a stretch injury of the brachial plexus, which has a much better prognosis. Brachial plexus avulsions usually result when a shoulder is violently depressed or from a hyperabducted arm.

Subsequent neurological deficit depends on which parts of the plexus are avulsed. Loss of abduction of the arm is associated with injury to the uppermost parts of the brachial plexus, while injury to the lowermost parts is associated with loss of motor function in the hand. Sometimes, the entire plexus is avulsed.

Neurological signs—in addition to loss of motor and sensory functions in the appropriate parts of the upper extremity—include Horner's syndrome, and there may be deficits in the paraspinal muscles as well. Confirmation of the injury is obtained by myelography, which usually demonstrates herniation of segments of the arachnoid around nerve roots. (This lesion will be further discussed in Chap. 20.)

☐ TREATMENT OF INJURIES TO THE SPINAL COLUMN BELOW THE NECK

Treatment of injuries to the spinal column has changed dramatically during the last half of this century. Beginning in 1947 and extending into the 1960s, Dr. Paul Harrington developed a set of metal rods, initially designed for the treatment of paralytic scoliosis.[49]

The fact soon became apparent that these rods could also be used in the treatment of spinal injuries and various other degenerative lesions of the spinal column.[50,51]

In the meantime, Hodgson had reported on the treatment of Pott's disease by debridement of infected segments of vertebrae and fusion through an anterior (transthoracic) approach. A number of investigations led to an understanding of influences on the anatomy of the spinal column and function of the spinal cord. These resulted in widespread incorporation of instrumentation into the treatment of a great percentage of cases of blunt trauma to the spinal column.[2,3,4,7,52]

The need for decompression of the spinal cord where it is compressed by bony elements has long been recognized. Historically, the simplest approach for providing decompression has been to "unroof" the spinal canal, i.e., laminectomy. This procedure relieves pressure on the posterior elements, and in many instances it allows the spinal cord to move away from elements anterior to it.

But even short laminectomies interrupt the interspinous ligaments and ligamentum flavum, and, in many instances, portions of whole facets must be removed as well. These interruptions have limited consequences when the bony elements of the vertebral bodies, the intervertebral disks, and their longitudinal ligaments remain intact. However, laminectomy may not decompress a spinal cord compromised by a mass that is compressing its anterior surface, and laminectomy may have devastating effects on the structural integrity of a spinal column when parts of the anterior and/or middle columns (vertebral bodies and longitudinal ligaments) are compromised or interrupted.

In his report in 1962, Harrington described both *compression* and *distraction rods* devised to straighten vertebral columns deformed by scoliosis.[49] Hooks for the distraction rods were designed to fit under laminae, while hooks for compression rods were usually applied to transverse processes in order to provide more leverage to straighten a scoliotic spine. The distraction rods incorporated a rachet system which provided the capability of separating vertebral elements that might be compressed or malaligned. Compression rods are threaded, providing the capability of progressive compression of vertebral column elements.

In addition to the standard system of distraction and compression rods, a *sacral bar* was devised that allowed implantation of the lower elements of the system onto the sacrum in the event of scoliosis extending so low on the vertebral column that adequate purchase could not be made in the vertebral column.

Since the Harrington system of rods was initially described, numerous adaptations of the rods themselves, as well as methods of implantation, have been made. For instance, it has been recognized that loss of normal lumbar lordosis results in an abnormal gait that is often painful. Assurance that lordosis is maintained is accomplished by the appropriate bending of rods, alignment of which is maintained by a hook that locks onto the rod, preventing rotation (Moe hook). Fixation of rods to the base of the spinous processes or to the laminae increases stability if a hook becomes displaced. This can be accomplished with Wisconsin wires passed through holes drilled at the bases of the spinous processes. Rods are fixed to the laminae by sublaminar wires.

Hooks for Harrington rods are usually inserted under laminae, at least two levels above and below the sites of injured vertebrae.[53] Insertion of the hooks into the spinal canal results in stenosis of the canal, which can compromise the neural elements. This narrowing may be minimized by removing all soft tissues between the dura and the lamina and by selecting the smallest appropriate hooks. Generally, hooks applied in the thoracic area should be smaller than those applied in the lumbar area and preferably applied about the facet joints. Space limitations may not be as great in the lumbar area as in the thoracic area. (See Fig. 19-24A through C.)

Instrumentation of the spinal column after trauma should reduce deformity and maintain stability. Fracture-dislocations are reduced by initial distraction and alignment. It may be necessary to remove a facet to allow realignment. For kyphotic deformities, alignment is accomplished from a posterior approach by a *three-point fixation*. Distraction hooks placed under the laminae two to three levels above and below the fracture site are forcibly separated while the lamina at the apex of the deformity is being displaced ventrally. Realignment is accomplished in mild kyphosis.

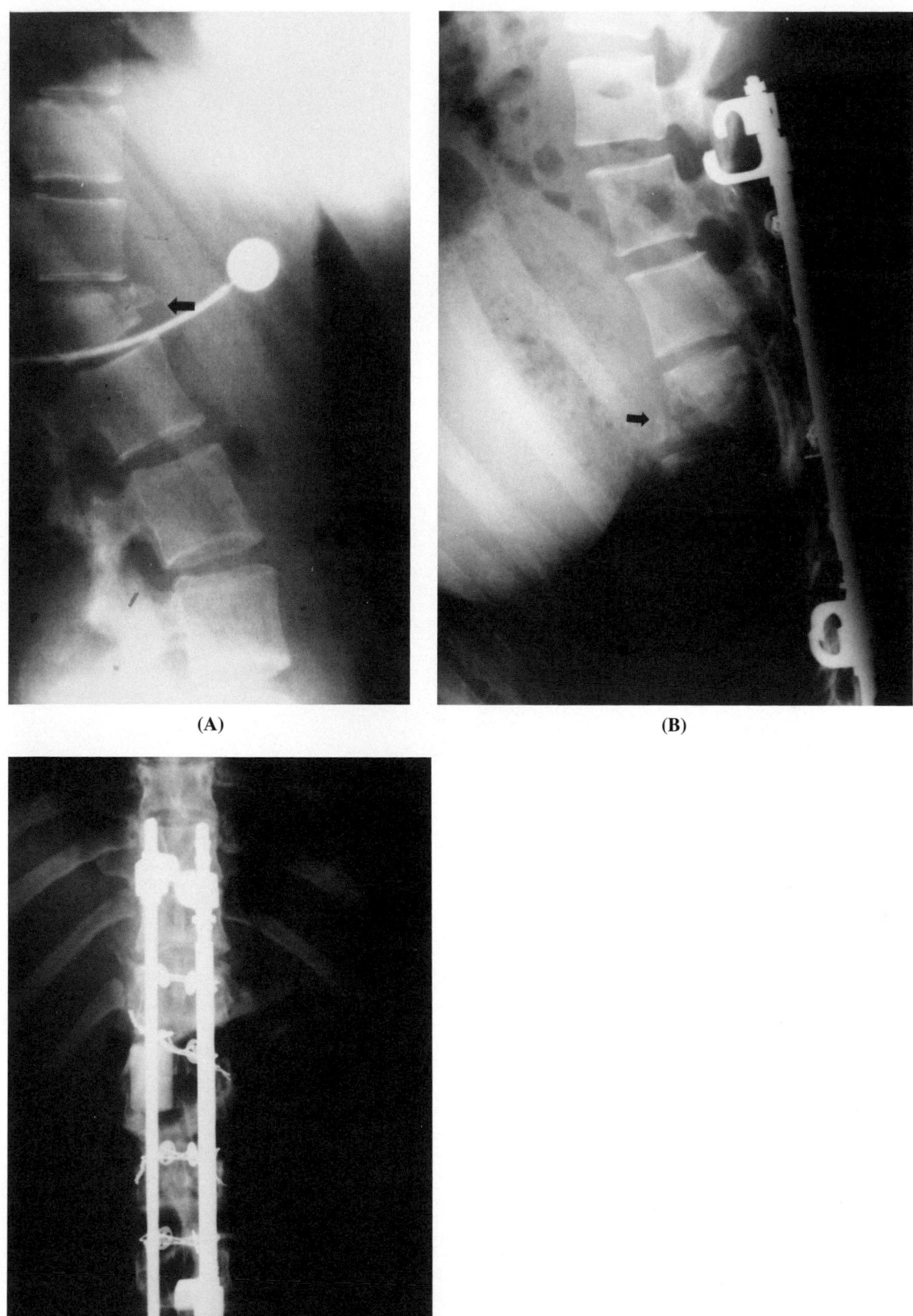

(A)

(B)

(C)

Figure 19–24   Compression fracture of L1 seen in the lateral radiographs before *(A)* and after *(B)* reduction with Harrington rods. The postoperative frontal view is also shown *(C)*.

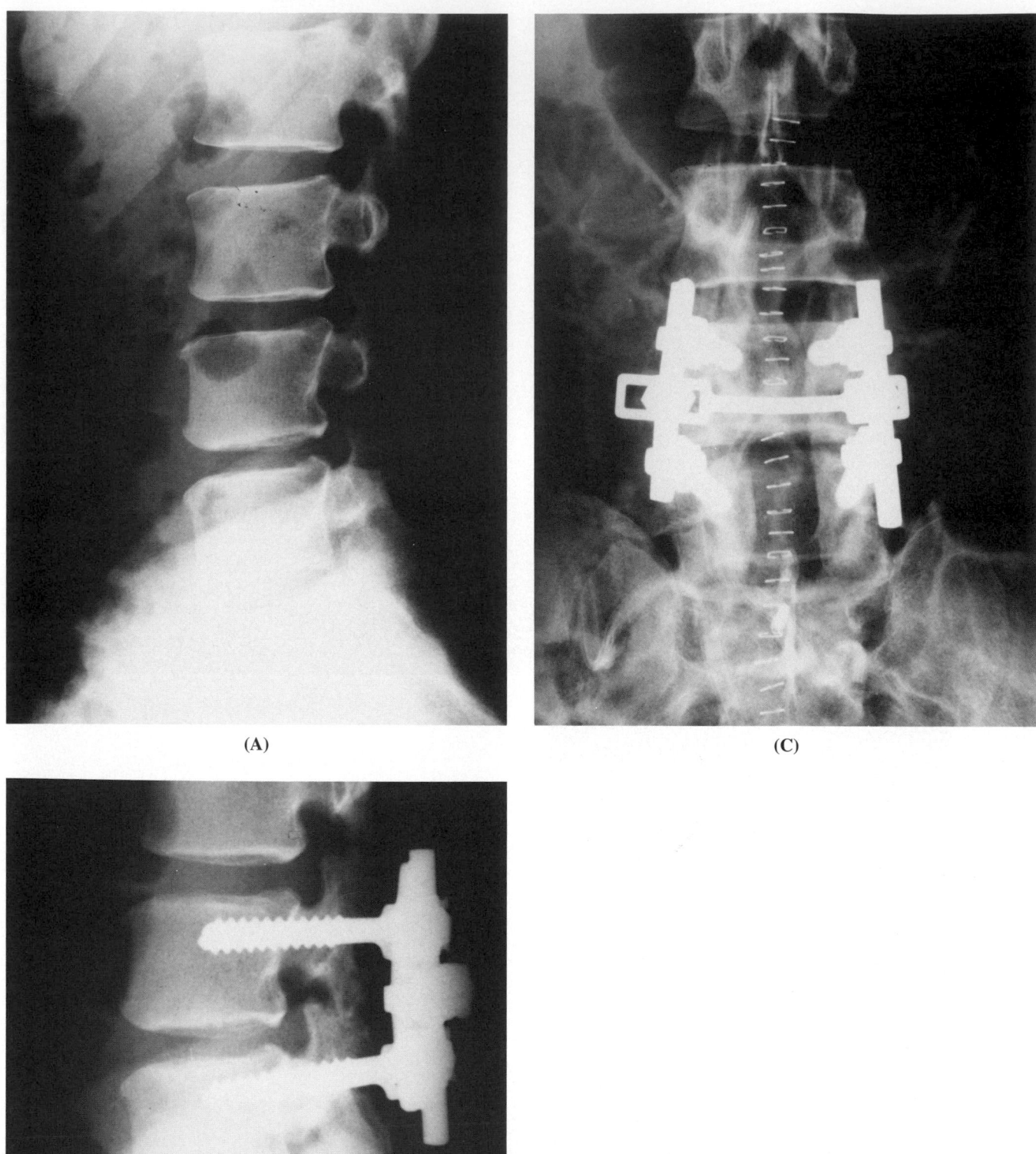

(A)

(C)

(B)

Figure 19–25   An iatrogenic fracture of the inferior facet of L4 seen in the lateral projection *(A)* is immediately immobilized with pedicle screws and connecting rods, using the Texas Scottish Rites Hospital system, shown in *B* and *C*. The patient's pain was relieved.

Use of polyethylene (Edwards) sleeves over the rods will assist in the realignment when rods are used over sites where the vertebrae are normally straight; however, rods can be bent to conform to any desired configuration in sites where the spine is normally lordotic. Maintenance of rods in their appropriate positions may require use of locking (Moe) rods and hooks so that rods will not rotate, reversing the curvature of the rod.

The possibility of compromise to the spinal canal by implantation of hooks beneath the laminae has already been mentioned. Implantation of sublaminar wires, as well as distraction of vertebrae, may likewise compromise neurological function. Monitoring of anatomical changes as well as neural function during the course of instrumentation of the spine is appropriate.

Anatomical changes can be monitored by fluoroscopy or serial radiographs. Neurological function may be monitored by evoked potential monitoring (EPM), or "wake-up" tests; that is, by awakening the patient after each step in instrumentation and asking the patient to move those parts that are potentially affected by instrumentation.[54,55,56,57]

Each of these tests has advantages and disadvantages. One disadvantage of EPM is that the neural pathways being tested are primarily the posterior columns, whereas it is the more anterior parts of the spinal cord which are of greatest concern. Another limiting factor is that in patients whose posterior columns have been damaged, evoked potentials may not be obtainable. Recent innovations in the procedure examine potentials obtained in response to cortical stimulations, which may improve monitoring capability. A practical problem relates to the need for a special team to administer EPM. Evoked potential monitoring also frequently requires modification of anesthetics.

The "wake-up" test necessitates cooperation of the patient at a time when he or she is quite drowsy—and when responses are considerably attenuated by anesthetics. The primary limitation of EPM, as well as the wake-up test, is that they determine a disability "after the fact" rather than at the time when alterations in neural function are occurring.

Distraction efforts using the Harrington rodding system may be amplified by a distractor, an offset-threaded bar which can provide tremendous force. The offset provides space for carrying out surgical manipulations at the site of injury. Primary concern centers around the distracting force that may be applied with this instrument. Distraction *must* be monitored.

Realignment of fragments of a vertebral body which have been displaced into the spinal canal as a result of a "burst" are of major concern. If the posterior longitudinal ligament remains intact, distraction of the vertebral column will provide force to relocate the fragments. If the posterior longitudinal ligament is incompetent, excessive distraction may be accomplished with minimal effort, and there will be no force to relocate the fragments and thus decompress the spinal canal. To determine the progress of realignment of the fragments, dissection down to the affected vertebral body can be accomplished through a pedicle, by which route the

anterior surface of the spinal canal may be examined. Displaced fragments of bone may be tapped into the longitudinally distracted vertebral body.

For patients with compression of the anterior half of the vertebral body but an intact middle column—and in patients with torn intraspinous ligaments and intact vertebrae—compression rods will provide stability by replacing the strength of the posterior ligaments and reducing the compression on the anterior portions of the vertebral bodies.[58] Compression rods are quite effective when applied to laminae adjacent to injured vertebrae.

In his initial reports describing rodding in scoliotic children, Harrington reported a high incidence of rod failures. The segment of the rod most likely to fail was the junction between its smooth and ratcheted segments. Much effort was directed toward improving the rods. The authors have not encountered rod failure in patients with spinal fractures, probably in part because we are dealing with an older population and also because many of our patients have severe neurological deficits. We have, however, experienced a significant incidence of displaced hooks in patients with distraction rods. Studies indicate that there is a progressive relaxation of ligaments under tension. We frequently utilize a compression rod with hooks located under the laminae on the side contralateral to a distraction rod in patients being treated for burst fractures or fracture-dislocations with a reduced incidence of dislodgment.

The Harrington rodding system works very well for injuries in the middle to lower thoracic and lumbar levels. It is not advised when fixation to cervical vertebrae is required. We have usually utilized the Luque system with sublaminal wiring when instrumentation must extend into the cervical area.[59] The system provides for alignment against a contoured rod and good fixation, but no distraction. Rods may be prepared to conform to the normal kyphotic and lordotic curves.

Use of sublaminar wires is necessary with the *Luque system.* They add strength to the Harrington system.[60] Alternate systems of fixing the rods to each other and to the vertebral column include *Wisconsin* wires and *Danek plates.* The *Cotrel-Debousset rodding system,* introduced in 1983, is more elaborate.[61] There are capabilities for numerous points of segmental fixation, and it has become very popular in the treatment of scoliosis.

One other form of instrumentation that should be mentioned is the *fixoteur interne,* a system which fixes vertebrae immediately above and below the sites of injury by transpedicular screws developed by Dick.[62] It may be used to alter relationships of vertebrae on-site. It has the advantage of providing specific manipulations and may provide for flexion or extension or unilateral repositioning of vertebral fractures. This system minimizes the number of functioning spinal segments that must be included in the orthodisis and maximizes fixation of the segments used. Several other systems using pedicle screws and rods are now in use. (See Fig. 19-25A through C.)

There are several rodding systems that can be applied to

the vertebral bodies through an anterior approach. Such equipment has the advantage of allowing reduction of fractures while the sites of injury are under direct vision. A big disadvantage to this approach is that instruments can erode great vessels if they come in contact. If this type of instrumentation is being used, one must make certain that implanted instruments are not left near great vessels.

Instruments implanted to treat traumatic lesions of the vertebral column are usually left in place indefinitely, and bony elements are often eroded. Permanent fixation can be assured only if a bony fusion is obtained. Therefore, the aligned laminae should routinely be decorticated, and cancellous bone, with or without finely divided cortical bone,

should be implanted over the decorticated laminae or vertebral bodies.

With the Harrington rodding system, an external orthosis, usually a thoracolumbosacral orthosis (TLSO) brace, is applied at the time of recovery from anesthesia. Ambulation is started in the immediate postoperative period if neurological status permits. If there is severe paresis, physical therapy is begun immediately. Discharge is usually accomplished within a week to 10 days. Orthoses are worn for about 3 months. Orthoses are considered unnecessary in cases of segmental fixation with Luque rods or pedicle screws and plates.

REFERENCES

1. Kirkaldy-Willis WH, Dupuis PR, Yong-Hing K: Biomechanics and aging of the spine, in Youmans JR (ed): *Neurological Surgery,* 3d ed. Philadelphia, Saunders, 1990, chap. 87, pp 2605–2628.
2. Holdsworth F: Fractures, dislocations, and fracture dislocations of the spine (review article). *J Bone Joint Surg* 52A:1534–1551, 1970.
3. Kelly RP, Whitesides TE Jr: Treatment of lumbodorsal fracture-dislocations. *Ann Surg* 167:705–717, 1968.
4. Denis F: The three-column spine and its significance in the classification of acute thoracolumbar spinal injuries. *Spine* 8:817–831, 1986.
5. Chance GQ: Note on a type of flexion fracture of the spine. *Br J Radiol* 21:452–453, 1948.
6. McAfee PC, Yaun HA, Fredricksonn BE, Lubicky JP: The value of computed tomography in thoracolumbar fractures: An analysis of one hundred consecutive cases and a new classification. *J Bone Joint Surg* 65A:461–472, 1983.
7. Ferguson RL, Allen BL Jr: A mechanistic classification of thoracolumbar spine fractures. *Clin Orthop Rel Res* 189:77–88, 1984.
8. Bracken MB, Shepard MJ, Collins WF, et al: A randomized controlled trial of methylprednisolone or naloxone in the treatment of acute spinal-cord injury: Results of the second national acute spinal cord injury study. *New Eng J Med* 322:1405–1411, 1990.
9. Schneider RC, Crosby EC, Russo RH, Gosch HH: Traumatic spinal cord syndromes and their management. Chap. 32, *Clin Neurosurg* 20:424–492, 1972.
10. Romanick PC, Smith TK, Kopmiky OR, et al: Infection about the spine associated with low-velocity-missile injury to the abdomen. *J Bone Joint Surg* 67A:1195–1201, 1985.
11. Venger BH, Simpson RK, Narayan RK: Neurosurgical intervention in penetrating spinal trauma with associated visceral injury. *J Neurosurg* 70:514–518, 1989.
12. Gardner WJ: The principle of spring-loaded points for cervical traction (technical note). *J Neurosurg* 39:543–544, 1973.
13. Koch RA, Nickel VL: The halo vest: An evaluation of motion and forces across the neck. *Spine* 3:103–107, 1978.
14. Chan RC, Schweigel JF, Thompson GB: Halo-thoracic brace immobilization in 188 patients with acute cervical spine injuries. *J Neurosurg* 58:508–515, 1983.
15. Jefferson G: Fracture of the atlas vertebra: Report of four cases and a review of those previously recorded. *Br J Surg* 7:407–422, 1920.
16. Schelihas KP, Latchaw RE, Wendling LR, Gold HA: Vertebrobasilar injuries following cervical manipulation. *J Am Med Ass* 244:1450–1453, 1980.
16a. Heller JG, Viroslav S, Hudson T: Jefferson fracture: The role of assessing transverse ligament integrity. Presented February 21, 1992, Paper 143, at the American Academy of Orthopedic Surgeons Meeting, Washington, DC.
17. Zimmerman E, Grant J, Vise WM, et al: Treatment of Jefferson fracture with a Halo apparatus: Report of two cases. *J Neurosurg* 44:372–375, 1976.
18. Spence KP, Decker S, Sell KW: Bursting atlantal fracture associated with rupture of the transverse ligament. *J Bone Joint Surg* 52A:543–549, 1970.
19. Dyck P: Os Odontoideum in children: Neurological manifestations and surgical management. *Neurosurgery* 2:93–99, 1978.
20. Scott EW, Haid RW Jr, Peace D: Type I fractures of the odontoid process: Implications for atlanto-occipital instability (case report). *J Neurosurg* 72:488–492, 1990.
21. Southwick WO: Management of fractures of the dens (odontoid process) [current concepts review]. *J Bone Joint Surg* 62A:482–486, 1980.
22. Cybulski GR, Stone JL, Crowell RM, et al: Use of Halifax interlaminar clamps for posterior C1-C2 arthrodesis. *Neurosurgery* 22:429–431, 1988.
23. Alexander E: Posterior fusions of the cervical spine. Chap. 17, *Clin Neurosurg* 28:273–296, 1981.
24. Borne GM, Bedou GL, Pinaudeau M, et al: Odontoid process fracture osteosynthesis with a direct screw fixation technique in nine consecutive cases. *J Neurosurg* 68:223–226, 1988.
25. Kornblum D, Clayton ML, Nash HH: Nontraumatic cervical dislocations in rheumatoid spondylitis. *J Am Med Ass* 149:431–435, 1952.
26. De Coster TA, Cole HC: Atlanto-axial dislocation in association with rheumatic fever (case report). *Spine* 15:591–595, 1990.

27. Greenberg AD: Atlanto-axial dislocations. *Brain* 91:655–685, 1968.
28. Jackson H: The diagnosis of minimal atlanto-axial subluxation. *Br J Radiol* 23:672–674, 1950.
29. Toolanen G, Larsson SE, Fagerlund M: Medullary compression in rheumatoid atlanto-axial subluxation evaluated by computerized tomography. *Spine* 11:191–194, 1986.
30. Miller J, Parent AD: Microscopic decompression of the anterior upper cervical spine: A case of odontoid malunion to the atlas. *Neurosurgery* 14:583–587, 1984.
31. Greenberg AD, Scoville WB, Davey LM: Transoral decompression of atlanto-axial dislocation due to odontoid hypoplasia. *J Neurosurg* 28:266–269, 1968.
32. O'Laoire SA, Thomas DGT: Transoral approach to the cervical spine: Report of four cases. *J Neurol Neurosurg Psych* 45:60–63, 1982.
33. Sukoff MH, Kadin MM, Moran T: Transoral decompression for myelopathy caused by rheumatoid arthritis of the cervical spine (case report). *J Neurosurg* 37:493–497, 1972.
34. Apuzzo MLJ, Weiss MH, Heiden JS: Transoral exposure of the atlantoaxial region. *Neurosurgery* 3:201–207, 1978.
35. Schneider RC, Livingston KE, Cave AJE, Hamilton G: "Hangman's fracture" of the cervical spine. *J Neurosurg* 22:141–154, 1965.
36. Levine AM, Edwards CC: The management of traumatic spondylolisthesis of the axis. *J Bone Joint Surg* 67A:217–225, 1985.
37. Mirvis SE, Geisler FH, Jelinek JJ, et al: Acute cervical spine trauma: Evaluation with 1.5-T MR Imaging. *Radiol* 166:807–816, 1988.
38. Gassman J, Seligson D: The anterior cervical plate. *Spine* 8:700–707, 1983.
39. Tippets RH, Apfelbaum RI: Anterior cervical fusion with the Caspar instrumentation system. *Neurosurgery* 22:1008–1013, 1988.
40. Bremer AM, Nguyan TO: Internal metal plate fixation combined with anterior interbody fusion in cases of cervical spine injury. *Neurosurgery* 12:649–653, 1983.
41. Goffin J, Plets C, Van den Bergh R: Anterior cervical fusion and osteosynthetic stabilization according to Caspar: A prospective study of 41 patients with fractures and/or dislocations of the cervical spine. *Neurosurgery* 25:865–871, 1989.
42. Baker R, Grubb RL Jr: Complete fracture dislocation of cervical spine without permanent neurological sequelae (case report). *J Neurosurg* 58:760–762, 1983.
43. Sonntag VKH: Management of bilateral locked facets of the cervical spine. *Neurosurgery* 8:150–152, 1981.
44. Maiman DJ, Barolat G, Larson SJ: Management of bilateral locked facets of the cervical spine. *Neurosurgery* 18:542–547, 1986.
45. Fried LC: Cervical spinal cord injury during skeletal traction. *J Am Med Ass* 229:181–183, 1974.
46. Tucker HH: Method of fixation of subluxed or dislocated cervical spine below C1-C2 (technical report). *Canad J Neurol Sci* 2:381–382, 1975.
47. Scoville WB, Palmer AH, Samra K, Chong G: The use of acrylic plastic for vertebral replacement or fixation in metastatic disease of the spine. *J Neurosurg* 27:274–279, 1967.
48. DeOliveira JC: Anterior reduction of interlocking facets in the lower cervical spine. *Spine* 4:195–202, 1979.
49. Harrington PR: Treatment of scoliosis: Correction and internal fixation by spine instrumentation. *J Bone Joint Surg* 44A:591–610, 1962.
50. Harrington PR: Instrumentation in spine instability other than scoliosis. *S Africa J Surg* 5:7–12, 1967.
51. Harrington PR: The history and development of Harrington instrumentation. *Clin Orth Rel Res* 227:3–5, 1988.
52. Hodgson AR, Yau A, Kwon JS, Kim K: A clinical study of 100 consecutive cases of Potts paraplegia. *Clin Orth Rel Res* 36:128–150, 1964.
53. Purcell GA, Markoff KL, Dawson EG: Twelfth thoracic first lumbar vertebral mechanical stability of fractures after Harrington instrumentation. *J Bone Joint Surg* 63A:71–77, 1981.
54. Engler GL, Spielholz NI, Bernhard WN, et al: Somatosensory evoked potentials during Harrington instrumentation for scoliosis. *J Bone Joint Surg* 60A:528–532, 1978.
55. Nuwer MR, Dawson EC: Intraoperative evoked potential monitoring of the spinal cord: A restricted filter, scalp method during Harrington instrumentation for scoliosis. *Clin Orthop Rel Res* 183:42–50, 1984.
56. Sudhir KG, Smith RM, Hall JE, Hansen DD: Intraoperative awakening for early recognition of possible neurologic sequelae during Harrington-rod spinal fusion. *Anesthes Anal* 55:526–528, 1976.
57. Hall JE, Levine CR, Sudhir KG: Intraoperative awakening to monitor spinal cord function during Harrington instrumentation and spine fusion: Description of procedure and report of three cases. *J Bone Joint Surg* 60A:533–536, 1978.
58. Nash CL, Schatzinger LH, Brown RH, Brodkey J: The unstable stable thoracic compression fracture: Its problems and use of spinal cord monitoring in the evaluation of treatment. *Spine* 2:261–265, 1977.
59. Luque ER: The anatomic basis and development of segmental spinal instrumentation. *Spine* 7:256–259, 1982.
60. Sullivan JA: Sublaminar wiring of Harrington distraction rods for unstable thoracolumbar spine fractures. *Clin Orthop Rel Res* 189:178–185, 1984.
61. Moreland DB, Egnatchik JG, Bennett GJ: Cotrel-Debousset instrumentation for the treatment of thoracolumbar fractures. *Neurosurgery* 27:69–73, 1990.
62. Krag MH, Beynnon BD, Pope MH, et al: An internal fixator for posterior application to short segments of the thoracic, lumbar, and lumbosacral spine: Design and testing. *Clin Orthop Rel Res* 203:75–93, 1986.

☐ STUDY QUESTIONS

I. A 23-year-old male, working on a construction job, is struck on his helmet by a falling timber. He complains of pain in the neck but exhibits no neurological deficits. On examination he is tender at the base of the skull posteriorly and movement of the neck causes pain.

Radiographs show that the lateral masses of C1 are separated by 7.1 mm, and the odontoid appears to be asymmetrically located within the ring.

1. What is the most likely diagnosis? **2.** What therapy should be applied? **3.** What was the mechanism of injury? **4.** What bony elements should be fused? **5.** Since there is no neurological deficit, does this imply that none will develop? If a neurological deficit did develop, what might it be?

II. A 25-year-old female is involved in a "head-on" collision while wearing her seat belt. She is paraparetic. She has dorsiflexion and plantar flexion of both feet and moderate rectal tone. Her quadraceps are weak. She cannot hold her knees extended against gravity, although she has severe back pain and the examiner cannot be certain that the patient is exerting full strength. Knee jerks are absent.

Radiography reveals a compression fracture of T12. The height of the anterior part of the body is about 40 percent of the height of the posterior segment of the body. A CT scan demonstrates that a fragment of the upper part of the vertebral body is displaced into the spinal canal.

1. What forms of treatment might be considered? **2.** What are the patient's chances for being able to walk? **3.** Will the neurological picture likely improve with conservative care (bed rest)? **4.** What are the chances for abdominal distension in the early post-injury period? **5.** Should laminectomy be considered? Why or why not?

III. A 35-year old male prisoner is thrown to the floor of his cell by a pair of irate cell mates. He sustains quadriplegia. His x-rays show an anterior dislocation of C5 on C6. The dislocation extends over half of the depth of the body. His only volitional movement of extremities is abduction of the shoulders and flexion of the elbows.

1. What should be the sequence by which this patient is evaluated and treated? **2.** How can the dislocation be reduced? **3.** What forms of fixation might be considered? **4.** What are the chances for recovery of motor function? **5.** On what type of bed should the patient be placed?

IV. The rifle of a deer hunter discharges when it is bumped, striking the hunter in the abdomen, the missile coming to rest in the spinal canal at the L2 level after the missile passes through the vertebral foramen. The patient is paraparetic, with minimal flexion and extension of the feet, weaker on the left than the right, weakness of extension of the knees, but some rectal tone still present.

1. What course of therapy should be followed? **2.** Should the spinal wound be explored? Why? **3.** If the wound is explored, what should be the objectives of therapy? **4.** Should there be concern over structural integrity? **5.** What type of urinary and bowel control problems might be expected and how should they be handled?

V. A 55-year-old male falls off his porch, striking his chin during an alcoholic binge. He is brought in on a spine board because of severe paresis. His legs are weak, although he has volitional activity in all muscle groups. However, he cannot flex or extend his fingers. He has flexion and extension of his elbows, although these movements are weak and there is a glove-type loss of sensation of pinprick in the hands and arms. Radiographs of the neck are made.

1. What is the most likely appearance on the x-rays? **2.** What part of the spinal cord is injured? **3.** What might an MRI of the cervical spinal cord be expected to show? **4.** What forms of therapy might be considered? **5.** What should be the anticipated outcome?

Degenerative Lesions of the Spine: Herniated Intervertebral Disks and Spondylosis

Marshall B. Allen, Jr.

J. Allan Goodrich

Herniations of intervertebral disks result from trauma or physical stress of varying degrees. Major trauma is usually the cause in children and young adults. Herniations in response to trauma may occur throughout life, but most disk herniations are associated with varying degrees of degeneration of the intervertebral disk and of the surrounding bony elements.

Frequently, the trauma that initiates symptoms seems almost incidental. Thus, it is appropriate to discuss disk herniations as a part of the overall degenerative processes of the vertebral column. Approaches to diagnosis and treatment are usually parallel, if not the same.

☐ PATHOGENESIS OF DEGENERATIVE CHANGES IN THE SPINE

Vertical strength of the spine is maintained by the column of *vertebral bodies* with its interspersed disks. Located on either side of the spinal canal are two columns of *facets* which contribute to maintenance of the vertebral alignment as well as vertical strength. The relationship of facets to vertebral bodies is assured by the *bony pedicles* and *laminae,* which also protect the neural elements. However, these fixed bony parts and the intervertebral disks contribute to neurological deficits as degenerative processes of the skeleton and the intervertebral disks develop.

Intervertebral disks are made up of a central core, the *nucleus pulposus,* surrounded by bands of fibrous tissue, the *annulus fibrosis.* (See Fig. 20-1.) Separating the soft parts of the disks from the vertebral bodies above and below are cartilaginous plates. Extending longitudinally along the vertebral column are the anterior and posterior longitudinal ligaments which blend with and strengthen the annulus fibrosis.

In infancy, and early childhood, the nucleus pulposus is gelatinous, containing hydrophilic polysaccharides, which are responsible for a water content in excess of 80 percent.[1,2] The annulus fibrosis is composed of concentric layers of collagenous fibers that are attached to the adjacent vertebrae.[3,4] The fibers are directed obliquely between the vertebrae in successive layers that are perpendicular to each other. Elasticity of the intervertebral disks is provided in large measure by the annulus fibrosis.

With aging, the intervertebral disk deteriorates. The structure of its polysaccharides undergoes change, and the disk loses much of its hydrophilic property. This results in loss of some of its water content. Fibers of the internal layers of the annulus fibrosis grow progressively into the nucleus pulposus. The disk becomes amorphous, sometimes discolored, and increasingly fibrotic.[2] (See Fig. 20-2.) It develops more tears,[5] loses height, and frequently breaks through cartilaginous plates into the vertebral body, protruding or expelling fragments out of the intervertebral spaces into surrounding areas. This results in pressure on adjacent structures and contributes to the development of hypertrophy of adjacent bone edges, producing *osteophytes,* a process that, in the extreme, results in "traction spurs."[5]

As the spinal cord passes through the spinal canal, it gives

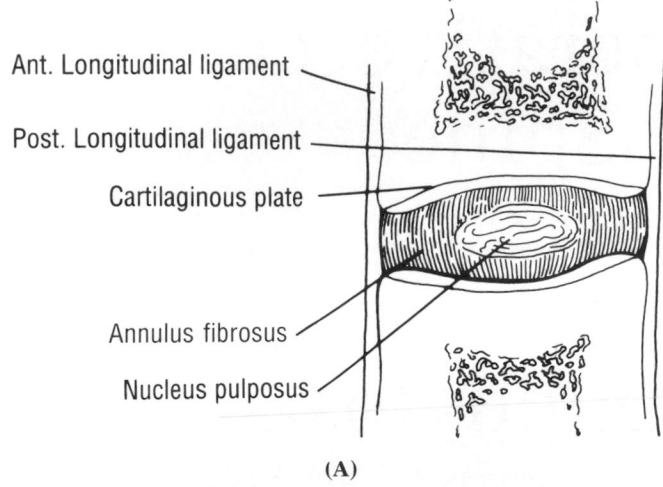

Ant. Longitudinal ligament

Post. Longitudinal ligament

Cartilaginous plate

Annulus fibrosus

Nucleus pulposus

(A)

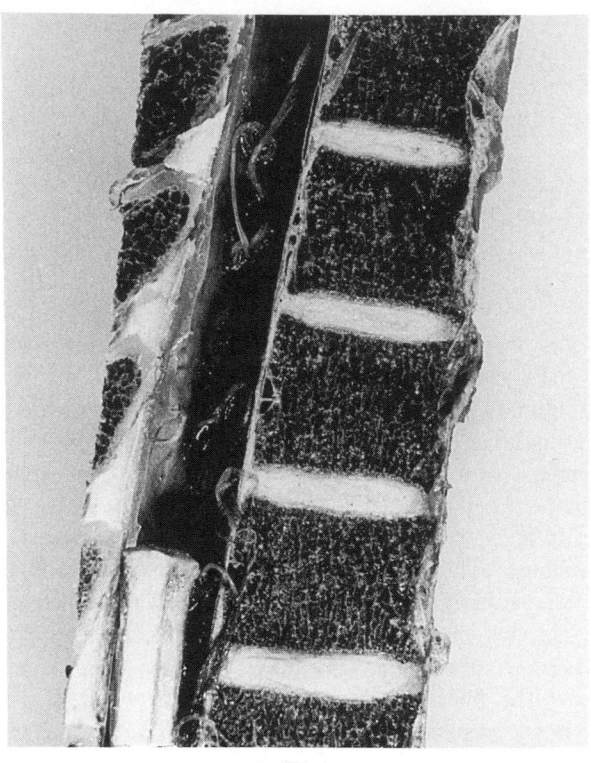

(B)

Figure 20–1 Diagrammatic illustration of lumbar intervertebral disk, showing central nucleus pulposus surrounded by annulus fibrosis and anterior and posterior longitudinal ligaments *(A)*. Photograph of an autopsied spine showing multiple disks and their relationships to the empty spinal canal, above, and the spinal cord, below *(B)*.

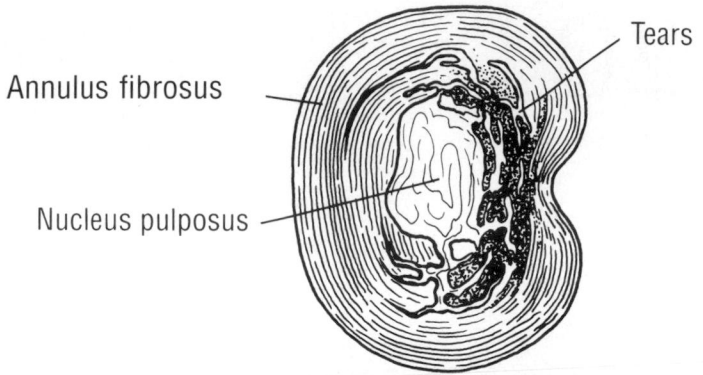

Annulus fibrosus

Nucleus pulposus

Tears

Figure 20–2 Diagrammatic illustration of degenerated disk showing the nucleus pulposus in the center surrounded by a degenerating annulus fibrosis.

off nerve roots which exit through the *neural foramina*— spaces delineated rostrally and caudally by pedicles, ventrally by the adjacent surfaces of the vertebral bodies and the interspaced intervertebral disks, and dorsally by the facets.

Degenerative changes of intervertebral disks and the adjacent vertebral bodies, or of the bony facets, compromise the spinal canal and the neural foramina. Disks protrude or herniate. Osteophytes develop at the edges of the vertebrae, or facets and bony malalignments occur. (See Fig. 20-3.)

Disk herniations and hypertrophy of bony elements appear along the anterior and lateral surfaces of the spinal column, ventral to the neural foramina. These produce dysphagia when they present in the neck[6,7] and back pain in lower segments, along with a number of symptoms that are less discrete than those related to compromise of the neural elements in the spinal canal.[8,9] Such changes are collectively referred to as *spondylosis*.

Disk herniations into the spinal canal may present medially, compressing the spinal cord or cauda equina, or laterally, under nerve roots approaching or in the neural foramina. Lateral herniations are notorious for producing pain with loss of motor function in the distribution of the affected nerve roots. Pain along the distribution of a compressed nerve root may be in part a result of edema.[10]

Spondylosis—most prominent at the epiphyseal plates of the vertebral bodies and the facets—represents degenerative changes that usually become apparent radiologically in young adults[11] and prominent in later life.

Exostoses of vertebral bodies adjacent to intervertebral disks are evident in areas of trauma or stress and thus more likely to occur in the cervical and lumbar areas than in the thoracic segments. Osteophytes may be related in part to the elevation of periosteum, with consequent stretching or displacement of the collagenous attachments to the vertebrae. Facets are likewise subject to hypertrophy of bony edges as well as degeneration of cartilaginous elements. Ligaments, which provide structural stability in young individuals, become lax as degeneration continues, partly a result of stretching or tearing and also a result of reduction in the height of intervertebral disks and degeneration of the cartilaginous plates in the facets.

Hypertrophy of the posterior edges of the vertebral bodies results in compromise of the anterior-posterior diameter of the spinal canal. This may add to any compromise produced by posterior protrusions of intervertebral disks. The anterior-posterior diameter of the canal is usually most severely compromised radiologically between the posterior-inferior edge of a vertebral body and the anterior-superior edge of a subjacent lamina. Narrowing of the canal may be further

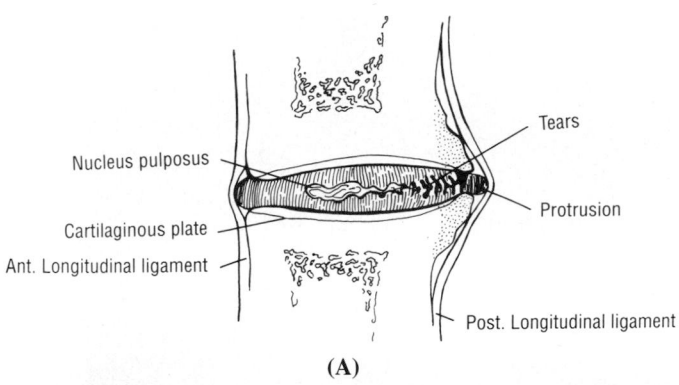

(A)

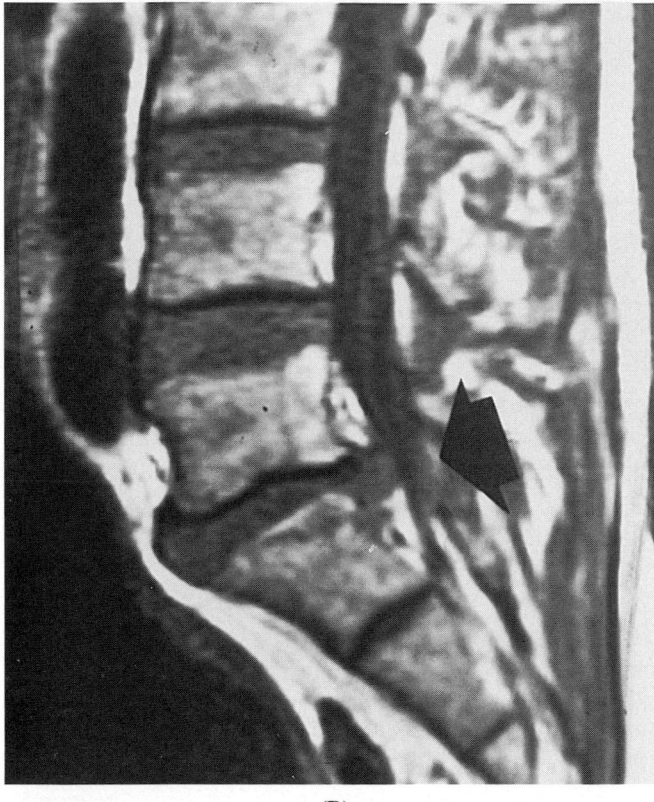

(B)

Figure 20–3 Diagrammatic illustration of sagittal view of spine showing disk protrusion anterior anteriorly and posteriorly with spondylosis posteriorly *(A)*. Photograph of a sagittal segment of the vertebral column shown by magnetic resonance imaging (MRI) with degenerative disks and an extrusion at the L5-S1 interspace, arrow *(B)*.

potentiated by infolding of the ligamentum flavum (often reported as "hypertrophy"), in large measure a result of reduction of the interlaminar spaces resulting from the degenerative changes described above.

Compromise of the lateral compartments of the spinal canal results from hypertrophy of the posteriolateral edges of the vertebral bodies and the facets.[12] Narrowing of the lateral compartments of the spinal canal usually produces symptoms related to nerve roots. Such symptoms are accentuated by soft disk protrusions whenever they are present. Consequently, these symptoms may be relieved by removal of

small fragments of disk material, even though large osteophytes may be the primary offending elements.

Compromise of the neural foramina by spondylosis is often produced by derangements of the facets.[5] Hypertrophy occurs in both the superior and inferior processes. In the lumbar area, hypertrophy of the superior process is likely to impinge on an exiting nerve root, while hypertrophy of the inferior facet is more likely to compress the posterior compartment of the spinal canal and, consequently, the central portion of the canal.[12]

Malalignment of facets adds to the compromise of the lateral compartments of the spinal canal, especially in the lumbar area. When a superior facet process of a lower vertebra moves cephalad to an inferior facet process of the superior vertebra, it can directly impinge on an exiting nerve root.[12] Such derangement is accentuated by standing or walking and reduced by sitting or lying down. Interestingly, there are usually very few associated neurological deficits or stretch signs—making the clinical diagnosis of this derangement difficult.

When degeneration of facets becomes severe and ligaments lax, *vertebrolisthesis* may result. In the lumbar area, *spondylolisthesis*, as a result of degenerative processes, is most likely to occur at the L4–L5 level, but it is also seen at the L5–S1 level. *Retrolisthesis* may appear at an adjacent level, but it is most likely to be found in the upper cervical levels, C3–C4 and C4–C5.[13] Such severe derangements compromise the spinal cord and nerve roots in the cervical area and nerve roots and distal cauda equina in the lumbar area.

Even more extensive derangements may be associated with scoliosis. (See Fig. 20-4.) In addition, the spinal canal may be compromised by ossification of the posterior longitudinal ligament, producing radiculopathies and/or myelopathy.[14,15,16,17] This lesion has been reported more frequently in Asians, but it is also seen in Caucasians. It is most commonly encountered in the neck but is reported at the thoracic and lumbar levels as well.[18]

Intervertebral disks can bulge or extrude fragments at any age, but herniations are most prevalent in the young to middle-aged adult. Osteoarthritic lipping, although commonly seen in radiographs of young adults, becomes more apparent in later years and is likely to be the primary basis of symptoms beyond the age of 40.

Acute herniations of intervertebral disks can occur at any level in the vertebral column but are more common in the lower lumbar and lower cervical levels. About 90 percent of herniations in the lumbar area occur at the L4–L5 and L5–S1 levels, with most of the remainder occurring at the L3–L4 level. Thoracic disks also herniate, but they do so less commonly than in the lumbar and cervical areas. Spondylosis occurs throughout the spinal canal; however, vertebral osteophytes are most prominent at the levels mentioned. Constrictions of the spinal cord and cauda equina may occur throughout the spinal canal, but they are most often encountered at C3–C4 and C4–C5, and L4–L5, respectively.[13] Cases of diffuse constriction of the thoracic spinal cord are also being reported.[19,20]

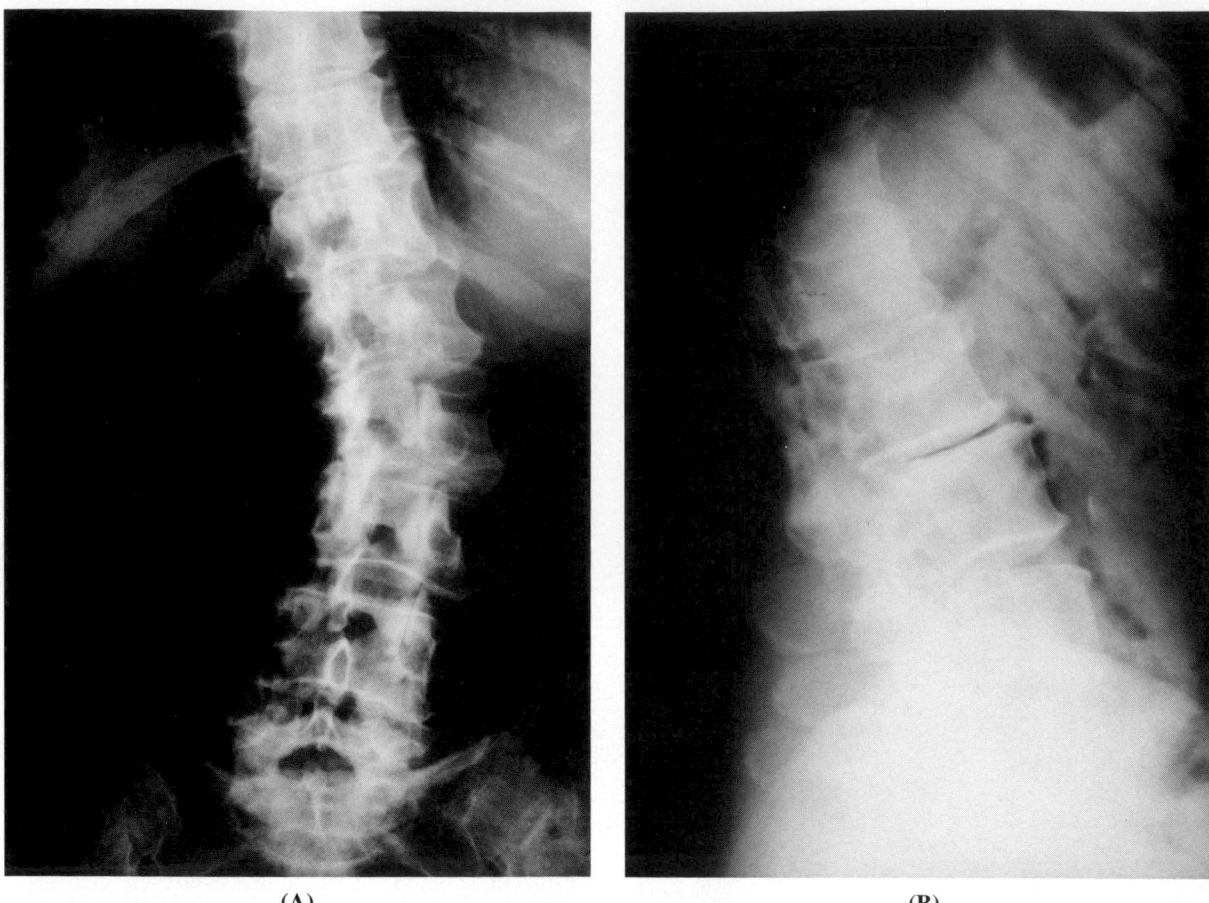

(A)   (B)

Figure 20–4   Photograph of x-ray of lumbar spine showing degenerative scoliosis of the lumbar spine. *A*. Frontal view. *B*. Lateral view.

☐ CLINICAL SIGNS AND SYMPTOMS

SIGNS AND SYMPTOMS OF HERNIATED INTERVERTEBRAL DISKS AND SPONDYLOSIS OF ADJACENT BONY ELEMENTS

Acutely herniated intervertebral disks in the lateral compartment of the spinal canal typically present with pain in the area of the herniation, with radiation in the distribution of the affected nerve root. (See Fig. 20-5.) Thus, pain from a herniated cervical disk radiates into the adjacent upper extremity, and pain from ruptured disks in the lumbar spinal canal radiates into the ipsilateral lower extremity. Onset of symptoms frequently follows trauma, which may vary in severity. A minor abnormal step or sudden rotation of the head will often set off acute symptoms. Alternatively, symptoms may begin spontaneously, especially from lesions in the cervical area. Another paradox is that pain in the site of the herniation may be insignificant or even absent in the face of acute radiating pain.

Often there is localized pain for weeks or months prior to the radiating pain, and the pain may radiate into the extremity episodically, extending further down the extremity with each episode. There may be pain in the paraspinal area for a few days or months, followed by pain radiating to the hip for another period, then it begins to radiate to the back of the knee and eventually to the ankle or foot. Symptoms are often intermittent, with pain being present either locally or in the distribution of the nerve root for a few days to weeks, following which there is often relief for weeks to months. The Valsalva maneuver usually exacerbates pain during acute episodes. Pain is relieved—or at least lessened—by bed rest. Persistent pain may demand aggressive therapy.

Signs of a laterally herniated intervertebral disk include hypalgesia in the cutaneous distribution of the nerve root, with weakness of the muscles innervated by that root. Atrophy of the innervated muscles occurs when the root compression persists. Specific signs related to herniations at common sites are described in subsequent paragraphs.

Major herniations in the lateral spinal canal or herniations into the medial portion of the spinal canal are likely to result from significant trauma. In the cervical area, the herniation may be the result of a vertebral dislocation. Major extrusions into the spinal canal produce paralysis below the level of the lesion. The spinal cord is compromised in the cervical area, and the cauda equina is affected in the lumbar area.

The anterior portion of the spinal cord can be severely compromised by extrusions in the cervical area. Such lesions cause paresis, with loss of pain and temperature sensations

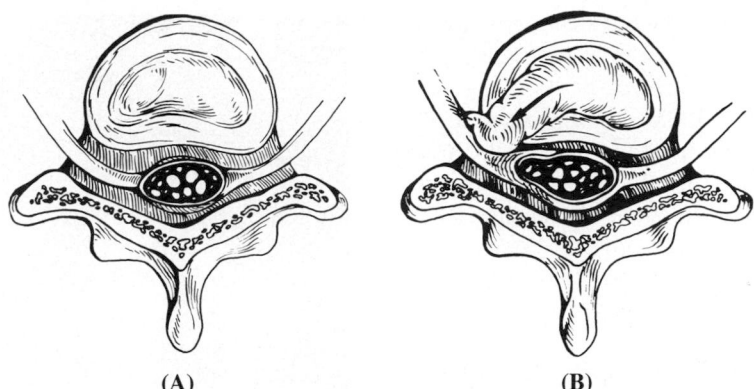

(A)   **(B)**

Figure 20–5 Diagrammatic illustrations of herniated intervertebral disk at lumbar level. Note relation of normal disk *(A)* compared to medial protrusion fragment *(B)*.

below the level of the lesion. Sensations of vibration and position are frequently retained. Compression of the cauda equina will produce paresis below the level of the lesion and loss of control of sphincters. Inability to urinate or defecate may accompany smaller lateral herniations because of the resulting pain.

A few reports have called attention to herniations of intervertebral disks from the anterior or lateral surfaces of the vertebral column. In the lumbar area, herniations produce symptoms by distortion of the fibers in the periphery of the annulus fibrosis and, perhaps, the sympathetic fibers.[9] Complaints of pain in the back, with radiation into the inguinal areas or the thighs, are common.[8,9] Spondylotic spurs are frequent.[21,22] In the cervical area, dysphagia may result from either acute herniation or spurs.[6,7]

Symptoms resulting from spondylotic lesions in the spinal canal often begin acutely, following injuries of varying severity, as do symptoms following acute herniations. However, symptoms of spondylotic lesions are usually more subtle in onset than those related to acute herniations. Likewise, symptoms may be intermittent for months or years. Signs of osteophytes located in lateral compartments of the spinal canal are frequently similar to those of acute lesions. However, signs of nerve root involvement in the lateral recesses may also be negligible for prolonged periods.[12] Spondylotic lesions compromising the spinal cord of the cervical and thoracic levels are often associated with minimal or no pain, resulting in the subtle onset of paresis and upper motor neuron signs below the level of the lesion.[23]

In asymmetric lesions there may be Brown-Séquard signs below the level of the lesion, with hyperactive reflexes on the ipsilateral side and loss of sensations of pain and temperature on the contralateral side below the lesion.[24] In other cases, the sensations of vibration and position may be impaired.[25] Hyperextension injuries in the presence of spondylotic lesions of the neck cause the "central cord syndrome," with disproportionate weakness and impairment of sensation in the upper extremities when compared to the lower extremities.[26] Frequently, there is quadriparesis, which may involve all extremities, but the lower extremities recover more rapidly than do the upper extremities.

Severe stenosis of the lumbar spinal canal usually causes paresthesias and claudication, which may be difficult to differentiate from claudication in the lower extremities due to ischemia. Paresis eventually results if the cauda equina is not decompressed.[27,28,29] The history is most important in differentiating vascular from neurogenic claudication. Vascular claudication is usually relieved almost immediately after cessation of walking. Neurogenic claudication, on the other hand, commonly requires 15 to 30 min of rest prior to improvement in symptoms. Also, patients with neurogenic claudication commonly find that a flexed posture relieves their symptoms. This is thought to be due to anatomically opening the neural foramina to their maximum capacity.

While spinal stenosis is divided into central and lateral types, the two coexist more often than not. Physical findings such as specific motor weakness and especially "stretch signs" by straight leg raising are often absent. The diagnosis should be suspected in the older patient with a history of pain and numbness in either or both legs which is exacerbated by activity and improved after a prolonged period of rest. The diagnosis is confirmed by appropriate x-rays, CT, or MRI scans, as well as by myelography.

SYMPTOM AND SIGN COMPLEX ASSOCIATED WITH THE MORE COMMONLY OCCURRING HERNIATED CERVICAL DISKS

The most commonly herniated disks in the neck are at the C5–C6 and C6–C7 levels. Laterally herniated disks at the C5–C6 level usually compress the C6 nerve root and produce paresthesias and numbness in its distribution. In the distal portion of the extremity, this includes the thumb and index finger. There is frequently demonstrable weakness of the biceps muscle, and the biceps and radial periosteal reflexes may be diminished or absent.

Herniation of an intervertebral disk at the C6–C7 level usually irritates the C7 nerve root and may produce hypalgesia and paresthesias in the middle finger. Objective evidence of involvement of the index finger, as well as the thenar side of the ring finger, is variable. The triceps muscle receives a large portion of its innervation through the C7 nerve root. It is often weak, a finding which is usually demonstrable if the reflex is depressed or absent.

A herniated disk at the C7–T1 level compresses the C8 nerve root and may be responsible for hypalgesia in the hypothenar portion of the ring and the fifth digits. Sensory changes extend up the forearm to about the junction of the middle and distal thirds. Hypalgesia in this distribution is helpful in distinguishing deficits resulting from compression of the C8 nerve root from those resulting from compression of the ulnar nerve at the elbow.

Signs may be absent or nonlocalizing.[30,31] One example relates to sensory changes in the C8 distribution, sometimes seen in association with herniated disks at higher levels. They may be the result of pressure on elements of the brachial plexus by muscles or bony structures in the area and could account for some cases of the "thoracic outlet syndrome." Some cases clearly resolve with treatment of herniated disks at higher levels. Muscle spasm is thought to be the cause. Apical lung tumors (Pancoast tumors) may also present with paresthesia in this distribution and should be considered, especially in patients with a long history of smoking. Chest x-rays with apical-lordotic views are helpful in the diagnosis of Pancoast tumors.

SIGNS AND SYMPTOMS OF COMMONLY HERNIATED LUMBAR INTERVERTEBRAL DISKS

The most commonly herniated disks in the lumbar area are at the L4–L5 and L5–S1 levels, with a smaller number of herniations at higher levels, usually at L3–L4.

A laterally herniated disk at the L3–L4 level usually impinges on the L4 nerve root, producing some weakness of extension of the knee and hypalgesia of the skin over the anterior surface of the knee which extends into the anterior and medial surfaces of the leg, frequently about halfway down the leg.

The knee jerk is usually diminished or absent. Since extension of the knee relaxes the nerve fibers to the extensor muscles of the thigh and sensory fibers crossing over the knee, straight leg raising may not produce pain. However, if the patient is placed in the lateral decubitus position with the affected side up, the hip hyperextended and the knee flexed, or if the patient is placed in the prone position and the knee flexed, pain may be severe, reproducing the patient's symptoms ("the reverse straight leg raising test" or "femoral stretch test"). Femoral neuropathy due to diabetes and retroperitoneal masses leading to compression of the L4 nerve root are to be considered in the differential diagnosis.

A disk herniation at the L4–5 level impinges upon the L5 nerve root, which usually produces decreased sensation to pinprick over the great toe and the medial one half to two-thirds of the dorsum of the foot. The pattern of hypalgesia over the anterior surface of the leg may vary. There is usually weakness of dorsiflexion of the great toe, and there may be atrophy of the intrinsic muscles of the foot. Walking

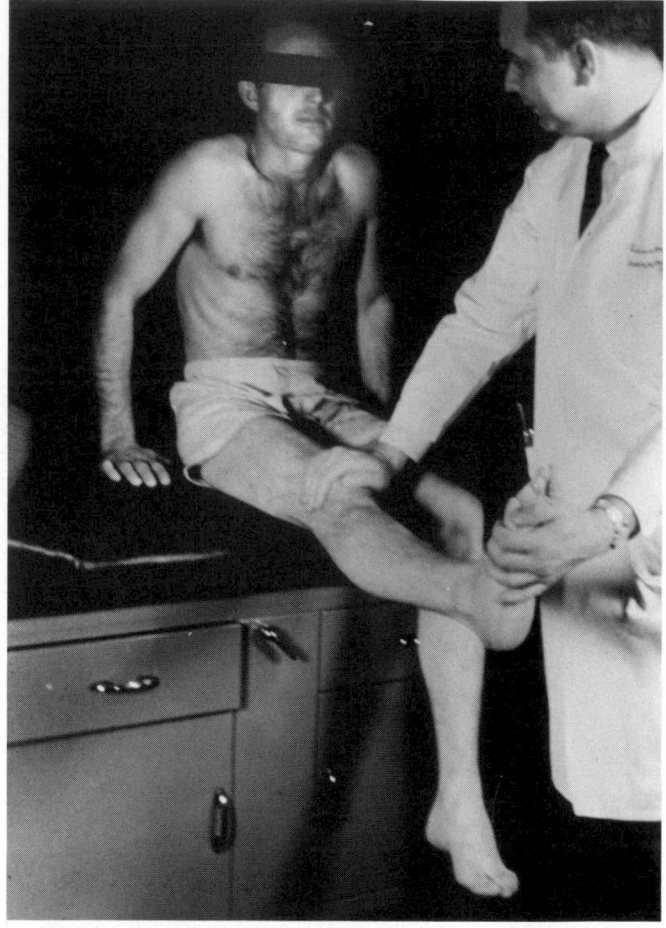

(A)

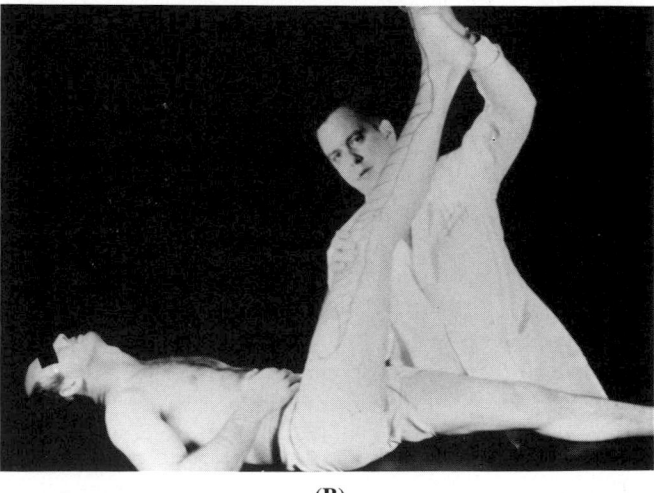

(B)

Figure 20–6   Examination of patient for pain on straight leg raising in sitting position *(A)* and while lying supine *(B)*.

on the heels may be impaired. Raising the leg, extended at the knee, usually reproduces the pain. (See Fig. 20-6*A* and *B*.) The pain can be exaggerated by dorsiflexion of the foot. There may be tenderness to palpation over the ipsilateral paraspinal muscles in the area of the L4–L5 interspace.

A herniated disk at the L5–S1 level usually compresses the first sacral nerve root and produces hypalgesia over the lateral aspect of the foot and ankle, extending onto the plantar surface of the foot. There may be weakness of eversion and plantar flexion of the foot, and the ankle jerk is usually depressed or absent. Since the gastrocnemius is a very strong muscle, testing of plantar flexion of the foot may require that the patient walk with his foot plantar flexed (on his "tip toes").

Straight leg raising usually reproduces the pain and this is increased by dorsiflexion of the foot. Tenderness is usually found at the lumbosacral junction over the paraspinal muscles. There may be reproduction of the pain by jugular compression in patients with extruded fragments of disk material at either lumbar interspace. Impairment of the anal sphincter and impairment of bladder function occur when a herniated disk compromises the cauda equina. However, lateral herniations may cause such severe pain that patients are unable to evacuate bowels or bladder.

☐ ELECTROMYOGRAPHY (EMG) AND NERVE CONDUCTION STUDIES

Electrodiagnostic investigations of patients with potential radiculopathies usually include determination of nerve conduction velocities and multiple needle insertions for evaluation of muscle action potentials. The purposes of the procedures are to determine evidence of radiculopathy that might not be apparent on physical examination and to rule out alternative lesions such as those along the course of peripheral nerves or neuropathies.

Compression of nerve roots at the neural foramina usually injures only a portion of fibers passing through. Initial symptoms result from impingement on sensory fibers, and the compression of those fibers is proximal to the dorsal root ganglia, which nurture the peripheral fibers. Even though peripheral motor neurons may be compressed, those axons which are divided degenerate, and surviving axons usually conduct normally distal to the site of compression. Consequently, nerve conduction studies along pathways distal to a root, compressed by a herniated disk or spondylitic spur, are usually normal. Findings on electromyograms indicating evidence of radiculopathy include fibrillation potentials and abnormal motor unit potentials.[32,33] Alterations of the H reflex may suggest a radiculopathy involving the S1 dermatome.

Fibrillation potentials are signals of contractions of single muscle fibers which may occur spontaneously or in response to insertion of needle electrodes. Such potentials usually fire at a constant rate, although they may be irregular. The potentials are biphasic spikes of short duration with an initial positive phase, or they may exhibit a positive sharp wave form. These potentials indicate denervation. They usually appear in proximal muscles within 7 to 10 days of injury to the nerve root but may not be seen in muscles supplied by more distal segments of the nerve fibers for 5 to 6 weeks. As they appear successively in proximal to distal segments of

nerve fibers, recovery occurs in a similar sequence, probably as a result of reinnervation.

Motor unit potentials showing evidence of denervation and reinnervation may show prolonged duration and be polyphasic. Such changes are evidence of chronic injury to innervating fibers. They are more likely to be associated with spondylosis, or they may be seen months to years after the occurrence of a herniated intervertebral disk.

The presence of fibrillations isolated to a nerve root is the most sensitive electrodiagnostic indicator of a radiculopathy. Diagnosis of a radiculopathy is based on the presence of abnormal firings in the distribution of a nerve root found in two or more muscles innervated by fibers from the same root, preferably passing through different nerves.

The "H wave" is a monosynaptic response which might be recorded from a number of muscles; practically, it is elicited from the gastrocnemius and soleus muscles in response to stimulation of the tibial nerve. Thus, fibers of the S1 root are being tested, and the H reflex is considered the electrodiagnostic equivalent of the ankle jerk. Its loss is therefore regarded as a sensitive indicator of an S1 radiculopathy. Unfortunately, the loss may result from many causes, including polyneuropathies and aging.

In summary, electromyographic activity is normal during the first few days after injury, and it may revert to normal months to years after injury as a result of reinnervation. Therefore, timing of an EMG is very important. The EMG must be considered a supplemental examination which adds in some cases to the sensitivity of the clinical examination. It should be noted that the presence of a normal electromyographic examination does *not* rule out a radiculopathy.

☐ NEURODIAGNOSTIC PROCEDURES FOR DEGENERATIVE LESIONS OF THE SPINE

Diagnostic investigations of degenerative lesions of the spine include: plain radiographs, tomograms, computerized tomography (CT), magnetic resonance imaging (MRI), myelography, and diskography. CT may be used to augment the outlines of the subarachnoid spaces after the injection of contrast material for myelography, and gadolinium may be used in conjunction with MRI investigations to help differentiate scarring in the epidural space from disk material in patients who have previously experienced surgery.

Plain radiographs demonstrate alignment of the vertebrae, as well as evidence of degenerative changes (including osteophytes), metabolic changes in the vertebrae, fractures, metastatic malignancies, and infection. (See Fig. 20-7.)

Straightening of the cervical and lumbar vertebral columns in the patient who is in an upright position or reversal of the lordotic curve seen on plain radiographs suggests muscle spasm. The apex of the reversal of the curve may point to the site of maximal spasm, which indicates the site of origin of pain. Narrowing of disk spaces, Schmorl's

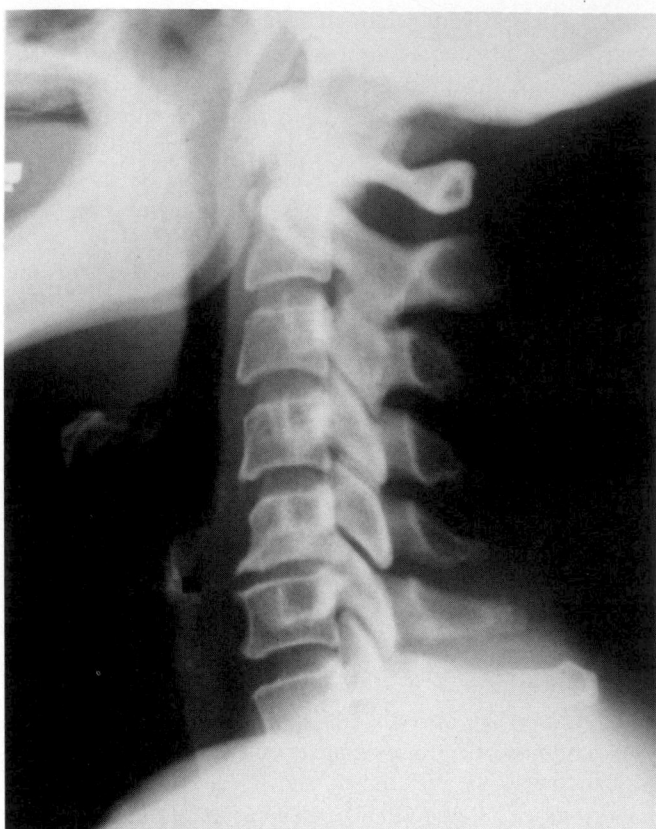

Figure 20–7 Plain radiograph and myelogram of cervical spine; lateral views showing positive osteophytes at the C5–C6 interspace.

nodes, calcification of intervertebral disks, and gas within intervertebral disks are indications of degenerative change. (See Fig. 20-8A to C.)

CT demonstrates fractures, stenosis of the spinal canal, hypertrophic changes in the facets, calcification of the posterior longitudinal ligament, and evidence of disk protrusions and/or disk extrusions. Reconstructions may be made to demonstrate malalignments.

The application of CT scanning to investigate degenerative lesions of the spine has emphasized the need for correlation with clinical signs and symptoms. (See Fig. 20-9.) One review of scans made in asymptomatic patients demonstrated abnormalities in over a third of all patients examined.[34] Nearly 20 percent of patients below the age of 40 had evidence of herniated disks, and half of the patients examined above the age of 40 had various degenerative lesions, including herniated disks, degeneration of facets, and stenosis of the spinal canal.

MRI has proved to be even more definitive than CT in the demonstration of defects of the vertebral column.[35,36] (See Fig. 20-10.) The vertical sagittal images demonstrate long segments of the spinal column, outlining the vertebral bodies and the intervertebral disks. (See Fig. 20-11A and B.) Cross sections reveal the relationships of the disks to the thecal sac and nerve roots. Even though bony elements are not as well delineated as on CT, evaluation of alignment is better. Spinal stenosis and arachnoiditis are also well outlined.[37]

The administration of gadolinium to patients having previously undergone surgery helps to differentiate disk herniations from scarring.[38] Dynamic MRI has revealed explanations for the development of myelopathy by demonstrating compression of the spinal cord when the neck is extended.[39] MRI, as well as CT, has emphasized the importance of clinical correlation. A recent study demonstrated progressively increasing numbers of degenerative lesions in the spine with increasing age.[40]

Myelography was developed over 70 years ago. Its clinical application was first reported a couple of years later.[36] It remains the standard for investigating etiologies of degenerative lesions of the spinal column. (See Fig. 20-12.) Initial myelograms were performed with air. Oil contrast media remained the standard for many years, but now most examinations are performed with water-soluble contrast media. These media are less toxic and provide discrete outlines of very small lesions. A disadvantage of water-soluble contrast media is that they are dissipated within a few minutes. However, CT imaging performed after the contrast material has been injected will show enhanced images for a longer period of time, and may reveal disk herniations isolated to the midportion of the spinal canal that can be missed without tomography. (See Fig. 20-13.)

Diskography, in which water-soluble contrast media is injected into intervertebral disks suspected of degeneration, was very popular in the 1960s, but the demonstration that degenerated disks were common and might not be associated with radiculopathies led to considerable skepticism regarding the examination. There has been a resurgence of interest in more recent years, probably at least in part as a result of the realization that the disks that received excessive quantities of dye and revealed extrusion into the epidural space were abnormal even though they were not associated with radiculopathies. Diskography is now performed in many centers, but a major part of the diagnostic evaluation is based on reproduction of the patient's symptoms by injection of contrast media into the affected disk space.[41] *Diskitis* is a known complication of the investigation, probably a result of organisms from the skin introduced via the needle used to inject contrast media.[42]

☐ TREATMENT OF HERNIATED INTEVERTEBRAL DISKS

The treatment for intervertebral disk disease has been subject to controversy. Opinions vary as to whether nonsurgical (conservative) or surgical treatment should be instituted and when. If surgical treatment is selected, there is consideration as to which form of surgery should be applied.

Early symptoms of herniated disks frequently begin with localized pain in the back or neck. These are common complaints, and the causes of such pain may be many. Often, episodes of localized pain have been diagnosed as "mechanical," "musculoskeletal strain," or "fascitis." Pain

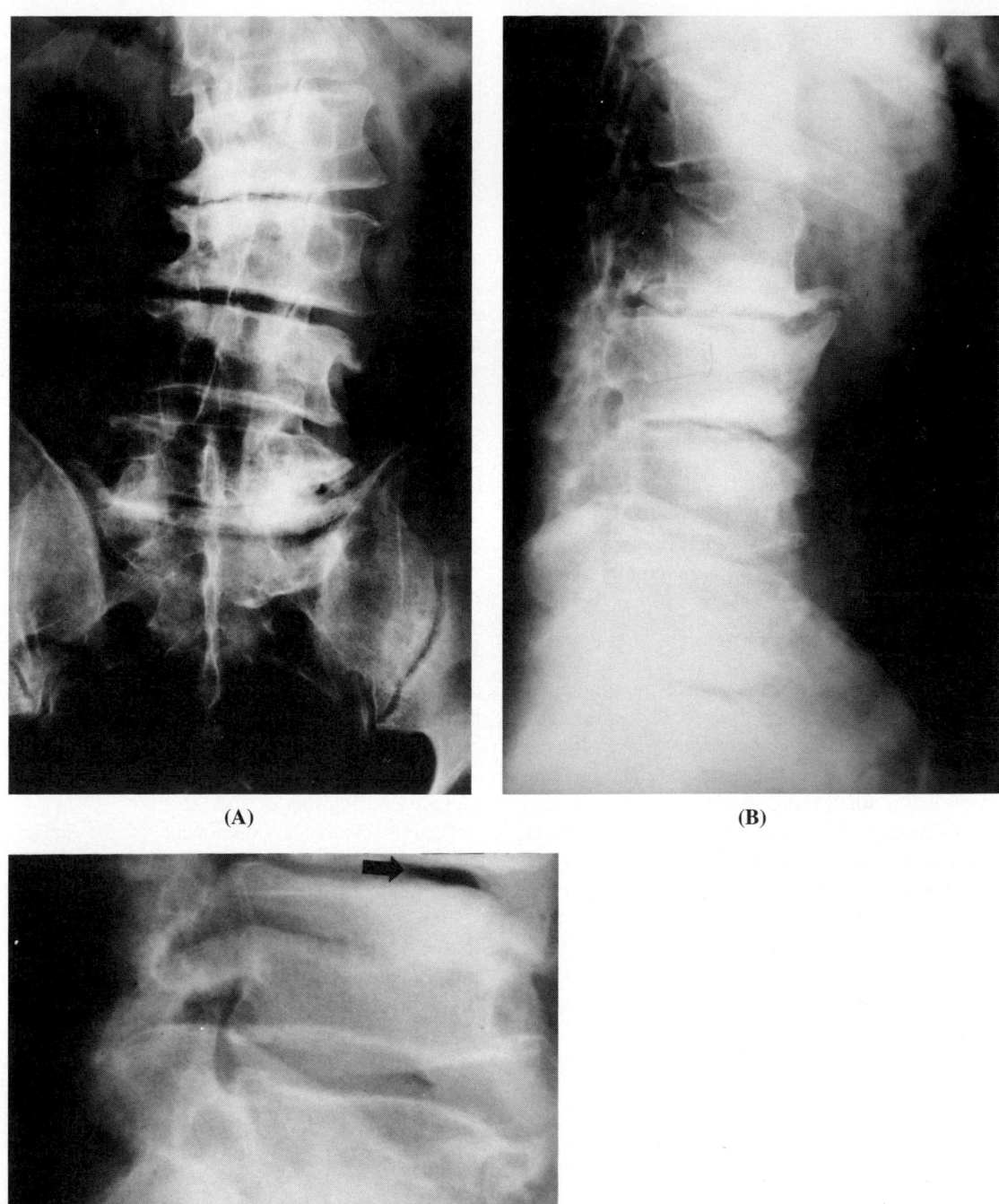

(A)

(B)

(C)

Figure 20–8 Spondylitic degenerative changes in lumbar spine. Note lateral osteophytes at each level but most marked at L2–L3 and L3–L4 in the frontal view, with narrowing of the disk space, most marked at L2–L3 in the frontal view *(A)*. The lateral view shows narrowing and irregularity of the disk spaces, large osteophytes anteriorly at L2–L5, and some in vertebrolisthesis views *(B)*. Gas shadows are identified by the arrows in *C*.

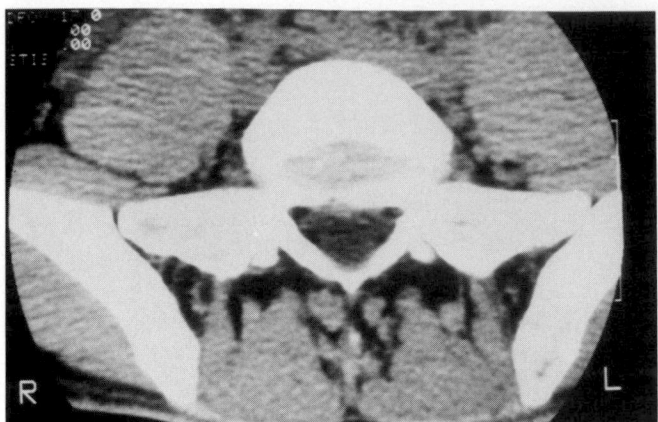

Figure 20–9 Computerized tomography of lumbosacral junction with contrast material in the spinal canal indicating herniated intervertebral disk.

may result from fracture, infection, arthritic involvement, or even vertebral abnormalities. Pain is often temporary and the symptoms will resolve with time, with or without bed rest, heat, massage, analgesics, sedation, or anti-inflammatory medications.

In the past, invasive techniques for investigating complaints referable to pain in the spine were performed only after the complaints had been unremitting for prolonged periods or neurological deficits were encountered. Imaging is currently done using much more liberal criteria. Degenerative changes of intervertebral disks that may be the basis for such complaints are often demonstrated.

Imaging reveals degenerative lesions of intervertebral disks and vertebrae in the spine even in the absence of symptoms, but it must be emphasized that pain in the back and neck often resolves, given time, even when radicular signs are present. Therefore, conservative treatment of such lesions must remain a serious consideration, even in the presence of a positively imaged lesion, unless symptoms persist or neurological deterioration is progressive. It must be emphasized that herniation of an intervertebral disk is *not* a life-threatening problem. Surgery should be considered only for severe or persistent pain, or neurological deficits.

Once a definitive lesion of an intervertebral disk or its adjacent bony elements has been demonstrated and a surgical procedure is indicated, controversies develop as to whether diskectomies in the neck should be performed through an anterior or posterior approach or whether, in association with an anterior approach, a fusion should be performed. Similarly, opinions vary on surgical approaches to the lumbar area as to whether fusion should be performed in association with diskectomies, and, if so, whether the fusion should be performed between the posterior or lateral elements of the spinal column or between the vertebral bodies.

Even the mechanism by which the disk is removed is subject to question in the lumbar area. Most diskectomies in the lumbar area are performed through laminotomies. This approach is used by many neurosurgeons in the cervical

area. Recent innovations have questioned whether diskectomies should be performed by needle aspiration, by open laminectomy, with magnification,[43] or with the use of an enzyme that digests the intervertebral disk.[44,45,46,47] In addition, with degenerative lesions of the vertebral column, questions arise as to (1) whether spondylitic lesions in the cervical area should be attacked through an anterior or posterior approach, (2) whether laminectomies in the lumbar area for spinal stenosis should be limited to one or two levels, and (3) whether such laminectomies should be accompanied by a fusion and/or the use of instrumentation to maintain alignment. Similarly, in the cervical area, controversies exist as to whether some form of prosthesis should be inserted to improve the structural integrity of the vertebral column.

For the purposes of this discussion, we will present the basically accepted techniques and mention some of the various alternatives that have been recommended.

CONSERVATIVE TREATMENT

A period of rest seems clearly indicated following the onset of acute pain in the neck or back before considering surgical therapy—unless there is indication of infection, vascular disease, tissue destruction, or significant neurological deficit. Opinions may differ as to the types of therapy that should be included during this period.

Pain is clearly a component of the muscle strain that occurs in association with strenuous exercise or blunt injury to a muscle. After a few days of rest, the pain resolves.

Bed rest is the mainstay of conservative treatment for pain in the neck or back, which could be temporary; pain and minor neurological deficits often resolve with time. Edema may play a significant role in radicular pain seen in association with herniated disks.[10] Reduction of edema of nerve roots could explain the remarkable clinical results that are often seen after the administration of steroids.

The administration of heat and massage provides some temporary relief of pain, and there does not appear to be any contraindication to their use in the treatment of radiculopathies. The authors have discouraged the use of vertebral manipulations in such cases, fearing the possibility of disk extrusions.

It has generally been our policy to maintain a period of bed rest for 2 weeks. During this time, radiographs of the structures in question can be obtained along with any ancillary laboratory studies where indicated, such as sedimentation rates and evaluation for arthritis. During this time, imaging is accomplished. Even if herniated intervertebral disks are demonstrated, we continue to rely on rest if pain is resolving.

In the past, the use of head halter or pelvic traction as a supplemental treatment for bed rest has been used, but anatomical justification cannot be demonstrated for the use of pelvic traction, and many patients abhor the use of head halters required for traction on the neck. As a result, the use

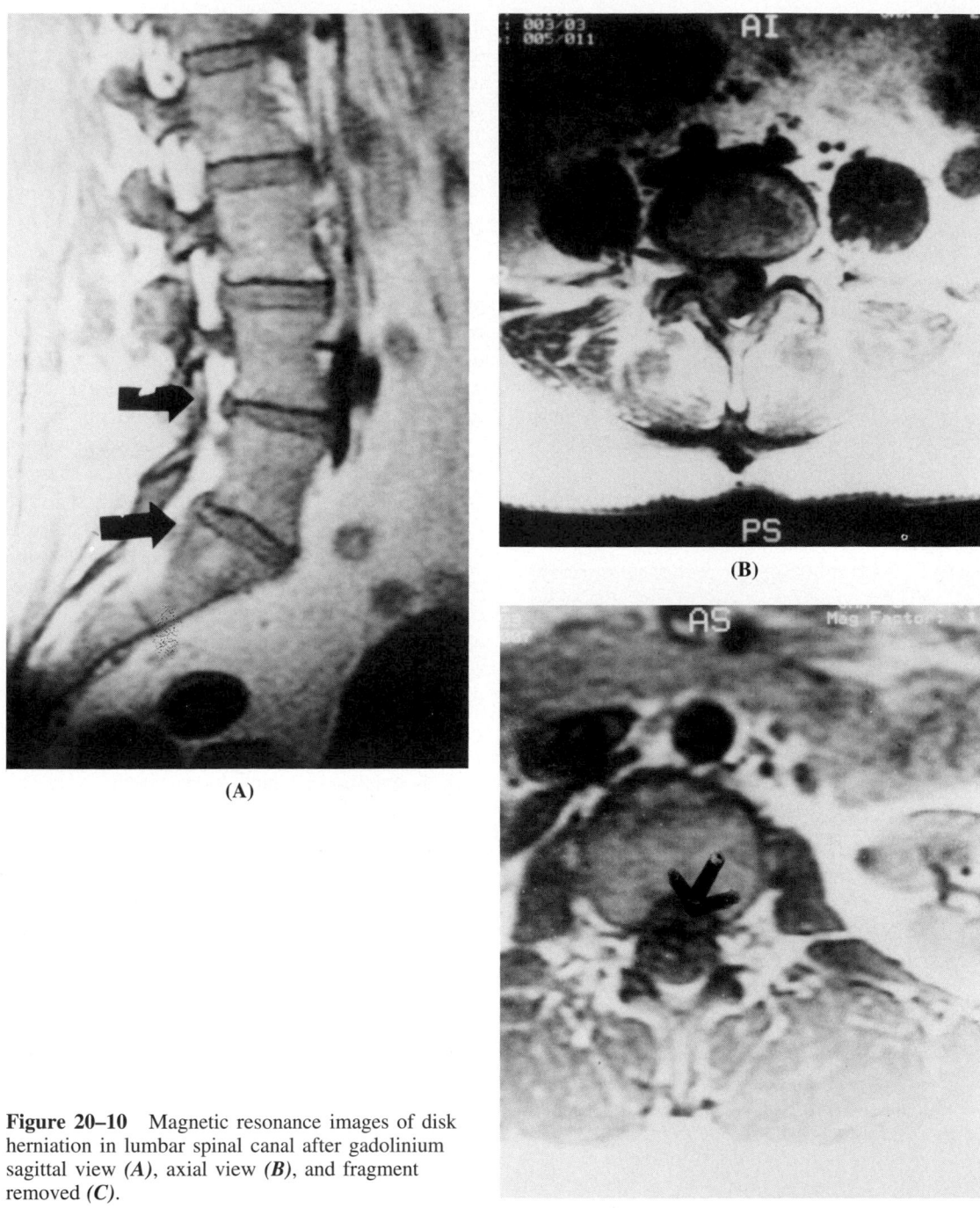

(A)

(B)

Figure 20–10 Magnetic resonance images of disk herniation in lumbar spinal canal after gadolinium sagittal view *(A)*, axial view *(B)*, and fragment removed *(C)*.

(C)

of traction as a form of therapy for temporary back and neck pain has been discontinued in many institutions.

The use of analgesics as a supplement to rest is often indicated, but one must be selective in the types of analgesics used. Narcotics are rarely necessary when patients remain at rest and should be avoided when treating chronic pain of benign etiology. Peripherally acting analgesics and nonsteroidal anti-inflammatory drugs are usually adequate. A temporary course of steroids may be helpful.

Sedatives have been administered in many cases when the pain is acute, especially if the patient is anxious. The administration of such drugs should be kept to a minimum.

Use of local anesthetics injected adjacent to nerve roots or into trigger points and in the epidural space has been advocated for many years. Infections in the epidural space can occur in conjunction with the administration of epidural anesthetics. The use of steroids has also been advocated, but while occasional administration of steroids may not be harmful, osteoporosis is exacerbated by their use. Cuckler concluded from his well-controlled, double-blind study that epidural steroid injections are of no value in the treatment of lumbar radicular pain.[48] White reported that variable results from epidural steroid injections were due to the finding that as many as 25 percent of injections were misplaced.[49] He

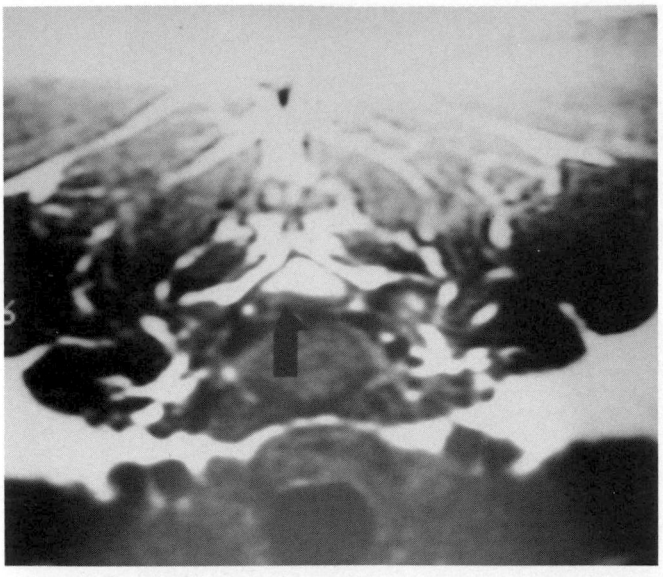

(A)

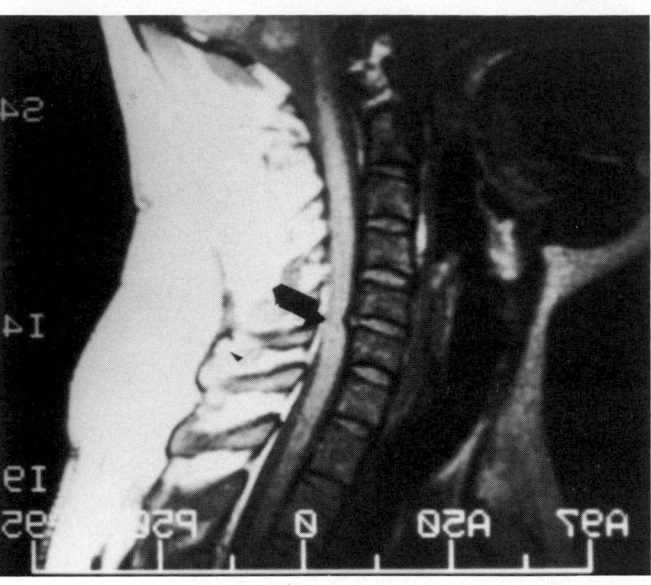

(B)

Figure 20–11 Sagittal MRI of cervical spine showing herniated cervical disk at the C5–C6 level in the sagittal *(A)* and axial *(B)* planes.

recommended injection under fluoroscopic control, using a small amount of contrast media to document location.

When definitive neurological deficits are apparent and imaging has demonstrated a protruding intervertebral disk as a cause and ruled out the presence of extruded fragments, some have suggested this is an indication for percutaneous diskectomy as the ultimate form of conservative care.[50,51,52,53] The authors' experience with this practice is limited, and we have met with limited success.

The procedure is carried out through a needle inserted through a cannula introduced about 10 cm lateral to the midline, directed toward the intervertebral space under fluoroscopic control. A curved cannula has been especially devised for insertion of a needle into the L5–S1 interspace. A diskogram

may exclude disruption of the annulus and posterior longitudinal ligament. Once the needle has been put in place, the disk material is aspirated with an ultrasonic aspirator. Many surgeons report a success rate for the relief of pain in the range of 70 to 80 percent; however, the authors' long-term success in a very small group of patients has been considerably less. A low rate of success has been reported in patients older than 50 years, and most authors have reported that pain from extruded fragments is exacerbated by such procedures.

In summary, it appears that patients seen with acute onset of pain in the neck or lumbar back—with or without a radicular component radiating into an upper or lower extremity—should be given a period of rest for at least 2 weeks. This may be done at home but is better administered in a controlled environment. We do not advocate use of traction but do use nonnarcotic analgesics and nonsteroidal anti-inflammatory drugs as well as, in some cases, mild sedation. We have not used injectable steroids. Heat and muscle massage are given to supplement bed rest, but we do not advocate manipulative therapy. If the symptoms appear to be resolving after 2 weeks, this conservative therapy is continued. Physical therapy along with muscle strengthening exercises is instituted as the pain resolves. If the pain persists despite therapy or if patients demonstrate neurological deficits, imaging is performed to determine indications for surgical therapy.

A definitive workup is indicated: for patients evaluated with symptoms that have persisted for several months, in patients who have evidence of spinal stenosis, long tract signs or lesions in the cervical or thoracic areas, or in patients who have claudication or pain on standing or walking with relief on sitting. This includes appropriate electrodiagnostic studies and imaging with surgical therapy as the ultimate objective.

SURGICAL THERAPY

Many factors enter into a decision as to whether, when, and what type of surgical therapy is indicated in a patient with a known herniated intervertebral disk. While a cure rate approaching 90 percent in patients with symptoms due to herniated disks has been reported in the past, residual pain persists for years in at least a third of patients treated surgically. Pain from compression of a nerve root is relieved in a high percentage of cases, but even when it is, there may be residual paresthesias, and relief of back pain is far from routine. Definitive indications for surgery are: (1) persistent pain of such a nature that the patient cannot pursue his or her livelihood or (2) a significant neurological deficit which is ascribed to the herniated disk.

OPERATIVE TECHNIQUE: LUMBAR

The standard surgical procedure for an uncomplicated herniated nucleus pulposus in the lumbar area is accomplished through a unilateral hemilaminotomy.

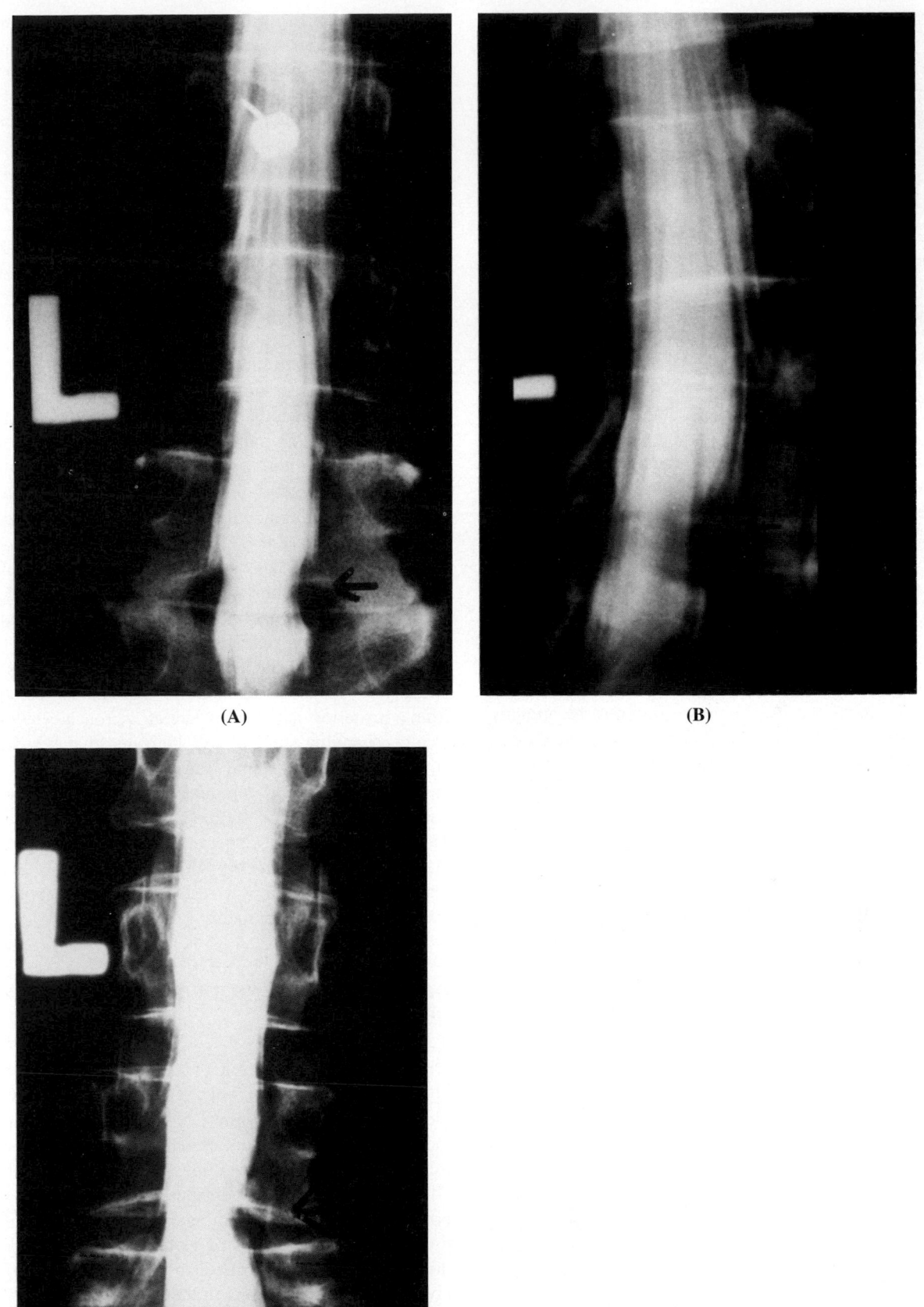

(A)

(B)

(C)

Figure 20–12   Myelograms showing lateral defects from herniated intervertebral disks at L5–S1 in the frontal view *(A)*, oblique view *(B)*, and a lateral defect in the frontal view at the L4–L5 level *(C)*.

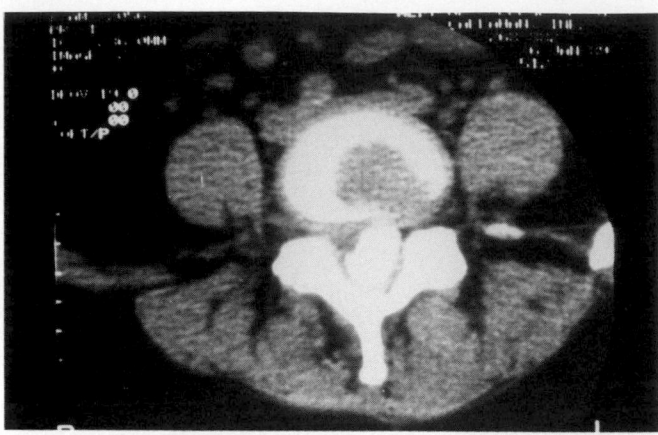

Figure 20–13 Computerized tomogram of lumbar spinal canal containing contrast media and showing laterally herniated nucleus pulposus.

The appropriate interspace is approached through a midline or paramedian incision. After the paraspinal muscles are separated from the adjacent spinous processes and laminae, the inferior margin of the lamina above the interspace is removed by rongeuring. The ligamentum flavum and medial margin of the adjacent facet may be removed, but the structural integrity of the facet should be preserved.

The spinal dura and the subjacent nerve root are usually retracted medially. In some instances, the disk herniation may present in the axilla between the nerve root and the adjacent dura, in which case the nerve root must be retracted laterally. (See Fig. 20-14.) Extruded fragments of disk material are removed with pituitary rongeurs. In the event of significant protrusions when the external fibers of the annulus are still intact, the annulus is incised or opened in a circular manner.

The inner portion of the disk is removed with rongeurs. The intervertebral disk space is curetted and fragments within the interspace removed, minimizing chances of extrusion of another fragment. The nerve root should be thoroughly decompressed, a search being made for additional fragments of disk material which might lie anterior to the nerve root and for osteophytes that might impinge on the nerve root in the neural foramen.

The presence of osteophytes that are likely to compromise

the neural foramen from the edges of the vertebral bodies or the facet may require a foraminotomy, that is, resection of the anterior and medial segments of the facet. If the stenosis compromises the spinal canal, a laminectomy must be performed. Intraoperative sonography may help locate disk fragments or osteophytes located anterior to the dura or nerve root.[54] Variations of diskectomy from a posterior approach have included use of the surgical microscope and resection through a large-bore needle.[43]

Instability following laminotomy or laminectomy in the lumbar area has been a concern for years.[55] In the past—and even continuing into the present on many services—fusions between adjacent posterior elements have been performed, often routinely, in association with diskectomies in the lumbar area.[56,57] This technique has been replaced by interbody fusion on many neurosurgical services.[58,59]

A radical diskectomy incorporating removal of the facet joints on either side may be followed by insertion of struts of bone between the adjacent vertebrae for an interbody fusion. When struts of bone are implanted, one must make certain that cartilaginous plates have been removed at the sties where struts are being incorporated. Fusions may be accomplished with bone removed from the iliac crest of the patient, or bank bone may be used with a high degree of success. Stabilization of sites of fusion is improved by the use of compression rods. (See Fig. 20-15.)

Excision of intervertebral disks herniated anteriorly or laterally to the vertebral column requires radical resection from a posterior, anterior, or lateral approach.[9,21,60]

When imaging studies have indicated that free fragments do not lie in the spinal canal, portions of the nucleus pulposus between the vertebrae can be removed by chemonucleolysis[44,45,46,47] or by percutaneous aspiration.[50,51,52,53] The authors' personal experience with these techniques has met with limited success. Diskitis is the most commonly reported complication;[61] it is a well-known complication of diskectomy by any approach.[62]

OPERATIVE TECHNIQUE FOR HERNIATED CERVICAL DISKS

Laminotomy and resection of disk fragments has been applied in the cervical as well as the lumbar area. The technique meets with the highest incidence of pain relief when there are uncomplicated herniations of soft disk material. Since disk herniations are commonly associated with osteophytic formations of the adjacent vertebral bodies and of the posteriorly placed facets, an anterior diskectomy with resection of adjacent segments of vertebrae above and below the disk space, as well as fusion of the adjacent vertebrae, is preferred for many lesions in the cervical area.[58,59,63,64,65]

For anterior cervical diskectomy, a transverse incision is usually made through a crease in the neck. An alternate incision may be made along the medial edge of the sternocleidomastoid muscle. After either incision, dissection separates the body of the sternocleidomastoid muscle and the

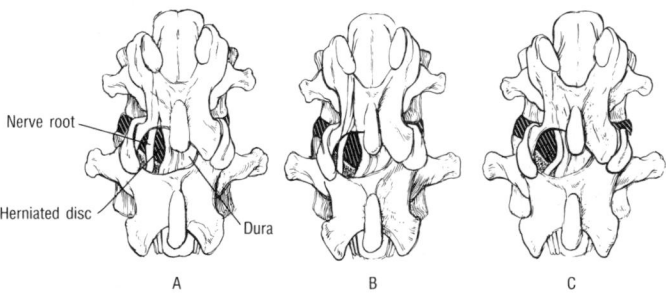

Figure 20–14 Schematic illustration of intervertebral disk impinging on the nerve root from directly anteriorly *(A)*, medially *(B)*, and laterally *(C)*. Disk excision is most often accomplished after moving the nerve root medially.

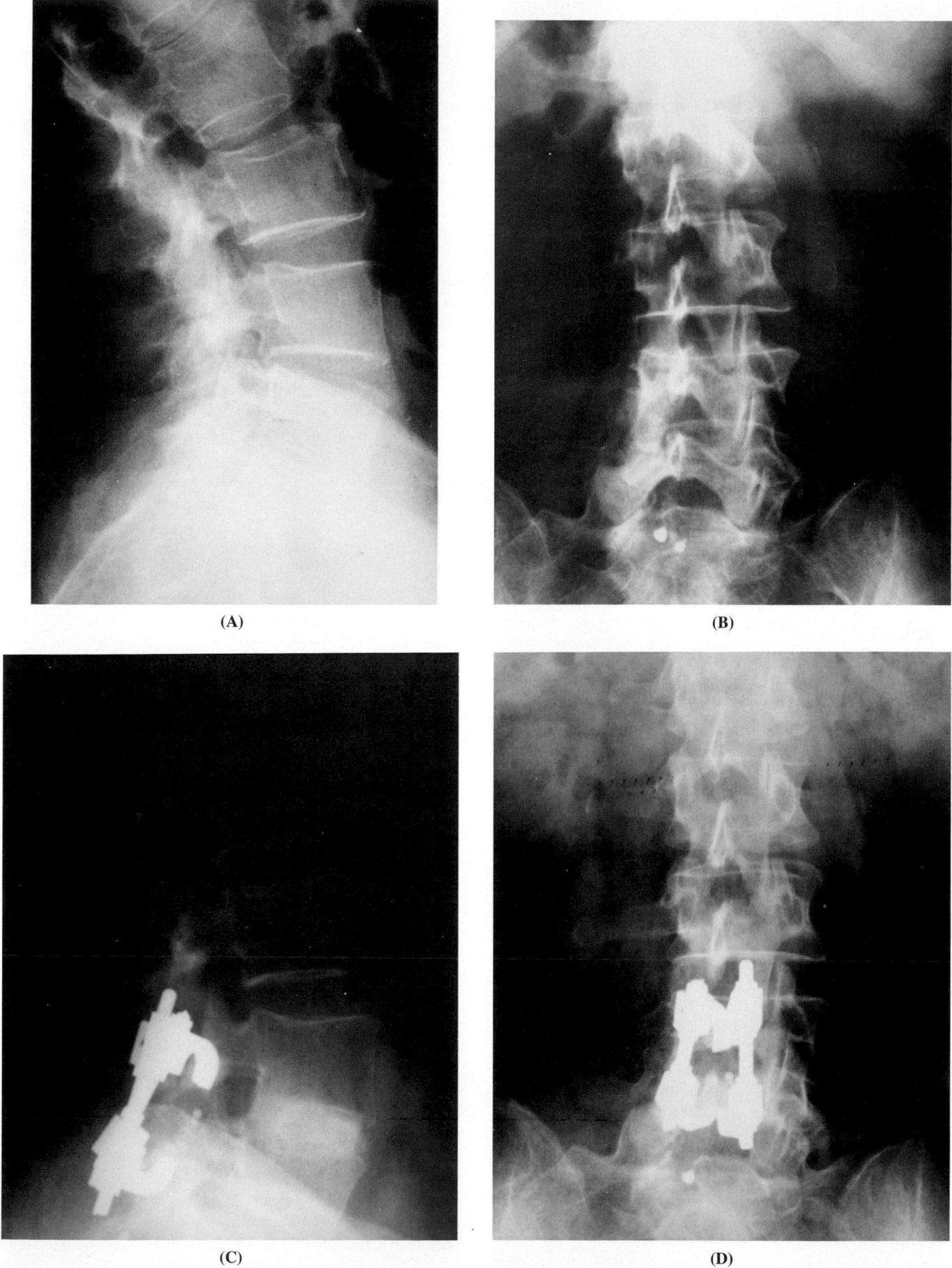

(A)

(B)

(C)

(D)

Figure 20–15 Recurrent herniated intervertebral disk at L4–L5 treated by excision and fusion, the latter aided by Harrington compression rods. Plain x-rays (A, B). For comparison with similar films after surgery (C, D).

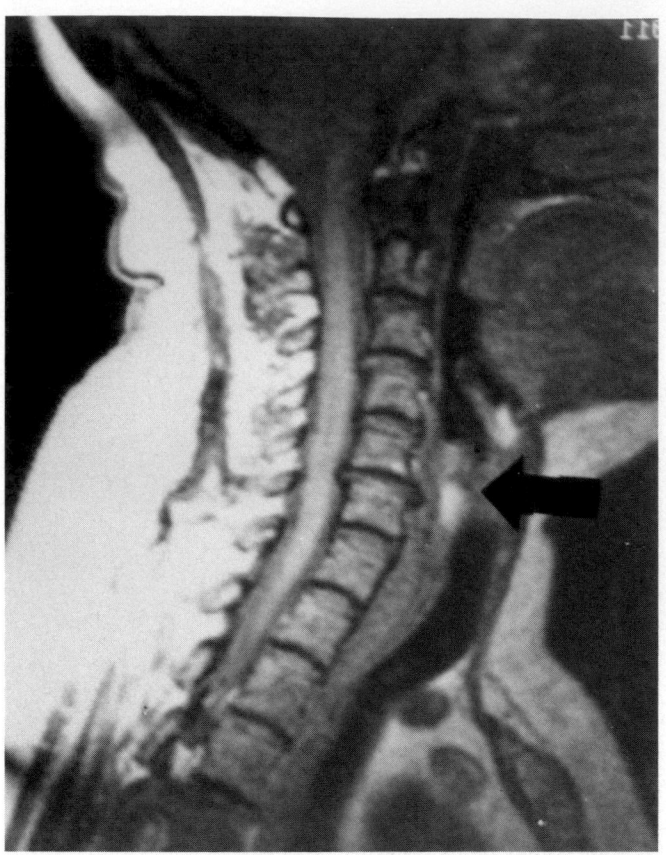
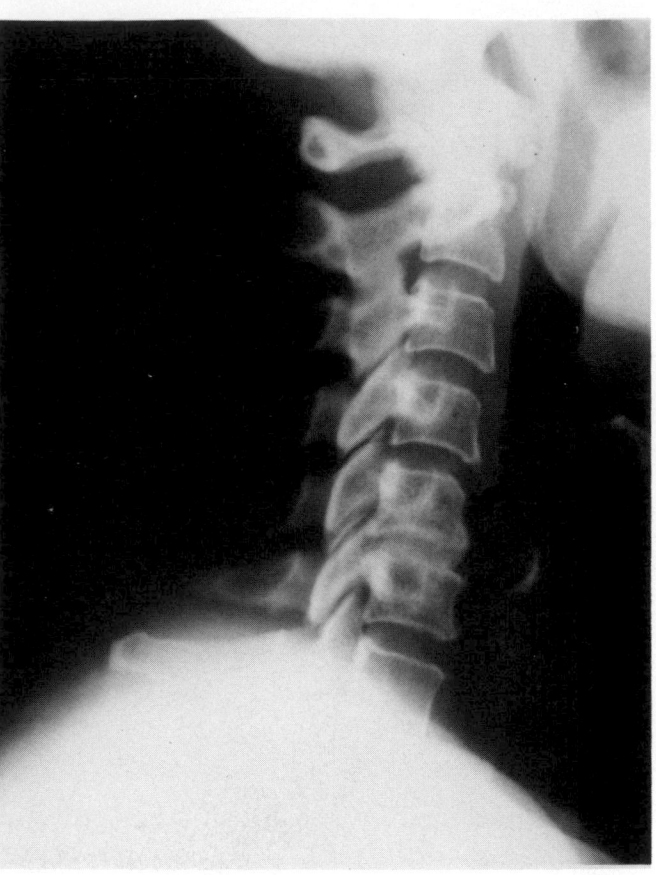

(A)   (B)

Figure 20–16   Magnetic resonance image *A*. Sagittal view of herniated disk, C5–C6. *B*. Lateral
view of x-ray neck after surgery, showing bone graft in place.

strap muscles of the neck. The sternocleidomastoid and
subjacent jugular vein, carotid artery, and vagus nerve are
retracted laterally, while the strap muscles, trachea, and
esophagus are retracted to the contralateral side. This bares
the anterior surface of the vertebral column with its intimately adherent longus coli muscles.

A lateral x-ray taken with a needle inserted into the
intervertebral disk identifies the level. After the vertebral
column has been bared of its soft tissues—including the
longus coli muscles on either side—a transverse incision is
made in the anterior longitudinal ligament and subjacent
annulus, and portions of the disk material are removed.

Varying techniques have been described for removing the
disk material and various portions of the adjacent vertebral
bodies by Cloward, by Smith and Robinson, and, more
recently, by other surgeons.[63,64,65]

Variations include: the use of a gas-powered burr for
removal of the adjacent portions of the vertebral bodies,
curettage and rongeuring of adjacent surfaces of the two
vertebral bodies, or simply curetting the disk material
without subsequent fusion. By any method, the nerve roots
are decompressed, care being taken not to injure the vertebral arteries or spinal cord. Through this approach, osteophytes on the adjacent vertebrae may be removed. (See Fig.
20-16.)

OPERATIVE TECHNIQUES FOR RESECTION OF HERNIATED THORACIC DISKS

For diskectomies in the thoracic area, alternative techniques
have been described. A direct approach through laminotomy
has met with complicating paresis in a high percentage of
cases. Therefore, an approach through thoracotomy has
gained popularity.[66,67,68] An alternative procedure is to remove a medial segment of the rib and transverse process,
exposing the appropriate intervertebral disk.[69] Using either
approach, a segment of rib is often implanted into the disk
space after the disk and cartilaginous plates have been removed.[70] (See Fig. 20-17.)

☐ SPONDYLITIC LESIONS OF THE SPINE

Spondylosis, the degeneration of bony and ligamentous elements of the spinal column, progresses with age. As with
lesions of intervertebral disks, neurological complications
may be related to involvement in the central portion of the
spinal canal, which impairs function of the spinal cord or
cauda equina, as distinct from involvement along the lateral
portions of the canal where lesions produce radicular signs

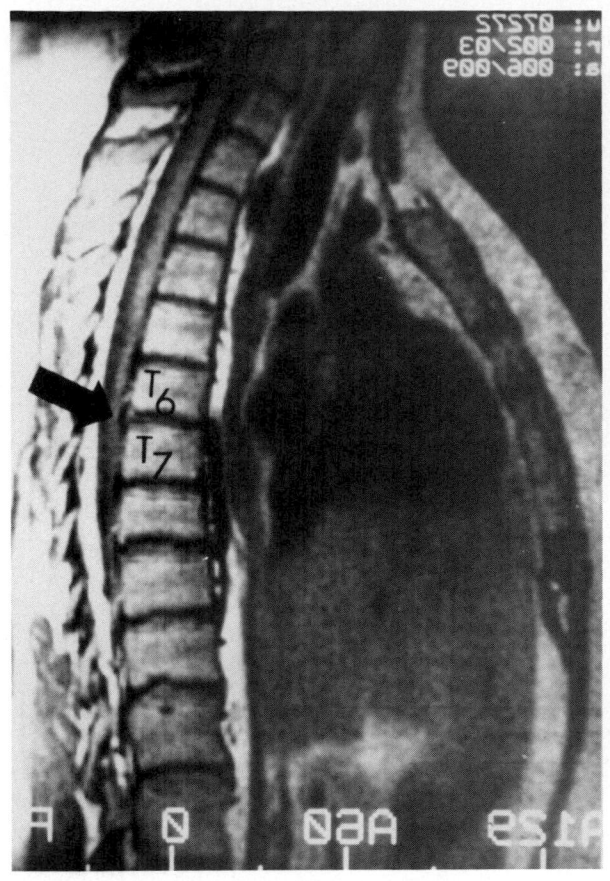
(A)

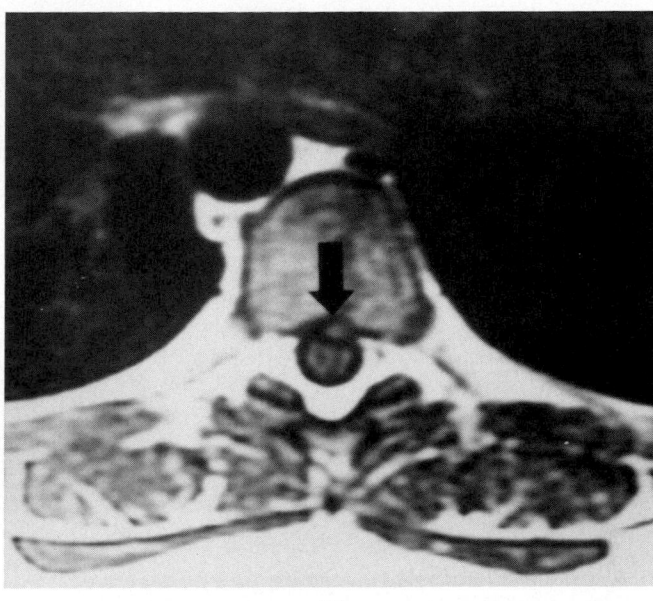
(B)

Figure 20–17   Herniated thoracic disk at T6–T7 seen on sagittal MRI *(A)* and axial views *(B)*.

and symptoms. In addition, severe derangement of the alignment of the spinal canal—which can be the result of deformation (compression) by part of a vertebral body, failure of pedicles or facets, or relaxation of ligaments—is often associated with pain locally. These are not necessarily associated with identifiable neurological deficits. (See Fig. 20-18.)

Hypertrophic changes of the superior and inferior edges of the vertebral bodies increase with age. Such changes are more prevalent in the cervical and lumbar areas than in the thoracic area, although they occur throughout the vertebral column. (See Fig. 20-19.) Hypertrophy is also a common degenerative feature of the facets.

Spondylitic spurs at the lateral parts of the vertebral bodies located within the spinal canal and hypertrophy of the superior facet are likely to impinge on exiting nerve roots. Hypertrophy of the more medial parts of the posterior vertebral bodies and hypertrophy of the inferior facet processes —at least in the lumbar area—decrease the volume of the spinal canal. Playing a role in ultimately determining the size of the spinal canal is the length of the pedicles and laminae as determined by development, as well as the presence of metabolic changes, which may result in thickening of all of these bony parts.

Relaxation of ligaments that may be a result of stretching or tears or, more often, degenerative processes may allow for malalignment and compromise in the diameter of the canal

or compromise of the neural foramina. Another feature that may add to compromise of the spinal canal is thickening of the posterior elements and thickening of the posterior longitudinal ligaments, which may be associated with calcification.[13,14,15,16,17]

☐ SPINAL STENOSIS

Stenosis of the spinal canal in the cervical and thoracic areas results in compressing the spinal cord, causing myelopathy that produces weakness and upper motor neuron signs. (See Fig. 20-20.) There are often posterior column signs as well, especially when there is retrolisthesis. Stenosis of the lumbar spinal canal is more likely to be associated with claudication on standing or walking, relieved by sitting with the back in a flexed position or by lying down. There are usually numbness and dysesthesias in the lower extremities. The symptoms of spondylotic lesions of the lateral parts of the spinal canal have been described earlier, and their treatment, discussed earlier, is primarily that of decompressing the lateral compartments of the spinal canal. It seems appropriate now to discuss treatment of lesions that affect the internal diameter of the canal.

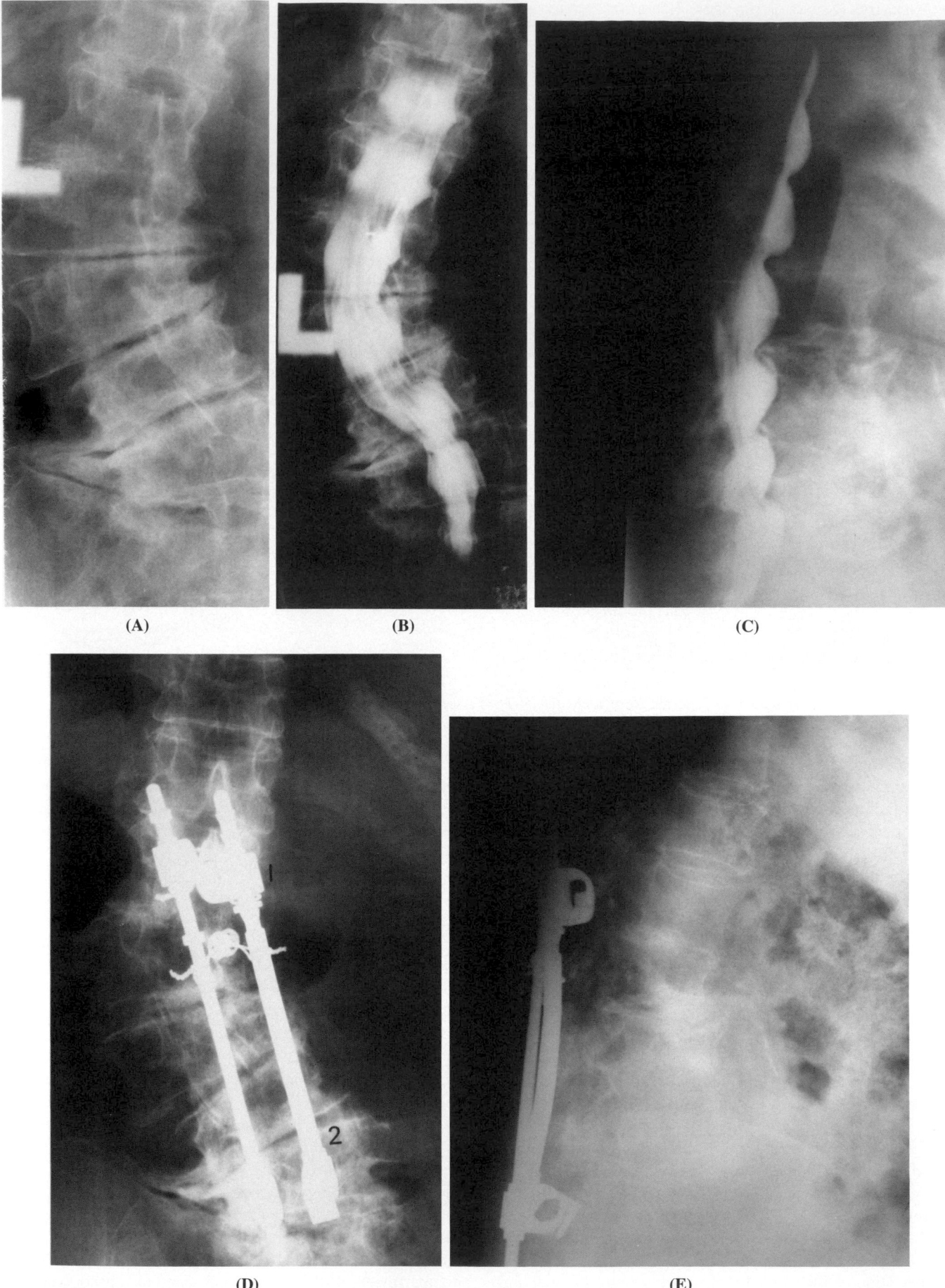

(A)   (B)   (C)

(D)   (E)

Figure 20–18   Severe spondylosis of the lumbar spine, showing narrowing of disk spaces, osteophyte formation, and scoliosis on the frontal views of the plain radiographs *(A)*. The myelogram shows narrowing of the spinal canal (stenosis) with indentations at every level *(B, C)*. The patient's pain was greatly reduced by internal fixation and fusion despite minimal anatomical improvement *(D, E)*.

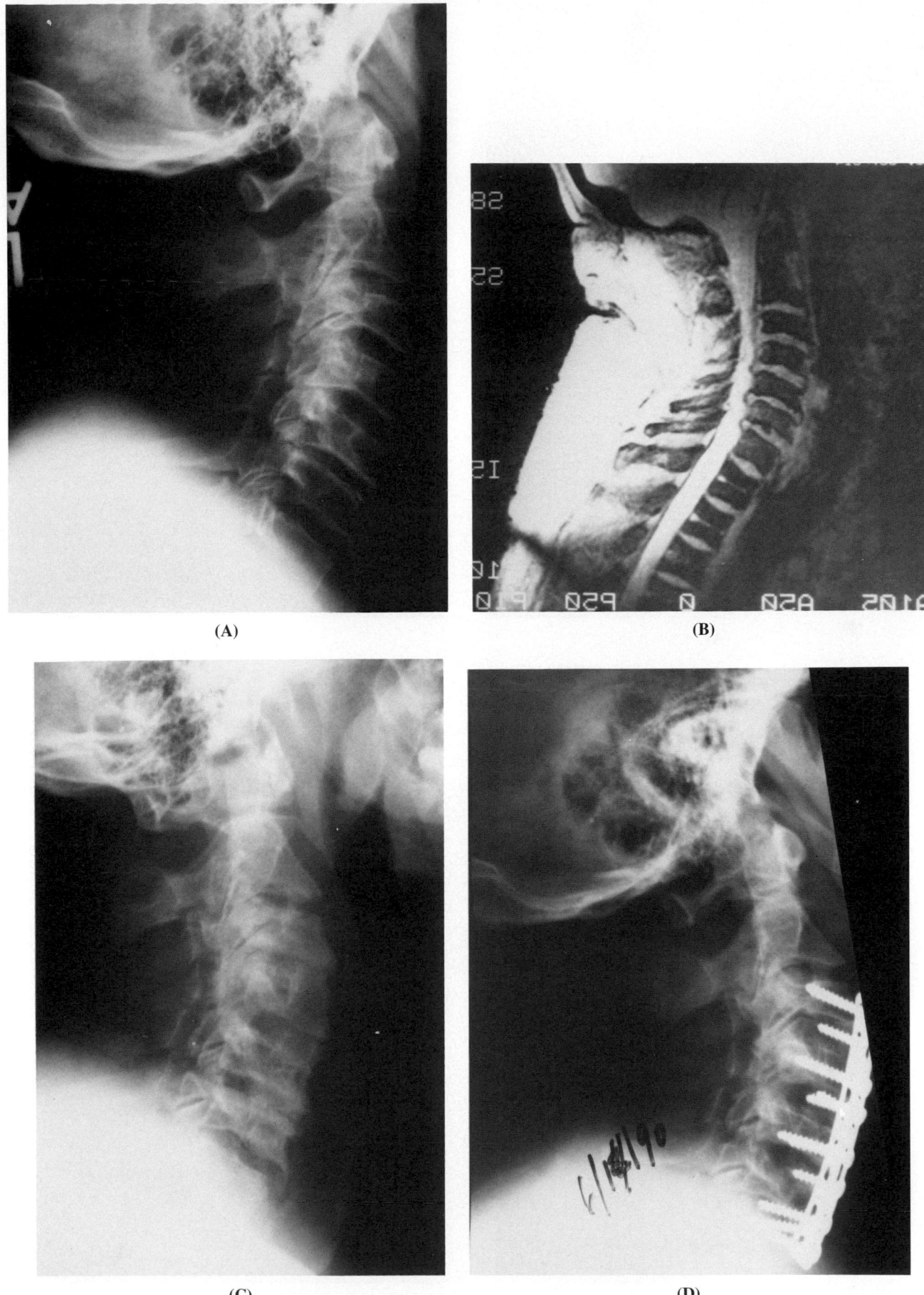

(A)

(B)

(C)

(D)

Figure 20–19 Cervical spondylosis with stenosis of the spinal canal and myelopathy treated by multiple diskectomies and fusion, and subsequent fixation with a Caspar plate. Note the osteophytic narrowing of the spinal canal *(A)* illustrated more graphically by the sagittal MRI *(B)*. A lateral radiograph *(C)* shows the multiple diskectomies and interbody fusions, held and internally fixed by the Caspar plates and screws *(D)*.

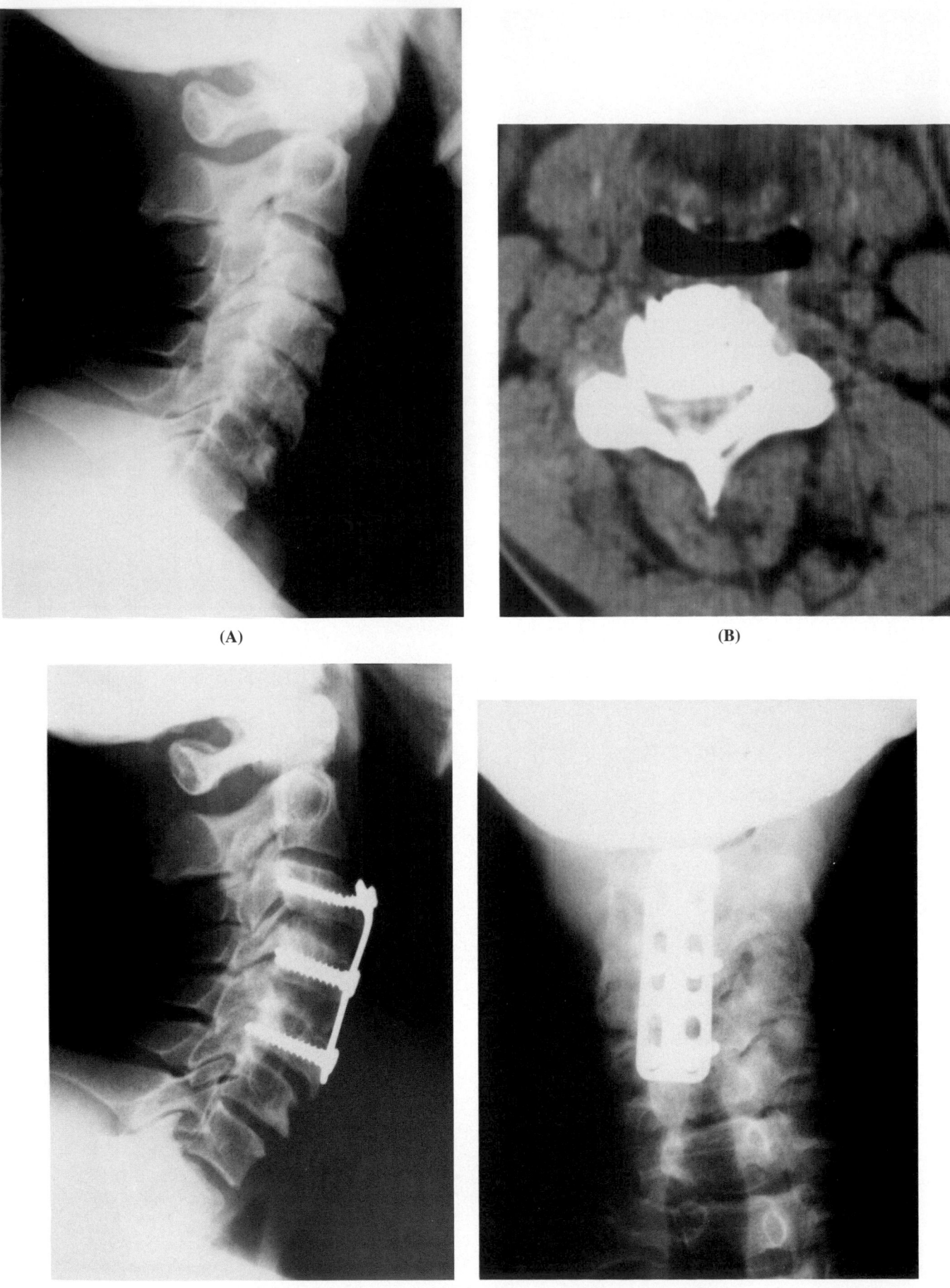

(A)

(B)

(C)

(D)

Figure 20–20 Cervical spondylosis and spinal stenosis, illustrated by a lateral plain radiograph *(A)* and myelogram *(B)*. Fixation with Caspar plates and screws is illustrated *(C, D)*.

TREATMENT OF SPINAL STENOSIS

Stenotic lesions occur at one or two levels or are more generalized, sometimes affecting an entire section of the spinal canal. Almost all of the cervical or lumbar spinal canal may be involved. On occasion, especially in achondroplastic patients or those with hypochondroplasia, the entire spinal canal is implicated.

OPERATIVE TECHNIQUE: CERVICAL AND THORACIC

In the cervical area, when one or two segments are involved, the spinal canal is usually decompressed by removing the offending hypertrophic bony lesions through diskectomy and fusion via an anterior approach. This proceeds in the same way it is described for performing an anterior diskectomy, but taking care to remove the offending osteophytes by drilling or rongeuring.

When multiple levels are involved, a laminectomy appears more appropriate, thus avoiding the need to immobilize a major part of the spinal canal. This is usually accomplished by exposing the spinous processes and laminae from C2 to C7 and drilling a trough through the lateral edge of the laminae with a power drill and burr. Such a technique allows the removal of spinous processes and laminae without compromising the spinal canal by the introduction of instruments.

Usually there is more space around the spinal cord at the levels of C2 and C7. When laminectomy has been extended to these limits, it has often gone beyond the area of constriction, and the normal lordotic curve tends to allow the spinal cord to move away from any ventral osteophytes. The facets should be preserved wherever possible in order to minimize the chances for deformity.[71,72,73,74,75] On occasion, disk herniations may occur after a decompressive laminectomy, in which case an anterior diskectomy might be required. However, such occurrences have been rare and limited to a single level in the authors' experience.

A refinement which has recently been recommended for use in cervical stenosis is the *suspension laminotomy,* in which the laminae are divided and separated from the lateral elements by fragments of bone held in place by sutures.[76] This technique adds significantly to the surgical procedure but reportedly reduces the incidence of complicating deformities, and the long-term neurological outcome is reportedly improved.[77] (See Fig. 20-21.)

For power drilling in laminectomy or laminotomy, a diamond burr is usually used to drill through the laminae in order to avoid leaving bits of metal in the wound. Retained metal produces artifacts on images performed with magnetic resonance.

Stenosis in the thoracic canal was thought to be rare in the past, but reports of such lesions have appeared in recent years.[19,20] It may be that more sophisticated and frequent imaging has resulted in better diagnosis of this entity. Treatment is similar to the treatment for stenosis in the cervical area.

Stenosis at a single level due to osteophytes is best treated by a diskectomy through an anterolateral approach through the chest, while narrowing over several segments is probably best treated by laminectomy through a posterior approach as described for the cervical area.

Stenosis in the lumbar area is usually limited to one or two levels—most commonly L4–L5 and, perhaps, L3–L4 or L5–S1. Decompressive laminectomy at the appropriate levels is the treatment of choice.[29] Fusion will reduce the chances for spondylolisthesis but is not routinely performed. Interbody fusions may be performed at one or two levels.[56,57] Lateral fusions, between the transverse processes may be used, or fusions may be performed in conjunction with use of screws inserted into the vertebral bodies through the associated pedicles and plates or rods.[69,70,78,79]

□ SPONDYLOLISTHESIS

Spondylolisthesis is malalignment of vertebral bodies where an upper body slips forward on its subjacent neighbor. The malalignment may be asymptomatic, but there may also be compression of nerve roots or the cauda equina with resultant severe pain. The pain is often localized, but it may be radicular, involving: the nerve root exiting at the level of the defect, the nerve root exiting at the level below the defect, or roots still retained within the cauda equina and located within the center of the spinal canal that are being compressed by the anteriorily displaced lamina.

Spondylolisthesis is classified as *dysplastic, isthmic, degenerative, posttraumatic,* or *pathological.*[80] Dysplastic cases occur in children, most often at the lumbosacral junction; there is a strong hereditary component. Isthmic spondylolisthesis is subdivided into (1) lytic, in which case there is a separation of the pars from a fatigue fracture, (2) elongation of the pars without separation, in which case there are frequently found fine fractures within the pars, and (3) acute fractures in the pars. Such lesions occur in young adults. Degenerative spondylolisthesis is found in adults, almost invariably above the age of 40, and cases are 6 times as common among women as men. Posttraumatic spondylolisthesis occurs when there is severe trauma. The fractures are found in structures other than the pars. Dislocations occur gradually in these cases.

Our experience with spondylolisthesis has been almost exclusively with adults of the isthmic type and in cases of the degenerative type. Most cases of spondylolisthesis in children are of the dysplastic variety, and the majority can be treated conservatively. In degenerative spondylolisthesis, pain is the indication for therapy. The pain follows a sciatic distribution in 70 percent of cases and a pattern of neurogenic claudication in 30 percent of patients.[80]

TREATMENT OF SPONDYLOLISTHESIS

Treatment consists of decompression and fusion using a posterior lumbar interbody fusion or lateral spinal fusion.

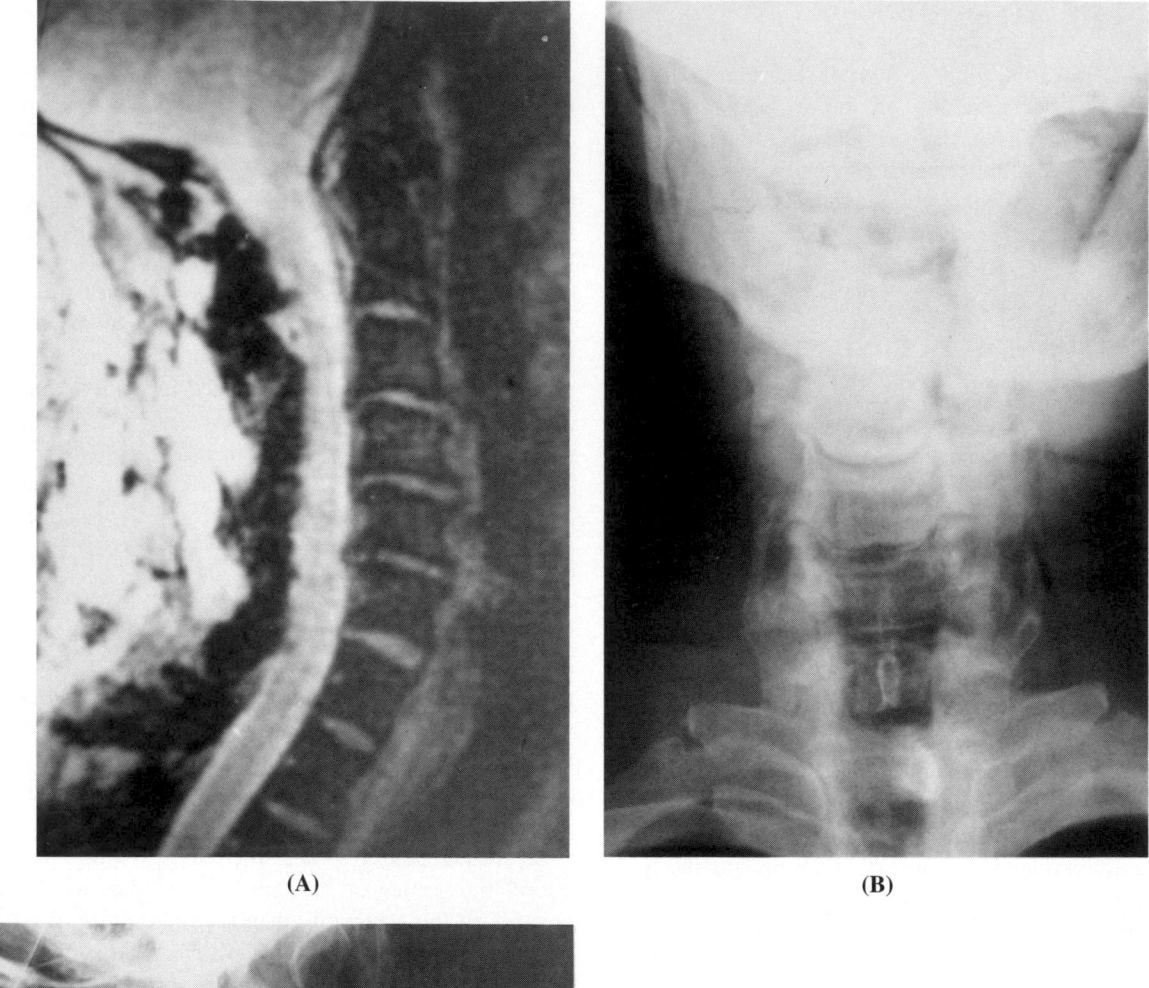

(A)

(B)

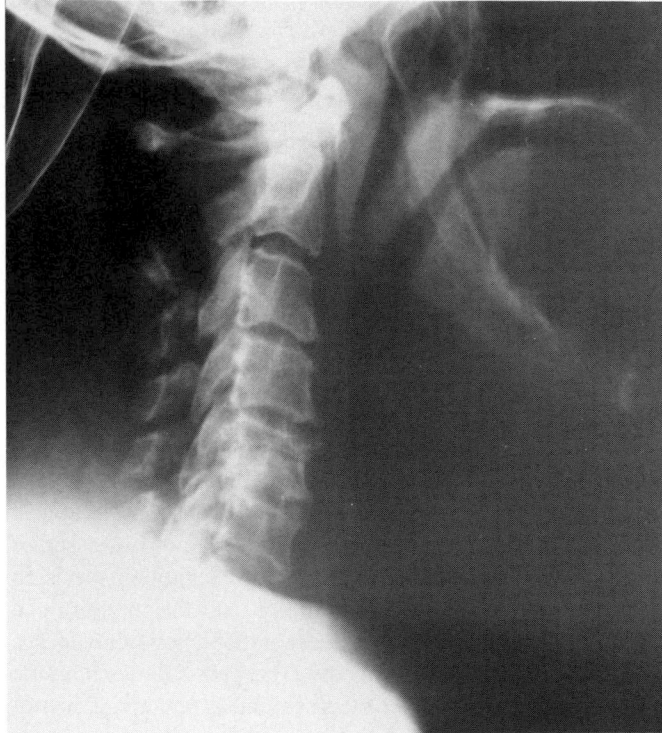

(C)

Figure 20–21 Cervical spondylosis and stenosis producing myelopathy, illustrated on the lateral MRI scan *(A)*, treated by suspension laminotomy. Postoperative radiographs are presented *(B, C)*.

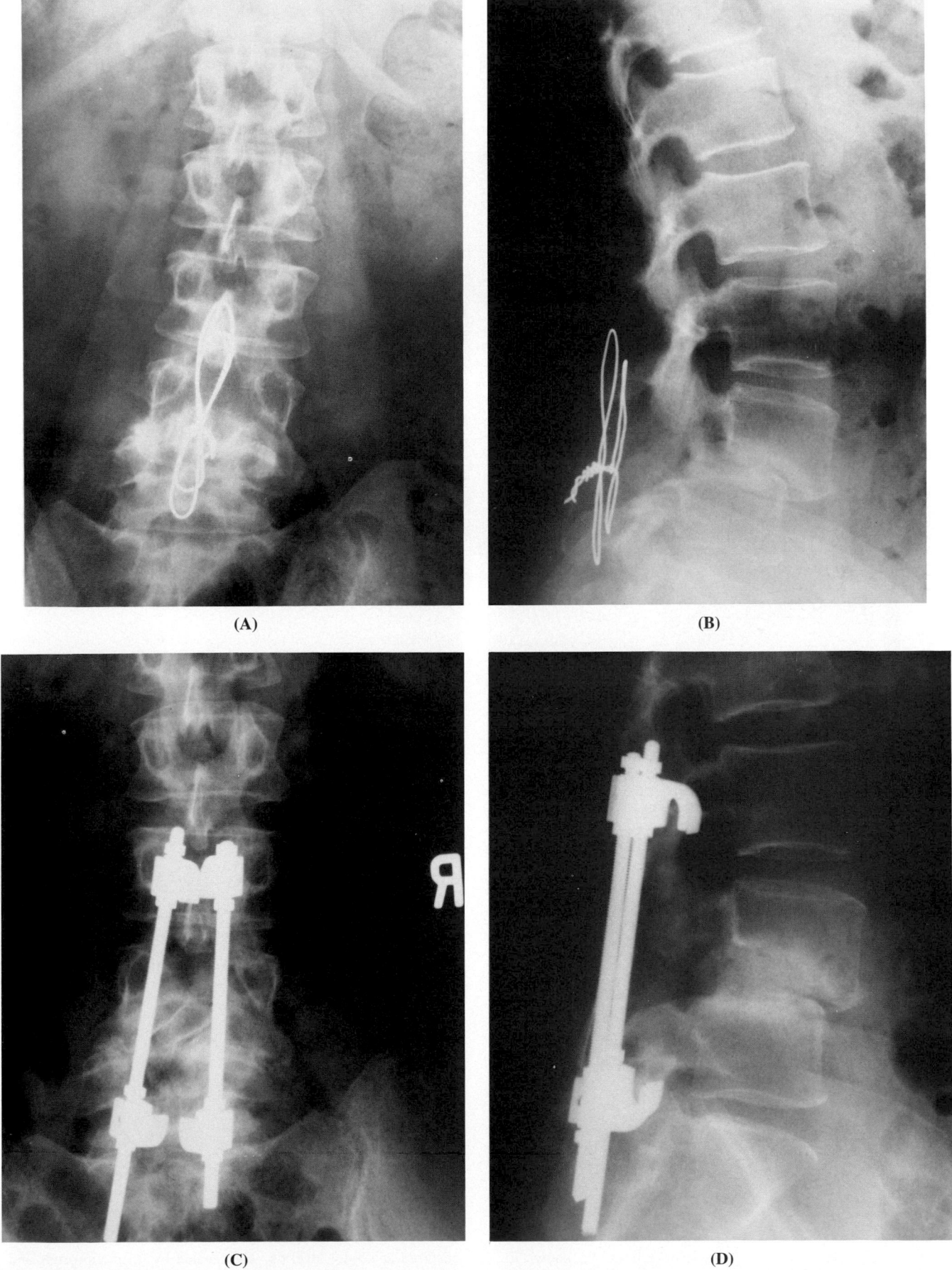

(A)

(B)

(C)

(D)

Figure 20–22 Spondylolisthesis treated by posterior lateral interbody fusion and subsequent intraspinous wiring because of failure
of the fusion at an outside hospital *(A, B)*. The bone grafts were
replaced and compression rods applied for greater stability *(C, D)*.

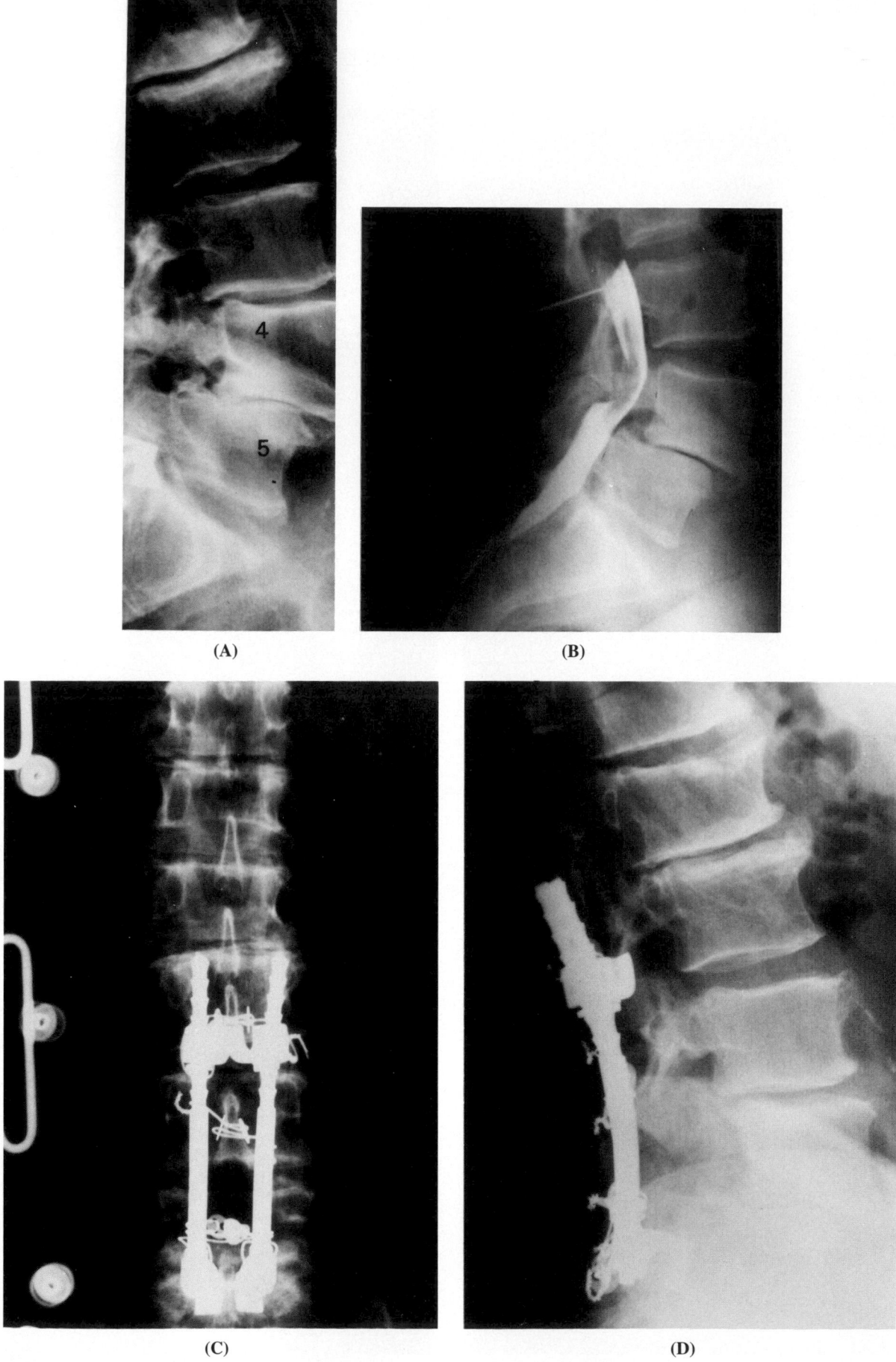

(A)

(B)

(C)

(D)

Figure 20–23 Degenerative spondylolisthesis L4–L5 known to have been present at least 5 years in a 63-year-old male who began experiencing severe back and radicular pain when retrolisthesis occurred at L3–L4 level *(A, B)*. Treated by distraction rods and fusion with excellent relief for 2 years *(C, D)*.

(See Figs. 20-22 and 20-23.) Most of the authors' cases in the past have been treated with posterior lumbar interbody fusion obtaining solid fusions and often with some residual localized back pain, which we ascribe to residual degenerative processes at adjacent levels. More recent cases have been treated with pedicle screws and rods. In his extensive review, Wiltse, combining decompression with a posterior lateral fusion, indicates that removal of all the posterior elements was associated with adequate relief of pain in about 30 percent of cases, whereas good results were obtained in about 70 percent of cases when the decompression was limited to the midline structures.[80] There was no good explanation for this paradoxical result.

A recently introduced procedure that is becoming a popular form of therapy for the treatment of spondylolisthesis of the more limited grades, is insertion of transpedicular screws in conjunction with segmental plates or rods.[78,79] The screws can be used to draw the vertebrae into alignment.

Patients may be ambulated very rapidly after spinal fusion of the interbody or intertransverse process variety or after fixation with pedicular screws. It has been recommended that if patients who have been fused by intertransverse process fusion experience progressive deformity during the early postoperative period, they should be returned to bed rest for 6 to 8 weeks. Progression of deformity is less likely following interbody fusions or treatment with pedicle screws.

☐ DEGENERATIVE SCOLIOSIS

Degenerative processes throughout the lumbar spinal column with relaxation of the ligaments may result in the development of *scoliosis*. Patients frequently complain of severe radicular pain. (See Fig. 20-24.) Myelography reveals evidence of stenosis and defects consistent with protrusions or extrusions of intervertebral disks. There are usually degenerative disk lesions with protrusions at multiple levels. Neurological deficits are variable.

Diskectomy often fails to relieve pain or may result in switching pain from one side to the other. Our most gratifying experience in the treatment of this lesion or series of lesions has been with the use of instrumentation (see Fig. 20-25), usually with distraction rods, although laminectomy and segmental plating appears to be equally promising, if not superior. Degenerative lesions of the spine can be expected to be more common in the future with an aging population. The salvage procedures described above show promise for making life more enjoyable for patients with progressive deterioration of the spinal column.

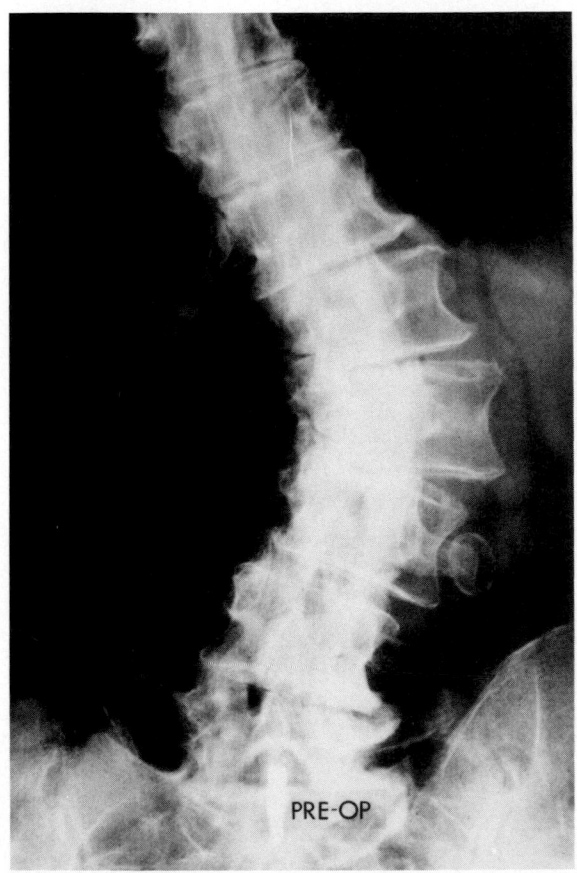

PRE-OP

(A)

Figure 20–24 Lumbar spondylosis with stenosis and scoliosis seen in the frontal radiograph and during myelography *(A)*. Treated by distraction rods and fusion with excellent relief of pain despite poor anatomical realignment *(B, C)*.

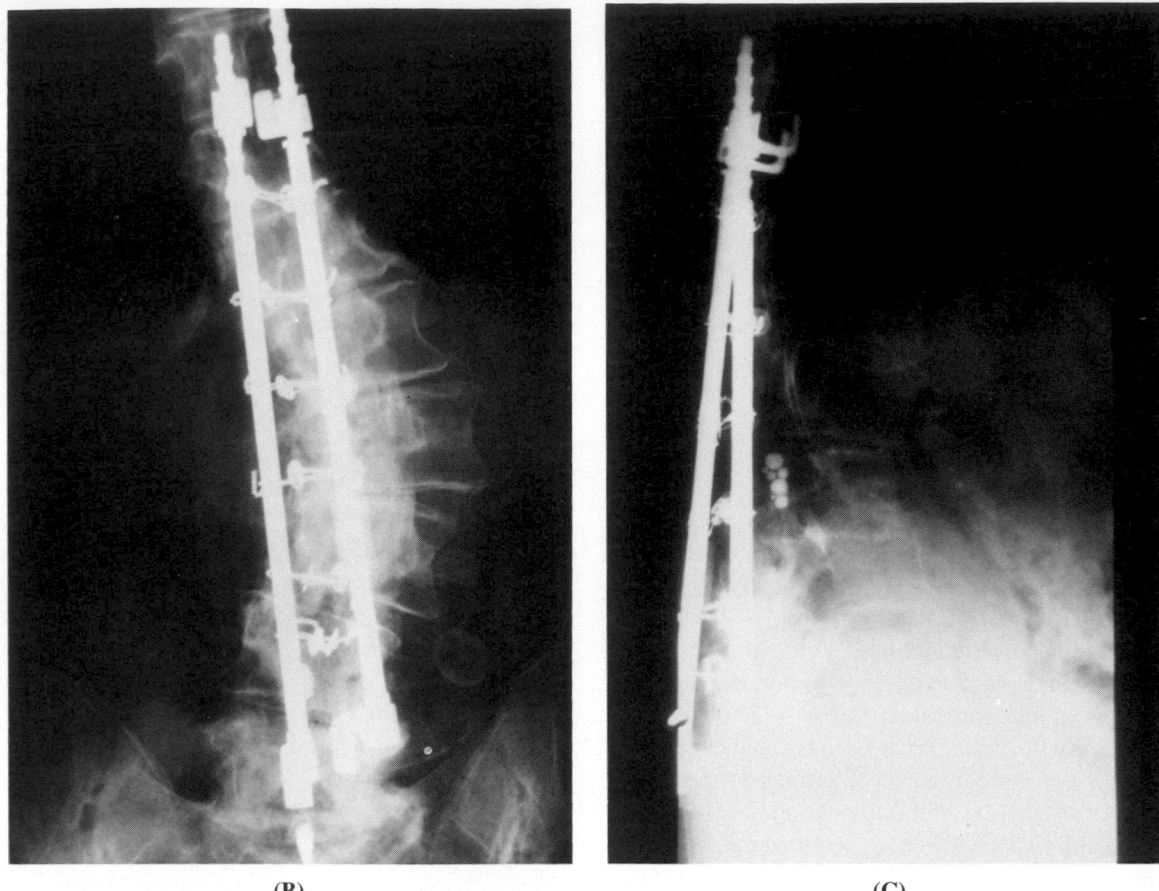

(B)   (C)

Figure 20–24 Continued

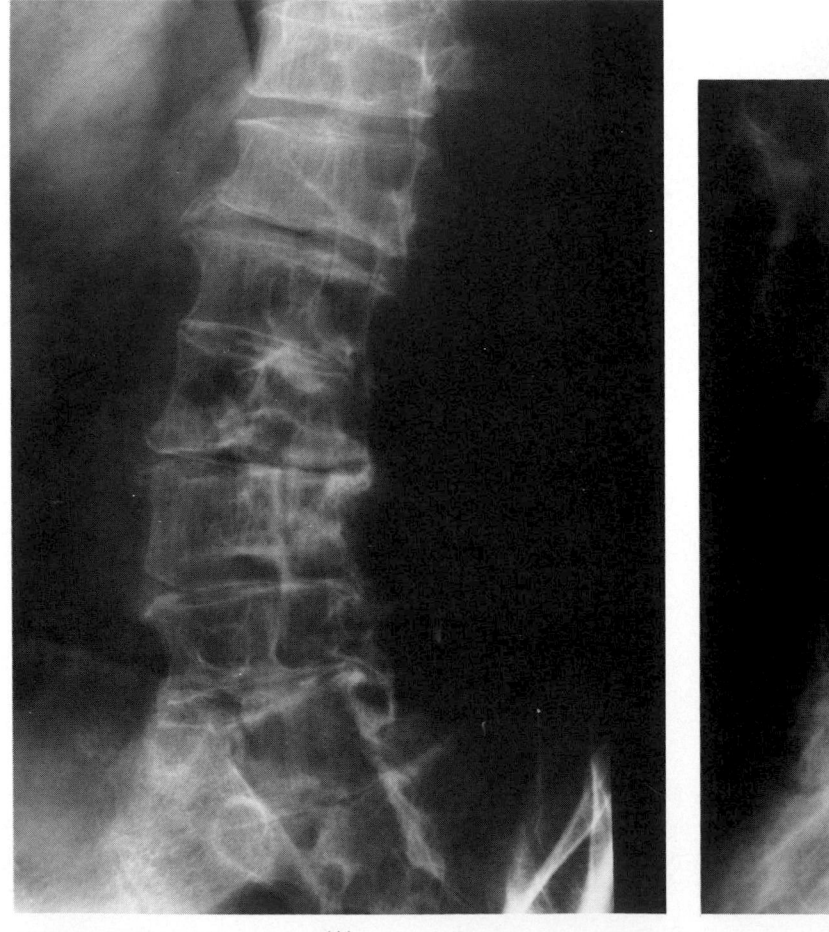

(A)

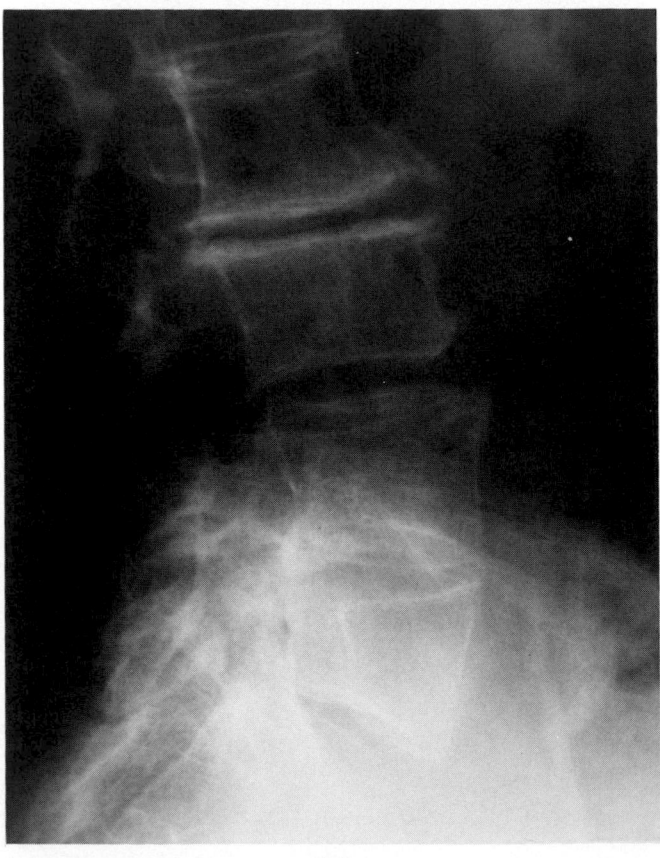

(B)

Figure 20–25 Lumbar spondylosis and scoliosis seen in frontal and lateral views, the lateral view from a myelogram *(A, B)*.

Treated with pedicle screw fixation and fusion *(C, D)*.

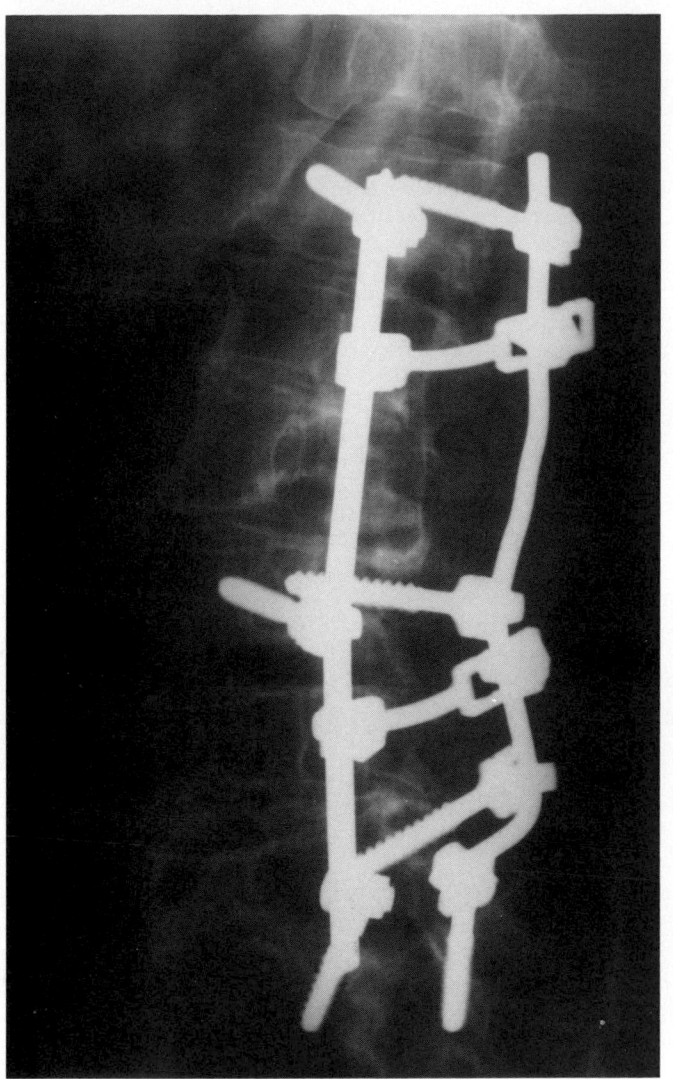

(C)

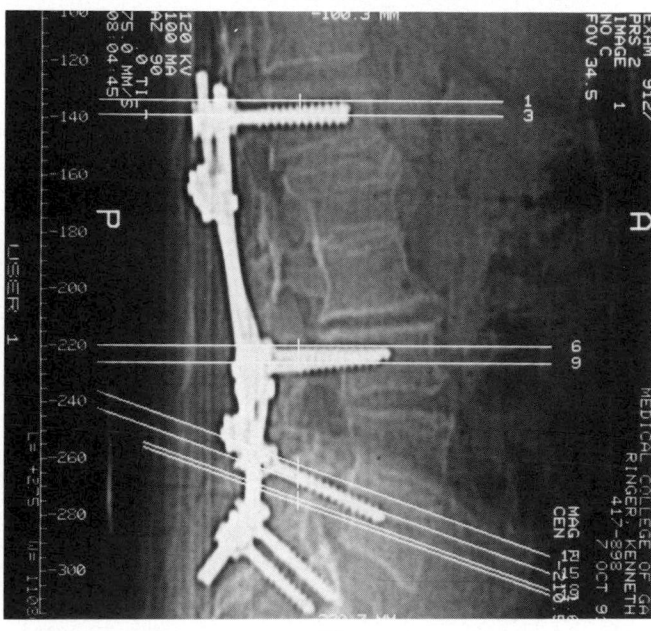

(D)

Figure 20–25   Continued

REFERENCES

1. Gower WE, Pedrini V: Age-related variations in proteinpoly-saccharides from human nucleus pulposus, annulus fibrosus, and costal cartilage. *J Bone Jt Surg* 51A:1154–1162, 1969.
2. Hendry NGC: The hydration of the nucleus pulposus and its relation to intervertebral disc derangement. *J Bone Jt Surg* 40B:132–144, 1958.
3. Markolf KL, Morris JM: The structural components of the intervertebral disc. *J Bone Jt Surg* 56A:675–687, 1974.
4. Eyring EJ: The biochemistry and physiology of the intervertebral disk: A study of their contributions to the ability of the disk to withstand compressive forces. *Clin Orth Rel Res* 67:16–28, 1969.
5. Kirkaldy-Willis WH, Wedge JH, Yong-Hing K, Reilly J: Pathology and pathogenesis of lumbar spondylosis and stenosis. *Spine* 3:319–328, 1978.
6. Bernardo KL, Grubb RL, Coxe WS, Roper CL: Anterior cervical disc herniation: Case report. *J Neurosurg* 69:134–136, 1988.
7. Brandenburg G, Leibrock LG: Dysphagia and dysphonia secondary to anterior cervical osteophytes. *Neurosurg* 18:90–93, 1986.
8. Cloward, RB: Anterior herniation of a ruptured lumbar intervertebral disk. *Arch Surg* 64:457–463, 1952.
9. Jinkins JR, Whittemore AR, Bradley WG: The anatomic basis of vertebrogenic pain and the autonomic syndrome associated with lumbar disk extrusion. *AJR* 152:1277–1289, 1989.
10. Takata K, Inoue S, Takhashi K, Ohtsuka Y: Swelling of the cauda equina in patients who have herniation of a lumbar disc. A possible pathogenesis of sciatica. *J Bone Jt Surg* 70A:361–368, 1988.

11. Edelson JG, Nathan H: Stages in the natural history of the vertebral end-plates. *Spine* 131:21–26, 1988.

12. Ciric I, Mikhael MA, Tarkington JA, Vick NA: The lateral recess syndrome: A variant of spinal stenosis. *J Neurosurg* 53:433–443, 1980.

13. Hayashi H, Okada K, Hamada M, Tada K, Ueno R: Etiologic factor of myelopathy. A radiographic evaluation of the aging changes in the cervical spine. *Clin Orthop* 214:200–209, 1987.

14. Kubota T, Sato K, Kawano H, et al: Ultrastructure of early calcification in cervical ossification of the posterior longitudinal ligament. *J Neurol* 61:131–135, 1984.

15. Lee BG, Fager CA, Freidberg SR, Tarlov E: Cervical myelopathy due to ossification of the posterior longitudinal ligament. *Neurosurgery* 19:154, 1986.

16. Klara PM, McDonnell DE: Ossification of the posterior longitudinal ligament in Caucasians: Diagnosis and surgical intervention. *Neurosurgery* 19:212–217, 1986.

17. Abo H, Tsuru M, Ito T, et al: Anterior decompression for ossification of the posterior longitudinal ligament of the cervical spine. *J Neurol* 55:108–116, 1981.

18. Yonenobu K, Ebara S, Fujiwara K, et al: Thoracic myelopathy secondary to ossification of the spinal ligament. *J Neurosurg* 66:511–518, 1987.

19. Barnett GH, Hardy RW Jr, Little JR, et al: Thoracic spinal canal stenosis: *J Neurosurg* 66:338–344, 1987.

20. Yamamoto I, Matsumae M, Ikeda A, et al: Thoracic spinal stenosis: Experience with seven cases. *J Neurosurg* 68:37–40, 1988.

21. MacNab, I: The traction spur: An indicator of segmental instability. *J Bone Jt Surg* 53A:663–670, 1971.

22. Rawat SS, Jain GH, Gupta HKD: Intra-abdominal symptoms arising from spinal osteophytes. *Br J Surg* 62:320–322, 1975.

23. Epstein JA, Epstein BS, Lavine LS, et al: Cervical myeloradiculopathy caused by arthritic hypertrophy of the posterior facets and laminae. *J Neurosurg* 49:387–392, 1978.

24. Hukuda S, Mochizuki T, Ogata M, et al: Operations for cervical spondylotic myelopathy: A comparison of the results of anterior and posterior procedures. *J Bone Jt Surg* 67B:609–615, 1985.

25. Valergakis FE: Cervical spondylosis: Most common cause of position and vibratory sense loss. *Geriatrics* 31:51–56, 1976.

26. Schneider RC, Cherry G, Pantek H: The syndrome of acute central cervical spinal cord injury with special reference to the mechanisms involved in hyperextension injuries of cervical spine. *J Neurosurg* 11:546–577, 1954.

27. Petropoulos BP: Lumbar spinal stenosis syndrome. *Clin Orthop* 246:70–80, 1989.

28. Alexander E Jr: Significance of the small lumbar spinal canal: Cauda equina compression syndromes due to spondylosis. *J Neurosurg* 31:513–519, 1969.

29. Ganz JC: Lumbar spinal stenosis: postoperative results in terms of preoperative posture-related pain. *J Neurosurg* 72:71–74, 1990.

30. Odom GL, Finney W, Woodall B: Cervical disk lesions. *JAMA* 166:23–28, 1958.

31. Williams JL, Allen MB Jr, Harkess JW: Late results of cervical discectomy and interbody fusion: Some factors influencing the results. *J Bone Jt Surg* 50A:277–286, 1968.

32. Nelson KR, Rivner MH: Electromyography and nerve conduction laboratory in clinical neurologic practice. *Semin Neurol* 10:131–140, 1990.

33. Wilbourn AJ, Aminoff MJ: The electrophysiologic examination in patients with radiculopathies. *Muscle Nerve* 11:1099–1114, 1988.

34. Wiesel SW, Tsourmas N, Feffer HL, et al: A study of computer-assisted tomography. I. The incidence of positive CAT scans in an asymptomatic group of patients. *Spine* 9:549–551, 1984.

35. Forristall RM, Marsh HO, Pay NT: Magnetic resonance imaging and contrast CT of the lumbar spine: Comparison of diagnostic methods and correlation with surgical findings. *Spine* 13:1049–1054, 1988.

36. Hesselink JR: Spine imaging: History, achievements, remaining frontiers. *AJR* 150:1223–1229, 1988.

37. Brown BM, Schwartz RH, Frank E, Blank NK: Preoperative evaluation of cervical radiculopathy and myelopathy by surface-coil MR imaging. *AJR* 151:1205–1212, 1988.

38. Hueftle MG, Modic MT, Ross JS, et al: Lumbar spine: Postoperative MR imaging with Gd-DTPA. *Radiology* 167:817–824, 1988.

39. Epstein NE, Hyman RA, Epstein JA, Rosenthal AD: Technical note: "Dynamic" MRI scanning of the cervical spine. *Spine* 13:937–938, 1988.

40. Boden SD, Davis DO, Dina TS, et al: Abnormal magnetic-resonance scans of the lumbar spine in asymptomatic subjects. *J Bone Jt Surg* 72A:403–408, 1990.

41. Antti-Poike I, Soini J, Tallroth K, et al: Clinical relevance of discography combined with CT scanning: A study of 100 patients. *J Bone Jt Surg* 72B:480–485, 1990.

42. Guyer RD, Collier R, Stith WJ, et al: Discitis after discography. *Spine* 13:1352–1354, 1988.

43. Thomas AMC, Afshar F: The microsurgical treatment of lumbar disc protrusions: Follow-up of 60 cases. *J Bone Jt Surg* 69B:696–698, 1987.

44. Gibson MJ, Buckley J, Mulholland RC, Worthington BS: The charges in the intervertebral disc after chemonucleolysis demonstrated by magnetic resonance imaging. *J Bone Jt Surg* 68B:719–723, 1986.

45. Chu KH: Collagen chemonucleolysis via epidural injection: A review of 252 cases. *Clin Orthop* 215:99–104, 1987.

46. Bouillet R: Treatment of sciatica: A comparative survey of complications of surgical treatment and nucleolysis with chymopapain. *Clin Orthop* 251:144–152, 1990.

47. Alexander AH, Burkus JK, Mitchell JB, Ayers WV: Chymopapain chemonucleolysis versus surgical discectomy in a military population. *Clin Orthop* 244:158–165, 1989.

48. Cuckler JM, Bernini PA, Wiesel SW, et al: The use of epidural steroids in the treatment of lumbar radicular pain: A prospective, randomized, double-blind study. *J Bone Jt Surg* 67A:63–66, 1985.

49. White, AH: Injection techniques for the diagnosis and treatment of low back pain. *Orthop Clin N Amer* 14:553–567, 1983.

50. Davis GW, Onik G: Clinical experience with automated percutaneous lumbar discectomy. *Clin Orthop* 238:98–103, 1989.

51. Hoppenfeld S: Percutaneous removal of herniated lumbar discs: 50 cases with ten-year follow-up periods. *Clin Orthop* 238:92–97, 1989.

52. Onik G, Maroon J, Helms C, et al: Automated percutaneous diskectomy: Initial patient experience. Work in progress. *Radiol* 162:129–132, 1987.

53. Stern MB: Early experience with percutaneous lateral discectomy. *Clin Orthop* 238:50–55, 1989.

54. Montalvo BM, Quencher RM, Brown MB, et al: Lumbar disk herniation and canal stenosis: Value of intraoperative sonography in diagnosis and surgical management. *AJR* 154:821–830, 1990.

55. Hopp E, Tsou PM: Post decompression lumbar instability. *Clin Orthop* 227:143–151, 1988.

56. Selby DK, Gill K, Blumenthal SL, et al: Fusion of the lumbar spine, in Youmans, JR (ed): *Neurological Surgery,* 3d ed. Philadelphia, Saunders, 1990, chap 95, pp 2785–2804.

57. Selby DK: Posterior lumbar fusion, in clinical entities, in Weinstein JN, Wiesel SW (eds): *The Lumbar Spine.* Philadelphia, Saunders, 1990, chap 7, pp 456–470.

58. Cloward RB: Posterior lumbar interbody fusion updated. *Clin Orthop* 193:16–19, 1985.
59. Lin PM: Posterior lumbar interbody fusion technique: Complications and pitfalls. *Clin Orthop* 193:90–102, 1985.
60. Maroon JC, Kopitnik TA, Schulhof LA, et al: Diagnosis and microsurgical approach to far-lateral disc herniation in the lumbar spine. *J Neurosurg* 72:378–382, 1990.
61. Blankstein A, Rubinstein E, Ezra E, et al: Disc space infection and vertebral osteomyelitis as a complication of percutaneous lateral discectomy. *Clin Orthop* 225:234–237, 1987.
62. Dall BE, Rowe DE, Odette WG, Batts DH: Postoperative discitis. Diagnosis and management. *Clin Orthop* 224:138–146, 1987.
63. Cloward RB: The anterior approach for removal of ruptured cervical disks. *J Neurosurg* 15:602–617, 1958.
64. Smith GW, Robinson RA: The treatment of certain cervical-spine disorders by anterior removal of the intervertebral disc and interbody fusion. *J Bone Jt Surg* 40A:607–624, 1958.
65. Robinson RA, Smith GW: Anterolateral cervical disc removal and interbody fusion for cervical disc syndrome. *Bull Johns Hopk Hosp* 96:223–224, 1955.
66. Hedge S, Staas WE Jr: Thoracic disc herniation and spinal cord injury. *Am J Phys Med Rehab* 167:228–229, 1988.
67. Perot PL Jr, Munro DD: Transthoracic removal of midline thoracic disc protrusions causing spinal cord compression. *J Neurosurg* 31:452–458, 1969.
68. Ransohoff J, Spencer F, Siew F, Gage L: Transthoracic removal of thoracic disc: Report of three cases. *J Neurosurg* 31:459–461, 1969.
69. Hulme A: The surgical approach to thoracic intervertebral disc protrusions. *J Neurol Neurosurg Psychiatr* 23:133–137, 1960.
70. Bohlman HH, Zdeblick TA: Anterior excision of herniated discs. *J Bone Jt Surg* 70A:1038–1047, 1989.
71. Lonstein JE: Post laminectomy kyphosis. *Clin Orthop* 128:93–100, 1977.
72. Lonstein JE: Post laminectomy kyphosis, in Chou SN, Seljeskog EL (eds): *Spinal Deformities and Neurological Dysfunction.* New York, Raven Press, 1978, pp 53–63.
73. Sim FH, Svien HJ, Bickel WH, James JM: Swan-neck deformity following extensive cervical laminectomy. *J Bone Jt Surg* 56A:564–580, 1974.
74. Yasuoka S, Peterson HA, Laws ER Jr, MacCarty CS: Pathogensis and prophylaxis of postlaminectomy deformity of the spine after multiple level laminectomy: Difference between children and adults. *Neurosurgery* 9:145–152, 1981.
75. Yasuoka S, Peterson HA, MacCarty CS: Incidence of spinal column deformity after multilevel laminectomy in children and adults. *J Neurosurg* 57:441–445, 1982.
76. Ohmori K, Ishida Y, Suzuki K: Suspension Laminotomy: A new surgical technique for compression myelopathy. *Neurosurg* 21:950–957, 1987.
77. Ishida Y, Suzuki K, Ohmori K, et al: Critical analysis of extensive laminectomy. *Neurosurg* 24:215–224, 1989.
78. Steffee AD, Biscup RS, Sitkowski DJ: Segmental spine plates with pedicle screw fixation: A new internal fixation device for disorders of the lumbar and thoraco lumbar spine. *Clin Orthop* 203:45–53, 1986.
79. Steffee AD, Sitkowski DJ: Posterior lumbar interbody fusion and plates. *Clin Orthop* 227:99–102, 1988.
80. Wiltse LL: Classification and treatment of spondylolisthesis, in Evarts CM (ed): *Surgery of the Musculoskeletal System.* New York, Churchill Livingstone, chap 19, pp 411–425.

☐ STUDY QUESTIONS

I. A 26-year-old policeman who has recently been appointed to the force is seen because of severe pain in the right lower extremity. The patient gives a history of having had sudden onset of lumbar back pain when helping to lift a refrigerator, while cleaning out his garage 2 years earlier. The pain persisted for 2 weeks then subsided.

He had two other occurrences of localized pain, radiating into the right hip in the interim, each resolving when he went to bed for 2 days. The episodes occurred while he was getting out of his automobile.

The latest episode of pain happened when he was taking calisthenics in training for his new position on the police force. On examination, the patient had hypalgesia over the dorsum of the foot with sensation to pinprick becoming normal at about the site of the metatarsal of the third toe. Knee and ankle jerks were normal but the patient dragged his right foot when he walked, and there was weakness of dorsiflexion of the right foot and some atrophy of the intrinsic muscles of the right foot.

1. What is the most likely diagnosis? **2.** What studies, if any, should be obtained? **3.** What treatment should be initiated? **4.** Should surgery be considered? If so, when? **5.** What might one expect to find on nerve conduction studies? On EMG the day after acute onset of pain? Two weeks later?

II. A 42-year-old housewife is referred because of pain in the neck and left upper extremity. The pain has been progressive for 6 months. The pain usually improves, although it is not absent when she gets up in the morning. It becomes worse as the day goes on. It is made much worse when she drives, especially as she turns her head. Indeed, she is unable to look behind her. Pain is exacerbated by coughing.

On examination, there is tenderness on palpation of the lateral surface of the neck. The neck is held quite straight. There is atrophy and weakness of the left biceps muscle, and the biceps reflex is absent, as is the radial periosteal reflex. There is hypalgesia over the thumb and index finger.

1. What is the most likely anatomical diagnosis? **2.** What might one expect to see on plain radiographs of the neck? **3.** What treatment(s) might be considered? **4.** What other studies might be considered? **5.** What might one expect to see on an EMG when the patient is seen first? Why?

III. A 48-year-old male laborer is seen because of progressive difficulty walking, which has worsened over the 3 months prior to his visit.

On examination, the patient has good strength in the upper and lower extremities. Deep tendon reflexes at the biceps and radial-periosteal sties are normal, but the triceps reflexes are quite fast. Deep tendon reflexes at the knees and ankles are brisk (4+), and clonus is present at each of these sites. Vibratory and position senses are slightly reduced in the lower extremities. The patient denies pain throughout the examination.

1. Where might a lesion be localized? **2.** What diagnoses should be considered? **3.** An MRI demonstrates a narrow spinal canal in the cervical area and impingement on the cord by slightly protruding disks at C3–C4, C4–C5, and C5–C6. What surgical treatments might be considered? **4.** Why is this patient not complaining of pain? **5.** What might one expect to be accomplished by surgery insofar as neurological disability is concerned?

IV. A 60-year-old postman has to stop working because of back pain and pain in the legs when he walks. While he has localized back pain at all times, the pain is much worse when he ambulates. Both the back and leg pain are much improved when the patient sits or lies down for 15 to 20 min. He always feels more comfortable when sitting in a flexed position.

Neurological examination is normal. Pulses in both lower extremities are normal. Plain x-rays of the lumbar spine demonstrate loss of lordosis on the lateral views and a mild scoliosis with concavity to the left on frontal views. There are degenerative changes at every level, most marked at L4–L5, with large osteophytes at that level.

1. What diagnoses should be entertained? **2.** What further studies should be considered? **3.** Assuming a myelogram shows failure of the contrast media to go below L4 when the patient is upright and that changes are indicative of extradural compression from anteriorly and laterally, what surgical therapy might be considered? **4.** What types of stabilization might be considered? **5.** Assuming that the patient had x-rays made 10 years earlier which show no evidence of scoliosis, what might be some explanations for the scoliosis?

V. A 35-year-old obese female nurse experiences mid-thoracic back pain after lifting a patient. Over a period of 3 months, the pain begins to radiate around the chest into the upper abdomen. She develops weakness and mild spasticity of her legs and decreased sensation to pinprick over the lower abdomen and lower extremities.

Plain radiographs of the thoracic spine reveal hypertrophic changes at the T8–T9 level and gas in the intervertebral disk at that level.

1. What diagnoses should be entertained? **2.** What investigations might be carried out? **3.** Assuming a midline herniated intervertebral disk is demonstrated at the T8–T9 level, how might it be treated? **4.** What might explain the hypertrophic changes in the bone surrounding the disk space? **5.** What nerve roots might be affected?

CHAPTER
21

Surgery of Peripheral Nerves

Geoffrey P. Cole
Joseph R. Smith

☐ BASIC ANATOMY AND METABOLISM OF PERIPHERAL NERVES

Peripheral nerves include *motor, sensory,* and *autonomic fibers.* Cell bodies for peripheral motor nerve fibers are located in the anterior horns of the spinal cord. The cell bodies of the preganglionic sympathetic nerves are located at the intermediolateral cell column from T1–L2. The cell bodies of the peripheral sensory nerve fibers are located in the dorsal root ganglia just outside the spinal canal.

Nerve fibers are composed of a central *axon* surrounded by a single layer of *Schwann cells.* (See Fig. 21-1.) About a fifth of the nerve fibers are *myelinated.*[1] The myelin is contained within the Schwann cells in a multilayered spiral concentric sheath. The outer basement membrane of the Schwann cell, seen only by electron microscopy, is referred to as the *endoneural sheath.* Schwann cells are sequentially located so that many may cover an individual axon.

Points of junction of Schwann cells are called *nodes of Ranvier,* where, in myelinated nerves, there is a brief segment of axon without myelin. (See Fig. 21-2.) This has physiological significance in that conduction along a myelinated nerve fiber is much more rapid because the nerve action potential in a myelinated nerve "jumps" from one node to another (*saltatory conduction*) rather than traveling directly along the entire length of the axon, as in the case of unmyelinated fibers.

Individual nerve fibers—and their Schwann cell sheaths in the case of myelinated axons—are surrounded by a thin tubule of collagen fibers, the *endoneurium.*

Groups of nerve fibers are collected into bundles, or *fascicles,* encircled by the *perineurium,* another collagen sheath. (See Fig. 21-3.) Variable numbers of fascicles will be collected together to form a nerve surrounded by an external *epineurium.*

Within the external epineurium and between the fascicles is the internal epineurium. There may be one, a few, or numerous fascicles within a nerve.

Peripheral nerves are supplied by external segmental blood vessels that give off segmental branches that supply intrinsic longitudinal vessels. (See Fig. 21-4.) Microvessels run within the epineurium and perineurium, but only capillaries are found in the endoneurium.[2] Preservation of the more complex external blood supply takes on considerable importance when one is attempting to develop free vascularized grafts.[3]

There is significant positional change in the fascicular pattern throughout the length of nerves, so that the cross-sectional localization of a given fascicle may change over just the course of a few millimeters.[4] This exchange in pattern is much more prevalent in proximal segments of nerves than distal.

There are also major positional changes in the motor and sensory fascicles that travel to various segments of the arm—within and just distal to the brachial plexus. Most of this cross-sectional positional change has occurred by the time the level of the elbow is reached. In fact, fascicles innervating a digit may travel for several centimeters in the forearm with very few positional changes.[5]

Metabolism of peripheral nerves is focused at the cell body, from which axoplasm and transmitter substances are transported toward the nerve terminals.[6,7] Similarly, unused transmitter substances are transported back to the cell body.[8]

Exact mechanisms of transport are unclear, but rates have been determined. Some materials prepared in the cell body are transmitted at a rate of 1 to 6 mm per day, whereas transmitter substances move much more rapidly, up to 410 mm per day.[9,10] Retrograde transport is reported to occur at a more constant rate of about 240 mm per day.[8,10]

Metabolism at the cell body increases significantly at the time of interruption of a peripheral nerve. The degree of augmentation depends, to some extent, on the distance of

419

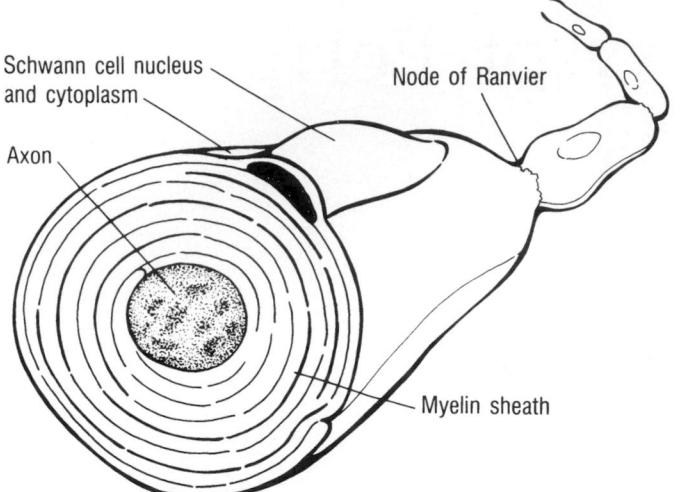

Figure 21–1 Microscopic anatomy of myelinated peripheral nerve fiber.

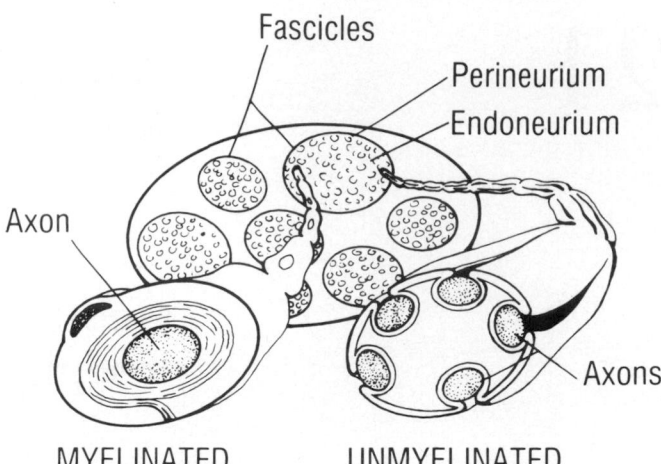

Figure 21–3 Anatomy of peripheral nerve. Note endoneurium within fascicles, between fibers. Fascicles bound by perineureum. Nerve bound by epineurium.

interruption from the cell body.[1,6] The rate of transport down the axon may not increase, but the amount of axoplasm will. The amount of transmitter substance decreases. However, if the axonal injury is proximate to the nerve cell, retrograde degeneration will involve the neuronal cell body and cell death will occur.

It is most likely that the trophic effects of a nerve depend to some extent on axonal transport.[11] Regeneration across a site of interruption also depends on the distance between the proximal and distal stumps, as well as on the trophic factors that direct axons into their appropriate distal neural tubes.[11,12]

☐ REACTION OF PERIPHERAL NERVES TO INJURY

Metabolism within the cell body of a nerve that has been injured is altered within hours.[1] The size of the cell body

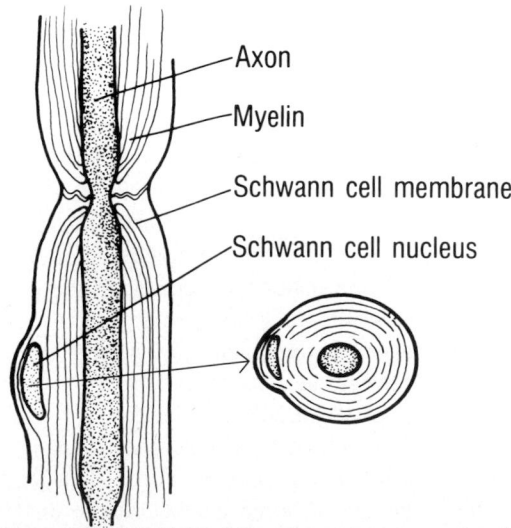

Figure 21–2 Node of Ranvier and cross-sectional view of myelinated axon.

increases, Nissl substance breaks up, and the nucleus migrates to the periphery of the cell body.

There is an increase in both ribonucleic acid (RNA) and the elements required for axon synthesis. Production of neurotransmitters decreases. Lipid synthesis increases significantly to reconstitute the Schwann cell membrane.

After injury to a peripheral nerve, some cells may die, depending in part on the distance of the injury from the cell body: the nearer the injury to the cell body the greater is the chance of cellular death.

Wallerian degeneration occurs in fibers distal to axonal interruption. Similar changes also occur retrograde for varying distances proximal to an injury, depending more on the severity of the injury than the location of the next proximal node of Ranvier.[13] This type of retrograde change may account for some cellular deaths.[1]

Multiple sprouts from a single severed axon occur within 24 h of transection of a peripheral nerve. These sprouts are initially unmyelinated, even when the axon of origin is myelinated. Growth cones that consist of filopodia develop on each axonal sprout.[14] They reach out for contact with an appropriate substrate—preferably fibronectin and laminin, both components of the basal lamina of Schwann cells.[15]

If the sprouts do not make appropriate contact, they will retract and advance again toward a more appropriate substrate. While there is usually loss of regenerating units at the site of a nerve repair, the multiplicity of sprouts results in an increased number of axons crossing a nerve repair.

The sprouts from myelinated nerve fibers eventually become myelinated, and the number of sprouts will decrease depending on whether contact is made with a distal tubule.[16] Eventually, this number approaches normal.[1] If the regenerating axons become lost in the extraepineural environment, a neuroma will form.

Following division of a nerve and wallerian degeneration of the distal segment, Schwann cells begin to proliferate and phagocytose debris, while myelin degenerates.[1] The endoneurial tubes collapse and are now merely stacked processes of Schwann cells known as *bands of Bungner.* The Schwann

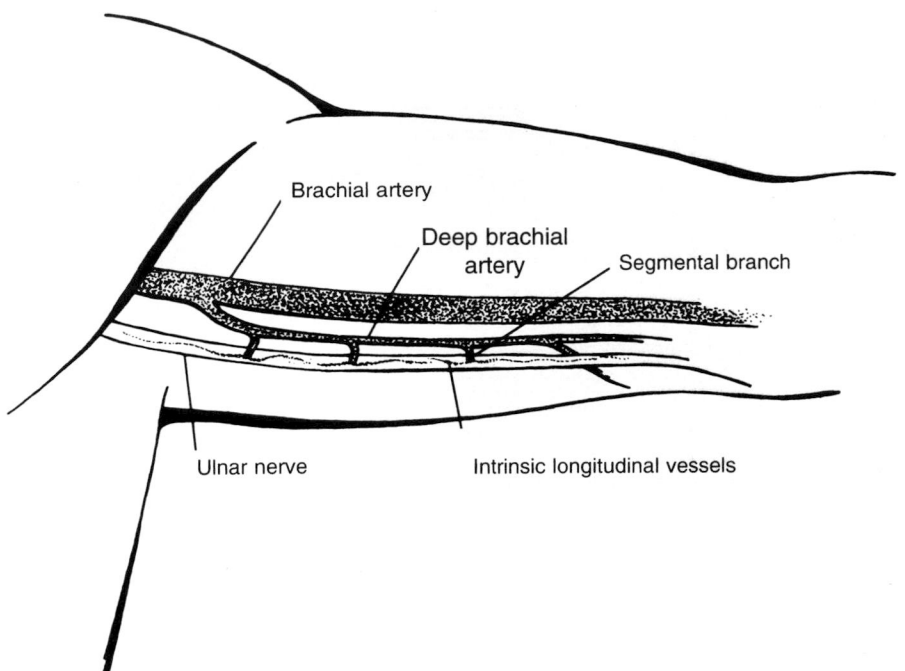

Figure 21–4 Vascular supply to peripheral nerve.

cells are organized into columns. The regenerating axons associate themselves with the layers of basal lamina, which may be considered potential tubes. Sprouts may enter inappropriate tubes, leading to misdirection and nonfunctional units.

The final result of reinnervation will depend on the number of axons that become associated with columns of Schwann cells to reinnervate appropriate end organs. Residual bands of Bungner are endoneural tubes that have failed to be reinnervated.

Muscle fibers undergo atrophy several weeks after denervation. The denervated fibers, on cross section, become rounded, and the nuclei, normally located at the periphery of muscle fibers, move to the center.[17] (See Fig. 21-5.)

Muscle fibers are normally typed I or II depending on whether they are "fast" or "slow," with variation in the amount of stain they take up. The type of nerve fiber innervating a muscle determines the type of the muscle fiber. After denervation, the types of muscle fibers become randomly distributed.

☐ REINNERVATION OF THE INJURED PERIPHERAL NERVE

Motor end plates are not altered for more than a year after denervation; however, the distribution of acetylcholine receptors changes markedly.[18] While acetylcholine receptors are normally located in the center of the length of muscle fibers, after denervation, fibers develop supersensitivity throughout their course. With reinnervation, motor fibers will reform neuromuscular junctions at the original end plates, but, in addition, innervating axons will send projections to adjacent muscle fibers so that a group of neighbor-

ing muscle fibers may receive innervation from the same axon. This will determine the type of muscle fibers demonstrated on histologic examination.

Questions have arisen about the feasibility of implanting transected ends of nerves into muscle. Studies demonstrate that this procedure results in reinnervation of some muscle fibers, but the reinnervation is not as efficient as reinnervation through distal segments of a motor nerve.[19]

There is no question about the effect trophic factors have on reinnervation. Implantation of a sensory nerve in a denervated muscle will result in axons of sensory fibers growing into muscle fibers; however, if the muscle is innervated, axonal growth of sensory fibers into nerve sheaths going to the muscle will be inhibited.[20,21]

Cutaneous sensation has a greater potential for recovery from denervation than does motor function. *Paccinian* and *Meissner corpuscles* are the receptors attached to quickly adapting nerve fibers mediating touch and vibration from glabrous (nonhairy) skin. Merkel neurites are more slowly adapting fiber receptors mediating touch and pressure. These undergo changes after denervation, but nonnervous elements survive and may be reinnervated years after denervation.[22,23] Sensory receptors of hairy skin are located at the base of hair follicles. Sensations of pain, touch, and temperature recover after denervation. Peripheral to central recovery of deafferented areas occurs if there is no axonal regeneration of the injured nerve elements. But if regeneration occurs, there should also be central-to-peripheral recovery of sensory function. Recovery begins at the edges of transplanted skin and proceeds toward the center.[24,25]

Transplanted digits may develop nearly normal sensation. The degree of recovery depends on the status of the donor nerve, the recipient nerves, and the type and quantity of sensory end organs.[26]

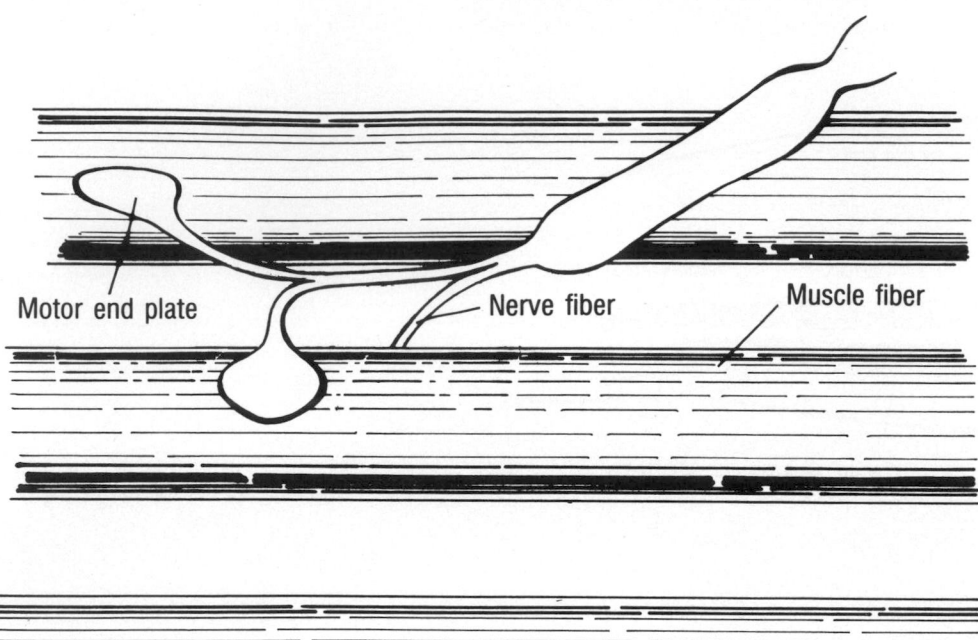

Figure 21–5 Motor end plates on muscle fibers.

THE EVOLUTION OF SURGERY ON PERIPHERAL NERVES

The evaluation and treatment of patients with peripheral nerve injuries has evolved and improved over the years. Quantum leaps in the clinical scientific basis for handling lesions of peripheral nerves have taken place at the time of great wars.

Weir Mitchell, while Commander of the United States Army Hospital for Injuries and Diseases of the Nervous System during the 1860s in the American Civil War, began his famous work on partial nerve injuries, out of which came his classical description of *causalgia*.[27]

World War II became the laboratory for Sidney Sunderland to advance the diagnosis and treatment of peripheral nerve lesions. Beginning in 1940 and lasting a decade, Sunderland was Professor of Anatomy at the University of Melbourne and Visiting Consultant of Peripheral Nerve Injuries to the 115th Australian General Military Hospital and the Commonwealth Repatriation Department in Melbourne. Here he was able to maintain a 10-year chain of unbroken records on 365 patients.[28] The American military contribution to peripheral nerve injury during World War II was led by Barnes Woodhall, who compiled and presented data from the Peripheral Nerve Registry.[29] Ducker, Kempe, and Hayes advanced the science of handling nerve injuries by including their experience from the Vietnam War and reviewing the metabolic basis for treatment of such lesions.[6]

INITIAL EVALUATION OF PERIPHERAL NERVE LESIONS

When a patient presents with a peripheral nerve lesion, three important factors should be noted in the first examination.

The physician must determine (1) the type of injury, (2) the time the injury occurred, and (3) the clinical condition of the patient at the time of the examination. Each of these components is essential to the understanding of what has happened to the nerve, how much deterioration has occurred, and how much recovery can be expected. This baseline examination is used to judge improvement or deterioration at subsequent evaluations. It also becomes the reference for determining improvement or deterioration after surgery involving the peripheral nerve.

CLASSIFICATION OF PERIPHERAL NERVE INJURY

TYPES OF INJURY

A peripheral nerve, or group of nerves, may be injured in many ways. A stab wound to the forearm resulting in a laceration of the ulnar nerve is a dramatic and obvious injury to the nerve, as opposed to the subtle and discrete nature of a slowly developing compression of a root or peripheral nerve. A nerve may also be crushed (acute severe compression), contused, stretched or avulsed, accidentally injected, thermally injured, damaged from shock waves (forces around a projectile), or rendered ischemic (e.g., Volkman's ischemic contracture). Examples of each type of injury include the following:

1. The median nerve is *compressed* by the flexor retinaculum, resulting in the clinical presentation of carpal tunnel syndrome.

The S1 nerve root is compressed with a herniation of the L5–S1 disk, resulting in a loss of the Achilles reflex, decreased sensation of the lateral aspect of the foot, and decreased plantar strength.

2. A nerve is *contused* by the sudden onset of blunt force. Trauma to the arm that may fracture the humerus may also contuse the radial nerve in the arm. Also, a severe crush injury to a nerve may occur in relation to massive limb trauma.

3. Peripheral nerves may be *lacerated* by an assortment of objects: a knife, the sharp edges of a broken window, unintentional laceration by an angiographer's needle or a surgeon's scalpel. The laceration may divide the whole nerve or divide only a portion of the fascicles.

4. Motorcyclists thrown from their vehicles and landing on the head and shoulder will *stretch* several roots or nerves within the brachial plexus. If the stretch injury to the brachial plexus is particularly severe, the nerve root(s) may be detached or *avulsed* from the spinal cord.

   Pelvic dystocia during delivery of an infant may result in an Erb's (C5–C6) palsy or, more rarely, both an Erb's and Klumpke's (C7–T1) palsy. Erb's palsy leaves the upper extremity adducted at the shoulder, extended at the elbow, and pronated. The biceps reflex is absent. Klumpke's palsy results in absence of flexion of the wrist and fingers and only minimal extension of the elbow.

5. Nerves are also affected by extreme *cold* and *heat.* Severe freezing (over a 2- to 3-day period) results in necrosis of the affected segment, with eventual regeneration of new, thinner fibers. This process of recovery takes approximately 3 months.[30] Transient freezing or cooling causes lesser degrees of disruption to nerve fibers that ranges from mild conduction blocks to interruption of the axons with wallerian degeneration.

   Severe burns may damage peripheral nerves at the time of the injury or lead to loss of function at a later date because of the constrictive fibrosis that is associated with destruction of adjacent tissues. This produces nerve lesions of varying severity.[28]

6. Even though a *missile* may not directly strike a nerve during its course through an extremity, the nerve may still be injured by the shock waves that spread out around the missile tract, thereby damaging tissue which may include the neural elements.

7. *Ischemic injury.* Limb trauma with sufficient hemorrhage or swelling may render nerves variably ischemic as they pass within involved muscles.

8. *Injection injury.* Improperly placed needles may enter the radial nerve in the arm or the sciatic nerve in the buttock. If the injection is not aborted when the patient reports pain with introduction of the needle, serious injury with painful neuroma may result.

ANATOMIC-PHYSIOLOGIC CLASSIFICATION

In 1943, Seddon described three classifications of nerve injury according to extent of disruption of axons and their supporting tissues: neurapraxia, axonotmesis, and neurotmesis.[31]

Neurapraxia is an injury to the nerve where the nerve tissue remains intact but the surrounding myelin sheath at the site of injury may be disrupted. The result is slowed conduction velocity lasting weeks to months. *Axonotmesis* is an injury where the axon and surrounding myelin are disrupted but the surrounding perineurium and epineurium remain intact. In order for this injury to recover, regeneration of the axon and resultant reinnervation of the target organ are necessary. *Neurotmesis* is a complete disruption of the nerve such as would result from a laceration. Recovery occurs only if the nerve ends are brought together and the neurons regenerate along their length and reinnervate the target organ.

Sunderland further categorized nerve injuries according to degree.[32] In a *first degree injury,* there is interruption of conduction at the site of injury, but preservation of the anatomical components of the nerve trunk, including the axon. This is equivalent to neurapraxia of Seddon. The block in conduction is fully reversible. Time of recovery of sensory and motor function is essentially the same for both proximal and distal function.

With *second degree injury,* the axon is severed or the axon below the level of the lesion fails to survive; however, the endoneurial tube is preserved despite wallerian degeneration. The end organ becomes isolated until the axon regrows, but the axon invariably returns to the end organ it originally innervated. Reinnervation follows a pattern determined by the distance the axon must regrow (i.e., proximal to distal, as opposed to neurapraxia).

Regrowth of sensory fibers may be followed by *Tinel's sign.* This sign is positive when tapping along the nerve elicits distal paresthesias in the sensory distribution of the nerve. But it is important to note that although a distally migrating Tinel's sign is evidence of functional recovery in a second degree injury, it is *not* necessarily a sign of functional recovery in the case of a more severe injury, because it may be elicited when only C fibers regenerate.

In *third degree injury,* the trauma is more severe. There is some disorganization of the internal structure of the fascicles. There may be intrafascicular fibrosis, which can prove an obstacle to regeneration. There may also be some loss of continuity of endoneural tubes so that some regenerating axons are no longer confined to the tubes they originally followed, and new anomalous patterns of innervation occur. Recovery may be incomplete.

A *fourth degree injury* results in bundles of nerve fibers being so disorganized that they are no longer sharply demarcated from the epineurium in which they are embedded. The continuity of the nerve trunk persists, but the involved segment is converted into a tangled strand of connective tissue, Schwann cells, and regenerating axons that may eventually form a neuroma. Recovery is often out of the question for that part of a nerve that undergoes fourth degree injury.

Fifth degree injury implies loss of continuity of the nerve

Type		Functional disorder	Anatomical/pathophysiological basis	Prognosis/recovery	Diagram (see footnote)
Physiological conduction block, type a[1]		Local conduction block.	Intraneural circulatory arrest. Metabolic (ionic) block with no nerve fibre pathology	Immediately reversible	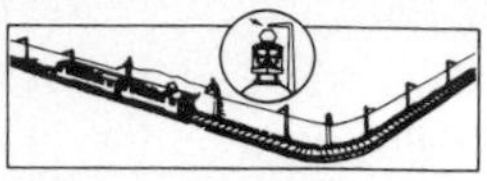
Physiological conduction block, type b[1]		Local conduction block.	Intraneural edema. Metabolic block with little or no nerve fibre pathology. Increased endoneurial fluid pressure (EFP)	Reversible within days or weeks	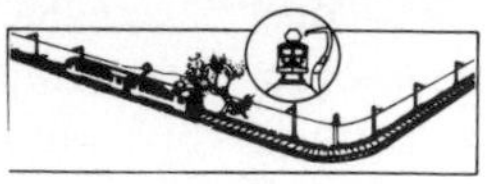
Seddon	Sunderland				
Neurapraxia	1	Local conduction block. Motor function and proprioception mainly affected. Some sensation and sympathetic function may be preserved[2]	Local myelin damage, primarily thick, myelinated fibres. Axonal continuity preserved. No wallerian degeneration	Reversible within weeks to months	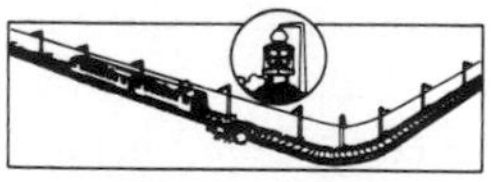
Axonotmesis	2	Loss of nerve conduction at level of injury and within distal nerve segment	Loss of axonal continuity, wallerian degeneration. Endoneurial tubes preserved	Recovery requires axonal regeneration. Correct orientation of growing fibres since endoneurial tubes are preserved. Correct targets will be reinnervated	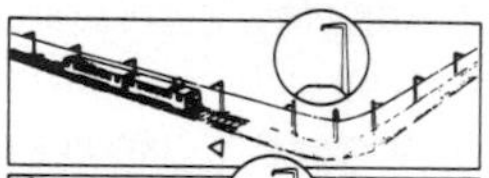 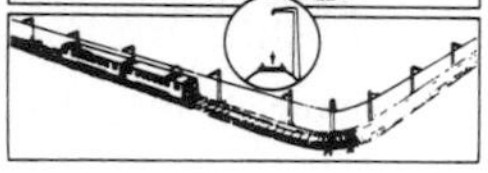
	3	Loss of nerve conduction at level of injury and within distal nerve segment	Loss of axonal continuity and endoneurial tubes; perineurium intact	Endoneurial pathways disrupted and disoriented, bleeding and oedema lead to scarring. Axonal misdirection. Poor prognosis. Surgery may be required	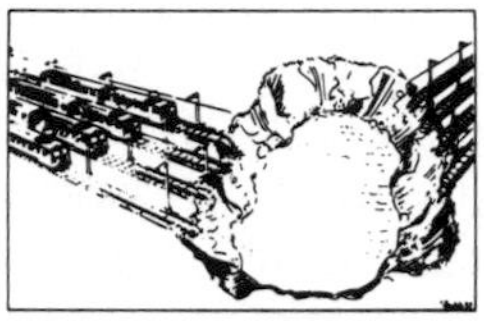
	4	Loss of nerve conduction at level of injury and within distal nerve segment	Loss of axonal continuity, endoneurial tubes and perineurium. Epineurium intact	Rupture and total disorganization of guiding elements of the nerve trunk. Intraneural scar formation. Axonal misdirection. Poor prognosis. Surgery required	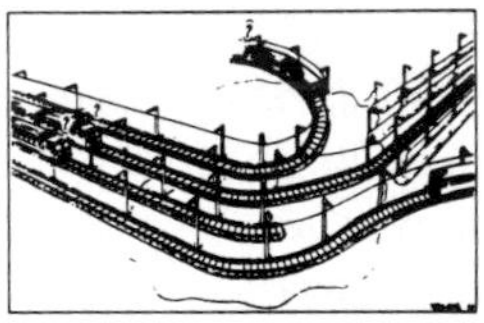
Neurotmesis	5	Loss of nerve conduction at level of injury and within distal nerve segment	Transection or rupture of entire nerve trunk	Recovery requires surgical adaptation and co-aptation of nerve ends. Prognosis dependent on the nature of the injury as well as local and general factors (cf ch. 6)	

[1]Not included in Seddon's or Sunderland's classifications.
[2]According to Seddon 1972.

Figure 21–6 Caricature of levels of nerve injury related to train. (*Reprinted with permission from the publisher, Churchill Livingstone, from* Nerve Injury and Repair *by Goran Lundborg, Table 31, pp 78–79, 1988.*)

trunk. Distances of interruption vary, but the nerve ends remain separated. Scar tissue and separation of the nerve ends provides a formidable barrier to spontaneous recovery.

A *sixth category of nerve injury* described by Sunderland—and emphasized by Mackinnin and Dellon in 1988—is a combination of the above injuries.[1,28] Some fibers escape injury while others experience various degrees of deterioration. Sunderland pointed out that it would be unlikely for all of a nerve to be crushed with a combination of first, and fourth, or fifth degree injuries to that same nerve, but that mixed injuries are common, especially with penetrating wounds.

Figure 21-6 is a visual analogy of the various levels of nerve injury to a train running along a track supplied by energy. The rails correspond to a nerve fiber, the track to the endoneural tube, and the train to the electric impulse traveling along the fiber. The electric wire corresponds to microvessels providing the blood supply to the nerve.

The physiological conduction block at the top of the page demonstrates what happens if the local energy supply is interrupted. The train cannot move in spite of an intact nerve fiber. The moment the energy supply is restored (electric wire repair), the train starts moving again, as in a first degree injury.

If the electric wire system is more severely damaged as in a second degree injury, illustrated by the falling tree, then the repair takes longer. Still, the rail is intact. In the example of neurapraxia, or Sunderland's first degree injury, the train is stopped because of local damage to the rail (demyelinating block), while more distal parts of the rail, as well as the energy supply system, remain intact. Repair of local damage takes up to 6 or 8 weeks.

In the illustration for axonotmesis, or Sunderland's second degree injury, the rail is damaged and has disappeared distal to the level of injury. The track is still intact and new rails can easily be laid in the correct position. In the example of neurotmesis, or Sunderland's third through fifth degree injuries, the rail as well as the track are destroyed. The result is a great deal of misdirection.[33]

☐ FACTORS INFLUENCING RECOVERY FROM PERIPHERAL NERVE INJURY

ESTABLISHING TIME AND NATURE OF INJURY

When evaluating the patient with a peripheral nerve injury, establishing the time of injury is important. This is usually easy to determine, but in some cases may not be clear. Symptoms of a compressive lesion may have an insidious onset which a patient only notices after several months. The deficits after a crush injury may not be present immediately but may present weeks to months later when scarring in the extremity renders the nerve dysfunctional. The same sort of delayed presentation may take place after a gunshot wound adjacent to a nerve.

Simple lacerations are injuries that usually do not present a problem in determining the time of the nerve injury. This is not, however, always the case. A large bloody laceration to the arm may result in injuries to many structures (skin, muscles, arteries, and veins) that require immediate attention. This may distract the physician from recognizing a possible deficit due to injury of a nerve. Only later may the deficit be recognized.

This can lead to a problem for a later examiner. Did the nerve lesion occur at the time of the accident, or was it an iatrogenic lesion that occurred during repair of the patient's other injuries? The question can have both legal and clinical implications.

Determination of the time of injury is essential in estimating the timing of recovery. The degree of recovery is also critical in determining the future management of a peripheral nerve injury. For example, recovery of sensory or motor function indicates continued conservative management, whereas a distally migrating Tinel's sign or recovery of autonomic function in the absence of sensory or motor recovery requires surgical exploration.

RATES OF REGENERATION

Axons of peripheral nerves regenerate at predictable rates. Various factors affect the rate of regeneration. After nerves are anastomosed, several days to weeks are required for an axon to cross the site of anastomosis, but once axons reach the distal nerve sheath, regeneration occurs at the rate of 1 to 1.5 mm per day or 2.5 to 4.5 cm per month, depending on the particular nerve and the distance of the injury from the cell body.[34,35,36] In general, axon regeneration near the cell body is more rapid than regeneration at greater distances.

IMPAIRMENT OF REGENERATION

If a transected nerve is not anastomosed with its distal sheath, axons will grow into surrounding tissue, but their growth is disorganized and individual axons rarely reach the appropriate end organ. Recovery will be slow and rarely functional. More devastating is the developing of scarring that may result in a painful neuroma at the proximal end of a lacerated nerve.

If a nerve trunk remains intact (in continuity) but its internal structure is severely disrupted (e.g., high velocity missile wound, severe compression, or other complex injury), then organized regeneration is unlikely.

TIMING OF SURGICAL INTERVENTION

Another factor important in determining whether reinnervation after injury will be successful is the timing of *surgical intervention*.

1. *Lacerations.* Repair within first 48 h. If injury is several days old, wait about 2 weeks for edema to subside.
2. *Blunt trauma.* Allow at least 6 weeks for evidence of recovery from a possible neurapraxic injury.

Since peripheral nerve regenerates about 1 in. per month and motor end plates are reinnervated with difficulty 1 year or more after denervation, surgery must be planned accordingly. For example, with a blunt injury to the sciatic nerve, surgical intervention should occur as soon as possible if no clinical evidence of recovery is seen within 6 to 8 weeks after injury. Early repair may provide recovery of plantar flexion of the foot and a very functional lower extremity. Delaying 3 or 4 months might result in diminished or absent recovery of plantar flexion of the foot. On the other hand, one can afford to observe a patient with distal median nerve injury for 3 or 4 months and still obtain a good surgical result.[37]

Denervated muscle fibers also degenerate. Although there may be fibrillations as long as 10 years after a human muscle has been denervated, thickening of the muscle sheath may cause difficulty with end-plate formation. In summary, the longer the period after an injury before repair, the poorer the results. Still, there are some rare exceptions when remarkable response to reinnervation has occurred 2 to 3 years after injury of a peripheral nerve.

In cases where the neurological deficit is initially incomplete—i.e., where motor function of all involved muscles is paretic but present and sensory function is diminished but present—the injury is most likely neurapraxic. If there is complete loss of function of the entire nerve or any of its divisions, the injury may be neurapraxic, axonotmetic, or neurotmetic.

A period of observation is required before one can conclude that exploration is indicated. During this time, neurological recovery in the case of Sunderland's first, second, and third degree injuries will occur. Proximal and distal recovery will be simultaneous in the case of neurapraxic injuries. If the injury is proximal to the next most distal muscle group, it may require several months of observation to distinguish between axonotmesis and neurotmesis; i.e., reinnervation will occur in the case of axonotmetic or second degree injuries.

If the distance between injury and the next most distal muscle group is greater than 12 in.—e.g., injury to the tibial division of sciatic nerve in the thigh—one might not have the luxury of 3 to 4 months for observation and might have to explore within 8 to 12 weeks after injury.

By the process of elimination, fourth degree injuries (where scarring fills the perineurium) and fifth degree injuries will not improve. In the case of neurotmetic (third, fourth, and fifth degree) lesions, a surgical approach is indicated either to (1) establish with nerve action potentials that there is physiological continuity and, in the latter case, remove the damaged segment and anastomose cleanly cut ends primarily or use an interposition graft, or (2) if the nerve is anatomically disrupted (fifth degree injury) to do a primary neurorrhaphy (repair) and place a cable graft between the proximal and distal nerve ends.[40]

☐ COMMON NERVE INJURY SYNDROMES

Specific syndromes of deficits due to peripheral nerve lesions have been selected for presentation because of their frequency, including carpal tunnel syndrome, ulnar neuropathy from compression at the elbow, radial nerve injury in the spiral groove, and peroneal nerve entrapment at the fibular head.

CARPAL TUNNEL SYNDROME

Carpal tunnel syndrome occurs when the median nerve is compressed beneath the flexor retinaculum. The anatomy of the median nerve is illustrated in Fig. 21-7. The carpal tunnel may be thought of as an inverted table—with the carpal bones forming the tabletop, and the hook portion of the hamate, the pisiform, the tubercle of the trapezium, and the distal pole of the scaphoid forming the table legs.[1] The flexor retinaculum is stretched over the legs of this metaphoric table.

Median nerve compression may occur in pregnancy, amyloidosis, diabetes, thyroid disease, and arthritis. The patient complains of pain at the wrist and into the thumb and index fingers. The pain usually occurs at night and may awaken the patient.

On examination, the thenar muscle group may demonstrate atrophy. The sensory deficit is over the palmar surface of the thumb, index, middle, and thenar half of the ring fingers. A Tinel's sign is present at the wrist approximately 50 percent of the time; therefore, it is of little diagnostic value. The nerve conduction velocity will slow as the first finding, and later, the EMG will show increased terminal latencies beyond the normal of 3.5 ms or a significant asymmetry on the two sides.

Conservative treatment may be effective. Placing the wrist at rest relieves the nocturnal pain of carpal tunnel syndrome in some patients with mild symptoms. Patients are placed in a "cock-up" splint that they may wear constantly or only at night. Relief may be temporary or continuous over a prolonged period. In patients with persistent symptoms and prolonged latency of the median nerve at the wrist by nerve conduction studies, decompression by division of the flexor retinaculum is indicated.

ULNAR ENTRAPMENT AT THE ELBOW

Ulnar entrapment at the elbow has also been called *tardy ulnar palsy*. The name originated from a paper written by Davidson and Horowitz in 1955 entitled "Late or Tardy Ulnar Nerve Paralysis." They wrote: "The classical picture of later ulnar neuritis occurs ten or more years after an injury to the elbow joints, usually in childhood."[38]

Patients present with pain and numbness in the ulnar side of the hand. Clinical examination reveals a Tinel's sign as the ulnar nerve travels over the medial epicondyle or as the nerve passes through the cubital tunnel. The cubital tunnel is defined by Mackinnon and Dellon as the fascial covering that is frequently loose and variable in its proximal extent at the level of the medial epicondyle and the olecranon—extending distally to a point between the two heads of the flexor carpi ulnaris, which is frequently tight.[1]

In the presence of appropriate physical findings, the diagnosis is confirmed by nerve conduction velocity studies and electromyography. The first findings are slowed conduction velocities followed by prolonged motor latencies. Neurotmesis can result from injury to the nerve. The ulnar nerve anatomy is illustrated in Fig. 21-8.

RADIAL NERVE INJURY

Fractures of the midshaft of the humerus sometimes result in a radial nerve injury as this nerve travels in the spiral groove of the humerus. The patient develops weakness in all muscles of the extensor compartment of the forearm. Characteristic wrist and finger drop makes the diagnosis fairly easy. Usually, function of the triceps muscle is normal, innervation to the triceps having exited from the radial nerve proximal to the spiral groove. Electromyography 2 to 3 weeks after the injury will aid in the diagnosis. The injury is usually neurapraxic or axonotmetic and will resolve. Exploration of the radial nerve is warranted in the injury that shows no improvement within 3 to 4 months following the humeral fracture.

PERONEAL NERVE INJURY

Compression of the peroneal nerve commonly occurs as the nerve crosses in the area of the fibular neck. The nerve is

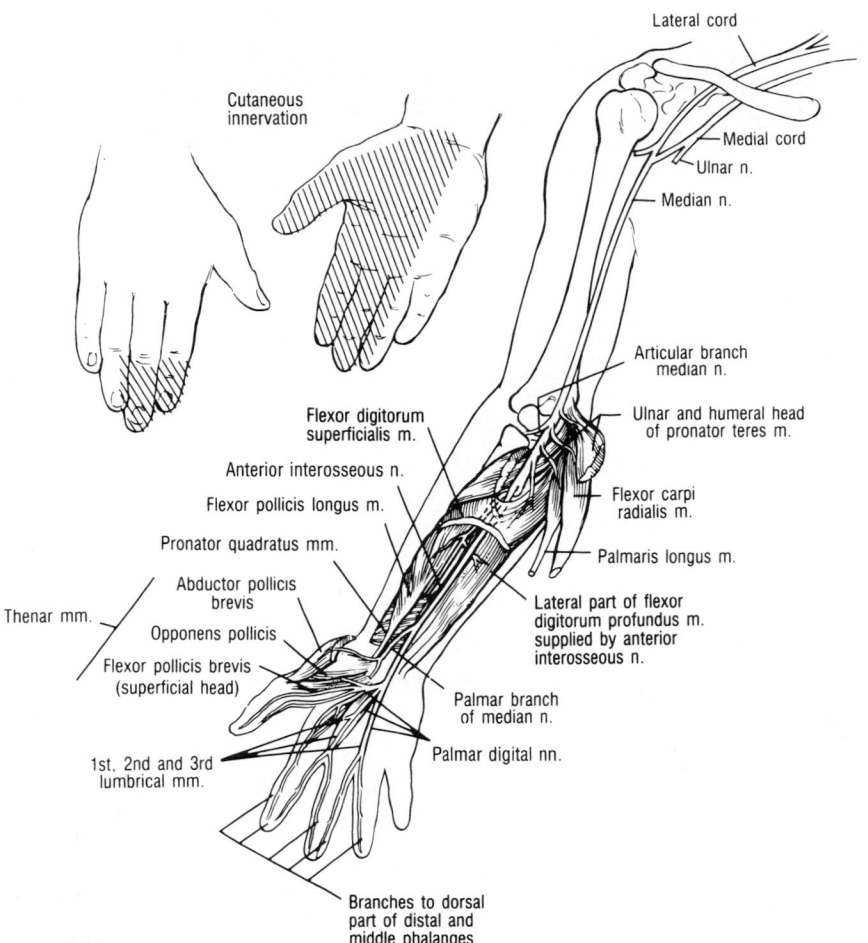

Figure 21–7   Anatomy of median nerve.

vulnerable to injury as it crosses the fibula through the opening in the peroneus muscle. Direct blunt trauma, fracture of the neck of the fibula, repeated compression from crossing the legs, or pressure from leaning on one side may cause paresis in the distribution of the peroneal nerve. Pain laterally in the leg and foot is a common symptom. Some patients may present with a painless foot drop, i.e., loss of motor function without sensory changes.

BRACHIAL PLEXUS INJURIES

The brachial plexus presents a challenge diagnostically and therapeutically. The anatomy is complex and has been illustrated in Fig. 21-9.

Table 21-1 provides a study guide that lists the branches of the brachial plexus and the muscles they innervate. With the exclusion of compressive injuries, the brachial plexus injuries may be classified as open or closed.

Open injuries may accompany serious, or even fatal, vascular or pulmonary injuries.[39] Management of these problems must precede surgery on the brachial plexus. The decision to explore the brachial plexus depends on several factors. If the injury is by a sharp object (knife, glass, needles, or other sharp object), it warrants early surgical

intervention as described in the section on timing of surgical intervention. Blunt injuries may be observed for a variable period of time, depending on the proximal or distal location of the injury. When repaired, a lesion to the upper or middle trunk, lateral cord, musculocutaneous nerve, posterior cord, or axillary nerve has the greatest chance for the return of useful function because of the proximal muscles they innervate.[40] Gun shot wounds in the region of the brachial plexus may require a waiting period of up to 3 months to help establish the degree of neural injury. When serial examinations during this time demonstrate persistent deficits, indicating type IV and V lesions, operative intervention is indicated. Evidence of lost neural tissue during an initial exploration for repair of other injuries is an indication for early grafting, after allowing local edema to resolve.

Closed injuries of the plexus can be further subdivided into *supraclavicular* and *infraclavicular* injuries. Infraclavicular injuries have a better prognosis and are usually the result of bony injuries in the shoulder region. Clavicular fractures or callus formation may compress the plexus. Supraclavicular injuries usually occur after high-speed motor vehicle accidents, often when a rider is thrown from a motorcycle, resulting in severe stretch injuries or avulsion of roots from the cord.

Damage ranges from nerve root avulsion through more

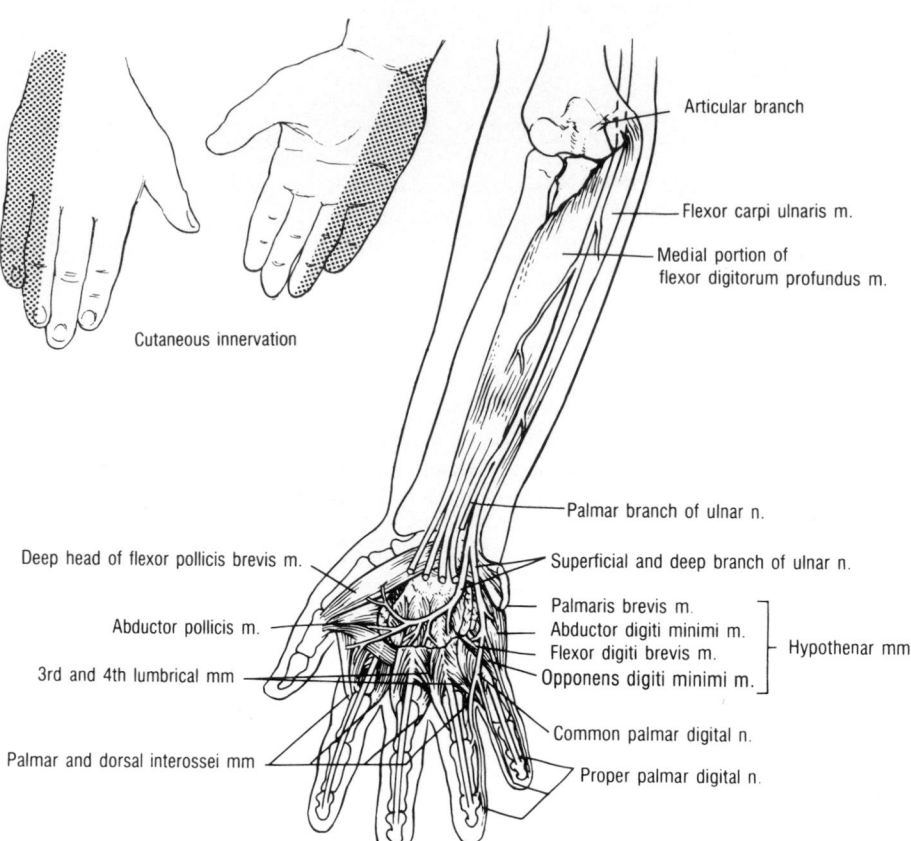

Articular branch

Flexor carpi ulnaris m.

Medial portion of
flexor digitorum profundus m.

Cutaneous innervation

Palmar branch of ulnar n.

Deep head of flexor pollicis brevis m.

Superficial and deep branch of ulnar n.

Palmaris brevis m.
Abductor pollicis m.
Abductor digiti minimi m.
Flexor digiti brevis m.   } Hypothenar mm.
Opponens digiti minimi m.

3rd and 4th lumbrical mm

Common palmar digital n.

Palmar and dorsal interossei mm

Proper palmar digital n.

Figure 21–8 Anatomy of ulnar nerve from elbow distally.

distal neurotmetic injuries to neurapraxic lesions. An upper plexus lesion that also presents with a Horner's syndrome (myosis, ptosis, and anhydrosis of the face) has a poor prognosis. The Horner's syndrome results from injury to the upper sympathetic chain located near the dorsal root ganglia of C8 through T2. In a blunt injury, this strongly suggests

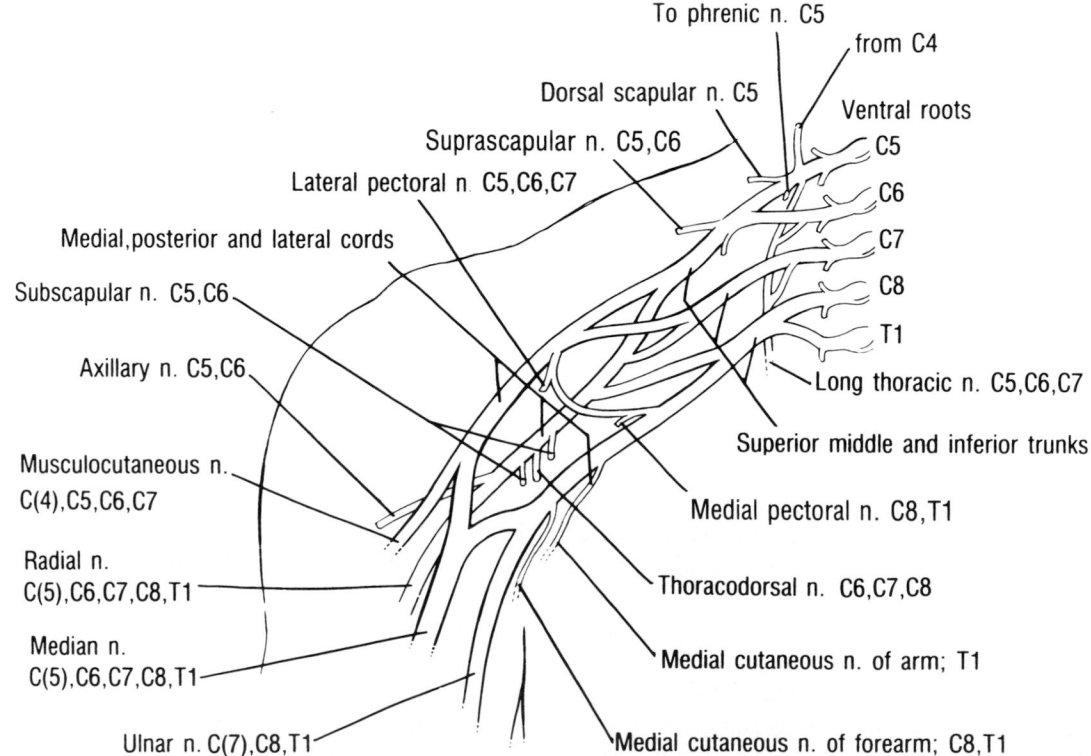

To phrenic n. C5

from C4

Dorsal scapular n. C5

Ventral roots

Suprascapular n. C5,C6

C5

Lateral pectoral n. C5,C6,C7

C6

Medial, posterior and lateral cords

C7

Subscapular n. C5,C6

C8

T1

Axillary n. C5,C6

Long thoracic n. C5,C6,C7

Superior middle and inferior trunks

Musculocutaneous n.
C(4),C5,C6,C7

Medial pectoral n. C8,T1

Radial n.
C(5),C6,C7,C8,T1

Thoracodorsal n. C6,C7,C8

Median n.
C(5),C6,C7,C8,T1

Medial cutaneous n. of arm; T1

Ulnar n. C(7),C8,T1

Medial cutaneous n. of forearm; C8,T1

Figure 21–9 Anatomy of brachial plexus.

Table 21-1
NERVE SUPPLY OF MUSCLES OF THE UPPER EXTREMITY

Nerve	Muscle
Axillary	Deltoid Teres minor
Long thoracic nerve	Serratus anterior
Dorsal scapular nerve	Levator scapulae Rhomboid minor Rhomboid major
Lower subscapular nerve	Teres major Subscapular (also from upper scapular nerve)
Suprascapular nerve	Supraspinatus Intraspinatus
Musculocutaneous	Biceps brachii Coracobrachialis Brachialis
Radial	Three heads of tricep Extensor pollicis brevis Extensor pollicis longus Extensor indicis Some branches of brachialis and brachioradialis Extensor carpi radialis longus Extensor carpi radialis brevis Extensor digitorum Extensor carpi ulnaris Anconeus Supinatus Abductor pollicis longus
Median	Pronator teres Pronator quadratus Flexor carpi radialis First and second lumbricalis Abductor pollicis brevis Flexor pollicis brevis (superficial head) Opponens pollicis Flexor digitorum Flexor pollicis longus Lateral half of flexor digitorum profundus
Ulnar	Flexor carpi ulnaris Medial half of flexor digitorum profundus Third and fourth lumbricalis Palmer interossei Dorsal interossei Adductor pollicis Abductor digiti minimi Flexor digiti minimi Opponens digiti minimi Flexor policus brevis (deep head)

avulsion. A flail or weak arm at the time of injury should be supported against gravity to prevent possible additional damage. In a complete brachial plexopathy, resulting from avulsions of the roots and causing a flail arm, grafting of intercostal nerves to the distal end of the musculocutaneous nerve may provide useful elbow flexion when combined with a distal limb prosthesis.[41]

Diagnostic evaluation after a brachial plexus injury should include plain cervical spine films. (Fractured cervical transverse processes provide good presumptive evidence of nerve injury.) Cervical myelography or magnetic resonance imaging of the cervical spine usually demonstrates traumatic pseudomeningoceles at the site of avulsed nerve roots. These studies should be carried out 2 to 4 weeks after the injury. Surgical management of pain in association with avulsion of the brachial plexus is discussed in Chap. 24.

Injury to the lumbar plexus is not as common as brachial plexus injury. This plexus is better protected in its retroperitoneal and pelvic location. It is most frequently involved in penetrating injuries. Fig. 21-10 demonstrates the nerves of the lumbar plexus.

☐ SURGICAL PROCEDURES

Nerve lesions of type IV in Sunderland's classification, or *neuromas in continuity*, are explored in order to determine the extent of that nerve's injury. Intraoperative action potentials on the isolated or individual fascicles will establish which fascicles are *not* functioning. Decompression or external neurolysis of a nerve may relieve entrapment. Examples of this are division of the flexor retinaculum overlying the median nerve at the wrist, transposition of the ulnar nerve, and peroneal nerve decompression.

A lacerated nerve is usually repaired primarily, or an autologous interposition graft may be needed if the repair is delayed. Prognosis for the extent of recovery is based on two factors: (1) At each site of anastomosis approximately 10 percent of the axons will not cross; therefore, in general, external recovery is better with primary neurorrhaphy compared to cable grafting. (2) Primary repair of the two ends of the injured nerve leads to better recovery if the anastomosis is not under tension. Tension can be released by the placement of an appropriate interposition graft, by rerouting of the anastamosed nerve, or by limb flexion.

There is debate as to whether *epineural* or *intrafascicular repair* is preferable.[42,43,44,45] (See Fig. 21-11.) Despite both laboratory and clinical investigations, neither technique has proven superior.[46] Fascicular repair is technically more challenging but is more traumatic to the nerve because of the necessary dissection. In a few instances, this technique may be better, but epineural repair appears appropriate for most cases. Fascicular repair should be used in a nerve that is cut distally where a clear distinction can be made between the sensory and motor divisions of the nerve.[46,47] This can only be done in the first 48 to 72 h. Surgery may be performed

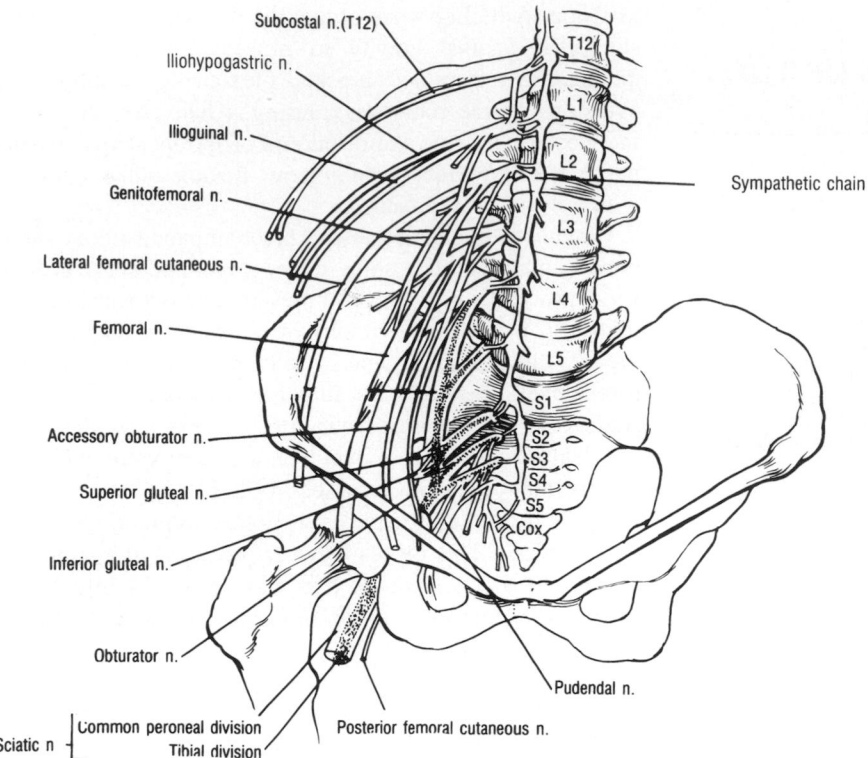

Figure 21–10   Anatomy of lumbosacral plexus.

under local anesthesia, with distal motor fascicles and proximal sensory fascicles identified by direct stimulation.

Nerves should be anastomosed primarily under minimal tension, using 7-0 to 10-0 prolene sutures through the epineurium alone. This technique requires magnification. The deep side of the anastomosis should be performed first, after two sutures are placed at each side of a line bisecting the horizontal axis for orientation. This also aids in rotation of the nerve, which is necessary for placement of the other sutures. The superficial repair is accomplished last.

A difficult and technically demanding technique using

vascularized nerve grafts has been developed by Julia Terzia. She recommends it for anastomosis of a nerve in an extremely scarred bed where vascularity is known to be poor.[48]

Interposition or cable grafts are used to repair an injured nerve when a length of the nerve has been destroyed. Sources for harvesting grafts include the sural nerve, the antebrachial cutaneous nerve, and occasionally the lateral femoral cutaneous nerve. Any extremity that the injured patient might have lost may be an excellent donor source.

Good material for grafting will support axon regeneration

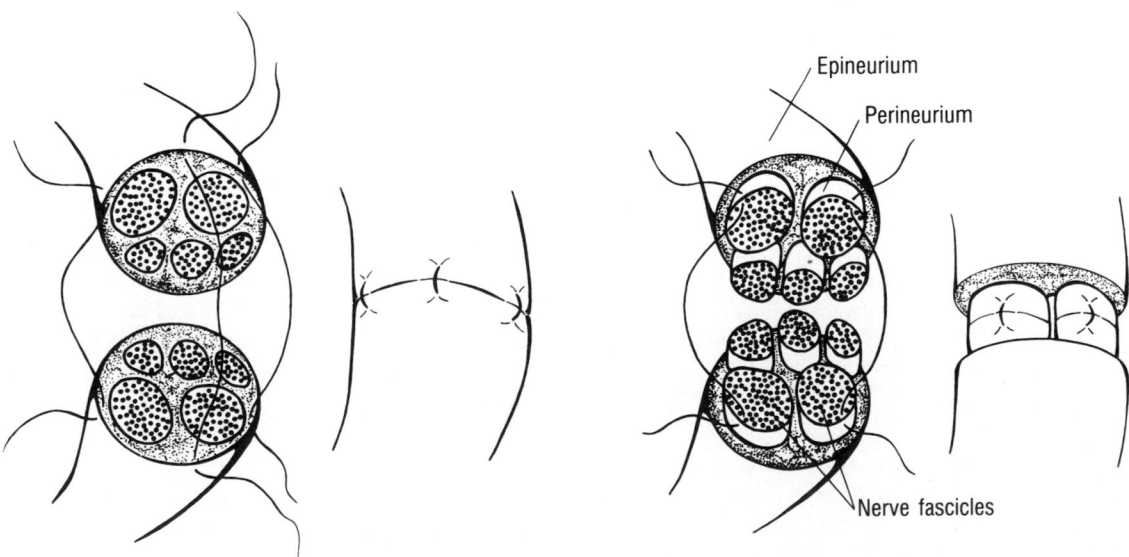

Figure 21–11   Epineural and intrafascicular repair.

while directing that growth toward the intended distal target nerve and, ultimately, its target organ. Functional recovery is the goal in all surgical repairs of peripheral nerves.

Other materials have proven effective in achieving that result. Sensory nerve repair has been accomplished using basal laminal grafts of muscle. The pectoralis muscle fibers are harvested, frozen in liquid nitrogen, thawed, and used to repair the injured digital nerve. Allograft (tissue from an unrelated donor) material has been used with limited success in rats. Mackinnon and Hudson have extended this work to human beings, but immunosuppression was used.[49] They subsequently discontinued the immunosuppression. The patient experienced excellent recovery of sensation but no return of motor function.

DECOMPRESSIVE PROCEDURES

A description of some of the decompressive nerve procedures follows.

Carpal Tunnel Release Anesthetic techniques which have been described for division of the flexor retinaculum include: axillary block, local nerve block, and the Bier block. Local infiltration with 0.5% lidocaine containing 1:200,000 epinephrine has been our most common choice. This may be supplemented with intravenous sedation in anxious patients.

The incision is located 6 mm to the ulnar or medial side of the thenar crease. A zigzag extension is used to carry the incision across the wrist in order to avoid a scar which restricts motion. The wound is held open with a self-retaining retractor. Subcutaneous fat is retracted and hemostasis obtained, using bipolar cautery. The palmar fascia is opened in the long axis of the hand, and the deep transverse carpal ligament is opened sharply with a scalpel, taking care to preserve the branches of the median nerve to the muscles at the base of the thumb. (See Fig. 21-12.)

The median nerve, once exposed, is protected with a no. 4 Penfield dissector as the incision is carried proximally to the distal portion of the antebrachial fascia and distally until the fat around the superficial palmar arch is encountered. A portion of the flexor retinaculum may be removed for pathologic examination.

The closure is accomplished in two layers, using absorbable sutures in the subcutaneous layer and nylon interrupted sutures on the skin. A bulky fluff gauze dressing is applied, along with an elastic wrap. The patient is instructed to move the fingers frequently but should not remove the dressing until the first postoperative visit, 10 to 12 days after surgery, when the sutures are taken out. If there is increasing pain or swelling, the patient should be seen as soon as possible. Patients are allowed to return to work 3 to 4 weeks after surgery. Postoperative visits should be scheduled for removal of sutures and at intervals of 3 months for up to a year.

Ulnar Nerve Transposition After the diagnosis of compression of the ulnar nerve at the elbow is made, a decision as to how to treat the lesion must follow. Treatment options include transposition of the nerve along with corrections of bony and ligamentous lesions at the elbow, medial epicondylectomy, removal of any compromising soft tissue mass, or simple transposition of the ulnar nerve. Transposition of the ulnar nerve will be described here.

Local infiltration, block, or general anesthesia may be used. The patient may be positioned supine with the arm outstretched while the surgeon and his assistant are on either side of the extremity. An alternative positioning is illustrated in Fig. 21-13. This is a more comfortable position for the patient who is awake, and it also makes accessible the entire segment of the ulnar nerve to be dissected. With the patient in the supine position, it is difficult to fully externally rotate the arm in order to dissect the ulnar nerve away from the medial epicondyle. The lateral decubitus position avoids this problem.

The "lazy omega" incision is used on the skin. (See Fig. 21-13.) This creates a skin flap that entirely covers the transposed nerve. Once the skin and subcutaneous tissues have been elevated, the fascia between the medial head of the triceps and the medial intermuscular septum is divided.

The ulnar nerve is dissected free, being retracted with a loop of umbilical tape or, preferably, a loop usually used for retraction of blood vessels. Dissection continues distally until the nerve is released from the cubital tunnel. Branches of the ulnar nerve, which innervate the proximal flexor carpi ulnaris, must be separated by interfascicular dissection and preserved.

The nerve may be transposed over the medial epicondyle to a bed fashioned in the flexor pronator fascia. (See Fig. 21-13.) The skin flap is then sutured to the fascia to act as a splint for the transposed nerve; 3-0 Vicryl sutures are used in this step. (See Fig. 21-13.) The skin is closed with interrupted sutures. A sterile dressing with an elastic bandage is applied. Sutures are removed 1 week later.

Peroneal Nerve Decompression Decompression of the peroneal nerve is illustrated in Fig. 21-14. The skin incision is carried out on the lateral aspect of the proximal leg. The common peroneal nerve is found proximal and posterior to the head of the fibula. The nerve is followed to its point of entrapment, which is usually where the nerve runs through a tunnel roofed by the peroneus longus muscle.

Swelling of the nerve is usually noted just proximal to the point of entrapment. The sharp edge of the arch of the peroneus longus is incised. The deep peroneal nerve is followed to the extensor digitorum muscle to ensure that it is free.

Harvesting of the Sural Nerve for Cable Graft The technique for harvesting the sural nerve is illustrated in Fig. 21-15. The lower extremity is positioned so that the lateral aspect of the leg is exposed. Once the leg is prepared, an incision is planned 1 cm lateral and parallel to the Achilles tendon.

The incision is begun 1 cm proximal to the lateral malleo-

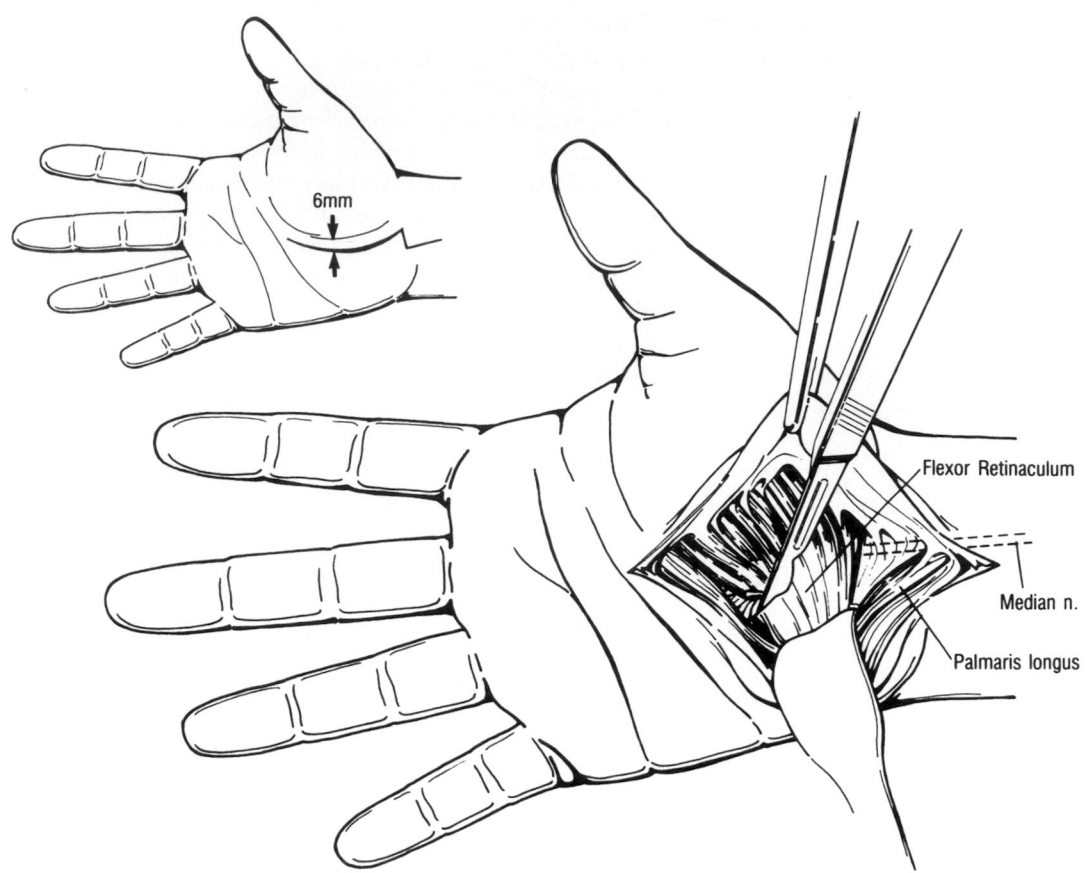

Figure 21–12
Carpal tunnel release.

lus and extended proximally. The sural nerve is found just superficial to the deep fascia and deep to the lesser saphenous vein. The nerve, once identified, is freed by sharp dissection. Proximal and distal ends are divided with a razor blade over a wooden spatula. If the patient is awake, a conduction block with xylocaine should be performed proximally before transecting the nerve, in order to prevent pain.

TUMORS OF PERIPHERAL NERVES

A classification of tumors of peripheral nerves has been provided by Harkin and Reed.[50] (See Table 21-2.) Surgeons who are planning an approach to neoplastic lesions of peripheral nerves should be familiar with schwannomas, neurofibromas, fatty infiltration of the median nerve, lipofibroma, intraneural lipomas, intraneural ganglia, and intraneural hemangiomas.

SCHWANNOMAS

Schwannomas arise from the Schwann cell sheath. They may occur on any nerve encased in a sheath of Schwann cells.

The microscopic pathology of these tumors has two characteristic patterns: Antoni A and Antoni B. Antoni A is the densely cellular form, with cells aligned in palisades. Antoni

B has a less cellular pattern, consisting of a loose arrangement of spindle cells and a watery, clear, mucinous matrix.

The eighth cranial nerve is involved more than all other cranial nerves. Schwannomas may be completely removed from peripheral nerves with minimal damage to the nerve. However, this is not the case when the tumor involves cranial nerve VIII. (See Chap. 11 on tumors of cranial nerves and coverings.)

NEUROMAS

Neuromas occur either as solitary tumors or as a part of neurofibromatosis. The neurofibroma is also a nerve sheath tumor but is differentiated from the schwannoma in that nerve fibers run through the tumor. Excision of this tumor routinely results in neurological deficits.

NEUROFIBROMATOSIS

Neurofibromatosis (von Recklinghausen's Disease) is an autosomal dominant genetic disorder that has varying degrees of manifestation. Its cardinal features include café-au-lait spots of the skin and neurofibromas within the peripheral, autonomic, and central nervous systems. Four types of the disease have been described, including central, peripheral, visceral, and forme fruste.[50]

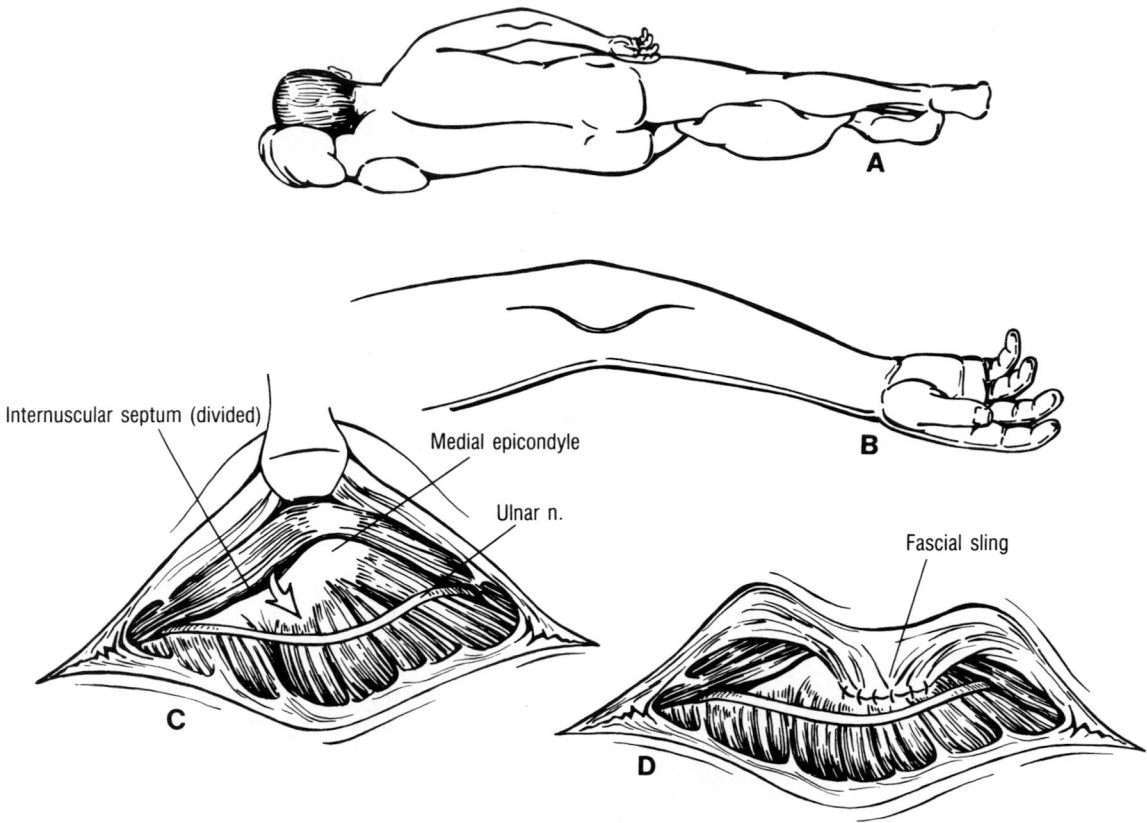

Internuscular septum (divided)

Medial epicondyle

Ulnar n.

Fascial sling

Figure 21–13   Transposition of ulnar nerve.

TUMORS OF NONNEURAL ORIGIN

Tumors of nonneural origin include *lipofibromatosis of the median nerve,* which usually presents as a soft mass in the palm during childhood or early adulthood. Carpal tunnel release offers only temporary relief. Extensive microsurgical neurolysis is more efficacious, since the tumor is outside the nerve. Removal of large amounts of the tumor may be accomplished with preservation of function. Intraneural lipomas, hemangiomas, and gangliomas have been described,

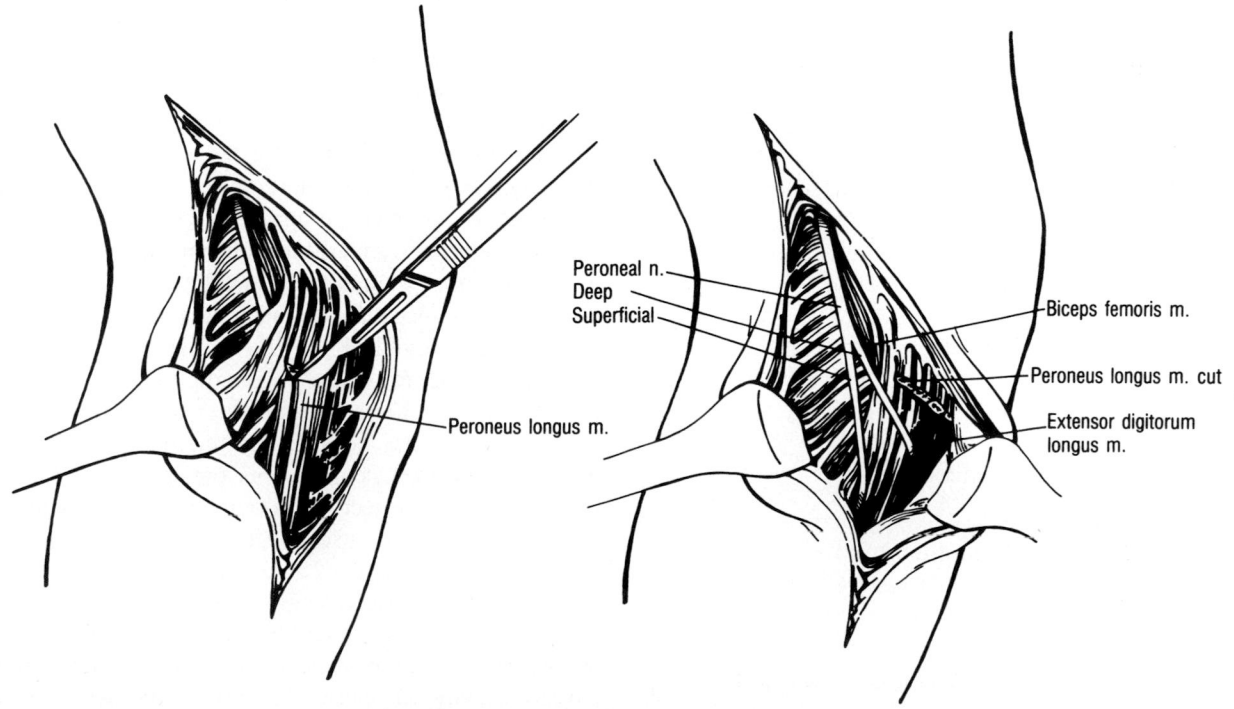

Peroneal n.
Deep
Superficial

Peroneus longus m.

Biceps femoris m.

Peroneus longus m. cut

Extensor digitorum longus m.

Figure 21–14   Decompression of peroneal nerve.

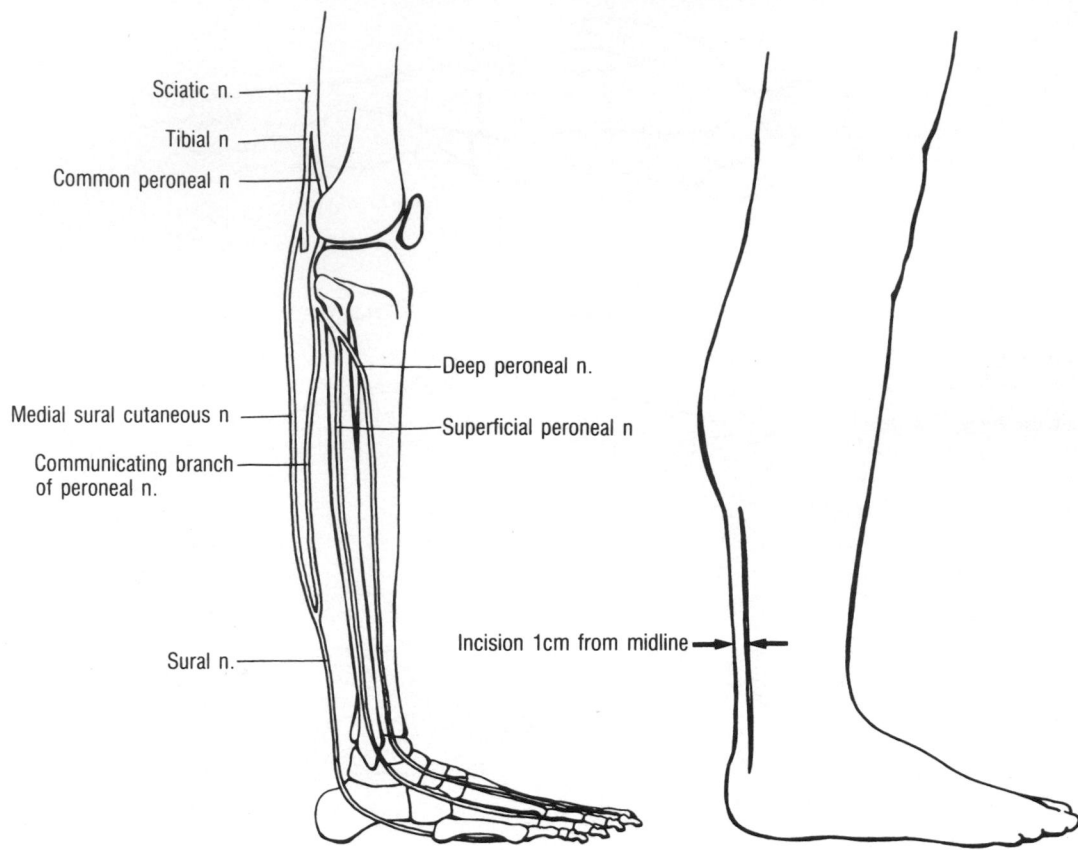

Figure 21–15   Harvesting sural nerve.

presenting as a mass, with neurological symptoms, or both.[51–56] Removal of these masses is possible without loss or interruption of function.

Table 21-2
CLASSIFICATION OF TUMORS OF PERIPHERAL NERVES

I.   **Neoplasms of nerve sheath origin**
  A. Benign primary nerve sheath tumors
    1. Schwannoma
    2. Neurofibroma
  B. Malignant primary nerve sheath tumors
    1. Malignant schwannoma
    2. Nerve sheath fibrosarcoma

II. **Neoplasms of nerve cell origin**
  A. Neuroblastoma
  B. Ganglioneuroma
  C. Pheochromocytoma

III. **Tumors metastatic to peripheral nerves**

IV. **Neoplasms of nonneural origin**
  A. Lipofibromatosis of the median nerve
  B. Intraneural lipoma, hemangioma, ganglion

V.   **Nonneoplasms**
  A. Traumatic neuroma
  B. Compressive neuroma (Morton's neuroma, Bowler's thumb)

☐ CAUSALGIA AND PAINFUL TRAUMATIC NEUROMAS

Injury to a peripheral nerve may result in loss of function supplied by the nerve, but it may also cause painful sequelae. The pain may result from a pressure-sensitive neuroma or an incomplete nerve injury that produces *causalgia* (from the Greek *kausis,* meaning "burning," and *algos,* meaning "pain").

Causalgia is an intense, constant, burning pain. The slightest movement of the affected extremities may cause paroxysms of the pain. Changes in the autonomic function to the affected extremity are apparent. The hand, for example, will be colder or warmer, bluer or pinker, and usually more moist than the contralateral, unaffected hand. In typical causalgia of the hand due to incomplete median nerve injury, a stellate ganglion block may be of diagnostic and therapeutic benefit. A series of stellate ganglion blocks may increase the duration of relief and even cause the condition to abate. However, there may be pitfalls to the interpretation of such blocks, and a short course of an oral alpha blocking agent may be equally effective in temporarily or permanently stopping such pain. (See section on sympathectomy in Chap. 24.)

If sympathetic blockade gives only temporary relief, surgical sympathectomy should be considered, provided a thorough psychological evaluation has ruled out any significant psychopathology. If causalgia involves the upper extremity, the lower half of the stellate ganglion and the upper two or three thoracic sympathetic ganglia are moved, using a trans-axillary or posterior approach (see Ref. 40 in Chap. 24).

In patients with painful neuromas, relief of the pain is sometimes difficult to achieve. For this reason, many treatment options have evolved. Kline and Nulson advocate sharply sectioning the nerve proximal to the neuroma and embedding the freshly sectioned nerve end in adjacent deep soft tissue.[40] This has, on occasion, led to reoperation to resect a new neuroma. Recurrence of the painful neuroma is less likely if the freshly sectioned nerve end is placed in a protective environment deep in the limb and surrounded by muscle.[40]

If the pain is related to a neuroma in continuity, there is complete loss of motor function of more than 3 but less than 12 mo duration, and intraoperative nerve action potentials indicate no regeneration across the site of injury, the neuroma should be excised and a primary neurorrhaphy or cable grafting performed. If there is intraoperative nerve action potential evidence of recovery of function, an external and

possibly an internal (interfascicular) neurolysis should be performed. If there is clinical or EMG evidence of recovery, adequate time for regeneration to complete itself should be allowed.[40] As in all cases of chronic pain, a thorough psychological evaluation should be done before finalizing plans for surgery.

☐ SUMMARY

In patients with peripheral nerve injuries, concurrent injuries that might be life-threatening must be treated first, and then the peripheral nerve injury approached systematically. The type of injury, its time of occurrence, initial deficit, and degree of recovery expected are important issues in establishing the treatment plan, which may range from skilled observation to extensive surgical intervention.

REFERENCES

1. Mackinnon SE, Dellon AL: *Surgery of the Peripheral Nerve.* New York, Thieme Medical Publishers, 1988, pp 638.
2. Lundborg G, Branemark PI: Microvascular structure and function of peripheral nerves. Vital microscopic studies of the tibial nerve in the rabbit. *Adv Microcirc* 1:66–88, 1968.
3. Breidenbach WC, Terzis JK: The blood supply of vascularized nerve grafts. *J Reconstr Microsurg* 3:43–58, 1986.
4. Sunderland S: The intraneural topography of the radial, median, and ulnar nerves. *Brain* 68:243–299, 1945.
5. Jabaley ME, Wallace WH, Heckler FR: Internal topography of major nerves of the forearm and hand: A current view. *J Hand Surg* 5:1–18, 1980.
6. Ducker TB, Kempe LG, Hayes GJ: The metabolic background for peripheral nerve surgery. *J Neurosurg* 30:270–280, 1969.
7. Droz B, Leblond CP: Migration of proteins along the axons of the sciatic nerve. *Science* 137:1047–1048, 1962.
8. Lubinska L, Niemierko S: Velocity and intensity of bidirectional migration of acetylcholinesterase in transected nerves. *Brain Res* 27:329–342, 1971.
9. Lasek RJ, Shelanski ML, Brinkley BR, et al: Cytoskeletons and the architecture of nervous systems. *Neurosci Res Program Bull* 19:1–153, 1981.
10. Droz B, Rambourg A, Koenig HL: The smooth endoplasmic reticulum: Structure and role in the renewal of axonal membrane and synaptic vesicles by fast axonal transport. *Brain Res* 93:1–13, 1975.
11. Weiss P: The technology of nerve regeneration: A review. Sutureless tubulation and related methods of nerve repair. *J Neurosurg* 1:400–450, 1944.
12. Brushart TM, Seiler WA IV: Selective reinnervation of distal motor stumps by peripheral motor axons. *Exp Neurol* 97:289–300, 1987.
13. Morris JH, Hudson AR, Weddell G: A study of degeneration and regeneration in the divided rat sciatic nerve based on electron microscopy. I: The traumatic degeneration of myelin in the proximal stump of the divided nerve. *Z Zellforsch* 124:76–102, 1972.
14. Yamada KM, Spooner BS, Wessells NK: Ultrastructure and function of growth cones and axons of cultured nerve cells. *J Cell Biol* 49:614–635, 1971.
15. Rogers SL, Letourneau PC, Palm SL, et al: Neurite extension by peripheral and central nervous system neurons in response to substratum-bound fibronectin and laminin. *Dev Biol* 98:212–220, 1983.
16. Sanders FK, Young JZ: The influence of peripheral connexion on the diameter of regenerating nerve fibres. *J Exp Biol* 22:203–212, 1946.
17. Cancilla PA: General reactions of muscle to injury, in Heffner RR (ed): *Muscle Pathology: Contemporary Issues in Surgical Pathology.* New York, Churchill Livingstone, 1984, pp 15–30.
18. Gorio A, Carmignoto G: Reformation, maturation and stabilization of neuromuscular junctions in peripheral nerve regeneration, in Gorio A, Millesi H, Mingrino S (eds): *Posttraumatic Peripheral Nerve Regeneration: Experimental Basis and Clinical Implications.* New York, Raven, 1981, pp 481–492.
19. McNamara MJ, Garrett WE, Seaber AV, Goldner JL: Neurorrhaphy, nerve grafting, and a neurotization: A functional comparison of nerve reconstruction techniques. *J Hand Surg* 12A:354–360, 1987.
20. Karpati G, Carpenter S, Charron L: Experimental reinnervation attempts of skeletal muscle cells by non-motor nerves, in Gorio A, Millesi H, Mingrino S (eds): *Posttraumatic Peripheral Nerve Regeneration: Experimental Basis and Clinical Implantations.* New York, Raven Press, 1981, pp 495–506.
21. Mackinnon SE, Dellon AL, Hudson AR, Hunter DA: Alteration of neuroma formation by manipulation of its microenvironment. *Plast Reconstr Surg* 76:345–352, 1985.

22. Dellon AL, Witebsky FG, Terrill RE: The denervated Meissner corpuscle. A sequential histological study after nerve division in the Rhesus monkey. *Plast Reconstr Surg* 56:182–193, 1975.

23. Dellon AL: Reinnervation of denervated Meissner corpuscles: A sequential histologic study in the monkey following fascicular nerve repair. *J Hand Surg* 1A:98–109, 1976.

24. Davis L: The return of sensation to transplanted skin. *Surg Gynecol Obstet* 59:533–543, 1934.

25. Kredel FE, Evans JP: Recovery of sensation in denervated pedicles and fres skin grafts. *J Neurol Neurosurg Psychiatry* 19:1203–1221, 1933.

26. Dellon AL: Sensory recovery in replanted digits and transplanted toes. A review. *J Reconstr Microsurgery* 2:123–129, 1986.

27. Mitchell SW: *Injuries of Nerves and Their Consequences.* Philadelphia, Lippincott, 1872, pp 266–273.

28. Sunderland S: *Nerves and Nerve Injuries,* 2d ed. Edinburgh, Churchill Livingstone, 1968, p vii.

29. Woodhall B: Peripheral nerve injuries. II: Basic data from the peripheral nerve registry concerning 7,050 nerve sutures and 67 nerve grafts. *J Neurosurg* 4:146–163, 1947.

30. Denny-Brown D, Adams RD, Brenner C, and Doherty MM: The pathology of injury to nerve induced by cold. *J Neuropath Exp Neurol* 4:305–323, 1945.

31. Seddon HJ: Three types of nerve injury. *Brain* 66:239–288, 1943.

32. Sunderland S: A classification of peripheral nerve injuries producing loss of function. *Brain* 74:491–516, 1951.

33. Lundborg G: *Nerve Injury and Repair.* Edinburgh, Churchill Livingstone, 1988, pp 78–79.

34. Seddon HJ, Medawar PB, Smith H: Rate of regeneration of peripheral nerves in man. *J Physiol* (Lond) 102:191–215, 1943.

35. Sunderland S: Rate of regeneration sensory nerve fibers. *Arch Neurol Psychiatr* 58:1–6, 1947.

36. Sunderland S: Rate of regeneration of motor fibers in the ulnar and sciatic nerves. *Arch Neurol Psychiatr* 58:7–14, 1947.

37. Yahr MD, Beebe GW: Recovery of motor function, in Woodhall B, Beebe GW (eds): *Peripheral Nerve Regeneration.* Washington, U.S. Government Printing Office, 1956, chap 3, pp 71–202.

38. Davidson AJ, Horwitz MT: Late or tardy ulnar-nerve paralysis. *J Bone Joint Surg* 17:844–856, 1935.

39. Nelson KG, Jolly PC, Thomas PA: Brachial plexus injuries associated with missile wounds of the chest: A report of 9 cases from Viet Nam. *J Trauma* 8:268–275, 1968.

40. Kline DG, Nulson FE: Acute injuries of peripheral nerves, in Youmans JR (ed): *Neurological Surgery,* 2d ed. Philadelphia, Saunders, 1982, chap 75, pp 2362–2429.

41. Yeoman PM, Seddon HJ: Brachial plexus injuries: Treatment of the flail arm. *J Bone Joint Surg* 43B:493–500, 1961.

42. Bora FW: Peripheral nerve repair in cats: The fascicular stitch. *J Bone Joint Surg* 49A:659–666, 1967.

43. Kutz JE, Shealy G, Lubbers L: Interfascicular nerve repair. *Orthoped Clin North Am* 12:277–286, 1981.

44. Kline DG, Hudson AR, Bratton BR: Experimental study of fascicular nerve repair with and without epineurial closure. *J Neurosurg* 54:513–520, 1981.

45. Edshage S: Peripheral nerve suture: A technique for improved intraneural topography. Evaluation of some suture materials. *Acta Chir Scand* (suppl) 331:1–104, 1964.

46. Orgel MG, Terzis JK: Epineural vs. perineurial repair: An untrastructural and electrophysiological study of nerve regeneration. *Plast Reconstruct Surg* 60:80–91, 1977.

47. Levinthal R, Brown WJ, Rand RW: Comparison of fascicular, interfascicular and epineural suture techniques in the repair of simple nerve lacerations. *J Neurosurg* 47:744–750, 1977.

48. Terzis JK, Smith KL: *The Peripheral Nerve: Structure, Function, and Reconstruction.* New York, Raven, 1990, pp 129–131.

49. Mackinnon SE, Hudson, AR: Clinical application of peripheral nerve transplantation. *Plast Reconstr Surg.* 90:695–699, 1992.

50. Harkin VC, Reed RJ: *Tumors of the Peripheral Nervous System.* Washington, Armed Forces Institute of Pathology, 1969, pp 67–97.

51. Morley GH: Intraneural lipoma of the median nerve of the carpal tunnel. *J Bone Joint Surg* 46B:734–735, 1964.

52. Mikhail IK: Meidan nerve lipoma in the hand. *J Bone Joint Surg* 46B:726–730, 1964.

53. Kojima T, Ide Y, Marumo E, et al: Hemangioma of median nerve causing carpal tunnel syndrome. *Hand,* 8:62–65, 1976.

54. Losli EJ: Intrinsic hemangiomas of the peripheral nerves: A report of two cases and a review of the literature. *Arch Pathol* 53:226–232, 1952.

55. Purcell FH, Gurdjian ES: Hemangiomata of peripheral nerves with report of a case of cavernous hemangioma of the sciatic nerve. *Am J Surg* 30:541–544, 1935.

56. Barrett R, Cramer F: Tumors of the peripheral nerves and so-called "ganglia" of the peroneal nerve. *Clin Orthop* 27:135–146, 1963.

☐ STUDY QUESTIONS

I. A 21-year-old male loses control of his motorcycle when it strikes a parked vehicle. He is thrown over the vehicle and hits a tree. He does not remember the accident, but when he regained consciousness, he has severe pain over the left clavicle. He can flex his fingers weakly but cannot flex his elbow or abduct or rotate his shoulder. He can hold his arm extended. He has anesthesia over the shoulder and down the lateral and thenar sides of his arm and forearm, respectively. X-rays reveal that the clavicle is fractured.

1. What is the differential diagnosis? **2.** How can the various diagnoses be determined? **3.** Assuming avulsion of the fifth and sixth cervical nerve roots, what might be done to reinnervate the shoulder and arm? **4.** Assuming avulsion of the upper roots of the brachial plexus, what might the EMG of the forearm show the day after the injury? A month later? **5.** When might one expect to see beginning recovery of motor function, assuming the injury is due to stretching of the upper brachial plexus?

II. A 45-year-old female falls on some ice, sustaining a Colles fracture of the right wrist, which is treated with reduction and a cast. After the cast is removed, the patient begins to notice numbness of the hand. She awakens at night with pain, gets up, and moves the hand about to be able to go back to sleep for a while.

She begins to notice atrophy of the muscles at the base of the thumb. Examination reveals hypalgesia over the palmar surface of the thumb, the adjacent two and a half fingers, and the corresponding part of the hand. Holding the wrist in flexion reproduces the nocturnal pain.

1. What is the most likely diagnosis? **2.** What forms of therapy might be considered? **3.** What would a nerve conduction study most likely show? **4.** If surgery on the median nerve is recommended, what structures might one expect to encounter? **5.** What is the likelihood of finding a Tinel's sign over the median nerve?

III. A 23-year-old male sustains a shotgun blast to the anterior surface of the elbow. The radial artery is injured, along with the superficial veins and the median nerve, which is not interrupted. The vessels are repaired. Initially, there is paralysis of flexion of the fingers, but there is gradual recovery. As sensation recovers, a severe burning pain develops in the forearm and hand.

1. What diagnoses might be considered? **2.** What are the possible therapies? **3.** What is the origin of the name "causalgia"? **4.** What determines the rate of recovery of sensation of the forearm and hand? **5.** What are the types of injury to the median nerve which might be considered?

IV. A 28-year-old male carpenter, who is known to frequent the bars in town, has a number of beers one Saturday night before he is taken home, where he falls asleep slumped in a large armchair. When he awakens, he cannot extend his wrist or fingers. He has some numbness in his hand.

1. What is his basic lesion and how did it occur? **2.** How is the lesion classified using Seddon's classification? **3.** What is the prognosis? **4.** What is the most likely distribution of sensory loss? **5.** What treatment should be instituted?

V. A 23-year-old male laborer sustains a laceration of the palmar surface of his forearm by a fragment of glass. The bellies of the flexor muscles are lacerated, as are the vessels and the median nerve. The neurological deficits are determined in the emergency room, following which the patient is taken to the operating room. The neurosurgeon is called after the blood vessels have been repaired, the request being for instructions as to what should be done with the median nerve.

1. What motor and sensory changes should be encountered in the emergency room? **2.** What instructions should be given to the surgeon regarding the nerve? **3.** Assuming the nerve is sutured that evening, what is the most likely first sign of a successful anastamosis, that is, axonal growth? **4.** How long is it likely to take for motor fibers to reach the muscles at the base of the thumb? **5.** How should the patient's arm and hand be treated in the interim?

Surgical Treatment of Epilepsy

Herman F. Flanigin
Joseph R. Smith

The prevalence of epilepsy is generally underestimated, as is the need for surgical treatment. The number of epileptics in the United States is estimated at well over 1 million. Approximately 800,000 of these suffer from *focal epilepsy*, the most common type being of temporal lobe origin. Only about 70 percent of patients with recurrent seizures are satisfactorily controlled by medication, while 10 to 20 percent are considered to have medically intractable epilepsy. Each year approximately 150,000 people in the United States develop epilepsy. It is estimated that 2000 to 5000 of these new patients might be candidates for surgery, but with only about 500 such operations annually, the surgical mode of treatment for epilepsy appears to be vastly underutilized.[1]

Lobectomy or *focal resection* is the procedure of choice for patients with a confirmed solitary focus. A single focus may not be identified in some patients who suffer from multiple types of convulsive and/or nonconvulsive generalized or partial seizures. Although such individuals are not candidates for focal resection of epileptogenic tissue, transection of the corpus callosum may control their seizures.[2]

Patients with infantile hemiplegia and with partial and secondarily generalized seizures whose foci cannot be isolated may benefit from physiological (or "functional") hemispherectomy.[3] In addition to improved seizure control and behavior, many experience improvement in cognitive and motor function.

A structural lesion of the brain in a seizure patient is another indication for evaluation. Even small tumors can produce seizures, as can nonneoplastic structural lesions. The seizures may lead to surgical removal of a structural lesion, resulting in control not only of the seizures but also of the neoplasm.

Patients whose seizures cannot be controlled by any other means may benefit from surgery, but if the protocol for surgical treatment establishes criteria so restrictive that only ideal candidates are selected for operation, many patients may be deprived of potentially beneficial surgery.[4,5] Justifiable reasons for rejection of patients for early resection have, however, been established.[5]

Two types of surgical procedures are utilized in the treatment of epilepsy: ablation of the seizure focus and disconnection of the focus from other functional parts of the brain. Ablation of the source of seizures may involve a small segment of brain tissue or the cortex of an entire hemisphere. The combination of ablation and disconnection in functional hemispherectomy is finding increased application.

Investigative Procedures

Patients with uncontrolled seizures are evaluated by an initial battery of investigative procedures. The multidisciplinary approach requires participation of several individuals with specific competence in selecting candidates for surgery. The following paragraphs review the salient features of such an investigation.

☐ HISTORY

The *seizure history* is the most important clinical feature in the initial evaluation. Age of onset should be obtained. Any history of neonatal or febrile seizures should also be recorded.

The "initial phenomenon" provides a correlation between the clinical focus and the focus verified at surgery.[6] The most useful localization data are those events consistently associated with the onset of a patient's attacks. Other successive phenomena may have value in defining pathways of spread or in establishing secondary generalization.[7,8] Adversive movements may be unreliable for determining the side of lateralization. Gustatory (chewing, mouthing, swallowing, savoring) movements or other automatisms are important. Postictal events, such as paresis, automatisms, confusion, memory, or personality changes should be noted.

identification of the structures removed.[27,28,29] In corpus callosotomy, the midsagittal image may be used for preoperative planning and for postoperative determination of the extent of resection.[30] In both instances the postoperative studies also are an aid in correlating neurological and neuropsychological outcome.

POSITRON EMISSION TOMOGRAPHY (PET)

The need for a cyclotron in the proximate area of the PET laboratory limits this technique to a few centers. Its contribution to the identification of seizure foci has, however, been recognized in many cases.[31,32,33]

In epileptic patients damaged regions of the brain which are epileptogenic may be found to be *hypo*metabolic in the interictal periods but *hyper*metabolic during seizures.[34] With rare exception there is a high correlation between these demonstrated changes and the epileptic foci demonstrated by depth electrode studies.[31]

Focal metabolic abnormalities on PET in children with epilepsy have corresponded to abnormal electrocorticographic areas which are presumably the epileptogenic regions. Such areas may appear normal on CT and MRI.[35]

SINGLE PHOTON EMISSION COMPUTED TOMOGRAPHY (SPECT)

SPECT provides the capability of examining brain metabolism by identifying areas of altered perfusion. Combined interictal and immediate postictal SPECT with 99mTc-HMPAO may provide an alternative to the use of depth electrode studies for confirmation of surface EEG findings in many patients with complex partial seizures.[33,36] A wide variation in the reliability of localization by interictal scans is noted, but when combined with postictal scans, the correlation with a demonstrable focus rises to 69 to 72 percent.[36,37] Reliability variation increases in the presence of structural lesions.

There may be differences in distribution of perfusion changes. Postictal hyperperfusion has been predominantly mesial temporal, and it is frequently associated with hypoperfusion of the lateral temporal cortex. Secondarily generalized seizures tend to show focal hyperperfusion less often than complex partial seizures.[36]

A high correlation of SPECT abnormality with memory function following surgery has been reported. In left temporal lobectomies postoperative verbal memory impairment occurred in only 8 percent of the patients if SPECT agreed with the side selected for surgery, but in 83 percent if it diverged from it. This gives strong support for the concept that demonstrable metabolic abnormalities reflect cerebral dysfunction associated with memory.[38] Of concern, however, is a finding that SPECT has revealed infrequent delivery of isotope to mesial temporal structures.[39]

ANGIOGRAPHY

Visualization of intracranial vessels is imperative in patients with vascular malformations being considered for surgery. It is also important to know the location of cortical vessels in patients undergoing depth electrode implantation. In an interhemispheric approach for corpus callosotomy, the position of the bridging cortical veins as they enter the superior sagittal sinus is a factor in planning,[40] as is the relationship between the anterior cerebral arteries, which may present problems in their separation during callosotomy. Occluded or atrophic vessels may provide etiologic information about hemispheric lesions and aid in their localization.

MAGNETOENCEPHALOGRAPHY (MEG)

Magnetoencephalography is emerging as a method for detection of epileptic foci. The electromagnetic fields in the brain produced by neuronal activity are recorded by arrays of detectors [Superconducting Quantum Interference Devices (SQUIDs)] placed over the scalp. The data may be displayed in a manner similar to EEG recordings or as graphic displays of the dipole.[33,41] Using stereotactic references, magnetic spike activity may be localized in three-dimensional stereotactic space and then onlayed over multiplanar MRI views in order to display anatomic location.

This method may have an advantage over EEG since the signals are detected directly rather than after volume conduction, and they are not attenuated by bone or altered by conflicting electrical signals. Therefore, multichannel MEG may have better potential for localizing, in three dimensions, foci from deep structures. Unfortunately, the strength of the signal diminishes with the square to cube of the distance, so that a signal 3 cm deep is attenuated by 80 percent. As with EEG, MEG detects signals in relation to the orientation of the recording sites, but magnetic dipoles are at right angles to their electrical dipoles. Also, as in EEG, a large number of recording points are necessary for localization.

Some studies of induced electrical dipoles in depth electrodes suggest that MEG has no significant advantage over EEG in localization of foci. The current role of MEG may be to provide complimentary information.[42] MEG can determine latency differences and propagation distances of spikes consistent with the conduction velocity of corticocortical fibers.[43] Noninvasive derivation of the cortical surface area of the spikes agrees with localization obtained by electrocorticography over the temporal neocortex.

Using replicated preoperative MEG studies with dipole electrical signals inserted through depth electrodes, spatial correlation has been found to be within 1 cm. These were localized within the area subsequently resected. The MEG localization was also in close agreement with intraoperative cortical recordings.[44]

ELECTROENCEPHALOGRAPHY (EEG)

EEG from scalp, sphenoidal, and intracranial electrodes remains the primary means of preoperative localization. There are two major types of electographic data useful in the preoperative localization studies: (1) interictal sharp waves and spikes (epileptiform discharges), and (2) the electrographic onset of ictal events.[5,45]

Following the development of EEG, interictal epileptiform discharges were the primary localizing tool for most of the early investigations for ablative surgery. The success of surgery in a large percentage of patients confirmed the validity of this method.[8,46,47,48] However, clinical seizures may begin in areas distant from or even contralateral to the location of interictal epileptiform activity.[5,48] Thus, interictal discharges without corroborating evidence should not be used as the sole means of localization.[5,48]

Interictal focal slow waves are valuable indicators of localized cerebral dysfunction. Alone, however, slow waves are not as useful as spikes in localizing the epileptic process.[48] While delta activity in scalp recordings reveals a high degree (92 percent) of lateralization and even lobar identification,[49] its use for seizure focus localization intraoperatively is not sufficiently reliable for ablative procedures.[50]

Ictal discharges are the most reliable means of localization and should be considered the most accurate method for determining the area for resection.[5] However, since it is impossible to record from all cortical and subcortical structures from which seizures may arise, the exact onset may not involve the recording electrodes until recruitment and spread of the discharge has occurred.[48]

Among surgical candidates the most common location for focal epileptiform discharges is the anterior to midtemporal area. Anterior temporal epileptiform discharges correlate well with "psychomotor" or complex partial seizures.[8,48,51] In patients with complex partial seizures, a well-localized anterior to midtemporal focus is indicative of a temporal lobe origin. Improvement in seizure control following surgery in numerous studies has confirmed the localizing significance of these discharges.[5,8,46,47,48,52]

Patients being evaluated for ablative surgery for seizures of temporal origin undergo needle placement of silver wire electrodes against the inferior surface of the greater wing of the sphenoid bone, beneath the mesial temporal lobe structures (sphenoidal electrodes). (See Fig. 22-1.)

Patients with complex partial seizures often show interictal epileptiform discharges which are maximal from the mesial temporal region; i.e., the primary phase reversal is recorded from the sphenoidal electrodes. Mesial temporal epileptiform discharges correlate with specific temporal pathological lesions, including hippocampal (mesial temporal-incisural) sclerosis and neoplasms.[48,53,54,55]

Sphenoidal electrodes are more effective than scalp electrodes in documenting the earliest evidence of onset of ictal activity in patients with seizures of mesial temporal origin.[31] Bilateral independent epileptiform activity from scalp recordings appears in up to 30 percent of patients with

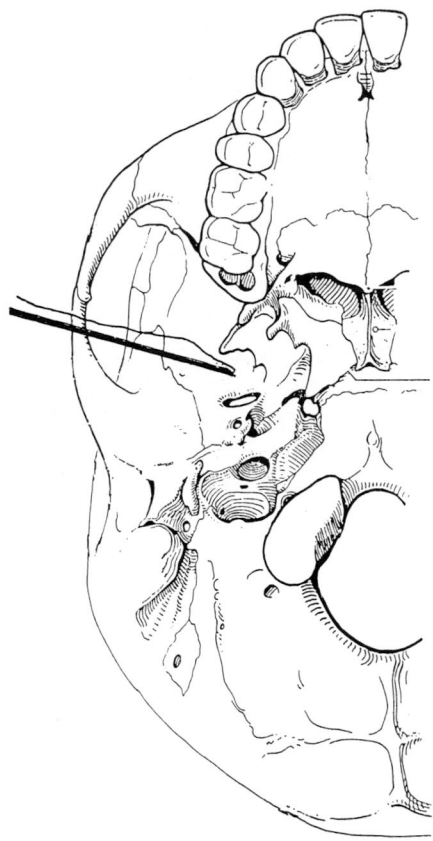

Figure 22–1 Schematic drawing of introducer placing sphenoidal electrode on the inferior surface of the greater wing of the sphenoid bone near the foramen ovale.

complex partial seizures and anterior to midtemporal foci.[48] Furthermore, even when scalp discharges are unilateral or one side clearly predominates, seizure onset may be contralateral to the side of surface-recorded epileptiform activity. This is due to the damaged temporal lobe structures not recruiting extensive synchronous activity compared with the opposite intact side. Confirmatory evidence by imaging, semiology, neuropsychological testing, or intracranial electrodes is required.[5,48] (See Fig. 22-2A and B.)

Interictal epileptiform discharges recorded from extratemporal regions are also useful in localizing an epileptogenic process.[8,48,56] Extratemporal spikes correlate well with the clinical ictal phenomena one might expect from seizures originating in these regions.[5,8] Because interictal discharges from extratemporal regions are often not as well localized as temporal foci, corroborating evidence from clinical phenomena, imaging studies, or invasive studies is required.

While data from a scalp-recorded ictal onset are useful in the localization process, there are disadvantages. Muscle artifact may obscure the most important electrographic changes. As a result, the initiating epileptic discharge may be in progress for several seconds before sufficient spread and recruitment present interpretable electrographic changes at the scalp.[57] Of more significance, the seizure onset in partial epilepsy often involves deep structures at some distance from scalp electrodes.

Thus, early ictal changes are often not identified in scalp

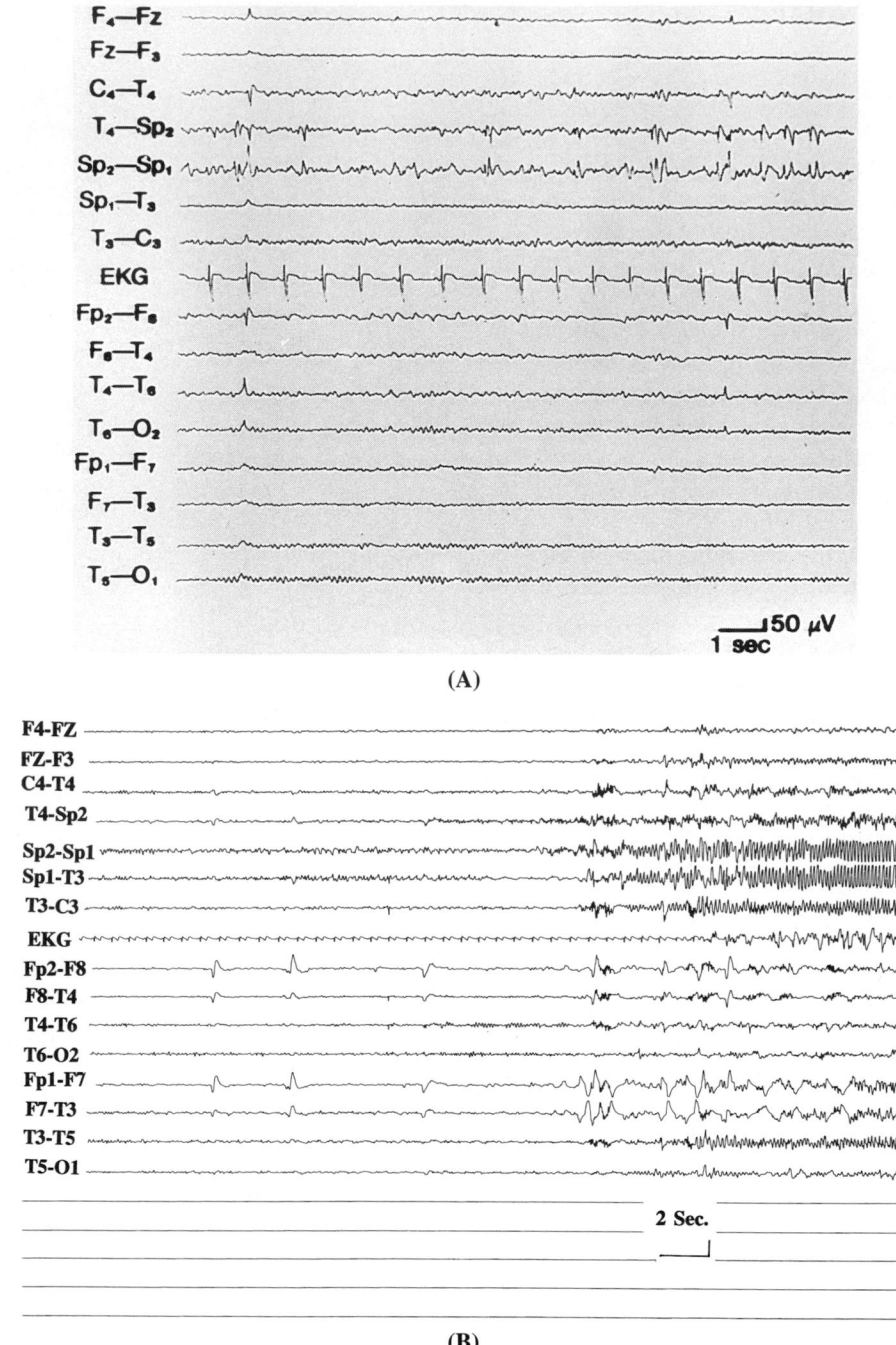

Figure 22–2 Abnormal activity recorded maximally from sphenoidal electrodes. (A) Spike discharge showing phase reversal at Sp2. (B) Seizure discharge originating at Sp1.

recordings.[48,58] In addition, although rare, false lateralization occurs[5,45,48] using scalp and sphenoidal studies. Even when sphenoidal electrodes are used, muscle artifact causes loss of signal clarity. Implantation procedures have been developed to address these problems.[5,40,57,58,59,60,61]

EPIDURAL AND SUBDURAL ELECTRODES.

Several types of epidural and subdural electrode implantation procedures have been developed in order to define more

accurately the epileptic focus prior to ablation. Multicontact strip or grid electrodes may be placed in the epidural space or in the subdural space for recording. (See Fig. 22-3.)

Operative Technique: Burr hole placement Electrodes may be implanted under local or general anesthesia. General anesthesia is required in children and uncooperative adults. Bilateral temporal incisions are positioned so that they can be used for a craniotomy later if needed. Burr holes are drilled and enlarged, permitting the dura to be incised in a cruciate manner. The brain is retracted from the dura,

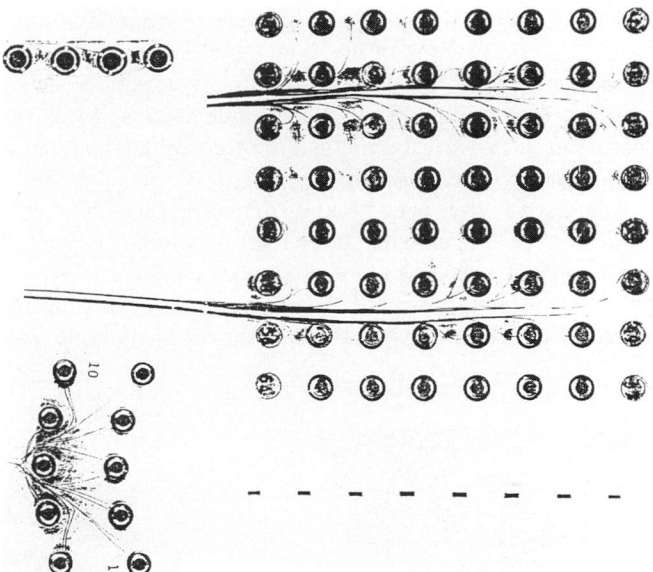

Figure 22–3 Examples of electrodes used for subdural strip, subdural grid, and interhemispheric and intracerebral implantation. Interelectrode spacing is 1 cm.

allowing the strip of electrodes to be passed inferiorly and anteriorly around the temporal tip. (See Fig. 22-4.)

A second strip may be passed inferiorly and posteriorly toward the uncus. Strips may also be passed beneath the frontal lobe and over its convexity using a pterional burr hole. By using burr holes placed in the parasagittal region, strips may be passed along the medial surface of the hemispheres. The leads from the strips are implanted beneath the scalp to exit through a stab wound 2 to 3 cm from the burr hole. They are held in place by sutures at the site of exit.

Operative Technique: Craniotomy placement Epidural and subdural electrode implantation, using a craniotomy, permits the extended recording of seizures as well as extensive mapping of sensorimotor cortex and speech areas. The operation is performed under general anesthesia, unless

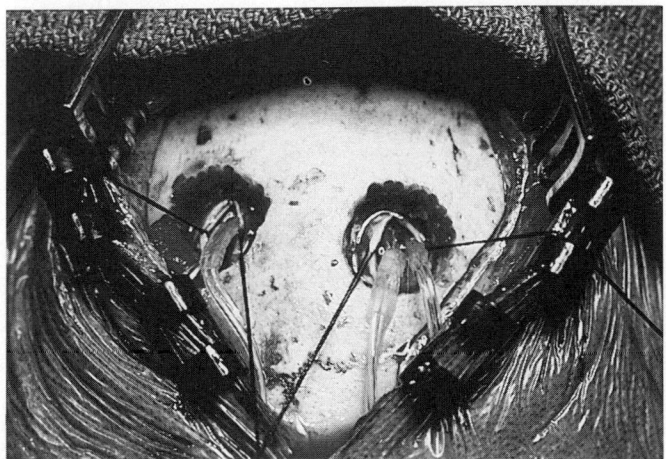

Figure 22–4 Bilateral parasagittal subdural electrode implantation. Electrodes have been inserted subdurally through burr holes.

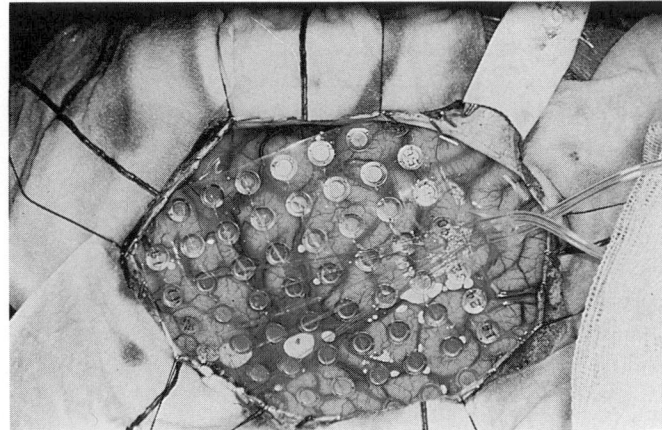

Figure 22–5 Subdural grid electrode array in place.

language or sensorimotor stimulation mapping is required as part of the implantation procedure.

The craniotomy is planned so that a definitive procedure will permit ablation or isolation of the focus at a second stage when the electrodes are removed. Photographic documentation of the anatomical position of the individual contacts permits correlation with electrophysiological data. Radiography of the strips or grids implanted permits further verification of position.[62,63,64] (See Fig. 22-5.)

Both of the above electrode implantation procedures permit extraoperative stimulation studies as well as video monitoring of clinical and cortical electrographic activity. The need for lead connections through the scalp does raise the issue of potential infection, and the duration of such studies is accordingly limited. Usually, the recording period may be extended for 7 to 10 days and occasionally up to 2 weeks. The strips and grids are removed at a second operation, and if a focus has been identified, definitive surgery may be accomplished at that time. The incidence of complications from implantation of epidural and subdural strips and grids is low.

INTRACEREBRAL ELECTRODES

Although epidural or subdural electrode studies add substantial information to the evaluation of many patients, the mesial, inferior cortical, and subcortical limbic structures and other areas deep within the brain may still be relatively inaccessible to recording. To gain access, multicontact depth electrodes located along the axis of the hippocampus are used to monitor structures in an anteroposterior orientation that otherwise would require several subdural strips.

Stereotactic instruments provide the means for accurate intracerebral electrode placement, but a limited number of electrodes can be placed, and these must be positioned in the structures most likely to be involved based on previous clinical and noninvasive studies.[45]

Patients considered for implantation are those with bilateral temporal abnormalities, as well as those with clinically focal seizures whose electrographic localization is indefinite.[5,64] Implantation use varies widely both in type and frequency. Intracranial electrodes may not even be necessary if scalp and sphenoidal EEG recordings are supported by semiology, imaging, and neuropsychological evaluation.[5,31,45]

Although false lateralization *can* occur when using only noninvasive means,[5,65] the adjunctive use of implantation raises other considerations. Serious complications, including hemorrhage, infection, and, rarely, transmission of viral disease occur in approximately 1 to 5 percent of cases when implanted electrodes are used.[60a] Fortunately, most complications are relatively minor and transient.

TECHNIQUE OF STEREOTACTIC ELECTRODE IMPLANTATION

See Chap. 23 for detailed information on stereotactic principles and techniques. (See Fig. 22-6.)

Operative Technique Targeted structures are defined preoperatively with CT or MRI. Angiography identifies avascular entry sites for trajectory planning. A vertex approach 10 to 14 cm posterior to the nasion and 2 to 3 cm lateral to the midline, or a posterior approach along the axis of the temporal lobe just inferior to the hippocampus, permits introduction of electrode contacts into the mesial temporal structures.

Using a technique modified from Crandall,[60] a stab wound is made in the scalp, and the skull is penetrated with a twist drill in the appropriate trajectory to—but not through—the dura. A specially designed hollow bolt is then placed in the bone and stereotactically aligned with the target point. A monopolar cautery tip penetrates the dura and controls dural and cortical bleeding. An insulated multiple lead electrode is inserted through the hollow bolt to the target. It is anchored by wrapping in the grooves of the bolt head and secured there by a plastic cap filled with liquid Silastic.

Successive placement to other targets is carried out in a similar manner. Placement positions are verified by intraoperative fluoroscopy, as well as subsequent x-ray and imaging studies. (See Fig. 22-7.)

A similar technique may be used to place single contact electrodes to, but not through, the dura, for epidural recording from selected sites over the convexity.

MONITORING

After recovery from the procedure, the patient is returned to the monitoring room and monitoring procedures are begun. Multifocal interictal discharges may be recorded from depth electrodes. As with surface recordings, interictal findings from depth structures are of limited value in localization decisions.[5]

The most reliable information *is* obtained from the ictal activity recorded at electrodes implanted in or adjacent to the

structures that are initiating the habitual seizures. The three most common patterns of electrographic change that signal seizure onset are: (1) voltage attenuation, (2) high-frequency rhythmic activity, and (3) high-amplitude spike and wave or sharp and slow-wave discharge followed by attenuation or high-frequency rhythmic discharges.

Attenuation has been found to be caused by rapid asynchronous neuronal discharges before organized synchronization develops.[66] A discharge confined to one or two contacts suggests a focal onset precisely localizing the origin of the seizure, whereas involvement of multiple con-

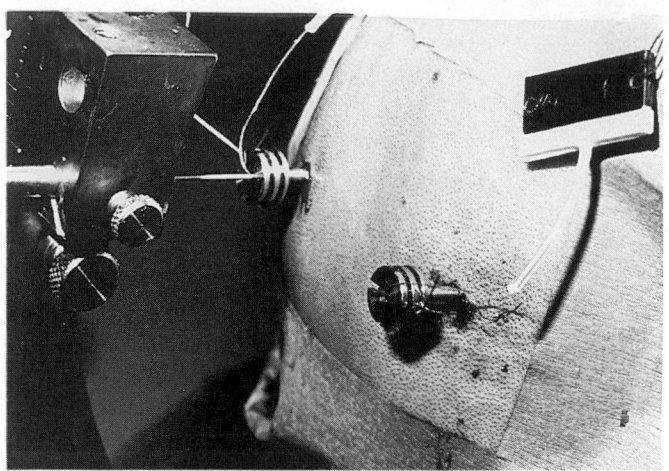

(A)

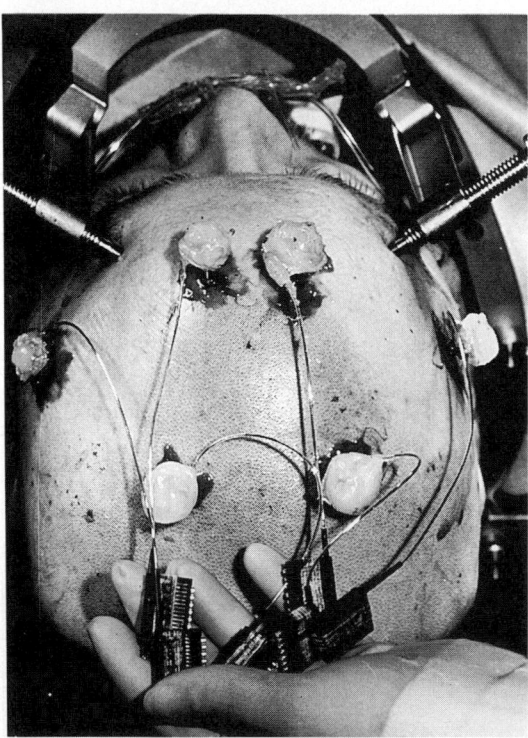

(B)

Figure 22–6 Stereotactic intracerebral electrode placement. *(A)* The electrode has already been placed through the special bolt on the right, and one is being inserted through the bolt on the left. *(B)* Vertex view after electrodes cemented in place in bolts.

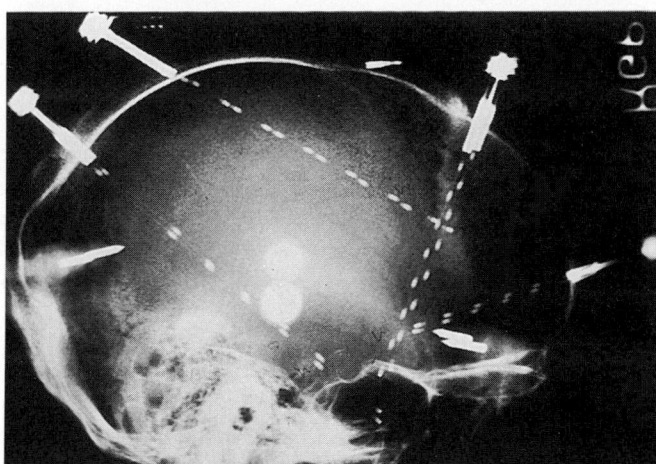

Figure 22–7 X-ray view of depth electrodes in place. Bilateral electrodes have been placed in mesial frontal, orbital frontal, cingulate, and axial temporal trajectories.

tacts indicates a regional onset that may be confined or that is itself indicating a more distant origin via the secondary activation of recording sites.

A precisely focal onset is *rarely* seen, during the use of two mesial temporal electrodes with multiple contact points, but in patients with seizures of mesial temporal origin a well-lateralized onset can be expected. Outcome following temporal lobectomy indicates that decisions based on these recordings have been correct. Most centers require recording and analysis of multiple seizures before making final recommendations for surgery. (See Fig. 22-8.)

PROLONGED MONITORING

Videotaping of the patient and his or her electrographic activity permits the simultaneous recording of the onset of multiple spontaneous seizures that correlate with observations of the patient during the attack. Montages can also be

reformatted—for replaying of data and extraction of maximum physiological information to correlate with such observations.

A localized electrographic change *preceding* the earliest clinical phenomena indicates the site of origin of the seizure. If electrographic changes *follow* the beginning of the clinical event, it is likely that the seizure has begun in a location distant to the site of the recording electrode.

In addition to reducing medications, it is frequently necessary during monitoring to resort to activation techniques in order to precipitate seizures. Activation may be produced by exercise, medications, alcohol, sleep deprivation, or induced sleep. Spontaneous spikes occurring during wakeful periods or during rapid eye movement (REM) sleep have more localizing value than those during slow-wave or barbiturate-induced sleep. Spikes under the latter conditions may be misleading. Also, ictal events recorded spontaneously appear to be more reliable than those provoked by convulsant drugs or electrical stimulation. The potential for false lateralization by drug withdrawal, sleep deprivation, and other routine procedures remains to be determined.[5]

STIMULATION STUDIES

Stimulation studies may be carried out using subdural or intracerebral electrodes.

It must be emphasized that electrical stimulation of the brain is not a truly physiological activation. The stimulating current produces responses in both activating and inhibiting neurons synchronous with the stimulus. The response perceived by the patient or an observer depends on the balance of activation and inhibition as well as on the area of the cortex stimulated. Activation is more evident, for example, in the primary projection (sensory, motor, visual) areas of the cortex. Inhibition may be "true" or a "busy line" impairment of cortical function. This is most evident in the testing of ongoing speech during stimulation of those corti-

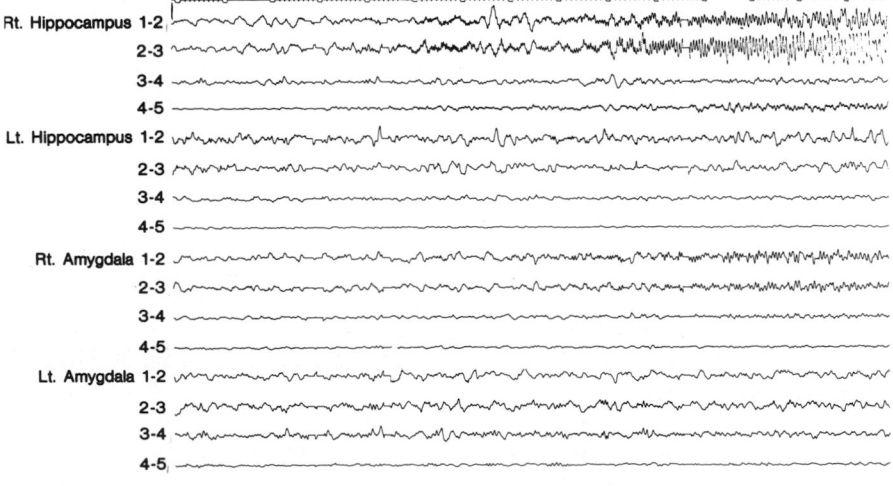

Figure 22–8 Depth electrode recording of a focal seizure onset in the right hippocampus.

cal areas representing language but it may also be present when stimulating the hippocampus during memory testing.

Responses to electrical stimulation in no way resemble voluntary movement initiated by the patient or normally perceived sensory experiences. Motor responses are contractions of muscle groups, and somatosensory responses are perceived as tingling, vibration, or other similar sensations. Likewise, visual and auditory responses are perceived as flashes of light or buzzing or ringing and not as normal perceptions of the normal environment. If a patient attempts to use an extremity involved in a motor stimulation sequence, the patient will be unable to do so. Likewise, availability of the sensory, visual, or auditory cortex for normal access is removed, and functional speech areas are inactivated. The stimulated cortex is so completely occupied with the electrical intrusion that it is not available for normal function, described by Penfield as the "busy line effect."

Stimulation of the normal association areas does not produce an activated response, but as in the primary projection areas, normal function is suppressed by the stimulus. In epileptogenic zones, however, stimulation of association areas may activate circuits habituated by the epileptic discharge. Such responses may be of perceptual illusions, "déjà vu," or even memory of previous events.[8]

These principles form the basis for *stimulation mapping* of the cortex for motor, sensory, and speech areas of the brain. They are also applicable to the study of the association areas for perceptual illusions—and even in the hippocampus for studies on memory.[40]

Following acquisition of spontaneous electrographic activity from intracranial electrodes, stimulation is begun. A two-channel stimulator with isolation and current control circuits provides balanced square wave bipolar stimuli of 60 Hz, with a 0.5 ms duration per phase and 1 to 12 mA. The stimulus train is usually applied for 3 s and passed between intracranial electrode contacts. Videotaping permits recording of electrographic, objective, and subjective phenomena.

When performing depth electrode stimulation, a threshold is established for after-discharge, and an attempt is made to reproduce a component of the patient's typical seizure. The highest threshold is frequently found at the site of major pathology. Thresholds are generally in the range of 1 to 6 mA. When thresholds are above 6 mA or when there is inability to establish a threshold for after-discharge in the amygdala or hippocampus, there is high correlation with localization of the pathological focus. A typical seizure may be produced in many patients.[40]

Therapeutic Operations

Criteria for the selection of candidates for epilepsy surgery were recently compiled in a report of the NIH Consensus Conference,[1] the recommendations of which are the following:

1. The diagnosis of epilepsy is established.
2. The type of epilepsy and syndrome is classified.
3. A metabolic or structural cause of the epileptic attacks has been diagnosed.
4. The patient has had a reasonable trial of appropriate antiepileptic drugs with adequate monitoring.
5. The patient and family have received detailed information about the specific seizure disorder, available drug treatment and side effects, and alternative treatments which include surgery.

In addition, the following questions should be addressed:

1. Is there evidence of structural lesion? If so, is special planning required for treatment?
2. Have the clinical and electrographic characteristics of the patient's seizures been sufficiently well-documented to recommend an ablative or other surgical procedure?
3. Are other investigative procedures (e.g., subdural or intracerebral electrodes) indicated for further evaluation?
4. What is the most appropriate surgical procedure, if any, for the patient?
5. Can the proposed surgery be performed without an unacceptable neurological or neuropsychological deficit?
6. What are the realistic expectations and outcomes of surgical treatment in this specific case?

Additionally, the patients who are *not* ideal candidates frequently benefit from operation. Because of this, if the criteria for selection are directed at the inclusion only of ideal candidates, they may exclude patients who otherwise might benefit from surgery.[4,5,67] In any case, the evaluation of each patient for surgery must be done with care. Engel has tabulated justifiable reasons for the exclusion of patients from resection.[5]

Young patients are treated surgically, even when only a few months of age.[4,49,68–71] Early operation is recommended if surgery is the treatment of choice. Intellectual requirements are flexible, leading at times to the selection of patients with low test scores. The requirement for preservation of memory must, however, be strictly maintained.

Using the guidelines recommended above, a procedure most applicable to the individual patient is selected, while maintaining fully realistic expectations of possible outcomes.

☐ ABLATIVE PROCEDURES

RESECTION OF TEMPORAL LOBE FOCI

Historically, ablative surgery for seizures arising in the temporal lobe involved the resection only of convolutions with

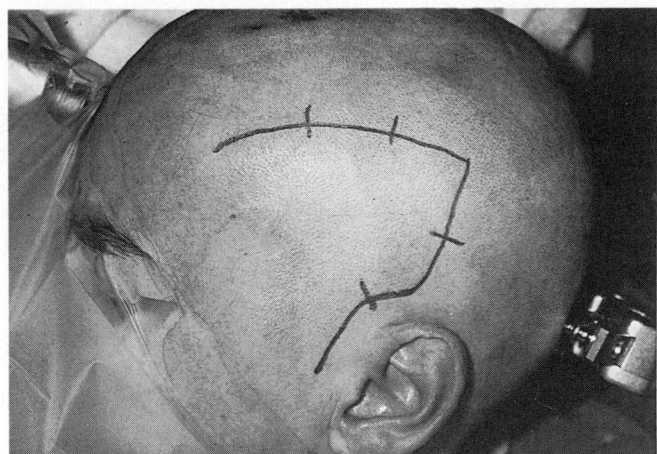

Figure 22–9 Position of incision for craniotomy for left temporal lobe resection.

evidence of a focus determined by a maximal abnormality that was apparent on electrocorticography or stimulation. Persistence of seizures in many patients after ablation indicated that the initial procedure had been inadequate, thus leading to resection of the entire anterior portion of the temporal lobe.[72] This usually includes the amygdala with or without the hippocampus.[69,73,74.]

In the dominant hemisphere, the value of operating under local anesthesia to permit stimulation mapping and identification of speech areas has been stressed.[8,11,40,73,75,76] Penfield and his coworkers used dissection and suction to remove tissue piecemeal, whereas Falconer[52] and Crandall[74] have advocated *en bloc* removal. The latter method provides opportunity for more extensive pathological study, but concern has been expressed about the risk of injury to structures medial to the temporal lobe such as the oculomotor nerve, optic tract, and posterior cerebral artery.

A more limited procedure is transtemporal resection of the amygdala and hippocampus, leaving the remainder of the temporal lobe intact.[77] This has recently been developed further using microscopic techniques.[78]

Operative Technique The head is placed in a pin-type headrest after the patient is in a comfortable lateral position on a well-padded operating table. An instrument table is attached to the operating table to provide adequate tenting of the drapes for visual access to the patient by the anesthesiologist and neuropsychologist. If depth electrodes are present, they are connected to the EEG monitor.

For proper flap placement, it is desirable to mark the proposed incision while the entire head can be viewed. Nonsurgical areas are walled off with adhesive plastic drapes prior to scalp preparation. The scalp is infiltrated along the incision line and across the base with 1 : 1 solutions of 0.5 lidocaine and 0.25 Marcaine, containing 1 : 200,000 epinephrine. A small "question mark" temporal incision is used for most anterior temporal lobe resections, but if a more extensive posterior exposure is required, the classic temporal craniotomy may be used.[73] (See Fig. 22-9.)

During incision, the motor branch to the frontalis muscle is preserved by careful dissection. The temporal squama and lateral sphenoid ridge anteriorly and inferiorly are removed to permit maximal exposure of the temporal tip. After tacking the surrounding dura to the pericranium at the periphery of the craniotomy, the dural flap is reflected superiorly.

Electrocorticography is carried out using strip electrodes or grids. If depth electrodes are present, simultaneous recording from both ipsilateral and contralateral depth electrodes is included. Cortical electrode placement is identified with lettered tickets. Tissue adjacent to a structural lesion may contain the epileptogenic focus, while the abnormal tissue is relatively silent or may show slow-wave activity.

In patients under local anesthesia, the neuropsychologist establishes communication for speech testing. Stimulation using balanced square wave pulses (60 Hz, 0.5 ms, and 2-10 mA per phase) is administered via a bipolar electrode with an interelectrode distance of 5 to 10 mm. The cortical threshold is determined by responses in the lower sensorimotor strip, after which the frontal speech area is located by having the patient count while intermittently stimulating the cortex. Interruption or perseveration of counting while stimulating anterior to the motor cortex is indicative of local cortical involvement in speech.

With these responses documented and the sites identified by numbered tickets, language tests for representation in the temporal lobe are performed. Recitation of a rhyme rather than counting gives more reliable results. Arrest, alteration of cadence, phonemic, semantic, or syntactic errors are indicative of speech representation in the stimulated area. A response cannot be considered negative unless the stimulation current threshold has been established by reproducibly positive responses elsewhere in the same patient.

Considerable disagreement exists regarding the need for stimulation mapping. Many surgeons feel safe in removing the anterior 4.5 cm of the left temporal lobe or resecting to the junction of the sylvian fissure with the inferior extent of the sensorimotor cortex. However, representation of language as far anterior as 2.5 cm from the temporal tip has been documented, and a persistent but slight speech deficit has resulted from resection of the anterior 4 cm of the dominant temporal lobe.[40] (See Fig. 22-10.)

The opportunity to elicit both recording and stimulation data from patients in whom subdural grids have been placed at an earlier procedure may provide sufficient physiological information so that definitive surgery can be performed under general anesthesia. This is advantageous in children and uncooperative adults.

Occasionally, there will be an isolated area of speech in the temporal cortex separate from, and some distance anterior to, the remainder of the temporal speech area. Interference with speech from stimulation of this area has been interpreted as being transmitted. Its importance can be tested by placing a cottonoid pledget soaked with 0.5 Xylocaine without epinephrine over the convolution at that point for 5 min. If there is no interference with spontaneous speech or recitation, the area may be safely resected.

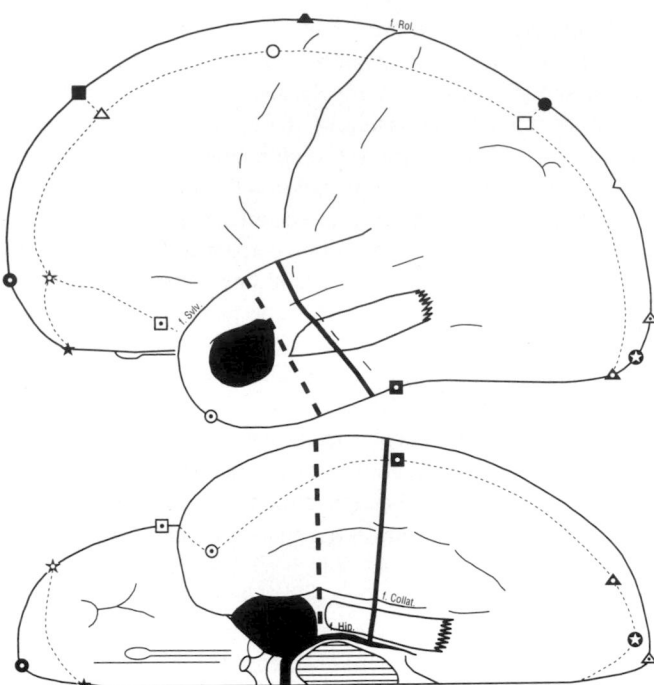

Figure 22–10 Schematized display of typical resection of anterior temporal lobe for seizures. Resection shown by dash line is used when the hippocampus must be spared. Resection shown by solid line permits removal of a varying extent of the hippocampus.

Based on preoperative and intraoperative clinical, imaging, and electrographic findings, the proposed cortical removal is outlined with a thin strip of cottonoid or a suture. (See Fig. 22-11.)

If a structural lesion is present, optimal results are obtained by resection of both the lesion and the epileptogenic focus.[79] The cortex surrounding the resection site is covered with a thin rubber sheet to protect the brain from trauma and

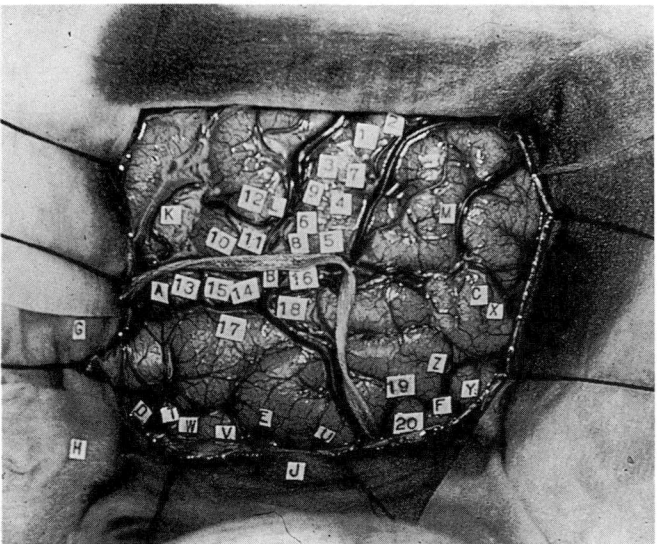

Figure 22–11 Stimulation mapping of cortex. Letters indicate recording electrode positions. Speech localized at positions 10–12. Auras reproduced at positions 13–18. Proposed resection indicated by umbilical tape.

drying. The cortical vessels are coagulated along the superior temporal convolution and across the temporal convolutions about 5 mm anterior to the desired extent of excision.

The convolutions are transected to the depth of the sulci and the pia arachnoid is incised over the superior convolution. The pia and the cortex of the superior convolution are then separated from posterior to anterior. In most instances the cortex will be gliotic and can be peeled away from the pia using a dissector.

Dissection is extended into the sylvian fissure and over the insula to the limbus, taking care to protect the middle cerebral vessels still covered by pia and arachnoid as the temporal operculum is reflected. Dissection is continued forward to the tip and inferiorly as far as the bulk of the temporal lobe permits.

Turning attention to the transected convolutions, dissection is continued down to the level of the insula and the floor of the middle cranial fossa. The subcortical white matter is then transected in a parasagittal plane, the inferior pia incised, and the lateral temporal lobe removed. Subsequently, the posterior white matter at the end of the second temporal convolution is transected to enter the temporal horn at the tip of the ventricle.

At the tip of the temporal horn, subpial dissection is continued inferiorly and posteriorly to free the amygdala, which can be removed by severing its connections to the temporal stem white matter. This provides an opportunity to verify the position of any implanted electrodes. Dissection is continued posteriorly, freeing the uncus from the pia. This structure is frequently quite gliotic and tough and held by adhesions within the incisura tentorii. The third nerve, neighboring vascular structures, optic tract, and upper brain stem should be protected.

At times, it is necessary to approach the uncus both anteriorly and posteriorly after removal of the hippocampus. The position of any electrode implanted in the hippocampus is observed, and if the hippocampus is to be removed, a transection is made at the appropriate level and continued inferiorly and medially to the pia of the parahippocampal gyrus. The hippocampus and gyrus are dissected free from the pia and removed en bloc.

At the choroid fissure there is an arcade of one to four small feeding arteries passing through the pia to the hippocampus. These must be isolated, coagulated, and then divided. Avulsion of these branches from the parent vessels in the incisura may result in infarction of the posterior limb of the internal capsule, with attendant hemiparesis. Any remaining uncus is then removed. Demonstrable herniation of the uncus mesially in the incisura has a high correlation with pathological change and with favorable outcome. This may add to the technical difficulty during removal. The edges of the transected gyri are debrided and any residual macerated cortical margins are removed. (See Fig. 22-12.)

Postexcisional recording is performed and, if necessary, additional tissue is removed. The wound and middle cranial fossa are irrigated with saline containing bacitracin and gentamicin prior to craniotomy closure.

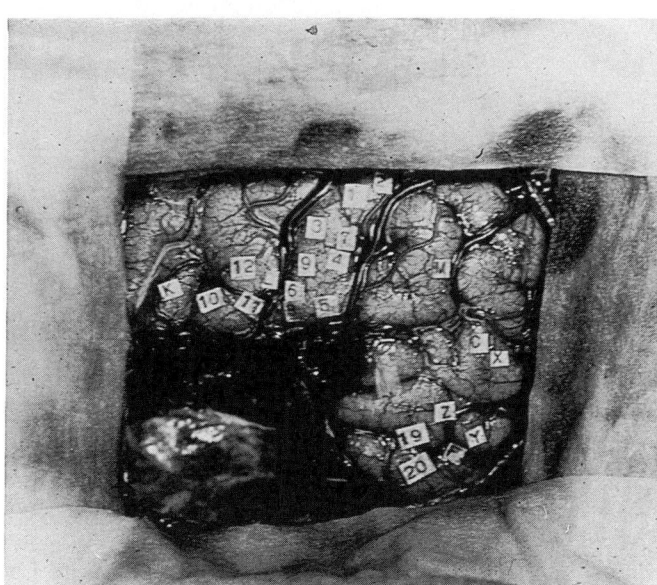

Figure 22–12 Postexcision view of case in Fig. 22–11.

RESECTION OF EXTRATEMPORAL FOCI

Extratemporal foci are localized by clinical, imaging, and EEG findings. A clearly defined surgical approach to encompass the focus is planned. In cases where noninvasive studies give no localizing or lateralizing information, an array of depth electrodes may provide localizing information.

When studies indicate a focus in one hemisphere but localization within the hemisphere cannot be determined, implantation of strip electrodes or a grid array of 16 to 64 contacts in the subdural space may give accurate localization. (See Fig. 22-13.)

The latter requires a craniotomy which is placed to provide optimal exposure of the most likely focal areas. Once the brain is exposed, if the operation is performed under

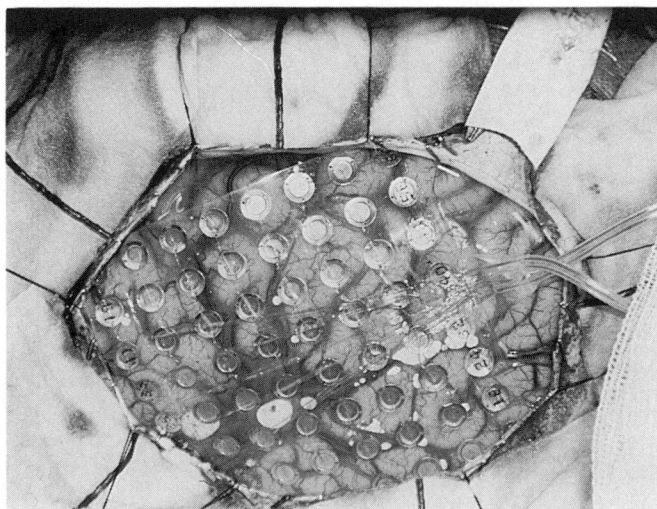

Figure 22–13 Subdural 64 contact grid electrode array placed over left hemisphere.

local anesthesia, cortical mapping by stimulation may be done, with photographic recording of response sites for reference at the time of resection. The grid array is then placed and additional photographic recordings made for documentation of the position of the individual contacts. The wound is closed with cables passed through the scalp by separate stab wounds. Over the next several days, both ictal and interictal activity are recorded from the contacts of the implanted array contacts. Stimulation mapping studies can be carried out extraoperatively during this period.[79] By reference to the recordings and photographs, a planned resection may be performed at a second stage, at which time the array is removed.

Since an epileptogenic focus may be at the margin of a damaged area of the brain, areas of structural alteration should be documented at the time of subdural implantation or resection. Spontaneous electrical activity in the form of interictal spikes or areas of slow-wave activity should be noted. Since inclusion of areas of interictal spikes in the resection is important to outcome,[79] intraoperative stimulation mapping may be indicated. Although simple motor responses can be obtained with the patient under light anesthesia, local anesthesia is required for mapping speech and subjective responses, particularly in searching for the site of an aura. The technique is similar to that described in temporal lobe cases, but more attention is directed to defining the sensorimotor strip and cortex adjacent to the area to be excised. In extratemporal cases subdural grid implantation for extraoperative evaluation provides an advantageous means of securing accurate information.

Operative Technique Excision of an extratemporal epileptogenic focus is performed by cortical resection. The pia-arachnoid over the gyrus to be resected is coagulated and incised, allowing subpial resection of the cortex to the bottom of the adjacent sulci using suction or dissectors. All larger arteries or veins adjacent to or crossing the gyri should be preserved.[8,80] Care should be exercised to avoid resection of deep fiber pathways in the white matter. (See Figs. 22-14 and 22-15.)

MODIFICATION OF ABLATIVE PROCEDURES

In temporal and extratemporal ablative procedures, epileptogenic foci may extend into a speech or sensorimotor area of cortex. Although language areas cannot be sacrificed without unacceptable deficits, the deficit from resection of other cortical areas must be weighed against the disability due to seizures. In the lower sensorimotor strip where face functions are located, bilateral cortical representation may minimize the deficit after unilateral resection of the face sensorimotor cortex.

A technique for gridding incisions of the gyri provides an option for dealing with foci in critical areas. When the focus occupies a nonexpendable area, a small opening in the pia at the margin of the gyrus permits insertion of a small blunt

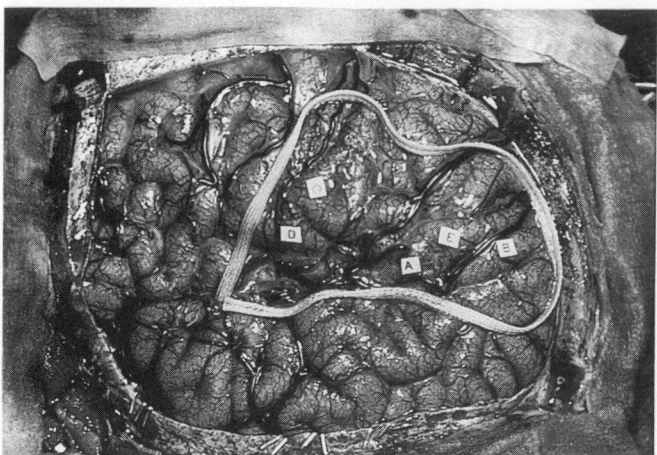

Figure 22–14 Parietal epileptogenic focus outlined prior to resection.

right-angled hook. This is then passed transversely across the gyrus and withdrawn superficially toward the pia, severing the horizontal connections in the cortex but leaving the vertically projecting subcortical connections and the pial nutrient vessels intact. The process is repeated at intervals of about 5 mm. (See Fig. 22-16A and B.) In a series of patients undergoing subpial cortical transection, speech and motor functions have been preserved and seizures reduced or eliminated.[81]

EFFECT OF ABLATIVE SURGERY ON SEIZURE FREQUENCY

Seizures in the immediate postoperative period are not necessarily indicative of eventual failure. Some may be due to irritation and edema of the tissues adjacent to resection (neighborhood seizures) and may be expected to subside.[8,82] The anticipation of continuing seizures is greater if postoperative attacks are identical to those occurring preoperatively. Many patients without motor attacks or loss of con-

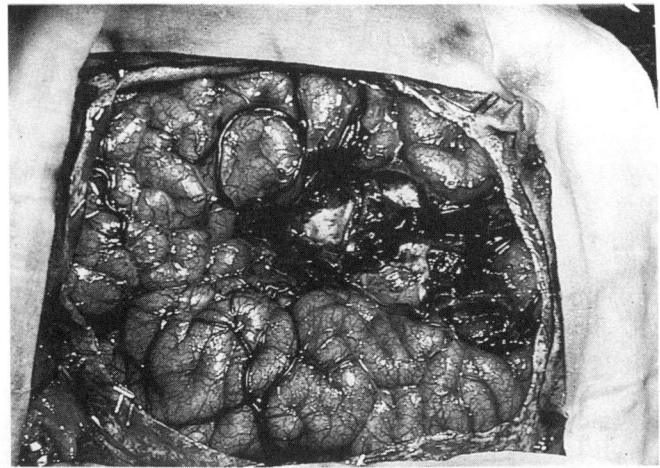

Figure 22–15 Postexcision view of case in Fig. 22–14. Note preservation of traversing vessels.

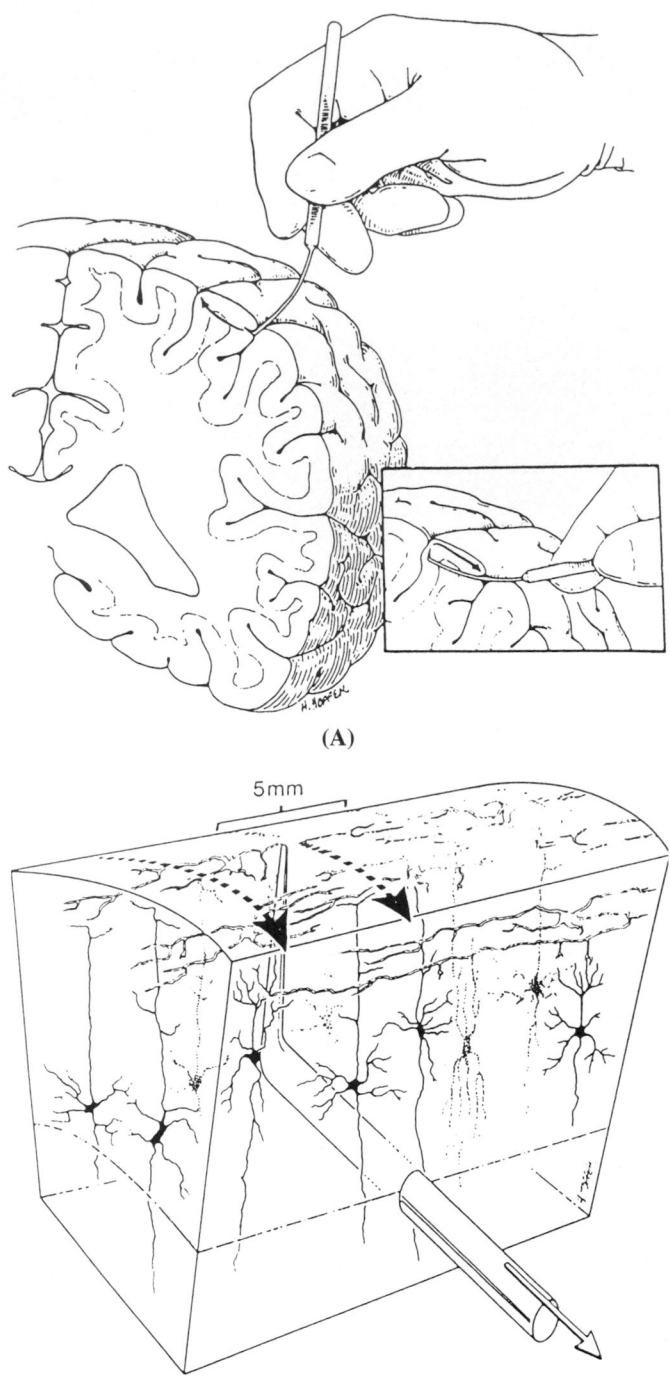

(A)

5mm

(B)

Figure 22–16A and B Method of gridding convolutions by multiple subpial cortical transections. (Morrell F, Whisler WW: Multiple subpial transection: A new approach to the surgical treatment of focal epilepsy. *J Neurosurg* 70:231–239, 1989. Reproduced with permission.)

sciousness may continue to have components of their preoperative auras. These episodes are not counted as seizures, although in the strictest sense they are. Some patients may have occasional seizures for a few years which then cease (wind down). Others may be seizure-free for a few years, then have recurrence.

Follow-up for at least 1 to 5 years is necessary before a

Table 22-1
SEIZURE OUTCOME FOLLOWING SURGERY

	Anterior temporal resection	Extra-temporal resection	Hemispher-ectomy
Total patients	2,336	825	88
Total centers	40	32	17
Number of seizure-free patients	1,296	356	68
% (range)	55.5 (26–80)	43.2 (0–73)	77.3 (0–100)
Number of improved patients	648	229	16
%	27.7	27.8	18.2
Number of patients not improved	392	240	4
% (range)	16.8 (6–29)	29.1 (17–89)	4.5 (0–33)

Adapted from Engel.[81] Survey data from 40 centers.

definitive determination of surgical outcome can be made. Data from the National Institutes of Health indicate that up to 50 percent of patients who are seizure-free during the first postoperative year again develop seizures, usually at a reduced frequency.[1]

In a series reported from the Montreal Neurological Institute, 1210 patients underwent temporal lobectomy for intractable seizures between 1928 and 1980. Of the 894 patients without tumors available for follow-up 2 to 44 years later, 22 percent have been seizure-free since surgery. Another 13 percent had occasional seizures in the first 1 to 2 years following operation but have since become seizure-free. Another 26 percent have had their seizure frequency reduced by 98 percent. Thus, 63 percent of the Montreal patients may be classified as having an excellent result. Even in the 144 patients with tumors and adequate follow-up, an excellent outcome was recorded in 76 percent.[83]

In a more recent survey of all known epilepsy surgery centers, the results of ablative surgery appear in Table 22-1.[82]

Patients undergoing ablative procedures for extratemporal foci also obtain worthwhile results, but to a slightly lesser degree than in temporal lobe resections.

Despite the marked improvement achieved by a majority of patients, some persons who meet acceptable criteria obtain minimal or no improvement following surgery. A number of factors may be responsible.

A review reveals that patients undergoing a complete temporal lobectomy, including resection of the three temporal gyri, fusiform and hippocampal gyri, uncus, amygdala, and anterior portion of the hippocampus, have significantly better results than those having partial resections in which one or more gyri or the mesial temporal structures are spared. Of these, the extent of mesial resection is more significant.[84] Likewise, 45 percent of 121 patients undergoing reoperation for focal epilepsy with additional resection have achieved excellent results.[83] These data suggest that more extensive resections are a key element in improved seizure control.

Inaccurate localization of the epileptogenic lesion accounts for some poor results. Absence of pathological abnormalities in resected temporal lobe tissue correlates with a poor surgical outcome.[54] In such patients, it is likely that the anatomic substrate responsible for the seizures was located elsewhere. Some of the traditional electrographic localization criteria may be falsely lateralizing.[5] A battery of test procedures to improve patient selection assesses both epileptic excitability and focal functional deficits. Early results using these methods appear promising. Newer imaging techniques—including MRI, SPECT, and PET[5,34,82]—combined with greater use of depth electroencephalography,[58,85,86] further improve localization. Improved selection criteria also make it possible to operate with beneficial results on patients previously rejected.[58,86]

Finally, it is likely that many patients with complex partial seizures who do not respond to temporal lobectomy have bilateral or multifocal disease not amenable to ablative surgery. More refined selection methods may prevent inappropriate surgery in these patients.

PATHOLOGICAL FINDINGS

The predominant pathological finding in temporal lobe epilepsy is hippocampal (or incisural-mesial temporal) sclerosis. There is direct evidence of the relationship between hippocampal sclerosis and the clinical features of temporal lobe epilepsy.[34,53,87,88]

These findings have been substantiated by studies of surgical specimens.[53,87,88,89,91] A high correlation exists between decrease in neuronal population in the hippocampus and epileptogenic activity.[55,87,89] (See Fig. 22-17.)

This appears to be most prominent in the Sommer sectors of Ammon's horn, with a gradient from anterior to posterior. Where marked cellular loss is found at the most posterior extent of the hippocampal resection, there is a high correlation with persistent seizures.[87]

The exact etiology of hippocampal sclerosis has not been established, but there seems to be a high correlation with neonatal and early childhood infections and convulsions. Other pathological processes associated with temporal lobe seizures are gliomas, meningiomas, hamartomas, tuberous sclerosis, and heterotopias. In all of these lesions, there has been some degree of cellular loss in the hippocampus.[87]

Regardless of the etiology of the hippocampal changes, it is evident that, as part of the development of the epileptogenic lesion, synaptic reorganization has taken place.[87]

EFFECT OF ABLATIVE SURGERY ON COGNITIVE FUNCTION, PSYCHIATRIC DISORDERS, AND SOCIAL AND VOCATIONAL STATUS

Ablative surgery has been associated with improvement in intelligence,[90] in psychiatric and behavioral disorders,[91,92,93] and in social and vocational function.[90,91] The mechanism of

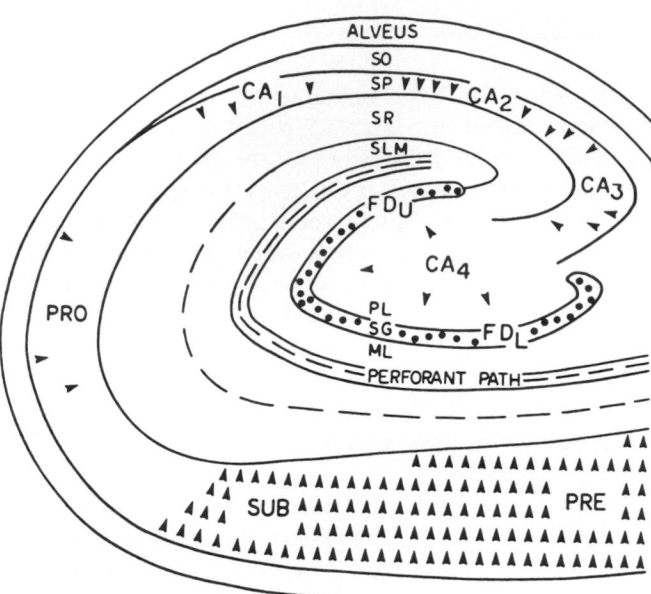

Figure 22–17 Sketch of cross section of hippocampus showing decreased cellular population in Sommer's sectors. (Babb TL, Brown WJ: Pathological findings in epilepsy, in Engel J Jr (ed): *Surgical Treatment of the Epilepsies.* New York, Raven Press, 1987, p 520. Reproduced with permission.)

improvement is not clear, but resection of abnormal epileptogenic brain tissue may remove the undesirable functional effects of abnormal tissue which are interfering with the function of other cortical areas.

Improved psychiatric and behavioral status usually parallels the degree of seizure control; however, frank preoperative schizophrenia does not respond to surgery.[21] Further studies, with more precise definitions of terms and quantification of multiple variables, will be necessary to determine the effect of ablative surgery on psychological and behavioral function. The suicide rate among postoperative patients, half of whom are free of seizures following surgery, is much higher than projected for the normal population. Personality disorders present in the preoperative state appear to have predictive value for socioeconomic outcome.[91]

The opportunity for postoperative social and economic rehabilitation is higher in children than in older age groups.[62,68,69] Improved seizure control after surgery is often accompanied by an improvement in social and vocational status.[89,91]

COMPLICATIONS OF ABLATIVE SURGERY

Mortality for ablative surgery has varied from 0 to 1.7 percent.[46,47,52,94] In the Montreal series, most deaths occurred in the early years. From 1957 to the end of 1973, there were only two operative deaths among 820 nontumorous patients. Falconer and Serafetinedes[52] had no deaths in their series of 100 temporal lobectomies, and Flanigin[40] reported 1 death in 200 ablative procedures.

The most common neurological deficit following temporal lobectomy is a contralateral superior quadrantanopsia that occurs in up to 75 percent of cases. The deficit is usually minor and rarely noticed by the patient.

Most reports of temporal lobectomies indicate a 5 to 10 percent incidence of more significant disability immediately following surgery.[46,47,52] Dysphasia may follow resections in the dominant hemisphere when margins of resection encroach on cortical speech areas. Transient dysphasia may result from edema and resolve. Rarely, permanent speech dysfunction is found and can usually be avoided by stimulation mapping extraoperatively using subdural electrodes or intraoperatively in the conscious patient.

The incidence of hemiparesis ranges from 0.39 to 3.0 percent.[94] It is usually transient, although it can be permanent. Posterior branches of the anterior choroidal artery may be injured, resulting in infarction of the posterior limb of the internal capsule. This may result in hemiparesis of varying degree, sometimes transient but possibly permanent.

Disturbance of memory function may follow temporal lobectomy.[90,91] After resection of the dominant temporal lobe, verbal memory is mildly impaired.[20,91] Visual memory following nondominant temporal lobectomy may be impaired.[91] These deficits are usually found only by formal testing. Rarely, memory deficits may be so severe and permanent that the patient is incapable of learning new material. This amnesic syndrome may occur when temporal lobectomy is carried out contralateral to an already severely damaged hippocampus and has been confirmed in one case.[19] Significant memory deficits occur in the range of 0.6 to 2.0 percent.

Transient third nerve palsy has occasionally been reported. It usually follows en bloc resections.

Neurological deficits following extratemporal surgery are dependent on the area of resection. The advantages of seizure control must be compared to the disadvantages of possible disability from resection of critical cortex.

HEMISPHERECTOMY

Hemispherectomy was first reported by Dandy for gliomas,[95] but McKenzie was the first to report its use in a patient with intractable seizures and infantile hemiplegia.[96] Several series reporting excellent results appeared later.[97,98]

Hemispherectomy is well-established as an effective treatment for seizures, with the ability of patients to function well after removal of a pathological hemisphere. A more accurate term is *hemicorticectomy,* since the basal ganglia are not usually removed. Motor function is retained and frequently improves with decrease in spasticity, although some spasticity may return later. Intellectual function continues at the preoperative level and frequently improves. Education and employment become realistic goals. (See Fig. 22-18.)

Beneficial effects on behavior are no less striking. Both improved seizure control and improved behavior in patients with Sturge-Weber disease have been reported.[91] Technical

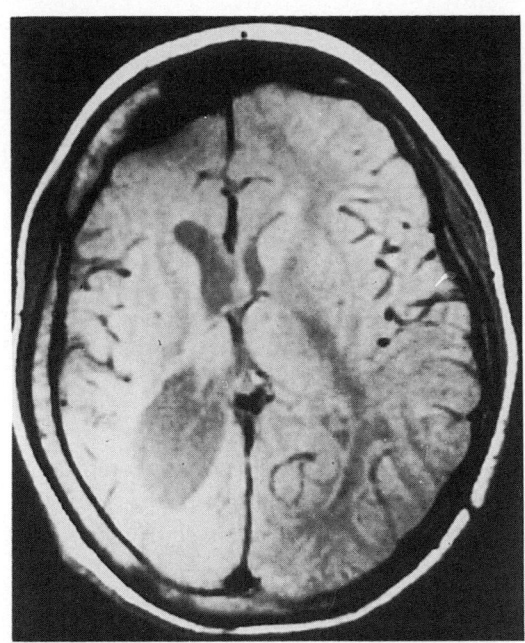

Figure 22–18 MRI showing atrophic hemisphere. Patients with this type of abnormality frequently respond well to hemispherectomy.

descriptions of anatomical hemispherectomy have been given by Ignelsi and Bucy[98] and by Green and Sidell.[69] Recently, functional hemispherectomy has been applied to patients with Sturge-Weber disease at an early age, with good seizure control and without evidence of progression of the disease 4 years after surgery.[70]

Following anatomical hemispherectomy, a late complication has added to the usual complications associated with craniotomy. Neurological function begins to deteriorate progressively years after surgery and eventually results in death. There is evidence of bleeding in the cerebrospinal fluid (CSF) pathways, and postmortem examination demonstrates hemosiderosis of the cavities in the brain which are lined with a granulomatous membrane indistinguishable from that of a chronic subdural hematoma. The contralateral foramen of Monro or the aqueduct of Sylvius becomes occluded, resulting in hydrocephalus and leading to herniation and death.[99,100] Incidence has been found to be 16 to 25 percent. Subtotal hemispherectomy (multilobe resection) reduces the incidence of hemosiderosis, but the percentage of patients experiencing seizure control is less.

Rasmussen[3] has developed a functional hemispherectomy in which the prefrontal and occipital lobes are left in place with an intact blood supply but are disconnected from the brain stem and contralateral hemisphere. The temporal lobe and the central suprasylvian part of the hemisphere are removed. Hemosiderosis has not been reported following this procedure.

Operative Technique Functional hemispherectomy[3] is the preferred procedure, combining ablation with disconnection. A large craniotomy flap is reflected over the central and temporal regions. Resection of the central cortex is

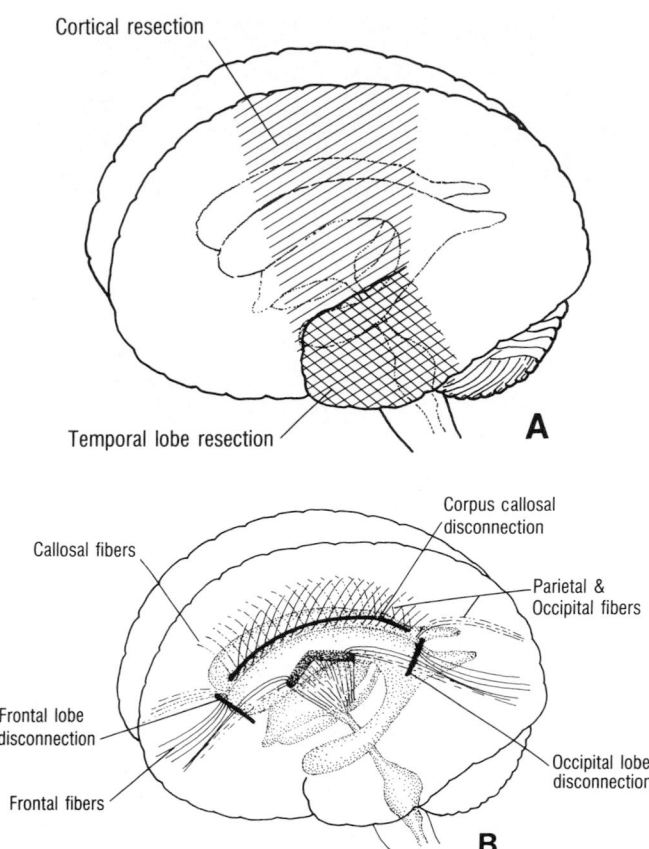

Figure 22–19 Schematic view of functional hemispherectomy. *(A)* Shaded area shows cortical resection in central region, crosshatched area shows temporal lobe resection. *(B)* Incisions in corpus callosum and deep projection fibers in white matter disconnecting remaining frontal and occipital lobes.

followed by a temporal lobectomy. Blood supply to the basal ganglia and the frontal and occipital lobes is preserved. After sectioning the corpus callosum, projection fibers to the frontal and occipital lobes are divided, isolating these structures but leaving them in place. (See Fig. 22-19A and B.)

The degree of resection or isolation may be modified to adjust to presenting pathological and electrocorticographic changes and the function to be preserved. Results in seizure control are comparable to anatomic hemispherectomy. (See Figs. 22-20, 22-21, and 22-22.)

☐ DISCONNECTION PROCEDURES

When an ablative operation is not indicated, disconnection may be an appropriate alternative. This is based on the concept of isolating the structures in which seizures originate.

CORPUS CALLOSOTOMY

Secondary generalized seizures spread through the corpus callosum.[101] Van Wagenen and Herren reported the first

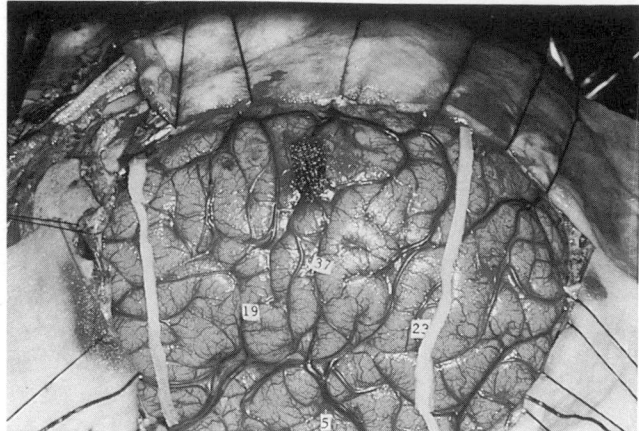

Figure 22–20 Preexcision view of structures outlined for ablation during functional hemispherectomy.

series of corpus callosotomy for control of seizures. Generalized convulsions were controlled, although minor seizures persisted.[102] Later series reported similar favorable results.[103,104] Psychological changes after section of the whole corpus callosum and anterior commissure prompted restriction of sectioning to the anterior two-thirds of the corpus callosum. Sparing the posterior body and splenium or at least the splenium avoided the undesirable effects of disconnection. Subsequent studies have shown that corpus callosotomy performed in two stages (anterior-posterior) avoids the acute prolonged apathy and confusion seen after complete division in a single stage.

Corpus callosotomy was initially applied to patients with bilateral electrographic abnormalities, but the procedure was later applied with excellent results to children who would otherwise have been considered for hemispherectomy.[105]

At least a 50 percent decrease in the frequency of atonic, tonic, and secondary generalized tonic-clonic seizures follows corpus callosotomy in about 75 to 80 percent of cases.[106] Corpus callosotomy may be offered to patients who are intractable to medical management and who have a

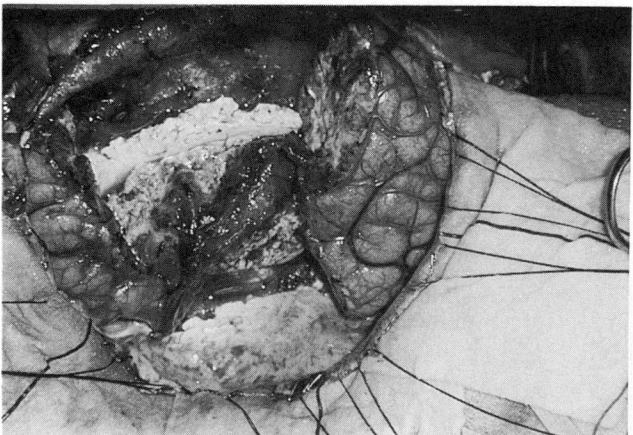

Figure 22–21 Postexcision view of ablation in Fig. 22–20. Sensorimotor cortex and temporal lobe have been removed. Sectioned corpus callosum, insula, and floor of middle cranial fossa are visualized.

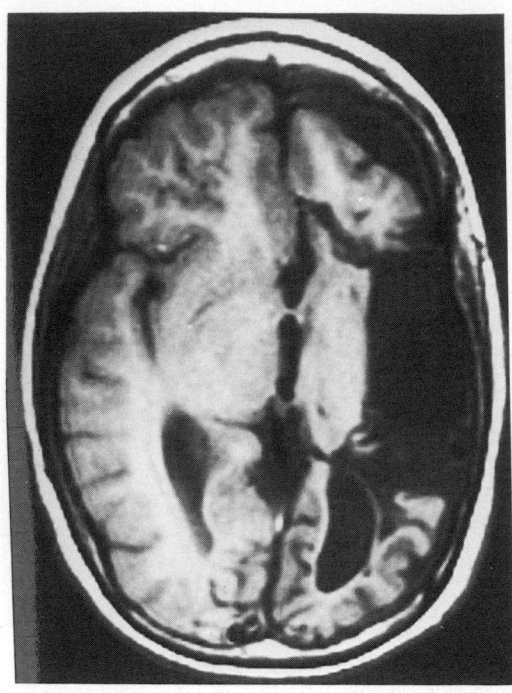

Figure 22–22 MRI image of patient following functional hemispherectomy. Note ablated area and disconnection incisions.

hemispheric abnormality not suitable for ablative surgery or who have bilateral or multifocal discharges.[2]

Operative Technique Initial surgery is usually limited to sectioning of the anterior two-thirds of the corpus callosum. Under general endotracheal anesthesia, the patient is placed in a lateral position in head pins, with the side for the craniotomy dependent. The vertex is elevated 30°. Using preoperative venous phase angiography as a guide, a flap is placed in the region of the coronal suture, permitting an approach between bridging cortical veins. In intact patients with a dominant left hemisphere, the approach is from the right, but if there is evidence of damage to the left hemisphere or if cortical vein position interferes with an approach from the right, an approach from the left is preferred. The "hanging hemisphere" approach permits access to the corpus callosum with little or no retraction of the dependent hemisphere once arachnoidal adhesions have been separated. It may be necessary to support the superior hemisphere by retractors when the falx does not extend far inferiorly between the hemispheres. Using magnification and microdissection, the anterior cerebral arteries are exposed. The lateralization of each artery is confirmed to avoid damage to the blood supply. The arteries are separated anteriorly to the genu, then posteriorly for the planned distance of the transection. A preoperative midsagittal MRI allows measurement of the anterior two-thirds of the corpus callosum. In retracting the anterior cerebral arteries, care should be exercised to avoid occlusion. The corpus callosum is identified as a white structure between the hemispheres and arteries. It is sectioned by a semisharp dissector or by suction. Transection should extend anteriorly around the genu. (See Figs. 22-23, 22-24, and 22-25.)

Preservation of the ependyma is advocated to reduce postoperative morbidity. An MRI-compatible clip may be applied at the posterior extent of the section for reference.

If a second stage is required, a posterior craniotomy is performed using a more posterior bone flap, and the remaining corpus callosum is sectioned. The extent of section may be recorded by MRI after each stage.

RESULTS OF CORPUS CALLOSOTOMY

Long-term postoperative undesirable sequelae after corpus callosotomy are infrequent, while acute disconnection phenomena occur more often. After an anterior two-thirds corpus callosotomy, transient mutism, apathy, confusion, and ideomotor apraxia of the nondominant hand may be observed for 3 to 4 days. Long-term sequelae with anterior corpus callosotomy are extremely rare. In the past, when complete callosotomy was done in a single stage, the above-mentioned disconnection phenomena were prolonged.[107] Occasionally, intermanual conflict following complete corpus callosotomy may be incapacitating. Cases of persistent severe aphasia have been reported with partial and total corpus callosotomies in right-handed patients with language function located in the right hemisphere.[108]

Generalized tonic-clonic, tonic, and, especially, drop attacks are significantly improved in one-third of the patients following anterior corpus callosotomy and in three-fourths of the patients following completion of the corpus callosotomy. In cases where significant improvement in seizure

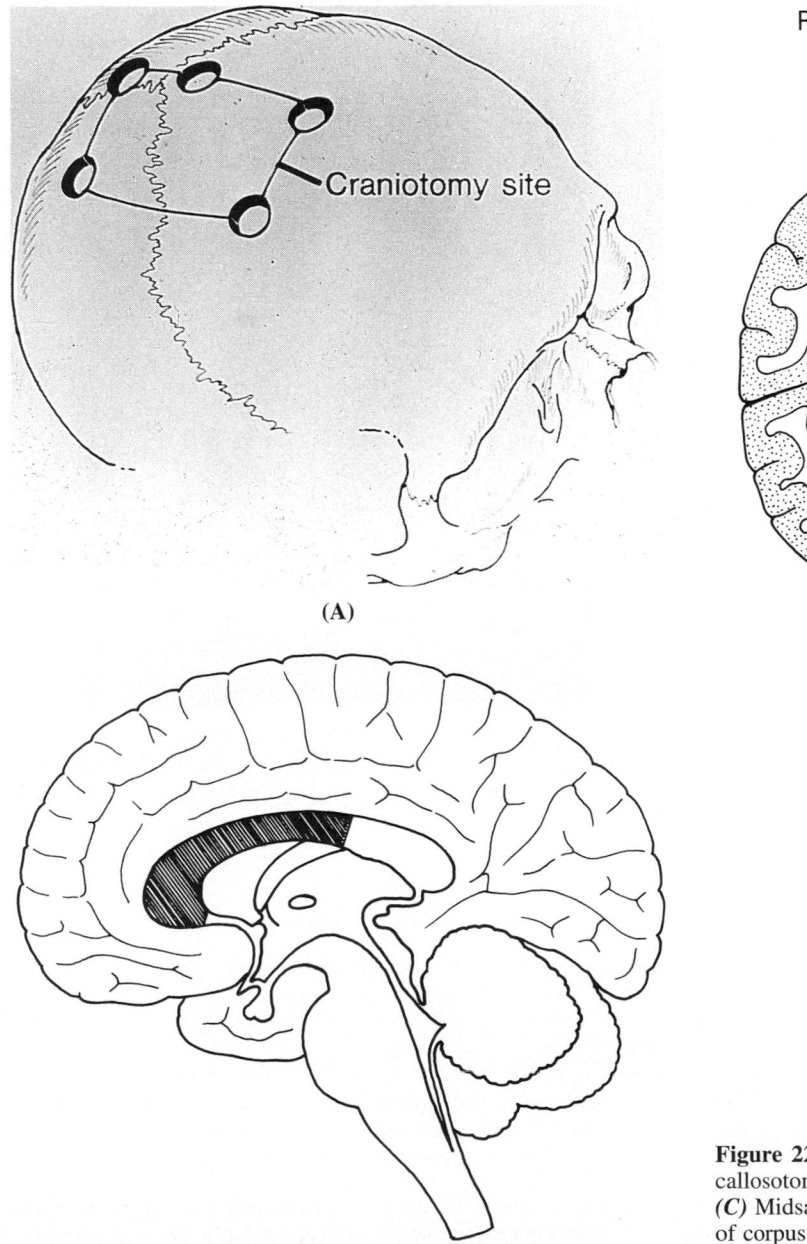

(A)

(C)

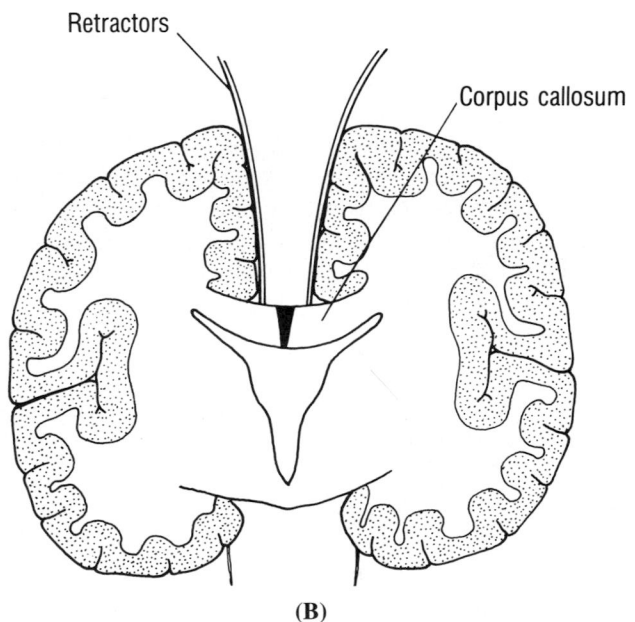

(B)

Figure 22–23 *(A)* Craniotomy site for anterior corpus callosotomy. *(B)* Coronal view of corpus callosal section. *(C)* Midsagittal view showing section of anterior two-thirds of corpus callosum.

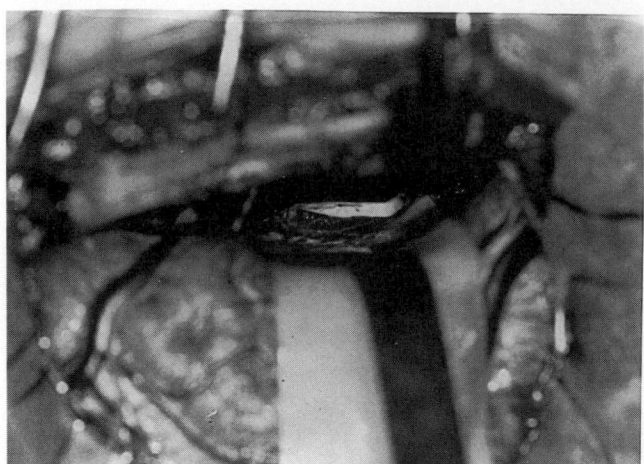

Figure 22–24 Operative photograph showing right (dependent) hemisphere retracted, exposing the corpus callosum between the anterior cerebral arteries.

control has been obtained, improvement in cognitive function has also been noted.

Although this operation has found favor in the management of intractable seizures, a definitive analysis of the role and indications for corpus callosotomy cannot yet be made. Such an analysis must address the various seizure types treated, the neurological and psychological conditions of the patients, and the variations in the operative procedures performed.

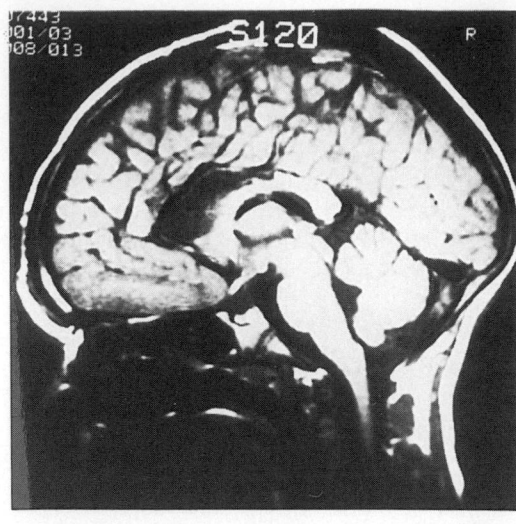

(A)

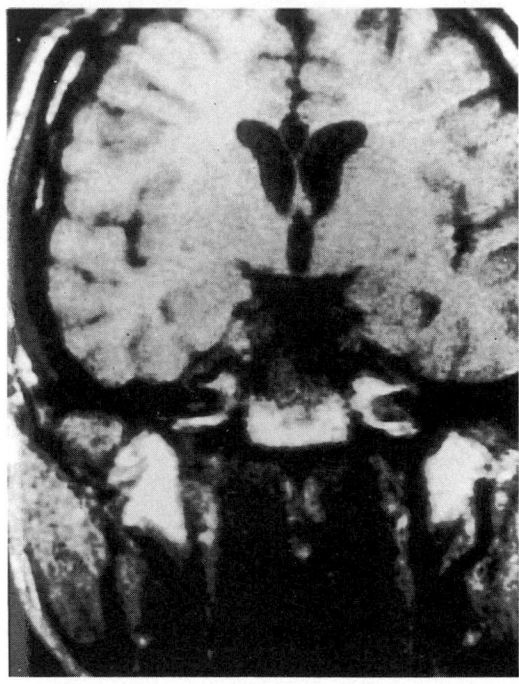

(B)

Figure 22–25 Postoperative MRI scans showing transected anterior corpus callosum in *(A)* midsagittal and *(B)* frontal planes.

REFERENCES

The wealth of material published in this field over the last 50 years had mandated the limitation of references to certain landmark publications and key sources.

1. NIH Consensus Conference: Surgery for Epilepsy. *JAMA* 264:729–737, 1991.

2. Williamson PD: Corpus callosum section for intractable epilepsy: Criteria for patient selection, in Reeves AG (ed): *Epilepsy and the Corpus Callosum*. New York, Plenum, 1985, pp 243–257.

3. Rasmussen T: Commentary: Extratemporal cortical excisions and hemispherectomy, in Engel J Jr (ed): *Surgical Treatment of the Epilepsies*. New York, Raven, 1987, pp 417–424.

4. Andermann F: Identification of candidates for surgical treatment of epilepsy, in Engel J Jr (ed): *Surgical Treatment of the Epilepsies.* New York, Raven, 1987, pp 51–70.

5. Engel J Jr: Approaches to localization of the epileptogenic lesion, in Engel J Jr (ed): *Surgical Treatment of the Epilepsies.* New York, Raven 1987, pp 75–95.

6. Penfield W, Kristiansen K: *Epileptic Seizure Patterns.* Springfield, Ill., Charles C Thomas, 1951, pp 3–9.

7. Ajmone-Marsan C, Ralston B: *The Epileptic Seizure: Its Functional Morphology and Diagnostic Significance.* Springfield, Ill., Charles C Thomas, 1957, pp 3–6, 187–230.

8. Penfield W, Jasper H: *Epilepsy and the Functional Anatomy of the Human Brain.* Boston, Little, Brown, 1954, pp 576–578.

9. Mullan S, Penfield W: Illusions of comparative interpretation and emotion. *Arch Neurol Psychiatry* 81:269–284, 1959.

10. Williamson PD, Wieser H-G, Delgado-Escueta AV: Clinical characteristics of partial seizures, in Engel J Jr (ed): *Surgical Treatment of the Epilepsies.* New York, Raven 1987, pp 101–120.

11. Sutherling WW, Risinger MW, Crandall PH, et al: Focal functional anatomy of dorsolateral frontocentral seizures. *Neurology* 40:87–98, 1990.

12. Swartz BE, Halgren E, Delgado-Escueta AV, et al: Multidisciplinary analysis of patients with extratemporal complex partial seizures: II. Predictive value of semiology. *Epilepsy Res* 5:146–154, 1990.

13. Newmark ME, Penry JK: *Genetics of Epilepsy: A Review.* New York, Raven, 1980, pp 21–86.

14. Penfield W, Robertson JSM: Growth asymmetry due to lesions of the parietal cerebral cortex. *Arch Neurol Psychiatry* 50:405–430, 1943.

15. Taylor LB: Localization of cerebral lesions by psychological testing. *Clin Neurosurg* 16:269–287, 1969.

16. Jones-Gotman M: Commentary: *Psychological evaluation—testing hippocampal function,* in Engel J Jr (ed): *Surgical Treatment of the Epilepsies.* New York, Raven, 1987, pp 203–211.

17. Bogen JE: The callosal syndrome, in Heilman KM, Valenstein E (eds): *Clinical Neuropsychology.* London, Oxford University Press, 1979, pp 308–359.

18. Wada J, Rasmussen T: Intracarotid injection of sodium amytal for the lateralization of cerebral speech dominance: Experimental and clinical observations. *J Neurosurg* 17:266–282, 1960.

19. Penfield W, Milner B: Memory deficit produced by bilateral lesions in the hippocampal zone. *Arch Neurol Psychiatry* 79:475–497, 1958.

20. Milner B, Penfield W: The effect of hippocampal lesions on memory. *Trans Am Neurol Assoc* 80:42–48, 1955.

21. Scoville WB: The limbic lobe in man. *J Neurosurg* 11:64–66, 1954.

22. Scoville WB, Milner B: Loss of recent memory after bilateral hippocampal lesions. *J Neurol Neurosurg Psychiatry* 20:11–21, 1957.

23. Jackson GD, Berkovic SF, Tress BM, et al: Hippocampal sclerosis can be reliably detected by magnetic resonance imaging. *Neurology* 40:1869–1875, 1990.

24. Bergen D, Bleck T, Ramsey R, et al: Magnetic resonance imaging as a sensitive and specific predictor of neoplasms removed for intractable epilepsy. *Epilepsia* 30:318–321, 1989.

25. Brooks BS, King DW, el Gammal T, et al: MR imaging in patients with intractable complex partial epileptic seizures. *AJR Am J Roentgenol* 154:577–583, 1990.

26. Heinz ER, Crain BJ, Radtke RA, et al: MR imaging in patients with temporal lobe seizures: Correlation of results with pathologic findings. *AJR Am J Roentgenol* 155:581–586, 1990.

27. Awad IA, Katz A, Hahn JF, et al: Extent of resection in temporal lobectomy for epilepsy: I. Interobserver analysis and correlation with seizure outcome. *Epilepsia* 30:756–762, 1989.

28. Katz A, Awad IA, Kong AK, et al: Extent of resection in temporal lobectomy for epilepsy: II. Memory changes and neurologic complications. *Epilepsia* 30:763–771, 1989.

29. Siegel AM, Wieser HG, Wichmann W, et al: Relationships between MR-imaged total amount of tissue removed, resection scores of specific mediobasal limbic subcompartments and clinical outcome following selective amygdalohippocampectomy. *Epilepsy Res* 6:56–65, 1990.

30. Harris RD, Roberts DW, Cromwell LD: MR imaging of corpus callosotomy. *AJNR Am J Neuroradiol* 10:677–680, 1989.

31. Engel J Jr, Henry TR, Risinger MW, et al: Presurgical evaluation for partial epilepsy: Relative contributions of chronic depth-electrode recordings versus FDG-PET and scalp-sphenoidal ictal EEG. *Neurology* 40:1670–1677, 1990.

32. Kuhl D, Engel J Jr, Phelps M: Patterns of local brain metabolism determined in epilepsy by positron emission computed tomography. *Arch Neurol* 38:735, 1981.

33. Sperling MR, Sutherling WW, Newer MR: New techniques for evaluating patients for epilepsy surgery, in Engel J Jr (ed): *Surgical Treatment of the Epilepsies.* New York, Raven, 1987, pp 235–257.

34. Engel J Jr, Brown WJ, Kuhl DE, et al: Patholgical findings underlying focal temporal lobe hypometabolism in partial epilepsy. *Ann Neurol* 12:518–528, 1982.

35. Olson DM, Chugani HT, Shewmon DA, et al: Electrocorticographic confirmation of focal positron emission tomographic abnormalities in children with intractable epilepsy. *Epilepsia* 31:731–739, 1990.

36. Rowe CC, Berkovic SF, Sia ST, et al: Localization of epileptic foci with postictal single photon emission computed tomography. *Ann Neurol* 26:660–668, 1989.

37. Shen W, Lee BI, Park HM, et al: HIPDM-SPECT brain imaging in the presurgical evaluation of patients with intractable seizures. *J Nucl Med* 31:1280–1284, 1990.

38. Grunwald F, Durwen HF, Bockisch A, et al: Technetium-99m-HMPAO brain SPECT in medically intractable temporal lobe epilepsy: A postoperative evaluation. *J Nucl Med* 32:388–394, 1991.

39. Jeffery PJ, Monsein LH, Szabo Z, et al: Mapping the distribution of amobarbital sodium in the intracarotid Wada test by use of Tc-99m HMPAO with SPECT. *Radiology* 178:847–850, 1991.

40. Flanigin HF, King DW, Gallagher BB: Surgical treatment of epilepsy, in Pedley TA, Meldrum B (eds): *Recent Advances in Epilepsy,* vol 2. London, Churchill Livingstone, 1984, chap. 16, 297–339.

41. Barth DA, Sutherling W, Engel J Jr, et al: Neuromagnetic localization of epileptiform spike activity in the human brain. *Science* 218:891–894, 1968.

42. Cohen D, Cuffin BN, Yunokuchi K, et al: MEG versus EEG localization test using implanted sources in the human brain. *Ann Neurol* 28:811–817, 1990.

43. Sutherling WW, Barth DS: Neocortical propagation in temporal lobe spike foci on magnetoencephalography and electroencephalography. *Ann Neurol* 25:373–381, 1989.

44. Eisenberg HM, Papanicolaou AC, Baumann SB, et al: Magnetoencephalographic localization of interictal spike sources: Case report. *J Neurosurg* 74:660–664, 1991.

45. Gloor P: Commentary: Approaches to localization of the epileptogenic lesion, in Engel J Jr (ed): *Surgical Treatment of the Epilepsies.* New York, Raven, 1987, pp 97–100.

46. Penfield W, Flanigin H: Surgical therapy of temporal lobe seizures. *Arch Neurol Psychiatry* 65:491–500, 1950.
47. Bailey P, Gibbs FA: The surgical treatment of psychomotor epilepsy. *JAMA* 145:365–370, 1951.
48. Quesney L-P: Extracranial EEG evaluation, in Engel J Jr (ed): *Surgical Treatment of the Epilepsies.* New York, Raven, 1987, pp 129–166.
49. Blume WT: Clinical profile of partial seizures beginning at less than four years of age. *Epilepsia* 30:813–819, 1989.
50. Panet-Raymond D, Gotman J: Can slow waves in the electrocorticogram (ECoG) help localize epileptic foci? *Electroencephalogr Clin Neurophysiol* 75:464–473, 1990.
51. Gibbs EL, Gibbs FA, Fuster B: Psychomotor epilepsy. *Arch Neurol Psychiatry* 60:331–339, 1948.
52. Falconer MA, Serafetinides EA: A follow-up study of surgery in temporal lobe epilepsy. *J Neurol Neurosurg Psychiatry* 26:154–165, 1963.
53. Earle KM, Baldwin M, Penfield W: Incisural sclerosis and temporal lobe seizures produced by hippocampal herniation at birth. *Arch Neurol Psychiatry* 69:27–42, 1959.
54. Engel J Jr, Driver M, Falconer MA: Electrophysiological correlates of pathology and surgical results in temporal lobe epilepsy. *Brain* 98:129–156, 1975.
55. Lieb JP, Engel J Jr, Brown WJ, et al: Neuropathological findings following temporal lobectomy related to surface and deep EEG patterns. *Epilepsia* 22:539–549, 1981.
56. Lesser RP, Luders H, Morris HH, et al: Commentary: Extracranial EEG evaluation, in Engel J Jr (ed): *Surgical Treatment of the Epilepsies.* New York: Raven, 1987, pp 173–179, 1987.
57. Lieb JP, Walsh GO, Babb TL, et al: A comparison of EEG seizure patterns recorded with surface and depth electrodes in patients with temporal lobe epilepsy. *Epilepsia* 17:137–160, 1976.
58. Ajmone-Marsan C: Depth electrography and electrocorticography, in Aminoff MJ (ed): *Electrodiagnosis in Clinical Neurology.* Edinburgh, Churchill Livingstone, chap. 4, pp 167–196, 1980.
59. King DW, Laxer KD: Postscript: Can the indications for specific invasive procedures be identified?, in Engel J Jr (ed): *Surgical Treatment of the Epilepsies.* New York, Raven, 1987, pp 371–376, 1987.
60. Brazier MAB, Schroeder H, Chapman WP, et al: Electroencephalographic recordings from depth electrodes implanted in the amygdaloid regions in man. *Electroencephalogr Clin Neurophysiol* 6:702, 1954.
60a. Smith JR, Flanigin HF, King DW, et al: Relationship of depth electrode complications to implant trajectory. *J Epilepsy* 5:253–260, 1992.
61. Bickford R, Dodge HW Jr, Peterson MC, et al: A new method of recording from subcortical regions of the human brain. *Electroencephalogr Clin Neurophysiol* 5:464, 1953.
62. Goldring S: Surgical management of epilepsy in children, in Engel J Jr (ed): *Surgical Treatment of the Epilepsies.* New York, Raven, 1987, pp 445–464.
63. Luders H, Lesser RP, Dinner DS, et al: Commentary: Chronic intracranial recording and stimulation with subdural electrodes, in Engel J Jr (ed): *Surgical Treatment of the Epilepsies.* New York, Raven, 1987, pp 297–321.
64. Ojemann GA, Engel J Jr: Acute and chronic intracranial recording and stimulation, in Engel J Jr (ed): *Surgical Treatment of the Epilepsies.* New York, Raven, 1987, pp 263–288.
65. Gloor P, Olivier A, Ives J: Prolonged seizure monitoring with stereotaxically implanted depth electrodes in patients with bilateral interictal temporal epileptogenic foci: How bilateral is bitemporal epilepsy?, in Wada JA, Penry JK (eds): *Advances in Epileptology, Xth Epilepsy International Symposium.* New York, Raven, 1978, pp 83–88.
66. Ward AA Jr: The epileptic neuron: Chronic foci in animals and man, in Jasper H, Ward AA, Pope A (eds): *Basic Mechanisms of the Epilepsies.* Boston, Little, Brown, 1959, pp 263–288.
67. Dreifuss FE: Goals of surgery for epilepsy, in Engel J Jr (ed): *Surgical Treatment of the Epilepsies.* New York, Raven, 1987, pp 31–49.
68. Glaser GH: Natural history of temporal lobe limbic epilepsy, in Engel J Jr (ed): *Surgical Treatment of the Epilepsies.* New York, Raven, 1987, pp 13–30.
69. Green JR, Sidell AP: Neurosurgical aspects of epilepsy in children and adolescents, in Youmans JR (ed): *Neurological Surgery.* Philadelphia, Saunders, 1982, chap 141, pp 3858–3909.
70. Villamure. Personal communication. 1991.
71. Falconer MA: The significance of surgery for temporal lobe epilepsy in childhood and adolescence. *J Neurosurg* 33:233–238, 1970.
72. Flanigin H, Hermann B, King D, et al: The history of surgical treatment of epilepsy in North America: Prior to 1975, in Leuders H (ed): *Epilepsy Surgery.* New York, Raven, 1991, chap 3, pp 19–35.
73. Penfield W, Baldwin M: Temporal lobe seizures and the technique of subtotal temporal lobectomy. *Ann Surg* 136:625–634, 1952.
74. Crandall PH: Cortical resections, in Engel J Jr (ed): *Surgical Treatment of the Epilepsies.* New York, Raven, 1987, pp 377–404.
75. Penfield W, Roberts L: *Speech and Brain Mechanisms.* Princeton, Princeton University Press, 1959.
76. Ojemann GA: Brain mechanisms for language: Observations during neurosurgery, in Lockard JS, Ward AA (eds): *Epilepsy: A Window to Brain Mechanisms.* New York, Raven, 1980, pp 243–260.
77. Niemeyer P: The transventricular amygdala-hippocampectomy in temporal lobe epilepsy, in Baldwin M, Bailey P (eds): *Temporal Lobe Epilepsy.* Springfield, Ill., Charles C Thomas, 1958, pp 461–482.
78. Wieser HG, Yasargil MG: Selective amygdalohippocampectomy as a surgical treatment of mesiobasal limbic epilepsy. *Surg Neurol* (United States) 17:445–457, 1982.
79. Awad IA, Rosenfield J, Ahl J, et al: Intractable epilepsy and structural lesions of the brain: Mapping, resection strategies, and seizure outcome. *Epilepsia* 32:179–186, 1991.
80. Penfield W, Steelman H: The treatment of focal epilepsy by cortical excision. *Ann Surg* 126:740–761, 1947.
81. Morrell F, Whisler WW: Multiple subpial transection for epilepsy eliminates seizures without destroying the function of the transected zone. *Epilepsia* 23:440–441, 1982.
82. Engel J Jr: Outcome with respect to epileptic seizures, in Engel J Jr (ed): *Surgical Treatment of the Epilepsies.* New York, Raven, 1987, pp 553–571.
83. Rasmussen TB: Surgical treatment of complex partial seizures: Results, lessons, and problems. *Epilepsia* 24(suppl 1): 65–76, 1983.
84. Van Buren JM, Ajmone-Marsan C, Mutsuga N, et al: Surgery of temporal lobe epilepsy, in Purpura DP, Penry JK, Walter RD (eds): *Advances in Neurology.* New York, Raven, 1975, vol 8, chap 8, pp 155–196.
85. Rayport M, Corrie WS, Ferguson SM: Contribution of stereoencephalographic studies to reduction of failure rates of cortical resection for seizure control. *Epilepsia* 22:244, 1981.
86. Spencer SS, Spencer D, Williamson D, et al: The localizing value of depth electroencephalography in 32 patients with refractory epilepsy. *Ann Neurol* 12:248–253, 1982.
87. Babb TL, Brown WJ: Pathological findings in epilepsy, in Engel J Jr (ed): *Surgical Treatment of the Epilepsies.* New York, Raven, 1987, pp 511–540.

88. Falconer MA: Mesial Temporal (Ammon's horn) sclerosis as a common cause of epilepsy: Aetiology treatment and prevention. *Lancet* 2:767–770, 1974.

89. Malamud N: The epileptic focus in temporal lobe epilepsy from a pathological standpoint. *Arch Neurol* 14:190–195, 1966.

90. Rausch R, Crandall PH: Psychological status related to surgical control of temporal lobe seizures. *Epilepsia* 23:191–202, 1982.

91. Taylor DC: Psychiatric and social issues in measuring the input and outcome of epilepsy surgery, in Engel J Jr (ed): *Surgical Treatment of the Epilepsies.* New York, Raven, 1987, pp 485–503.

92. Falconer MA: Reversibility by temporal-lobe resection of the behavioral abnormalities of temporal-lobe epilepsy. *N Engl J Med* 289:451–455, 1973.

93. Serafetinides EA: Psychosocial aspects of neurosurgical management of epilepsy, in Purpura DP, Penry JK, Walter RD (eds): *Advances in Neurology.* New York, Raven, 1975, vol 8, chap 16, pp 323–332.

94. Van Buren JM: Complications of surgical procedures in the diagnosis and treatment of epilepsy, in Engel J Jr (ed): *Surgical Treatment of the Epilepsies.* New York, Raven, 1987, pp 465–475.

95. Dandy WE: Removal of right cerebral hemisphere for certain tumors with hemiplegia: Preliminary report. *JAMA* 90:823–825, 1928.

96. McKenzie KG [cited by Williams DJ, Scott JW (1939)]: The functional responses of the sympathetic nervous system of man following hemidecortication. *J Neurol Psychiatry* 2:313–322, 1938.

97. Krynauw RA: Infantile hemiplegia treated by removing one cerebral hemisphere. *J Neurol Neurosurg Psychiatry* 13:243–267, 1950.

98. Ignelzi RJ, Bucy PC: Cerebral hemidecortication in the treatment of infantile cerebral hemiatrophy. *J Nerv Ment Dis* 147:14–30, 1968.

99. Falconer MA, Wilson PJE: Complications related to delayed hemorrhage after hemispherectomy. *J Neurosurg* 30:413–426, 1969.

100. Wilson PJ: Complications related to delayed hemorrhage after hemispherectomy. *J Neurosurg* 30:413, 1969.

101. Erickson TC: Spread of the epileptic discharge. *Arch Neurol* 43:429, 1940.

102. Van Wagenen WP, Herren RY: Surgical division of commissural pathways in the corpus callosum. Relation to spread of an epileptic attack. *Arch Neurol Psychiatry* 44:740–759, 1940.

103. Geoffroy G, Lassonde M, Delisle F, et al: Corpus callosotomy for control of intractable epilepsy in children. *Neurology* 33:891–897, 1983.

104. Bogen JE, Vogel PJ: Cerebral commissurotomy in man: Preliminary case report. *Bull Neurol Soc* 27:169–172, 1962.

105. Luessenhop AJ: Interhemispheric commissurotomy: As an alternative to hemispherectomy for control of intractable seizures. *Am Surg* 36:265, 1970.

106 Gates JR, Rosenfeld WE, Maxwell RE, et al: Responses of multiple seizure types to corpus callosum section. *Epilepsia* 28:28–34, 1987.

107. Bogen JE: The callosal syndromes, in Heilman KM, Valenstein E (eds): *Clinical Neuropsychology,* 2d ed. New York, Oxford, 1985, chap 11, pp 295–338.

108. Sass KJ, Novelly RA, Spencer DD, et al: Post callosotomy language impairments in patients with crossed cerebral dominance. *J Neurosurg* 72:85–90, 1990.

☐ STUDY QUESTIONS

I. A 30-year-old female is referred because of uncontrolled seizures. Her seizures began when she was 12 years of age. They were described as beginning with the illusion of a cloud coming over the right field of vision, followed by a "strange" feeling, as though the patient has visited her current location before, no matter where she was.

She subsequently developed some chewing actions and lost memory during a generalized seizure, usually lasting for 1 to 5 min. Anticonvulsant medications had included phenobarbital, phenytoin, carbamazepine, and valproic acid—each to therapeutic levels. Seizures had continued at the rate of two to three per week.

She had a history of a difficult birth with a delivery by forceps. She failed to breath for several minutes after birth, and respirations were slow for several hours. She subsequently developed normally but was left-handed. Examination revealed that the right arm and leg were slightly smaller than the left, and radiographs revealed a smaller left hemicranium than right. Angiogram was normal. There was slow-wave activity throughout the left hemisphere and numerous spikes recorded from the left spenoidal electrodes.

1. What was the most likely anatomical origin of her seizures? **2.** What surgical procedure(s) might be considered to alter the course of seizures? **3.** What might be the cost in terms of intellect, social and psychological behavior to not having surgical therapy accomplished? **4.** What further diagnostic tests might be considered to determine location and pathological cause for the seizures? **5.** What procedures might be accomplished to determine whether speech would be affected by any surgical procedure which might be performed?

II. A 4-year-old girl is referred because of continuing focal seizures in the right side of the face and arm. The patient had a history of normal birth and development until 2 years of age, when she had an episode involving the onset of a high fever which lasted for 3 to 4 days and during which she developed generalized convulsions that were controlled only with large doses of phenobarbital and dilantin.

The fever and seizures gradually subsided, but 2 months later, the patient began to experience frequent seizures in the right side of the face and arm. Prior to the original episode, it was thought that the patient showed a preference for use of her right arm, but afterward she performed almost all functions with the left hand, using the right upper extremity as a "club." She would not use it at all when she was having seizures.

The seizures became more frequent, and for the past 6 months it has been impossible to stop the seizures unless she was sedated enough to put her to sleep. An EEG showed diffuse slow-wave activity over the left hemisphere with active seizure activity over the motor strip. An MRI showed a diffusely enlarged ventricle on the left with shift of the right cerebral hemisphere to the left.

1. What was the likely event that occurred at 2 years of age? 2. What might be the indications for surgical therapy? 3. When should surgical therapy be considered? Why? 4. What surgical procedures might be considered? 5. What would be the patient's prognosis after surgery?

III. An 8-year-old boy is referred because of frequent seizures, focal to the left side of the body. The patient had been born with a "birth mark" on the right face and upper lip. He had a number of generalized seizures as an infant but these have remained focal to the left side of the body for the last 4 years. Despite anticonvulsant medications, the seizures are of such frequency as to deter progress in school. The patient's IQ measures 90, however. His only neurological deficit is a left homonymous hemianopsia. Plain x-rays and CTs show strips of calcification along the cortical edges of the right occipital lobe. The right hemicranium is smaller than the left.

1. What is the most likely diagnosis? 2. What might an angiogram show? 3. What surgical therapy might be considered? 4. What permanent neurological deficits might be anticipated? 5. What are the likely consequences of no therapy?

IV. A 24-year-old male is seen because of frequent seizures, beginning with visual hallucination and "lip smacking," followed by a generalized seizure—usually, although not invariably. Anticonvulsant therapy has been unsuccessful. An EEG shows many spikes over the right temporal area and constant slow-wave activity over the left temporal area.

Surgery was being contemplated, but the patient has a very peculiar personality. He is obsessive in several areas and most difficult to get along with, but reveals no features of schizophrenia.

1. What is the most likely diagnosis? 2. Would the personality features contraindicate surgery? 3. Which side would the seizures most likely be coming from? 4. How would you prove the origin of the seizures? 5. What surgical procedures might be considered?

V. A 31-year-old man began to have partial complex seizures at age 29. Initially, the seizures were controlled with tegretol, but they began to be unresponsive to this therapy.

Plain skull x-rays showed some questionable calcification in the right temporal area that was confirmed by CT. Between the spicules of calcification, the attenuation is decreased. MRI shows the temporal horn to be displaced and deformed, and there are mixed increased and decreased signals throughout the anterior temporal area. Angiography suggests increased vascularity in the area.

1. What diagnoses might be considered? 2. What surgery should be considered? 3. What should control the limits of surgery? 4. When should the surgery be performed? 5. What would be the undesirable effects of radical surgery in this area?

Stereotactic Neurosurgery

Joseph R. Smith
Herman F. Flanigin

☐ DEFINITIONS

Stereotactic neurosurgery utilizes an aiming device to guide a probe or beam to a predetermined intraspinal or intracranial target which has been defined in a 3-dimensional space that is referable to a stereotactic apparatus.

The primary goal of *functional neurosurgery* is to alter the activity of an area of the nervous system either ablatively, electrically, or pharmacologically in order to establish more normal overall patient function. Modern stereotactics has its origins in functional neurosurgery.[1] In fact, many current surgical techniques for the management of intractable pain, disorders of movement and tone, and epilepsy are stereotactic.

This chapter will deal with the principles of morphological (as distinct from functional) stereotactic procedures, those that are involved in the diagnosis and treatment of structural lesions of the central nervous system (CNS).

Stereotactic Principles and Instrumentation

☐ PRINCIPLES

TARGET IMAGING AND LOCALIZATION IN 3-DIMENSIONAL STEREOTACTIC SPACE

Prior to the introduction of computerized tomography (CT) and, subsequently, magnetic resonance imaging (MRI), target localization most frequently involved cannulating the lateral ventricle through a burr hole and injecting air or a positive contrast substance in order to outline third ventricular structures adjacent to diencephalic targets (Fig. 23-1A and B). The target areas were then lesioned to control movement disorders, pain, or psychoaffective disorders.[1]

Such procedures required careful collimation or aiming of anteroposterior (AP) and lateral x-ray beams relative to the stereotactic apparatus in order to avoid x-ray parallax error when localizing the target with AP and lateral x-rays. It was also necessary to correct for x-ray magnification and for tilt or rotation of the patient's head. This technique had the further disadvantage of not directly imaging the target.[2] It is now being replaced by image-guided stereotaxis.

CT and MRI have the advantage of directly imaging CNS structures, and both techniques provide a 3-dimensional data base which can then be translated into stereotactic space in several ways. One method of target localization uses the lateral CT scout view (Fig. 23-2A). The base plane and the plane containing the target are identified and drawn on a stereotactic lateral scout x-ray (Fig. 23-2B). The distance between the two planes defines the depth (z coordinate) of the target in stereotactic space. The x and y coordinates are obtained from an axial CT view showing the target or lesion (Fig. 23-2C).

Most current scanners have software that allows metric measurement, and the x, y data can be transferred to the lateral and AP intraoperative x-rays respectively after correcting for magnification of the intraoperative x-rays. The shortcoming of this method is that it assumes no patient movement between acquisition of the base reference and target scan views as reconstructed on the preoperative lateral CT scout (Fig. 23-2B). Also, it does not take into account head tilt. Either of these two factors can introduce several millimeters of error in the depth of target position. This procedure should probably be reserved for biopsy or aspiration of lesions of greater than 1 cm in diameter.

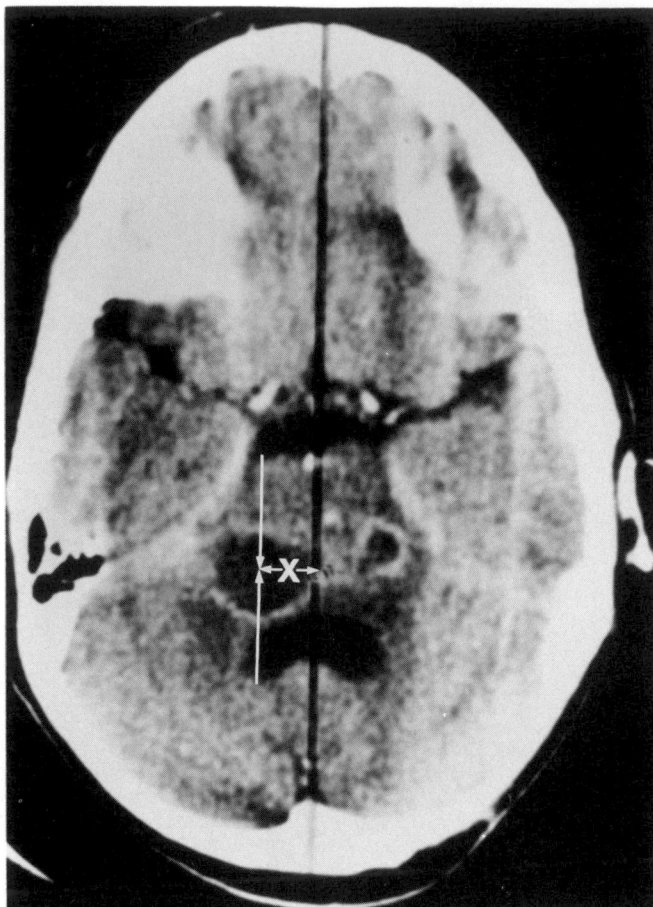

Figure 23–2 *C.* Target plane axial CT view. Line drawn in the midsagittal plane defines *x* = 0, since the patient's skull midline is positioned with x-ray control in the stereotactic midline. Using conversion measurements, the laterality (*x* coordinate) of one of the tumor cysts is determined. Target position in the AP plane (*y* coordinate) is determined by measuring the target position along the midsagittal plane. Using a conversion factor, that point is then defined on the target plane drawn on the lateral stereotactic x-ray (Fig. 23-2*B*).

probe position, not only in the operative notes but also with x-rays, computer printouts, or on magnetic tape.

STEREOTACTIC FRAME TYPES

Some commonly used stereotactic instruments and their function will be discussed in this section. Other types of instruments are discussed elsewhere.[4]

In a *target-centering arc-radius* stereotactic instrument, the patient's head is fixed in a base ring that is separate from but attached to the same platform as the aiming arc. The arc rotates around a horizontal axis, and the probe holder may be moved to any position along the arc. The trunions on which the arc rotates and the arc itself have angular calibrations so that any procedure can be performed using an entry-point or angles-of-entry technique (see section on trajectory planning). The focal point of the arc remains fixed in

3-dimensional stereotactic space. It is the patient's head with its intracranial target that is moved in any of the three orthogonal planes to the focal point of the instrument. Vernier scales calibrated in millimeters allow accurate measurement of head movement in each of the three planes. The radius of the arc system as well as its focal point remain fixed. Therefore, the distance of the target from the arc is always known, regardless of where the burr hole or twist drill hole entry point is placed. The Todd-Wells (Fig. 23-8) and Kelly instruments are examples.

In *arc-centering arc-radius* instruments, the arc, which is fixed to the base ring on the patient's head, is moved in order to bring its focal point to the target, previously defined in stereotactic space. An entry point or angles-of-entry technique may also be used here. The Cosman-Roberts-Wells (CRW) instrument (Fig. 23-9) and Leksell apparatus fall into this category.

In the past, both types of arc-radius systems have been used for ventriculography-guided procedures; they are currently being used in image-guided, computer-assisted procedures. In the latter case, both base ring and localizer must be compatible with the imaging modality (CT, MRI, and so forth).

Target coordinates for *polar-coordinate instruments* (Brown-Roberts-Wells, Reichert-Mundinger) may be determined utilizing either ventriculograms or computerized imaging studies. If an entry-point technique is chosen, trajectory construction depends on a phantom device (Fig. 23-10*A*). The base ring of the phantom corresponds to the patient base ring, and therefore any rectilinear or 3-dimensional coordinates referable to the stereotactic apparatus are identical to the same coordinates defined by the phantom.

Using the Brown-Roberts-Wells (BRW) instrument (Fig. 23-10*B*) for a computer image–guided stereotactic procedure as an example, the 3-dimensional coordinates of the entry point are defined as follows. The arc is first locked on the base ring fixed on the patient's head. A guide tube is then passed through the guide block down to the chosen entry site. The arc system with the guide tube firmly fixed in position is then transferred to the phantom. The target simulator of the phantom is moved into contact with the tip of the guide tube (Fig. 23-10*A*). The 3-dimensional coordinates are then read from the three vernier scales of the phantom, thereby giving the coordinates for the entry point. These are entered into a computer which has previously calculated the coordinates for the target. It then calculates the four angular settings (polar coordinates) of the arc guidance system (Fig. 23-10*B*) as well as the distance from the target to the arc. In this instance, the procedure is *phantom-dependent.*

If an angle-of-entry technique is used, the azimuth (horizontal angle) and declination (vertical angle) are entered into the computer after deriving the coordinates. The computer then calculates the four arc angles and the depth of the target. Here the phantom apparatus is used subsequently to check the accuracy of the probe trajectory and depth (Fig. 23-10*A*). This technique is *phantom-assisted* but not phantom-dependent.

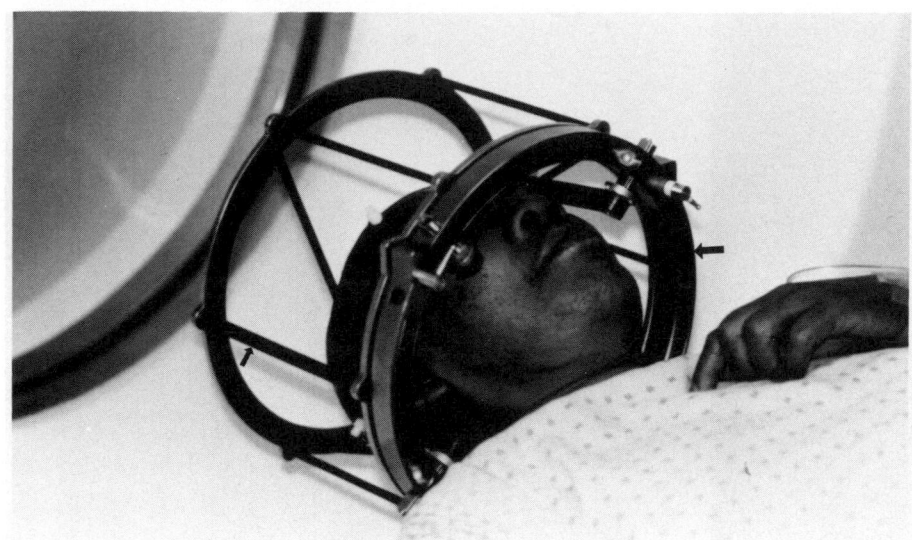

Figure 23–3 The patient's head is fixed in the base ring (large arrow), which is clamped to the CT scan table. The CT localizer (small arrow) is fixed to the base ring. The CT gantry is in the background.

☐ INDICATIONS

There are two categories of stereotactic procedures. *Morphological (anatomical) stereotaxis* includes biopsy, stereotactically guided endoscopic and open craniotomies, interstitial and intracavitary irradiation of selected cerebral neoplasms, and radiosurgery, which involves the application of the principles of stereotactic surgery to convergent beam–ionizing irradiation therapy of vascular and neoplastic lesions that would otherwise be difficult to treat by open craniotomy.

Functional stereotaxis includes procedures used to treat intractable movement disorders, pain, and epilepsy. These topics are covered in other chapters.

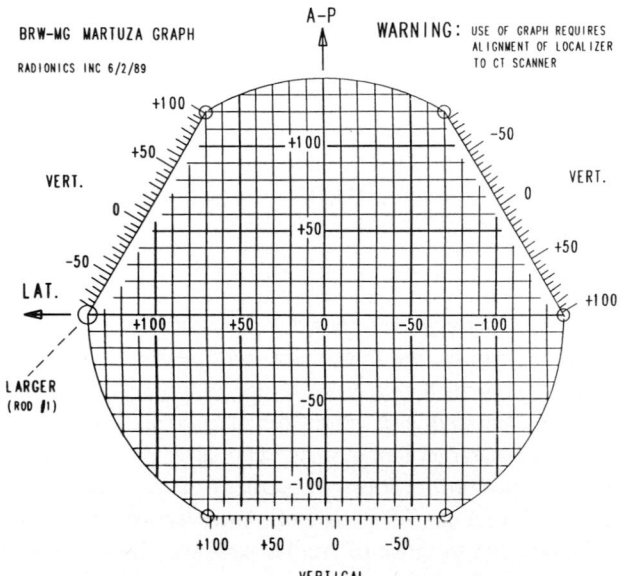

Figure 23–4 Grid localizer. When the transparent grid is overlaid on a CT scan, the six vertical fiducial rods (see Fig. 23-6A) directly underlie the six circles seen at the perimetry of the grid. The x, y, and z coordinates for any intracranial point can then be read from the grid.

☐ MORPHOLOGICAL (ANATOMIC) STEREOTACTICS

STEREOTACTIC BIOPSY

Small and deep-seated lesions are ideally suited to stereotactic technique where an open craniotomy would be more likely to produce morbidity. Since the introduction of image-guided stereotactics, deep lesions that might have previously been treated without diagnosis are now biopsied.

The diagnostic rate of some biopsy series has ranged from 91 to 100 percent, and in some series results have been different from the initial clinical diagnosis in up to 50 percent of the cases.[5] The type of biopsy instrument used will depend on the consistency of the tissue and where it is located. The Nashold side-slotted instrument (Fig. 23-11A and B) will yield a specimen, approximately 1 × 7 mm, that can be removed with little likelihood of morbidity from a subcortical lesion. Removal of a 1 × 2 mm specimen with microalligator forceps (Fig. 23-11A and B) passed through a

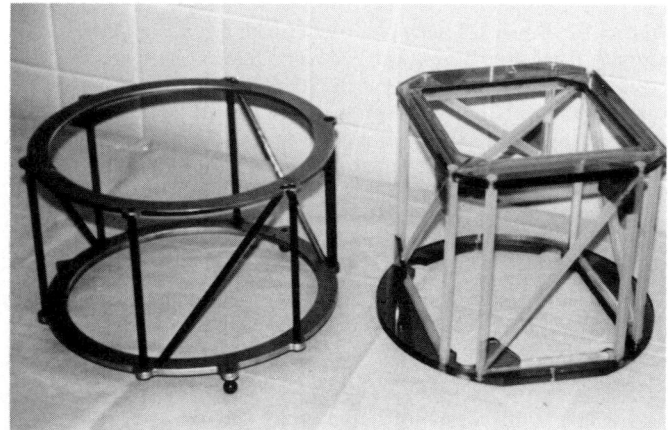

Figure 23–5 CT-compatible localizer (left) and MRI-compatible localizer (right).

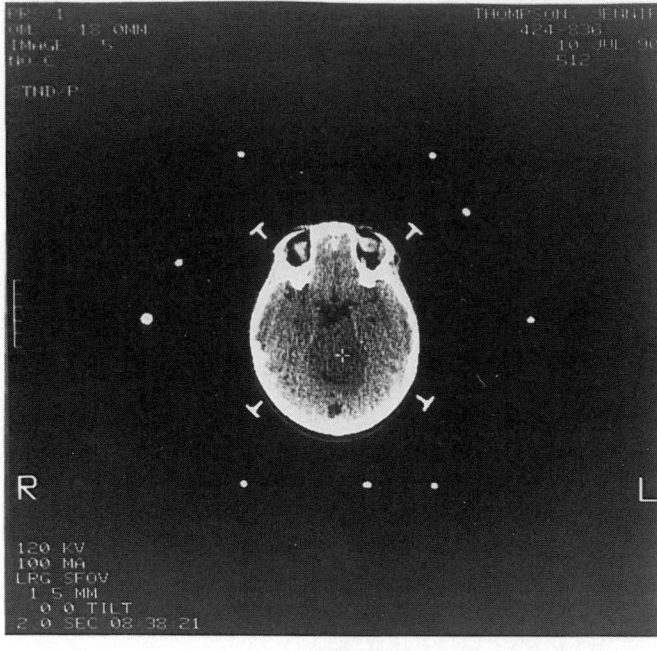

(A)

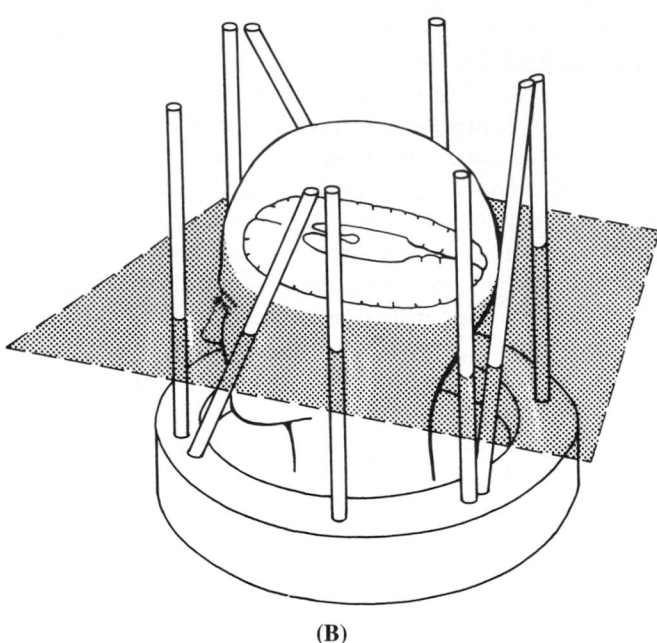

(B)

Figure 23–6 *A.* CT scan of a patient with a pontine glioma. Cursor defines the biopsy site. The nine fiducial rods are seen as white dots surrounding the patient's head. *B.* Drawing showing the CT scan "cutting" through the three sets of vertical and diagonal fiducial rods in the target plane. The *x, y* coordinates of each of the nine rods are entered into the computer, which calculates the distance from each of the three diagonal rods to the base ring, based on the proportionate distance of each diagonal rod from its associated vertical rods in that plane. These three points define the plane of the target relative to the base ring, and from this the 3-dimensional coordinates of the target are calculated.

guide cannula is much safer for a lesion in the brainstem. Solid acute intracerebral hematomas can be evacuated with instruments such as the Higgins-Nashold device (Fig. 23-11*A* and *B*).

```
TRENTWELLS
BRWT PROGRAM

12.15.89.
PATIENT:
██████████████

SCAN(R/S) OR TARGET(STO)
                    RUN

X1=
          -13.77   RUN
Y1=
           2.44    RUN
X2=
          -10.25   RUN
Y2=
           8.48    RUN
X3=
          -6.63    RUN
Y3=
          14.70    RUN
X4=
           7.39    RUN
Y4=
          14.61    RUN
X5=
          10.83    RUN
Y5=
           8.48    RUN
X6=
          14.36    RUN
Y6=
           2.35    RUN
X7=
           7.22    RUN
Y7=
          -9.83    RUN
X8=
           1.18    RUN
Y8=
          -9.74    RUN
X9=
          -6.80    RUN
Y9=
          -9.74    RUN
XTG=
           1.85    RUN
YTG=
           1.18    RUN

CORRECTIONS?
                    RUN

TARGET:
A-P=-12.4
LAT=-15.7
VERT=2.9
```

Figure 23–7 Thermal paper printout of *x, y* data for the nine fiducial localizer rods and the target. The 3-dimensional target data are printed out at the bottom of the sheet.

Although satisfactory debulking of larger intracerebral hematomas can be accomplished,[6] with about 60 percent of the clot removed, the overall results appear to be about the same for operated and nonoperated patients.[7] In general, patients with large hematomas who also present in poor clinical condition do poorly regardless of the type of intervention. The results of stereotactic intervention at this stage are comparable to those of similar patients whose clots have been evacuated at open craniotomy.

The authors have observed rapid reversal of clinical signs after stereotactic aspiration of a chronic brainstem hematoma performed with gentle aspiration through a small-diameter stereotactic biopsy needle. One should be aware of the

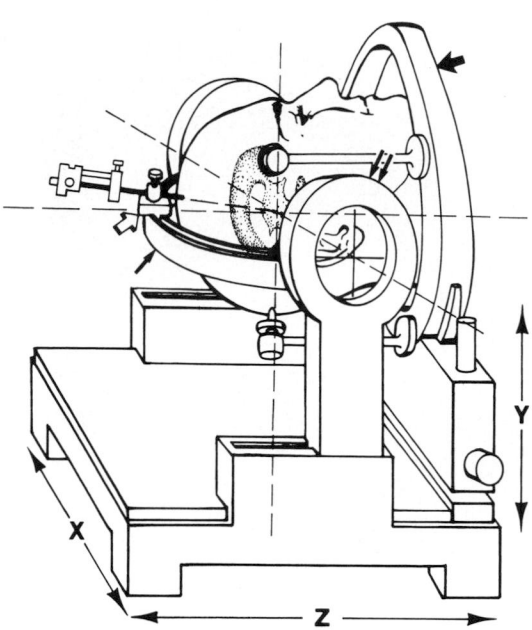

Figure 23–8 Todd-Wells stereotactic instrument. The skull is fixated in the base ring (large white arrow) which can be moved along any of the three rectilinear directions. The arc (small white arrow) can rotate on the trunions (large black arrow), but its base (marked with vertical white labels) does not move. The guide block (small black arrow), through which the probe passes, can be moved to any point along the arc.

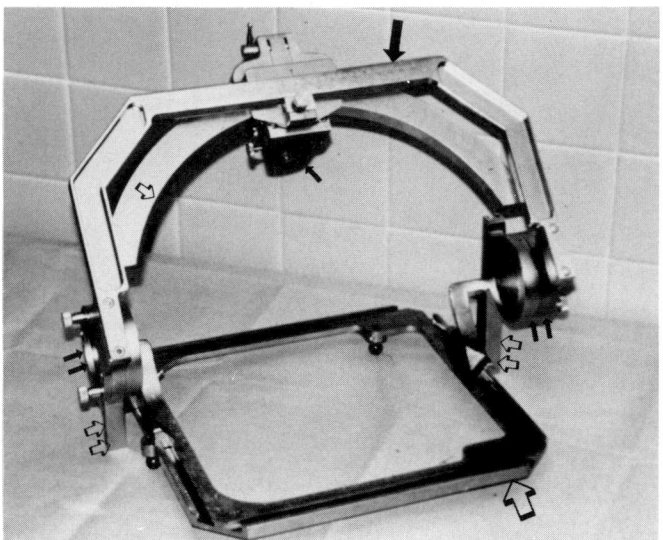

Figure 23–9 CRW stereotactic instrument. The base plate (large white arrow) attaches to the base ring (see Fig. 23-3). The arc (small white arrow) can be moved in the AP direction along grooves in the base plate and superior-inferior along the vertical bars (small double white arrows). The arc moves laterally along the U bar (large black arrow), which is attached to the trunions. The arc rotates on the trunions. The guide block (small black arrow) can be moved to any position along the arc. Millimeter vernier scales are located along the base plate, vertical bars, and the U bar for precision placement of the focal point of the arc in 3-dimensional stereotactic space.

possibility of an underlying neoplasm or vascular malformation when approaching intracerebral hematomas operatively. Stereotactic aspiration is ideally suited to the diagnosis and drainage of deep-seated and multiple intracranial abscesses. The technique of gentle aspiration through a small blunt-tipped needle is the same as for liquefied intracerebral hematomas. Patients who are quite ill will tolerate this procedure under local anesthesia better than under general endotracheal anesthesia. General anesthesia is usually reserved for children.

STEREOTACTICALLY GUIDED ENDOSCOPIC OR OPEN CRANIOTOMIES

Stereotactically guided endoscopic or open craniotomies are indicated in cases where the neurosurgeon's goal is removal or debulking of deep-seated lesions with minimal manipulation of overlying tissue.[2,8,9] Examples would be an endoscopic approach to a small ventricular tumor such as a colloid cyst of the third ventricle or a transcortical approach to a subcortical tumor for the purpose of removal or debulking. Figure 23-12 shows an endoscopic kit. Figure 23-13*A* to *C* shows the steps in a stereotactically guided craniotomy and tumor removal.

A technique referred to as *interactive volumetric stereotactics,* which involves utilization of the carbon dioxide laser, has added a new dimension to the stereotactic approach to deep-seated intracranial lesions.[2,8] These procedures are accomplished as follows. As previously described,

a CT- or MRI-compatible stereotactic base ring and localizer are applied. Imaging is performed and selected views are transferred to the computer. The CT or MRI localizer is then replaced with an angiographic localizer, after which digital subtraction angiography is performed and selected views are transferred to the computer.

The lesion border is digitized by the computer on individual thin-cut CT or MRI scans, after which a computer volumetric reconstruction of the lesion is obtained. Using these images, an optimal approach, usually along the long axis of the tumor, is selected. The computer will also derive the stereotactic coordinates of an avascular cortical entry point as defined on the digital subtraction angiogram.

Next, a trephine craniotomy is performed, and through a relatively small cortical incision, the deep-seated lesion is approached using a specially designed cylinder-shaped retractor that passes through the guide block of the primary stereotactic arc in the planned trajectory of the procedure. The laser and the microscope are mounted on a larger 400-mm secondary stereotactic arc and adjusted so that the axis of vision through the microscope and the laser beam pass directly through the cylindrical retractor.

Reformatted sequential images, from superficial to deep, are brought up on the operating room computer monitor, as is a cursor that corresponds to the position of the laser beam in the operative field. The laser beam is controlled by a joystick, attached to the laser microslad, which transmits the position of the laser beam in the surgical field to the

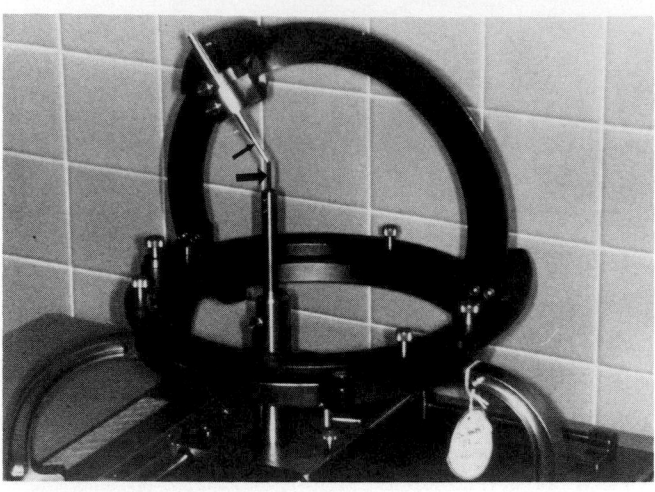

(A)

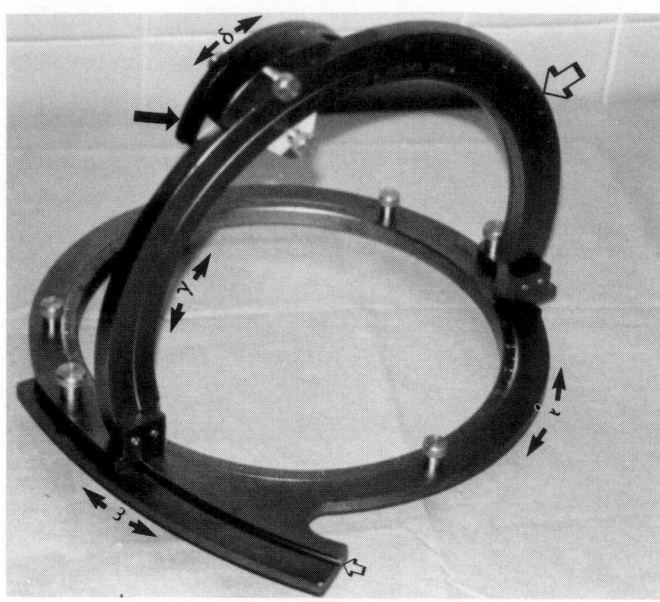

(B)

Figure 23–10 *A.* The BRW arc apparatus is locked onto the phantom apparatus. The entry point 3-dimensional coordinates are determined by moving the phantom pointer (large white arrow) to the guide tube (small white arrow), the tip of which had previously been passed through the arc-guide block apparatus onto the actual entry point. The 3-dimensional coordinates that are read from the phantom represent the 3-dimensional coordinates of the entry point. These data are then entered into the computer, which has already calculated the target coordinates. It will then calculate the four angular settings for the arc as well as the depth of the target. After this, a probe is passed through the guide tube with the phantom pointer repositioned at the target point. If the probe tip touches the phantom pointer, this verifies the accuracy of the four angular settings and the depth reading. *B.* BRW stereotactic instrument. The main arc (large white arrow) rotates 360° (computer read out for this setting is alpha). The main arc can be moved eccentrically (beta setting) using the accessory base plate groove (small white arrow). Adjusting both these components of the main arc will bring the target and entry point into the same vertical plane, which is designated by the horizontal angle or azimuth. The secondary arc-guide block (large black arrow) travels along the main arc (gamma setting) and has a second component which rotates around a pin in the secondary arc-guide block (delta setting). This secondary arc system brings both the target and entry point into the same diagonal plane, forming an angle with the horizontal plane that is referred to as *declination.*

computer monitor by optical encoders located in the joystick assembly.

The computer monitor displays the position of the cursor relative to the tumor as the surgeon guides the focused laser beam around the margin of the tumor. After cutting around the periphery of the tumor at a given depth, the surgeon uses the defocused laser to evaporate that "slice" of tumor. The next deeper slice of tumor is then brought up on the monitor, and the surgeon then repeats the process at that next deeper level. Vessels are coagulated with long forceps under microscopic control.

INTERSTITIAL AND INTRACAVITARY IRRADIATION

While external-beam irradiation is the most effective means of irradiating malignant brain tumors, the amount delivered to the neoplasm is limited by the tolerance of the surrounding tissues to the effects of ionizing irradiation.[10] *Interstitial irradiation* is a means of circumventing this limiting factor. It involves stereotactically implanting multiple sources of ionizing irradiation into specified areas of a tumor. This allows additional irradiation of the tumor while minimizing irradiation of the surrounding brain. High-dose I-125 is often

used because of its lower energy emission compared to other available isotopes. This allows for limited postoperative shielding. The patient wears a lead-lined helmet when others enter his or her private room. Typically, the sources along with the stereotactically placed afterloading catheters are removed after 5 or 6 days of treatment.[10]

Ideally, planning placement of the afterloading catheters and sources is done by computer. The first step involves volumetric reconstruction of the tumor from multiple 2-dimensional axial CT views. Subsequently, the trajectories are planned and the catheters stereotactically implanted. The source or sources are then loaded into each afterloading catheter. The planned position of each source within the afterloading catheter will determine the depth of implantation of the catheter.

The calculated dosimetry or dose delivery of each source will determine its position relative to other sources, both within its afterloading catheter as well as in surrounding catheters.

Graphic simulation of the procedure at the computer workstation confirms the dosages to the tumor and surrounding brain (Plate 13). Any necessary modifications in the position of afterloading catheters or isotope seeds can then be made before the actual procedure. Because reactive edema in the surrounding brain may occur, steroids are

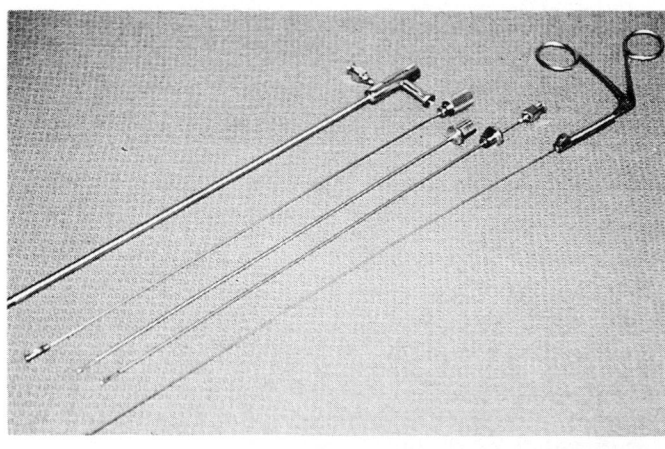

(A)

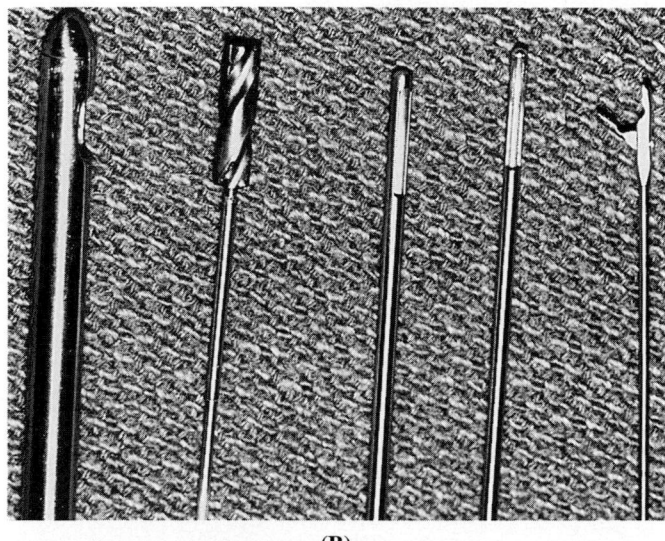

(B)

Figure 23–11 *A.* Stereotactic instruments. *Upper left corner.* Nashold-Higgins clot evacuator has suction and irrigation ports at its proximal end. The inner Archimedes screw, to the right of the outer cannula, is rotated during suction to draw out fragments of clot. Next is the Nashold side-slotted biopsy probe to the right of the clot evacuator. *Far right.* Alligator forceps, which is passed through an outer cannula, and is used to obtain small biopsy specimens. *B.* Close-up of the distal ends of the instruments shown in Fig. 23-11*A.*

given during the period of treatment. The size of treatable tumors is limited to those of a 5-cm diameter or less because treatment of larger tumors can lead to life-threatening edema.

Current controlled studies indicate that interstitial radiation used as a supplement to debulking surgery and external beam irradiation prolongs survival of patients with glioblastoma and anaplastic astrocytoma. However, chemotherapy has recently been reported to be superior to interstitial irradiation in the case of anaplastic astrocytomas.[10]

Radiation necrosis is a common complication, which presents with evidence of increased intracranial pressure or neurological deterioration several months to more than a year after interstitial irradiation. The appearance on a contrast-enhanced CT scan may be indistinguishable from that

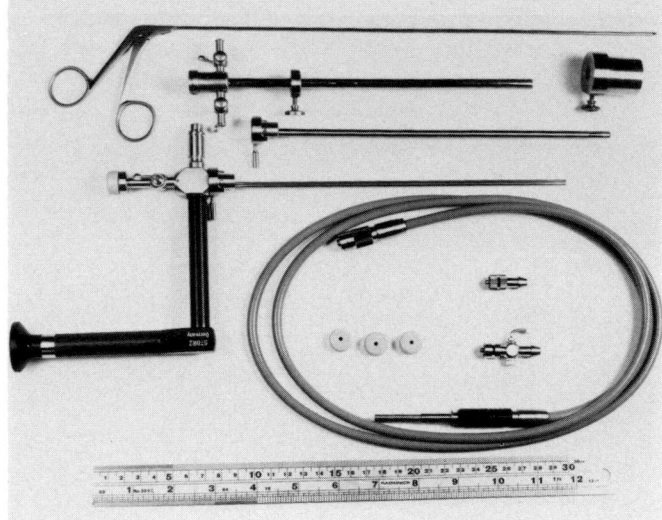

Figure 23–12   Stereotactic endoscopy kit. *(Courtesy of Radionics, Inc.)*

of recurrent tumor. Although there may be symptomatic improvement with systemic steroids, as many as 35 percent may require craniotomy for debulking.[10]

While interstitial irradiation is useful for selected solid tumors, *intracavitary irradiation* may be of benefit for some primarily cystic tumors, e.g., craniopharyngioma. Typically, one of several isotopes in a colloidal suspension is injected into a subgaleal reservoir connected to a catheter which has been stereotactically implanted into the cyst previously. The suspension is aspirated after several days. P-32 and Y-90 have been used. Both have limited tissue penetrance, and therefore only the cellular wall of the cyst that produces the fluid should receive significant irradiation. This is not always the case, and radiation damage to the hypothalamus, optic nerves and chiasm, and oculomotor nerves has occurred. However, serious complications are not common and the cysts are often reduced in size.[12]

☐ RADIOSURGERY

Radiosurgery utilizes multiple converging beams of ionizing irradiation to deliver a single-fraction high dose of irradiation to a small circumscribed volume of CNS tissue previously defined in 3-dimensional stereotactic space. By using multiple beams or arcs of treatment, a high dose of ionizing irradiation is given to a lesion with a rapid falloff or steep gradient of dosage at the lesion edge. This maximizes protection to surrounding brain.

Regardless of the type of ionizing energy and instrument that is used, derivation of target location and volume as well as dosimetry planning are very similar. Prior to the treatment, the patient is placed in a stereotactic base ring, and a CT scan or angiogram is obtained with the appropriate localizer attached. After deriving the shape and volume of

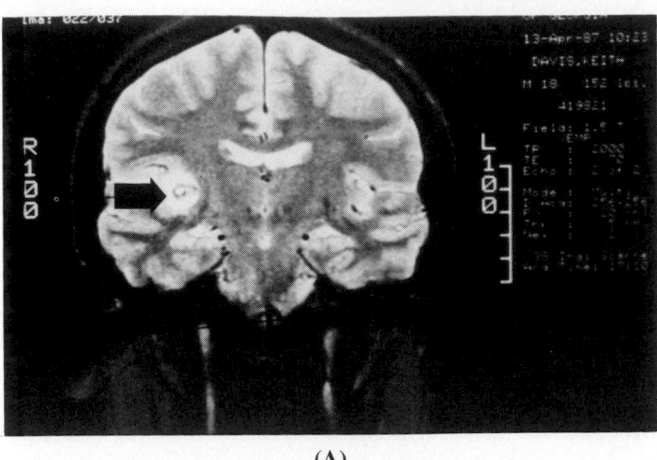

(A)

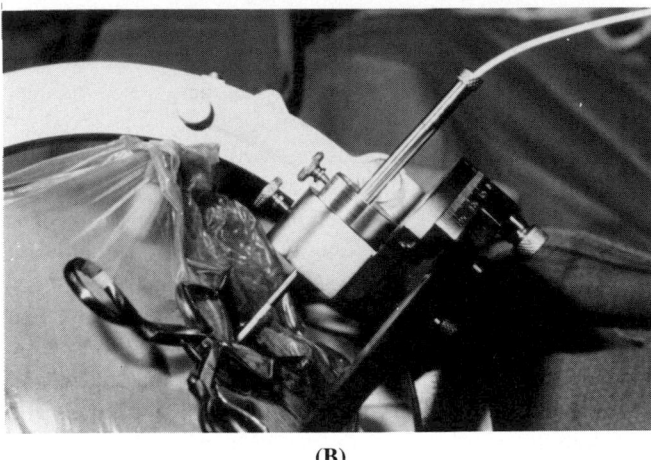

(B)

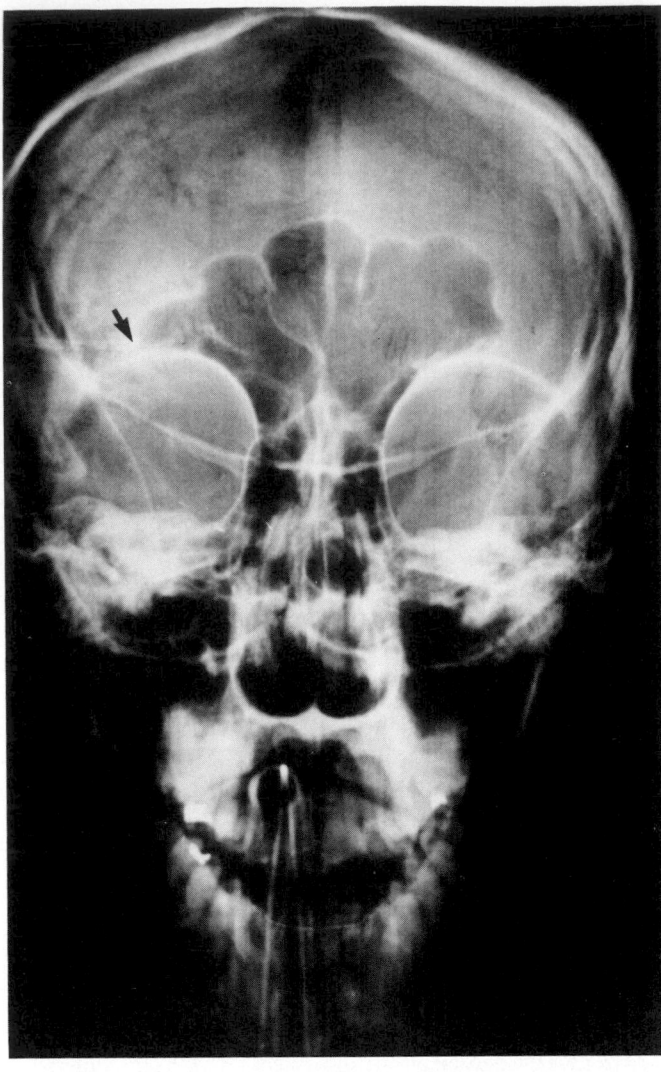

(C)

Figure 23–13 *A.* Right insular glioma (arrow). *B.* Stereotactic placement of catheter tip through superior temporal gyrus down to the lateral aspect of the glioma. *C.* Catheter tip (arrow) placed into area of right insular glioma.

the arteriovenous malformation (AVM) or tumor, dosimetry planning is carried out. Lesion size, shape, and location will determine dosimetry, which must be calculated to encompass as much of the lesion as possible while minimizing dosage to any adjacent functional structures or areas. Dose must also be limited to minimize the possibility of postoperative radiation necrosis. Regardless of the type of radiosurgical device, the stereotactic base ring in which the patient's head is fixed is positioned so that the intracranial target is at the isocenter of the radiosurgery device during treatment.

CYCLOTRON

Three different types of instruments are currently in use. Because of their prohibitive expense (approximately 20 million dollars), cyclotrons are available at only several centers in the United States. They operate on the principle of focusing a circumscribed heavy particle beam approximately 10 mm in width. The shape and circumference of the beam are determined by a series of collimators through which the cyclotron beam passes.[13] The proper depth of radiation occurs as a result of focusing the Bragg peak phenomenon at the target point. Multiple treatment ports are created by rotating the patient, or more precisely the intracranial target, a predetermined number of degrees and then carrying out the next segment of the treatment. If a lesion is more than 10 mm thick relative to an individual port of treatment, beam lamination or refocusing at different depths of the lesion will be required in order to have homogeneous dose distribution to the lesion for that port.[13] Dosimetry planning may be more complex when the lesion is less spherical or when a sensitive functional structure such as the optic chiasm or nerve is nearby.

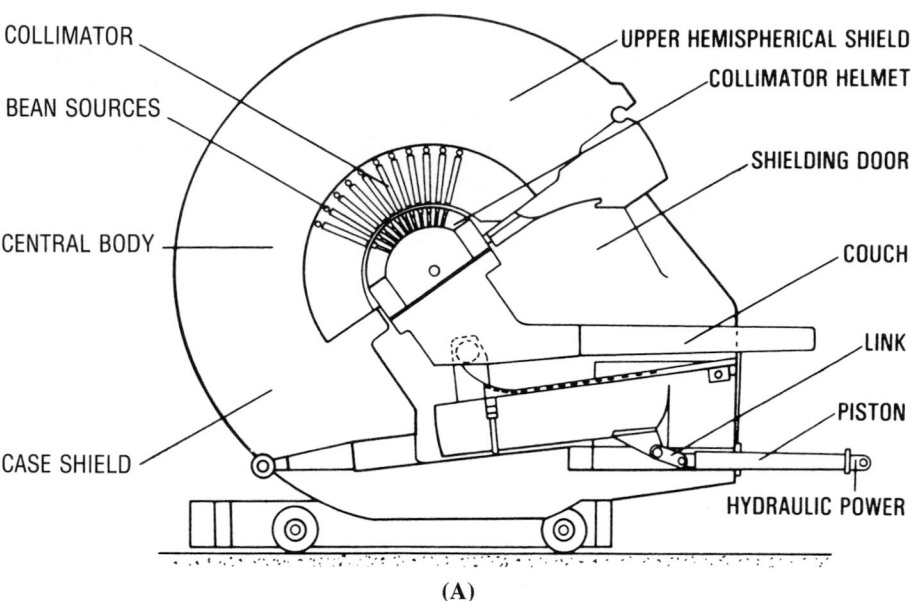

(A)

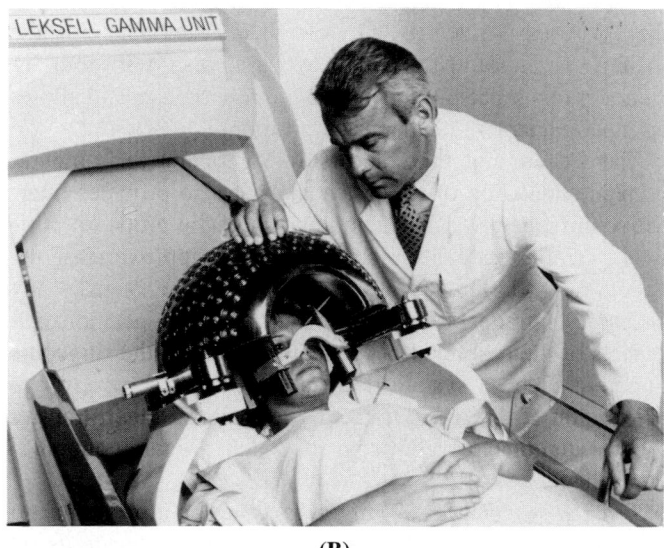

(B)

Figure 23–14 *A.* Cross-section illustration of the gamma knife showing cobalt 60 sources in the central body aligned with the primary collimators and collimator helmet. Also shown are the treatment couch and hydraulic system. *(Courtesy of Elekta Instruments, USA.)* *B.* The patient is fixed in the stereotactic frame with the intracranial target centered at the isocenter of the collimator helmet. The shield and shielding door are seen immediately behind the patient. *(Courtesy of Elekta Instruments, USA.)*

GAMMA KNIFE

The *gamma knife,* although less expensive than the cyclotron, requires about 4 million dollars for equipment and on-site expenditures. This elegant instrument consists of a heavily shielded central body containing 201 sources of Co-60 radially distributed over a sphere (Fig. 23-14*A*). Each source is individually collimated to the focal point of the instrument, which has a mechanical accuracy of +/− 0.1 mm.

The size of the treatment beam will depend on the size of the collimator helmet. Helmets come with four standard size collimators: 4, 8, 14, and 18 mm. One helmet contains 201 collimators, each of which is coaxial with the cobalt sources (Fig. 23-14*B*).

Once imaging and dosimetry planning have been completed, the patient and stereotactic frame are fixed in position under the collimating helmet. Head position is adjusted in the three rectilinear coordinates to bring the intracranial target to the focal point of the instrument. All personnel then leave the room, after which the door of the shielded radiation sources in the central body opens, and the hydraulic system moves the patient and collimator helmet into position (Fig. 23-14*A*).

Once the patient and collimator helmet are locked in position, the cobalt sources in the central body become coaxial with each of the collimators in the helmet. The length of the procedure will depend partly on the number of targets. A multitarget treatment may be required for a nonspherical lesion. The length of an individual treatment will also depend on the age of the decaying cobalt sources, which are usually replaced every 5 to 10 years.

LINEAR ACCELERATORS (LINACs)

Linear accelerators (LINACs) are designed to deliver ionizing irradiation to small areas as they rotate around an isocenter. Because the isocenter of a LINAC may move several millimeters during an arc of treatment and because the isocenter of a stereotactic apparatus may move when the patient is rotated into a new position for the next arc of treatment, unmodified LINACs and stereotactic devices are usually not suitable for radiosurgery.

Many institutions have modified LINACs for radiosurgery, and some systems have achieved a mechanical accuracy comparable to the gamma knife.[13,14] Special modifications of the LINAC and the stereotactic base stand that holds the patient's head are necessary to ensure that there is no movement of either the LINAC isocenter during arcs of treatment or the isocenter of the stereotactic apparatus from one arc of treatment to the next. Secondary collimators of different sizes are fitted to the primary LINAC collimator system to focus the beam for treatment of lesions of different sizes.

Many LINAC-based radiosurgery centers perform recollimation before each procedure. This consists of passing an x-ray beam from the LINAC through a phantom pointer fixed at the isocenter of the stereotactic instrument. X-rays are obtained with the LINAC and an x-ray film at four to eight different positions. Ideally, the round phantom pointer tip should be centered in each of the x-rays.

In order to achieve a satisfactory dose gradient between lesion and surrounding tissue, multiple arcs of treatment (usually five) are necessary. As in the case of the cyclotron, the patient is rotated into another position for each arc of treatment while maintaining the target at the isocenter of the LINAC (Fig. 23-15).

Since the early 1970s, radiosurgery has been used to treat AVMs and certain CNS neoplasms. In general it is indicated in situations where the risk of an open craniotomy would be unacceptable or when the patient otherwise refuses surgery. This includes such examples as deep, inaccessible brainstem AVMs or remnants of an AVM previously incompletely resected and bilateral acoustic neuromas in which unilateral resection has resulted in unilateral deafness. (Chances of hearing preservation are approximately 25 percent after radiosurgery but are much lower after open resection.) AVM occlusion occurs within 2 years in over 85 percent in cases when the lesion has been entirely encompassed by the field of radiation.[16] There is a decrease in size of 43 percent of acoustic neuromas and arrest in 42 percent.[17]

Radiosurgery is also being used in the treatment of malignant gliomas and metastatic brain tumors. Many of the indications for radiosurgery are not yet well-established, nor is optimal dosimetry. Computers with the capability of rapid volumetric lesion reconstruction and dosimetry optimization will increase the speed and accuracy of such procedures. Plate 14 is an example of a type of graphic rendering of a simulated radiosurgical procedure that can be done with state-of-the-art computer hardware and software.

☐ FUTURE DEVELOPMENTS

With the resurgence of stereotaxis in the last decade, there has been a shifting toward utilization of less-invasive techniques, e.g., stereotactically guided biopsies and craniotomies and stereotactic radiosurgery. The most recent technologies introduced to stereotactics are robotics[18,19] and frameless stereotaxis.[20]

Robotics[18,19] involves replacing the aiming device or arc system of the stereotactic apparatus with a robotic arm. Instead of transferring 3-dimensional stereotactic target coordinates to an arc system, the computer calculates these coordinates and transfers them to the robotic arm. Special computer software is used to translate the target and entry-point data into angular settings for each of the moving joints of the robotic arm, and it also programs the depth of penetration of the probe.

Each of the joints of the robotic arm contains a servomotor. The servomotor houses an optical incremental encoder, which provides position and velocity feedback to the robot servosystem. In this way, the position of the probe tip can be displayed relative to the lesion on an operating room computer monitor in real time. By mounting the robotic arm to the stereotactic base ring which is fixed to the patient's head, the base ring serves as the reference base plane for the system, as in standard stereotactic systems. A custom-designed probe holder is attached to the robotic arm and allows for fine adjustment of the probe position.

The system not only allows for preoperative computer graphic simulation of the procedure but also provides interactive intraoperative real-time imaging of the probe-tip position overlaid on a scan slice that best approximates the operative field. This allows the neurosurgeon to make any necessary intraoperative adjustments in probe position. All aspects of the robotic arm's function are under the surgeon's direction. Such a system decreases the chance for error in calculation of target and trajectory as well as in their transfer to the stereotactic robotic arm, which are all computer-controlled.

Frameless stereotaxis[20] involves a sensor arm similar to that used in robotics. The arm may be used to locate its tip in an open operative field or may be programmed to reach a target through a twist drill hole. Rather than using a stereotactic frame as a reference, the sensor arm locates three points on the patient's head (which defines a plane) after its proximal segment is fixed in position for the procedure. Each of these points is touched with the tip of the multi-jointed sensor arm to establish the reference plane for subsequent spatial calibration. The locations of the fiducial markers at each of these same three points as seen on the imaging study are also transferred to the computer. The computer then calculates the 3-dimensional relationship and also the scaling factor between the patient's head and the images. This bypasses the use of a stereotactic frame, which might interfere in the subsequent turning of a craniotomy flap.

The detection devices (e.g., potentiometers, optical encoders) at each of the joints give continuous feedback information to a computer. The computer monitor then displays the probe-tip location on single or multiplanar image slices of interest. This type of system is used interactively by the

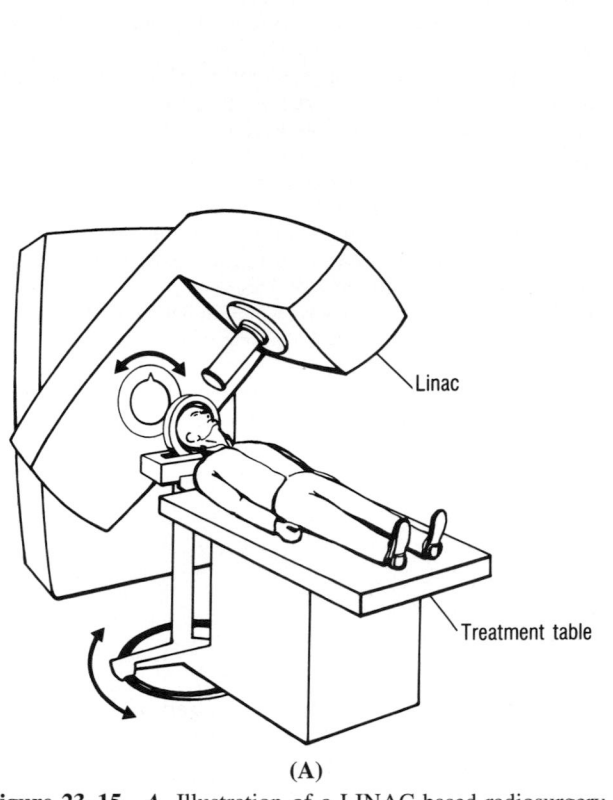

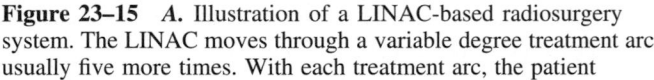

(A)

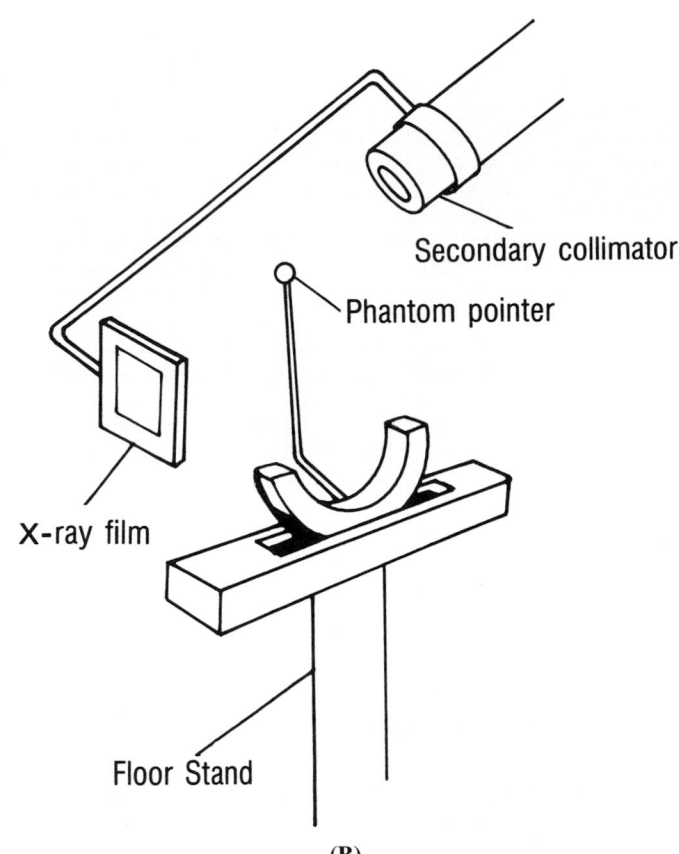

(B)

Figure 23–15 *A.* Illustration of a LINAC-based radiosurgery system. The LINAC moves through a variable degree treatment arc, usually five more times. With each treatment arc, the patient and treatment table are rotated into a different position. **B.** X-ray film is fixed to an extension of the secondary collimator. The phantom pointer is at the isocenter of the stereotactic instrument.

neurosurgeon in open craniotomies where continuously updated graphic displays of a small operative field and its associated critical vascular and anatomical structures provide for a safer and faster operation. Such systems will probably see more extensive use in the future for guidance of some open craniotomies, e.g., localizing deep-feeding vessels to arteriovenous malformations.

One limiting factor in any of the previously described computer-assisted stereotactic systems is that although 3-dimensional data may be displayed on a computer monitor, the individual images are viewed in only 2 dimensions at any one time. However, real 3-dimensional computer displays exist, and it is conceivable that high-resolution *computer-generated 3-dimensional holograms* might be utilized in interactive stereotactic neurosurgery in the future.[21]

REFERENCES

1. Spiegel EA: *Guided Brian Operations.* Basel, S Karger, 1982.
2. Kelly PJ: Principles of stereotactic surgery, in Youmans J (ed): *Neurological Surgery,* 3d ed. Philadelphia, Saunders, 1988, chap 162, pp 4191–4194.
3. Kelly PJ: Principles of stereotactic surgery, in Youmans J (ed): *Neurological Surgery,* 3d ed. Philadelphia, Saunders, 1988, chap 162, pp 4197–4198.
4. Gildenberg PL: General concepts of stereotactic surgery, in Lunsford LD (ed): *Modern Stereotactic Neurosurgery.* Boston, Nijhoff, 1988, chap 1, pp 3–11.
5. Coffey RJ, Friedman WA: Stereotactic applications: General overview, in Heilbrun MP (ed): *Stereotactic Neurosurgery.* Baltimore, Williams & Wilkins, 1988, chap 2, pp 17–53.
6. Kandel EI, Peresedov VV: Stereotactic evacuation of spontaneous intracerebral hematomas. *Stereotact Funct Neurosurg* 54 and 55:427–431, 1990.
7. Niizuma H., Yonemitsu T, Jokura H, et al: Stereotactic aspiration of thalamic hematoma: Overall results of 75 aspirated and 70 nonaspirated cases. *Stereotact Funct Neurosurg* 54 and 55: 438–444, 1990.

8. Kelly PJ: Volumetric stereotaxis and computer-assisted stereotactic resection in subcortical lesions, in Lunsford LD (ed): *Modern Stereotactic Neurosurgery*. Boston, Nijhoff, 1988, chap 12, pp 169–184.

9. Jacques S, Shelden CH, Lutes HR: Computerized microstereotactic neurosurgical endoscopy under direct 3-dimensional vision, in Lunsford LD (ed): *Modern Stereotactic Neurosurgery*. Boston, Nijhoff, 1988, chap 13, pp 185–194.

10. Barbaro NB, Leibel SA, Gutin PH: Interstitial brachytherapy for malignant brain tumors: Technique and results, in Lunsford LD (ed): *Modern Stereotactic Neurosurgery*. Boston, Nijhoff, 1988, chap 18, pp 235–243.

11. Gutin PH: Brachytherapy. Address to the American Society of Stereotactic and Functional Neurosurgery, Pittsburgh, Pa., June 19, 1991.

12. Sturm V, Wowra B, Clorius J, et al: Intracavitary irradiation of cystic craniopharyngiomas, in Lunsford LD (ed): *Modern Stereotactic Neurosurgery,* Boston, Nijhoff, 1988, chap 17, pp 229–233.

13. Kjellberg RN, Masamitsu A: Stereotactic Bragg Peak proton beam therapy, in Lunsford LD (ed): *Modern Stereotactic Neurosurgery*. Boston, Nijhoff, 1988, chap 36, pp 463–470.

14. Winston K, Lutz W. Linear accelerator as a neurosurgical tool for stereotactic radiosurgery. *Neurosurgery* 22: 454–464, 1988.

15. Friedman WA, Bova FJ: Stereotactic radiosurgery, in Tindall GT (ed): *Contemporary Neurosurgery*. Baltimore, Williams & Wilkins, 1989, vol 11 (12), pp 1–7.

16. Steiner L: Radiosurgery in cerebral arteriovenous malformations, in Flam E, Fein J (eds): *Textbook of Cerebrovascular Surgery*. New York, Springer-Verlag, 1986, vol 4, pp 1161–1215.

17. Leksell DG: Stereotactic radiosurgery: Present status and future trends. *Neurolog Res* 9:60–68, 1987.

18. Young RF: A robotic system for stereotactic neurosurgery, in Lunsford LD (ed): *Modern Stereotactic Neurosurgery*. Boston, Nijhoff, 1988, chap 20, pp 259–266.

19. Drake JM, Joy M, Goldenberg A, Kriendler D: Computer- and robot-assisted resection of thalamic astrocytomas in children. *Neurosurg* 29: 27–33, 1991.

20. Watanabe E, Mayanagi Y, Kosugi Y, et al: Open surgery assisted by the neuronavigator, a stereotactic, articulated, sensitive arm. *Neurosurg* 28: 792–800, 1991.

21. Kelly PJ. *Tumor Stereotaxis*. Philadelphia, Saunders, 1991.

☐ STUDY QUESTIONS

I. A 38-year-old right-handed male has a generalized seizure, following which he is given a CT scan that demonstrates a nodule measuring 1.5 cm in diameter located in the posterior temporal lobe within the transverse gyrus of Heschl on the left. The nodule enhanced with IV contrast and an MRI reveals mild edema around it.

1. How might this lesion be biopsied? **2.** What are the alternative stereotactic methods? **3.** What are the advantages and disadvantages of each technique? **4.** Assuming this to be a malignant lesion, how might it be treated? **5.** Assuming it to be a capillary hemangioma, how should it be treated?

II. Using the case described in question 1:

1. What entry techniques might be considered? **2.** How would the location of the lesion play a part in the type of entry technique which might be considered? **3.** What type of stereotactic frame(s) might be indicated? **4.** What are the advantages to the various frames? **5.** What types of biopsy devices are available for obtaining specimens?

III. An 18-year-old girl develops a left hemiparesis. A CT scan reveals an area of decreased attenuation measuring $3^1/_2$ cm in diameter in the right parietal lobe. MRI reveals the lesion to be about $4^1/_2$ cm in diameter, overlying the lateral ventricle, situated at its nearest point about 2 cm lateral to the midline (corpus callosum).

1. What considerations might be required for a stereotactically guided resection? **2.** What could be accomplished by such a resection? **3.** How is the technique performed? **4.** What are the advantages of the laser in such a procedure? **5.** How is bleeding controlled?

IV. A 14-year-old girl has a sudden onset of right hemiparesis following which CT reveals a small hemorrhage in the left thalamus. Further investigation reveals a nidus of an arteriovenous malformation (AVM) in the thalamus measuring about 1 cm in diameter.

1. How should the hematoma be evacuated? **2.** What noninvasive techniques might be considered for treating the AVM? **3.** What advantages might these techniques have over a direct attack? **4.** What concerns might the surgeon have? **5.** How would dosimetry be determined?

V. Further considering the case described in IV, above:

1. At what time might one expect the AVM to be occluded assuming the use of a gamma knife? **2.** What percentage of AVMs would be occluded using this technique? **3.** What are the advantages of the gamma knife over LINAC. **4.** What advantages might LINAC have over the gamma knife? **5.** How do these forms of radiation compare to heavy particle radiation?

CHAPTER
24

Surgical Management of Intractable Pain

Joseph R. Smith
Herman F. Flanigin

Pain surgery involves both stereotactic and open operative techniques. The basic principles of stereotactic surgery have already been discussed in Chap. 23. Although there are no absolute criteria for the timing of surgical intervention in cases of intractable pain, final consideration of surgery should occur only when it is clear that all attempts at conservative management have failed to provide adequate pain relief. It should also be established that there are no significant psychological contraindications to surgical intervention.

Transcutaneous nerve stimulation (TENS) is sometimes forgotten as a method of conservative management for both acute and chronic pain; it is all but totally free of side effects, and virtually nothing is lost if it is ineffective. As is the case with many analgesic medications, TENS is usually given an adequate trial of several weeks before making any conclusions regarding further use.

Choice of surgical procedure will be based not only on the location of the pain but also on the pain's basic pathophysiological mechanism. Pain of a continuous, burning, or intermittent and sharp shooting character which occurs in an area of neurological deficit is referred to as *deafferentation* or *neuropathic pain.*[1] It is important to distinguish such pain from *nociceptive pain,* which is due to potentially tissue-damaging stimulation of peripheral nociceptors.

The type of pain includes acute pain and most cases of pain as a result of cancer. It should be noted that patients with nociceptive cancer pain may develop superimposed deafferentation pain if the neoplasm invades a local nerve or plexus.

As the mechanism of deafferentation pain differs from that of nociceptive pain, both its medical and surgical management will differ also. For instance, deafferentation pain may respond poorly to narcotics and to ablative procedures involving the central or peripheral pathways, whereas chronic nociceptive pain may respond quite well to these modalities. A careful history and physical examination may help to differentiate between the two types. With proper patient and procedure selection good results will be obtained in a majority of cases.

Surgical Procedures

☐ **CANCER PAIN**

In cancer, conservative management of pain includes the use of narcotics on a non-prn (noncontingent) schedule as well as the administration of nonsteroidal antiinflammatory agents, as tolerated to control local inflammation. Antidepressants may also control the depression that often accompanies severe cancer pain. In instances where surgery incompletely relieves pain, the supplemental use of a combination of these drugs can yield excellent overall results.

INTRAVENTRICULAR AND INTRASPINAL MORPHINE (MS)

Procedures to introduce MS into the cerebrospinal fluid (CSF) have become standards for the surgical treatment of cancer pain. The main advantage of these modalities is pain control with micro quantities of morphine, which thereby avoids systemic side effects. The efficacy of such treatment is based on the binding of MS to stereospecific receptor sites in the superficial portion of the posterior horns, the nucleus caudalis of the trigeminal nerve, and the brainstem receptor sites. In fact, this modality may be effective for nociceptive pain in any anatomic distribution.

Intrathecal MS in a hyperbaric solution of 7% dextrose may be effective for control of pain in the lower trunk, pelvis, and legs. Intrathecal MS in isotonic saline solution may provide analgesia up through the caudal cervical segments.[2] *Intraventricular MS* has been used for head and neck as well as diffuse pain.[2,3] One comparative study[4] suggests that intraventricular MS gives more profound analgesia, and another study[3] has noted that intraventricular MS may be effective in patients with lower body pain who no longer respond to intraspinal MS.

In general, about 80 percent of patients will obtain significant relief.[3,4] Cases of tolerance have been observed,[4] and this has been linked to bolus administration (versus continuous infusion) as well as to patients on higher doses of systemic opiates prior to MS pump implantation.

As long as proper dosage is adhered to, the incidence of side effects is low and short-lived. Urinary retention and pruritus occur with intraspinal MS. Confusion, dysphoria, hallucinations, dizziness, nausea, and vomiting have been observed commonly with intraventricular MS, but respiratory depression is unusual.[2-4] Occasionally, these side effects have been severe enough to warrant discontinuing treatment.

Implantation of opiate delivery devices requires that one or several test injections first be done to establish subsequent dosage and concentration and observation for any serious side effects. The test dose of MS should be hyperbaric MS—via lumbar puncture if the pain involves the lower body and via a subgaleal Ommaya reservoir connected to a ventricular catheter if the pain is diffuse or cervicofacial. Neither analgesia nor side effects develop until there is some degree of receptor saturation (after 30 to 45 min), and patients receiving test injections should be observed overnight in an intensive care or stepdown unit for any side effects and to document the extent of pain control.

After candidacy is established, a percutaneous intrathecal thoracolumbar or ventricular catheter is implanted. The tubing is passed subcutaneously and attached to an implanted subclavicular or subcostal infusion device, respectively. This may be a commercially available bolus pump or a continuous infusion apparatus, either of which must be refilled every few weeks to months, depending on patient usage and drug concentration.

Contraindications to implanation include: significant side effects related to a test injection of proper dose, high risk of infection or hemorrhage, the patient's inability to comprehend the need for periodic refilling of the drug reservoir, and lack of available local medical resources for refilling the reservoir. Another contraindication is a history of prolonged use of high-dose opiates, in which case tolerance to intrathecal or intraventricular morphine may develop rapidly.

Ablative procedures are effective alternatives in cases of intractable, nociceptive cancer pain, in which intraspinal or intraventricular morphine might be contraindicated for reasons mentioned previously.

INTRATHECAL ALCOHOL

Intrathecal alcohol can effectively alleviate pain that is confined to one or two unilateral segments. Absolute alcohol is hypobaric relative to CSF and is instantaneously neurolytic; therefore, the instillation is performed with the patient in the decubitus position with the painful side up and on a table or bed with Trendelenburg controls (which should always be tested before injection).

The patient is placed so that the roots to be irrigated are in the least-dependent position; e.g., for left S1 pain the patient should be in right decubitus with head down and buttocks up. Further, the patient should be rotated slightly prone. This will facilitate irrigation of the posterior roots in their least-dependent position so that the alcohol will stratify, protecting the anterior roots. The spinal tap should be performed with a 22-gauge needle. Some texts[5] recommend that the needle be positioned where roots exit the cord, but for lumbar and S1 injections, one may position it in the midline at or near the foraminal exit site, with the bevel pointing toward the root (e.g., lumbar puncture at L5–S1 for an L5 or S1 rhizolysis).

One cm^3 of absolute alcohol is drawn into a tuberculin syringe before the lumbar puncture. After the needle penetrates the dura, it is rotated several times to allow arachnoid membrane to move away from the needle tip. This decreases the likelihood of a subdural injection. The needle is advanced several more millimeters and rotated a few times again. Injection is begun only after good CSF flow is assured and then only in 0.1-mm increments.

After the initial injection, if the patient complains of stinging, burning pain anywhere other than at the site of pain, he or she is instructed to cough (in order to break up the small volume of alcohol) and is then repositioned immediately. For example, if a patient undergoing an S1 rhizolysis complains of pain in the left L5 distribution after 0.1 cm^3 of alcohol, he or she is asked to cough and is then repositioned with the head in Trendelenburg position. Given proper technique, after injection of 0.2 to 0.3 cm^3 both the stinging pain of injection and the cancer pain should begin to subside. Usually about 0.5 cm^3 will give a satisfactory block.

An effective method of treating bilateral sacral pain in patients with total lower motor neuron paralysis of bowel and bladder function is injection of approximately 3 cm^3 of absolute alcohol in small increments into the caudal thecal sac through an L5–S1 LP with the patient in a prone Trendelenburg position. The patient should be left in the same position for at least 30 min after the block to allow the alcohol to bind to local tissue. Relief may last up to 6 months. Earlier pain recurrence can herald extension of the cancer beyond the initially involved segments.

As is true for many other ablative procedures, patient cooperation is imperative in this procedure. Phenergan 25 mg IM or IV is an effective anxiolytic for such procedures.

CORDOTOMY

This is an effective procedure for unilateral multisegmental cancer pain. The lateral spinothalamic tract can be transected with either a radiofrequency current passed through an electrode [as in high-percutaneous radiofrequency (RF) cervical cordotomy] or with a cordotomy knife or the tip of a No. 11 blade (as in high-thoracic cordotomy).

Either technique will give effective analgesia for cancer pain in the contralateral lower torso or leg. It must be mentioned, however, that the level of thermanalgesia will descend a variable number of segments within 2 to 3 weeks after surgery. It is reasonable to expect a level at C5 after percutaneous high-cervical lesioning[6] and a T8 level after high thoracic cordotomy.[7]

Preoperatively, not only must deafferentation pain be ruled out but also it must be determined whether there is any pain on the side opposite the severe pain. In the latter instance, the patient may complain that the milder preexisting pain ipsilateral to the cordotomy has become more severe after an otherwise successful procedure. In certain patients with bilateral pain, consideration of bilateral high thoracic cordotomy or midline myelotomy (see section on commissural myelotomy) may be appropriate. Performing a cordotomy on someone with preexisting deafferentation pain invites worsening of an already intractable pain since most postcordotomy dysesthesias (burning pain) occur in areas of preexisting neurologic deficit with or without sensory loss.[7]

There are several relative contraindications to cordotomy. Respiratory compromise applies particularly to high cervical cordotomy. The voluntary control of respiration is located in fibers in the lateral corticospinal tracts which would be spared by transection of the anterolateral quadrant of the cord containing the lateral spinothalamic tract. However, the involuntary pathway is located in the anterolateral quadrant immediately medial to the cervical spinothalamic fibers.[8] A unilateral ablation in someone with significant ipsilateral or generalized pulmonary dysfunction, although not affecting voluntary respiratory effort, might have a significant indirect effect on automatic respiration during sleep, resulting in a sleep apnea that might prove fatal. Candidates with respiratory compromise are not necessarily ruled out for unilateral cordotomy, but they must have a careful preoperative evaluation which includes pulmonary function tests, arterial blood gases, and, in cases where phrenic nerve dysfunction is suspected, fluoroscopy of the diaphragm.

Patients with sacral pain or preexisting bowel or bladder dysfunction are at risk for developing increased dysfunction. The ascending pathways responsible for the sensation of fullness of the bladder—which gives rise to the desire to urinate, as well as sensations of pain and temperature in the lower urinary tract—are located in the anterolateral quadrant just medial to the sacral spinothalamic fibers. The risk of permanent bowel or bladder dysfunction is particularly high after bilateral cordotomy.[7]

Either high cervical or high thoracic cordotomy may be effective for unilateral leg pain. Although there is some patient stress involved in performing the high cervical percutaneous cordotomy under local anesthesia with sedation, this technique is far less injurious than open high thoracic cordotomy done under general anesthesia. The latter involves a laminectomy and has the additional disadvantage of the surgeon not being able to locate the lateral spinothalamic tract with intraoperative stimulation.

The *high cervical percutaneous RF cordotomy* begins with fixation of the patient's head in a stereotactic device (Fig. 24-1A). Corrections in head tilt or rotation are made based on anteroposterior (AP) scout skull films. Lateral scout x-rays are made to assure that the patient is positioned

with the upper cervical spinal canal horizontal. Rigid head fixation is preferable, because if there is head rotation during fluoroscopic localization of the needle tip, the resultant parallax may lead to inaccurate positioning of the electrode (see text following).

The patient is medicated with enough intravenous (IV) narcotic and sedatives so that he or she is comfortable but still cooperative. The side of the neck opposite the pain is prepared with povidone-iodine. Using a C-arm image intensifier, a point at the C1–C2 intralaminar space halfway between the anterior and posterior limits of the spinal canal is identified with a radiopaque marker. This point is usually just caudal to the tip of the mastoid process.

The area is infiltrated with 1% Xylocaine with epinephrine and a small stab incision is made with a No. 11 blade. A 9-cm thin-walled 18-gauge needle is inserted and guided with lateral fluoroscopy to the C1–C2 interspace. Additional local anesthesia is injected through the guide needle as it is advanced in order to control local pain.

When the needle tip is appropriately positioned at a depth of about 3 cm and halfway between the anterior and posterior limits of the spinal canal, the anesthesiologist is instructed to give enough IV pentothal to provide brief general anesthesia when the guide needle penetrates the dura. Once a flow of CSF is established, the needle is rotated gently and inserted an additional 1 to 2 mm. Several cm³ of CSF are then withdrawn and mixed with an equal volume of Pantopaque. One cm³ of this emulsion is injected to outline the anterior margin of the dentate ligament, which usually—but not always—marks the equator of the cord (Fig. 24-1B).

If the patient's head is not rotated, the right and left dentate ligaments should superimpose, and the guide needle will be properly positioned just anterior to the ligament. If the patient is initially positioned with the upper cervical canal horizontal, the emulsion will remain stratified on the anterior surface of the dentate ligament. Injection of 5 to 10

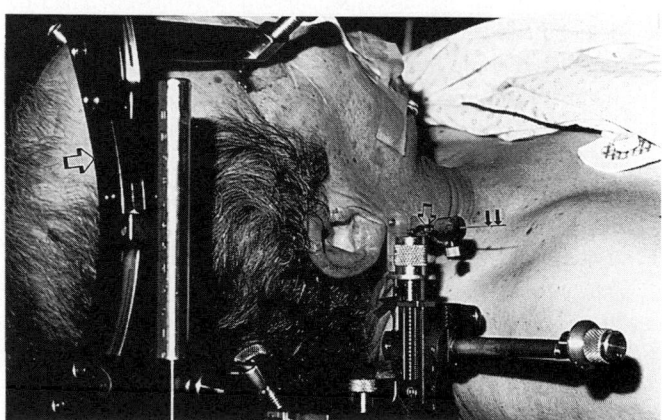

Figure 24-1A The patient's head is fixed in a Todd-Wells base ring (large white arrow). The cordotomy electrode passes through a guide needle (small white arrow), which is held in the vertical arm (black arrow) of the microdrive apparatus. The guide needle and electrode enter the C1–C2 interspace slightly caudal to the mastoid tip.

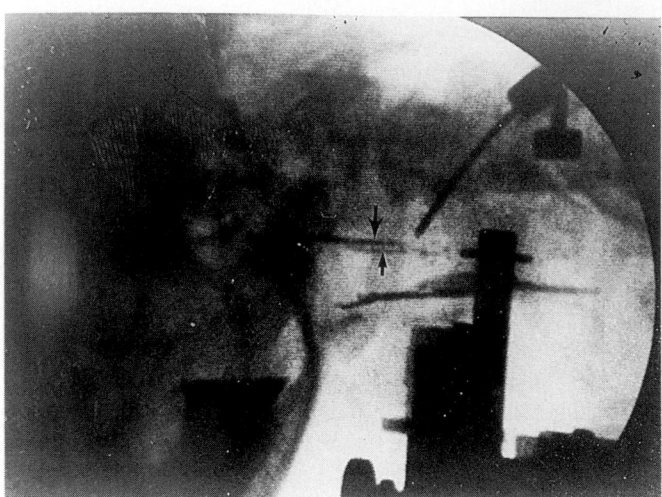

Figure 24-1B Lateral radiograph displays oil-soluble contrast medium, outlining the ipsilateral (large arrow) and contralateral (small arrow) dentate ligaments. The cordotomy electrode enters the cord slightly anterior to the dentate ligament.

cm³ of filtered room air to outline the anterior margin of the cord is optional.

The next step is fixation of the guide needle in the microdrive apparatus. The needle is slowly advanced and intermittently checked for cessation of CSF flow, which indicates that it is contacting the cord. Once this occurs, the stylet is replaced with a cordotomy needle which has an approximately 2-mm uninsulated thermocoupled tip with temperature monitoring capability. This is advanced while maintaining continuous impedance monitoring until there is a rapid change of impedance from approximately 500 to 1000 ohms, indicating that the cord has been penetrated.

At this point physiological testing begins. Initially, low frequency stimulation of 2 to 5 Hz is carried out. Contraction of ipsilateral nuchal muscles at such a frequency indicates that the electrode is probably too anterior, and contraction of ipsilateral leg muscles suggests that the electrode is too far posterior. In either case the electrode should be removed. Then the guide needle is withdrawn 1 mm at a time.

As soon as there is the slightest flow of CSF, the butt end of the needle should be repositioned up or down, e.g., needle butt end up to direct the guide needle tip more posteriorly. When lateral fluoroscopy confirms proper repositioning, the needle is advanced until CSF flow stops. The electrode is then reinserted. Impedance is rechecked but may be a less-accurate indicator of cord penetration after reinsertion.

The process of stimulation is begun again. When little or no motor response is obtained at low frequency and stimulation at 50 to 100 Hz produces a warm or cool thermal sensation or, less likely, pain or paresthesias on the contralateral body side, this confirms proper electrode position. Sensory responses which involve the entire contralateral body below the neck level or the hand suggest that satisfactory analgesia below C5 will be obtained.

At this point lesioning is begun. All lesions are performed for 60 sec to allow the tissue surrounding the electrode to reach thermal equilibrium in order to ensure a uniform lesion. Lesioning is initiated at temperatures barely above those causing reversible damage (42.5° to 44°C), and the patient is checked continuously during lesioning for development of contralateral thermanalgesia or for ipsilateral paresis indicating extension of the lesion into the corticospinal tract. In the latter case the procedure is stopped immediately and may be attempted again another day. If only hypalgesia or incomplete analgesia is obtained, the lesion temperature is increased 5°, and lesioning repeated until a satisfactory or best possible result is obtained. Figure 24-1C shows the topographic arrangement of the various pathways in the upper cervical cord.

Initially, 80 to 90 percent of patients will experience satisfactory pain relief, but this may decrease to 50 percent by the end of 1 year. The operation usually provides satisfactory relief for patients with limited life expectancy. Deaths are very rare even when temporary respiratory failure occurs after uni- or bilateral operations. However, most neurosurgeons will not perform bilateral staged high cervical cordotomies for fear of fatal sleep apnea. Persistent paresis or persistent worsening of bladder function occurs in at least 5 percent of bilateral cases.[6]

High thoracic cordotomy is usually performed under general anesthesia and is reserved for those patients with pain caudal to T8 who cannot comply with percutaneous cervical cordotomy under local anesthesia. A T2 to T3 laminectomy is performed. In the case of bilateral cordotomy, a T2 to T4 laminectomy is executed since the two cuts are performed with one as far rostral and the other as far caudal as possible. The dura is opened in a modified U incision for unilateral lesions or an H-shaped incision for bilateral lesions. Dural tack-up stitches are placed. The dentate ligament is identified, at its dural attachment, and retracted posteriorly and medially. It is essential that the ligament be retracted at the point where it joins the cord. If it is grasped too far laterally and the equator of the cord misidentified, then the posterior limit of the cord incision may be in the lateral column with an attendant ipsilateral paresis of the leg.

An avascular area of the anterolateral quadrant is identified. Bipolar cautery at low power is used to coagulate small

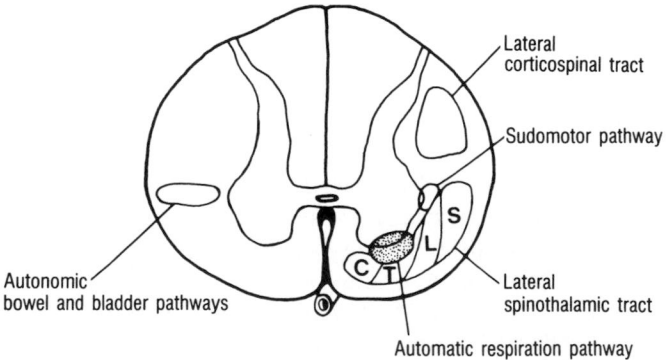

Figure 24-1C Cross-sectional drawing of the upper cervical spinal cord displaying the position of ascending and descending tracts that may be transected during cordotomy.

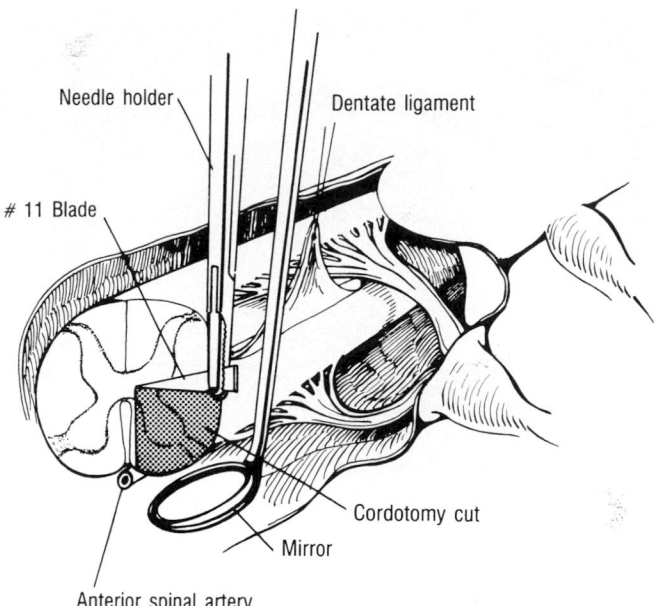

Needle holder

Dentate ligament

11 Blade

Cordotomy cut

Mirror

Anterior spinal artery

Figure 24-2 The dura is opened, and the dentate ligament is cut and retracted. A small dental mirror is positioned anterior to the cord in order to visualize the anterior spinal artery. The end of a No. 11 blade no more than 5 mm in length is held in a needle holder and inserted into the cord at the point where the dentate ligament attaches to the cord. It is then drawn anteriorly so that its tip exits the cord just lateral to the anterior spinal artery.

pial vessels. The pia-arachnoid is divided in an axial plane, beginning at the point of attachment of the dentate ligament and extending to a point about 2 mm medial to the anterior root. After measuring half the width of the cord (usually no more than 5 mm), an equal length of No. 11 blade is measured and grasped by a needle holder. It is inserted at the level of the dentate ligament and then drawn anteriorly, with a dental mirror held anterior to the cord to assure that the tip of the blade avoids the anterior spinal artery as the cut is completed anteriorly. (See Fig. 24-2.) Lastly, a microinstrument with a blunt curved tip is drawn through the incision to make sure no fibers have been left intact. The dura is closed watertight with a fine braided filament suture in a running interlocking stitch.

The results and complications, except for absence of neurogenic respiratory complications, are very similar to those for high cervical cordotomy. Most neurosurgeons do not do bilateral high cervical cordotomies because of the risk of postoperative sleep apnea, but they will do a staged high cervical and contralateral high thoracic cordotomy for control of bilateral multisegmental nociceptive cancer pain.

COMMISSURAL MYELOTOMY

Commissural myelotomy, which is done in a single stage, is useful for treatment of bilateral pain located below the neck. It has successfully controlled deep paramedian pain, pain of somatic or visceral origin, and deafferentation pain. Its mechanism is unknown but is assumed to be related to

destruction of a central multisynaptic pathway that courses in the area of the central grey commissure.

Until 1968 this procedure consisted of longitudinally incising in the midsagittal plane all cord segments involved in the pain transmission as well as the next three rostral segments. This required a multilevel laminectomy and general anesthesia. Frequently, the operation was done for cancer pain involving the lower abdomen, pelvis, perineum, and lower extremities.[9] The microscopic technique involved inserting a No. 11 blade to a depth of approximately 6 to 7 mm until the anterior sulcus was entered and then drawing the blade caudally the length of the planned incision. About 60 percent of patients obtained complete relief, and an additional 30 percent obtained partial relief. However, persistent bladder dysfunction or motor loss occurred in about 10 percent of patients (about the same as with bilateral high thoracic cordotomy), and over 25 percent had persistent leg dysesthesias with or without loss of position sense. Curiously, objective loss of pain and temperature sensation did not always accompany pain relief.

Stereotactic high cervical commissural myelotomy was introduced in 1968.[10] The procedure is performed under local anesthesia with the patient's head well flexed in the stereotactic apparatus in order to fix the upper cervical cord. A guide needle is introduced posteriorly in the midline through the occiput–C1 interspace under fluoroscopic guidance. After penetrating the dura and obtaining CSF, the needle is advanced until flow stops, after which the electrode is introduced and advanced until impedance changes from 500 to 1000 ohms. Stimulation at 50 Hz and approximately 1.0 volt is carried out as the electrode is advanced. Symmetrical paresthesias should be obtained in the legs and perineum and subsequently in both arms as the electrode is advanced.

After arm responses are no longer obtained, the electrode is advanced another 2 mm. Radiofrequency coagulation with temperature monitoring is then carried out in increments up to 75°C until significant hypalgesia or analgesia occurs or unwanted neurologic deficit begins to develop. With this technique, pain relief rarely occurs without significant loss of pain sensation, but 80 percent of those with sensory loss will obtain good relief.

No weakness, sphincter disturbances, or respiratory dysfunction has been reported. This is consistent with the more peripheral location of the voluntary and involuntary pathways for such functions (see Fig. 24-1C). This procedure, which has been used for both lower and upper body cancer pain, is an alternative to bilateral cordotomy.

More recently, a limited open technique of midline or commissural myelotomy, which may be nearly as successful as the original open technique, has been introduced as a treatment for midline pelvic pain.[11] This involves a T9 or T10 laminectomy, after which a 5-mm segment of the cord is opened in the midline. A blunt microdissector is then used to dissect in the midline along this exposed segment to a depth of approximately 6 mm. Usually the pial fold of the anterior sulcus can be palpated with the dissector. The technique has also been used at the C1 level with limited

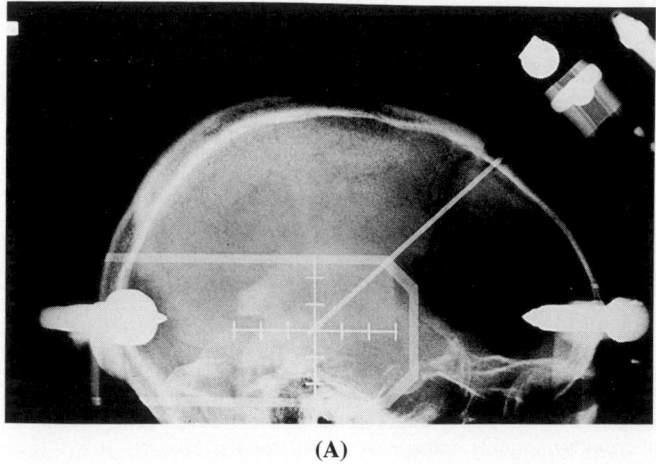

(A)

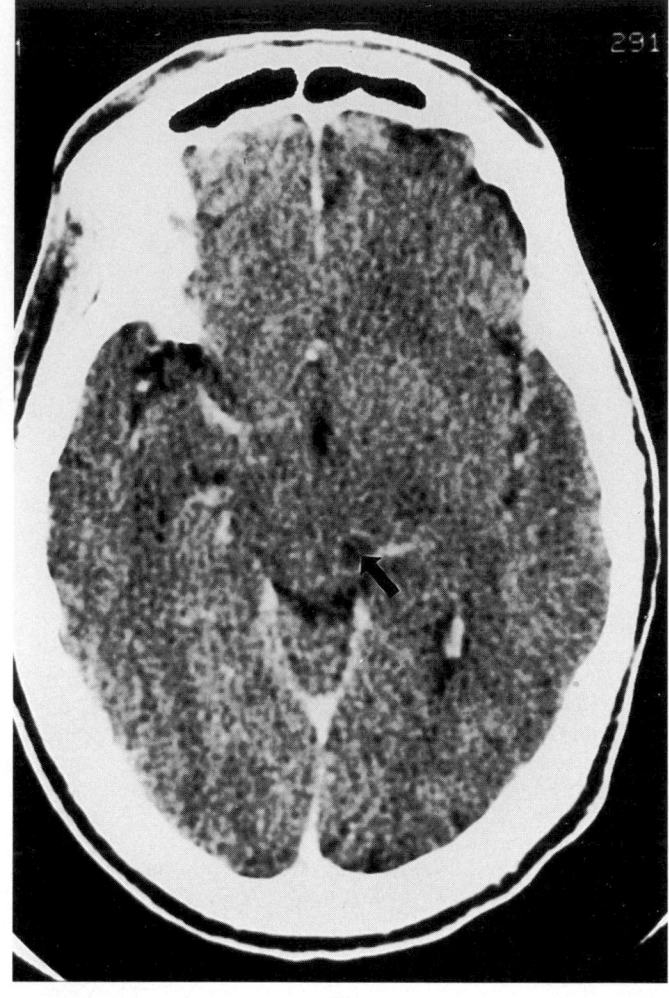

(B)

Figure 24-3 *A.* The electrode tip is positioned 5 mm inferior to the posterior commissure (not seen) and 8 to 9 mm lateral to the midline. *B.* Left mesencephalic tractotomy (arrow) 3 weeks after surgery.

success. Alternatively, a small RF lesion can be made, essentially the same as with the stereotactic high cervical commissural myelotomy. No demonstrable sensory loss, weakness, or sphincter dysfunction has been reported.

RF TRIGEMINAL RHIZOTOMY

This procedure is a simple, effective means of alleviating nociceptive cancer pain of the face confined to the trigeminal distribution. It can be used if the region of the ipsilateral foramen ovale or the planned guide needle tract is free of tumor. As opposed to trigeminal neuralgia where a hypalgesic lesion is sufficient for prolonged relief, in the case of cancer pain profound hypalgesia or analgesia must be attained to achieve adequate pain relief. This technique is described in the section on the treatment for trigeminal neuralgia.

STEREOTACTIC MESENCEPHALIC TRACTOTOMY/THALAMOTOMY

In cases of cancer pain of the face where trigeminal rhizotomy can't be performed for the technical reasons just men-

tioned or in cases where nociceptive pain also involves the region of the ear, oropharynx, neck or shoulder, these two operations may be effective. An image-guided, computer-assisted technique is used, the basics of which are described in Chap. 23. The use of computer resident stereotactic brain atlases, which assist in the anatomic localization of the target, is discussed in the section on thalamotomy for movement disorders in Chap. 25.

The procedures may be performed with either CT or MRI guidance; however, the latter allows for target imaging in two additional planes and therefore gives a better localization of target depth provided there is minimal geometric distortion of the image. After computer acquisition of selected views, the appropriate computer resident stereotactic atlas views are superimposed on those image views that best display the target. The computer is then used to calculate the 3-dimensional target coordinates and the AP and lateral angles of trajectory.

Following this, the awake patient is then transferred from the scan suite to the operating room and positioned supine just as during the scan. This avoids any movement of target coordinates that might occur with positional changes. The target coordinates and angles of trajectory are transferred to the stereotactic arc, which is fixed to the base ring on the patient's head. The entry point is infiltrated with local anesthesia and a ¼-inch incision made with a No. 15 blade. A 7⁄64-inch twist drill hole is then made in the trajectory of the electrode and the underlying dura and pia-arachnoid are cauterized with a monopolar electrode. A stimulating-lesioning electrode is then inserted.

The *mesencephalic tractotomy* target is approximately 5 mm posterior and inferior to the superior aqueduct and 9 mm lateral to midline. If the electrode is properly positioned in the spinothalamic tract, stimulation will usually produce a contralateral thermal sensation. If it is too medial, near the medial lemniscus, contralateral paresthesias or electric shock sensations may be reported.

Lesion size will be a function of electrode temperature and of electrode tip dimensions. Lesioning is begun at 50°C for 60 to 90 sec. The patient is repeatedly checked for evidence of position sense loss. Loss of upward gaze and at least temporary diplopia are expected. Lesioning is increased in 5° increments until side effects or contralateral thermanalgesia occur.

A 4 mm lesion will usually suffice. Over 90 percent of patients have satisfactory relief. Permanent ocular palsies occur in under 10 percent and are easily compensated with eye patching.[12] Figure 24-3A and B display the electrode positioning and lesion dimensions. A target point 5 mm off midline, which lesions the multisynaptic pain pathway, may be effective in alleviating deafferentation pain involving the head, neck, or shoulder.

Thalamotomy involves lesioning in the area of the centromedian nucleus, which is a relay for the slower-conducting multisynaptic pain pathway that transmits poorly localized pain. The thalamic target is located posteriorly about nine-tenths of the total distance from anterior to posterior commissure, 4 mm above the intercommissural line, and 9 mm lateral to the midline. The target nucleus is more accurately located in individual cases by computer graphic overlay of a digitized thalamic nuclear map scaled to the dimensions of the patient's thalamus (see Chap. 25, section on thalamotomy).

This lesion has been used with limited success for both nociceptive cancer and deafferantation pain. Physiological localization has been verified by high-threshold stimulation, which produces a vibrating sensation in the contralateral arm.[13] A more accurate method may be that of using low-amplitude stimulation, exploring with a side-extruding electrode (see Chap. 25, section on thalamotomy) to find the junction of the centromedian and ventralis posteromedialis nuclei (personal observation), after which the location of the centromedian nucleus can be inferred. When using ventriculography for target localization, this technique has produced pain attenuation in slightly over 50 percent of patients. Complications such as aphasia and hemiparesis have been rare.[12]

STEREOTACTIC FRONTOLIMBIC DISCONNECTION PROCEDURES

It has been known since shortly after the introduction of frontal lobotomy that frontolimbic disconnection will allay

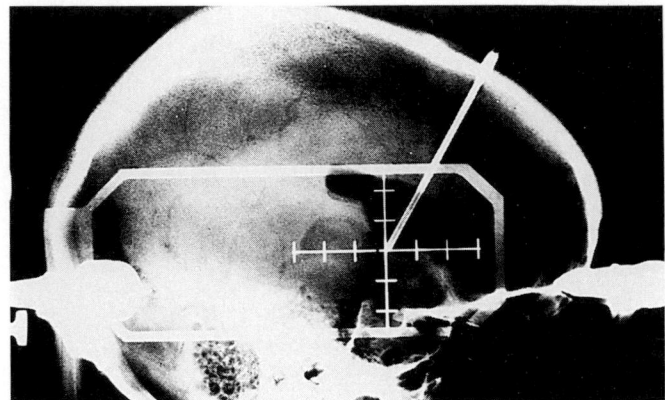

Figure 24-4A Electrode positioning for frontothalamic tractotomy, slightly anterior to the foramen of Monro.

the severe anxiety that can accompany chronic pain. With the development of more limited lobotomies and, subsequently, the introduction of stereotactic techniques for frontolimbic disconnections at various sites, disconnections have been reported to alleviate suffering associated with cancer pain. There is no loss of intellect and little long-term personality alteration. It should be pointed out, however, that this type of operation does not alter the pain threshold and will not be particularly effective for stoic patients who display little suffering. Its use should also be avoided in sociopathic or hysteroid individuals in whom it may abolish what little social inhibition they possess.

Our experience and that of others indicates that up to 80 percent of properly selected patients will obtain relief until the time of death. Bilateral lesions located either in the frontothalamic tracts or subcaudate area or combined lesions in the subcaudate white matter and the cingulum may be effective.[14] (See Fig. 24-4A to C and Plate 15.) These same techniques are less commonly used to treat certain medically intractable psychoaffective disorders.

STEREOTACTIC ALCOHOL HYPOPHYSECTOMY

This procedure has been used effectively for the alleviation of diffuse cancer pain due primarily to hormonally sensitive tumors, e.g., breast and prostate.[15] In such cases intraspinal or intraventricular morphine might be used and would avoid the utilization of postoperative hormone replacement therapy.

☐ CHRONIC NONCANCER PAIN

In some types of chronic noncancer pain such as trigeminal neuralgia the syndrome is clear-cut. The medical and surgical modes of management are well-established and effective in the majority of patients. In such pain syndromes the results of psychosocial evaluations usually will not alter medical or surgical management. However, in many other types of pain discussed in this section, even though the

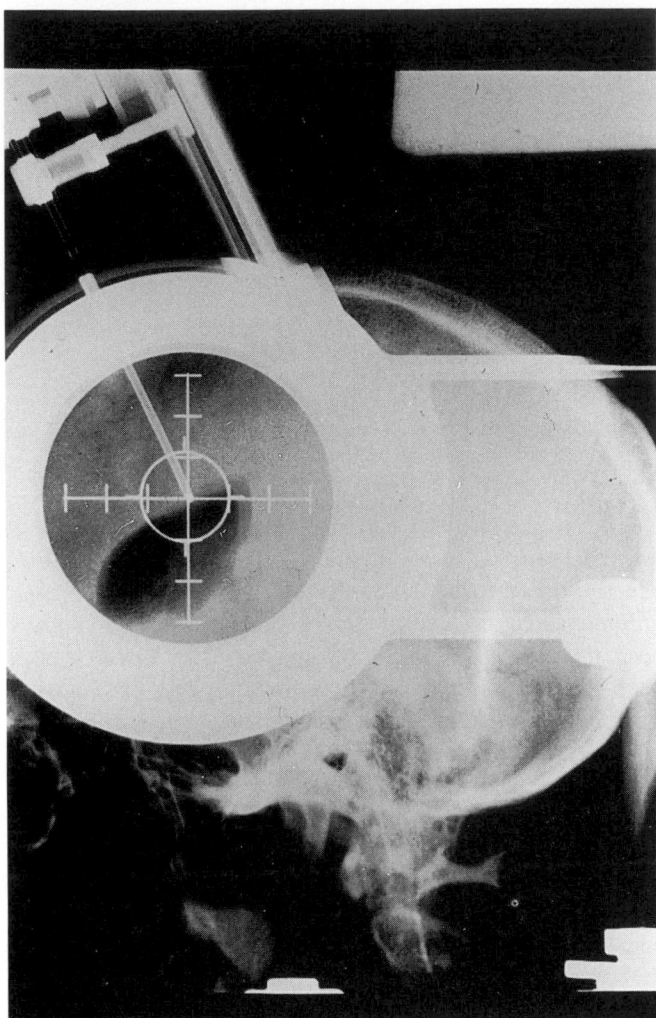

Figure 24-4B Probe positioning for stereotactic cingulumotomy, approximately 2 cm posterior to the tip of the frontal horn.

etiology of the pain may be clear, there will be psychological factors involved that may sabotage what would otherwise be effective medical or surgical management. For this reason, it is recommended that patients undergo psychological evaluation, including Minnesota Multiphasic Personality Inventory (MMPI), and that the evaluating psychologist address the issue of the appropriateness of medical or surgical management. Patients with significant psychological factors involved in their chronic pain behavior are better off if referred to a multidisciplinary pain center for further evaluation and therapy. This text will not discuss such therapy and will assume that anyone deemed a candidate for surgical management has undergone appropriate psychological screening and that all attempts at medical management, short of addiction, have been exhausted.

PERCUTANEOUS TRIGEMINAL RHIZOTOMY AND MICROVASCULAR DECOMPRESSION (MVD)

The mechanism of *trigeminal neuralgia* is not entirely understood, but demyelination of the axons in the root entry

zone at the pons is thought to play a role. The two techniques most commonly used in the surgical management of trigeminal neuralgia are percutaneous rhizotomy and microvascular decompression (MVD). Neither of these operative procedures is curative, although MVD has longer-lasting results. Each has its advantages and drawbacks. The majority of cases undergoing MVD will be found to have a loop of superior or anterior inferior cerebellar artery compressing the root at its entry zone. Surgically displacing the vessel loop with a piece of synthetic material will usually give prolonged relief. However, such a vascular loop is not found in all cases, and its exact role in pain generation is unknown.

The diagnosis of trigeminal neuralgia (also called *tic douloureux* or *tic pain*) is based on a history of intermittent lancinating pain—often electric shock–like—that is confined to one or more divisions of the trigeminal nerve and is often triggered by nonnoxious external stimuli or patient-generated stimuli, e.g., chewing and talking. Some patients may develop a continuous background aching pain of lesser intensity later in the course of the disease. Also, some patients display mild sensory deficits in the distribution of the pain. Patients with continuous background pain or significant sensory deficit in a trigeminal distribution are referred to as having *atypical trigeminal neuralgia*.

Pain that does not fit these criteria is not trigeminal neuralgia. Patients presenting with tic pain or other types of facial pain with neurological deficits should undergo an MRI

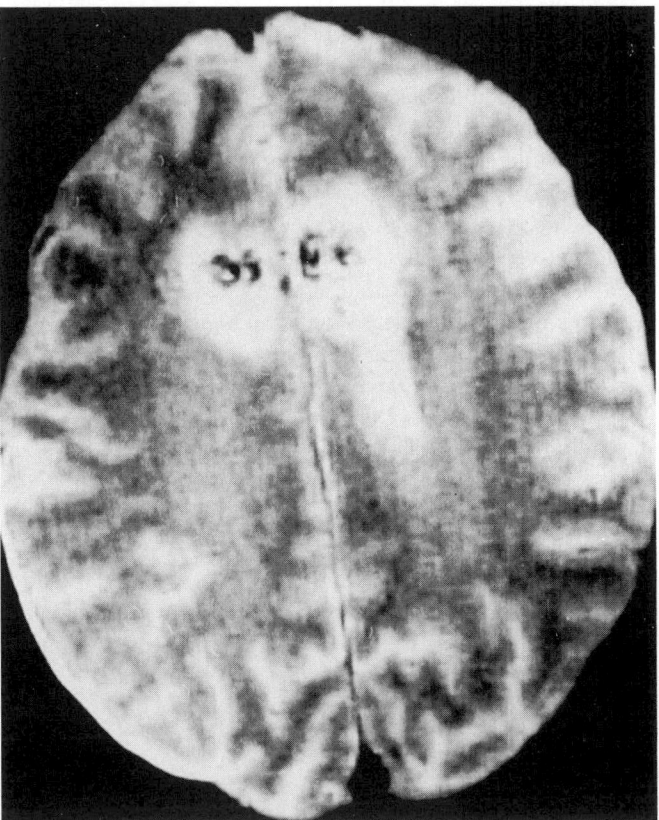

Figure 24-4C One week postoperative axial MRI scan displaying bilateral lateral and medial cingulumotomy lesions with residual surrounding edema.

scan to rule out a possible intra- or extra-axial posterior fossa structural lesion, e.g., tumor or arteriovenous malformation.

Percutaneous trigeminal rhizotomy[16,17] may be accomplished by lesioning trigeminal rootlets either with glycerol or radiofrequency (RF) current. The advantage of glycerol is that it may give relief for many months without any significant neurological deficit. However, the onset of relief may be delayed up to several weeks, and occasionally unexpected deficits occur. Selective lesioning of specific divisions is difficult. Also, deficits are more likely to occur if the patient has undergone previous RF or glycerol rhizotomy.

The effectiveness of RF rhizotomy depends on the production of some degree of sensory deficit in the distribution of the pain. Control over the level and distribution of deficits is greater with RF lesioning, and the time period over which relief lasts will be proportional to the degree of sensory loss. However, the risk of postoperative anesthesia dolorosa (severe pain of a continuous burning nature in the area of sensory loss) is greater with complete anesthesia, particularly when the first division or the entire face is involved. Therefore, analgesia and hypesthesia in the distribution of the pain are preferred. Glycerol rhizotomy may be reserved for first division cases and those cases where repeated attempts at RF lesioning have not produced an adequate lesion in spite of anatomic and physiologic verification of proper electrode position.

The technique is as follows. Submentovertex and lateral x-rays or fluoroscopy are performed to verify the location of the foramen ovale and to define the angle created by the clivus and the petrous ridge. An IV rapid-acting narcotic drip is supplemented with droperidol sedation. This neuroleptic analgesia should be limited so that the patient is always easily arousable. Guide needle placement is the same for both types of rhizotomy. A point approximately 2 cm lateral to the corner of the mouth and a second point about 3 cm anterior to the external auditory canal at the level of the zygoma are marked. This area is prepped with betadine and the entry point lateral to the corner of the mouth is infiltrated with 1% Xylocaine with epinephrine. (See Fig. 24-5A.)

If an RF procedure is planned, the surgeon should verify that the electrode protrudes through the guide needle 1 to 2 mm beyond the insulated collar of the electrode. If a curved tip electrode is being used, the surgeon should confirm the direction of the curve before insertion. Before guide needle insertion, a small incision with a No. 11 blade is made at the entry site.

The surgeon inserts a gloved index finger in the patient's mouth so as to palpate the guide needle tip through the mucosa as it is advanced, making certain it does not breech the mucosa. The thumbs and other index finger are used to advance the needle. The needle should be aimed so that it points toward the medial aspect of the patient's ipsilateral iris and toward the previously marked point 3 cm anterior to the external ear canal. When the patient shows evidence of pain, the surgeon stops and instructs the anesthetist to give a bolus of brevital (thiopental lasts too long in our experience) sufficient for brief general anesthesia.

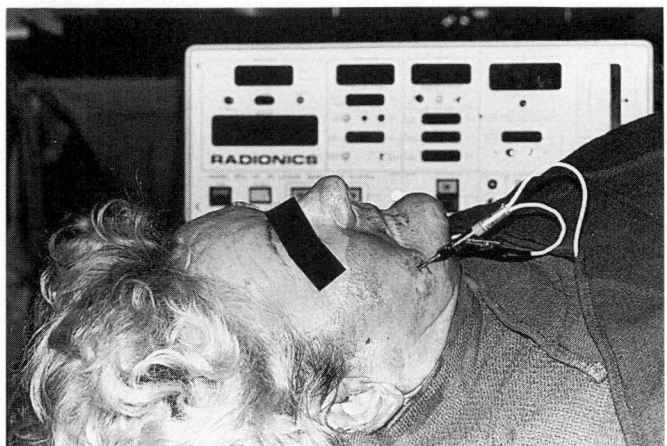

Figure 24-5A Guide needle enters approximately 2 cm lateral to the corner of the mouth. It is aimed at the inner aspect of the ipsilateral pupil and at a point approximately 3 cm anterior to the external ear canal.

As soon as the patient's corneal reflex is abolished, the surgeon advances the needle through the foramen ovale. There is some resistance and a feeling of a pop as the foramen is penetrated, and the patient may grimace or moan. The needle is slowly advanced until a slight release is felt, signaling penetration through the Gasserian ganglion. The stylet is then withdrawn to check for CSF, verifying that the needle tip is within the trigeminal cistern.

At this point repeat x-rays or fluoroscopy are used to check the needle position (Fig. 24-5B). Rarely is it necessary to advance the guide needle posterior to the clivus, even for a first-division lesion. The needle should be withdrawn or advanced several millimeters, depending on which division is to undergo RF lesioning. If there is a flow of CSF, the guide needle is usually satisfactorily positioned in the cistern; however, if the needle passes through the foramen ovale very far off center, it may enter the subtemporal subarachnoid space as it is advanced. If it penetrates into the temporal lobe, a life-threatening temporal lobe hematoma could occur or an epileptic focus might later develop. If the needle trajectory is too vertical and anterior, it may enter the inferior orbital fissure, in which case optic nerve damage could occur. If the needle is oriented too horizontally, it may hang up on the posterior rim of the foramen. When initial x-rays or fluoroscopy indicate improper guide needle position, it is usually better to completely withdraw the needle, pick a new entry point to appropriately alter the trajectory, and then repeat the above process.

If the patient has previously undergone an open rhizotomy, MVD, or multiple RF procedures, CSF flow may be minimal or absent, and one will have to rely on imaging and stimulation to assess proper electrode placement. By the time the RF electrode is inserted through the guide needle, the patient should be recovering from the brief brevital anesthesia. This recovery will be slower in older patients and when multiple brevital injections are necessitated by multiple attempts to penetrate the foramen ovale.

A thermocoupled, curved electrode may be used to obtain

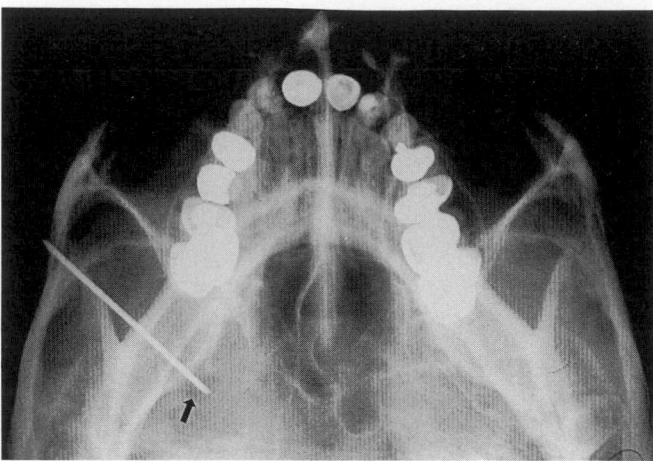

Figure 24-5B Submentovertex skull radiograph showing guide needle passing through the foramen ovale (arrow).

localizing paresthesias and lesioning confined to a single division of the trigeminal nerve (Fig. 24-5C). In a "virgin" case paresthesias should be obtainable at 0.1 V and at no more than 0.25 V. Electrode position should be manipulated until the paresthesias are confined to the distribution in which the pain is located.

At this point lesioning is begun with the patient awake if possible, using a very low lesioning current until the patient begins to complain of pain. When that pain subsides, the current is slowly increased. Sensory testing is carried out repeatedly so that a sensory deficit extending beyond the desired distribution can be detected almost immediately. Unfortunately, some patients cannot tolerate the local pain accompanying this technique and the lesioning must be performed under brief general anesthesia with additional IV

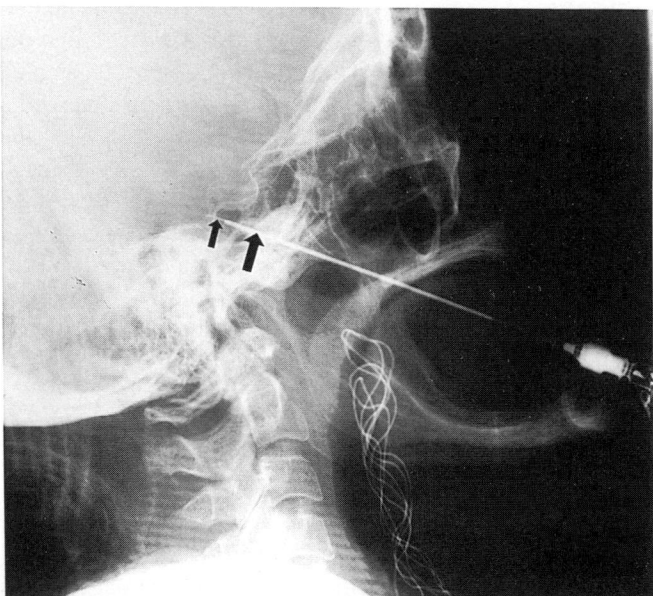

Figure 24-5C Lateral radiograph showing guide needle (large arrow) and curved-tipped electrode (small arrow) positioned for a second-division trigeminal radiofrequency rhizotomy.

brevital. In such a case, as soon as the corneal reflex is abolished, a lesion is made at 70°C for 90 s.

The patient is assessed after the general anesthesia subsides. Lesioning is repeated with temperature increases in 5° increments until the desired level of sensory deficit is obtained. Unwanted deficits are more likely to occur when using the latter technique since results of prelesion stimulation are not absolutely reliable in predicting the distribution of sensory deficit.

It should be emphasized that there are several commercially available tic electrodes that have different uninsulated tip dimensions that will create lesions of different sizes at given temperatures. Therefore, particularly if the lesion is performed with the patient under brevital anesthesia, a lower initial temperature (50°C) should be used if a large diameter tic electrode is employed.

Greater sensory deficits are more effective in the case of MS patients with tic pain, as is the case when the face pain is due to cancer. Lesions producing lesser sensory deficit are less likely to produce satisfactory long-term results. Lesser sensory deficits may still give satisfactory results in cases of idiopathic tic pain.

Up to 80 percent of patients with idiopathic trigeminal neuralgia will retain pain relief at 1 year, but by the fifth year up to 65 percent may experience recurrence of tic pain.[18] Deaths are extremely rare, and serious morbidity such as anesthesia dolorosa, corneal anesthesia with keratitis, oculomotor palsy, and masticator paralysis are infrequent.

For *glycerol rhizotomy,* once proper guide needle placement has been verified with imaging and flow of CSF, the patient is placed in a semisitting position with the neck moderately flexed and the head slightly tilted ipsilaterally. The head is supported by taping it up against a horseshoe headrest (Fig. 24-6A). Omnipaque-300, 0.5 cm³ is injected, and fluoroscopy is used to see if it is in the trigeminal cistern (Fig. 24-6B). The cistern may be difficult to visualize, and some prefer to rely on presence of CSF flow, needle placement as seen on fluoroscopy or x-ray, and results of stimulation (done before the patient is brought into the semisitting position) to check for proper needle placement. If cisternography is performed, the Omnipaque is subsequently removed by allowing fluid to flow from the guide needle, then temporarily releasing the patient's head and extending the neck to allow any residual Omnipaque to exit the trigeminal cistern. No dye should be left behind since it is hyperbaric relative to glycerol and can prevent the glycerol from penetrating the most dependent rootlets, i.e., V3. Next, a tuberculin syringe with 0.5 cm³ of sterile anhydrous glycerol is attached to the guide needle and sterile anhydrous glycerol is injected in 0.1-cm³ increments to a maximum of 0.4 cm³. The patient is left in the sitting position for about 30 min to allow the glycerol to bind to local neural tissue. The needle is then removed and the entry site covered with a betadine-bandaid dressing.

Microvascular decompression, once thought to be potentially curative, more recently has been found to provide a

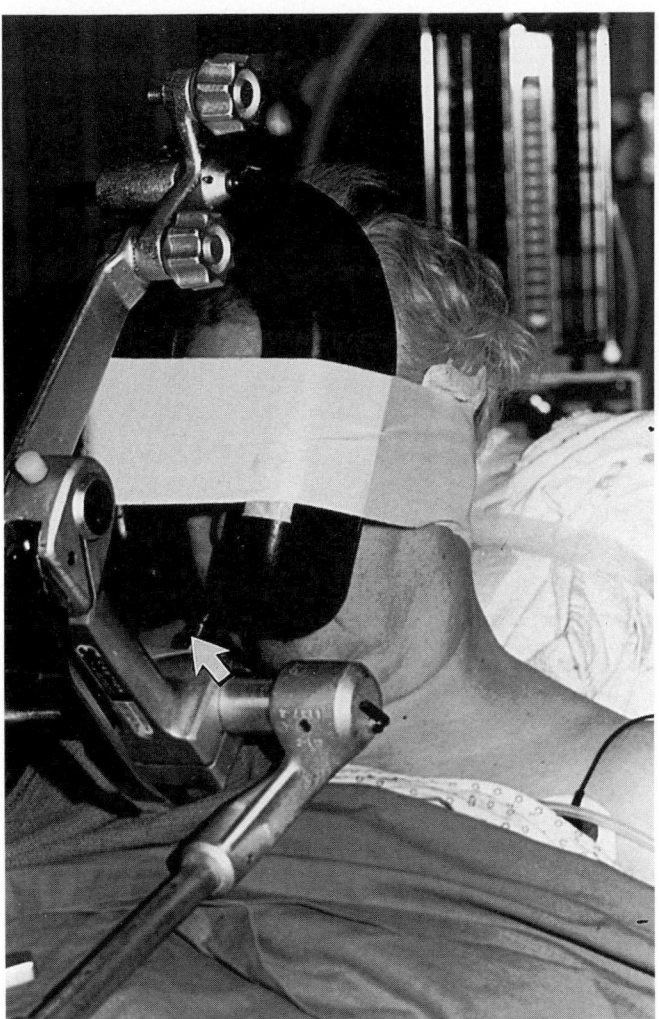

Figure 24-6A Patient in a semisitting position with head taped to a horseshoe headrest. The guide needle (arrow) is passing through the right cheek.

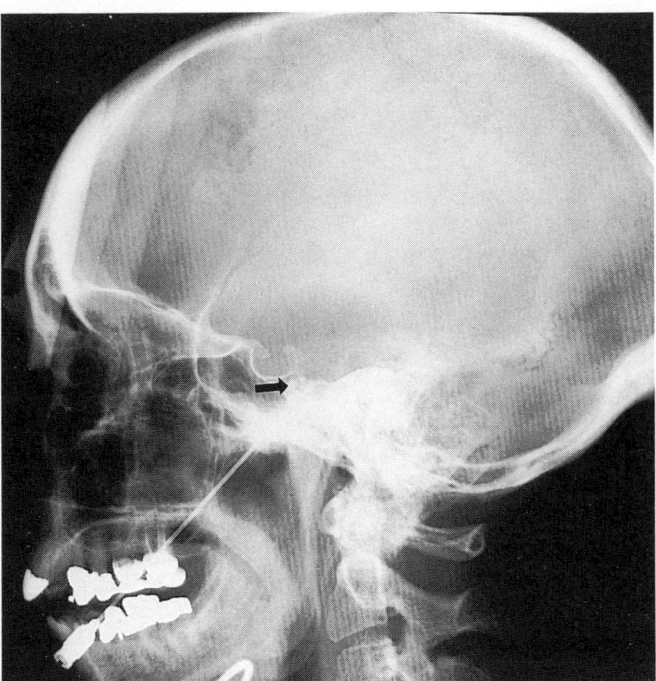

Figure 24-6B Arrow points to meniscus of 0.4 cm³ of water-soluble contrast agent injected into the trigeminal cistern.

finite period of complete pain relief with a recurrence rate of 3.5 percent per year.[19] This is a longer period of relief than can be expected from percutaneous rhizotomies. Some patients prefer percutaneous procedures with shorter hospitalizations, lower morbidity, and mortality. Many elderly patients simply are not candidates for MVD. However, the operation offers prolonged satisfactory relief for younger patients and those with more robust overall health.[19] Approximately 10 percent of patients will experience complications such as ipsilateral hearing loss, temporary vertigo, ataxia, trochlear or facial nerve palsy, or CSF fistula. Deaths, though infrequent, are more often associated with MVD than rhizotomy.

The operation[20] is performed under general endotracheal anesthesia. The patient is in a semisitting position with the neck flexed and the face rotated away from the side of surgery. This should position the ipsilateral tentorium parallel to the floor. A lazy-S incision is outlined two finger breadths behind the hairline with the central third of the incision behind the ear and the upper and lower thirds superior and inferior to the ear, respectively (Fig. 24-7A).

The incision area is prepped and draped, after which the incision is infiltrated with 1% Xylocaine with epinephrine. Incisional skin bleeding is controlled with bipolar cautery. A monopolar cutting current is used to expose the occipital bone, including its more inferior retromastoid portion. A 3 × 3 cm craniectomy is performed by making multiple burr holes and thinning the interspersed bone with a high-speed drill, after which the remaining inner table is rongeured away.

The craniectomy should extend laterally and superiorly, exposing the inferior margin of the lateral sinus and the medial margin of the sigmoid sinus. When the dura is opened, in cruciate fashion, the lateral and superior surfaces of the cerebellar hemisphere are exposed (Fig. 24-7B). After tacking up the dural flaps, the sterilely-draped microscope is

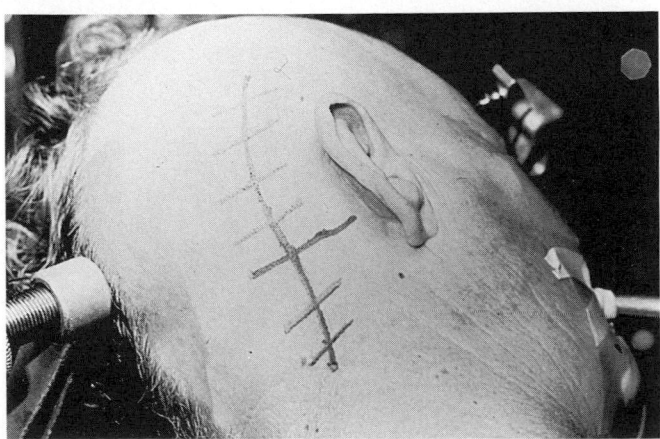

Figure 24-7A Incision for retromastoid craniectomy for microvascular decompression.

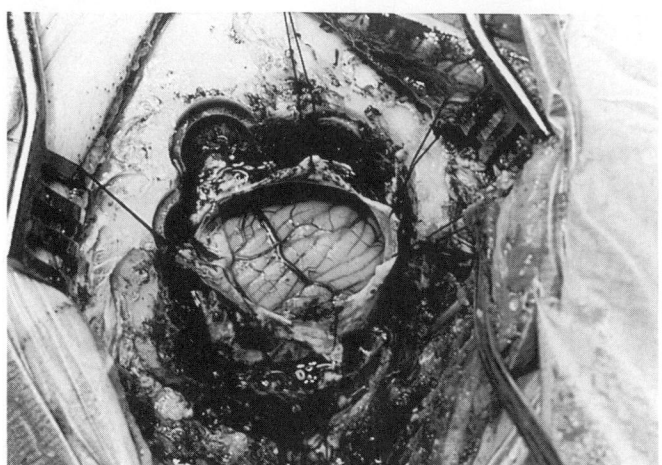

Figure 24-7B Patient orientation is the same as in Fig. 24-7A. The dura is opened, exposing the junction of the lateral and superior surfaces of the cerebellar hemisphere.

brought into the field and a self-retaining retractor blade is inserted to retract the cerebellum inferiorly and medially. Usually, the lateral portions of the fifth and eighth nerve complex will be seen, after opening a film of arachnoid. The petrosal vein will be visible also.

After the petrosal vein is coagulated and divided, the retractor blade is inserted deeper, keeping a thin sheet of telfa between retractor and cerebellar hemisphere. At this point the fifth nerve should be visible, and with slightly more retraction its entry zone into the pons can be seen. Visual examination usually reveals a loop of the superior or anterior inferior cerebellar artery impinging on the nerve at this root entry zone (Fig. 24-7C).

The vessel is dissected away from the nerve. One or more pieces of shredded Teflon sheeting are wrapped circumfer-

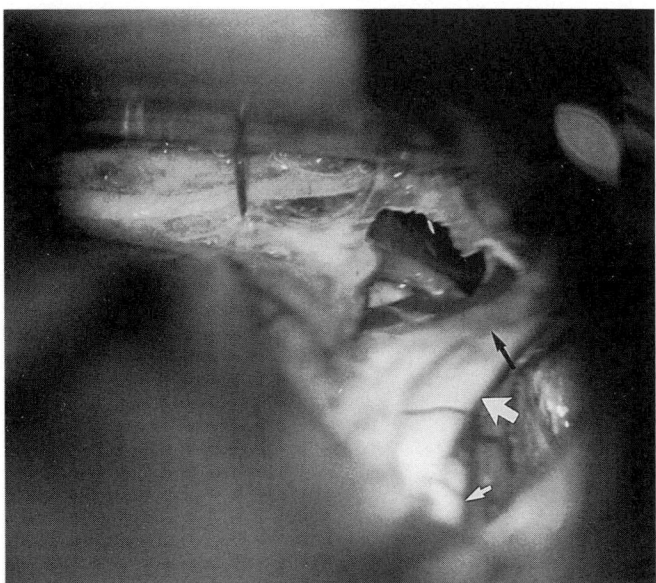

Figure 24-7C Trigeminal nerve (large white arrow) is seen entering the pons (small white arrow). A segment of the anterior inferior cerebellar artery (black arrow) is seen indenting the nerve.

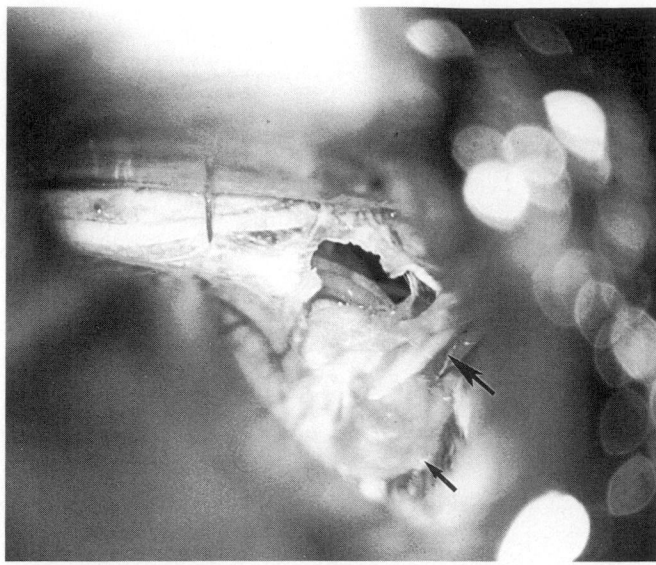

Figure 24-7D The trigeminal nerve (large arrow) is seen wrapped in shredded polytetrafluoroethylene (Teflon) (small arrow) at its root entry zone.

entially around the nerve at the entry zone (Fig. 24-7D. This tends to keep the Teflon cushion from dislodging and protects the nerve from any retracted additional vascular loops that might impinge on the nerve after removal of the retractor. The anesthetist is instructed to perform a Valsalva maneuver on the patient twice as the surgeon watches the nerve and implant under the microscope to be sure that there is no movement of the implant. After that the retractor is removed, the area is irrigated with antibiotic solution, the dura is closed with a watertight running interlocking suture, and the rest of the incision is closed in anatomic layers.

RF rhizotomy and MVD have been used for glossopharyngeal neuralgia, a condition very similar to tic, with similar success. Also, MVD has been employed successfully in the treatment of hemifacial spasm, Meniere's disease,[21] and selected cases of spasmodic torticollis (see Chap. 25, section on torticollis).

DREZ (DORSAL ROOT ENTRY ZONE) LESIONING

Although ablative procedures may be contraindicated in cases of deafferentation pain, this procedure is one exception to that rule, as is rhizotomy for trigeminal neuralgia. DREZ lesioning has been effective for plexus avulsion pain, phantom limb pain, postparaplegia end-zone pain, and selected cases of postherpetic neuralgia.[22,23] Although DREZ lesioning was originally designed to destroy the superficial layers of the posterior horn, recent experimental evidence suggests that it should destroy layers I to V. Lesions may be produced by RF current, laser,[22] or by incision and microbipolar coagulation.[24] The mechanism of destruction may not be as important as the accuracy and completeness of destruction.

Plexus avulsion pain occurs in at least 20 percent of patients suffering hyperabduction or hyperadduction injuries of the brachial or lumbosacral plexus and is usually immediate in onset. There may be a constant burning, crushing type of pain as well as an intermittent shocklike pain. In the past, myelography was used to image pseudomeningoceles at levels of root avulsion though there was no 1:1 correlation with segments involved with pain. Subsequently, CT was used postmyelographically to check for posttraumatic pseudomeningocele or syrinx. MRI is now becoming the modality of choice for imaging pseudomeningoceles and syringes.

Electrodiagnostic studies may be used to distinguish between plexus stretch injuries and avulsion injuries. Pure root injuries will leave the dorsal root ganglion intact and, therefore, distal nerve conduction velocities (NCVs) should be intact. Also, the N9 dorsal root ganglion evoked potential will be preserved with a pure root avulsion injury. This differentiation is not insignificant since avulsion injuries respond well to DREZ lesioning whereas peripheral stretch injuries do not.[25] Plexus avulsion pain patients undergoing DREZ lesioning will have fair-to-good pain relief in over 80 percent of cases.[26] Patients with distal stretch injuries may respond to spinal cord or deep brain stimulation.

Pain of spinal cord injury may occur in either of two distributions. *End-zone pain* begins at the physiological level of cord injury and occupies variable portions of dermatomes immediately caudal to the level of sensory loss. Pain in this location may be constant and aching or burning, or it may be paroxysmal and cramping, lasting up to 5 min. This pain may be triggered by local nonpainful stimuli such as rubbing or touch applied within the painful area or just rostral to it, and it responds well to DREZ lesioning in about 80 percent of cases.[26] The second distribution of pain is also caudal to the level of injury but more diffuse and nondermatomal in distribution. It is usually burning, constant, and often most intense in the saddle area. This pain is not evoked by nonpainful stimuli, and it responds poorly to DREZ lesioning even when the lesions are extended into the sacral cord segments.[26]

In general, evokable pain responds well to DREZ lesions and nonevokable burning or shooting pain does not.[27] Shooting, nonevokable pain may respond well to cordotomy or to cordectomy.[27] *Cordectomy* has been particularly effective for such episodic pain when it has been located caudal to the hips and the vertebral injury has been at or below the T11 vertebra. Laminectomy at the level of injury with excision of the damaged area of the cord is the procedure of choice.[28] This area of vertebral trauma should be stabilized prior to cordectomy. At least 70 percent of the pain can be relieved in 90 percent of cases.

Burning, nonevokable pain does not respond well to any type of surgery, although approximately one-third of such patients have responded to thalamic or spinal cord stimulation.[27]

Some spinal cord injury patients will develop delayed-onset pain or progressive neurological deficits due to a posttraumatic syrinx. If accompanying pain is due to the syrinx, it should be brought on by Valsalva maneuvers. Shunting of the syrinx is the treatment of choice. However, if there is coexisting so-called end-zone pain, this may respond to DREZ lesioning but will not respond to shunting of the syrinx.[27]

Phantom limb pain should be clearly distinguished from stump pain when considering surgical management. In the former, the pain is clearly located in the phantom limb, whereas in the latter, the pain is confined to the amputation stump. True phantom limb pain responds to DREZ lesioning in about 75 percent of cases,[23] but stump pain does not.[29] If there is a stretch injury associated with the phantom limb pain, DREZ lesioning may be of limited benefit. Although NCVs might be difficult or impossible to do in such cases, an absent or diminished N9 evoked potential would suggest the presence of a stretch injury. Magnetic stimulation (see Chap. 28) of involved nerve stumps might effectively generate evoked potentials in such cases, whereas it might require painful electrical stimulation to activate such potentials.

Postherpetic neuralgia was initially thought to respond to DREZ lesioning, but follow-up studies suggest that only about 25 percent of patients obtain prolonged relief. The best results occur in patients with superficial burning, itching pain with hyperalgesia, and absence of sensory deficits. Patients with deep, aching pain and associated segmental sensory deficits have obtained less satisfactory results.[26] Since up to 25 percent of such patients undergoing thoracic DREZ lesioning require mechanical assistance with ambulation postoperatively, nondestructive modalities such as spinal cord or deep brain stimulation (see following section) may be safer and as effective in such cases. Patients suffering from deep, continuous postherpetic pain might also respond to spinal cord stimulation or deep brain stimulation.

The technique of RF DREZ lesioning involves exposure of the involved segments by laminectomy.[22] In the case of root avulsions, the involved cord segments are easily visualized. In cases of phantom limb pain or end-zone pain of paraplegia the involved segments may be identified by following one of the roots to its foramen, and then obtaining intraoperative x-rays to confirm the level. In the case of avulsion[25] and phantom pain the segments involved with pain as well as one segment rostral and caudal are lesioned. In the case of post spinal cord injury pain, two segments rostral and one segment caudal to the physiological transection are lesioned.[26] Individual lesions are immediately adjacent to each other.

A commercially available thermocoupled temperature monitoring electrode with a 2-mm uninsulated tip is used. It is inserted into the root entry zone approximately 30 degrees off the vertical plane, and a lesion is made at 75°C for 15 sec. This is not enough time for thermal equilibrium to be reached, but experience has determined that these lesioning parameters produce a satisfactory result. Lesioning of the nucleus caudalis for selected types of facial pain—e.g., superficial postherpetic facial pain—requires an especially designed thermocoupled electrode that is described elsewhere.[30]

SPINAL CORD STIMULATION (SCS) AND DEEP BRAIN STIMULATION (DBS)

These are nonablative techniques of pain control. Candidates for these procedures have usually failed all other attempts at treatment. The term *spinal cord stimulation* is used instead of *dorsal column stimulation* since there is clinical and experimental evidence that the therapeutic response may be due to stimulation of one of several tracts.[31] There is a general tendency for neurostimulation-induced pain relief to be less effective with time.[32,33] Counseling patients on limiting the use of SCS or DBS can sometimes prevent this tolerance from occurring.

Deep brain stimulation involves stimulation of the ascending or descending systems that modulate pain. One is the *descending endorphin system,* which passes through the periventricular and periaqueductal gray matter. Although it was initially thought that stimulation of this system alleviates pain by way of an increased output of endogenous opiates, there is now conflicting evidence.[34] The other system is the *ascending lemniscal system,* which is stimulated by implantation in the somatosensory ventrocaudal thalamic nucleus (VPM-VPL) or in the sensory portion of the posterior limb of the internal capsule. The exact mechanism of pain relief produced by activation of this system is also unknown.[35]

Spinal cord stimulation has been shown to have long-term effectiveness in the treatment of postherpetic neuralgia and ischemic or vasculopathic pain,[32] but this has not been the case with phantom limb pain.[35] DREZ lesioning is effective for phantom limb pain,[22] and SCS may be effective in the alleviation of stump pain or pain due to peripheral stretch injuries. Previous studies have indicated that SCS was not effective in the long term for patients with the "failed back surgery syndrome," i.e., recurrent pain after multiple low back operations, usually multiple lumbar diskectomies.[32] However, more recent experience[37,38] indicates that utilization of properly placed multicontact epidural-stimulating electrodes may give effective long-term relief of leg and back pain in such cases. SCS may also be effective in some cases of painful peripheral neuropathy.

It has been stated that SCS can only be effective when the induced paresthesias cover the area of pain. Although this is usually the case, relief of deafferentation pain has been reported when paresthesias could only be produced in the area surrounding the pain.[36]

The technique of SCS varies. Multicontact electrodes allow the option of using various contacts as the cathode or anode during the period of trial stimulation. There is recent evidence that multicontact implants provide better pain control than bipolar implants.[37] Cylindrically shaped multicontact electrodes may be inserted percutaneously through a large-bore needle with a curved tip, into the posterior epidural space (Fig. 24-8A). The distal end of the electrode is externalized, and a period of several days of trial stimulation follows. The electrode is later internalized and connected to an RF receiver or an internalized pulse generator if trial stimulation has been effective.

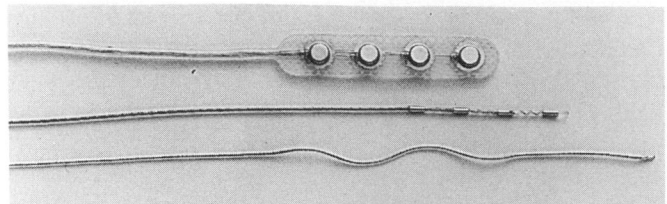

Figure 24-8A   *Top:* flat four-contact electrode, which is implanted through a laminotomy. *Middle:* cylindrical four-contact electrode, which is implanted percutaneously through a guide needle. *Bottom:* cylindrical single-contact electrode, which is implanted percutaneously. (Courtesy of Medtronic, Inc., Minneapolis, MN.)

It may require weeks of testing of various pulse widths, frequencies, and amplitudes, as well as careful logging of the results before successful parameters of stimulation are established. For that reason the option to implant the entire device in one stage may be preferred.

Irrespective of whether the procedure is performed in one or two stages, another option is to implant a multicontact electrode of flat design with flat disk-shaped electrodes (Fig. 24-8A). A two-level midline laminotomy is performed. The electrode is inserted in the midline in the posterior epidural space at the caudal level and advanced to the level of the rostral laminotomy. The polyurethane insulating coat of the electrode is sutured to the dura rostrally and caudally to prevent migration.

Both the open and percutaneous techniques are performed under local anesthesia and sedation so the patient can be awakened for testing after initial electrode placement. Every effort is made to place the electrode so that paresthesias superimpose over the area of pain or surround it, as in the case of some deafferentation pains. The electrode should be positioned so that its most rostral contact is no more than several cord segments above the most rostral level of pain. Placing the electrode too far rostral might result in difficulty in activating axons of more caudal origin located deeper within the posterior columns at the point of stimulation. In the case of deafferentation pain involving a large area, it may require two multicontact electrodes to activate the cord segments rostral and caudal to the deafferented cord segments in order to produce paresthesias entirely surrounding the pain.[36]

Once the electrode is satisfactorily positioned, its cable is tunneled subcutaneously toward a subcutaneous pocket created for the receiver or pulse generator. The cable of the receiver or pulse generator is tunneled toward the electrode cable. They are connected at the site of an incision placed somewhere between the laminotomy and the pulse generator or RF receiver site incisions. The subclavicular and subcostal abdominal areas are the usual sites for implanting the receiver or pulse generator. The technique involves inserting the electrode with the patient in a sitting position for a cervical implant or prone for a thoracic implant. In the latter case the patient is subsequently rolled into a lateral decubitus position and reprepped for implanting the receiver or pulse generator subcostally.

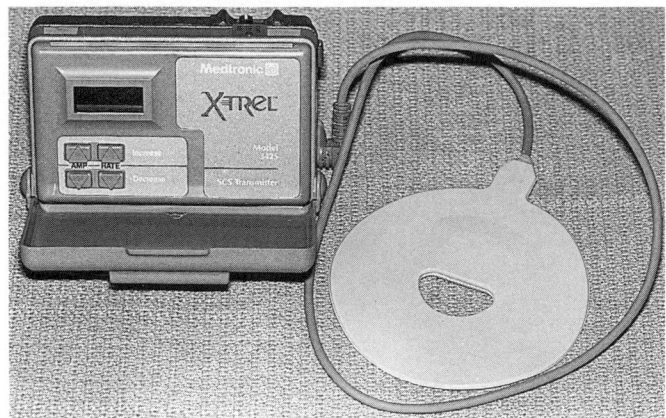

Figure 24-8B Frontal view of an external RF transmitter and transmitting antenna.

If a passive receiver is connected to the electrode and implanted, an external RF transmitter will be used to activate it (Fig. 24-8B). A transmitting antenna connected to the transmitter is taped over the receiver site when the system is in use. Inductive coupling occurs at the transmitter and receiver antennas, and the previously programmed parameters of stimulation are then transmitted to the activated electrode contacts (Fig. 24-8C). The patient can control both amplitude and frequency, but usually the surgeon adjusts the internal settings to control pulse width, on-off cycling of stimulation, amplitude range, signal ramping, and electrode contact activation and polarity.

If an internalized pulse generator (Fig. 24-9A) is used, the patient controls on-off function with a ring-shaped magnet temporarily placed over the internalized pulse generator, or a hand-held programmer can be used to control both amplitude and frequency (Fig. 24-9B). The surgeon is able to control these parameters, as well as pulse width, ramping, on-off cycle, individual contacts activated, and contact polarity with a desktop programmer.

There is some evidence that implantation of multiple percutaneous multicontact electrodes, adjacent to each other at the same level or separated by a short AP distance, may be more effective in the treatment of bilateral multi-segmental leg and back pain.[38] Others[37] have observed that a single multicontact electrode of flat design may produce a pattern of paresthesias covering the low back and both lower extremities, resulting in pain relief in that distribution.

Complications include early electrode migration or fracturing of insulation or leads, either of which will require surgical revision. Infection and local skin breakdown may also occur. Either of these complications may require removal of the entire implanted system. Serious complications are rare.

Deep brain stimulation has been shown in a multicenter study to alleviate effectively deafferentation pain in over 40 percent of cases and to give effective relief in up to 60 percent of cases of nociceptive pain.[33] In the study, most patients with nociceptive pain had cancer pain or low back and leg pain related to multiple failed low back operations. They responded to *periventricular gray (PVG)* stimulation.

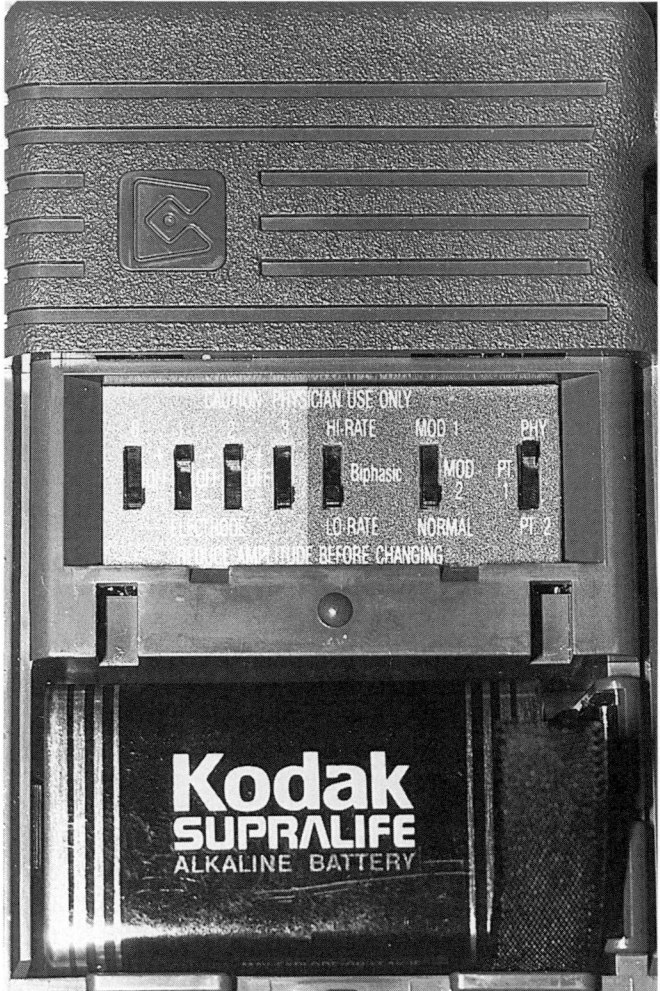

Figure 24-8C Opened rear compartment of an RF transmitter. The four switches to the left control activation and polarity of the four electrode contacts. The next switch to the right controls the frequency range. (One of the two patient-controlled external dials regulates the programmed frequency range.) The next switch to the right modifies pulse sequencing. The switch to the far right is used to regulate patient and physician-controlled stimulation parameters.

Thalamic or *capsular* stimulation was more successful in the treatment of deafferentation pain related to arachnoiditis resulting from multiple myelographies and lumbar disk surgeries, as well as some peripheral neuropathies, including postherpetic facial pain but not phantom limb pain.[33,34] Thalamic stimulation may help some cases of deafferentation pain due to central lesions, e.g., burning pain related to cord trauma,[27] but in general it has not been successful in the treatment of deafferentation pain of central origin.[33]

Electrodes (or DBS) are inserted stereotactically. The 3-dimensional coordinates for PVG and thalamic targets have already been described.[33,34] Proper electrode placement is verified with intraoperative stimulation. The PVG target is within several millimeters of the wall of the third ventricle and slightly anterior to the posterior commissure. Brief test stimulation usually produces a sensation of warmth referable to midline structures such as the face or trunk and may give

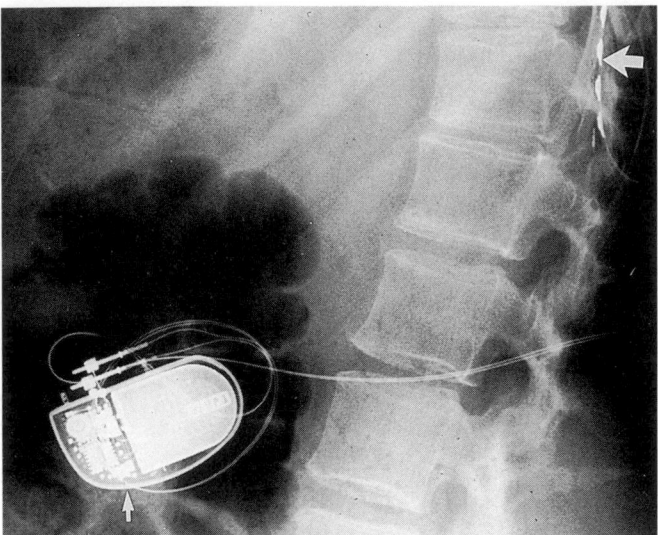

Figure 24-9A Lateral radiograph showing laminotomy design four contact SCS electrode (large arrow) connected to an internalized pulse generator (small arrow).

some relief of pain. (Periaqueductal grey stimulation produces similar pain relief but also may cause oscillopsia or severe anxiety.) CT or MRI scanning is used to define the PVG target, thalamic target, or the capsular target in the posterior third of the posterior limb of the internal capsule. A resident computer stereotactic atlas map and previously archived sensory responses to somatosensory thalamic and capsular stimulation assist in anatomic localization of these

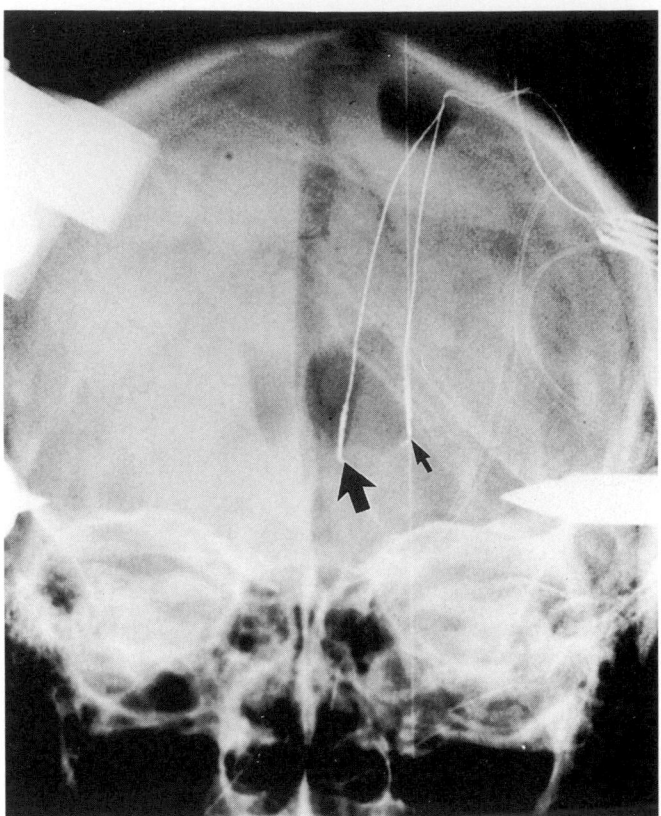

Figure 24-10A AP radiograph of implanted PVG (large arrow) and capsular (small arrow) DBS electrodes.

targets (see section on image-guided, computer-assisted stereotactic thalamotomy in Chap. 25).

Once imaging is completed, the patient is transferred to the operating room (OR), where the previously placed stereotactic base ring is secured to the OR table with the patient supine. Sedation is given if necessary. The computer-derived 3-dimensional target coordinates and angles of trajectory are transferred to the stereotactic arc system, which will guide the electrode. After injecting a local anesthetic, a curved scalp incision is made around the proposed twist drill hole site to make room for the electrode anchoring device. A twist drill hole is made in the trajectory of the electrode.

After coagulating both dura and pia-arachnoid, a special 16-gauge cannula with blunt stylet is passed to the target to create a tract. Once its position is confirmed with intraoperative fluoroscopy, the 3-contact electrode with a central stylet is introduced. Stimulation is performed to confirm proper positioning. Following this, the electrode is secured in position by some type of anchoring device. Figure 24-10A and B shows examples of PVG and capsular implants.

Lastly, with the use of additional sedation and local anesthesia a subclavicular subcutaneous pocket is made for the programmable pulse generator. Subcutaneous and subgaleal tunnels are created and the cables joined at a small retroauricular incision. The procedure is repeated if additional implants are indicated. Complications include stimulation tolerance, hemorrhage, infection, and electrode migration.

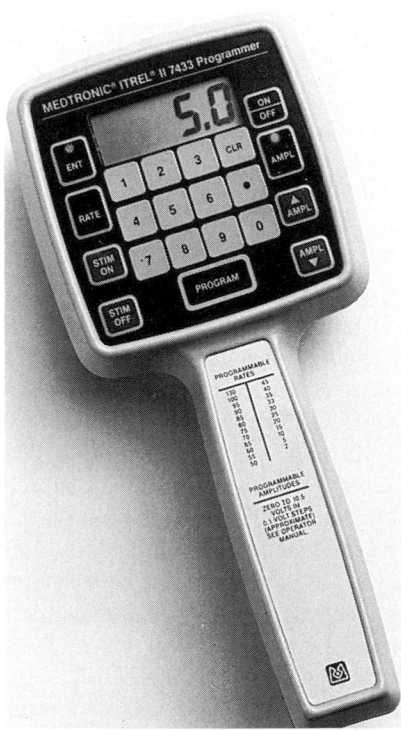

Figure 24-9B Hand-held programmer which patient can use to reprogram rate and amplitude as well as stimulation on-off. (Courtesy Medtronic, Inc.)

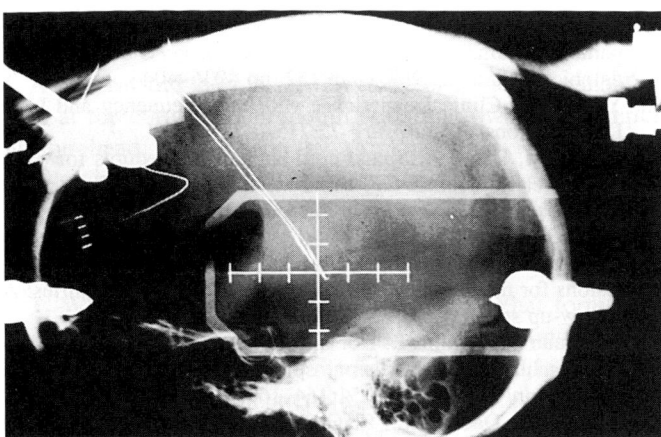

Figure 24-10*B*   Lateral radiograph of PVG and capsular electrodes.

SYMPATHECTOMY

Sympathectomy has been successful in the treatment of causalgia and other *reflex sympathetic dystrophies*. Recently, this type of pain has been referred to as *sympathetically mediated pain*. The pathophysiology is thought to involve local sympathetic hyperactivity which releases norepinephrine peripherally, activating or perpetuating impulses. These impulses travel over large-diameter peripheral axons and are encoded as pain centrally. Presently much of this type of pain is managed and sometimes cured with conservative treatment,[39] such as serial sympathetic or regional guanethidine blocks, or an alpha-blocking agent such as phenoxybenzamine.

For diagnosis, some prefer alpha-1 blockers such as phenoxybenzamine because of their specific sympatholytic effect. If a high concentration of local anesthetic has been used, a sympathetic block might also affect transmission over larger-diameter fibers, as would be the case with guanethidine regional infusion performed with proximal tourniquet. In the latter two instances the mechanism of temporary pain relief might not be due to sympathetic blockade, and misinterpretation of the results could lead to a subsequently failed sympathectomy.

Causalgia, which often has its onset within 24 h of a partial injury, usually to the sciatic or median nerve, is most often located in the hand or foot.[39] The pain is usually described as burning, but it may also be characterized as throbbing, aching, or stabbing. With time, the pain may spread proximally and outside the distribution of the injured nerve. Typically, non-noxious stimuli such as touch or cold may trigger or aggravate the pain. Initially the limb may be warm, dry, and pink, but within several weeks, sweating, cyanosis, and coolness appear. The magnitude of the autonomic changes usually parallels the severity of the pain. Trophic changes include joint stiffening, finger tapering, hair loss, and local muscular atrophy.

Other sympathetically mediated pains often referred to as *sympathetic dystrophies* or *minor causalgia* result from minor limb trauma, but the pain is similar to causalgia.[39] These disorders show similar trophic changes as well as local osteoporosis. In such cases the results of chemical or pharmacological sympathetic blockades must be interpreted carefully. If the results of psychosocial evaluation are questionable, sympathetic placebo blocks should be included in a series of sympathetic blocks. Alternatively, a short course of sympatholytic and placebo drugs should also be administered before final consideration of surgical sympathectomy.

Sympathectomy may effectively alleviate the pain of peripheral vascular occlusive disease, but it will not be effective in cases of intermittent claudication. Sympathectomy can also alleviate postamputation pain of digits but is not effective in the case of amputations proximal to the ankle or wrist.[39]

At present, most surgical sympathectomies are performed for causalgic limb pain or pain of peripheral vascular occlusive disease and only occasionally for distal stump pain or pain of chronic pancreatitis. However, none of these procedures is commonly performed, and the reader is referred for descriptions of those techniques.[40,41]

Future Developments

Tissue transplantation of adrenal medulla into the subarachnoid space and periaqueductal gray of rats[42] has been shown to diminish responsiveness to acute pain. More recently, adrenal medullary subarachnoid implants in rats previously rendered arthritic has also been shown to decrease pain behavior.[42] Stimulation of local release of catecholamines and opioid peptides is thought to be the underlying mechanism since the analgesic effect was reversible with naloxone and sham implants had no effect on pain behavior. If such implants were able to provide long-term pain relief, this would become a viable alternative, not only to DBS and intrathecal-intraventricular MS but perhaps also to certain ablative pain procedures.

REFERENCES

1. Tasker RR, Tsuda T, Hawrylyshyn P: Clinical neurophysiological investigation of deafferentation pain, in Bonica JJ, Lindblom U, Ainsley I (eds): *Advances in Pain Research and Therapy,* vol 5. pp 713–738.

2. Nurchi G: Use of intraventricular and intrathecal morphine in intractable pain associated with cancer. *Neurosurgery* 15:801–803, 1984.

3. Poletti CE, Sweet WH, Schmidek HH, Pilon RN: Intraspinal

denervation of both the sternomastoid and trapezius muscles. This may leave the patient with residual paresis of arm abduction due to the decreased ability of the paretic trapezius to fix the scapula.

The posterior rami of the fifth through seventh roots on the side of the anterior rhizotomy of the first to fourth cervical roots, as well as the posterior rami of the fourth through seventh cervical roots on the opposite side, may be coagulated at the point where they pass around the associated cervical facet joint. This further denervates the posterior paraspinal muscles while leaving the anterior cervical rami intact.

The majority of patients with torticollis display various forms of the disorder, i.e., involvement of different cervical muscle groups to different degrees. Therefore, the rhizotomy-myotomy operation is tailored to the individual patient. Operations are based upon the analysis of individual muscles or muscle groups involved. Preoperative videotaping of the patient during electromyogram (EMG) is performed for archiving and to determine further which muscles are to be sectioned or denervated.

The scalene muscles are transected when they produce anteflexional or lateroflexional torticollis. These muscles are innervated by lower cervical roots which cannot be transected without producing paresis of the associated upper extremity. Pure retrocollis is rare and may be best managed by selective myotomy.[10] Figure 25-3 shows a unilateral resection of splenius and semispinalis muscles.

Regardless of the procedure chosen, one can expect patients to benefit in about 80 percent of cases. Aggressive physical therapy is a necessity in the correction of reversible postural deformities that have occurred prior to surgery. Strengthening of the muscles left intact must also be undertaken so that the patients will be able to position their heads properly, execute swallowing, and avoid the pain that may accompany limited use of poorly conditioned muscles.

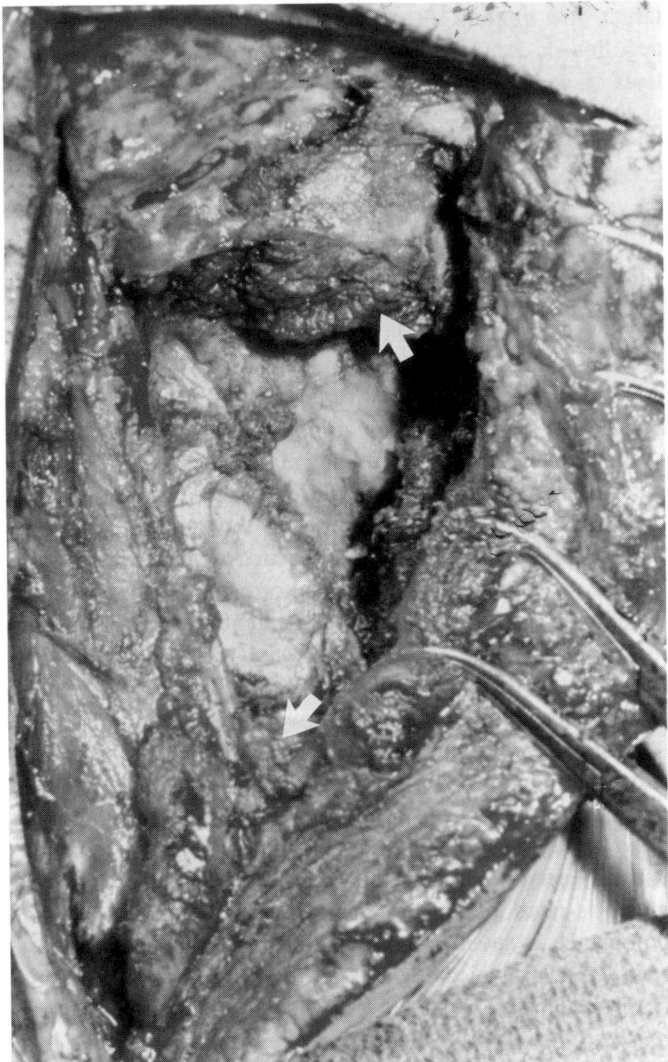

Figure 25-3   A segment of the more superficially located right spenius has been resected, as has a segment of the deeper semispinalis, whose cut ends are seen (arrows).

INTRATHECAL BACLOFEN (ITB), SPINAL CORD STIMULATION (SCS), BISCHOF MYELOTOMY, PERCUTANEOUS SPINAL RADIOFREQUENCY (RF) RHIZOTOMY, DENTATOTOMY

Lesions of the spinal cord, particularly those of incomplete traumatic injury or involvement by multiple sclerosis, may result in the appearance of uncontrollable spasms of the extremities and of the bladder. Spasms of extremities are usually flexor but may also be extensor. If the lesion involves the upper cervical cord, the spasms may involve all four extremities, the trunk, and the bladder. *Intrathecal baclofen (ITB), spinal cord stimulation (SCS), Bischof myelotomy,* and *percutaneous spinal radiofrequency (RF) rhizotomy* have each been used to control such spasms. Although these procedures are more often utilized for intractable flexor spasms, ITB and RF spinal rhizotomy have also been used to decrease the tone of spasticity and its associated postural abnormalities, e.g., adduction posturing of the lower

extremities and flexor posturing at the elbow. This implies similar pathophysiological mechanisms for both conditions.

Bischof myelotomy (longitudinal myelotomy) and percutaneous RF spinal rhizotomy are destructive procedures which may be associated with loss of sensory and motor function, and they are probably best reserved for patients with extensive or complete loss of cord function. Bischof myelotomy involves dividing the cord into anterior and posterior halves over the segments involved in the flexor spasms, typically L2–S1, in order to interrupt the local reflex arcs. Bischof myelotomy[11] may not prevent spasms triggered by stimuli from segments rostral to L2 or caudal to S1.

Percutaneous spinal RF rhizotomy,[12] theoretically, may be performed at any segment, but if many segments are involved bilaterally, this can be a very time-consuming procedure which must utilize both fluoroscopy and stimulation to verify electrode positioning at each level. The procedure is performed under local or general anesthesia, using low-frequency stimulation to obtain motor responses as an indication of proper positioning of the lesioning electrode. Debilitated patients who would have high risks under general anesthesia (e.g., Bischof myelotomy) can better tolerate this percutaneous procedure under local anesthesia (if any anesthesia is necessary). Lesions are usually made at temperatures of 70 to 90°C. This can produce a therapeutic response that lasts several years. If the patient survives long enough, in all probability the procedure will require repeating.

ITB and SCS are nondestructive procedures. ITB is administered in much the same way as intrathecal morphine for cancer pain. Baclofen's mechanism of action appears to be inhibition of excitatory neurotransmitters of Ia afferents on anterior horn cells. Patients are very sensitive to small changes in the microdoses of baclofen, and a telemetrically programmable pump may be implanted so that the dosage can be regulated without having to replace the entire contents of the reservoir with a different concentration. For example, the patient can decrease the flow rate if the ongoing flow rate is causing excessive decrease in muscle tone. The other available and totally implanted pump uses a passive bellows system with a fixed flow rate, and dosage can only be changed by replacing the entire contents of the reservoir with a different concentration. ITB is still in an investigational phase, but early reports suggest dramatic reductions in both spasticity and spasms.[13]

Although well-controlled studies are lacking, there are reports of SCS decreasing flexor spasms in patients with spinal cord injury.[14] Results seem to be better when the stimulating epidural electrode is implanted caudal to the level of the injury. SCS has also been shown to benefit reflex and voluntary bladder control in patients with multiple sclerosis.[15] The degree of benefit may be related to the amplitude of stimulation.[14] The parameters of stimulation are in the frequency range of 30 Hz, pulse width of 200 μs, and amplitudes ranging from 2 to 12 mA.[14] The technique of implantation has already been described in Chap. 24.

When spasticity or spasms are confined to the bladder or to a single limb, limited ablative procedures may be of benefit. *Posterior root ganglionectomy* of sacral segments has been effective in increasing the capacity of the spastic bladder.[16] *Selective peripheral neurotomy* involves sectioning those nerve fascicles—identified by intraoperative stimulation—which maintain spastic tone and posturing—e.g., the tibial nerve at the popliteal region for spastic foot and the musculocutaneous nerve for elbow flexion. This procedure has provided long-term relief in over 80 percent of cases.[17]

Selective posterior rhizotomy has become the surgical procedure of choice in the treatment of those cases of spasticity due to cerebral palsy uncomplicated by other associated movement disorders.[18] The surgical technique involves exposure of the cauda equina through an L2–L5 laminectomy. After anatomic identification of the L2 root at its exit foramen, the S1 anterior root is identified by low-frequency stimulation. Fascicles of each of the posterior roots from L2–S1 are isolated and stimulated. Those fascicles, stimulation of which causes ipsilateral tetanic or multisegmental motor responses or any contralateral motor responses, are sectioned. The intraoperative clinical responses are correlated with intraoperative changes in the EMG. Usually, 60 to 80 percent of the fascicles are sectioned, which results in diminished sensation lasting no longer than several weeks. If the patients are young and have adequate cognitive function and aggressive physical therapy is carried out postoperatively, the results are excellent in nearly all cases. However, nonambulatory patients cannot be expected to become ambulatory, though reduction of adductor spasms may facilitate their overall care. Complications directly related to the procedure are rare.

Stereotactic dentatotomy has been of limited usefulness in the management of spasticity.[19] The best surgical results have been obtained in patients with congenital spasticity. About 50 percent of these have experienced worthwhile improvement. Today, many of them would be candidates for selective posterior rhizotomy, which provides a much higher success rate. There are, however, occasionally patients with congenital choreoathetosis and spasticity who still would not qualify as candidates for selective posterior rhizotomy, but who might benefit from dentatotomy. Some of these undergo thalamotomy to control the choreoathetosis. If they subsequently develop worse spasticity as a result of the thalamotomy, ipsilateral dentatotomy may be considered.

This operation has previously been performed using pneumoencephalography or ventriculography to guide anatomic localization of the target.[19] The current availability of MRI-guided, computer-assisted stereotaxis should facilitate anatomic localization, though intraoperative stimulation for target verification is recommended.

☐ FUTURE DEVELOPMENTS

With the resurgence of stereotactic techniques in the last decade, there seems to have been a shifting of neurosurgical procedures toward less-invasive techniques, such as stereotactically guided biopsies and craniotomies and stereotactic radiosurgery. The majority of current neurodiagnostic procedures (such as CT, MRI, SPECT, and PET) are noninvasive.

Two recently introduced diagnostic technologies are *magnetic stimulation* and *magnetoencephalography* (*MEG*). Both are completely noninvasive modalities, and future refinements of them may position them to play key roles in the surgical management of movement disorders, epilepsy, and even pain.

Transcranial magnetic stimulation has been used to stimulate the motor cortex, frontal language cortex, and visual cortex.[20] Localizing functional areas noninvasively may be of use in the preoperative assessment of language lateralization in candidates for epilepsy surgery; however, highly focal stimulation with present-generation magnetic stimulation coils is not possible.[21] Currently, stimulation is limited to cortical structures because of the widening and weakening of magnetic current with increasing depth.[21] This modality may have much broader applications in functional neurosurgery with development of accurate focal stimulation, both superficial and deep.

MEG is used for recording electromagnetic potentials from epileptic foci,[22] as well as evoked potentials from functional cortex, such as auditory cortex.[23] Presently, MEG provides limited spatial accuracy,[24] but the newly introduced generation of 37-channel MEG units and improved mathematical localization formulas may lead to more accurate localization of epileptic foci and evoked potentials.[25]

The use of a stereotactic fiducial reference marker[23] allows localization of magnetic dipoles within stereotactic space (Plate 19). Stereotactically localized interictal epileptic magnetic dipoles defined with a 37-channel MEG unit have also recently been used to assist in the planning and execution of stereotactic radiosurgery on a small series of patients with intractable focal epilepsy.[26] The preliminary results are encouraging.

It may be possible in the future to use the noninvasive modality of stereotactic radiosurgery to perform other functional neurosurgical procedures, with the target physiologically defined by transcranial magnetic stimulation or by evoked magnetic potentials detected by MEG.

REFERENCES

1. DeJong RN: Abnormal movements, in *The Neurologic Examination,* 3d ed. New York, Harper & Row, 1969, chap 31, pp 534–536.
2. Ojemann GA, Ward AA Jr: Abnormal movement disorders, in Youmans JR (ed): *Neurological Surgery,* 3d ed. Philadelphia, Saunders, 1988, chap 163, pp 4227–4262.
3. Hardy TL: Stereotactic CT atlases, in Lunsford LD (ed): *Modern Stereotactic Neurosurgery.* Boston, Nijhoff, 1988, chap 34, pp 425–439.
4. Brierley JB, Beck E: The significance in human stereotactic brain surgery of individual variation in the diencephalon and globus pallidus. *J Neurol Neurosurg Psychiatry* 45:815–819, 1959.
5. Cosman ER, Nashold BS, Bedenbaugh P: Stereotactic radiofrequency lesion making. *Appl Neurophysiol* 46:160–166, 1983.
6. Mohadjer M, Goerke H, Milios E, et al: Long-term results of stereotaxy in the treatment of essential tremor. *Stereotact Funct Neurosurg* 54–55:125–129, 1990.
7. Olson L: Grafts and growth factors in CNS—basic science with clinical promise. *Stereotact Funct Neurosurg* 54–55:250–267, 1990.
8. Madrazo I, Franco-Bourland R, Ostrosky-Solis F, et al: Fetal homotransplants (ventral mesencephalon and adrenal tissue) to the striatum of parkinsonian subjects. *Arch Neurol* 47:1281–1285, 1990.
9. Shima F, Fukui M: Clinical picture and surgical treatment of spasmodic torticollis of eleventh nerve origin. *Stereotact Funct Neurosurg* 54–55:223, 1990.
10. XinKang C: Selective resection and denervation of cervical muscles in the treatment of spasmodic torticollis: Results in 60 cases. *Neurosurgery* 8:680–688, 1981.
11. Ivan LP: Longitudinal (Bischof's) myelotomy, in Schmidek HH, Sweet WH (eds): *Operative Neurosurgical Techniques,* 2d ed. Philadelphia, Saunders, 1988, chap 106, pp 1177–1184.
12. Kasdon DL, Lathi ES: A prospective study of radiofrequency rhizotomy in the treatment of posttraumatic spasticity. *Neurosurgery* 15:526–529, 1984.
13. Broseta J, Garcia-March G, Sanchez-Ledesma MJ, et al: Chronic intrathecal baclofen administration in severe spasticity. *Stereotact Funct Neurosurg* 54–55:147–153, 1990.
14. Campos RJ, Dimitrijevic MR, Sharkey PC, Sherwood AM: Epidural spinal cord stimulation in spastic spinal cord injury patients. *Appl Neurophysiol* 50:453–454, 1987.
15. Abbate AD, Cook AW, Atallah M: Effect of electrical stimulation of the thoracic spinal cord on the function of the bladder in multiple sclerosis. *J Urol* 117:285–288, 1977.
16. McGuire EJ, Savastano JA: Urodynamic findings and clinical status following denervation procedures for control of incontinence. *J Urol* 132:87–88, 1984.
17. Sindou M, Mertens P, Jeanmonod D: Microsurgical ablative procedures in the peripheral nerves and dorsal root entry zone for relief of focal spasticity in the limbs. *Stereotact Funct Neurosurg* 54–55:140–146, 1990.
18. Peacock WJ, Arens LJ, Berman B: Cerebral palsy spasticity. Selective posterior rhizotomy. *Pediatr Neurosci* 13:61–66, 1987.
19. Siegfried J: Stereotaxic cerebellar surgery for spasticity, in Schaltenbrand G, Walker AE (eds): *Stereotaxy of the Human Brain.* New York, Georg Thieme Verlag, 1982, chap 37, pp 562–564.
20. Maccabee PJ, Amassian VE, Cracco RQ, et al: Stimulation of the human nervous system using the magnetic coil. *J Clin Neurophysiol* 8(1):38–55, 1991.
21. Cohen D, Cufin BN: Developing a more focal magnetic stimulator. Part I: Some basic principles. *J Clin Neurophysiol* 8(1):102–111, 1991.
22. Sato S, Smith PD: Magnetoencephalography. *J Clin Neurophysiol* 2:173–192, 1985.
23. Papanicolaou AC, Baumann S, Rogers RI, et al: Localization of auditory response sources using magnetoencephalography and magnetic resonance imaging. *Arch Neurol* 47:33–37, 1990.
24. Barth DS, Sutherland W, Broffman J, Beatty J: Magnetic localization of a dipole source implanted in a sphere and a human cranium. *EEG and Clin Neurophysiol* 63:210–273, 1986.
25. Rose DF: Magnetoencephalography–technology and equipment review. *J Clin Neurophysiol* 8(2):238, 1991.
26. Lindquist C: Stereotactic localization of epileptic foci by magnetoencephalography and MRI followed by gamma knife surgery. Presented at the 10th meeting of the American Society for Stereotactic and Functional Neurosurgery, Pittsburgh, 1991.
27. Laitinen LV, Bergenheim AT, Hariz MI: Leksell's posteroventral pallidotomy in the treatment of Parkinson's disease. *J Neurosurg* 76:53–61, 1992.

☐ STUDY QUESTIONS

I. A 39-year-old female is referred for treatment of a familial movement disorder. The patient has rapid irregular movements of the facial muscles and throughout the extremities. The movements have been progressively increasing for 20 years. There is a family history of similar movements, progressive intellectual deterioration, and early death. Two members of the family have committed suicide. The patient is depressed and her intelligence quotient is recorded as being mildly retarded.

1. What is the most likely diagnosis? 2. Could these abnormal movements be helped by a thalamotomy? 3. In what part of the thalamus might a lesion be most helpful? 4. What parts of the syndrome might be most positively affected by a thalamotomy? 5. What genetic advice might be offered this patient?

II. A 45-year-old male is referred because of difficulty writing. He has a "pill-rolling" tremor in the right hand. Movements of the arm are slowed. The patient is alert and there is no indication of intellectual deterioration. He has not been on any psychotropic drugs but he has been on levodopa, which initially relieved the tremor but has been associated with some athetoid movements.

1. What is the most likely diagnosis? 2. What surgical treatment might be considered? 3. What would be the most likely outcome of a thalamotomy? 4. What would be the most likely complications? 5. Assuming the disorder was bilateral, what would be the objection to bilateral thalamotomies?

III. A 50-year-old male began to experience ataxia and intention tremor such that he was unable to continue his occupation as a draftsman. MRI showed evidence of atrophy of the cerebellum. There are no other neurological deficits.

1. Would this patient be a candidate for thalamotomy? 2. What part of the thalamus should be targeted? 3. How would a thalamotomy affect the basic disease? 4. What imaging techniques might be used to direct probes? 5. For how long might surgical therapy be effective?

IV. A 16-year-old male, who began having difficulty keeping up with his playmates at age 10, is becoming more ataxic. His deep tendon reflexes are absent, but he has arched feet and his toes move upward when the plantar surface of the foot is stroked.

1. What is the most likely diagnosis? 2. Would this patient's deficits be improved by thalamotomy? 3. What treatments might be helpful? 4. What is the outlook for this patient? 5. What other neurological conditions should be differentiated?

V. A 55-year-old male experienced a turning motion to the head, the head tilting to the left, the chin rotating to the right. The neck has become progressively more painful.

1. What is the most likely diagnosis? 2. What surgical therapies might be considered? 3. Assuming rhizotomy and peripheral nerve fiber divisions are selected, what roots should be divided and where should one divide the nerve fibers peripherally? 4. What complications might be anticipated from such procedures? 5. What therapies might be provided to reduce these complications?

☐ NOTE

Since this article was written, posteroventral pallidotomy has been reintroduced and appears to be effective in treating some signs of Parkinson's disease.[27]

CHAPTER
26

Infectious Processes Affecting the Nervous System

Ross H. Miller

Infections involving the intracranial and intraspinal spaces are caused by microorganisms. These organisms reach the central nervous system (CNS) via the bloodstream and/or invade the spaces directly following penetrating wounds or surgery. Infections may enter the skull by direct extension from the mastoid air cells (to the temporal area) or paranasal sinuses (frontal area) of the intracranial cavity.[1] A congenital dermal sinus may become infected and the infection extend into the intracranial and intraspinal spaces.

Infections become disseminated by the cerebrospinal fluid (CSF) once the organisms reach the CSF. Treatment of infections of the CNS involves: (1) identification of the organism and its source, (2) selection of appropriate antimicrobials (see Table 26-1),[2] (3) removal of any collection of purulent material (abscesses, empyema), (4) treatment of the sources of the infection, and (5) control of any complications that may occur as a result of infection.

☐ GENERALIZED INFECTIONS OF THE NERVOUS SYSTEM

MENINGITIS

Bacterial infections When an infectious process invades the leptomeninges, headache, fever, and stiff neck indicate irritation of the structures. Organisms responsible for meningitis vary with the age of the patient. *Escherichia coli, β-hemolytic streptococci,* and *Haemophilus influenzae* are most common in pediatric patients. *Streptococcus pneumoniae* and *Neisseria meningitidis* are more common in adult patients. Fungi and *Mycobacterium* tuberculosis produce chronic meningitis.

Headache, fever, sensitivity to light, nausea, and vomiting are the most common symptoms of meningitis. Seizures may occur with cortical irritation by the inflammatory process. Invasion of the brain by the infection will produce focal neurological defects. Cranial nerve palsies occur with exudates over the base of the brain and are more common in chronic meningitis caused by tuberculosis or fungi.[3,4] Upon examination, the patient may be irritable and drowsy, and the neck will be stiff. Papilledema may be present.

Examination of CSF will confirm the diagnosis of meningitis in most patients. A lumbar puncture (LP) should be postponed when papilledema is present. Herniation of a temporal lobe into the tentorial notch or herniation of the cerebellar tonsils into the foramen magnum may occur with release of CSF from the lumbar area. It is important to obtain a computerized tomogram (CT) or magnetic resonance image (MRI) to rule out a mass lesion as a cause for the papilledema before a decision is made to perform an LP.

Meningitis is confirmed if the CSF contains large numbers of polymorphonuclear or mononuclear cells. CSF glucose is decreased in pyogenic infections; CSF protein, as well as pressure, is elevated.

The organism is usually identified in the CSF by direct smear and culture. Following its identification, its sensitivity to antibiotics is determined and the appropriate antibiotic prescribed.[2] In some cases, it may be necessary to place antibiotics directly into the CSF if they do not effectively cross the blood-brain barrier. Some antibiotics (e.g., penicillin) may produce convulsions when introduced in large concentrations in the CSF, and this should be avoided.[5]

Fungal Infections Fungal infections are usually treated with amphotericin B.[3] Intraventricular catheters may be used to place antibiotics directly into the ventricles. Prolonged therapy can be obtained by attaching a reservoir to the catheter, enabling the physician to repeat treatments without repeated ventricular puncture. In selected patients, a lumbar subarachnoid catheter may be used for repeated injections of antibiotics into the lumbar CSF.

Table 26-1
INFECTIONS OF THE CENTRAL NERVOUS SYSTEM AND THEIR TREATMENT

Causative Bacteria	Antimicrobial Agent
A. *Staphylococcus aureus*	Oxycillin Nafcillin Cefazolin Vancomycin Amoxicillin Clindomycin
B. *Streptococcus*	Penicillin G Penicillin V Amoxicillin Cefazolin Erythromycin Chloramphenicol
C. *Pneumococcus*	Erythromycin Penicillin G Amoxicillin
D. *H. influenza*	Cefuroxamine Ampicillin Cefotaxime Chloramphenicol Ceftriaxone
E. *Pseudomonas aeruginosa*	Gentamicin Amikacin Imipenem-cilastatin Ceftazidime + amino glycoside
F. *E. coli*	Gentamicin Amikacin
G. *Mycobacterium tuberculosis*	Streptomycin Isoniazid Rifampin Ethambutol

H. *Viral Infection*
  Herpes
  AIDS
  Influenza A
	Amantadine
	Vidarabine
	Acylovir (most often used)
	Ribavirin
	Zidovudine (AIDS)

I. *Fungal Infections*
  Cryptococcus neoformans
  Histoplasma capsulatum
  Coccidioides immitis
  Aspergillus fumigatus
	Amphotericin B
	Flucytosin
	Ketoconazole
	Miconazole

Cryptococcosis *Cryptococcus neoformans* is a widespread mycotic infection of the CNS, most often seen in immunosuppressed patients with AIDS. It may invade the meninges or present with symptoms of diffuse encephalitis. Cryptococcus causes severe thickening of the meninges, followed by hydrocephalus and cranial nerve dysfunction.

Diagnosis is confirmed by culturing this mycotic organism from CSF, its presence confirmed by India ink preparation, in addition to positive cryptococcal antigen and antibody tests. Treatment of cryptococcal infection is with amphotericin B, 5-fluorouracil, and ketoconazole.[3]

ACQUIRED IMMUNODEFICIENCY SYNDROME (AIDS)

The proliferation of AIDS in the population is reaching disastrous proportions.[6,7] A wide variety of central and peripheral nervous system abnormalities occurs during the course of HIV infection.

Direct infiltration of the nervous system is common in patients with HIV. The infection produces clinical manifestations that include AIDS dementia complex (ADC), secondary meningoencephalitis, and peripheral mono- and polyneuropathies, including peripheral facial nerve palsy and brachial plexopathy. A Guillain-Barré syndrome and myelopathy may develop.

Examination of CSF in patients with HIV infection shows mononuclear pleocytosis with elevation of CSF protein but normal levels of glucose. The HIV is detected by culture and anti-HIV specific antibody can be demonstrated in the CSF. CSF findings may subside if the patient becomes asymptomatic.

AIDS Dementia Complex This is the most frequent clinical feature of the CNS in a patient with AIDS. Pathological abnormalities are found mainly in the basal ganglia and hypothalamus, with mononuclear cell infiltrates. Reactive gliosis, atrophy of white matter, loss of myelin, and brain cell vacuolation also occur. HIV can be detected in the affected brain tissue.

Principal symptoms of ADC include impairment of memory, concentration, and intellectual performance. Motor responses are delayed and there is decreased response to verbal and visual stimuli. Patients with ADC progress to total immobility, mutism, and loss of sphincter control.

Electroencephalography (EEG) may show diffuse slowing. Brain CT is normal in the early stages of ADC, while MRI shows multifocal areas of increased signal in the white matter, basal ganglia, and thalamus on T2-weighted images.

HIV Myelopathy Changes in spinal cord function may or may not occur in patients with ADC. Vacuolation of the posterior and lateral columns of the spinal cord occur. Patients with myelopathy will present with ataxia, spasticity, and weakness of the lower extremities, as well as hyporeflexia, paraparesis, and sphincter dysfunction.

CT and MRI may be helpful in the diagnosis of AIDS myelopathy, but in patients with AIDS the diagnosis is made primarily by exclusion of other lesions which could cause the presenting symptoms: e.g., vitamin B_{12} deficiency, spinal cord tumor, multiple sclerosis.

Acute transverse myelitis may be secondary to lymphoma

or herpes zoster, but it can also be due to direct infection of neurons in the spinal cord by HIV.

Peripheral Neuropathy Distal sensory neuropathy occurs during the early stages of HIV infection. Initial symptoms include paresthesias of the hands and/or feet, pain, and progression to muscle weakness. All abnormalities are more frequent in the lower extremities, but slow progression may reach the girdle muscles and muscles supplied by the sacral or brachial plexus.

Nerve conduction velocities, EMG, and sural nerve biopsy show abnormalities consistent with axonal neuropathy with secondary demyelinization.

Treatment with antidepressants, salicylates, anticonvulsants, and analgesics may relieve some of the symptoms. Specific treatment of HIV infection of the CNS is still in the early stages of development.[8] Zidovudine may help reverse or halt progression of some neurological symptoms. Side effects of zidovudine may be confused with progression of the disease, and patients who respond to therapy may have significant exacerbation of their symptoms if medications are discontinued.

Other Manifestations of HIV Other diseases of the meninges and CNS may accompany HIV. Patients with diffuse neurological dysfunctions have neurological symptoms that present with fever, headache, nausea, and vomiting secondary to an associated infection of the CNS. Diseases presenting with focal neurological defects include: single or multiple brain abscesses, herpes encephalitis, fungal infections, and malignancies. Lymphoma of the brain is the most commonly associated tumor with HIV.

Acute vascular events have been described in patients with AIDS; these may be caused by necrotizing vasculitis due to secondary bacterial,[9,10] fungal,[6] or viral[8] infection.

Progressive multifocal leukoencephalopathy (PMLE) may occur because of papovavirus infection of the brain. Focal signs associated with PMLE depend on the area of the brain affected by the changes in the site of greatest involvement.

Meningeal diseases associated with AIDS usually are subacute or chronic in course. Headache and fever are early symptoms, followed by slow development of focal and diffuse signs.

The diagnosis of CNS dysfunction as a result of HIV may be difficult. Awareness or suspicion of HIV is the most important indicator.[7]

Neurological examination of the patient reveals diffuse and focal changes caused by lesions of the nervous system and it provides a baseline for future reference to assess the effectiveness of treatment and progression of disease.

CT and MRI aid in the diagnosis of patients with AIDS. Lesions seen on CT and MRI may be similar to those in patients who do not have HIV, but infections are often more severe because of AIDS.

Guillain-Barré syndrome can occur at any time in the course of AIDS. Treatment with corticosteroids will often aggravate symptoms, due to their added immunosuppressive effect.

Cytomegalovirus will produce a cauda equina syndrome with flaccid paralysis, absent reflexes, and loss of bladder and bowel control.

Brachial and sacral plexopathies arise during the acute phases of the disease. They may resolve spontaneously, although recurrence of symptoms develops with disease progression, in spite of treatment with azidothymidine (zidovudine).

The localization and extent of the neuromuscular disease associated with HIV infection requires a thorough neurological examination, CT and MRI of the spinal cord, EMG, CSF analysis, nerve and muscle biopsies.

The diagnosis of AIDS and associated diseases of the CNS requires awareness on the part of the physician that AIDS may be present in *any* patient with symptoms of infection in the CNS and peripheral nerves. Recognition of the potential for HIV is mandatory to protect the patient as well as those involved in the treatment of that patient.[7]

☐ LOCALIZED BACTERIAL INFECTIONS

Subgaleal abscess usually occurs secondary to scalp trauma.[10] Suppuration develops between the skull and galea. Purulent material may spread to involve the skull (osteomyelitis) and extend into the subdural space.

Treatment is early aspiration for drainage and antibiotics appropriate for the bacteria causing the infection.

Osteomyelitis of the skull is associated with subgaleal infection. It can result from skeletal traction, trauma, or infection at the site of a craniotomy or cranioplasty. It may result from direct extension of infection of any of the paranasal sinuses or mastoid air cells, or it may be the result of hematogenous spread.[1]

Symptoms include pain and swelling over the site and drainage of purulent material if an open wound is present, as well as low-grade fever, and edema of surrounding tissue. Diagnosis is made by x-ray and CT of the skull.

Treatment is drainage of purulent material and excision of infected bone, followed by appropriate antibiotic therapy.[2,5,11,12,13] Repair of the cranial defect, if needed, should be deferred until several months after the infection has resolved.

Osteomyelitis of the skull base and petrous bone, known as *Gradenigo's syndrome,* is difficult to treat because of extensive involvement of the bone. Extensive multidisciplinary surgery may be required.

Epidural abscess may develop following trauma to the skull, osteomyelitis of the skull, or mastoiditis; most commonly it follows craniotomy. The dura presents a barrier protecting the brain parenchyma; however, if venous drainage is compromised and becomes infected, there may be spread of the infection into the subdural space and brain parenchyma as well—or into the CSF, producing acute meningitis, cerebritis, and abscess. Diagnosis is confirmed with CT.

Treatment is drainage of the abscess and antibiotic therapy.[2,5,11,12,13]

Subdural empyema can be lethal if not treated early. Infection produces early venous thrombosis and proceeds to fulminating meningitis and brain abscess. It spreads most commonly from the paranasal sinuses, producing thrombosis of the cortical veins and venous sinuses and extensive cerebral edema.

Symptoms include headache, lethargy, cranial nerve palsies (most commonly the third cranial nerve), and papilledema. Hemiparesis, convulsions, and coma complete the syndrome. Infants may develop subdural effusions secondary to influenzal meningitis, with signs of increased intracranial pressure (enlarged fontanel and spreading of suture lines). Subdural taps confirm the diagnosis.

Appropriate antibiotic therapy (usually ampicillin) is instituted. If the effusion does not subside, craniotomy and removal of the membranes or subdural-peritoneal shunting may be necessary. Chloramphenicol may be used in patients beyond the neonatal age.[14,15]

Brain abscess is a purulent infection of the brain parenchyma. Abscesses develop following direct extension of bacteria from the mastoid or paranasal sinuses, or they may develop from hematogenous spread from the lungs, heart, or kidneys. Children with congenital heart disease are prime candidates for brain abscesses. Patients with HIV infection (AIDS) are also candidates.[6,9]

Cerebritis forms secondary to the invading organisms, with cerebral edema and loss of structure of the white matter of the brain secondary to focal vasculitis and thrombosis. The brain tissue liquefies, and the glial cells and phagocytes attempt to contain the infection by developing a capsular wall around the diseased tissue.

If the brain is successful in containing the infection, a firm capsule filled with degenerated brain and purulent material develops. The abscess is surrounded by edema, which adds to the size of the lesion, producing increased intracranial pressure and shifting of the cranial contents. Herniation of the uncus of the medial temporal lobe into the tentorial notch is a frequent consequence.

Brain abscesses may be single or multiple. If multiple in a patient who is not immunocompromised, the cause is most likely from hematogenous spread (congenital heart disease or endocarditis). Patients infected with HIV are prone to multiple abscesses. Frontal lobe abscesses are usually extensions of paranasal sinus infections, and a search for middle ear or mastoid infections is indicated in patients with a temporal lobe abscess.[1] Brain abscess may be secondary to dental infections. (See Figs. 26-1 and 26-2A and B.)

The symptoms of brain abscess are determined by its location and size. Headache, fever, nausea, and vomiting occur early, followed by papilledema, lethargy, convulsions, and hemiparesis. Abscesses occurring in the posterior fossa produce cerebellar signs of ataxia and dysmetria, nystagmus, and papilledema early in the illness, with rapid deterioration of the patient's clinical status.

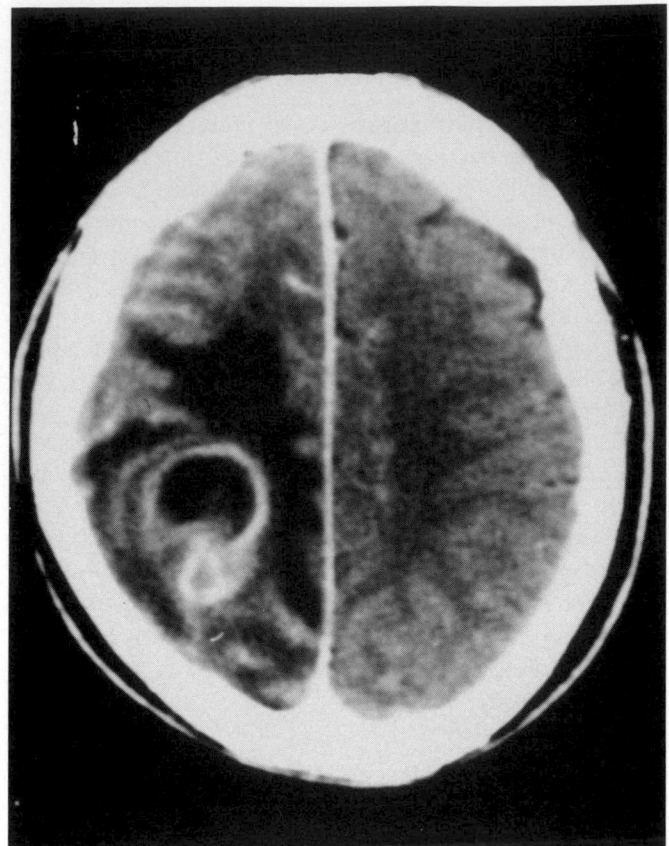

Figure 26-1 Computerized tomography scan, axial view (enhanced). Brain abscess, multiloccular right parietal lobe secondary to Pseudomonas petrous bone infection. The abscess is surrounded by cerebral edemas.

The diagnosis is made by neurological examination, x-rays of the skull, CT, and MRI. Spinal puncture is contraindicated in a patient suspected of having a brain abscess because of the danger of precipitating an acute herniation of the medial surface of the temporal lobe into the tentorial notch, thus compromising the brain stem, or because of the danger of a herniation of the cerebellar tonsils into the foramen magnum, thus compromising the medulla.

Chest x-rays and blood cultures suggest possible sources of the cause of the abscess. Cerebral angiography will reveal a large avascular mass. However, CT and MRI suggest the diagnosis by showing the mass lesion, often incapsulated, and the extent of cerebral edema. (See Fig. 26-3.) There may be multiple lesions.

Treatment of brain abscess is directed to drainage of the abscess to reduce increased intracranial pressure and to determine the etiological organisms, which will indicate the type of antibiotic therapy to be used. In recent years, aspiration of the abscess by stereotactic means to reduce the size of the lesion has been popular. Most abscesses will respond to this therapy, followed by long-term antibiotic therapy.

Large abscesses located in the frontal or temporal lobes of the brain, may be excised with removal of the abscess capsule and its contents. This procedure must also be followed by antibiotic therapy. The adjacent infected tissues

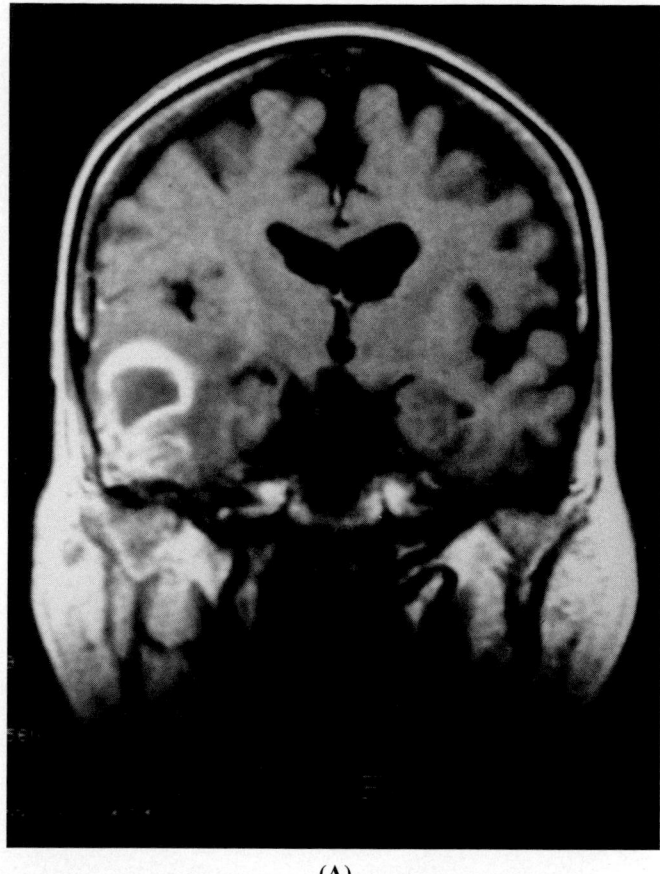

(A)

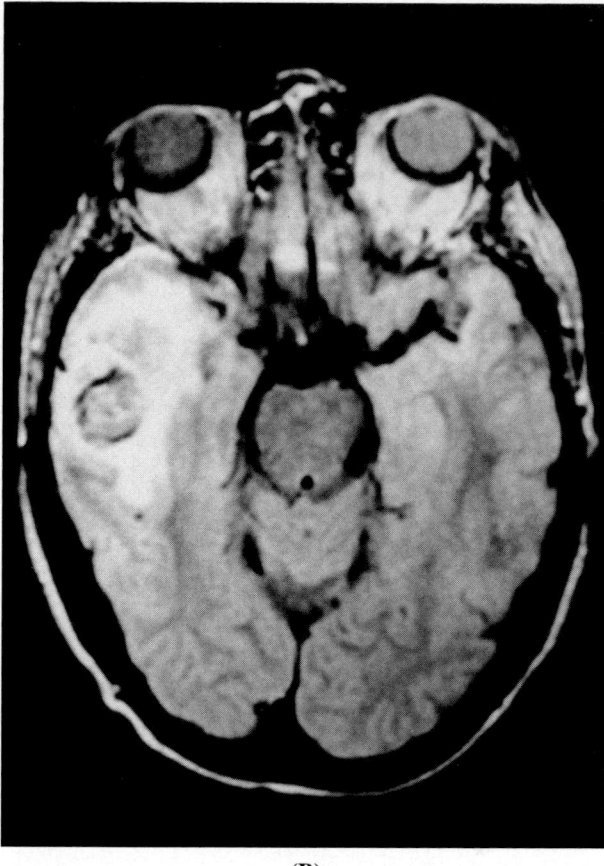

(B)

Figure 26-2 *A.* Magnetic resonance image coronal view. Brain abscess, right temporal lobe. The abscess extends from the petrous bone into the right temporal lobe. *B.* Magnetic resonance image, axial view. Brain abscess, right temporal lobe, secondary to Pseudomonas infection of petrous bone. Note extensive edema secondary to the abscess.

and bone involved in mastoiditis or sinusitis must also be treated surgically to prevent reoccurrence of the abscess. It is important to treat a brain abscess as soon as it is recognized because the lesion will otherwise enlarge and rupture into the ventricular system, producing an overwhelming infection and death.

☐ VIRAL INFECTIONS

Viral encephalitis develops as an extension of mumps or herpes simplex infection. The viral infection produces diffuse edema and meningeal inflammation. There is swelling and disintegration of the cortical neurons, perivascular inflammation, and focal hemorrhages of the cortex and white matter.

Early, or prodromal, symptoms of viral encephalitis include fever, malaise, nausea and vomiting, as well as symptoms of upper respiratory disease.

There is a sudden onset and rapid progression of encephalitis with convulsions, drowsiness, and focal weakness. Diagnostic studies should include EEG, which will show focal slow waves in the area of the lesion but also some diffuse slow waves over the brain. CT will reveal a large

mass, most often of the temporal lobe, but it can extend into the frontal lobe, with decreased attenuation and occasional hemorrhage within the lesion. (See Fig. 26-4*A* and *B*.) MRI will reveal evidence of edema and mass effect and, possibly, hemorrhage.

Treatment includes biopsy and microscopic examination of the lesion. Specimens of the issue are cultured to isolate the offending virus. In some patients, the virus may be cultured from the spinal fluid. It is also possible to demonstrate a specific antigen for herpes virus with immunofluorescence studies. After diagnosis of herpes simplex viral encephalitis, the specific treatment is cytosine arabinoside and adenosine arabinoside, which are usually started immediately after biopsy of the lesion.[8,16]

☐ PARASITIC AND FUNGUS INFECTIONS

Parasitic and fungal infections of the brain are being seen more frequently in the United States because of the great amount of international travel. The presence of AIDS and patients undergoing immunosuppressive therapy add to the number of patients found with fungal infections.[6,3,17]

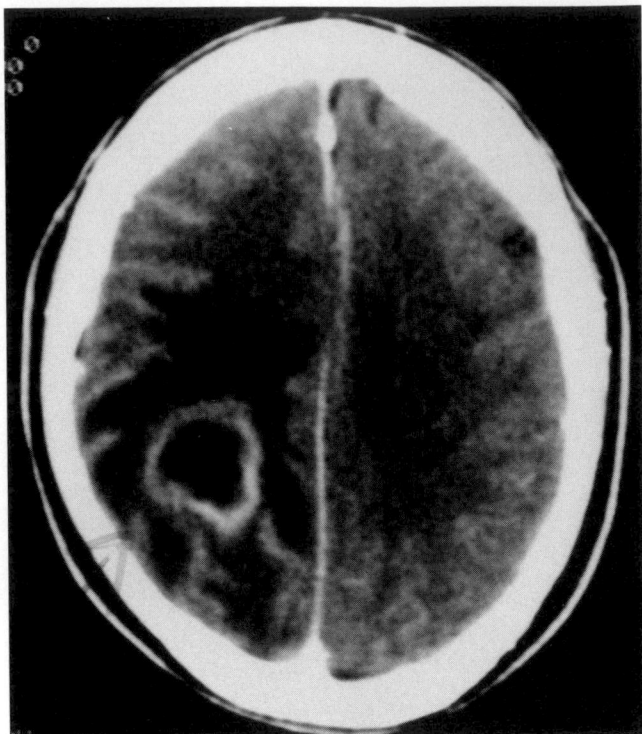

Figure 26-3 Computerized tomography (enhanced) of cerebral hemisphere. Brain abscess, right parietal area, secondary to *Streptococcus viridans* septicemia.

Fungal and parasitic infections should be considered in any patient with CNS symptoms.

Amebiasis (Entamoeba histolytica) is present in a small portion of the general population of the United States, but it is a common infection in Central America. The *E. histolytica* trophozoite is ingested, it passes to the bloodstream, and seeds to the liver and on to the brain as an embolus via the bloodstream. The parasite produces confluent hemorrhagic areas and infarction in the brain. Multiloculated cysts most often occur in the frontal lobes and basal ganglia.

Symptoms include headache, seizures, and facial spasms, and cranial nerve palsies are frequently found. Anatomic diagnosis is made by CT examination. The lesions may be small, with little evidence of surrounding inflammatory response. Serum complement fixation associated with immunofluorescence antibody is diagnostic.

Treatment is directed to drainage of abscesses and drug therapy with emetine HCl, chloroquine, tetracycline, and metronidazole. Corticosteroids are contraindicated in these patients.

Toxoplasmosis gondii is found worldwide. It is usually asymptomatic but most often causes symptoms in patients who are immunosuppressed with AIDs or its therapy.[6]

Symptoms and signs of diffuse encephalitis develop as the disease becomes active. Antibody titers are increased on complement fixation examination. The CSF reveals that protein content is elevated, and there is an increase in mononuclear cells. The CSF glucose is usually normal.

Roentgenograms and CT reveal multiple areas of irregular

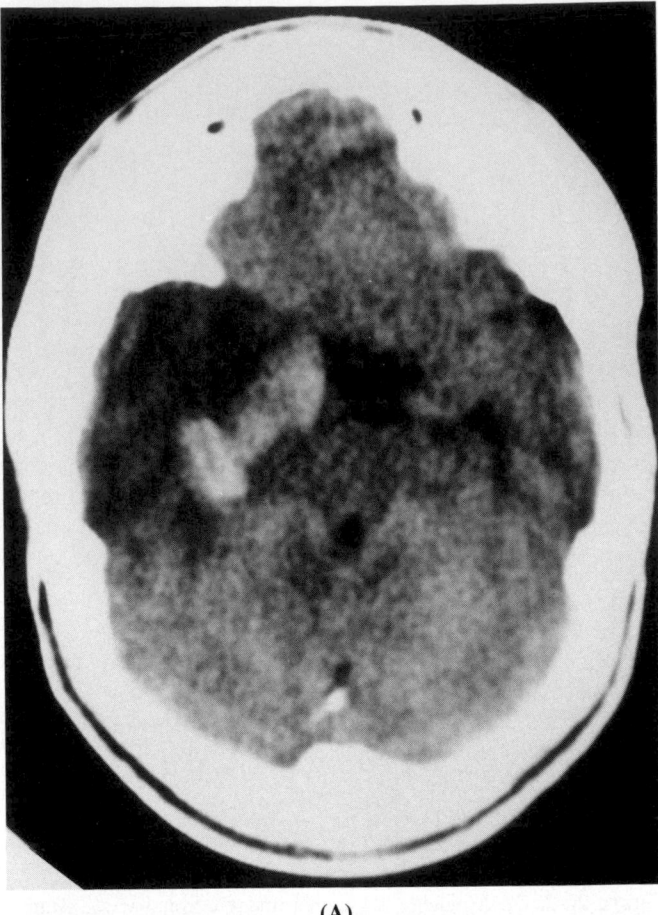

(A)

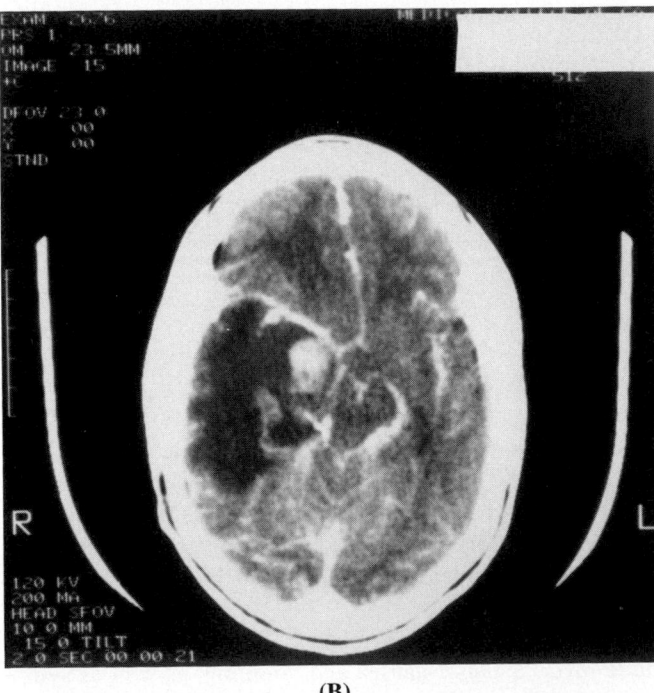

(B)

Figure 26-4 *A.* Computerized tomography scan (enhanced) of herpes encephalitis showing a large area of edema and intracerebral hemorrhage of the right temporal lobe. *B.* Magnetic resonance image, T2-weighted sequence, of the brain showing herpes encephalitis with extensive edema and intracerebral hemorrhage in the right temporal lobe.

nodular calcification, most often surrounding the ventricular system.

The usual treatment of toxoplasmosis includes sulfadiazine and pyremethamine.[2] Corticosteroids should not be given.

Cysticercosis (Taenia solium), or pork tapeworm, enters the patient who eats raw or poorly cooked pork products. The disease is prevalent in much of the world. It is rare in most of the United States and Canada but is seen in southern United States and California.

Cysticercosis may involve any part of the CNS. Small cystic lesions produce multiple symptoms, depending on the location. The basilar cisterns are frequently involved.

Diagnosis is made by identification of the parasite in the tissue and by complement fixation tests on the CSF. No medications will eradicate the disease. Treatment is directed toward excision of lesions of the brain and spinal cord and shunting any associated hydrocephalus.

Hydatid cysts are lesions occurring in the human as intermediate host of the dog tapeworm. They should be distinguished from cysticercosis both in cause and treatment. Treatment is removal by large craniotomy, being careful not to rupture the cyst. This is best accomplished by careful corticotomy down to the cyst, which is expelled by cerebral pulsation and irrigation. The lesions are common in southern United States and California.

Trichinosis (Trichinella spiralis) also occurs with the ingestion of raw or poorly cooked pork. The nervous system is affected in a small number of patients infested with this parasite. CNS symptoms are those of meningoencephalitis with cranial nerve dysfunction and progression to major neurological deficits. Diagnosis is made by the bentonite-flocculation immunofluorescent antibody and latex agglutination tests.

Treatment is with corticosteroids and thiabendazole. Prognosis is good with the therapy.[17]

Mucormycosis is a clinical syndrome, which usually begins in the paranasal sinuses and extends into the orbit, causing headache, pain in one eye and the face, with periorbital edema, commonly ophthalmoplegia, and proptosis. Blindness may result from occlusion of the retinal artery.

This syndrome is caused by various genera of fungi, usually *Mucor, Rhizopus,* or *Absidia.* The organisms are nonpathogenic except in patients with diabetic ketoacidosis. In clinical settings the organisms are likely to cause occlusion of blood vessels, resulting in infarction. Bones at the base of the skull are usually invaded.

Involvement of the eye may be followed by symptoms of encephalitis, with headache and lethargy from subsequent abscess formation.

Aggressive surgical treatment in the form of block excision of infarcted areas is followed by intense medical therapy with amphotericin B and 5-fluorocytosine. Mortality rates are high.

Aspergillosis (Aspergillus fumigatus) is a commonly encountered mycotic infection of the CNS. The organism is opportunistic and frequently occurs in patients with low host

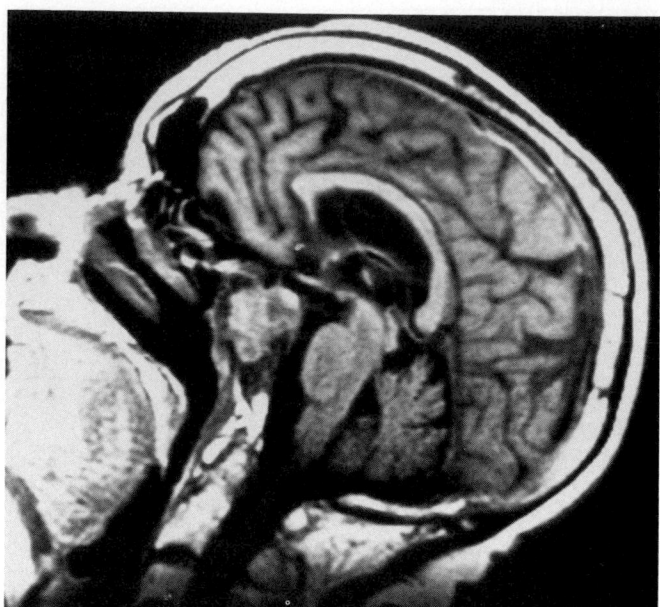

Figure 26-5 Magnetic resonance image of skull, sagittal view. Large aspergillosis granuloma involving the sphenoid sinus, clivus, and encasing the right carotid artery. Note the irregular enlargement of the carotid artery within the granuloma.

resistance. Patients with leukemia, AIDS, or neoplastic diseases or those on steroids or immunosuppressive therapy are particularly susceptible.[6,18]

Exclusive involvement of the brain is rare, but the kidneys and brain are often involved in this systemic disease. The respiratory tree is the common source of infection, and the brain receives the infection, most often, via the bloodstream. This mycotic pathogen can enter the CNS through the paranasal sinuses by contiguous spread or by iatrogenic spread through contaminated needles or neurosurgical procedures

Aspergillus may produce symptoms consistent with meningitis, encephalitis, or granuloma. The infection may extend from the paranasal sinuses or mastoid bone into the intracranial cavity. Abscesses occur as an extension of meningeal infections. (See Fig. 26-5.)

Granulomas are more common in patients with chronic infection. CNS symptoms are related to the location of the infection. The granuloma produces a sclerosing vasculitis after invasion of the artery of the lesion. Transient ischemic attacks occur secondary to septic emboli and may progress to infarction. The invasion of the wall of the carotid artery may produce mycotic aneurysms. (See Fig. 26-6A and *B.*)

Treatment includes decompression of the intracranial cavity—with removal of the lesions if possible—and drug therapy with amphotericin B and 5-fluorouracil and itraconozale.[3]

Tuberculosis of the intracranial cavity is rare in the United States, but tuberculosis of the parenchyma, particularly the posterior fossa, is common in third world countries. Tuberculosis also causes subdural or epidural granulomas. Isolated brain abscesses without edema are the common CT findings. Streptomycin, ethambutol, isonicotinic acid hydrazide, and

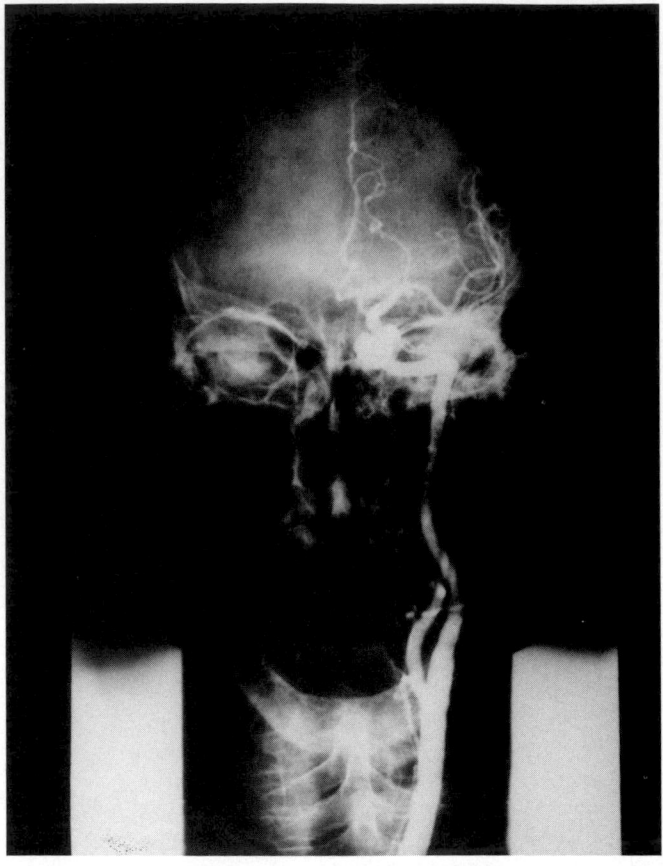
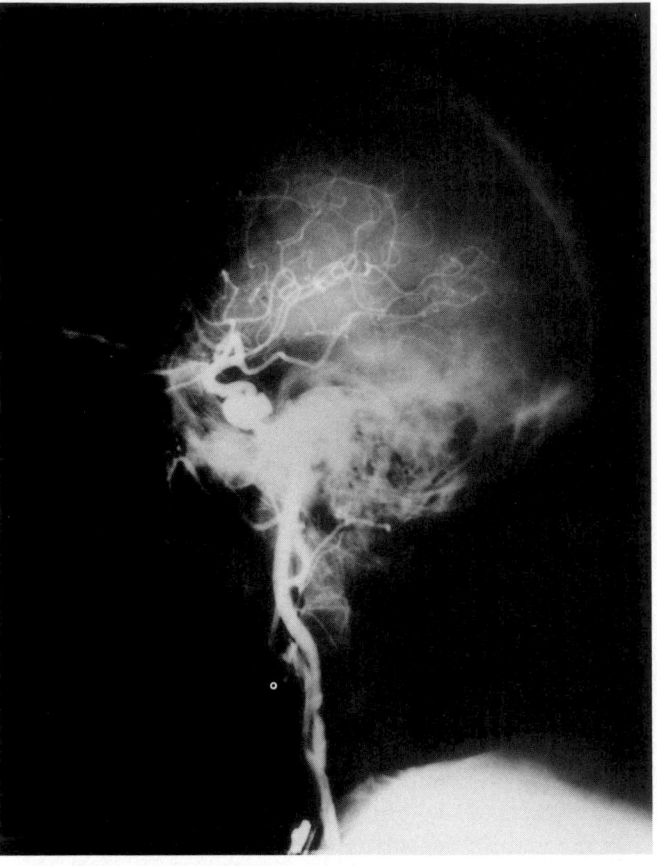

(A)   **(B)**

Figure 26-6 *A.* Right carotid angiogram, frontal view. Large multilobular mycotic aneurysm of the infraclinoid portion of the right carotid artery, secondary to aspergillosis invading the artery.

B. Lateral view of the multilobular aneurysm of the right carotid artery.

rifampin are used in combination to treat tuberculosis of the central nervous system.[4,13,20]

Sarcoidosis produces multiple granulomatous lesions and is of unknown etiology. This reticulosis is more common in blacks and forms noncaseating granulomatous lymphoid tissue. The granulomatous lesions are found throughout the CNS and may involve the peripheral nerves. Involvement of the base of the brain and the cranial nerves is frequent.

Patients develop meningitis, seizures, hydrocephalus, and dysfunction of the pituitary gland. Alterations in mental function are common. The diagnosis can be made by chest x-ray because the lungs are commonly involved. The only treatment is corticosteroids and control of hydrocephalus if it is present.

☐ BACTERIAL INFECTIONS OF THE SPINE

Epidural abscesses of the spine are usually the result of blood-borne bacteria or occur postoperatively following laminectomy. The abscess can be related to previous spinal puncture or an infected congenital dermal sinus.

Symptoms of spinal epidural abscess are severe back pain,

fever, and progressive compression of the spinal cord, resulting in progressive paresis from compression of the neural elements. The sedimentation rate is usually quite elevated. Granulation tissue is commonly found in association with epidural abscesses and may require excision during the course of decompression.

The diagnosis is confirmed with x-ray of the spine, which will show early osteomyelitis of the vertebra and presence of a localized extradural collection of material shown on CT or MRI.

Treatment is immediate decompression of the spinal cord by laminectomy and removal of the abscess, followed by appropriate antibiotic therapy.[2] Spinal puncture should be avoided, as infection may be transferred from the extradural space to the subarachnoid space and result in meningitis.

Subdural abscesses of the spinal canal are rare, and they are usually extensions of extradural infection. Diagnosis is made by MRI or CT scan.

Osteomyelitis of the vertebra develops from hematogenous spread of infection to the vertebrae, but it may occur by direct extension from a disk space infection or from an intraabdominal or thoracic infection.

Deep back pain, aggravated by movement and often relieved by recumbency, fever, and increased sedimentation rate, point toward infection in a vertebral body.

X-rays of the spine may be normal early in the course of the disease, but later films will show collapse of the body. Infections of the vertebrae usually involve the intervertebral disk space while malignant lesions do not. Diagnosis can be made readily by CT scan, and a bone scan with gallium will help in many cases.

Treatment of osteomyelitis of the spine is directed toward control of the infection, comfort for the patient, and measures to prevent further collapse and deformity of the vertebral canal. If no deformity exists in the vertebral body, diagnosis may be secured by CT-directed needle biopsy of the affected vertebrae. Complications may result from misdirected needles, with perforation of a major blood vessel, the spinal canal, the subarachnoid space, or the spinal cord. Needle biopsy of the vertebrae should therefore be approached with caution.

Open biopsy may be necessary to obtain adequate tissue for culture and correction of vertebral deformity. Correction with corpectomy may be indicated. If instrumentation is required, the implanted instruments should be isolated from the site of infection.

Appropriate antibiotics are administered, depending on the type of bacteria isolated.[2,5,11,19]

Disk space infection is usually a complication of previous surgery or needle puncture of intervertebral disks.

The infection develops 6 to 8 weeks post-surgery, and it produces severe pain in the area of the previous surgery, aggravated by palpation and pressure and partially relieved by recumbency. Fever and muscle spasm are evident in patients with disk space infection, and their sedimentation rates are elevated.

X-rays of the spine and CT scan are normal early in the course of this condition. Interpretation of gallium scans is difficult as the scan may be positive because of the recent surgery. Later in the course, destructive changes will appear along the edges of the intervertebral disk space, and a CT scan *will* demonstrate these changes early. Narrowing of the intervertebral space occurs.

Treatment involves bed rest and mild medication for pain and muscle spasms. Needle biopsy of the involved inter-space identifies the causative bacteria—most often staphylococcus—and antibiotic therapy will then be started.[2,5,11] Cultures are often sterile, in which case a direct surgical biopsy may be required. Some surgeons prefer to give an elective trial of antibiotics selected for treatment of staphylococcal organisms.

Patients who do not respond to conservative therapy may need to undergo open surgery to remove the infected material from the interspace. Interspace infections *must* be observed closely, since extradural abscesses develop with spinal cord compression. When the infection is controlled, the interspace will eventually narrow, and spontaneous fusion will occur.

Tuberculous infection of the spine with spinal cord compression is a common disease in third world countries.

Tuberculosis is found most frequently in the lower thoracic and upper lumbar vertebrae. Usually, multiple vertebral bodies are involved, but posterior elements rarely show evidence of infection.

The disease starts early in life (first decade); symptoms, however, are most obvious in young adults between 30 and 40 years of age.

Decalcification of the vertebral body occurs, followed by vertebral collapse. Paravertebral abscess usually develops. CT is most accurate in diagnosis. Medical treatment includes streptomycin, para-aminosalicylate, and isoniazid.[13] Surgical correction by debridement and corpectomy is appropriate if there is collapse of the vertebral body or compression of the spinal cord.

☐ FUNGAL INFECTIONS OF THE SPINE

Epidural granulomas may cause compression of the spinal cord with paraparesis or transverse myelitis following vascular occlusion secondary to arterial invasion by a granuloma. Treatment is decompression of the spinal cord, if necessary, and drug therapy with amphotericin B and 5-fluorouracil, and itraconazole.[3]

REFERENCES

1. Nager GT: Mastoid and paranasal infections and their relation to the central nervous system. *Clinical Neurosurgery* 14:288–313, 1967.
2. Wilkowske CJ, Hermans PE: General principles of antimicrobial therapy. *Mayo Clin Proc* 62:789–798, 1987.
3. Terrell CL, Hermans PE: Antifungal agents used for deep seated mycotic infections. *Mayo Clin Proc* 62:116–1128, 1987.
4. Van Scoy RE, Wilkowske CJ: Antituberculous agents. *Mayo Clin Proc* 62:1129–1136, 1987.
5. Wright AJ, Wilkowske CJ: The penicillins. *Mayo Clin Proc* 62:806–820, 1987.
6. Florida Medical Association: *Clinical Manual on HIV and AIDS.* Jacksonville, Florida Medical Association in Conjunction with the Florida Dept. of Health and Rehabilitation Services, 1989, pp 53–59.

7. Schiff SJ: A surgeon's risk of AIDS. *J Neurosurg* 73:651–660, 1990.

8. Hermans PE, Cockerill FR III: Antiviral agents. *Mayo Clin Proc* 62:1108–1115, 1987.

9. Cockerill FR III, Edson RS; Trimethoprim and sulfamethoxazole. *Mayo Clin Proc* 62:921–929, 1987.

10. Tindall GT, Flanagan JF, Nashold BS: Brain abscess and osteomyelitis following skull traction. *Arch Surg* 79:638–641, 1959.

11. Edson RS, Terrell CL: The aminoglycosides: Streptomycin, kanamycin, gentamicin, tobramycin, amikacin, netilmicin, and sisomicin. *Mayo Clin Proc* 62:916–920, 1987.

12. Hermans PE, Wilhelm MP: Vancomycin. *Mayo Clin Proc* 62:901–905, 1987.

13. Wilson WR, Cockerill FR III: Tetracyclines, chloramphenicol, erythromycin, and clindamycin. *Mayo Clin Proc* 62:906–915, 1987.

14. Rhodes KH, Johnson CM: Antibiotic therapy for severe infections in infants and children. *Mayo Clin Proc* 62:1018–1024, 1987.

15. Thompson RL: Cephalosporin, carbapenem, and monobactam antitiotics. *Mayo Clin Proc* 62:821–834, 1987.

16. Whitely RJ, Soong SJ, Dolin R, Galasso GJ, Ch'ien LT, Alford CA, and the Collaborative Study Group: Adenine arabinoside therapy of biopsy-proved herpes simplex encephalitis: National Institutes of Allergy and Infectious Diseases Collaborative Antiviral Study. *N Engl J Med* 297:289–294, 1987.

17. Martz RD, Hoff T: Parasitic and fungal diseases of the central nervous system, in Youmans JR (ed): *Neurologic Surgery,* 3d ed. Philadelphia, Saunders, 1990, chap 134, pp 3742–3751.

18. Piotrowski WP, Pilz P, Chuang I-H: Subarachnoid hemorrhage caused by a fungal aneurysm of the vertebral artery as a complication of intracranial aneurysm clipping: Case report. *J Neurosurg* 73:962–964, 1990.

19. Walker RC, Wright AJ: The Quinolones. *Mayo Clin Proc* 62:1007–1012, 1987.

20. Carey ME: Infections of the spine and spinal cord, in Youmans JR (ed): *Neurologic Surgery,* 3d ed. Philadelphia, Saunders, 1990, chap 136, pp 3759–3781.

☐ STUDY QUESTIONS

I. A 28-year-old diabetic male complains of nasal congestion and frontal headaches for about 6 weeks before he becomes drowsy and has a series of generalized seizures. On examination, he is drowsy and has a left hemiparesis and bilateral papilledema. His scalp is "boggy." There is fluctuation beneath it and pitting edema. Palpation produces severe pain. His temperature was 39°C. Skull x-rays show clouded frontal sinuses, and the frontal bone on the right is "moth-eaten." CT scan shows a large mass in the right frontal area.

1. What is the most likely cause of the mass? **2.** What surgical therapy should be administered? When? **3.** How should the diabetes be controlled? **4.** When should a cranioplasty be performed? **5.** Assuming smears and cultures indicate *Mucor* as the etiologic agent, should the surgical therapy be altered in any way?.

II. A 37-year-old female who has experienced weight loss and night sweats for about a month, has a sudden onset of severe headache, nausea, vomiting, and drowsiness with a left hemiparesis. CT shows evidence of subarachnoid hemorrhage in the right parietal area. An arteriogram shows an aneurysm on a distal branch of the ascending frontoparietal branch of the right middle cerebral artery. The patient has a temperature of 38°C. A Westergren sedimentation rate is 115, and there is a variable systolic murmur.

1. What is the most likely cause of the aneurysm? **2.** What diagnostic procedures should be accomplished? **3.** What treatment should be instituted for the aneurysm? For infection? **4.** How long should medical treatment be continued? **5.** What antibiotics might be administered before organisms are identified?

III. A 34-year-old heterosexual male who is addicted to heroin is admitted with chief complaints of headache and drowsiness. The family is aware that the patient has been deteriorating intellectually for 4 months. He has a right hemiparesis. CT reveals multiple round "cystic" areas throughout the brain, and there are two larger ones over the vertex on the left at the frontoparietal junction.

1. What diagnoses should be considered? **2.** What is the most likely diagnosis? **3.** What tests should be performed? **4.** What therapy should be administered? **5.** What diagnostic or therapeutic procedures might a neurosurgeon have to offer?

IV. A 39-year-old black male is hospitalized because of progressive weakness in his lower extremities for 2 weeks. He has been losing weight and has had night sweats for 3 months. He has a productive cough. The patient noted generalized weakness a month earlier but has developed lower thoracic back pain and a bandlike pain around the lower chest and abdomen. He has been unable to walk because of weakness for the past 2 days. Chest x-ray shows bilateral diffuse infiltrates, more in the upper fields, and there is cavitation in the right apex. X-rays of the thoracic spine show collapse of the lower half of T8 and the upper half of T9. The disk space is eroded.

1. What diagnoses should be entertained? **2.** What diagnostic studies should be performed? **3.** Assuming acid-fast organisms are obtained from the sputum, how should the lesion of the thoracic spine be approached? **4.** What antibiotics should be instituted? When? **5.** What is the prognosis for the neurological deficits?

V. A 31-year-old female undergoes a diskectomy at the L4–L5 interspace for pain in the right buttock, radiating into the right foot. The pain is relieved except for localized back pain when she awakens from anesthesia, but 2 weeks later, the patient begins to have increasing back pain and excruciating pain in the right lower extremity in the same distribution as the pain the patient had postoperatively; but 2 days later, the patient's temperature is 102°. However, this pain is much more severe and exacerbated by any movement.

1. What is the most likely diagnosis? **2.** What is the most likely offending organism? **3.** What tests (procedure?) might be considered? **4.** What therapy might be instituted? **5.** Assuming the patient had a disk space infection, which resolves on therapy, what might one expect to see on radiographs taken a year later?

CHAPTER
27

Rehabilitative Therapy for Patients with Neurological Deficits

Ross H. Miller

The term *rehabilitation* derives from the Latin *re* plus *habilitas,* meaning "return to ability." It is used in many contexts today, including restoration of "good repute."

Medically, rehabilitation indicates a return to function and applies to restoration of patients with physical disorders to a level of ability to care for themselves and be productive. It is also used to indicate the therapy that is applied to children whose abilities have been limited from birth, as well as the therapy of patients with chronic pain, emotional disorders, or those whose dependence on chemicals has been such that they have been unable to adapt appropriately to society.

Historically, perhaps one of the most common applications of rehabilitative therapy in learning to adapt to society has been the instruction of individuals having undergone the loss of body parts causing limitations of specific function.

Rehabilitation plays a major role in the adaptation of individuals with neurological deficits to society. In many instances, its purpose is to teach patients to attend to their personal needs; indeed, this may be the extent of their capabilities. In other instances, rehabilitation is directed toward adapting to a former career in the presence of imposed limitations—or, in many instances, the development of a new career.

Thus there are many types of rehabilitation, depending upon a patient's age, experience, and deficits. This chapter will deal primarily with rehabilitation of the patient with neurological deficits. Experiences and problems in rehabilitation of patients with head injuries vary widely, depending upon the patient's deficits and emotional status. The needs of patients with head injuries differ from those with injuries to the spinal cord or peripheral nerves. Needs of patients with neurologic disabilities will also vary with age, those in children being quite different from the needs of mature adults.

A framework for identifying and solving the many problems associated with rehabilitation of the patient with neurological injury was introduced by Umphred in 1985[1] in a comprehensive treatise. References to specific resolutions for problems recommended by other authors will also be made in the text following.

☐ PLANNING REHABILITATIVE THERAPY

Planning for rehabilitation and the administration of physical therapy should begin as soon as feasible after injury and/or surgical therapy—often the day of injury or the day after surgery. In cases of elective surgical therapy, rehabilitative considerations may play a major role in the planning of surgical therapy. Ideally, the team treating the acute injury and the team directing the rehabilitation should be one and the same. However, for practical reasons, specialized units have been instituted for rehabilitation according to the type of neurologic deficit: severe head injury, injury to the spinal cord, chronic pain disorders, and the like.

Rehabilitative therapy should have specific goals that aim toward optimum levels of achievement but are also realistic. They must be within the medical, physical, and intellectual capabilities of the patient. Objectives that are unrealistically high will be recognized as such and, at the least, result in withdrawal—at the worst, in emotional depression. Goals that are too limited will end in loss of interest. The objectives of rehabilitation therapy are usually set by a rehabilitation team.[2,3]

☐ THE REHABILITATION TEAM

The rehabilitation team consists of many trained professionals: nurses; physical, speech, and occupational therapists;

psychologists; social workers; and vocational counselors. Members of the patient's family are also very important. The team is usually coordinated by a physician and may include other health-care professionals such as respiratory therapists, dieticians, and nutritionists. The physician is primarily responsible for the physical well-being of the patient. It is necessary for each member of the team to evaluate the patient to determine his or her capabilities, following which, goals will be set at a coordinated policy meeting.

The *nursing staff* play a most important role in the rehabilitation effort. They are often the most knowledgeable about the patient, have the most personal contact of all the professional team, and are essential in the encouragement of patients, helping them to understand their problems.[3]

Physical therapists provide expert care in evaluating the degree of disability of the disabled patient. They carry out evaluations and treatments aimed at optimizing the use of disabled muscles. This includes passive and active exercises designed to prevent contractures and increase strength in paretic muscles. Strengthening normal muscles that may be required for use with crutches or prostheses, day-to-day activities such as using wheelchairs, and making transfers from chair to bed are emphasized. Physical therapists maintain muscle activity with electrical stimulation during periods of denervation, and they maintain the positioning of extremities to prevent contractures or excessive stretching of muscles. They determine timing and train patients in ambulation. They also may play a role in pain relief through the application of heat and stimulation.

Occupational therapists are vital to the disabled patient's development of complex skills that may be required for daily living, in helping the patient with perceptual problems, and in the development of weakened extremities. During the course of evaluation, occupational therapists may call attention to the possibility that patients may not be able to develop certain skills a specific job will require. By tradition, occupational therapists have also become expert in the preparation of splints to maintain proper positioning of limbs during the period of rehabilitation.

Speech therapists are particularly helpful in determining capabilities of communication that patients possess. Speech may be impaired by loss of organs, i.e., the larynx or muscles of mastication or loss of innervation of some of these structures. Alternatively, speech may be impaired by injury to the brain in Broca's area or Wernicke's area. Loss of hearing may be a major factor in loss of communication skills. Speech therapists can differentiate these problems and develop compensatory skills utilizing those organs or capabilities still present.

The role of *psychologist* will depend in large measure on the type of injury that the patient has experienced. Evaluation by a neuropsychologist will be very important in determining the capabilities of a patient who has sustained a head injury involving specific parts of the brain, whereas a clinical psychologist may play a more important role in the evaluation and therapy of a patient who has sustained neurological deficits from extracranial injuries. Depression is a common prob-

lem in patients who have recently sustained paraplegia or loss of a limb or its function. Psychiatric support may be required when problems of adjustment are severe enough to require medication.

Social workers play a major role in evaluating or renewing family ties or in determining other external relationships for patients who have recently experienced injury to the nervous system. They play a major role in developing possible sources of financial support or in determining the possibilities for such external support as living quarters.

Vocational guidance counselors are helpful in developing capabilities for patients who have sustained injuries such that they are unable to return to former occupations but may be able to find future employment in another area. More or new education may be required.

The *physician* maintains a leadership role throughout the period of rehabilitation. Medical problems may be residual from the injury or even preexist it. There may be medical complications such as infections of the urinary tract or lungs. Medications may be required. Generally, the physician's role is assumed by a physiatrist in a specialized rehabilitation center, but in the presence of complicated injuries of the head or spine, the original treating physician may be the best-qualified person to oversee rehabilitation.

☐ INJURIES TO THE NERVOUS SYSTEM

The most common injuries to the nervous system requiring rehabilitation therapy are injuries to the brain and spinal cord. Injuries in either of these structures may result from trauma, ischemia (stroke in the case of the brain), other vascular insults, mass lesions, or other mishaps. In the case of children, many of the injuries may be congenital or a result of insults occurring at birth. Thus, trauma accounts for only a part of the lesions for which rehabilitative therapy is required.

☐ REHABILITATION OF PATIENTS WITH BRAIN INJURY

The first objective of rehabilitation of a patient with a head injury is the development of physical and cognitive independence, leading to becoming a contributing member of society. This may require relearning old skills or learning methods to compensate for skills that may have been lost. Rehabilitation is a creative, cooperative effort of the health-care team, the patient, and the family to optimize mental, social, and vocational aptitudes. Most specialized rehabilitation units dispense an assessment team to acute care hospitals to evaluate patients with head injuries and to determine whether they are candidates for transfer to a rehabilitation unit.

Rehabilitation should begin as soon as the patient is stable. Efforts are made (1) to prevent contractures, (2) to keep joints mobile, (3) to prevent decubiti, and (4) to avoid pulmonary and urinary tract infections. It is at this time that patients are fully evaluated, and the rehabilitation team develops a comprehensive plan. Education of the patient and family is imperative.

Guidelines for treatment published by the Texas Head Injury Foundation are the following:[4]

1. Treatment should be adjusted to the patient's level of function.
2. Treatment should be consistent, repetitious, and structured.
3. As the patient's ability improves, the difficulty of the task should be increased and the degree of structure should be decreased.
4. Results of performance should be consistently provided to the patient.
5. Information should be presented via more than one sensory avenue.
6. Information and tasks should be relevant to the needs and interests of the patient.

These guidelines of therapy provide the basis for progressive cognitive growth. Progress is largely dependent upon the patient's ability to cooperate. While the physical consequences and recommended medical and surgical therapy for patients having sustained head injury have been presented in Chap. 18, rehabilitation therapy must continue until optimum training has been achieved or the patient has become independent and, optimally, is able to contribute to society.

The rate and course of recovery from a head injury vary according to the severity of the injury and structures most severely injured. Rehabilitation therapists at Rancho Los Amigos Hospital in Downey, California, have categorized levels of recovery of cognitive functioning.[5,6] The categories have been utilized as a guide to indicate the level and type of activity in which a therapist or family member might realistically expect to engage the patient who has experienced a severe head injury.[4]

I. *No response.* Patients appear to be in a deep sleep and do not respond to stimulation.
II. *Generalized response.* Patients appear to be sleeping and respond inconsistently to stimuli. They may withdraw to painful stimuli or pull at catheters, but once the stimulus is removed they will remain stuporous. Patients in this state may show a bias toward family members, responding to them but not to others.
III. *Localized response.* Patients react more specifically toward stimuli, but responses are still inconsistent. Patients may vocalize to painful stimuli and they may follow commands, but slowly and inconsistently. They are unable to cooperate and do not discriminate. Verbalization is incoherent and/or inappropriate.
IV. *Confused-agitated.* At this point, patients are in a heightened state of activity, but behavior is frequently bizarre, often inappropriate, and sometimes aggressive. Patients are unable to cooperate with treatment.

They lack recall in the short term, although they may continue to react to past events.

V. *Confused, inappropriate, and nonagitated.* Patients are alert and respond to simple commands, but responses break down with more complex commands. They may show some agitated behavior as a result of external stimuli. Their attention is focused on the environment but they are unable to remain focused on a task for a prolonged period. Verbalization may be inappropriate, and confabulation may occur. Memory is severely impaired and such patients are unable to learn new information. They respond best to themselves, their bodies, comfort, and family members. They can usually perform self-care. They may be irresponsible in that they may wander off the ward.
VI. *Confused-appropriate.* At this point, patients may show goal-directed behavior, but they are still dependent on external direction. They follow simple commands consistently and carry out relearned tasks. There are still memory problems, and this may lead to incorrect responses. However, responses may be appropriate to situations. The responses may be delayed and patients show decreased ability to process information. Patients may be demonstrating awareness to situations, recognizing when they do not know answers. Selective attention to tasks may be impaired. They may perform common daily duties.
VII. *Automatic-appropriate.* Patients appear appropriate and oriented in hospital and home settings but are frequently "robot-like." They have shallow recall. There is increased awareness to self and the environment but these patients lack insight into their condition. They learn, but at a reduced rate. They become independent in self-care and require minimal supervision. They are able to initiate tasks but judgment is impaired. They should not drive.
VIII. *Purposeful and appropriate.* At this point, patients are alert and oriented, able to recall and integrate events, and they are aware of and responsive to their culture. They may be independent within limits of physical capabilities. It is at this point that vocational rehabilitation counseling is indicated. There may still be decreased ability when compared to abilities prior to injury, such as reasoning, tolerance, stress, and judgment in new situations. Patients are functional in society.

While these categories retrace the progressive growth in a patient's cognitive skills, neurological deficits require specific therapy, the timing of which will depend on the patient's ability to cooperate. The type of therapy is indicated by the category of recovery the patient has reached. For instance, paresis or paralysis may require frequent passive, and ultimately active mobilization of affected extremities.

Details of specific goals and neurologic rehabilitation treatment procedures have been provided by Smith in her comprehensive review of the evaluation and therapy for patients with traumatic head injuries.[7] Progressive ambulation is required in virtually all patients. Nutrition must be maintained, and other bodily functions addressed. (See Chap. 18.) When spasticity is a problem, appropriate medications such as baclofen or dantrolene sodium may be prescribed.[4]

We have been reluctant to prescribe diazepam over prolonged periods because of experiences with dependency. Appropriate anticonvulsants must be administered in the presence of seizures.

Throughout the rehabilitation process, the family remains a primary part of the program. Members must be kept informed of the progress. They will usually wish to learn techniques, and instruction should be provided. When discharge planning is begun, it is the family who will assume primary responsibility in most cases. This can be accomplished most efficiently if family members have been receiving instruction all along and feel they are a part of the program throughout the recovery period. It may be necessary for them to assume responsibility for feedings, for catheters, for physiotherapy, and for further development of communication skills. Their efforts will be more rewarding if they are aware of the general development of cognitive skills. It is often the family who will have to assume responsibility for obtaining further outpatient therapy. They will be more capable if they can communicate with the rehabilitation team and know the purposes of further treatments.

☐ SPINAL CORD INJURY

An estimated 11,000 cases of spinal injury causing some degree of neurological deficit occur in the United States each year, of which 7000 to 8000 are the result of trauma.[8] Costs run to billions of dollars annually.

Patients with quadriplegia or paraplegia secondary to spinal cord injury offer the greatest challenge for the rehabilitation team. Patients with neurological deficits following spinal cord injury must receive intensive nursing care. The presence of vertebral fracture and/or dislocation requires immediate immobilization and stabilization of the patient. Beds must provide for this stabilization as well as for the relief of pressure on the skin and soft tissues. Halo traction and immobilization are used on patients with cervical fractures to prevent any movement in the spinal canal that might exacerbate spinal cord injury. If surgical intervention for decompression and/or stabilization is indicated, it should be integrated with an overall management plan.

Complications other than those arising within a few hours or days of the injury include the potential for contracture of muscles, ankylosis of joints, osteoporosis, hypercalcemia, and fractures—all of which may result from long-term immobilization. (This has been discussed in Chap. 19.) Some degree of prevention must be accomplished whenever possible by early and intensive activation of muscles.[7]

The high excretion of calcium in the urine may lead to formation of stones in the urinary tract.

Spinal deformities may complicate spinal injuries at the time of the injury or at a later date, often adding to the prior incompetence of the posterior ligaments of the spine (described in Chapter 19). Heterotopic ossification or bone formation may occur in collagenous elements within or around paralyzed muscles. The etiology is not clear, but there is usually clinical evidence of an initial inflammatory process. Although the ossification does not originate in the joints, ankylosis occurs in about 20 percent of cases. Decubitus ulcers frequently complicate the ectopic calcification. Diphosphonates may be administered to prevent the crystallization of calcium phosphate, but they have no effect on mature ectopic bone.[7] Surgical resection may be the only applicable therapy once the bone has matured.

Pain, most commonly perceived at the site of the spinal injury, and spasticity are two of the most severe complications of spinal injury. (Therapy is discussed in Chap. 24.) There are other serious difficulties as well. Loss of sensation of pain and proprioception and also failure of motion make the patient liable to decubitus ulcerations. Daily inspection of the skin is necessary. Ulcerations are prone to occur when the skin is moist. Prevention of ulcers requires frequent change in position on a bed designed and operated in such a fashion as to remove pressure from any point of the skin, at least every 2 hours. This may be accomplished with beds that rotate from side to side or on mattresses that alternate sites of pressure on the skin periodically. The skin must be kept dry, requiring diversion of urine and the absorption of fluids from other sources such as perspiration or spillage. Ring supports are to be avoided as they restrict circulation. Sheepskin sheets may be helpful.

The occurrence of decubitus ulcers requires excision and coverage with skin flaps if the lesion extends below the skin surface. Early irritation may be treated by keeping pressure off the wound and keeping the wound dry.

Urinary bladder and bowel care will prevent urinary retention and infection. Intermittent catheterization helps to develop an automatic bladder. Subsequently, condom catheters may be used on the male to collect urine, but in the female intermittent catheterization on a long-term basis may be required. Specialized diets and scheduled routines for enemas and/or laxatives may be necessary in order to train the bowels.

The patient's bed should be fitted with footboards to keep ankles and toes in a neutral position. Soft braces are used to fix the lower extremities in a neutral position and to prevent contractures. The skin beneath the braces and footboards must be inspected daily for "pressure areas" and early decubiti.

Exercises to strengthen unaffected muscles are started as soon as possible to enable patients to maintain and increase their strength for use in daily activities. Gradual progression toward a vertical position should be begun as soon as spinal stability is achieved. Maintaining the horizontal position for a prolonged period will result in loss of sympathetic tone and consequent hypotension when the patient does eventually assume the upright position. Therefore, initial efforts toward the upright position should be made slowly and deliberately, with simultaneous monitoring of systemic blood pressure in case the patient develops symptoms of hypotension, such as vertigo, diaphoresis, or decrease of vision.

Paraplegics and quadriplegics should be given training and exercises such that they are able to use a wheelchair. Training for walking in braces and use of crutches are appropriate for some paraplegics.

Development of specialized (computerized) devices that stimulate denervated muscles to augment walking is under way in some spinal treatment centers and may provide additional support for victims of spinal injury in the future, but such devices are not routinely used today. Motorized wheelchairs requiring minimal effort for direction are available to increase the mobility of patients with severe limitations of locomotion. Intrathecal administration of baclofen may be helpful.

The treatment of chronic spinal cord injury with spasticity is difficult. Patients with this condition should be given muscle-stretching exercises to maintain range of motion. Baclofen and dantrolene sodium are often helpful in reducing nocturnal spasms.

Those patients with extreme flexion contractures may be surgical candidates for a destructive lesion of the spinal cord to convert the spastic into a flaccid paralysis, thus allowing easier rehabilitation of the patient. These destructive lesions are carried out only after a prolonged period of unsuccessful rehabilitation. Surgical procedures used to convert spastic to flaccid paralysis include spinal cordectomy, myelotomy, alcohol or phenol destruction of the intraspinal elements, and, in some patients, anterior rhizotomy, which has been helpful for focal control of spastic muscles. (See Chap. 25.)

NEUROGENIC BLADDER

Early in the course of spinal cord injury, the urinary bladder is flaccid and becomes distended. The distension, if chronic, will destroy autonomic nerve fibers in the bladder wall. This can be prevented by keeping the bladder small, using indwelling catheters or by intermittent catheterization every 4 to 6 hours. Such measures will allow the bladder to fill and be emptied on a regular basis, and they must continue indefinitely. Female patients may use indwelling catheters to keep bladder residual to 100 cm^3 or less.

Transurethral resection in males and urethral sphincterotomy in female patients can help lower residual urine levels. The small spastic bladder is difficult to treat and is annoying to the patient. Involuntary loss of urine occurs with flexor spasms of the extremities, at which time the bladder detrusor muscles also contract. Renal stones occur frequently in spinal cord–injured patients. These may be prevented by acidifying the urine.

☐ PERIPHERAL NERVE INJURY

The evaluation and surgical therapy of patients with injuries to peripheral nerves have been reviewed in Chap. 21. It may

be helpful to note as well that after surgery, bracing of affected joints will be necessary often in order to prevent contractures. Daily passive motion of joints which have been immobilized will prevent fixation, and stretching of muscles may be necessary to prevent deformities, particularly of the fingers. Periodic transcutaneous stimulation will prevent muscles from deteriorating and will help to maintain functional capability of the motor endplates. Early passive motion and active exercises are applied to those muscles with partial function. Electromyograms reveal the extent of denervation of muscles and repeat examinations demonstrate rates of reinnervation.

Denervation pain may be a major problem in patients with peripheral nerve injury. Rehabilitation of such patients with chronic pain following a peripheral nerve injury may be difficult. Antidepressant medications have proven helpful in many cases. Surgical therapy usually involves the production of destructive lesions at the dorsal root entry zone. (See Chap. 24.)

Causalgia is common following partial nerve lesions, most commonly involving the median nerve, and may be seen with ulnar and posterior tibial nerve lesions. In selected patients, blocking of the injured nerve or the sympathetic ganglia with a short-acting local anesthetic may help control the pain and confirm the diagnosis of causalgia. Occasionally, interruption of the sympathetic innervation to the painful area is indicated for permanent relief of the pain. (See Chap. 21.)

☐ CERVICAL AND LOW BACK PAIN

Patients with cervical and lumbar back pain are frequently seen on rehabilitation services for heat and massage. This may relieve pain, at least temporarily. The hope is that relief of pain with these forms of conservative therapy will defer and possibly remove the need for surgical treatment of a protruded cervical or lumbar disk.

Patients referred for treatment must have an initial neurological examination, roentgenograms, and computerized tomography (CT) or magnetic resonance imaging (MRI) of the spine to exclude a tumor or extruded disk material which, if not removed surgically, could cause deterioration of the neurological status of the patient.

Patients seen for acute lumbar pain as a result of strain are treated with heat and massage to the area of pain and to the muscles which are in spasm. After some improvement is seen for lumbar pain, the therapy will progress to instructions in the use of a firm bed for rest and relaxation of the lumbar muscles. William's exercises are also demonstrated and patients are instructed in their daily use. These movements will help decrease the lumbar muscular pain and often provide enough relief to exclude surgery.

Pain in the cervical area secondary to nerve compression by an osteophyte or protruded cervical disk is treated first with heat and massage to relax the cervical muscles, followed by mild cervical traction.

If there is an increase in the patient's pain and/or a neurological deficit occurs during treatment, the neurological surgeon should reevaluate the patient for surgical treatment of the offending lesion. Daily neurological examination is important to evaluate the progress the patient is making with nonsurgical treatment.

REFERENCES

1. Umphred DA: Conceptual model: A framework for clinical problem solving, in Umphred DA (ed): *Neurological Rehabilitation,* vol 3. St. Louis, Mosby, 1985, chap 1, pp 3–25.
2. Kottke FJ, Lehmann JF, Stillwell GK: Preface to the third edition, in Kottke FJ, Lehmann JE (eds): *Krusen's Handbook of Physical Medicine and Rehabilitation,* 4th ed. Philadelphia, Saunders, 1990, pp xxvii–xxxviii.
3. Anderson TP: Rehabilitation management and the rehabilitation team in medical rehabilitation, in Basmajian JW, Kirby RL (eds): *Medical Rehabilitation.* Baltimore, Williams & Wilkins, 1984, chap 9, pp 144–151.
4. Lehmkuhl LD: *Comprehensive Rehabilitation of the Head Injured Person. A Family Manual.* Houston, The Texas Head Injury Foundation, 1985, pp 74.
5. Hagen C, Malkmus D, Durham P: Levels of cognitive functioning, in *Rehabilitation of the Head Injured Adult*: *Comprehensive Physical Management.* Downey, Rancho Los Amigos Hospital, 1972, pp 13–17.
6. Malkmus D, Stenderup K: Levels of cognitive functioning (revised), in *Rehabilitation of the Head Injured Adult*: *Comprehensive Physical Management.* Downey, Rancho Los Amigos Hospital, 1974, pp 14–17.
7. Smith SS: Traumatic head injuries, in Umphred DA (ed): *Neurological Rehabilitation.* St. Louis, Mosby, 1985, chap 10, pp 249–288.
8. Schneider FJ: Traumatic spinal cord injury, in Umphred DA (ed): *Neurological Rehabilitation.* St. Louis, Mosby, 1985, chap 12, pp 314–373.

☐ STUDY QUESTIONS

I. John is a 13-year-old male who sustained an extradural hematoma on the left when he was struck by an automobile while riding his bicycle. The hematoma was evacuated, but the injury left him with a right hemiparesis and great difficulty speaking. He seems to understand quite well and follows directions but can utter only a few words a week after the injury.

1. What steps should be taken toward getting John back to school? **2.** Who should participate in John's care? **3.** What evaluations should be made? **4.** What expectations might be considered? **5.** What goals should be set?

II. A 6-year-old boy is referred to the pediatric neurosurgeon because of spastic diplegia, present from birth. The child is alert and intellectually near normal, but he cannot walk and can barely hold food in his hands because of the spasticity. He had had lengthening of his Achilles tendons and division of the adductors of his thighs in the past. He has minimal deformities because of the excellent care he has experienced. He is scheduled for interruption of abnormally firing motor fibers intradurally.

1. When should the rehabilitation team be called into this case? **2.** Who should participate in the team for this patient? **3.** When should physical therapy be begun? **4.** What part might occupational therapy play in this patient's therapy? **5.** What drugs might be used to reduce spasticity?

III. A 22-year-old right-handed male draftsman sustains a missile injury to the left cerebral hemisphere. Wounds are debrided and closed as an emergency. When the patient awakes, he cannot speak and has a severe right hemiparesis.

1. When should the rehabilitation team be assembled to begin evaluation and therapy of the patient? **2.** When should physical therapy begin passive exercises? Active exercises? **3.** What is the likelihood that this patient will be able to return to his former occupation? **4.** How might a speech therapist participate in the rehabilitation? **5.** What medications are likely to play a role in this patient's rehabilitation?

IV. A 26-year-old female sustains a head injury from a head-on collision in her automobile. When admitted to the emergency room she has a Glasgow coma scale rating of 8. After 25 h, this had advanced to 11. CT reveals no hematomas. There are normal cisterns, and she has no lateralizing signs.

1. What is the anticipated neurological progress? **2.** What stages of recovery might she be expected to pass through?

3. At what point might one expect the patient to become responsible for her actions? **4.** When could this patient drive? **5.** What advice and instructions might the family be given assuming the patient is discharged 4 days after injury?

V. A 40-year-old male sustains a compression fracture of T11 in a motor vehicle accident. He is rendered immediately paraplegic. He has no voluntary activity of his lower extremities and no sensation to pinprick, deep pain, or position from T12 distally. He has no rectal tone. The body of the T11 vertebra is collapsed and the core of the vertebra is displaced into the spinal canal, almost completely occluding it.

1. What objectives might be formulated for surgical therapy? **2.** What type of bed might this patient be placed on? **3.** What type of care should be administered for evacuation of urine? For bowels? **4.** What goals would be appropriate for rehabilitation? **5.** What concerns might be maintained for skin care?

CHAPTER 28

Future Developments in Neurosurgery

Marshall B. Allen, Jr.

When this book was being planned, there was a consensus among the authors that a chapter should be devoted to anticipated developments in neurosurgery. One objective might be to give the resident, the future neurosurgeon, some background and ideas for subjects that might be fruitful for investigation; another might be to help orient special training.

A logical approach to such an endeavor might be to review current literature. Since it is impossible to survey every area that might offer future contributions to neurosurgery, five topics have been selected because of their exceptional promise—in some cases because development in a given area appears to be complete but applications to clinical neurosurgery have not yet been generally instituted, and in other cases because preliminary reports suggest promise but techniques in the area have yet to be developed.

Without question, much of what is presented here will prove to have been guesswork ten years from now, but at this time some areas that appear promising include: (1) the use of magnetic impulses to stimulate and record the nervous system, (2) fetal surgery, (3) treatment of vasoconstriction from vasospasm and arteriosclerosis, (4) transplantation of neural tissue, and (5) computer-assisted stereotactic procedures that may be applied to open surgery and radiotherapy.

One area that will not receive attention in this review is the manipulation of genes, which in the future will play without doubt a major role in the approach of the physician to the diagnosis and management of patients who are or might be candidates for certain neoplasms and degenerative diseases. Genetic research and manipulation will influence the course of neurosurgery, as well as oncology and medicine in general. The implications of genetic manipulation appear to have such a broad and profound impact that a meaningful discussion in this text is not possible. For the same reason, anticipated developments in reconstruction of the spine will not be discussed either. Current developments have been reviewed elsewhere in this text; future developments will depend on types of instrumentation that have yet to be developed. Present-day technology and technique is progressing so rapidly that it is difficult to remain current, and it is equally difficult to analyze definitively the results of any particular type of instrumentation. For future developments in reconstruction of the spine the reader is referred to Chaps. 19 and 20.

This chapter ends with some general comments on the use of computers in making clinical decisions. At present, computers play a major role in imaging, orientation of stereotactic probes, planning radiation therapy, and many administrative hospital operations—to say nothing of the parts they play in teaching and institutional accounting. Doubtless, in future, computers will play an even greater part in the planning and selection of therapies for patients, as well as in the evaluation of physician services. The human elements of judgment, ability, and experience must not be abandoned, however.

☐ THE USE OF MAGNETIC IMPULSES TO STIMULATE AND RECORD NERVOUS SYSTEM FUNCTION

Magnetic impulses may be used to stimulate and record the electrophysiologic activity of the nervous system.[1,2] Probes emitting such magnetic impulses can deliver stimuli to either peripheral nerves or the brain with effects similar to those set off by electrical stimulation. One advantage of magnetic stimulation is activation of the nervous system—either peripheral nerves or brain—without penetration of the skin; the stimulation is virtually painless. Transcutaneous stimuli may be used to provide evoked responses of the sensory and motor pathways.

Magnetic impulses are generated by passing large electrical currents through a coil.[3] The strongest magnetic stimuli are produced by loops at the periphery of the coil.[1] Weaker impulses are generated by loops near the center of the coil, and no energy is generated at the coil's center. This effect within the coil results in imprecise sites of stimulation, which is of significance in the stimulation of peripheral nerves and functional cortical areas.

Peripheral nerve stimulation is accomplished with round coils which have an outside diameter of up to 9.2 cm or with pointed probes, which measure 8.6 × 10.6 cm.[4] They may be applied to the skin overlying the nerve that is to be stimulated in one of several different ways: orthogonally, longitudinally, tangentially, off-center, symmetrically, obliquely, or transversely. Coils do not require the use of substances to connect them to the skin. They do not penetrate the skin, although, for convenience, they usually are applied to the skin surface. It is not necessary to remove clothing for stimulation.[5]

Magnetic impulses travel through body tissues painlessly and without attenuation between the probe and the nervous tissue being stimulated.[3] Stimulation may be applied to peripheral nerves, nerve roots in the spinal canal, at the base of the brain, or to the motor or sensory cortex....[1,3–12] Magnetic stimuli penetrate to considerable depths without causing large electrical fields at the surface. By contrast, electrical stimulation does cause pain, and impulses obtained by recordings are attenuated and distorted, as are electrical impulses applied for stimulation.

Magnetic impulses decrease in magnitude in relation to the inverse square of the distance from the coil. Currents induced at the surface of the skin by magnetic stimulation will be oriented parallel to the skin and will thus activate structures from a different orientation than that of electrical stimuli.[3] Use of magnetic stimulation provides the capability of obtaining evoked responses to percutaneous stimulation of nerve roots as well as stimulation of the motor cortex.[12,13] Interestingly enough, latencies before motor responses evoked by stimulation of the motor cortex are shortened when muscles are slightly contracted voluntarily.

The capabilities of magnetic stimulation have already demonstrated their usefulness in the diagnosis of multiple sclerosis, degenerative ataxic disorders, and nerve root compression by herniated intervertebral disks.[12,14,15] Latencies are significantly prolonged in patients with multiple sclerosis, and the degree of prolongation is greatest in patients who have the most severe clinical involvement.[15]

Significant abnormalities are found in patients with Friedreich's ataxia and other conditions involving demyelination or degeneration of the CNS.[16] Stimulation of lumbosacral roots by stimulation in the central sacral region reveals reduction in the compound muscle action potentials and prolongation of the latencies in patients with radiculopathies proved by surgery or imaging studies.[12]

Cerebral stimulation for evoked potential monitoring to identify sites of involvement with spondylosis and use of electrical current during the course of intraspinal surgery are currently recommended. Cortical stimulation is thought to be superior to somatosensory evoked potential monitoring since motor pathways may be monitored.[17,18] Activation of the motor cortex with magnetic stimuli should prove superior in this type of monitoring since the stimulation is more easily applied and painless, but responses evoked in the lower extremities by transcranial stimulation with magnetic stimuli are of smaller amplitude and more difficult to elicit than evoked responses in the hand.[3]

Stimulation probes are bulky and the points of activation of peripheral nerves are imprecise, rendering the use of magnetic stimulation impractical for nerve conduction studies, except in those cases where proximal nerve trunks or nerve roots are stimulated.[1,6,12] However, sites of stimulation of peripheral nerves are not imprecise enough to influence significantly the determination of latencies of evoked potentials.

Magnetoencephalography (MEG) is the recording of magnetic signals from the brain. Electrical activity at the junction of the dendrite with the body of the neuron produces a magnetic field.[19] Magnetic signals are weak, about 10^{-13} tesla when compared to the normal geomagnetic field of 5×10^{-8} tesla.[2] Typical urban noise is recorded as about 5×10^{-7} tesla/Hz. Thus, magnetic signals from the brain are about one billionth the strength of the earth's magnetic field.[19] MEG became feasible with the development of sensitive superconducting quantum interference devices (SQUIDS) and gradiometers, systems of detector coils that filter signals originating within the body from distant sources of noise.[2,19,20] Since 1975 there has been a steady development of MEG systems, evolving from single-channel probes to current systems that comprise up to 37 channels. It is speculated that future systems may have as many as 100 channels, allowing for monitoring of the entire brain with a single probe placement.[1,21]

Scalp electroencephalographic recordings indirectly reflect the electrical activity of the brain: Electrical currents are transmitted and their volume conducted through the brain, skull, and scalp, which are sources of inhomogeneous impedance that result in attenuation and distortion of electrical activity. MEG has the theoretical advantage that magnetic signals are not significantly affected by the medium through which they pass.[2]

Magnetic potentials are recorded from the cranial surface as two finite regions of opposite polarity (extrema) that are juxtaposed. The generator of these extrema lies deep along the bisection of the line joining the extrema, and its direction is perpendicular to the line. Its depth is linearly related to the distance between the extrema.[2]

The location of the generator is found by an inverse solution. A number of spheres of known radii are used to approximate mathematically the patient's recorded extrema. The radius of whichever sphere most closely approximates the measured extrema is then used to calculate the source location.[22] The head is not an absolute sphere, particularly in low-convexity regions such as the temporal. This renders the inverse solution potentially less accurate in these areas. However, comparison of the spatial resolution of electrically and magnetically recorded epileptiform and evoked potentials indicates that the inverse solution usually localizes magnetic dipoles to within approximately 1 cm of electrically recorded potentials.

MEG compares well with other functional imaging techniques and depth electrode recordings for determining sites of epileptic foci.[23,24,25] EEG and MEG recordings of interictal events often show quite different wave forms and different temporal relations, which may reflect different physiological processes or generators. Single-channel MEG recordings have demonstrated abnormal signals from epileptic patients, even when abnormal signals were not present on EEG.[23] Neuromagnetic signals have proven to be sufficient to establish the location, depth, orientation, and polarity of currents underlying paroxysmal discharges.[24,25] An orderly magnetic field pattern accompanies interictal spikes.[26] Simultaneous multichannel MEG recordings (e.g., 37-channel MEG) may resolve some of the spatiotemporal discrepancies between EEG and limited-channel MEG recordings.

EEG and MEG compliment each other in the investigation of sources of epilepsy. In both EEG and MEG, the signal recorded depends on the relative orientation of the discharging dipole and the recording apparatus. When combined, the EEG and MEG offer good possibilities for localizing sites of cerebral activity, either spontaneous or induced.

MEG recordings of evoked responses may aid in the localization of segments of the somatosensory cortex activated by peripheral stimulation.[27] Various components of the somatosensory response to stimulation of nerves in the arms or legs provide different dipole sources in the projection areas. Both ipsilateral and contralateral responses are recorded from secondary somatosensory areas.[28]

Neuromagnetic recordings of the human auditory cortex have demonstrated that sounds of different frequencies produce responses at different sites in the primary auditory cortex.[29] There is an orderly progression in the tonographic map within the auditory cortex. This finding supports the hypothesis that there is a direct mapping of the cochlea on the cortex. Responses vary in amplitude according to the alertness of the subject.

MEG studies of patients during attacks of migraine have shown changes similar to those of spreading depression in laboratory animals, causing a biphasic slow wave followed by reduction of activity for as much as 10 min.

This brief review concludes that magnetic stimulation will provide an effective means of obtaining evoked potentials in alert patients being investigated for various CNS diseases, particularly multiple sclerosis, and other degenerative disorders in the future. Magnetic stimulations may also be used increasingly as a means of investigating radiculopathies. If the instrumentation can be significantly improved, magnetic stimulations will surely play a major role in nerve conduction studies. Magnetoencephalography shows great promise as a complimentary modality for the localization of sources of epileptic activity, and it may play a role in diagnosing a number of other illnesses such as migraine. It presents a most valuable research tool for the topographic localization of various functional areas of the human cerebral cortex.

☐ FETAL SURGERY

Major changes in pediatric neurosurgery during the next decade will involve the delineation of indications and the development of techniques for the general institution of surgery in the correction of congenital defects in fetuses. A review of fetal surgery with its expectations during the current decade has been published recently, and this section will draw heavily from that review.[30]

Hydrocephalus and myelomeningoceles are the two most common congenital defects involving the nervous system. There are indications that the earlier hydrocephalus is treated, the less severe the deficits may be. It could be that prenatal treatment of dysraphism could reduce the consequent deformities since a more physiological development might result.

Prenatal detection of abnormalities in the development of the neural tube has been made possible by the availability of ultrasound and examinations of amniotic fluid for karyotypes, alphafetoprotein, and acetylcholinesterase—techniques which are relatively common now; however, it must be recognized that even with detailed examination 20 to 40 percent of abnormalities will be missed.[30]

There have been reports of attempts to treat hydrocephalus in utero since 1981.[30–35] These have primarily consisted of inserting ventriculostomies so that fluid from the ventricles can drain into the amniotic cavity—the hypothesis being that the earlier the intraventricular pressure is reduced, the less damage there will be to the cerebral mantle.

Evans et al. indicate that as of July 1, 1989, there had been 45 cases reported to the international registry, the shunts being performed at 25 ±2.73 weeks with a range of 18 to 31 weeks of gestation.[30] Thirty-four out of forty-one treated fetuses had survived. Of the seven fetal deaths, four were due to trauma at the time of surgery or the onset of premature labor, which occurred within 48 hours of the operative procedure. Of the 38 survivors with a follow-up of 12.2 ±5.8 months (range, 6–36 months), 14 are reported to be normal. The remaining 24 have varying degrees of neurological deficits with 18, or 53 percent, of the survivors having severe handicaps. This indicates that about one-third of the entire series was normal; however, ventriculostomies have allowed the remainder of the abnormal fetuses to survive.

Most of the intellectual and neurological deficits were due to associated lesions, cortical blindness, seizure disorders, and spastic diplegia.[30] In this series of patients there were cases which could have been rejected for shunting had selection criteria been more rigidly followed. Individuals with holoprosencephaly and autosomal trisomies should have been excluded from surgery. All were late in reaching their developmental milestones and had tested less than 60 in developmental quotients. The conclusion is that the results have been quite disappointing, but efforts should continue with stricter selection criteria since the history of untreated hydrocephalus is so poor. There should be continued attempts at refining techniques in the selection and treatment of these devastating lesions.

There are reasons to believe that at least some of the severe effects of myelomeningocele might be reversed by prenatal repair. For the selection of cases for fetal surgery there must be a knowledge of the natural history of the lesion which is being treated, an assessment of the danger to the mother and infant, and a practiced team with good equipment for carrying out the surgical procedure in utero. One of the greatest problems with such prenatal surgery is the induction of premature labor. A combination of sedatives and prostaglandin inhibitors is used to suppress uterine contractions.

Much experience and success in the treatment of diaphragmatic hernia in utero is being accumulated despite an exceptionally high mortality rate in the initial tries.[38] Normally, there is a very high postnatal mortality rate with this lesion.

Since these are such complex procedures with so many implications—including the lives of two individuals—and since the candidates for fetal surgery are so rare, institutions offering such therapies will surely be limited, but fetal surgery for congenital defects will undoubtedly become available in this decade.[30,38]

TREATMENT OF IMPAIRED CEREBRAL PERFUSION FROM CHRONIC VASOSPASM AND ARTERIOSCLEROTIC NARROWING

CEREBROVASCULAR SURGERY

For many years chronic vasospasm has presented a great challenge to surgeons treating subarachnoid hemorrhage. The incidence of neurological deficits and even mortality in patients who have recently experienced subarachnoid hemorrhage has been disappointing and has rendered surgery hazardous during the period between 2 days and 2 weeks following a subarachnoid hemorrhage. An almost incalculable number of drugs have been tried in the treatment of chronic vasospasm, without success. The only therapy that has enjoyed consistent success has been the use of artificial hypertension and volume expansion, approaches that would appear to be contraindicated while defects in vessel walls are present.[39–43] Treatment of ruptured aneurysms in the early period after hemorrhage is now common.

The pathophysiology of chronic vasospasm has been debated, with many contending that the clinical state is due to muscle contraction, but growing evidence suggests that the basic lesion is a pathological state. Recent reports indicate

that cerebral vasospasm due to subarachnoid hemorrhage and trauma to the vessel walls responds to transluminal dilatation of the vessels by microballoons. This is encouraging and consistent with the reports which suggest that vasospasm is a pathological condition of the vessel walls.[44,45] Evaluation of cerebral vasospasm by use of transcranial Doppler techniques offers hope that we will soon have specific indications for such therapy.[46]

The finding that anastomosis of extracranial blood vessels to branches of a middle cerebral artery does not provide statistically significant evidence of clinical improvement was a disappointment to most surgeons who were charged with the care of stroke patients.[47,48] Other techniques designed for revascularization or for interrupting the relentless course of degenerative lesions of blood vessels supplying the brain must be analyzed for effectiveness in preventing cerebral ischemia. Techniques that have appeared include (1) omental transplantation, (2) laser angioplasty, and (3) balloon dilitation.

Goldsmith, Chen, and Duckett recommended revascularization of the brain by intact omentum almost 20 years ago.[49] Through a series of subsequent reports Goldsmith has presented a strong case for the use of such techniques to prevent or treat cerebral ischemia.[50–53] On superficial observation, there is a strong reason to question whether this technique offers much that has not been offered by the by-pass procedure. The technique has been supported by the Chinese efforts and certainly deserves comprehensive evaluation.[54–57]

Of considerable interest, also, are a series of reports indicating success with the use of lasers in transluminal angioplasty. Most of these reports are related to angioplasty in coronary vessels, but the techniques have been applied to other vessels and may be applicable to vessels supplying the brain.[58–60]

TRANSPLANTATION OF NEURAL TISSUES

The history of transplantation of neural tissues in mammals extends over a hundred years.[60,61] Thompson reported on the implantation of a segment of cortex in a dog's brain in 1890.[62] He speculated that transplantation of neural tissues would have a place in future research. The first well-documented survival of a graft to the CNS in newborn rats was reported in 1917 by Dunn.[63] In 1930, May reported on intraocular grafts of tissue removed from the CNS, and in 1940, Le Gros Clark gave detailed descriptions of the survival of cortical transplants.[64,65]

The anterior chamber of the eye became a favorite target for implanting grafts since the transplanted tissues could be observed there. This was the site that Greene and Arnold chose to transplant embryonic grafts of CNS tissue, which they reported in 1945,[66] and in 1970, it was the site that Olson and a subsequent cadre of colleagues used.[67] In another report of the same year Olson also demonstrated axonal growth and secretion of neurotransmitters by the transplanted neurons.[68] It was this series of reports that sparked great interest and investigation into the possibilities of neural tissue transplantation.

Lund and Hauschka, using fetal transplants of CNS tissue, reported on the synaptic specificity in mammalian brain, and Stenevi, Bjorklund, and Syendgard demonstrated that neurons taken from fetal brains could survive transplantation into adult mammalian brains. They outlined the factors important for successful neural transplantation in adult host rat brains.[69,70] Perlow et al., shortly thereafter, showed that the transplanted fetal neurons could survive, grow axons, and produce neurotransmitters with resultant reversal of motor abnormalities in host animals with movement disorders that resembled Parkinson's disease.[71] In subsequent reports, evidence has been presented that animal models with lesions resulting in learning deficits somewhat resembling Alzheimer's disease would respond to the implantation of dopaminergic and cholinergic neurons, and they reported significant improvement in swimming performance in old animals that had undergone grafting.[72]

These and many other reports of experimental successes in the treatment of animal models with lesions of the septohippocampal system by grafting with monoaminergic and cholinergic neurones lead to interest in clinical trials.[73–75] Even more dramatic successes in the treatment of animals having experienced lesions in the nigrostriatal pathways by grafting with mesencephalic-dopamine-rich neurons taken from 16–17 day old fetuses support this.[71,76]

Evidence is that tissues most likely to provide appropriate neurotransmitters leading to improvement in learning or the treatment of movement disorders would be those that contain monoaminergic or cholinergic neurons or neurons capable of producing dopamine or acetylcholine.[61] Sources for donor cells which have shown promise are: (1) the septum or brain stem of fetuses, from which most experimental material has come; (2) the peripheral nervous system; and (3) cell lines.

There is evidence that the sympathetic ganglia and adrenal medulla of mature individuals produce the neurotransmitters necessary for successful reimplantation, and that mature neurons from these organs would grow axons and produce neurotransmitters. Thus the peripheral nervous system provides for the capability of making autologous grafts. Neuroblastomas, tumors of immature cells of the nervous system, reportedly, can be converted into mature cells in culture, and it is possible to differentiate some lines of cells which are cholinergic, others which are adrenergic, and still other lines which are mixed. Thus it is theoretically possible to develop lines of cells which might be selected for maturation and implantation.[77,61]

While animal fetal tissues may be easy to obtain, many ethical and moral questions are raised when one considers using cells of aborted human fetuses for transplantation. Chances for a successful program using such tissues would appear to be remote. Transplantations using adrenal medulla have been attempted in many patients with varying degrees of success reported. There have been major complications, resulting in part from the fact that two major operative procedures are being performed on a debilitated patient. The procedure has been abandoned in most centers in the United States at present. So far, there has been very little success in the development of a cell line from neoplasms suitable for transplantation, and we are aware of very few attempts to implant such cells. However, the technique is appealing, and we are anticipating some continued experimental trials if a suitable cell line becomes available.

In summary, it appears likely that neural tissue transplantation may have much to offer in the treatment of degenerative lesions of the nervous system, and it would appear that alternative sources of transplantable tissue should be investigated.

NEW DIRECTIONS FOR STEREOTAXIC SURGERY USING COMPUTER ASSISTANCE

The association of late-generation computers, computerized tomography (CT), magnetic resonance imaging (MRI), and lasers as well as radiation therapy with stereotaxis has revitalized and expanded the capabilities for stereotactic surgery. The first stereotactic instrument for use in animals was described by R.H. Clarke and V. Horsely in 1906,[78] and this was followed 2 years later by the classic investigation in which they reported on their examination of deep cerebellar nuclei in small animals.[79] Stereotactic instruments for animals were designed so that measurements were based upon a reference plane connecting the external auditory meatus and the inferior rims of the orbit. After considerable success with their anatomical studies, Clarke concluded that stereotaxic methods might be applied to human beings. A disagreement with Horsley over this recommendation ended their long and productive relationship.

Other devices and instruments for use in animals and humans were eventually developed. In 1947 Drs. Speigel and Wycis and their associates reported on the application of an instrument for stereotactic operations in humans.[80] Several different instruments were developed.[81,82] Stereotactic surgery became very popular, primarily for the treatment of movement disorders but also for the treatment of pain and psychiatric conditions. Stereotactic biopsies of brain substance and the production of lesions deep within the brain were possible even from the time instruments were first developed. Initially, human stereotactic atlases related deep cerebral target structures to anatomic landmarks in the diencephalon identified by ventriculography.[83–85]

Problems arose relating to the ethics of treating psychiatric disorders. With the use of levodopa for the treatment of Parkinson's disease in the 1960s, there was a great decline in the numbers of stereotactic procedures performed.

The development of computerized tomography (CT) led

to the adaptation of stereotactic instruments using CT guidance.[86–88] This provided the capability of localizing lesions deep within the cerebral tissue, open biopsy of which might produce increasing neurological deficits.[88–90] Biopsy of such lesions, using stereotactic methods for precision, became commonplace.[91,92] This increased the number of indications for stereotactic procedures.

Development of the carbon dioxide laser has added new capabilities to the stereotactic approach to deep-seated intracranial lesions. Now neoplasms could be treated.[93] Kelly and his associates have reported on the treatment of large series of patients with deep—and even superficial—intracranial lesions treated with stereotactic instrumentation, resections being accomplished with the carbon dioxide laser.[94–97] Kelly has also used these techniques to resect vascular lesions, radiation necrosis, and epileptic foci. Details of the technique as used for volumetric resection of neoplasms are discussed in Chap. 23.

Other areas of development in stereotactic surgery such as stereotactic robotics, frameless stereotaxis, and holographic guidance of stereotaxis are also discussed in Chap. 23.

☐ THE ROLE OF COMPUTERS IN CLINICAL DECISIONS

The past decade has witnessed a phenomenal growth in the role of computers in daily life. In hospitals, computers are indispensable in imaging, teaching, the distribution of information, and in accounting. Computers are playing an ever-increasing role in teaching, especially in teaching us how to make decisions. Now computers are assisting in the clinical decision-making process.

Computers have the ability to expand the basis upon which decisions are made and to separate facts from emotions. In a recent series of reports, emanating from the Department of Surgery at the Riyadh Armed Forces Hospital in Saudi Arabia, patients who were considered possible candidates for termination of life support were evaluated by their physicians, their nurses, and by a computer program based upon an "acute physiology and chronic health evaluation" (APACHE II).[98] A false positive anticipation of death of between 6.7 percent and 16.7 percent occurred among the human evaluators, but never by the computer analysis.[99] Use of daily APACHE II scores improved the predictive capability of the computerized system by a factor of 4. The system was not recommended for clinical decisions at the time of publication, but one could clearly envision benefits from utilizing computers in decision-making processes.

Similarly, cardiologists have reported that:

Computers can aid in avoiding distorting influences to which clinicians are subjected: (1) by placing the clinician's limited personal experience into broader perspective through comparison with a larger repository of clinically relevant information; (2) by making explicit the assumptions implied by his or her decisions; and (3) by alerting the clinician whenever the decisions made do not appear consistent with these assumptions, with the available information or with the conventional rules of logic.[100]

Experiences relating to the prediction of deaths are clearly applicable to the practice of neurosurgery in critical care units at the present, especially where trauma patients are involved. Similarly, computerized predictions could be applicable to the indications for surgery, and for the selection of pre- and postoperative care. While the institution of computerized systems in decision making might be slower in coming about and would obviously require updating almost on a daily basis, it is clear that computers will play an ever-increasing role in physicians' decision-making processes in the future, and, equally important, they will play a major part in the evaluation of the services that physicians deliver.

It is imperative that physicians who will be practicing medicine 5 to 10 years from now become thoroughly acquainted with the computer's capabilities and that the programs for their applications be developed.

REFERENCES

1. Hallett M, Cohen LG: Magnetism: A new method for stimulation of nerve and brain. *JAMA* 262:538–541, 1989.
2. Editorial: Magnetoencephalography. *Lancet* 335:576–577, 1990.
3. Barker AT, Freeston IL, Jalinous R, Jarratt JA: Magnetic stimulation of the human brain and peripheral nervous system: An introduction and the results of an initial clinical evaluation. *Neurosurgery* 20:100–109, 1987.
4. Maccabee PJ, Amassian VE, Cracco RQ, Cadwell JA: An analysis of peripheral motor nerve stimulation in humans using the magnetic coil. *Electroencephalogr Clin Neurophysiol* 70:524–533, 1988.
5. Barker AT, Jalinous R, Freeston IL: Noninvasive stimulation of human motor cortex. *Lancet* 2:1106–1107, 1985.
6. Evans BA, Litchy WJ, Daube JR: The utility of magnetic stimulation for routine peripheral nerve conduction studies. *Muscle Nerve* 11:1074–1078, 1988.
7. Schriefer TN, Mills KR, Murray NMF, Hess CW: Evaluation

of proximal facial nerve conduction by transcranial magnetic stimulation. *J Neurol Neurosurg Psychiatry* 51:60–66, 1988.

8. Maccabee PJ, Amassian VE, Cracco RQ, et al: Intracranial stimulation of facial nerve in humans with the magnetic coil. *Electroencephalogr Clin Neurophysiol* 70:350–354, 1988.

9. Rothwell JC, Day BL, Thompson PD, et al: Some experiences of techniques for stimulation of the human cerebral motor cortex through the scalp. *Neurosurgery* 20:156–163, 1987.

10. Amassian VE, Quirk GJ, Stewart M: Magnetic coil versus electrical stimulation of monkey motor cortex. *J Physiol* (Lond) 349:119, 1987.

11. Mills KR, Murray NM, Hess CW: Magnetic and electrical transcranial brain stimulation: Physiological mechanisms and clinical applications. *Neurosurgery* 20:164–168, 1987.

12. Chokroverty S, Sachdeo R, Duvoisin RC: Magnetic stimulation of the lumbosacral roots: A new diagnostic technique. *Neurology* 38:387, 1988.

13. Hess CW, Mills KR, Murray NMF: Responses in small hand muscles from magnetic stimulation of the human brain. *J Physiol* (Lond) 388:397–419, 1987.

14. Hess CW, Mills KR, Murray NMF, Schriefer TN: Magnetic brain stimulation: Central motor conduction studies in multiple sclerosis. *Ann Neurol* 22:744–752, 1987.

15. Ingram DA, Thompson AJ, Swash M: Central motor conduction in multiple sclerosis: Evaluation of abnormalities revealed by transcutaneous magnetic stimulation of the brain. *J Neurol Neurosurg Psychiatry* 51:487–494, 1988.

16. Claus D, Harding AE, Hess CW, et al: Central motor conduction in degenerative ataxic disorders: A magnetic stimulation study. *J Neurol Neurosurg Psychiatry* 51:790–795, 1988.

17. Abbruzzese G, Dall'Agata D, Morena M, et al: Electrical stimulation of the motor tracts in cervical spondylosis. *J Neurol Neurosurg Psychiatry* 51:796–802, 1988.

18. Boyd SG, Rothwell JC, Cowan JMA, et al: A method of monitoring function in corticospinal pathways during scoliosis surgery with a note on motor conduction velocities. *J Neurol Neurosurg Psychiatry* 49:251–257, 1986.

19. Rose DF, Smith PD, Sato S: Magnetoencephalography and epilepsy research. *Science* 238:329–335, 1987.

20. Romani GL: Superconducting instrumentation for biomagnetism. *Int J Refrigeration* 2:215–219, 1979.

21. Ricci GB, Romani GL, Salustri C, et al: Study of focal epilepsy by multichannel neuromagnetic measurements. *Electroencephalogr Clin Neurophysiol* 66:358–368, 1987.

22. Cuffin BN: The role of model and computational experiments in the biomagnetic inverse problem. *Phys Med Biol* 32:33–42, 1987.

23. Modena I, Ricci GB, Barbanera S, et al: Biomagnetic measurements of spontaneous brain activity in epileptic patients. *Electroencephalogr Clin Neurophysiol* 54:622–628, 1982.

24. Barth DS, Sutherling W, Beatty J: Neuromagnetic localization of epileptiform spike activity in the human brain. *Science* 218:891–894, 1982.

25. Rose DF, Sato S, Smith PD, et al: Localization of magnetic interictal discharges in temporal lobe epilepsy. *Ann Neurol* 22:348–354, 1987.

26. Barth DS, Sutherling W, Engel J: Neuromagnetic evidence of spatially distributed sources underlying epileptiform spikes in the human brain. *Science* 223:293–296, 1984.

27. Sutherling WW, Crandall PH, Darcey TM, et al: The magnetic and electric fields agree with intracranial localizations of somatosensory cortex. *Neurology* 38:1705–1714, 1988.

28. Hari R, Hamalainen M, Kaukoranta E, et al: Neuromagnetic responses from the second somatosensory cortex in man. *Acta Neurol Scand* 68:207–212, 1983.

29. Romani GL, Williamson SJ, Kaufman L, Brenner D: Characterization of the human auditory cortex by the neuromagnetic method. *Exp Brain Res* 47:381–393, 1982.

30. Evans MI, Drugan A, Manning FA, Harrison MR: Fetal surgery in the 1990s. *Am J Dis Child* 143:1431–1436, 1989.

31. Birnholz JC, Frigoletto FD: Antenatal treatment of hydrocephalus. *New Engl J Med* 303:1021–1023, 1981.

32. Clewell WH, Johnson ML, Meier PR, et al: A surgical approach to the treatment of fetal hydrocephalus. *New Engl J Med* 306:1320–1325, 1982.

33. McCullough DC, Balzer-Martin CA: Current progress in overt neonatal hydrocephalus. *J Neurosurg* 57:378–383, 1982.

34. Harrison MR: Congenital hydrocephalus, in Harrison MR, Globus MS, Filly RA (eds): *The Unborn Patient.* New York: Grune & Stratton, 1984, chap 12, pp 349–377.

35. Glick PL, Harrison MR, Halks-Miller M, et al: Correction of congenital hydrocephalus in utero: II. Efficacy of in utero shunting. *J Pediatr Surg* 19:870–881, 1984.

36. Bovicelli L: Management of pregnancies complicated by fetal central nervous system abnormalities. *Fetal Therap* 1:80–82, 1986.

37. Clewell WH, Manco-Johnson ML, Manchester DK: Diagnosis and management of fetal hydrocephalus. *Clin Obstet Gynecol* 29:514–522, 1986.

38. Harrison MR, Adzick NS, Longaker MT, et al: Successful repair in utero of a fetal diaphragmatic hernia after removal of herniated viscera from the left thorax. *New Engl J Med* 322:1582–1584, 1990.

39. Espinosa F, Weir B, Noseworthy T: Nonoperative treatment of subarachnoid hemorrhage, in Youmans, JR (ed): *Neuro-Surgery*. Philadelphia, Saunders, 1991, chap 54, pp 1661–1688.

40. Pritz MB, Giannotta SL, Kindt GW, et al: Treatment of patients with neurological deficits associated with cerebral vasospasm by intravascular volume expansion. *Neurosurgery* 3:364–368, 1978.

41. Kosnik EJ, Hunt WE: Postoperative hypertension in the management of patients with intracranial arterial aneurysms. *J Neurosurg* 45:148–154, 1976.

42. Giannotta SL, McGillicuddy JE, Kindt GW: Diagnosis and treatment of postoperative cerebral vasospasm. *Surg Neurol* 8:286–290, 1977.

43. Kassell NF, Peerless SJ, Durward QJ, et al: Treatment of ischemic deficits from vasospasm with intravascular volume expansion and induced arterial hypertension. *Neurosurgery* 11:337–343, 1982.

44. Higashida RT, Halbach VV, Cahan LD, et al: Transluminal angioplasty for treatment of intracranial arterial vasospasm. *J Neurosurg* 71:648–653, 1989.

45. Newell DW, Eskridge JM, Mayberg MR, et al: Angioplasty for treatment of symptomatic vasospasm following subarachnoid hemorrhage. *J Neurosurg* 71:654–660, 1989.

46. Seiler RW, Grolimund P, Aaslid R, et al: Cerebral vasospasm evaluated by transcranial ultrasound correlated with clinical grade and CT-visualized subarachnoid hemorrhage. *J Neurosurg* 64:590–600, 1986.

47. Barnett HJM, Sackett DL, Taylor DW, et al: Failure of extracranial-intracranial arterial bypass to reduce the risk of ischemic stroke: Results of an international randomized trial. *New Engl J Med* 313:1191–1200, 1985.

48. Barnett HJM, Sackett DL, Taylor DW, et al: Are the results of extracranial-intracranial bypass trial that generalizable? *New Engl J Med* 316:820–824, 1987.

49. Goldsmith HS, Chen WF, Duckett SW: Brain vascularization by intact omentum. *Arch Surg* 106:695–698, 1973.

50. Goldsmith HS, Duckett S, Chen WF: Prevention of cerebral infarction in the dog by intact omentum. *Am J Surg* 130:317–320, 1975.

Index

Page numbers in **boldface** indicate tables or illustrations.